Nutrition and Integrative Medicine

A Primer for Clinicians

Nutrition and Integrative Medicine

A Primer for Clinicians

Edited by
Aruna Bakhru

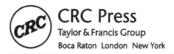

CRC Press
Taylor & Francis Group
Boca Raton London New York

CRC Press is an imprint of the
Taylor & Francis Group, an **informa** business

CRC Press
Taylor & Francis Group
6000 Broken Sound Parkway NW, Suite 300
Boca Raton, FL 33487-2742

Printed in Canada on acid-free paper

International Standard Book Number-13: 978-1-4987-5948-9 (Hardback)

Library of Congress Cataloging-in-Publication Data

Names: Bakhru, Aruna, editor.
Title: Nutrition and integrative medicine : a primer for clinicians / [edited by] Aruna Bakhru.
Description: Boca Raton : Taylor & Francis, 2018. | Includes bibliographical references.
Identifiers: LCCN 2017057584 | ISBN 9781498759489 (hardback : alk. paper)
Subjects: | MESH: Integrative Medicine--methods | Nutrition Therapy |
Nutritional Physiological Phenomena | Complementary Therapies--methods
Classification: LCC RM217 | NLM WB 113 | DDC 615.8/54--dc23
LC record available at https://lccn.loc.gov/2017057584

Visit the Taylor & Francis Web site at
http://www.taylorandfrancis.com

and the CRC Press Web site at
http://www.crcpress.com

This book is dedicated to my mother, Gita Bakhru, who is the embodiment of unconditional love in my life. Ultimately, it is love that heals. It is the love within the physician that heals the patient, and it is love, loving kindness that will heal our planet.

Aruna Bakhru, MD, FACP

Disclaimer

The purpose of this book is to educate the reader. The publisher, editor, and the authors have no liability or responsibility to any person(s) or entity with respect to any alleged loss or damage or injury caused directly or indirectly by information contained in this book. The information presented here is not a substitute for medical consultation or treatment.

Aruna Bakhru, MD, FACP

Contents

Preface...xi
Acknowledgments...xv
Editor xvii
Contributors xix

SECTION I   Nutritional and Functional Medicine

Chapter 1   The Role of the Microbiome on Human Health..3

Rodney R. Dietert and Janice M. Dietert

Chapter 2   Nutritional Approaches to Chronic Illness 19

Miriam Maisel

Chapter 3   Orthomolecular Parenteral Nutrition Therapy..39

Arturo O'Byrne-Navia and Arturo O'Byrne-De Valdenebro

Chapter 4   Toxicology: Exploring the Concept of Exogenous and Endogenous Toxins............ 121

Stevan Cordas

Chapter 5   Environmental Toxins and Chronic Illness: Clinical Management Using Traditional and Allostatic Load-Based Approaches 149

Jeffrey Moss

Chapter 6   Neuroprotection, Aging, and the Gut–Brain Axis: Translating Traditional Wisdom from the Mediterranean Diet into Evidence-Based Clinical Applications 177

Miguel A. Toribio-Mateas

Chapter 7   The Dental Connection to Health: Dental and Gingival Health and Its Relation to Chronic Illness...205

Alyse Shockey, Lisa Marie Samaha, and Dawn Ewing

Chapter 8   The Crucial Role of Craniofacial Growth on Airway, Sleep, and the Temporomandibular Joint 227

Mayoor Patel and Julia Worrall

Chapter 9   The Role of the Clinical Laboratory in Nutritional Assessment............................ 261

Harvey W. Kaufman

SECTION II *Integrative Medicine*

Chapter 10 Revisioning Cellular Bioenergetics: Food as Information and the
Light-Driven Body 291
Sayer Ji and Ali Le Vere

Chapter 11 The Scientific Basis of Ayurvedic and Chinese Medicine 319
Peter Eckman

Chapter 12 Ayurvedic Medicine: An Integrative Approach 329
Vasant Lad

Chapter 13 An Introduction to Ayurveda: Marma Therapy 347
Shekhar Annambhotla

Chapter 14 Chinese Medicine and Acupuncture 357
Yemeng Chen

Chapter 15 Yoga and Healing: Yogic Asanas, Breath, Mudras, and Their Relation to
Human Anatomy and Subtle Anatomy 363
Virender Sodhi

Chapter 16 Mind–Body Medicine 393
Jacqueline Proszynski and Darshan H. Mehta

Chapter 17 Meditation, Neurobiological Changes, Genes, and Health: A New Paradigm
for the Healthcare System 423
Marjorie H. Woollacott

Chapter 18 The Fourth Phase of Water: Implications for Energy, Life, and Health 439
Gerald H. Pollack

Chapter 19 Sound Healing, Theory, and Practice 449
John Beaulieu and David Perez-Martinez

Chapter 20 Healing with Light 473
Anadi Martel, Wesley Burwell, and Magda Havas

Chapter 21 The Role of Light and Electromagnetic Fields in Maintaining Vascular Health 501
Stephanie Seneff

Chapter 22 Electromagnetic Hygiene 523

Magda Havas

Chapter 23 Identifying Pharmaceutical-Grade Essential Oils and Using Them Safely and Effectively in Integrative Medicine..551

Joshua Plant and Scott Johnson

Chapter 24 On the Sophistication of Herbal Medicines 571

Stephen Harrod Buhner

Chapter 25 Psychological Trauma: Integrating Somatic and Psychological Methods to Treatment 591

Leslie Korn

Chapter 26 Anti-Aging and Regenerative Medicine..609

Adonis Maiquez

Chapter 27 Overcoming Chronic and Degenerative Diseases with Energy Medicine...............641

James L. Oschman

Chapter 28 Non-Invasive Early, Quick Diagnostic Methods of Various Cancers (Part I) and Safe, Effective, Individualized Treatment of Cancer (Part II).........................687

Yoshiaki Omura

Chapter 29 Low Doses Big Effects: Application to Pediatrics 713

Michel Bouko Levy

Chapter 30 Nutritional and Alternative Medicine: Legal and Ethical Considerations...............745

Peter A. Arhangelsky, Esq.

Index...771

Preface

As a practicing internist for over 25 years, I realized long ago that standard medical care did not have all the answers. There were many times that I found myself unable to help chronically ill patients. Over the years of my practice, chronic illness and the toll it has taken on the population of the United States and the rest of the world, the cost of care, and the burden on the caregivers has only continued to increase. The financial ramifications for the industry, government, society, and families are unsustainable in the long term. We can kick the can down the road only for so long. Amazingly, the answers are available but in separate pieces: the ancient healing sciences of Ayurveda, yoga, Chinese medicine, nutrition, homeopathy, plant essential oils, the use of light and sound in healing, mind–body medicine, the detrimental effects of toxins and electromagnetic/microwave frequencies on the human body. I could go on, but the list is in the book. Even as a trained physician, I did not understand the value, the importance, and the absolute imperative of nutrition. Vitamins were something you took as a kind of insurance in case you were missing something in your diet. The USDA food groups were what you explained to your patients, before sending them off to the dietician as you certainly did not, and still do not, have the time to go over what they were eating. I recall being taught that Vitamin B12 levels should be checked only in the elderly, what I found in actual practice was that a great number of my patients complaining of fatigue had low B12 levels, even though they were young. I eventually, as a standard practice, started getting baseline B12 levels in all of my patients and discovered that almost half of them were deficient in B12. Of course, I did not check the entire spectrum of B vitamins as that was not cost-effective; however, I did recommend that in addition to B12 injections, they take organic, whole food-based B complex vitamins. To this day, I am not certain what is causing this. I suspected the environment and recently read that autoimmune disease was exploding possibly as a result of EMF exposure. Then came the 1-25 hydroxyvitamin D3; again I found that almost a majority of my patients were deficient and those who were not, did not seem to get sick. To my amazement, I found that most over-the-counter vitamins were petroleum-based and actually harmful and I had to seek out organic, non-GMO, whole food-sourced vitamins.

The cell membrane is mainly comprised of fatty acids. An imbalance or a deficiency of essential fatty acids causes the cell membrane to lose its flexibility and become stiff and impermeable. Paradoxically, the diet and nutrition industry has exploded into a billion-dollar business. Yet, the American population is more obese than ever. People obsess over their carbohydrate, fat, and protein intake without realizing the subtle component of food. Where was it grown? How was it treated, what chemicals were used? What kind of seeds, what were the soil conditions? What additives were added? Excitotoxins added to processed food have now been demonstrated to cause inflammation in the body and the vascular system resulting in a whole host of problems ranging from migraines to restless leg syndrome and more. It is the responsibility of the food industry to pay attention to the health ramifications of their additives, beyond taste and food preservation.

Now research is coming out that epigenetics rather than genetic factors are the major cause of chronic disease. From Chapter 10 we learn, "In effect, the epigenetic effects of diet, via the many activators and suppressors of chromatin remodeling enzymes that food contains, can deprogram or reprogram vast quantities of genes regulating metabolic pathways, which in turn can influence the development of chronic, long-latency, and degenerative diseases." Also, "Food, when not artificially sterilized, is comprised of other organisms, that is, all food has a microbiome." This is powerful information indeed! Chapter 1 is entirely devoted to the microbiome of the human superorganism while Chapter 10 is devoted to the microbiome of our food and food as information. Research is now beginning to show that bacteria, fungi, and parasites in our gut actually effect our brain and thought process, causing a craving for the type of food that the parasite requires, rather than what is healthy for our body and mind.

Then, there is water—water that composes over 75% of our bodies. Research, as is being done at the Pollack laboratories, is desperately needed, yet is not a priority for funding. A deep understanding of water is essential. What kind of water are we putting into our body? Microwaved? Chemically treated? All water is not equal. We know that healing springs and waters exist. Why is it that some waters are healing and others not? It is not simply a matter of toxins in the water. Water seems to act as a source of information. The best analogy that I can think of is, imagine water as a blank computer disc upon which information can be imprinted. This water then, if assimilated by our body carries information into our system, which as we know consists of over 75% water as stated earlier. Yet, if you drive down our highways, what do you see? Water towers with Cell towers wrapped around them! Imagine the consequences of drinking, showering, washing clothes in this water? Also, there is not a remote corner of our world's oceans that you could go to, dip a slide or test tube in, and not come up contaminated with PCBs and dioxins. Our enzymatic systems and pathways are overwhelmed by the unprecedented toxic chemicals they are faced with in this century.

We are heading blindly toward more and more technology, 4G now 5G wireless networks, tethered to our cell phones, unable to exist without them. Getting more disconnected from nature, from the Earth, from each other. Over 500 Facebook friends but no one to talk to, families pull out their phones and everyone is immersed in their own phone as they sit together but are not together. Cell phones have added much value to our lives no doubt, but cautious responsible use is recommended. They have become a source of addiction, not to mention that as electromagnetic beings we need to be mindful of the unknown effects that these invisible waves are having on us. The scanner at the grocery checkout emits a red beam at the level of the groin! What effects could that be having on our human system and what can be done to mitigate their harmful effects?

The teeth are approached as inert objects, sitting in our gums that help us to chew food. If there is a cavity, it is drilled and filled, or God forbid a root canal is performed causing the bacteria to proliferate throughout the dentinal tubule system of the teeth, then into the bloodstream and spreading through the body, changing the microbiome, causing disease in the areas of weakness, where they settle. We have forgotten that our teeth are made of cells and respond to good nutrition as well as a supportive environment. Thankfully, I read that work is being done regarding filling cavities with the person's own stem cells, which is a much better approach.

Homeopathy is decried as placebo medicine because we do not understand it. A lack of understanding does not invalidate the reality that it is, in fact, an elegant system of vibrational medicine. A dead body is dissected in medical school, but the living vibrationally alive human is not yet fully understood. Jacques Benveniste was a French immunologist who was the head of INSERM's Unit 200, performing research on immunology and allergy. In 1988, he published a paper in the journal *Nature* that caused an international controversy. The research was co-authored by four laboratories worldwide in Canada, Italy, Israel, and France. He diluted a solution of human anti-IgE antibodies in water so that there was no possibility that even a molecule of the antibody remained in the water solution. Human basophils still responded to the solution as though they had encountered the original antibody. This effect was reported only when the solution was shaken violently during dilution. This heretical view cost Jacques his laboratory, his funding, and his reputation. The journal retracted the paper. Later, a Swiss chemist Louis Rey published a paper in *Physica A*, 2003 claiming to show that "even though they should be identical, the structure of hydrogen bonds in pure water are very different from that in homeopathic dilutions of salt solutions." Luc Montagnier, a Nobel prize laureate whose research paper on "Electromagnetic Signals Are Produced by Aqueous Nanostructures Derived from Bacterial DNA Sequences" 2009 was also questioned on his beliefs about homeopathy, to which he replied: "I can't say that homeopathy is right in everything. What I can say now is that the high dilutions are right. High dilutions of something are not nothing. They are water structures which mimic the original molecules. We find that with DNA, we cannot work at the extremely high dilutions used in homeopathy; we cannot go further than a 10^{-18} dilution, or we lose the signal. But even at 10^{-18}, you can calculate that there is not a single molecule of DNA left. And yet we detect a signal" (Enserink, December 2010).

Another interesting finding regarding water came from The University of Michigan astronomers, Cleeves and Bergin published in *Science* 2014, that about half the water on Earth may be older than the solar system. I could not but help draw a parallel to the legend of the river Ganges in India which is said to have originated from the "heavens" and not of this Earth. I could be wrong, but it is a curiously interesting study. The Ganges river water has been extensively studied for its unique bacteriostatic properties.

We know there is electricity running in the body as evidenced by the brain waves, the EKG, the muscle action potential, and in fact, science has now shown that there is electrical as well as neurotransmitter activity at the neuromuscular junction. In a study published in the *Proceedings of the National Academy of Sciences*, January 2007, UC San Diego said that "modifying electrical activity in the adult brain can alter neurotransmitters and receptors." We already know, of course, that messages are conducted along nerve fibers in the form of electrical activity (Seethaler 2006).

According to Ayurveda, marmas (similar to acupuncture points in Chinese Medicine) are vulnerable or sensitive spots that have a specific use in diagnosis and healing. They connect with nadis (energetic nerves) and chakras (energetic centers). They manage the interaction between the physical and the subtle bodies. They are like windows on the skin surface acting as junction points between body, mind, and spirit. I recall a teacher, who was training me on these points, saying to me, "Think of them as geysers where energy comes close to the surface and can be measured." The leaky gut syndrome was first described in Ayurveda. It arises from the presence of "ama," which is a toxic byproduct of poor digestion. One of the features of "ama" is that when it enters the "dhatu" (dhatu means tissue—plasma, blood, muscle, fat, bone marrow, reproductive tissue, etc.) cycle, it disrupts the nutrition and function of the tissues. It has an affinity for tissues that are weak and tends to accumulate there. Once lodged there, it causes increased congestion followed by inflammation and finally degeneration. Sushruta, one of the original Ayurvedic physicians, pioneered rhinoplasty and the surgeons of the East India Company learned the procedure from watching Ayurvedic surgeons. Dr. Peter Eckman's chapter talks about the differing approaches towards the definition of science between Eastern and Western Medicine. While Western Medicine is predominantly focused on the material aspect, Eastern Medicine also focuses on that which is nonmaterial. Dr. Marjorie Woollacott's research has shown that meditation affects our genetics and has proven neurobiological changes as well.

Dr. Valerie Hunt was a Professor Emeritus of Physiological Sciences at UCLA. She is best known for her pioneering research into vibrational medicine. She discovered that neuromuscular ennervation patterns were foundational to non-verbal communication. She proved that energy radiating from the body's atoms gives off frequencies 1000 times faster than the electrical activity of the body. Using fractal mathematics, her energy field data showed dramatic chaos patterns in human biological systems, and she showed that it did not take much beyond a homeopathic dose to convert the chaos into a beautiful, symmetrical pattern.

According to Deepak Chopra, M.D., "We can trace the physical structure of the body, down to the molecular level and still have no explanation for beliefs, desires, memory, and creativity."

The SQUID Magnetometer, Super Conducting Quantum Interference Device, can detect biomagnetic fields associated with physiological activities in the body. David Cohen of MIT used it to measure fields around the heart and the head in the 1970s. Dr. John Zimmerman studied therapeutic touch at The University of Colorado School of Medicine in the 1980s. He found pulsating biomagnetic fields emanating from the hands of healers with different healers having differing results. Cohen is currently on the faculty at Harvard Medical School and a mentor at MIT's Martinos Imaging Center (Wikipedia).

If we are to change course and have a balanced medical care system, then we need to extend our understanding to the so-called CAM modalities that have in actual fact existed for thousands of years before modern medicine and continue to exist. The ancient healing modalities are there, the cutting-edge research into nutrition, the microbiome, biophotons, epigenetics is all there, just not within the pages of our medical textbooks yet. We treat the mind as though the body does not exist, and we treat the body as though the mind does not exist. The powerful effects of the mind on the body are dismissed as the placebo effect. It is as though we are missing the forest for the trees. The human body, capable of amazing feats of healing, is not a machine. All of us went into medical school with dreams of helping people, then the reality of the system hit, onerous burdensome regulations, up late at night, poor lifestyle, no time to eat well, to exercise. Who are we, as doctors, to tell people how to live, when our own lifestyles are not healthy? Doctors have a deep desire to heal others, they are intelligent, driven people. This book is an effort to bring another perspective that was perhaps not noticed, yet has much to offer.

Therefore, this book is offered to clinicians, their patients, families, and loved ones everywhere as a source of information and knowledge of a science-based understanding, regarding healing modalities that have much to offer humanity and to those that are the guardians of health.

Aruna Bakhru, MD, FACP

REFERENCES

Cleeves, L. I. et al. "The ancient heritage of water ice in the solar system." *Science*, vol. 345, no. 6204, 2014, pp. 1590–1593, doi: 10.1126/science.1258055.

Enserink, M. "Newsmaker interview: Luc Montagnier. French Nobelist Escapes "Intellectual Terror" to pursue radical ideas in China." *Science*, 24 December 2010, 1732. doi: 10.1126/science.330.6012.1732. Full article mirror Source Wikipedia.

Rey, L. "Thermoluminescence of ultra-High dilutions of lithium chloride and sodium chloride." *Physica A: Statistical Mechanics and its Applications*, vol. 323, 2003, pp. 67–74, doi: 10.1016/s0378-4371(03)00047-5.

Seethaler, S. *Electrical Activity Alters Language Used by Nerve Cells.* 2006 December 19, http://ucsdnews.ucsd.edu/archive/newsrel/science/snervact.asp

Acknowledgments

This book would not have been possible without the expertise of each of the contributing authors. It is thanks to their dedication to their chosen field as well as their generous willingness to share the information that has brought this book into existence.

Special thanks also to Ms. Randy Brehm, Senior Editor at Taylor & Francis, who has been my rock throughout the editing process. Without her helpful advice and expedient replies to my queries, I do not think that I would have been able to navigate the editing process. Thanks are also due to Sylvester O'Gilvie, who despite being quite buried under so many manuscripts was ever helpful and prompt in his replies to my emails. Thanks also to my Acquisitions Editor, Ingrid Kohlstadt, MD, MPH, FACH, whose faith in my abilities as an editor I will ever be grateful for. She was also instrumental in introducing me to Dr. Yoshiaki Omura, a physician and physicist.

Many thanks to Shayna Murry for her creative expertise in bringing the vision that I had for the book cover to life. Thank you to Jonathan Pennell for creating the social media images. Samantha Holt and everyone else in Marketing for working hard to ensure that the book is successful. Thanks also to my Project Editor, Marsha Hecht, for helping make the production process seamless and efficient. Kudos to Annie Lubinsky, Teena Lawrence, and the entire team at Nova Techset for their attention to detail and patience during the process.

My husband, Sushil Dhawan, MD, and my sons, Nikhil and Rahul, who have tolerated all my traveling, being away from home, taking courses, and my forays into the unknown.

My brothers, Umesh and Dinesh Bakhru, for their never ending support and my late father Govind Bakhru who always wanted me to be a writer.

Editor

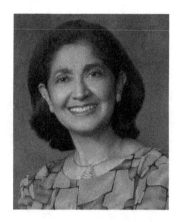

Aruna Bakhru, MD, FACP, is Board Certified in Internal Medicine and a Fellow of The American College of Physicians. She graduated in Medicine and Surgery from Lady Hardinge Medical College, New Delhi, India and completed her residency in internal medicine at Prince George's Hospital and Medical Center in Maryland. She also conducted research with Valerie Johnson, MD, PhD, at New York Medical College, Lincoln Hospital and Medical Center. Currently, she is affiliated with Vassar Brothers Medical Center, Poughkeepsie, New York.

A respected and long-standing figure in her field, Dr. Bakhru currently serves as a physician with a focus on integrative and internal medicine at her private practice, which she has maintained for over 25 years.

Dr. Bakhru has held numerous appointments over the course of her career, serving as the Young Physician Section Representative of The Dutchess County Medical Society and as the Chair of the Integrative Medicine Subcommittee of The Dutchess County Medical Society. She has also served on the Ambulatory and Emergency Services Committee at Vassar Brothers Medical Center, the Medical Audit Committee of Vassar Brothers Medical Center, and the Complementary Care Committee at Vassar Brothers Medical Center, as well as on the Utilization Review and Quality Assurance Committee of Mohawk Valley Plan Health Plan.

Dr. Bakhru has over 20 years of experience and training in many other modalities such as nutrition, functional medicine, Ayurvedic medicine, herbal medicine, and bioenergetic medicine, as well as the efficacy of sound and light as healing modalities. She trained with The American Academy of Environmental Medicine, learning to treat twenty-first century problems caused by our lifestyle and environmental issues. She has also been involved with numerous community service activities, volunteering at the medical clinic for the indigent at Vassar Hospital and serving as a volunteer physician for the summer camp run by SVSC, a nonprofit group. She has also written for numerous publications, appeared on radio and television, and lectured on medically related topics.

Dr. Bakhru has been endorsed as a leader in the healthcare industry by *Marquis Who's Who*, the world's premier publisher of biographical profiles, and recently was named a Lifetime Achiever by that publisher. As in all *Who's Who* volumes, individuals profiled are selected based on current reference value. Factors such as position, noteworthy accomplishments, visibility, and prominence in a field are all considered during the selection process.

In addition to her status as Lifetime Achiever, Dr. Bakhru has previously received the Excellence in Integrative Medicine Award from Emord and Associates and was honored by The Holistic Doctors Recognition Board as one of the Top Ten doctors in New York State. Additionally, she received awards in Pathology and Forensic Medicine from the University of Delhi as well as the Certificate of Excellence from many insurance groups. Furthermore, Dr. Bakhru has been a featured listee in *Who's Who in America*, *Who's Who in Medicine and Healthcare*, *Who's Who in the World*, and *Who's Who in Science and Engineering.* She also volunteers on Cyber Safety India International Board of Advisors and is an Executive Committee member of the Dutchess County Regional Science Fair. She has also published various articles in her local newspapers as well as appeared on public television in White Plains, and radio talk shows for WKIP and WVKR 91.3 FM out of Vassar College.

Her website is www.centerforenergymedicine.com. She currently practices in New York and believes that treating the patient as a whole leads to better outcomes and satisfaction for both the physician and patient.

Contributors

Shekhar Annambhotla, BAMS (Ayurved)
Director
Ojas, LLC—Ayurveda Wellness Center
and
President
Association of Ayurvedic Professionals of
    North America
Coopersburg, Pennsylvania

and

Director
Global Ayurveda Academy and Conferences
Pennsylvania

Peter A. Arhangelsky, Esq.
Principal Attorney
Emord & Associates, P.C.
Gilbert, Arizona

John Beaulieu, ND, PhD
Founder of BioSonic Enterprises, Ltd.
Stone Ridge, New York

and

Professor of Integrative Health
Zentrum für Inner Ökologie
Zürich, Switzerland

Stephen Harrod Buhner
Senior Researcher
Foundation for Gaian Studies
Silver City, New Mexico

and

Fellow
Schumacher College
Totnes, United Kingdom

Wesley Burwell, CBS, LHSC
PLT Coach and Instructor
Certified Stress Management–Polychromatic
    Light Therapy
Tillsonburg, Ontario, Canada

Yemeng Chen, PhD, LAc, FICAE
President
New York College of Traditional Chinese
    Medicine
Mineola, New York

Stevan Cordas, DO
Adjunct Assistant Professor
Texas College of Osteopathic Medicine
Fort Worth, Texas

Janice M. Dietert, MASS
Performance Plus Consulting
Lansing, New York

Rodney R. Dietert, PhD
Professor of Immunotoxicology
Department of Microbiology and
    Immunology
Cornell University
Ithaca, New York

Peter Eckman, MD, PhD
Private Practice
San Francisco, California

Dawn Ewing, RDH, PhD
International Academy of Biological Dentistry
    and Medicine (IABDM)
Spring, Texas

Magda Havas, PhD
Trent School of the Environment
Trent University
Peterborough, Ontario, Canada

Sayer Ji, BA
Director
GreenMedInfo.com
Naples, Florida

Scott Johnson, AMP, CEEOS, CCMA, CPC
Founder and President
Research and Development
    at Zija International
and
Integrative Essential Oils
    Certification Program
Orem, Utah

Harvey W. Kaufman, MD, MBA, FCAP
Senior Medical Director
Quest Diagnostics
Secaucus, New Jersey

Leslie Korn, PhD, MPH
Core Faculty
Capella University
Private Practice
Minneapolis, Minnesota

Vasant Lad, BAM&S, MASc
Director
The Ayurvedic Institute
Albuquerque, New Mexico

**Ali Le Vere, BS (Human Biology), BS
(Psychology)**
Senior Researcher
GreenMedInfo
Naples, Florida

Michel Bouko Levy, MD
President and Founder
l'Institut d'Homeopathie de Provence
Marseille, France

and

Founder
Homeopathic Medical Association
    of Canada
Ontario, Canada

Adonis Maiquez, MD, ABAARM
Medical Director
Carillon Miami Wellness Resort
Miami Beach, Florida

Miriam Maisel, MD
Family Practitioner
Nutrition and Lifestyle Intervention
Tel Aviv, Israel

and

General Practitioner
Dumfries and Galloway
    Royal Infirmary
Scotland, United Kingdom

Anadi Martel, MSc
Physicist
Sensortech Inc.
Ste-Adele, Quebec, Canada

Darshan H. Mehta, MD, MPH
Medical Director
Benson-Henry Institute for Mind Body
    Medicine
Massachusetts General Hospital
and
Associate Director of Education
Osher Center for Integrative
    Medicine
Harvard Medical School and
    Brigham and Women's Hospital
Boston, Massachusetts

Jeffrey Moss, DDS, CNS, DACBN
President
Moss Nutrition Products, Inc.
Hadley, Massachusetts

Arturo O'Byrne-De Valdenebro, MD
Biological Medicine Private Practice
and
Director
Academic Affairs at Sociedad
    Argentina de Medicina
    Biológica y Homotoxicología
    (SAMByH)
Buenos Aires, Argentina

Arturo O'Byrne-Navia, MD
Medical Director
Centro de Medicina Biológica
and
Professor
Integrative Medicine Chair at Pontificia
    Universidad Javeriana
Cali, Colombia

**Yoshiaki Omura, MD, ScD, FACA,
FICAE, FAAIM, FRSM**
Adjunct Professor
Department of Family and Community
    Medicine
New York Medical College
Valhalla, New York

and

President and Professor
International College of Acupuncture and
    Electro-Therapeutics
New York City, New York

and

Editor-in-Chief
Acupuncture and Electro-Therapeutics
    Research
International Journal of Integrated Medicine
Valhalla, New York

James L. Oschman, PhD
Nature's Own Research Association
Dover, New Hampshire

Mayoor Patel, DDS, MS
Private Practice
Craniofacial Pain and Dental Sleep Center
    of GA
Atlanta, Georgia

and

Adjunct Clinical Instructor
Dental College of Georgia
Augusta, Georgia

and

Tufts University
Boston, Massachusetts

David Perez-Martinez, MD
Founder of TuneUpRx
Faculty
Sound and Music Institute
New York Open Center
New York, New York

Joshua Plant, PhD
Chief Scientific Officer
Pharmatech Labs
Lindon, Utah

Gerald H. Pollack, PhD
Professor of Bioengineering
University of Washington
Seattle, Washington

Jacqueline Proszynski, BS
Clinical Research Program Coordinator
The Benson-Henry Institute for Mind Body
    Medicine
Massachusetts General Hospital
Boston, Massachusetts

Lisa Marie Samaha, DDS, FAGD
Private Practice Owner
Port Warwick Dental Arts
and
Founder, Researcher and Professor
Perio Arts Institute, PerioPassion Dental
    Seminars
and
International Academy for Ozone in
    Healthcare
Newport News, Virginia

Stephanie Seneff, PhD
Senior Research Scientist
MIT Computer Science and Artificial
    Intelligence Laboratory
Cambridge, Massachusetts

Alyse Shockey, RDH, CMT, CHHP
HH Wellness, LLC
Baltimore, Maryland

Virender Sodhi, MD (Ayur), ND
Ayurvedic & Naturopathic Physician
CEO, Ayush Herbs Inc.
Director, Ayurvedic and Naturopathic Medical
    Clinic
Bellevue, Washington

Miguel A. Toribio-Mateas, BSc (Hons), MSc
School of Health and Education
Middlesex University
London, United Kingdom

Marjorie H. Woollacott, PhD
Faculty
Institute of Neuroscience
and
Professor
Human Physiology
and
Director
Motor Control Laboratory
University of Oregon
Eugene, Oregon

Julia Worrall, RN
Certified Critical Care Nurse Specializing
   in Sleep and Craniofacial Growth and
   Development
Founder and Executive Director
The Foundation for Airway and Craniofacial
   Excellence (FACE)
Toronto, Ontario, Canada

Section I

Nutritional and Functional Medicine

1 The Role of the Microbiome on Human Health

Rodney R. Dietert and Janice M. Dietert

CONTENTS

Introduction 3
A Different Patient 4
The Noncommunicable Disease Epidemic 5
The Problem with Many Existing Drugs 5
Managing the Microbial Ecology of the Patient 7
Complementary Therapies: Rebiosis 8
    Antibiotic Adjunct Therapies 9
    Postoperative Recovery 9
    Protection against Stress-Induced Dysbiosis 9
    Correction of Depression and Anxiety 11
    Anti-Aging Effects 11
    Protection against Recurrent *Clostridium difficile* Infection 11
    Protection against Environmental Toxicants 11
    Treating Metabolic Syndrome 12
    Potential Help for Infantile Colic 12
Biofilms 12
Conclusions 13
References 14

INTRODUCTION

Much of allopathic medicine today is based on a process for treating medically coded conditions with a specified regime of diagnostic tests, procedures, and the administration of pharmaceutical agents. Efficacy and safety of these agents is determined by a regulated procedure of phased evaluation, usually first in laboratory animal models and then, subsequently, in humans. Individual variation based on age, genetic background, sex, and existing diseases and conditions can influence efficacy and safety. However, the predictability of adverse outcomes among subpopulations has been highly imprecise if not largely unknown.

The assumption was that, with the advent of the human genome program and the complete sequencing of the human gene sequence, individual patient variation could be fully accounted for, and what has been envisioned as precision or individualized medicine would be the foundation for the future. However, the recent realization that the human patient is actually a majority microbial based on cell number and gene number, and that human metabolism and physiology reflects this chimeric reality, has changed how health and wellness is most effectively approached. No longer is it only the mammalian part of humans that can be medically treated with expectation that the overall health of the patient will be optimized. In fact, via both special issues and recognition of significant breakthroughs, *Science Magazine* has focused on the microbiome as a pivotal factor when considering human health versus disease (Pennisi and Mueller 2016).

This chapter describes a landscape in which integrative medicine can utilize the microbiome, the microbial part of humans, for more effective disease prevention, treatment, and care of patients. The foundational message is that species purity is unhealthy, and that it is not possible to have a truly healthy patient unless the microbiome is also well diversified and healthy. Early life attention to the microbiome is emphasized since we now know that our microbes developmentally program our physiological systems for later-life function. A dysfunctional microbiome in childhood has been connected to elevated risk of numerous serious childhood and adult diseases (Dietert 2016a). Both infectious and noncommunicable diseases (NCDs) are included in the discussion. However, given the fact that NCDs are the overwhelming majority killer globally, are stressing healthcare systems, and are more often managed across a lifetime rather than cured (Dietert 2016b), an emphasis is placed on them.

A DIFFERENT PATIENT

The human superorganism patient presents both challenges and new opportunities for both disease prevention and integrative therapies. Approximately 99% of the genes in humans are microbial. A recent cataloguing of all microbial genes in humans estimated that just under 10 million microbial genes exist (Li et al. 2014). By comparison, the human chromosomal genes are estimated to be in the range of 22,000–25,000 (International Human Genome Sequencing Consortium 2004).

In utero exposure of the fetus to microbes occurs via the placental microbiome (Aagaard et al. 2014). Interactions between the trophoblast layer, the outer layer of the blastocyst, and the microbiome (Mor and Kwon 2015) affect both fetal immune development and immunoregulation in the mother that is needed to maintain the pregnancy to term (Zheng et al. 2015). Management of the pregnancy needs to include management of the mother's microbiome including that of the placenta. Researchers have suggested that the placental microbiome profile is a driver of both pregnancy outcome and the future destiny for the fetus (Cao et al. 2014; Fox and Eichelberger 2015).

The primary microbial seeding event for the baby occurs at birth during vaginal delivery and via skin-to-skin contact (Mueller et al. 2015). However, Cesarean delivery interrupts the primary seeding event leaving the baby's microbial seeding to come largely from outside or beyond the mother. Antibiotics and other drugs given during pregnancy, as part of the C-section procedure, or immediately during infancy can also deplete the baby's microbiome and alter the course of infant microbial and physiological maturation (Bokulich et al. 2016; Stokholm et al. 2016; Yassour et al. 2016). When a newborn has a depleted microbiome, it has been represented as a type of birth defect in that there are known, predictable physiological alterations, anatomical changes (e.g., barrier function), and health risks associated with the continuation of this infant state (Dietert 2014). In fact, the early life events relative to the infant microbiome shape both subsequent immune and metabolic functions (Wang et al. 2016).

While attention to a healthy microbiome is beneficial at any age, there is particular benefit during pregnancy and early infant life. Attention to the microbiome during pregnancy has the potential to improve the health of both mother and baby (Isolauri et al. 2015). This affords a new, important opportunity for health professionals involved with pregnancy management. Likewise, attention to microbiome status of the newborn is critical, since the newborn's microbiome and physiological systems (e.g., the immune system and brain) co-mature together (Wopereis et al. 2014; Diaz Heijtz 2016). Breast feeding offers another window of opportunity both for microbiome seeding and for introduction of specific complex carbohydrates designed exclusively as an energy source for the microbiome (Bashiardes et al. 2016).

There is evidence that elements of modernization (urbanization, processed non-local food, elective C-sections), antibiotic overuse, and Westernized diets low in fiber have contributed to the degradation of the human microbiome and loss of diversity. Recent studies suggest that within-generation improvement of microbiome diversity is possible through rebiosis and dietary change. However, continued transmission of a degraded, unhealthy microbiome across multiple generations can blunt the capacity for us to use dietary changes as a strategy to correct problems with the microbiome

(Sonnenburg et al. 2016). For this reason, we may have little generational time to medically address microbial degradation in humans. The current generation of children is at risk from a deficient microbiome; but, based on the recent findings of Sonnenburg and colleagues (Sonnenburg et al. 2016), failure to act on the current generation of children could make microbiome corrections in future generations more difficult.

While the gastrointestinal microbiome has the most extensive research, it is important to recognize that many different tissues have their own microbiome and that these are distinct from that of the gut. Each body site such as the airways, skin, breast tissue, placenta, and urogenital tract has its own healthy and dysfunctional microbiome profiles. For example, Yu et al. (2016) recently described the human lung microbiome and reported that the lung microbiota are distinct from the microbial communities in oral, nasal, stool, vagina, and skin. In lung, Proteobacteria were the dominant phylum (60%).

THE NONCOMMUNICABLE DISEASE EPIDEMIC

Noncommunicable diseases (NCDs), also called chronic diseases, are the scourge of the twenty-first century. As recently as the early-mid twentieth century, infectious diseases were the primary concerns with first influenza and polio viruses as well as the tuberculosis-causing bacterium grabbing both medical and institutional public health focus. Asthma, type 1 and 2 diabetes, heart disease, obesity, cancer, autism spectrum disorders, Alzheimer's disease, Parkinson's disease, and the myriad of autoimmune and inflammatory conditions were but blips on the healthcare radar.

All that changed within mere decades and a couple of generations. In many ways, the battle against infectious diseases has been highly successful. New pandemics continue to emerge, and they present challenges; but their global impact pales in comparison to the toll of NCDs.

One of the challenges with NCDs is that few are actually cured. More often, the symptoms of these diseases and conditions are medically managed. In some cases, this can last for a lifetime resulting in decades of ever-increasing needs for prescriptions drugs. Such ongoing medical and drug dependency can take a toll not only on the patient but also on family members (Stuckey et al. 2016). Currently, the only exception to this trend of lifelong prescription drugs for certain NCDs is that drugs may be removed for patients near the end of life (Nishtala et al. 2016).

Another problem is that extensive co-morbidities exist for NCDs. The diagnosis of any one NCD automatically means that the individual is at an elevated risk of additional NCDs with aging (Dietert et al. 2010). With increased medical diagnoses, healthcare costs, and pharmaceutical burdens, and the likelihood of restrictions on function and/or activities, quality of life often degrades (De Maeseneer and Boeckxstaens 2011). Additionally, the risk of drug incompatibilities and problematic side effects increases, and the number of diseases and required medications increases accordingly.

Because of the importance of early life programming of later life NCDs, or what is known as the Barker Hypothesis, the earlier prevention and intervention measures can be taken, the greater the likelihood of reduced NCDs across an individual's life course. This was emphasized recently by Roura and Arulkumaran who stressed that to fully address the NCD epidemic, the frontline of the battle is *in utero* (Roura and Arulkumaran 2015) given the importance of fetal programming of later life disease (Morton et al. 2016).

THE PROBLEM WITH MANY EXISTING DRUGS

One problem with existing drugs and many of those about to be released is that the benefit-risk determination is likely to be flawed. Most of these drugs were never vetted for safety of the microbiome. In fact, they were vetted for safety under a rubric that was mammalian-centric and never considered whether the drugs could damage the microbiome or required specific microbes to work. This is likely part of the explanation for the frustratingly long list of side effects that are associated with many of today's drugs (see Table 1.1). However, beyond those known side effects (e.g., drug-induced

TABLE 1.1

Examples of Drugs Whose Efficacy and/or Safety Depend on Microbiome Status

Drug	Treatment Use	Reported Effect	References
Berberine	Metabolic disorders	Gut microbiota are required for drug absorption and microbiome status determines efficacy	Feng et al. (2015)
Amlodipine (a calcium channel blocker)	Hypertension	Therapeutic potency is affected by status of the gut microbiota	Yoo et al. (2016)
Cyclophosphamide	Cancer Autoimmune disease Transplantation	Requires specific microbes for efficacy, treatment alters the microbiome	Xu and Zhang (2015)
Digoxin	Cardiovascular disease	Both safety and efficacy depend upon the microbiome profile	Haiser et al. (2014)
Lovastatin (a statin)	Elevated cholesterol	Status of the gut microbiota affects the conversion of the prodrug lovastatin to the active form	Yoo et al. (2014), Klaassen and Cui (2015)
Metformin	Diabetes	Efficacy improved by co-administration of probiotic *Bifidobacterium animalis* ssp. *lactis* 420 in mice	Stenman et al. (2015)
Nitrazepam	A benzodiazepine used for anxiety and insomnia	Production of a teratogenic metabolite is affected by gut microbiota status	Klaassen and Cui (2015)
Non-steroidal anti-inflammatory drugs (NSAIDs)		Ibuprofen and naproxen both skew the gut microbiome vs. controls but they also enrich different families of bacteria	Rogers and Aronoff (2016)
Proton pump inhibitors	Excess gastric acid production, peptic ulcers, and gastro-esophageal reflux disease (GERD)	Long-term use produces a skewing in microbiome composition and an increased risk of *C. difficile* infection	Clooney et al. (2016), Imhann et al. (2016), Jackson et al. (2016)
Tempol	Anti-oxidant, prevention of weight gain	Tempol appears to require gut microbiota alterations for pharmacological activity	Cai et al. (2016)

gut symptoms or diarrhea), drug-induced microbial dysbiosis can eventually lead to other NCDs (e.g., inflammation-driven diseases) that are unlikely to be noted as a drug-induced "side effect."

In a recent comprehensive review of microbiome-associated drug and chemical metabolism, Klaassen and Cui (2015) describe how our microbes can drive numerous drug and chemical metabolic pathways. For example, bacteria can biotransform drugs and chemicals affecting the spectrum and relative amounts of metabolites that an individual produces and, thereby, affect drug efficacy and safety. This microbe-mediated transformation occurs through the following chemical reactions: acetylation, amine formation and hydrolysis of amide bond, azoreduction, deconjugation, deglycosylation, dehydroxylation, denitration, isoxazole scission, N-demethylation, N-oxide bond bond cleavage, proteolysis, reduction, hydrolysis, succinate group remover, and thiazole ring opening.

Additionally, our microbes can both produce and regulate the levels of certain super families of genes encoding inducible metabolic enzymes. One prominent family is the cytochrome P (CYP) 450 enzymes. CYP450 enzymes are so designated because 450 nm is the wavelength of light they maximally absorb when they are in a reduced state and complexed with carbon monoxide. By affecting CYP gene activity in the liver, the status of the microbiome can exert a significant influence on the metabolism of all xenobiotics. Among the most significant CYP450 for drug metabolism is the group known as 3A, which is prominent in the liver and intestines. CYP450 3A enzymes metabolize most drugs and eventually help with detoxification of the body (Klaassen and Cui 2015; Selwyn et al. 2015, 2016).

Drugs are not the only chemicals metabolized by the microbiome. Health safety from environmental chemicals is also affected by microbiome status. As with drug metabolism pathways there are many ways that our microbes can affect the delivered internal dose of environmental chemicals (Dietert and Silbergeld 2015). Among these is the capacity of gut microbiota to activate a cell transcriptional factor known as the aryl hydrocarbon receptor (AHR). Microbes can do this through the metabolism of tryptophan (Zelante et al. 2013). AHRs are important because they bind flavonoids, polyphenolics and indoles, as well as synthetic polycyclic aromatic hydrocarbons and dioxin-like compounds. They are also important in the body's detoxification process, and the fact that microbes can control AHR expression as well as other biological processes determining our internal exposure to toxicants means that they play a significant role in our environmental health protection.

Susceptibility to toxic chemicals in the environment and food can be affected by microbiome status. For example, the status of the gut microbiota can affect the internal burden from oral exposure to heavy metals such as cadmium and lead (Breton et al. 2013). In the case of the toxic metal arsenic, gut microbes affect which of several different forms of arsenic will exist in the body. Some gut microbes have the capacity to produce the most toxic forms while others lack those genes. As a result, the specific profile of the microbiome can determine the risk to the individual from a given exposure to arsenic (e.g., via drinking water) (Dc-Rubin et al. 2014).

Finally, the industrial chemical melamine is a toxicological risk for both humans and animals. This was a recent problem when melamine contaminated both infant formula and pet food produced in China (Dalal and Goldfarb 2011; Wang et al. 2011). Melamine toxicity results in crystal formation in the kidneys. However, the extent of crystal formation after melamine exposure is affected by the presence of and levels of specific gut microbes (Zheng et al. 2013; Klaassen and Cui 2015). It is another example where the profile of gut microbes determines the actual individual health risk.

MANAGING THE MICROBIAL ECOLOGY OF THE PATIENT

A recent view of human biology is that we are a collection of thousands of different species that all fit together to the benefit of the whole. Our closest models for this are the living coral reef and tropical rainforests. Much is known about the ecological management of a coral reef or tropical rainforest, and they are appropriate models when it comes to the design of integrative health approaches for humans. The challenge will be to shift our basic thinking about the nature of the human patient.

As in the coral reef, risk to any of the species (mammalian and microbial) contributing to overall human integrity and health needs to be considered before pursuing treatment options. The benefit of the whole is the goal. In essence, the physician becomes a superhuman ecologist with the task of managing the microbial ecology of the patient so as to "do no harm." Either ignoring the status of a patient's microbiome or operating without a clear understanding of risk-benefit for all the patient's species can result in unintended adverse consequences.

Just as with the coral reef, the patient's total ancestral, environmental, and medical experiences play a role in the status of the microbiome. Modulators of the microbiome start with the chemicals and other environmental factors to which a human is exposed (e.g., diet, environmental pollutants, radiation, and drugs). Because the microbiome sits at our portals of exposure to the external environment (e.g., skin, gastrointestinal tract, airways, urogenital tract), the microbiome is exposed to, filters, deals with, and responds to these factors before our mammalian cells ever encounter them (Dietert and Silbergeld 2015). In effect, the internal exposure dose to a dietary component, environmental chemical, or drugs is heavily regulated by our microbiome. The particular composition and richness of an individual's microbiome can affect human health risk (Dietert and Silbergeld 2015).

Chemical factors are not the only considerations. Risk factors for the microbiome include physical and psycho-social factors as well. For example, undue stress is a known health risk. It is also a significant factor in microbiome balance. For example, maternal stress during pregnancy has been implicated in changes in the vaginal microbiome as well as vaginal protein profiles that are associated with the first wave of microbial colonization in the offspring and subsequent programming of both metabolism and neurological development (Jašarević et al. 2015). One of the ways that stress and other environmentally induced changes in the microbiome are thought to influence neurological development and behavior is through changes in epithelial barriers that separate the microbiome from immune cells. Increased permeability and loss of tight junction function among epithelial cells allow microbial signaling of immune cells that predispose for inflammation. John and colleagues (John et al. 2015) have suggested that the subsequent proinflammatory state that is created by the dysfunctional microbiome leads to brain alterations signaled though the vagus nerve such as cytokine-induced alterations of the HPA axis and shifts in tryptophan metabolism. One of the molecular pathways involved appears to be the inflammasome, which is a go-between for microbial disruption and immune establishment of a proinflammatory state (Wong et al. 2016).

Within the brain there are ultrastructural changes that reflect the state of the microbiome. For example, it appears that the level of myelination in the pre-frontal cortex region of the brain is directly related to the sufficiency of the microbiome (Hoban et al. 2016). Additionally, distinct gut-to-brain and brain-to-gut pathways linking anxiety/depression and irritable bowel syndrome (IBS) were recently described by researchers from Australia. In some cases, the neurologically related symptoms preceded the gastrointestinal distress and in many others, this relationship was reversed with IBS arising before anxiety or depression (Koloski et al. 2016). Recent studies of gut microbiota both in animal models as well as human patients have shown a link between gut microbiome status and the neuroinflammatory autoimmune disease, multiple sclerosis (Glenn and Mowry 2016). Similarly, gut microbiota dysbiosis has been demonstrated in patients with the debilitating condition myalgic encephalomyelitis (previously known as chronic fatigue syndrome) (Giloteaux et al. 2016). Finally, the outcome of ischemic stroke appears to be affected by the composition of the gut microbiota via their impact on immune regulatory cell activities (Benakis et al. 2016).

While more information on specific regulators of microbially driven, gut-brain alterations will be useful, it is increasingly clear that healthy neurological and psychiatric function is difficult if not impossible to maintain in the absence of a healthy microbiome. Additionally, there is a golden opportunity to use microbes and/or their metabolites as therapeutics for mood, depression, and psychological problems (Sherwin et al. 2016).

Recently, new adaptive tests to examine data sets for microbiome composition and physiological as well as health outcomes have provided new insights into the ecology of the human microbiome. For example, application of these multivariate data analyses has led to better insights into the role of gender in differences among specific bacterial families (Wu et al. 2016).

COMPLEMENTARY THERAPIES: REBIOSIS

Complementary strategies to achieve a better balance within the microbiome at various body sites involve the process known as rebiosis. This takes several forms: (1) consumption of fermented foods with active cultures, (2) consumption of or topical application of probiotic formulations containing missing or deficient microbes, (3) consumption of prebiotics (food/energy sources for specific microbes) often given with probiotics, and (4) the more comprehensive microbiota alteration called fecal microbiota transplantation (FMT). To facilitate the likelihood that the microorganism will take up residence in the patient, the nutrient tailored to support the growth of the probiotic microorganisms (called prebiotics) is often used either in the same formulation as the live microbial cultures or separately. Ideally, consumed probiotics can take up residence at the desired body site (part of the GI tract, skin, mouth, nose, urogenital tract). But even in cases where the microbes are only transient, there can be some metabolic benefit by the application and the presence of probiotic metabolites (Guo et al. 2016). Table 1.2 illustrates some of the examples in which rebiosis has been used in the treatment of disease. Among the examples shown are allergic, inflammatory, behavioral, autoimmune, and infectious diseases and conditions.

Fecal microbiota transplantation involves a more comprehensive alteration of the gut microbiome than might be expected from consumption of probiotic-containing foods or probiotic formulations. Importantly, donor selection is important in FMT. As discussed by Fuentes and de Vos (2016) FMT is not really a radical idea. They argue that the most significant transplantation event is via natural childbirth when the mother donates her microbiota to seed the baby. FMT can lead to a complete change in the gastrointestinal microbiota such that it more closely resembles the donor profile than the recipient microbiome. However, while the impact on existing diseases such as *Clostridium difficile* infections can be prompt, complete changes in the microbiome profile may not be evident for months and could take years (Broecker et al. 2016).

In addition to the information in Table 1.2, many preventative and therapeutic applications involving probiotics and FMT are introduced in the following section.

ANTIBIOTIC ADJUNCT THERAPIES

Overuse of antibiotics is recognized as a major factor in the depletion of the human microbiome and even when they are needed, these drugs are likely to kill commensal bacteria along with the pathogen (Blaser 2016). Investigators have argued that it is time to consider probiotics as an adjunct therapy for antibiotic administration. In particular, this has been advocated in the treatment of *Clostridium difficile* infection (Spinler et al. 2016). However, given the impact of antibiotics on the microbiome, adjunct therapies could help avoid the destruction of the microbiome and subsequent altered physiology, barrier function, and risk of inflammatory-driven diseases. A recent trial in children looked at the adjunct administration of yogurt containing three probiotic bacteria versus control pasteurized yogurt for children receiving prescribed antibiotics. The study reported that the probiotics group had a lower and less severe incidence of antibiotic-associated diarrhea (Fox et al. 2015).

POSTOPERATIVE RECOVERY

The postoperative phase of major surgical procedures is receiving additional attention as that can affect the subsequent health trajectory of patients (Fujikuni et al. 2016). There are opportunities for this to move beyond pain management to include attention to microbiome status, probiotics, and the use of prebiotics and functional foods. Mizuta et al. (2016) examined the effects of daily *Bifidobacterium longum* BB536 administration preoperatively (preoperatively for 7–14 days and then postoperatively for 14 days) among patients undergoing colorectal surgery. The clinical investigators found that probiotic supplementation resulted in both an improved balance of gut microbes following surgery and reduced levels of inflammatory biomarkers (e.g., C-reactive proteins).

PROTECTION AGAINST STRESS-INDUCED DYSBIOSIS

Preventative application of probiotics to avoid the damage of environmental changes can be beneficial. For example, Kato-Kataoka et al. (2016) reported that daily ingestion of milk-borne *Lactobacillus casei* strain Shirota by healthy medical students preparing for examinations led to an increased diversity of gut microbiota, reduced abdominal distress, reduced salivary cortisol levels, and reduced stress-induced changes in leukocytes in the probiotic-supplemented test group versus the placebo group. Early life stress can produce developmental impairment in learning. Researchers showed that a probiotic formulation of *Lactobacillus rhamnosus* and *L. helveticus* given to rat dams corrected maternal separation-induced developmental impairment of the pups (Cowan et al. 2016).

TABLE 1.2
Some Examples of Microbiome Rebiosis to Treat Diseases and Conditions

Medical Condition	Microbial Intervention	Reported Outcome	References
Atopy and food hypersensitivity	Meta-analysis of 17 human studies on consumption of probiotics during pregnancy and early childhood and risk of childhood atopy and food hypersensitivity	Probiotics administered both during pregnancy and early childhood could reduce the risk of childhood atopy and food hypersensitivity	Zhang et al. (2016)
Atopic dermatitis	Meta-analysis of 25 studies with 1599 participants concerning probiotics in the treatment for atopic dermatitis	Probiotics could be a useful treatment option for children and adults	Kim et al. (2014)
Bacterial vaginosis	In a multicenter study, 160 participants with at-risk vaginal environment profiles were randomly assigned to test and placebo groups. The test group was given a 7-day regimen of a probiotic mix with *Lactobacillus fermentum* 57A, *Lactobacillus plantarum* 57B, and *Lactobacillus gasseri* 57C	As a preventative measure for at-risk populations, probiotics restored the microbial profile and pH to normal ranges reducing the risk of bacterial vaginosis	Tomusiak et al. (2015)
Depression	Supplementation with *Lactobacillus helveticus* R0052 and *Bifidobacterium longum* R0175	Decreased scores for anxiety and depression	Messaoudi et al. (2011)
Depression	Eight-week supplementation with *Lactobacillus acidophilus* *Lactobacillus casei* and *Bifidobacterium bifidum*	Beneficial effects on Beck Depression Inventory	Akkasheh et al. (2016)
Late-onset sepsis in preterm neonates	Meta-analysis of 17 trials with enteral probiotic supplementation examining risk of sepsis in neonates	Significant reduction in risk of any sepsis, bacterial sepsis and fungal sepsis that also included low birth weight babies	Zhang et al. (2016)
Gingivitis and peridontitis	Meta-analysis of 50 studies with 3247 participants involving use of probiotics in oral disease management	Treatment with probiotics bacteria such as lactibacili and bifidobacteria was effective in managing both gingivitis and peridotitis	Gruner et al. (2016)
Pathogenic bacterial biofilms	Probiotic bacteria (combinations of *Lactobacillus plantarum* SD5870, *Lactobacillus helveticus* CBS N116411 and *Streptococcus salivarius* DSM 14685) used to inhibit biofilm formation and disrupt existing biofilms	Overlay and co-culture experiments showed that the probiotics disrupted biofilm formation, disrupted existing biofilms and inhibited gene expression in *Candida albicans* that was required for the formation of biofilms by the opportunistic pathogen	James et al. (2016)
Recurrent *Clostridium difficile* infection	Fecal microbiota transplantation (FMT), including in the form of frozen preparations, has been shown to be effective at treating this condition at least in part by changing bile acid composition	FMT not only corrects this condition but also reduces the burden of antibiotic resistant genes in the microbiome of patients	Lee et al. (2016), Weingarden et al. (2016), Millan et al. (2016)
Rheumatoid arthritis	Sixty patients (30 test and 30 control) took probiotics (capsules of *Lactobacillus acidophilus*, *Lactobacillus casei* and *Bifidobacterium bifidum* for 8 weeks	Significant probiotic-associated clinical and metabolic improvement was found for the Disease Activity Score of 28 joints, as well as for metabolic and inflammatory biomarkers	Zamami et al. (2016)
Ulcerative colitis	Meta-analysis of 25 studies including 234 ulcerative colitis patients who received fecal microbiota transplantation (FMT)	Overall results were 41.6% with clinical remission and 65.3% with useful clinical outcomes	Shi et al. (2016)

Correction of Depression and Anxiety

Gut microbiota can communicate with the brain using immune, neuro, and endocrine pathways (Slyepchenko et al. 2014). Probiotics are becoming a useful tool in the treatment of depression and anxiety. Vlainić et al. (2016) described the value in probiotic adjunct therapy for treating major depressive disorder (MDD). Part of the basis for microbiome adjustments in MDD is the fact that the gut microbiome plays a major role both directly and indirectly in the production of neurotransmitters, neuroactive peptides, and glutamatergic and GABAergic transmission (e.g., GABA, serotonin, norepinephrine, dopamine) (Cryan and Dinan 2015). Additionally, the microbiome profile largely determines the balance of pro- and anti-inflammatory cytokines that play a role in MDD (Dinan and Cryan 2016). The control of mood and behavior is so extensive that researchers recently coined the term psychobiotics to refer to mind altering probiotics (Wall et al. 2014). Some gut microbes have the potential to regulate myelination in the prefrontal cortex via changes in gene expression (Hoban et al. 2016). Among the potential candidate probiotics to treat depression and anxiety are: *Bifidobacterium longum* (B.) 1714 and *B. breve* 1205 (Savignac et al. 2014).

Additionally, the immune system can be involved in the connection between social behavior and the microbiome. A recent study by Filiano et al. (2016) found that meningeal immunity, particularly interferon-gamma-driven signaling, is key to the level of GABAergic (γ-aminobutyric-acid) responses in neural circuits. Immune dysfunction can act as a pathway to social dysfunction.

Anti-Aging Effects

Oxidative damage in body sites such as the skin is a major part of the aging process (Poljšak et al. 2012; Rinnerthaler et al. 2015). Probiotics appear to offer promise in protecting the skin from both intrinsic and extrinsic aging (Sharma et al. 2016). Importantly, not only is oxidative stress attenuated, but barrier function can be improved via a microbial strategy. Among the probiotics that have shown promise for the skin are: *Lactobacillus plantarum*, *Lactobacillus paracasei*, and *Bifidobacterium breve*.

Protection Against Recurrent *Clostridium difficile* Infection

Clostridium difficile infection presents a significant, largely hospital borne, health risk. One of the problems with antibiotic therapies is that while they may control the pre-existing infection, they invariably put the patient at an elevated risk for recurrent *C. difficile* infection. This appears to occur because of the existence of antibiotic-resistant *C. difficile* spores, which have an advantage to reinfect the patient due to the antibiotic-induced general disruption of the gut microbiota (Sbahi and Di Palma 2016). An effective tool against recurrent infection with *C. difficile* is FMT (Sbahi and Di Palma 2016). While this has been historically done by colonoscopy installed transplantation of fecal microbiota, more recent developments have allowed frozen oral capsules to be the route of administration (Youngster et al. 2014).

Protection Against Environmental Toxicants

Because the microbiome resides largely at the site of the body's exposure to the external environment, the microbes receive the bolus of most drugs and environmental chemicals before the human mammalian cells. Risk of human toxicity is, therefore, affected by the diversity, richness, and composition of the microbiome in different sites (e.g., skin, GI tract). Heavy metals such as cadmium are neuro- and immuno-toxicants and have the capacity to disrupt barrier function at least in part via oxidative damage. A recent study in mice on cadmium exposure found that treatments with the probiotic *Lactobacillus plantarum* CCFM8610 increased excretion rather than absorption of cadmium, reduced disruption of intestinal barrier tight junctions, reduced inflammation, and decreased the intestinal permeability of mice (Zhai et al. 2016). The discovery of the importance of certain probiotics on both barrier function and levels of inflammation is consistent with the recent focus on the microbiome, host defense barrier, and immune system complex termed the microimmunosome (Dietert 2016a).

TREATING METABOLIC SYNDROME

Rebiosis approaches appear promising when it comes to treating metabolic syndrome. A course of *Bifidobacterium lactis* HN019 (in fermented milk) was administered to a subgroup of Met S patients for 45 days and lipid metabolism plus inflammatory biomarkers were evaluated in probiotic-administered versus control patients (Bernini et al. 2016). The investigators found that ingestion of the probiotics-laden milk resulted in a significant reduction in body mass index, total cholesterol, and low-density lipoprotein when compared with the baseline and control group results. Additionally, levels of two proinflammatory cytokines (tumor necrosis factor alpha and interleukin 6) were significantly decreased with the supplementation. Based on these results, the conclusion was that probiotic supplementation may reduce the risk of cardiovascular disease among MetS patients.

A key target in the treatment of metabolic syndrome via the microbiome involved the bacterial species *Akkermansia muciniphila*. *A. mucinphila* is a key bacterium involved with regulation of the mucus layer in the gut and, as a result, integrity of the gut barrier and protection against inappropriate and/or excessive inflammation. To date, prebiotics have been used to modulate the size of the *A. muciniphila* population in the patient's gut. However, next generation probiotic formulations including *A. muciniphila* are on the horizon pending safety evaluations, and these may be useful against metabolic syndrome linked conditions (Cani and Van Hul 2015; Gómez-Gallego et al. 2016).

POTENTIAL HELP FOR INFANTILE COLIC

A randomized double-blind study in Canada using *Lactobacillus reuteri* DSM 17938 found that daily administration of the probiotic to breastfed infants significantly reduced the crying time and fussiness in babies when compared to the placebo group (Chau et al. 2015).

BIOFILMS

Biofilms are community level organizations of microbial species that stick to each other, thereby forming a superstructure and usually also adhering to host tissue. The superstructure organization allows the microbes to change metabolism, producing an almost impenetrable matrix of extracellular polymeric substance (EPS) that protects this specialized microbial form from many traditional antimicrobial agents.

As a result, pathogenic biofilm can be comparatively resistant to both host defenses and normal medical treatments such as dosing with antibiotics. Some pathogens are more likely than others to form biofilms. Additionally, they can be associated with many different tissues including the oral and urogenital cavities and hair follicles. A further concern is the ability of biofilms to form on implanted medical devices.

Biofilm formation is affected by specific gene expression, which is affected by several factors including the surface to which bacteria attach (Watnick and Kolter 2000). It is also thought that biofilms are more likely to form in response to local ecological competition and changes such as cellular damage regardless of the instigating factor (e.g., bacterial-derived toxins such as pyocins as well as antibiotics) (Oliveira et al. 2015).

An example of biofilms is the three-dimensional biofilms formed by *Propionibacterium acnes* during acne vulgaris in sebaceous follicles (Jahns et al. 2012; Jahns and Alexeyev 2014). However, not every comedone contains *Propionibacterium acnes*, and some clinicians have suggested that inflammatory imbalances in the follicle may be the actual initiating factor for the condition (Shaheen and Gonzalez 2013). Similarly, clinical presentation of Hidradenitis Suppurativa (HS) is also associated with bacterial biofilms potentially involving several different species. However, it is not clear whether the biofilms are involved with disease induction or reflect the disturbance of the local hair follicle environment once the condition has become established (Ring and Emtestam 2016).

While biofilms can prevent a significant health challenge in any tissue, their consideration is particularly important in managing oral hygiene and preventing oral disease. Biofilms are readily formed in the mouth as part of the regular community microbial structure (Arweiler and Netuschil 2016) However, if not managed, caries and oral disease can result. There is evidence that biofilm formation in the mouth can occur in stages during which facultative anaerobic bacteria can become replaced by gram-negative anaerobic bacteria (Wake et al. 2016).

Evidence suggests that probiotics can offer part of an integrative health strategy for prevention and reduction of biofilms. However, the specific selection of the probiotic bacteria, the genes they carry relative to the pathogens involved in the biofilm and the stage of development of the biofilm appear to be important considerations. Vuotto et al. (2014) recently reviewed the use of probiotics in the prevention and treatment of specific biofilms. Much of the most extensively studied examples involve *Bifidobacterium* spp.—and *Lactobacillus* spp.—containing probiotics. Combinations of *Lactobacillus plantarum* SD5870, *Lactobacillus helveticus* CBS N116411, and *Streptococcus salivarius* DSM 14685 bacteria or their supernatants have been found to significantly reduce oral biofilm formation by *Candida albicans* (James et al. 2016).

While biofilms are generally thought to be detrimental to the patient, there are several examples where biofilms involving keystone commensal species of bacteria are actually required to support fundamental human biological functions. Among these is the maintenance of the microimmunosome, the microbiome-host defense barrier-immune complex, and balanced physiology. For example, biofilm formation in the colon appears to be required to support normal mucus production. This is often disrupted with colitis. Restoration of the biofilm using a hydrogen sulfide donor chemical (diallyl disulfide) in experimental animals and in human *ex vivo* tissues can restore mucus production and reduce inflammation (Motta et al. 2015). This example of useful biofilm formation suggests that alterations of microbiota for improved health do not require elimination of all biofilms. Instead, changes in the microbial species composition of biofilms may be a more unifying strategy when patient barrier function is an issue.

CONCLUSIONS

Integrative medicine is likely to focus increasingly on the microbiome as biomarkers of future health risks, targets of therapeutic strategies, and indicators of the effectiveness of medical treatments. This is because the microbiome is a dominant and integral component of the newly envisioned human superorganism patient. Human mammalian-centric approaches treat only a portion of the patient and, while there is still much to be learned about the microbiome and microbiome-based medicine, it represents the path to truly holistic and integrative medicine.

The ongoing NCD epidemic is this century's health crisis and current approaches most often manage disease symptoms rather than provide cures. Microbiome profiling of patients is likely to become routine as physicians will need to know those parameters before determining the most useful therapeutic approaches. In fact, recent knowledge that some drug prescriptions pose an unacceptable risk for individuals with certain microbiome imbalances (e.g., digoxin) will drive the need to monitor a patient's microbiome profile (Haiser et al. 2014).

Rebiosis at any age can be a useful part of integrative therapies. But the range of effects is likely to most significant during pregnancy (which can affect both the mother and child) and in the young. Changes in diet with the inclusion of prebiotics to feed desired microbes, consumption of fermented foods, use of probiotic supplements, and fecal microbiota transplantation are among the options currently available to shift the patient's microbiome profile. Finally, newly envisioned drugs are likely to work with and through the microbiome.

REFERENCES

Aagaard, K., Ma, J., Antony, K.M., Ganu, R., Petrosino, J., and Versalovic, J. 2014. The placenta harbors a unique microbiome. *Sci Transl Med* 6(237):237–65.

Akkasheh, G., Kashani-Poor, Z., Tajabadi-Ebrahimi, M., Jafari, P., Akbari, H., Taghizadeh, M., Memarzadeh, M.R., Asemi, Z., and Esmaillzadeh, A. 2016. Clinical and metabolic response to probiotic administration in patients with major depressive disorder: A randomized, double-blind, placebo-controlled trial. *Nutrition* 32(3):315–20.

Arweiler, N.B. and Netuschil, L. 2016. The oral microbiota. *Adv Exp Med Biol* 902:45–60.

Bashiardes, S., Thaiss, C.A., and Elinav, E. 2016. It's in the milk: Feeding the microbiome to promote infant growth. *Cell Metab* 23(3):393–4.

Benakis, C., Brea, D., Caballero, S., Faraco, G., Moore, J., Murphy, M., Sita, G. et al. 2016. Commensal microbiota affects ischemic stroke outcome by regulating intestinal γδ T cells. *Nat Med* 22:516–23.

Bernini, L.J., Simão, A.N., Alfieri, D.F., Lozovoy, M.A., Mari, N.L., de Souza, C.H., Dichi, I., and Costa, G.N. 2016. Beneficial effects of *Bifidobacterium lactis* on lipid profile and cytokines in patients with metabolic syndrome: A randomized trial. Effects of probiotics on metabolic syndrome. *Nutrition* 32(6):716–9.

Blaser, M.J. 2016. Antibiotic use and its consequences for the normal microbiome. *Science* 352(6285):544–5.

Bokulich, N.A., Chung, J., Battaglia, T., Henderson, N., Jay, M., Li, H., D Lieber, A. et al. 2016. Antibiotics, birth mode, and diet shape microbiome maturation during early life. *Sci Transl Med* 15;8(343):343–82.

Breton, J., Daniel, C., Dewulf, J., Pothion, S., Froux, N., Sauty, M., Thomas, P. et al. 2013. Gut microbiota limits heavy metals burden caused by chronic oral exposure. *Toxicol Lett* 222(2):132–8.

Broecker, F., Klumpp, J., Schuppler, M., Russo, G., Biedermann, L., Hombach, M., Rogler, G., and Moelling, K. 2016. Long-term changes of bacterial and viral compositions in the intestine of a recovered *Clostridium difficile* patient after fecal microbiota transplantation. *Cold Spring Harb Mol Case Stud* 2(1):a000448.

Cai, J., Zhang, L., Jones, R.A., Correll, J.B., Hatzakis, E., Smith, P.B., Gonzalez, F.J., and Patterson, A.D. 2016. Antioxidant drug tempol promotes functional metabolic changes in the gut microbiota. *J Proteome Res* 15(2):563–71.

Cani, P.D. and Van Hul, M. 2015. Novel opportunities for next-generation probiotics targeting metabolic syndrome. *Curr Opin Biotechnol* 32:21–7.

Cao, B., Stout, M.J., Lee, I., and Mysorekar, I.U. 2014. Placental microbiome and its role in preterm birth. *Neoreviews* 15(12):e537–45.

Chau, K., Lau, E., Greenberg, S., Jacobson, S., Yazdani-Brojeni, P., Verma, N., and Koren, G. 2015. Probiotics for infantile colic: A randomized, double-blind, placebo-controlled trial investigating *Lactobacillus reuteri* DSM 17938. *J Pediatr* 166:74–8.

Clooney, A.G., Bernstein, C.N., Leslie, W.D., Vagianos, K., Sargent, M., Laserna-Mendieta, E.J., Claesson, M.J., and Targownik, L.E. 2016. A comparison of the gut microbiome between long-term users and non-users of proton pump inhibitors. *Aliment Pharmacol Ther* 43(9):974–84.

Cowan, C.S., Callaghan, B.L., and Richardson, R. 2016. The effects of a probiotic formulation (*Lactobacillus rhamnosus* and *L. helveticus*) on developmental trajectories of emotional learning in stressed infant rats. *Transl Psychiatry* 6(5):e823.

Cryan, J.F. and Dinan, T.G. 2015. More than a gut feeling: The microbiota regulates neurodevelopment and behavior. *Neuropsychopharmacology* 40(1):241–2.

Dalal, R.P. and Goldfarb, D.S. 2011. Melamine-related kidney stones and renal toxicity. *Nat Rev Nephrol* 7(5):267–74.

Dc-Rubin, S.S., Alava, P., Zekker, I., Du Laing, G., and Van de Wiele, T. 2014. Arsenic thiolation and the role of sulfate-reducing bacteria from the human intestinal tract. *Environ Health Perspect* 122(8):817–22.

De Maeseneer, J. and Boeckxstaens, P. 2011. Care for noncommunicable diseases (NCDs): Time for a paradigm-shift. *World Hosp Health Serv* 47(4):30–3.

Diaz Heijtz, R. 2016. Fetal, neonatal, and infant microbiome: Perturbations and subsequent effects on brain development and behavior. *Semin Fetal Neonatal Med* 21(6):410–7.

Dietert, R. 2016a. The microbiome-immune-host defense barrier complex (microimmunosome) and developmental programming of noncommunicable diseases. *Reprod Toxicol* 68:49–58.

Dietert, R. 2016b. *The Human Superorganism*. New York: Dutton Penguin Random House.

Dietert, R.R. 2014. The microbiome in early life: Self-completion and microbiota protection as health priorities. *Birth Defects Res B Dev Reprod Toxicol* 101(4):333–40.

Dietert, R.R., DeWitt, J.C., Germolec, D.R., and Zelikoff, J.T. 2010. Breaking patterns of environmentally influenced disease for health risk reduction: Immune perspectives. *Environ Health Perspect* 118(8):1091–9.

Dietert, R.R. and Silbergeld, E.K. 2015. Biomarkers for the 21st century: Listening to the microbiome. *Toxicol Sci* 144(2):208–16.

Dinan, T.G. and Cryan, J.F. 2016. Microbes, immunity and behaviour: Psychoneuroimmunology meets the microbiome. *Neuropsychopharmacology* doi: 10.1038/npp.2016.103.

Feng, R., Shou, J.W., Zhao, Z.X., He, C.Y., Ma, C., Huang, M., Fu, J. et al. 2015. Transforming berberine into its intestine-absorbable form by the gut microbiota. *Sci Rep* 5:12155.

Filiano, A.J., Xu, Y., Tustison, N.J., Marsh, R.L., Baker, W., Smirnov, I., Overall, C.C. et al. 2016. Unexpected role of interferon-γ in regulating neuronal connectivity and social behaviour. *Nature* 535(7612):425–9.

Fox, C. and Eichelberger, K. 2015. Maternal microbiome and pregnancy outcomes. *Fertil Steril* 104(6):1358–63.

Fox, M.J., Ahuja, K.D., Robertson, I.K., Ball, M.J., and Eri, R.D. 2015. Can probiotic yogurt prevent diarrhoea in children on antibiotics? A double-blind, randomised, placebo-controlled study. *BMJ Open* 5(1):e006474.

Fuentes, S. and de Vos, W.M. 2016. How to manipulate the microbiota: Fecal microbiota transplantation. *Adv Exp Med Biol* 902:143–53.

Fujikuni, N., Tanabe, K., Tokumoto, N., Suzuki, T., Hattori, M., Misumi, T., and Ohdan, H. 2016. Enhanced recovery program is safe and improves postoperative insulin resistance in gastrectomy. *World J Gastrointest Surg* 8(5):382–8.

Giloteaux, L., Goodrich, J.K., Walters, W.A., Levine, S.M., Ley, R.E., and Hanson, M.R. 2016. Reduced diversity and altered composition of the gut microbiome in individuals with myalgic encephalomyelitis/ chronic fatigue syndrome. *Microbiome* 4:30.

Glenn, J.D. and Mowry, E.M. 2016. Emerging concepts on the gut microbiome and multiple sclerosis. *J Interferon Cytokine Res* 36(6):347–57.

Gruner, D., Paris, S., and Schwendicke, F. 2016. Probiotics for managing caries and periodontitis: Systematic review and meta-analysis. *J Dent* 48:16–25.

Guo, S., Gillingham, T., Guo, Y., Meng, D., Zhu, W., Walker, W.A., and Ganguli, K. 2016. Secretions of Bifidobacterium infantis and lactobacillus acidophilus protect intestinal epithelial barrier function. *J Pediatr Gastroenterol Nutr* 64(3):404–12.

Gómez-Gallego, C., Pohl, S., Salminen, S., De Vos, W.M., and Kneifel, W. 2016. *Akkermansia muciniphila*: A novel functional microbe with probiotic properties. *Benef Microbes* 7(4):1–14.

Haiser, H.J., Seim, K.L., Balskus, E.P., and Turnbaugh, P.J. 2014. Mechanistic insight into digoxin inactivation by Eggerthella lenta augments our understanding of its pharmacokinetics. *Gut Microbes* 5(2):233–8.

Hoban, A.E., Stilling, R.M., Ryan, F.J., Shanahan, F., Dinan, T.G., Claesson, M.J., Clarke, G., and Cryan, J.F. 2016. Regulation of prefrontal cortex myelination by the microbiota. *Transl Psychiatry* 6:e774.

Imhann, F., Bonder, M.J., Vich Vila, A., Fu, J., Mujagic, Z., Vork, L., Tigchelaar, E.F. et al. 2016. Proton pump inhibitors affect the gut microbiome. *Gut* 65(5):740–8.

International Human Genome Sequencing Consortium. 2004. Finishing the euchromatic sequence of the human genome. *Nature* 431(7011):931–45.

Isolauri, E., Rautava, S., Collado, M.C., and Salminen, S. 2015. Role of probiotics in reducing the risk of gestational diabetes. *Diabetes Obes Metab* 17(8):713–9.

Jackson, M.A., Goodrich, J.K., Maxan, M.E., Freedberg, D.E., Abrams, J.A., Poole, A.C., Sutter, J.L. et al. 2016. Proton pump inhibitors alter the composition of the gut microbiota. *Gut* 65(5):749–56.

Jahns, A.C. and Alexeyev, O.A. 2014. Three-dimensional distribution of Propionibacterium acnes biofilms in human skin. *Exp Dermatol* 23(9):687–9.

Jahns, A.C., Lundskog, B., Ganceviciene, R., Palmer, R.H., Golovleva, I., Zouboulis, C.C., McDowell, A., Patrick, S., and Alexeyev, O.A. 2012. An increased incidence of Propionibacterium acnes biofilms in acne vulgaris: A case-control study. *Br J Dermatol* 167(1):50–8.

James, K.M., MacDonald, K.W., Chanyi, R.M., Cadieux, P.A., and Burton, J.P. 2016. Inhibition of *Candida albicans* biofilm formation and modulation of gene expression by probiotic cells and supernatant. *J Med Microbiol* 65:328–36.

Jašarević, E., Howerton, C.L., Howard, C.D., and Bale, T.L. 2015. Alterations in the vaginal microbiome by maternal stress are associated with metabolic reprogramming of the offspring gut and brain. *Endocrinology* 156(9):3265–76.

John, R., Kelly, P., Kennedy, J., Cryan, J.F., Dinan, T.G., Clarke, G., and Hyland, N.P. 2015. Breaking down the barriers: The gut microbiome, intestinal permeability and stress-related psychiatric disorders. *Front Cell Neurosci* 9:392.

Kato-Kataoka, A., Nishida, K., Takada, M., Kawai, M., Kikuchi-Hayakawa, H., Suda, K., Ishikawa, H. et al. 2016. Fermented milk containing *Lactobacillus casei* strain Shirota preserves the diversity of the gut microbiota and relieves abdominal dysfunction in healthy medical students exposed to academic stress. *Appl Environ Microbiol* 82(12):3649–58.

Kim, S.O., Ah, Y.M., Yu, Y.M., Choi, K.H., Shin, W.G., and Lee, J.Y. 2014. Effects of probiotics for the treatment of atopic dermatitis: A meta-analysis of randomized controlled trials. *Ann Allergy Asthma Immunol* 113(2):217–26.

Klaassen, C.D. and Cui, J.Y. 2015. Review: Mechanisms of how the intestinal microbiota alters the effects of drugs and bile acids. *Drug Metab Dispos* 43(10):1505–21.

Koloski, N.A., Jones, M., and Talley, N.J. 2016. Evidence that independent gut-to-brain and brain-to-gut pathways operate in the irritable bowel syndrome and functional dyspepsia: A 1-year population-based prospective study. *Aliment Pharmacol Ther* 44(6):592–600.

Lee, C.H., Steiner, T., Petrof, E.O., Smieja, M., Roscoe, D., Nematallah, A., Weese, J.S. et al. 2016. Frozen vs fresh fecal microbiota transplantation and clinical resolution of diarrhea in patients With recurrent *Clostridium difficile* infection: A randomized clinical trial. *JAMA* 315(2):142–9.

Li, J., Jia, H., Cai, X., Zhong, H., Feng, Q., Sunagawa, S., Arumugam, M. et al., and MetaHIT Consortium. 2014. An integrated catalog of reference genes in the human gut microbiome. *Nat Biotechnol* 32(8):834–41.

Messaoudi, M., Violle, N., Bisson, J.F., Desor, D., Javelot, H., and Rougeot, C. 2011. Beneficial psychological effects of a probiotic formulation (*Lactobacillus helveticus* R0052 and *Bifidobacterium longum* R0175) in healthy human volunteers. *Gut Microbes* 2(4):256–61.

Millan, B., Park, H., Hotte, N., Mathieu, O., Burguiere, P., Tompkins, T.A., Kao, D., and Madsen, K.L. 2016. Fecal microbial transplants reduce antibiotic-resistant genes in patients with recurrent *Clostridium difficile* infection. *Clin Infect Dis* 62(12):1479–86.

Mizuta, M., Endo, I., Yamamoto, S., Inokawa, H., Kubo, M., Udaka, T., Sogabe, O. et al. 2016. Perioperative supplementation with bifidobacteria improves postoperative nutritional recovery, inflammatory response, and fecal microbiota in patients undergoing colorectal surgery: A prospective, randomized clinical trial. *Biosci Microbiota Food Health* 35(2):77–87.

Mor, G. and Kwon, J.Y. 2015. Trophoblast-microbiome interaction: A new paradigm on immune regulation. *Am J Obstet Gynecol* 213(4 Suppl):S131–7.

Morton, J.S., Cooke, C.L., and Davidge, S.T. 2016. In utero origins of hypertension: Mechanisms and targets for therapy. *Physiol Rev* 96(2):549–603.

Motta, J.P., Flannigan, K.L., Agbor, T.A., Beatty, J.K., Blackler, R.W., Workentine, M.L., Da Silva, G.J., Wang, R., Buret, A.G., and Wallace, J.L. 2015. Hydrogen sulfide protects from colitis and restores intestinal microbiota biofilm and mucus production. *Inflamm Bowel Dis* 21(5):1006–17.

Mueller, N.T., Bakacs, E., Combellick, J., Grigoryan, Z., and Dominguez-Bello, M.G. 2015. The infant microbiome development: Mom matters. *Trends Mol Med* 21(2):109–17.

Nishtala, P.S., Gnjidic, D., Chyou, T., and Hilmer, S.N. 2016. Discontinuation of statins in a population of older New Zealanders with limited life expectancy. *Intern Med J* 46(4):493–6.

Oliveira, N.M., Martinez-Garcia, E., Xavier, J., Durham, W.M., Kolter, R., Kim, W., and Foster, K.R. 2015. Biofilm formation as a response to ecological competition. *PLoS Biol* 13(7):e1002191.

Pennisi, E. and Mueller, K. 2016. The microbes that make us. *Science* 352(6285), http://www.sciencemag.org/topic/microbiome.

Poljšak, B., Dahmane, R.G., and Godić, A. 2012. Intrinsic skin aging: The role of oxidative stress. *Acta Dermatovenerol Alp Pannonica Adriat* 21(2):33–6.

Ring, H.C. and Emtestam, L. 2016. The microbiology of hidradenitis suppurativa. *Dermatol Clin* 34(1):29–35.

Rinnerthaler, M., Bischof, J., Streubel, M.K., Trost, A., and Richter, K. 2015. Oxidative stress in aging human skin. *Biomolecules* 21;5(2):545–89.

Rogers, M.A. and Aronoff, D.M. 2016. The influence of non-steroidal anti-inflammatory drugs on the gut microbiome. *Clin Microbiol Infect* 22(2):178.e1–9.

Roura, L.C. and Arulkumaran, S.S. 2015. Facing the noncommunicable disease (NCD) global epidemic–the battle of prevention starts in utero–the FIGO challenge. *Best Pract Res Clin Obstet Gynaecol* 29(1):5–14.

Savignac, H.M., Kiely, B., Dinan, T.G., and Cryan, J.F. 2014. Bifidobacteria exert strain-specific effects on stress-related behavior and physiology in BALB/c mice. *Neurogastroenterol Motil* 26(11):1615–27.

Sbahi, H. and Di Palma, J.A. 2016. Faecal microbiota transplantation: Applications and limitations in treating gastrointestinal disorders. *BMJ Open Gastroenterol* 3(1):e000087.

Selwyn, F.P., Cheng, S.L., Klaassen, C.D., and Cui, J.Y. 2016. Regulation of hepatic drug-metabolizing enzymes in germ-free mice by conventionalization and probiotics. *Drug Metab Dispos* 44(2):262–74.

Selwyn, F.P., Cui, J.Y., and Klaassen, C.D. 2015. RNA-seq quantification of hepatic drug processing genes in germ-free mice. *Drug Metab Dispos* 43(10):1572–80.

Shaheen, B. and Gonzalez, M. 2013. Acne sans P. acnes. *J Eur Acad Dermatol Venereol* 27(1):1–10.

Sharma, D., Kober, M.M., and Bowe, W.P. 2016. Anti-aging effects of probiotics. *J Drugs Dermatol* 15(1):9–12.

Sherwin, E., Rea, K., Dinan, T.G., and Cryan, J.F. 2016. A gut (microbiome) feeling about the brain. *Curr Opin Gastroenterol* 32(2):96–102.

Shi, Y., Dong, Y., Huang, W., Zhu, D., Mao, H., and Su, P. 2016. Fecal microbiota transplantation for ulcerative colitis: A systematic review and meta-analysis. *PLoS One* 11(6):e0157259.

Slyepchenko, A., Carvalho, A.F., Cha, D.S., Kasper, S., and McIntyre, R.S. 2014. Gut emotions—Mechanisms of action of probiotics as novel therapeutic targets for depression and anxiety disorders. *CNS Neurol Disord Drug Targets* 13(10):1770–86.

Sonnenburg, E.D., Smits, S.A., Tikhonov, M., Higginbottom, S.K., Wingreen, N.S., and Sonnenburg, J.L. 2016. Diet-induced extinctions in the gut microbiota compound over generations. *Nature* 529(7585):212–5.

Spinler, J.K., Ross, C.L., and Savidge, T.C. 2016. Probiotics as adjunctive therapy for preventing *Clostridium difficile* infection—What are we waiting for? *Anaerobe* 41:51–7.

Stenman, L.K., Waget, A., Garret, C., Briand, F., Burcelin, R., Sulpice, T., and Lahtinen, S. 2015. Probiotic B420 and prebiotic polydextrose improve efficacy of antidiabetic drugs in mice. *Diabetol Metab Syndr* 7:75.

Stokholm, J., Thorsen, J., Chawes, B.L., Schjørring, S., Krogfelt, K.A., Bønnelykke, K., and Bisgaard, H. 2016. Cesarean section changes neonatal gut colonization. *J Allergy Clin Immunol* 138(3):881–9.e2.

Stuckey, H.L., Mullan-Jensen, C., Kalra, S., Reading, J., Wens, J., Vallis, M., Kokoszka, A. et al. 2016. Living with an adult who has diabetes: Qualitative insights from the second Diabetes Attitudes, Wishes and Needs (DAWN2) study. *Diabetes Res Clin Pract* 116:270–8.

Tomusiak, A., Strus, M., Heczko, P.B., Adamski, P., Stefański, G., Mikołajczyk-Cichońska, A., and Suda-Szczurek, M. 2015. Efficacy and safety of a vaginal medicinal product containing three strains of probiotic bacteria: A multicenter, randomized, double-blind, and placebo-controlled trial. *Drug Des Devel Ther* 9:5345–54.

Vlainić, J., Šuran, J., Vlainić, T., and Vukorep, A.L. 2016. Probiotics as an adjuvant therapy in major depressive disorder. *Curr Neuropharmacol* 14(8):952–8.

Vuotto, C., Longo, F., and Donelli, G. 2014. Probiotics to counteract biofilm-associated infections: Promising and conflicting data. *Int J Oral Sci* 6(4):189–94.

Wake, N., Asahi, Y., Noiri, Y., Hayashi, M., Motooka, D., Nakamura, S., Gotoh, K. et al. 2016. Temporal dynamics of bacterial microbiota in the human oral cavity determined using an in situ model of dental biofilms. *NPJ Biofilms and Microbiomes* 2:16018.

Wall, R., Cryan, J.F., Ross, R.P., Fitzgerald, G.F., Dinan, T.G., and Stanton, C. 2014. Bacterial neuroactive compounds produced by psychobiotics. *Adv Exp Med Biol* 817:221–39.

Wang, M., Monaco, M.H., and Donovan, S.M. 2016. Impact of early gut microbiota on immune and metabolic development and function. *Semin Fetal Neonatal Med* 21(6):380–7.

Wang, Z., Luo, H., Tu, W., Yang, H., Wong, W.H., Wong, W.T., Yung, K.F. et al. 2011. Melamine-tainted milk product-associated urinary stones in children. *Pediatr Int* 53(4):489–96.

Watnick, P. and Kolter, W. 2000. Biofilm, city of microbes. *J Bacteriol* 182(10):2675–9.

Weingarden, A.R., Dosa, P.I., DeWinter, E., Steer, C.J., Shaughnessy, M.K., Johnson, J.R., Khoruts, A., and Sadowsky, M.J. 2016. Changes in colonic bile acid composition following fecal microbiota transplantation are sufficient to control *Clostridium difficile* germination and growth. *PLoS One* 11(1):e0147210.

Wong, M.L., Inserra, A., Lewis, M.D., Mastronardi, C.A., Leong, L., Choo, J., Kentish, S. et al. 2016. Inflammasome signaling affects anxiety- and depressive-like behavior and gut microbiome composition. *Mol Psychiatry* 21(6):797–805.

Wopereis, H., Oozeer, R., Knipping, K., Belzer, C., and Knol, J. 2014. The first thousand days—Intestinal microbiology of early life: Establishing a symbiosis. *Pediatr Allergy Immunol* 25(5):428–38.

Wu, C., Chen, J., Kim, J., and Pan, W. 2016. An adaptive association test for microbiome data. *Genome Med* 8:56.

Xu, X. and Zhang, X. 2015. Effects of cyclophosphamide on immune system and gut microbiota in mice. *Microbiol Res* 171:97–106.

Yassour, M., Vatanen, T., Siljander, H., Hämäläinen, A.M., Härkönen, T., Ryhänen, S.J., Franzosa, E.A. et al., and DIABIMMUNE Study Group. 2016. Natural history of the infant gut microbiome and impact of antibiotic treatment on bacterial strain diversity and stability. *Sci Transl Med* 8(343):343–81.

Yoo, D.H., Kim, I.S., Van Le, T.K., Jung, I.H., Yoo, H.H., and Kim, D.H. 2014. Gut microbiota-mediated drug interactions between lovastatin and antibiotics. *Drug Metab Dispos* 42(9):1508–13.

Yoo, H.H., Kim, I.S., Yoo, D.H., and Kim, D.H. 2016. Effects of orally administered antibiotics on the bio-availability of amlodipine: Gut microbiota-mediated drug interaction. *J Hypertens* 34(1):156–62.

Youngster, I., Russell, G.H., Pindar, C., Ziv-Baran, T., Sauk, J., and Hohmann, E.L. 2014. Oral, capsulized, frozen fecal microbiota transplantation for relapsing *Clostridium difficile* infection. *JAMA* 312(17):1772–8.

Yu, G., Gail, M.H., Consonni, D., Carugno, M., Humphrys, M., Pesatori, A.C., Caporaso, N.E., Goedert, J.J., Ravel, J., and Landi, M.T. 2016. Characterizing human lung tissue microbiota and its relationship to epidemiological and clinical features. *Genome Biol* 17:163.

Zamani, B., Golkar, H.R., Farshbaf, S., Emadi-Baygi, M., Tajabadi-Ebrahimi, M., Jafari, P., Akhavan, R., Taghizadeh, M., Memarzadeh, M.R., and Asemi, Z. 2016. Clinical and metabolic response to probiotic supplementation in patients with rheumatoid arthritis: A randomized, double-blind, placebo-controlled trial. *Int J Rheum Dis* 19(9):869–79.

Zelante, T., Iannitti, R.G., Cunha, C., De Luca, A., Giovannini, G., Pieraccini, G., Zecchi, R. et al. 2013. Tryptophan catabolites from microbiota engage aryl hydrocarbon receptor and balance mucosal reactivity via interleukin-22. *Immunity* 39:372–85.

Zhai, Q., Tian, F., Zhao, J., Zhang, H., Narbad, A., and Chen, W. 2016. Oral administration of probiotics inhibits heavy metal cadmium absorption by protecting intestinal barrier. *Appl Environ Microbiol* 82(14):4429–40.

Zhang, G.Q., Hu, H.J., Liu, C.Y., Zhang, Q., Shakya, S., and Li, Z.Y. 2016. Probiotics for prevention of atopy and food hypersensitivity in early childhood: A PRISMA-compliant systematic review and meta-analysis of randomized controlled trials. *Medicine (Baltimore)* 95(8):e2562.

Zheng, J., Xiao, X., Zhang, Q., Mao, L., Yu, M., Xu, J. 2015. The placental microbiome varies in association with low birth weight in full-term neonates. *Nutrients* 7(8):6924–37.

Zheng, X., Zhao, A., Xie, G., Chi, Y., Zhao, L., Li, H., Wang, C. et al. 2013. Melamine-induced renal toxicity is mediated by the gut microbiota. *Sci Transl Med* 5:172ra22.

2 Nutritional Approaches to Chronic Illness

Miriam Maisel

CONTENTS

Introduction: Perspectives, Problems, Priorities 19
The Heart of the Matter 21
    Nutritional Intervention in Cardiovascular Disease 21
    Nutritional Interventions in Diabetes 23
    Nutritional Interventions in Hypertension 24
        Salt and DASH 24
        Other Dietary Approaches to Hypertension 25
Selected Mechanisms Underlying the Effect of Food on Cardio-Metabolic Parameters 29
    Endothelial Function 29
    Modification of Trimethyl-n-Oxide Levels 30
Nutritional Treatment of Selected Inflammatory and Auto-Immune Conditions 30
    Nutritional Treatment of Multiple Sclerosis (MS) 30
    Nutritional Treatment of Rheumatoid Arthritis (RA) 31
    Nutritional Treatment of Fibromyalgia Syndrome (FMS) 33
Summing Up: The Common Ground 33
Ethical Aspects and Iatrogenics 34
Conclusion: "Mind the Gap" 35
References 36

Nutritional treatment of selected chronic conditions, emphasizing published research on interventions proven to prevent and reverse cardio-metabolic disease, and slow down progression and achieve remission in selected autoimmune conditions. Focusing on the efficacy of whole food plant-based nutrition, and water-fasting, as safe and effective therapeutic modalities. Ahead of the guidelines but not ahead of the evidence.

INTRODUCTION: PERSPECTIVES, PROBLEMS, PRIORITIES

As clinicians it is our duty to preserve human life and reduce human suffering. In good faith we commit years of our own lives to education and training, years when we are tasked with absorbing and integrating imponderable quantities of information. All this information should be the means by which the wish to make a difference matures into the power to do so. Our profession is privileged to live where the warmth of humanitarian values can meet the cool clarity of rigorous science. At least, in an ideal world this would be so. Regarding the science aspect, however, things may not be as clear as we would like to believe. On the whole, doctors are passive and very indirect consumers of science, and culturally indoctrinated simply to adhere to "best practice," defined by guidelines, produced by panels of experts, who rely on meta-analyses of the published peer-reviewed literature. This is very indirect indeed, and depends on implicit trust in the filtering process by which the guideline reaches the working doctor. Yet, how can working doctors look at the staggering numbers of published papers and decode all the statistics about all the medical problems that we see every day? Guidelines are established, and then change, and even if our extensive medical training had really provided the tools to challenge any part of this process, where would we find the time? How many clinicians really read and understand medical research papers? How many of us even know what to read, or even how to choose what to read?

The area of nutrition is probably one of the most challenging. We all know that apart from the original zygote, formed from the union of sperm and egg, the mass of every human body is entirely formed from ingested and reassembled food. And this body is not just a static mass, but a highly complex and dynamic system where countless enzymatic reactions take place simultaneously, every millisecond. Food itself is not much less complex: even simple foods such as an apple or a lettuce leaf are virtual miracles of complexity, containing macronutrients, vitamins, minerals, fiber, and a huge variety of phytochemicals, many of which have yet to be defined. Having said that, how many physicians have learned during training and education that "most deaths in the United States are preventable" (Greger and Stone 2015, Lenders et al. 2013) or that "our diet is the number one cause of death and the number one cause of disability" (Greger and Stone 2015, Murray et al. 2013)?

In medical education and training we learn to target a single problem or aspect of a problem using a point to point approach. There is a pill for high blood pressure, a different pill for diabetes, a different pill for cholesterol, and a different pill for pain and inflammation, as if they were magic bullets. However, the term "magic bullet" comes from a different context. This term was first used by Nobel Prize winner Paul Ehrlich, at the end of the nineteenth century, and referred to the search for specific substances that would go straight to the major killers of the day, pathogens such as diphtheria and syphilis (Auterhoff 1967). The magic bullet approach is appropriate for acute infectious diseases, should prevention fail. But in the case of our modern Western chronic diseases, the equation changes. For chronic conditions, medications are prescribed long term and it is well known that the cholesterol lowering medications can promote diabetes, the various blood pressure medications can cause diabetes, gout, or depression, the anti-gout medications can damage the stomach and kidneys, and the antidepressants can cause weight gain and impair sexual functioning (British National Formulary 2016), although fortunately there are other pills to address the new problems. It is clear that whatever benefits conventional pharmacotherapy may have with respect to such chronic conditions, it does not provide magic bullet solutions. The situation may be more reminiscent of the mythical nine-headed hydra, a monstrous serpent. When one head was cut off, two would grow in its place.

The magic bullet idea seems also to exist with respect to the popular approach to nutritional supplements. U.S. law permits manufacturers to make health claims such as "supplement X will preserve heart health" as long as the claims are accompanied by a disclaimer, to the effect that the health claims have not been evaluated by the FDA (Cohen 2016). As there are now an estimated 55,000 supplements in the U.S. marketplace, and 52% of U.S. adults take supplements (Kantor 2016), one can probably assume that many people are convinced by these highly qualified health claims, at least sufficiently convinced to support a $32 billion industry (Cohen 2016).

The saving grace of the supplement phenomenon may be the public perception that such quasi-natural products are less dangerous than pharmaceuticals, an idea which speaks of an aspiration to attain health through more natural means. The popularity of supplements implies a deeply buried idea that nutrition, and perhaps even food, could be important for health. This phenomenon also demonstrates the willingness of a large proportion of the population to spend its own money on products of perceived benefit to health.

Certainly, no doctor could be expected to be fully conversant with the claims and effects (or lack thereof) of 55,000 different supplements, and it is indeed questionable how much a busy clinician should be interested in a manufacturer's claim on a little bottle which is followed by a disclaimer. But if patients show their doctor what supplements they are taking, and the doctor responds with shrugged shoulders and a glazed expression, this may only reinforce the notion that doctors neither know nor care about "nutrition."

How can responsible clinicians find a way through this jungle of "too much information," or too much so-called information? Is it possible to come to a better and more useful understanding of the role of food, of nutrition, which will inform our clinical practice and which will be of significant benefit to our patients? In other words, what approach can we use to find information that is true and that matters (Campbell and Jacobson 2013)?

In this chapter, many studies will be presented, studies that demonstrate the potential of nutrition (food) as a therapeutic tool in some of the conditions that matter the most—major causes of death and disability in our society, now, at the beginning of the twenty-first century. A case could be made to say that awareness of at least some of these pioneering studies should be a cornerstone of medical education and should form part of the common knowledge base of clinicians, including not only physicians and surgeons, but also osteopaths, naturopaths, homeopaths, herbalists, practitioners of traditional Chinese medicine, Ayurvedic medicine, and so on. This is because the findings are so positive, and matter so much, that for clinicians not to share them with their patients is arguably unethical, since it constitutes a failure to inform patients of treatment choices that are highly effective and benign. If clinicians themselves are not exposed to these studies during their education and training, then a definite onus falls on the educating and training institutions and their standards. Hopefully, the findings presented in this chapter will inform the guidelines of the future. It is to be noted, however, that the landmark studies on cigarette smoking and carcinoma of the lung were first published in the 1950s (Hutchinson 2006). Yet it took a long time for perceptions to change and it required up to five decades for laws to be passed banning smoking in public places. A follow-up report by the original authors 50 years after the first evidence was presented concluded that prolonged smoking was likely to shorten life by a decade (Doll et al. 2004). Nowadays, it would be unthinkable not to address patients' smoking, since the research evidence has been incorporated into guidelines and has become part of accepted good practice. In the case of nutrition, as will be seen, much evidence exists in the literature but has not (yet) become part of standard guidelines. This should not prevent thoughtful and caring clinicians from applying safe and effective nutritional interventions that are not "ahead of the evidence" but only ahead of the guidelines.

THE HEART OF THE MATTER

NUTRITIONAL INTERVENTION IN CARDIOVASCULAR DISEASE

The CDC ranked "diseases of the heart" as the top leading cause of death in 2014, accounting for 23.4% of U.S. deaths, over 614,000 deaths in that year. Cerebrovascular disease is listed as the fifth leading cause of death, accounting for 5.1% of all U.S. deaths in 2014, over 131,000 deaths (Heron 2016). Considering these together would attribute 28.4% of all U.S. deaths in 2014 to diseases of heart and cerebrovascular disease combined, for a total of just over 747,000 deaths. Further, an earlier CDC analysis ascribes 10.9% of disability to these two entities, with 6.6% ascribed to "heart trouble," 2.4% to stroke, and 1.9% to high blood pressure, out of a total of 45 million adults reporting a disability in that year (Brault et al. 2009). This equates to upward of 4.9 million Americans living with disabilities broadly attributed to vascular or cardiovascular disease. In yet another analysis using data from the Global Burden of Disease 2010 Study, ischemic heart disease and stroke rank as the first and third causes of years of life lost to premature mortality, together accounting for 735,000 deaths deemed to be premature. These entities also contribute very significantly to the number of years lived with disability (Murray et al. 2013).

Any discussion of nutrition and coronary artery disease would be incomplete without including the pioneering clinical studies of Dr. Dean Ornish and Dr. Caldwell Esselstyn, which were published in the 1990s and which demonstrated symptomatic improvement of coronary artery disease, improved heart function, and angiographic regression of severe stenoses. Both trials used a low-fat vegetarian diet.

Dr. Esselstyn's study aimed to reduce total cholesterol to below 3.88 mmol/L (150 mg/dl) and used a core diet based on whole grains, legumes, vegetables, and fruit, excluding meat, fish, fowl, added oils, excess salt, nuts, and avocados. Initially, non-fat milk and yoghurt were allowed in small amounts but these were later excluded along with caffeine and fructose. After 1987, lipid lowering medications were used to attain the desired cholesterol value if this had not been attained by diet alone (Esselstyn 1995, 2014).

Dr. Ornish's trial used a broadly similar diet but restricted salt only for hypertensive patients. Initially a small amount of egg white and a small amount of non-fat dairy were allowed, maintaining dietary cholesterol intake below 5 mg per day. The diet provided approximately 10% of calories from fat, 15%–20% from protein, and 70%–75% of calories from complex carbohydrates. Smoking cessation (for the one patient who smoked), stress management training, and moderate exercise were included. Vitamin B12 supplementation was used, but not lipid lowering medications (Ornish et al. 1990).

Dr. Ornish's study was randomized, and the control group followed "usual care" as provided by their own physicians. The recommendations current at the time were to consume "less red meat, more fish and chicken" aiming for a "low fat diet" in which 30% of dietary calories came from fat (Ornish 1990). In Dr. Ornish's study, The Lifestyle Heart Trial, in the experimental group, results at one year showed dramatic improvement (reduction) in angina frequency and duration, as well as an average change toward angiographic regression of coronary artery stenosis. In the control group, there was, on average, worsening of both symptoms and angiographic severity of lesions. The degree of improvement in the experimental group correlated with the degree of adherence to the diet and other components of the program. Dr. Ornish concluded that while his experimental diet was able to reverse coronary artery disease, the prevailing dietary recommendations current at the time (30% of calories from fat) did not go far enough to achieve reversal of disease (Ornish 1990).

Dr. Esselstyn's initial study followed a small group of cardiac patients from the Cleveland Clinic, all of whom had severe progressive triple vessel coronary artery disease, for a period of 5 years. The structure of the study did not involve a formal control group but patients who did not adhere to the dietary guidelines, or left the study, became a de facto control group. The 11 patients who completed the study had collectively experienced 37 cardiac events in the 8 years prior to the study. At the end of the 5 years of following the protocol, there were no new infarctions, and analyses of coronary lesions by percent stenosis showed that 100% of lesions had stabilized and 83% had regressed. Angina symptoms, present in 10 of the patients at the beginning of the study, decreased in all cases and were completely eliminated in 30% of cases. All five of the patients who dropped out of the study and resumed their former diet experienced new cardiac events, including worsening angina symptoms, disease progression requiring angioplasty or coronary artery bypass graft, ventricular tachycardia, and an arrhythmia related death (Esselstyn 1995). A larger study followed 198 patients for a mean of 3.7 years with the same dietary interventions, with the 21 patients who did not adhere to the program constituting a de facto control group, as in the earlier study. In the group of 177 patients who adhered to the dietary intervention, 81% improved and there were no cardiac deaths. Approximately 27 of these patients were able to avoid coronary artery stenting or bypass grafts that had previously been recommended. In the non-adherent group of 21 patients, 62% got worse, none experienced symptom reduction, and 2 died (Esselstyn 2014).

As previously noted, Dr. Ornish's study included formal stress reduction training and support groups. Dr. Esselstyn's study ostensibly included only a pure nutritional intervention (with some pharmacotherapy) to reduce total cholesterol to 3.88 mmol/L (150 mg/dL). However, in the original 5-year study, Dr. Esselstyn himself met with each participant twice a month to discuss the patient's food diary and blood test results. There were also gatherings of all the participants several times a year. These meetings, as well as other intensive educational inputs, were broadly understood to have a positive effect on adherence of patients to the prescribed regime (Esselstyn 1995).

Dr. Esselstyn points out that myocardial reperfusion and reduction of angina symptoms was documented to occur sometimes after a matter of only weeks of adherence to the very low-fat plant-based diet. This is attributed to the restored ability of endothelial cells to produce the vasodilator nitric oxide, as well as a reduced production of endothelin, a vasoconstrictor produced by damaged endothelial cells (Esselstyn 2014). This and other mechanisms of interest will be discussed in a subsequent section.

There were other useful and positive findings in the studies described above, but the crucial take-home message is the answer to the question posed by Dr. Ornish: "Can lifestyle changes reverse coronary heart disease?" (Ornish 1990). The answer is a resounding yes. If this information alone were understood and internalized by doctors, and applied to patient care, a great many patients could benefit, since heart disease is a prime cause of death and disability (Brault et al. 2009, Heron 2016).

NUTRITIONAL INTERVENTIONS IN DIABETES

The CDC lists diabetes as the seventh leading cause of death, accounting for 2.9% of total U.S. deaths in 2014 (Heron 2016). This number does not consider the known contribution of diabetes to other leading causes of death such as heart disease, strokes, and end stage renal disease (CDC 2014). Diabetes also confers significantly higher risk for certain cancers including cancers of bowel, endometrium, and pancreas, and cancer mortality is also increased for diabetics. This implies that deaths due (or partly due) to diabetes are probably underestimated (Giovannucci et al. 2010). CDC statistics show an exponential rise in the number of diagnosed cases, from approximately 5 million in 1990, doubling to 10 million in 1999, and further doubling to 20 million cases in 2009 (CDC 2014).

A 22-week trial comparing a low-fat vegan diet (10% of energy from fat, 15% from protein, and 75% from carbohydrate) with the American Diabetes Association (ADA) diet (15%–20% calories from protein, <7% calories from saturated fat, and 60%–70% of calories from combined carbohydrate and monounsaturated fat) showed overall greater reduction of glycated hemoglobin (HbA1c) in the low-fat vegan group. The overall average drop in the vegan group was 1.0 percentage points compared with 0.6 percentage points in the ADA group. In participants who did not require medication adjustment during the study, the differences were greater, with a 1.23 percentage drop in HbA1c in the vegan group compared to a 0.38 percentage drop in the ADA group. The vegan group also experienced greater weight loss than the ADA group and also showed greater reductions in total and LDL cholesterol than the ADA group (Barnard et al. 2006).

A second study continued to follow the same group of participants for a total of 74 weeks. Here also the low-fat vegan diet improved glycemic and plasma lipid values more than the ADA diet, while weight loss did not vary significantly between the groups by the end of the 74-week study (Barnard et al. 2009).

The vegan group overall consumed 50% more fiber than the ADA group, and participants on average consumed 8.5 total servings of fruits and vegetables, compared to 5.6 servings for the ADA group.

The recommended macronutrient composition of the vegan diet was very similar to the diet in the Ornish and Esselstyn studies cited above, with 10% of overall calories from fat. However, analysis of the diet actually consumed by the vegan group Barnard study showed that approximately 22% of calories were derived from fat, with 5% of total calories from saturated fat. In the final analysis, these patients' total cholesterol dropped by 10.9%. In the ADA group, fat calories consumed slightly exceeded 30% of total dietary calories (similar to the recommendations followed by the control group in the Ornish study described above), and saturated fat consumed comprised 9.9% of calories consumed, and these patients' total cholesterol dropped only slightly (3.4%) (Barnard et al. 2009).

The lipid lowering effect of the vegan diet was noted to be particularly important, since cardiovascular complications are a primary cause of morbidity and mortality in diabetics.

The Ornish study, described in the previous section, demonstrated the superiority of the experimental (low-fat vegetarian) diet as compared to the standard recommendations at the time (reduction of red meat, consumption of 30% of dietary calories from fat) (Ornish et al. 1990). Not only did the experimental group in general reverse established coronary artery disease, the control group experienced progression of lesions and worsening of symptoms. Here, in the Barnard study, the experimental (low fat vegan) diet is shown to be superior to the ADA diet in terms of improvement in glycemic parameters and the "side effect" of improvement in serum lipids (Barnard 2009).

In support of the low-fat vegan diet, Dr. Barnard notes that intramyocellular lipid is associated with insulin resistance and that vegans have been found to have lower intramyocellular lipid than age and weight matched omnivores (Goff et al. 2005).

Nutritional Interventions in Hypertension

Salt and DASH

In a major analysis, high blood pressure appears as the third leading risk factor for death and the fourth leading risk factor for disability adjusted life years in the United States (Murray et al. 2013). Yet in a recent CDC document discussing the leading cause of death, "hypertension" as such is not listed among the top 10 causes. But, given that the first and fifth leading causes of death appear as heart disease and cerebrovascular disease (Heron 2016) and, worldwide, hypertension is responsible for at least 45% of heart disease deaths and 51% of stroke deaths (World Health Organization 2013), there can be no doubt that high blood pressure is a major killer. In addition, hypertension contributes to heart failure, aneurysms, renal failure, blindness, and cognitive impairment (World Health Organization 2013).

Mean blood pressure rises with age but it has long been known that this age-associated rise in blood pressure is not seen in societies where dietary consumption of salt is very low (Intersalt 1988). "Moderate" dietary sodium restriction is recommended by international (World Health Organization 2013) and national bodies, from 2.0 to 2.3 grams of sodium (5.1–6.0 grams of salt) for all individuals, down to 1.5 grams of sodium (3.8 grams of salt) for individuals who are black, over age 51, diabetic, or diagnosed as hypertensive (Kaplan 2015).

In most countries, average per capita daily salt intake, at 9–12 grams (World Health Organization 2013) is roughly double the general recommended intake and three times the more stringent recommended intake noted above. Multiple sources note that most dietary sodium is found in processed foods and therefore the approach of reducing the salt content of processed foods is regarded as a useful public health measure (Kaplan 2015, World Health Organization 2013). Another way, of course, would be for individuals to avoid processed food and limit the amount of salt which they themselves add to food to stay within the relevant daily guidelines ranging between 2300 mg sodium (6 grams or one teaspoon of salt) and 1500 mg of sodium (3.8 grams or 3/5 teaspoon of salt, just over half a teaspoon). This is a clear instruction that could be communicated easily by doctors to patients. For those choosing to consume processed foods, a helpful strategy for controlling sodium intake looks at "sodium density" favoring foods which contain no more than 1 milligram of sodium per calorie (Novick 2013), information which is readily available on food labels where the caloric and sodium content are both listed. In this way, a person eating 2000 calories per day would not consume more than 2000 mg of sodium (2 grams of sodium or 5.2 gram of salt, about 4/5 of a teaspoon) so that even if processed foods comprised the whole of their diet, they would remain within the general WHO guidance (World Health Organization 2013).

Salt restriction alone (to 2.4 grams of sodium or 6 grams of salt) is credited with producing an average 2–8 millimeters of mercury reduction in systolic blood pressure (NIH 2003). The Dietary Approaches to Stop Hypertension diet (DASH), in addition to limiting sodium, encourages a diet rich in fruit and vegetables (NIH 2003), which are good dietary sources of potassium (McGuire and Beerman 2013). Potassium deficiency can increase sensitivity to the blood pressure raising effect of dietary sodium, and correction of deficiency reduces this sodium sensitivity (Kaplan

2015). The DASH diet is credited with an average 8–14 millimeter of mercury reduction in systolic blood pressure (NIH 2003) and the increase of dietary potassium in this diet may account for the increased efficacy of the DASH diet over simple sodium restriction. More recent guidelines continue to support a combination of the DASH diet along with lowered sodium intake (Eckel et al. 2013).

Lifestyle management was at the top of the 7th JNC guideline but is preceded by the statement that most patients will require two medications to reach their blood pressure treatment goal (NIH 2003). In a similar vein, although the updated version of the JNC in 2014 places lifestyle interventions at the top of the treatment algorithm (with lifestyle interventions to be continued throughout management), the bulk of the guideline deals with pharmaceutical management of hypertension. This guideline is described as being based on an extensive evidence review by a panel of experts in hypertension, primary care, cardiology, pharmacology, epidemiology, and related fields. The evidence considered was initially restricted to randomized controlled trials (RCTs) and then further restricted to trials involving at least 2000 participants (James et al. 2014). Drawing conclusions from this evidence, it could seem that lifestyle measures have but a small part to play in the management of hypertension given the modest blood pressure lowering effect of the DASH. If one relies exclusively on the JNC 8 evidence, one is left with the impression that dietary intervention is relevant, but not powerful enough to achieve adequate change in blood pressure for patients who require lowering of systolic blood pressure by more than the 8–14 mm Hg expected from the DASH diet. One may be left with the implication or tacit assumption that before the advent of the anti-hypertensive medications, hypertension could not be effectively treated. The very fact of selection of only large RCTs as in the JNC 8 report (James et al. 2014) focuses attention on drug trials (for which RCTs are the agreed standard) but at the same time, as a result, focuses attention away from trials of nutritional interventions, which may be smaller or not randomly controlled, and yet, the excluded trials may well produce valid, beneficial, and even astonishing findings, like the studies of Drs. Ornish, Esselstyn, and Barnard cited above. These trials would have been automatically excluded from any meta-analysis which used the kind of criteria employed in the JNC 8, in effect throwing out the baby with the bath water.

Other Dietary Approaches to Hypertension

There are indeed trials involving nutrition, which have produced impressive blood pressure lowering results, but which would have been excluded from the JNC 8 analysis due to their size or design. Several of these trials provide evidence of more potent blood pressure lowering effect than simple sodium restriction or the DASH diet, using a variety of nutritional approaches.

Dr. Walter Kempner and the Rice Diet

The work of Dr. Walter Kempner is a case in point. Dr. Kempner, a physician and physiology researcher born and trained in Germany, took up a post at Duke University in North Carolina in 1934, when Hitler's anti-Jewish laws made it impossible for him to continue to be employed in the country of his birth (Newborg and Nash 2011). With his physiology background and after close observations of kidney tissue in vitro, Dr. Kempner reasoned that renal dysfunction could be ameliorated through reducing the workload of the kidneys, by reducing protein and fat in the diet, and that these interventions, along with reduction of sodium in the diet, would reduce edema, improve renal blood flow, and allow viable kidney tissue to heal. In 1939, he first used the later to be famous "rice and fruit diet" to treat patients hospitalized at Duke with severe kidney disease and edema. In the transcript of a lecture in which he described the logic that led him to this specific choice of diet, Dr. Kempner mentions as an aside that ideally one could substitute extracts of animal kidneys, or synthetic substances, for the "ferments" which had been destroyed in diseased kidneys. (This would have been, in effect, a magic bullet approach.) However, as such a solution was not yet available, he went on to his "less perfect approach," which he termed "the compensation of renal metabolic dysfunction with the rice diet" (Kempner 1946).

In an extensive report summarizing observations of 500 patients who were treated with the diet, Dr. Kempner describes the rice diet as containing 250–350 grams of white rice (uncooked weight), to be cooked in water or fruit juice. Fruits were allowed as well as fruit juice, but not vegetables, nuts, and so on. White sugar was allowed. Sodium intake was not greater than 150 mg per day (380 mg salt, about 1/16 tsp in kitchen terms), and this was mainly the sodium naturally present in foods. This was the whole of the diet. Many of the patients were suffering from severe hypertension with systolic pressures well over 200 mm Hg and diastolic pressures well over 100 mm Hg. Average blood pressure was 199/117 mm Hg. These 500 patients were described as seriously ill individuals who had not responded to other forms of treatment. Many had cardiac enlargement and EKG abnormalities such as T wave inversion and axis deviation. Retinal changes with papilledema, hemorrhages, and exudates were present in many of the patients (Kempner 1948). Such findings are characteristic of hypertension with multiple organ damage, or malignant hypertension (Cremer 2016), a condition which, in the 1950s, carried a very poor prognosis. How poor? One study of 211 British hypertensive patients who had diastolic blood pressures over 100 mm Hg (but who were considered unsuitable for sympathectomy) constituted a no-treatment group which was followed for 13 years. At the end of the 13 years, 106 patients (50%) were dead. Of the 106 patients who had died, 92 (87%) were under the age of 60. Of the 59 untreated patients with initial diastolic blood pressures above 130 mm Hg, 43 patients (72%) died. Within that group of 59, there were 21 patients with initial diastolic blood pressure over 150 mm Hg, all of whom died (100%). Of the 20 patients diagnosed with malignant hypertension, all died (100%). The deaths were recorded as due to cerebral hemorrhages, uremia, myocardial infarctions, aneurysms, and so on. Among the 105 survivors in the series of 211 patients, 37 (35%) had suffered strokes or myocardial infarctions, or were living with heart failure or angina. In a parallel series where 114 patients were treated with lumbodorsal sympathectomy, it was reported that 10 patients (9%) did not survive the operation itself. Of the 82 sympathectomy patients who met the criteria of diastolic blood pressure greater than 120 mm Hg prior to the operation, and who did not die from the procedure itself, 65 (80%) were judged to have been successfully treated with average reductions of 40 and 46 mm Hg for men and women, respectively. These 65 "successful" patients represent 57% of the original cohort of 114 patients (Leishman 1959).

The data presented above are meant to convey an impression of the seriousness of hypertension in Kempner's day, as well as the high risk of available treatment at the time. This should provide the context for understanding the ethical correctness of Dr. Kempner's decision not to have a control group in his rice diet studies (McDougall 2013). Untreated patients with severe hypertension, and, in addition, target organ damage, had little hope in those days.

In Kempner's study 500 patients were followed for an average of 85 days, or just under 3 months. In the original group of 500 patients, there were 26 patients (5%) who were critically ill at the onset of the diet, and who died within an average of 39 days. All but one of these had been deemed to have secondary renal involvement prior to commencing the diet. Kempner defined "improvement" in this study as a drop of 20 mm Hg in "mean arterial pressure" (MAP), the sum of systolic and diastolic pressures divided by 2. By these criteria, 311 (62%) of 500 patients improved, with average drops in MAP of 33 mm Hg and average drops in systolic pressure of 46 mm Hg. The "not improved" group included 163 (33%) patients who had a drop in MAP of "only" 11 mm Hg, and a drop in systolic blood pressure of "only" 17 mm Hg (Kempner 1948).

It is noteworthy that the "not improved" group in the rice diet experiment in the 1940s achieved a greater reduction of systolic blood pressure than is expected with the modern DASH diet where 8–14 mm Hg systolic blood pressure reduction is anticipated (NIH 2003). By current criteria, therefore, Kempner's "not improved" group would be deemed to have improved, meaning that out of the original patient group of 500, 474 (95%) experienced improvement.

In addition, dramatic improvements in retinopathy were seen, as well as resolution of EKG abnormalities including T wave inversion. Heart size, as measured by x-ray, was seen to be reduced in many cases. Glycemic control improved in diabetic patients with reduced need for insulin. Serum cholesterol values also improved (Kempner 1948). Total cholesterol data from a prior series showed a reduction from an average of 6.28 mmol/l (243 mg/dl) to 4.7 mmol/l (183 mg/dl), a drop of 24% (Kempner 1946). Thus, while blood pressure was the main factor under consideration, other important parameters improved as well.

This diet required frequent checks of patients' blood and urine chemistry, and was recommended by Kempner for use in hypertensive vascular disease with cardiac, renal, and retinal involvement as well as in uncomplicated hypertension "when a more liberal regime has failed." Kempner recommended continuing the diet "without modification until the conditions which were the indication for its use have disappeared," at which point specific modifications could be made. Kempner did not oppose the use of lumbodorsal sympathectomy, but tactfully advised a trial of the rice diet before proceeding to a surgical option (Kempner 1948).

The Nutrient Dense Plant-Rich (Nutritarian) Dietary Protocol

The nutrient dense plant-rich (nutritarian) dietary pattern is similar in many ways to the research protocols of Ornish, Esselstyn, and Barnard described above. This diet is based on consumption of fresh and cooked vegetables, fruits, legumes, and whole grains, excluding dairy, refined oils, refined carbohydrates such as white flour, white rice, and sugar, and limiting salt to 1000 milligrams per day. It differs from the Ornish, Esselstyn, and Barnard vegan diets in encouraging the consumption of 30 grams (an ounce) of seeds or nuts daily and in permitting up to 240 grams (8 ounces) of animal products per week.

In one study (Fuhrman and Singer 2015), 2273 outpatients in a single-family practice were followed for an average of 3.8 years. There were 1759 patients (77%) who reported being at least 80% compliant with the nutritarian recommendations. Among 443 hypertensive patients, the average reduction in systolic blood pressure was 26.4 mm Hg and average reduction in diastolic blood pressure was 14.7 mm Hg. Of these 443 patients, 316 patients were on medication at the beginning of the study. Of these, 136 patients (43%) were able to discontinue their medication while still demonstrating an average reduction of systolic blood pressure of 28.6 mm Hg and an average reduction of diastolic blood pressure of 11.9 mm Hg. These improvements exceed those attributed to the DASH diet (NIH 2003) and compare favorably with results of the rice diet study described above (Kempner 1948).

Other parameters observed were weight and serum lipids. Within the group of 1759 adherent patients, 685 patients had a body mass index greater than 30 kg/m^2 at the beginning of the study. After one year of the nutritarian diet, average weight loss in this group was 22.3 kg (49 pounds). Large drops in serum lipids were also observed in this study. Thus, in this study, blood pressure was affected significantly and favorably, along with other important parameters.

Selected Special Foods

Linseeds (Flax Seed)   The FLAX effects in Peripheral Arterial Disease (FLAX-PAD) study was a prospective double blinded placebo controlled randomized trial involving 110 patients with peripheral arterial disease and hypertension. The patients in the experimental group consumed 30 grams (1 ounce) of milled flaxseed daily over a period of 6 months. Alpha linoleic acid (ALA) and enterolignan levels in plasma were checked to evaluate compliance. Fish consumption was not allowed in either the treatment or placebo group for the duration of the study. In the treatment group, blood pressure declined throughout the 6-month study, and at the end of the 6-month study period, patients in the treatment group had an average reduction of 10 mm Hg in systolic blood pressure and 7 mm Hg in diastolic blood pressure. Patients whose initial systolic blood pressure exceeded 140 mm Hg experienced sustained reductions of 15 mm Hg in their systolic blood pressure. There was an overall absence of adverse effects in both the treatment and placebo group. There was 1 stroke in the treatment group compared with 2 strokes in the placebo group. There were 2 myocardial infarctions in the treatment group compared with 4 in the placebo group. Serum ALA levels correlated well with the blood pressure reductions noted above (Rodriguez-Leyva et al. 2013).

Hibiscus   A 6-week double blind placebo controlled trial of hibiscus tea was carried out, in which the subjects were mildly hypertensive patients. The treatment group received 3 servings of hibiscus tea daily, while the placebo group drank a preparation with similar appearance and taste. In the treatment group, systolic blood pressure was reduced by 7.2 mm Hg and diastolic blood pressure was reduced by 3 mm Hg. In the placebo group, small reductions of 1.3 mm Hg and 0.5 mm Hg were seen, for systolic and diastolic blood pressure, respectively. Compared to the placebo beverage the hibiscus tea contained at least 10 times the amount of phenols, and had a 10 times greater oxygen radical absorbance capacity (ORAC) value. In addition, the hibiscus tea contained anthocyanins, which were not found in the placebo beverage. No adverse effects were reported. The authors propose that drinking a cup of hibiscus tea 3 times a day may be an intervention that would elicit better compliance than more comprehensive dietary interventions (McKay et al. 2009).

Medically Supervised Water-Only Fasting

A study of 174 consecutive patients with essential hypertension employed water-only fasting in a medically supervised environment. In this study "water-only fasting" is defined as "complete abstinence from…food, tea, juice, non-caloric beverages, etc., with the sole exception of distilled water ad libitum." Initial mean blood pressure was 159.1/89.2 mm Hg. Prior to the fasting period, participants were instructed to eat a diet consisting exclusively of steamed vegetables and fresh raw vegetables and fruits for at least two days. Participants fasted for an average of 10 to 11 days. The fasting period was followed by several days of supervised refeeding, initially with fresh raw fruit and vegetable juice, then with solid raw fruits and vegetables, after which a diet of whole natural foods was introduced. This diet consisted of fresh fruit, fresh, steamed, and baked vegetables, cooked whole grains and legumes, and small quantities of nuts and seeds. The whole natural food diet excluded meat, fish, fowl, eggs, and dairy as well as any added sugar, salt, or oil. The average length of the refeeding period was one half that of the fasting period. Participants were monitored with twice weekly blood and urine testing, and, where clinically indicated, EKG. Apart from mild nausea and orthostatic hypotension during the fasting period, no adverse effects were observed.

Blood pressures dropped during the pre-fasting and water-only fasting periods, and continued to drop during the refeeding period. The overall mean blood pressure drop was 37.1/13.3 mm Hg. Approximately 89% of subjects achieved normotensive status with a final mean blood pressure of 117.5/78.7. Patients with stage 3 hypertension (mean baseline blood pressure 193.8/96.4) achieved the greatest blood pressure reduction, with a mean drop in systolic blood pressure of 59.6 mm Hg and a mean drop in diastolic blood pressure of 16.9 mm Hg.

Given the continued drop in blood pressure during the refeeding period, the authors reasoned that the results might be sustainable with a low sodium vegan diet. In support of this, it was found that 42 of the original 174 hypertensive subjects, who were followed up after an average post-treatment period of 27 weeks, had a mean blood pressure of 123/77 at the time of follow-up (Goldhamer et al. 2001).

A further series of 68 patients with borderline hypertension was later studied, under the same conditions. Approximately 82% of patients achieved blood pressures under 120/80 mm Hg by the end of the supervised refeeding period (Goldhamer et al. 2002).

Natriuresis is cited as one of the likely mechanisms, but probably not the sole mechanism since the blood pressure reductions in the study were greater than those seen with salt restriction alone. Physiological changes during water-only fasting include natriuresis of 3.5–5.8 grams of sodium (9–15 grams of salt) per day, early in the fast (Goldhamer et al. 2013).

The authors point out that the water-only fasting period may provide an opportunity to resensitize the taste faculty in persons who had previously been accustomed to consuming a typical diet of high sodium and high fat foods, thus increasing the palatability of the low sodium, low fat, high potassium plant foods, which comprise the recommended follow-up diet.

SELECTED MECHANISMS UNDERLYING THE EFFECT OF FOOD ON CARDIO-METABOLIC PARAMETERS

ENDOTHELIAL FUNCTION

The endothelium has several relevant functions, including regulation of vascular permeability and tone. It is described as the body's largest endocrine organ. It brings about short-term vasodilation through nitric oxide and other mediators, and vasoconstriction through thromboxane and other factors including oxygen-free radicals. There is an ongoing balance between vasoconstriction, which is pro-atherosclerotic, and vasodilation, which is anti-atherosclerotic. It has been asserted that "every risk factor that is associated with atherosclerosis also impairs endothelial function." These risk factors include, among others, cigarette smoking, hypertension, diabetes, and increased cholesterol (Vogel 1999). Endothelial injury is also one of the main microscopic pathological changes seen in malignant hypertension (Kitiyakara and Guzman 1998).

Endothelial function can be assessed clinically by measuring flow mediated dilation, using brachial artery ultrasound. The diameter of the brachial artery is measured by ultrasound at baseline, the artery is then occluded, and the diameter of the artery is measured again after occlusion is released. The percent difference in the two measurements is the flow mediated dilation, or FMD (Vogel 2000).

FMD has been used to study the post-prandial effects of different foods. In one study, comparing a high-fat meal to a low-fat meal, following a typical 900-calorie fast food meal composed of eggs, fried potatoes, and sausage, and containing 50 grams of fat and 225 mg of cholesterol, FMD was reduced by 50% at 3 hours and was still reduced by 25% at 6 hours. The 900-calorie low-fat meal of cereal with skimmed milk, juice and coffee, containing 0 grams of fat and 13 mg cholesterol, did not reduce FMD (Vogel et al. 1997).

Another study compared effects of ingesting 60 ml of different oils on FMD. The oils used were olive, soybean and palm oils, both fresh and at two different deep-frying levels. All meals showed acute endothelial impairment with FMD reduced by 32% at 3 hours, independently of the type of oil or deep-frying level (Rueda-Clausen et al. 2007).

Yet another study compared effects of three different 900-calorie 50-gram fat meals: olive oil and bread, canola oil and bread, and salmon and crackers. Contrary to the expectations of the researchers, FMD was reduced by 31% in the olive oil group, 10% in the canola oil group, and only minimally in the salmon group. Interestingly, the reduction in FMD in the olive oil and canola oil groups was significantly attenuated (but not abolished) when antioxidants in the form of salad and balsamic vinegar, or vitamins C and E, were consumed with the meal (Vogel et al. 2000). In the light of other studies showing benefits of a Mediterranean diet style on cardiovascular health, it had been broadly assumed that olive oil contributed to that benefit. The authors propose that the heart health benefits of a Mediterranean eating style are more likely due to consumption of anti-oxidant rich foods, such as fruits and vegetables, and omega-3 rich fish, noting as well that olive oil itself contains 17% saturated fat, and saturated fat consumption was shown to impair endothelial function in the earlier study (Vogel et al. 1997, 2000).

The Lifestyle Heart Trial (Ornish et al. 1990), described in a previous section, demonstrated improvement in angina symptoms, myocardial perfusion, functional status, and other parameters, with a very low fat vegetarian diet along with other lifestyle measures. In a small study aiming to elucidate mechanisms behind these improvements, participants in the experimental group adhered to the components of the lifestyle change program including vegetarian diet with fewer than 10% of calories from fat. FMD was observed to improve by 20%, and markers of inflammation and endothelial dysfunction, human high sensitivity CRP and human interleukin 6, were reduced at 3 months. The authors asserted that endothelial dysfunction constitutes an important factor in the pathogenesis of atherosclerosis, as it predisposes blood vessels to constriction and promotes inflammation and platelet activation (Harvinder et al. 2010). Dr. Esselstyn has repeatedly asserted that when foods that cause endothelial dysfunction are avoided, the capacity of the endothelium to pro-duce the vasodilator nitric oxide will be restored (Esselstyn et al. 2014). Given the duration of reduced FMD after a single high fat meal (Vogel et al. 1997), it is very plausible that with a diet where a high fat meal follows a high fat meal, the endothelium is continually assaulted and does not have the time to recover fully from each temporary impairment.

MODIFICATION OF TRIMETHYL-N-OXIDE LEVELS

Elevated plasma levels of trimethylamine-n-oxide (TMAO) are associated with atherosclerosis and cardiovascular adverse events. While the precise mechanism has not been fully elucidated, platelet activation is likely to be involved. In the human body, gut flora convert dietary choline, phosphatidyl choline (lecithin), and carnitine to TMAO. Dietary sources of these TMAO precursors include red meat, eggs, dairy, and salt water fish. The authors of a review article on TMAO note that altering the gut microbiome by antibiotic treatment has been shown to reduce TMAO during treatment, but do not regard this as a viable long-term approach. Instead, the authors propose reducing dietary intake of TMAO precursors (Velasquez et al. 2016).

NUTRITIONAL TREATMENT OF SELECTED INFLAMMATORY AND AUTO-IMMUNE CONDITIONS

NUTRITIONAL TREATMENT OF MULTIPLE SCLEROSIS (MS)

This debilitating progressive neurological disease is understood to be an immune condition, but little is understood about its causation and factors that may contribute to exacerbations or deteriora-tion (Jelinek and Hassed 2009). Can food have a role to play?

Consulting the NICE guidelines, which provide the treatment standard for the United Kingdom, one finds no recommendations relating to food, and a brief statement saying that Vitamin D and omega-3 fatty acids should not be used to treat MS (NICE 2014). The Mayo Clinic succinctly denies that a special diet can treat MS, but gives a nod to a low fat and high fiber eating pattern, which is described as the recommended diet for the general population, and not specific for MS (Mayo Clinic 2016).

If one is satisfied with the views of these two authorities, one may be inadvertently doing a great disservice to one's patients.

The neurologist Dr. Roy Swank published a study in which 144 multiple sclerosis patients fol-lowed a "low fat" diet for 34 years. Patients were instructed to reduce dietary saturated fat to 15 g per day, mainly by cutting down on milk and fat from other animal sources. The diet included 5 g per day of cod liver oil. Unsaturated oils were used but hydrogenated and saturated plant oils (palm, coconut) were not (Swank and Duggan 1990). The full diet plan can be found in Swank's book (Swank and Duggan 1987). Patients were categorized at the outset of the study as having minimal, moderate, or severe disability, based on the standard grading correlated with the Kurtzke scale. Later, patients were categorized as "good dieters" or "poor dieters" based on self-reported con-sumption of less than, or more than, 20 grams of fat daily. At the end of 34 years, it could be seen that the patients classed as "good dieters" showed less neurological deterioration than the poor diet-ers. This was true at all three levels of initial disability, but the difference was most striking in the group that had minimal disability at the beginning of the study. At the end of 34 years, the surviving "poor dieters" were confined to bed and chair. Of the initial group of "poor dieters," 80% had died of MS related causes. By contrast, only 5% of the "good dieters" had died of MS related causes. The remaining "good dieters" in this group of survivors had an average Kurtzke grade of 1.1 at the end of the 34-year study. These patients were ambulatory and able to work, in contrast with the severely disabled "poor dieters" (Swank and Duggan 1990). This was a small but highly meaningful study, and as seen above, its results are not reflected or even mentioned in the MS guidelines.

In a discussion paper citing Swank's work, the point is made that there is presently enough evidence for lifestyle therapies to be a standard part of primary care management of MS. It is further stated that "many people are searching for the advice from complementary practitioners which they should possibly be receiving from their GPs" (Jelinek 2009). As seen above in the studies by Barnard, Fuhrman, and Kempner, lifestyle interventions may affect multiple health parameters in a positive manner. In citing Ornish's lifestyle approach to treating heart disease, which has also been shown to be associated with reduced progression of prostate cancer (Ornish 2005), it is affirmed that "the lifestyle approach in primary care, especially for chronic diseases, should be first line therapy and not an afterthought" (Jelinek 2009).

Inspired by Swank's work, a 1-year trial of a low-fat plant-based diet in multiple sclerosis studied a group of 61 participants diagnosed with relapsing remitting MS. There were 32 patients assigned to the diet group. Given the short duration of the study and the fact that most of the patients in both groups were taking disease modifying treatment (DMT), relapse rate was expected to be very low in both groups. This was in fact the case. At the end of one year, the two groups did not differ significantly in terms of new lesions on MRI. However, the treatment group experienced significant improvement in fatigue ratings, a meaningful benefit, since fatigue is one of the chief symptoms affecting quality of life in MS, even when DMT is used (Yadav et al. 2016). It is possible that given more time, outcomes in the two groups would diverge in other significant ways. Larger and longer-term outcome trials will be the final arbiter of effectiveness (Jelinek 2009), but while the results of such trials are awaited, there is Swank's study with outcomes showing that a dietary intervention sustained over decades was associated with the difference between nearly full functioning and severe disability or death (Swank 1990).

Nutritional Treatment of Rheumatoid Arthritis (RA)

A rheumatoid arthritis guideline by the Royal College of Physicians contains over 200 pages of evidence and recommendations, 5 pages of which are devoted to diet. While acknowledging evidence for various benefits from various diets, the guideline states that no modifications demonstrate global improvements in measures of disease activity and function, and that "there was no consistent evidence of benefit from any one particular diet" although research results showing some benefits from gluten free, elemental, and vegan diets were presented. It was further stated that some diets, such as vegetarian diets, might be unpopular with some patients. The ultimate recommendation was to encourage clinicians to advocate the principles of the Mediterranean diet for people with RA who "wish to experiment with their diet." Here the Mediterranean diet was described as having more bread, fruit, vegetables, and fish, and having less meat, and replacing butter and cheese with products based on vegetable and plant oils. This recommendation was made mainly based on the increased cardiovascular disease risk experienced by RA patients, and on the possibility that such a diet "might be beneficial to musculoskeletal symptoms." It was also asserted that the Mediterranean diet would more likely elicit better adherence than "more unpalatable alternatives" (National Collaborating Centre 2009). It should be noted that no evidence was presented for unpalatability of any specific eating pattern, or degree of patients' willingness or unwillingness to follow any particular diet, so that the remarks about potential compliance and palatability could be seen to reflect mere assumptions or prejudices of the guideline authors.

Published research on the treatment of rheumatoid arthritis with fasting followed by vegetarian diet is of interest in this context. This was a prospective single blind randomized trial with 53 subjects, of which 27 were randomized to the diet group. All subjects had rheumatoid arthritis with active disease, most were taking nonsteroidal anti-inflammatory drugs (NSAIDS), and many were taking corticosteroids, antimalarial drugs, gold, penicillamine, sulfasalazine, or cytostatic drugs. Only three patients in the treatment group were not on any medications at study entry. About half of patients reported specific food intolerances.

The regime for the treatment group was to a degree inspired by previously existing regimes at Scandinavian health farms (Kjeldsen-Kragh 1991). The initial fast of 7–10 days was not a water fast as described above (Goldhamer et al. 2001, 2002), but a "subtotal fast" where intake was limited to herbal teas, garlic, vegetable broth, decocted potatoes and parsley, and juices of carrots, beets, and celery. Patients' medications were not altered. Following the sub-total fast, patients were fed with a basic diet which initially included only the elements listed above. On the principle used in elimination diets, a single new food item was introduced every second day. If symptoms worsened within the subsequent 2–48 hours, the item was excluded for that individual and only reintroduced one week later. If exacerbation occurred again, the food was not reintroduced. The first 3.5 months which followed the modified fast were defined as the "vegan phase." During this period, all dairy products and gluten were excluded along with meat, fish, eggs, refined sugar, citrus, salt, strong spices, preservatives, alcohol, coffee, and tea. Oils were permitted. The vegan phase was followed by a further 9 months where dairy and gluten were allowed; these were introduced one at a time and were not continued if they were seen to exacerbate arthritis symptoms (Kjeldsen-Kragh 1999).

Clinical indices such as pain, duration of morning stiffness, and joint swelling and tenderness improved markedly after only one month in the treatment group. At the end of 13 months, 12 of the 27 patients in the experimental group were categorized as "improvers" contrasted with only 2 of 26 patients in the control group. At the end of the 13-month trial, participants were free to change their diets. One year later, follow-up of 22 patients in the experimental group revealed that all the diet responders had continued the diet of their own accord. These responders continued to have reductions of clinical disease variables, as well as reduction of erythrocyte sedimentation rate (ESR) (Haugen 1999). Of note, about one-third of patients had reported exacerbations of symptoms with specific foods.

The authors credit the improvements among the responders to several characteristics of the diet, including immunosuppression due to decreased energy intake, identification and removal of individual aggravating elements of the diet through the protocol described above, differing proportions of fatty acids altering the inflammatory process, and changes in fecal flora (Kjelsden-Kragh 1999). Another factor of interest was the potentially protective role of natural antioxidants (Haugen et al. 1999).

The subtlety of a trial which individualizes dietary intervention while staying within the parameters of an overall vegan or vegetarian pattern is worth noting. Insisting on a totally uniform diet for all in the treatment group, or an immediate transition to a general vegan or vegetarian diet, might not have produced as much clinical improvement. This kind of individualized approach seems worthy of emulation both in research and clinically. However, the subtlety of the intervention in the study may have made it difficult to categorize and compare with other studies. While the above-mentioned guideline document did include this study in the evidence base, and even recognized the benefits in the treatment group, the experimental dietary pattern was merely described as "gluten free followed by vegetarian" (National Collaborating Centre 2009). This description clearly does not capture important features of the dietary intervention. The guideline had indeed stated that "there was no consistent evidence of benefit from any one particular diet" (National Collaborating Centre 2009), and in a sense that was not incorrect. However, the guideline did not mention the methodically individualized feature of the diet in this study. Guidelines purport to look for "best treatment," but in this case, if one were only to read the guideline and not the actual study, one could conclude that diet is not likely to be of much benefit for RA sufferers. This would be unfortunate, since patients in this particular study improved clinically and maintained the diet and improvements one year later, as described. The fact that patients continued the diet on their own also challenges the guideline assumptions of unpopularity and unpalatability which were, in any case, not supported by evidence. This is not to deny the usefulness of meta-analyses and guidelines, but such tools, in seeking the big picture (populations), may lose sight of the small picture (individuals and individual variation).

Remission of rheumatoid arthritis and other autoimmune conditions is described in a set of case reports where the therapeutic intervention was a combination of water-only fasting and diet. Brief case reports of three RA patients, one systemic lupus erythematosus patient and one patient with mixed connective tissue disease were provided, along with a case report from one fibromyalgia patient. These patients each underwent a period of water-only fasting, preceded by a high nutrient density vegan diet (Fuhrman et al. 2002). Prior to the water-only fasting, patients had been weaned off their medications. The water-only fasting protocol with gradual refeeding was essentially the same as described in the blood pressure studies cited above (Goldhamer et al. 2001, 2002). The high nutrient density vegan diet was followed again after the refeeding period. These individuals were reported to have achieved remission from their autoimmune disease (or from fibromyalgia), and the remissions were reported to be maintained at follow-up months and even years later. In one case, when a flare of disease activity recurred, a second fast was able to produce remission again, and that remission was subsequently maintained (Fuhrman 2002). It should not be forgotten that a true remission of a painful and disabling autoimmune condition not only improves quality of life, but also spares the patient iatrogenic complications of the medical regimes which are usually used, regimes which carry significant toxicity.

NUTRITIONAL TREATMENT OF FIBROMYALGIA SYNDROME (FMS)

This condition produces chronic pain, but unlike known autoimmune diseases, lacks unique pathophysiological characteristics. A major clinical review describing a stepwise approach to FMS did not mention diet at all (Goldenberg et al. 2004). In the case report studies above (Fuhrman 2002), one of the patients had fibromyalgia, and obtained remission through the protocol of water-only fasting preceded and followed by a nutrient dense vegan diet. In a 3-month study of 30 fibromyalgia patients, a dietary intervention was used which consisted of a mostly raw vegan diet, which included flax seed and olive oils, but excluded alcohol, caffeine, refined sugar, refined and hydrogenated oils, dairy, eggs, and all meat. There were 19 of the 30 subjects who were classified as responders and had significant improvement in clinical measures of pain, fatigue, and quality of life (Donaldson et al. 2001).

A causative or contributory role in fibromyalgia pain symptoms has been hypothesized for dietary glutamate and aspartate, two non-essential amino acids which function as excitatory neurotransmitters. Bound forms of these exist in meat, whereas free forms of these amino acids are found in the diet as additives. Examples include monosodium glutamate (MSG), hydrolyzed protein, protein concentrate, aspartame, fish sauces, and aged cheeses. The author of a review of this subject advises using a whole food diet without additives, to adequately test for sensitivity to these agents (Holton 2016).

It should be noted that several of the regimes described in the preceding section would have also eliminated food additives, though this was not specifically addressed in the modified fast/vegetarian protocol (Kjelsden-Kragh 1999, Kjelsden-Kragh et al. 1991) or in the water-fasting/nutrient dense vegan protocol (Fuhrman 2002).

SUMMING UP: THE COMMON GROUND

With the exception of Dr. Kempner's rice diet and Dr. Swank's low-fat diet, all of the interventions described in this chapter utilized a broadly similar approach. They emphasized the consumption of cooked and raw vegetables, fruits, legumes, grains and seeds, while excluding meat, dairy, and eggs, and minimizing or excluding oils, sugar, and salt. All the regimes resulted in marked reduction of saturated fat (also a feature of the Kempner and Swank diets).

Calling these regimes "vegetarian" or "vegan" addresses only the exclusion aspect whereby meat, or all animal products, respectively, are excluded. Yet a vegan diet, thus defined, could be composed entirely of highly processed nutrient-poor elements such as sodas, candy, cakes, potato chips, doughnuts, and fake meats and cheeses laden with salt, oil, and additives. Without a fruit or vegetable in sight, it would still be, strictly speaking, a vegan diet (Maisel 2015b).

The term "whole food plant-based diet" has much to recommend it. This term, coined by the nutritional biochemist researcher and author of The China Study (Campbell and Campbell 2006), refers to a diet composed of plant-based foods in forms as close to their natural state as possible, including vegetables, fruits, nuts, seeds, legumes, and whole grains, and avoiding heavily processed foods, animal products, salt, oil, and sugar (Campbell and Jacobson 2013, Maisel 2015a).

A look back at the various regimes cited in this chapter shows that they generally conform to this description. This is the essence of the regimes used to reverse atherosclerotic heart disease, improve diabetes, and reduce blood pressure, often extending beneficial influence on parameters other than the main target pathology. This is also the essence of the regime which brought about clinical improvement and even remission in rheumatoid arthritis and fibromyalgia. Further studies will better elucidate mechanisms behind the clinical improvements seen here and in the considerable body of evidence favoring a whole foods, plant-based diet (Campbell and Campbell 2012a,b).

In the real world, many smokers still opt to continue smoking. Similarly, many patients may not be interested in exploring dietary change. This should not prevent clinicians from recommending diet, and specifically, some form of a whole food plant-based diet, as first line treatment in many conditions, and as an adjunct to conventional therapy. Whether to follow such advice will, of course, be the patient's own responsibility.

For added reassurance, a recent position paper of the Academy of Nutrition and Dietetics asserts that appropriately planned vegetarian and vegan diets are healthful and nutritionally adequate (Academy of Nutrition and Dietetics 2016).

ETHICAL ASPECTS AND IATROGENICS

Earlier this year, the Centers for Disease Control (CDC) was challenged to list medical error as the third leading cause of death in the United States. A composite figure of 251,454 deaths per year was projected onto the total number of deaths in 2013 (2,596,993 deaths) which would mean that deaths due to medical error would account for 9.7% of all deaths. This composite figure was composed of a sum of deaths due to errors in judgment, skill, or coordination of care, diagnostic errors, system defects resulting in failure to rescue a patient from death, and preventable adverse events. The author therefore argues that medical error should be listed as the third leading cause of death, and further notes his view that the estimate derived from the literature represents an underestimate, since the studies did not include outpatient deaths or deaths at home due to medical error (Makary 2016).

This is not an entirely new observation. Nearly two decades ago, a figure of 225,000 iatrogenic deaths per year was quoted and similarly presented as the third leading cause of death. This figure was the sum of 12,000 deaths per year from unnecessary surgery, 7000 deaths per year from medication errors in hospitals, 20,000 deaths per year from other errors in hospitals, 80,000 deaths per year due to nosocomial infections in hospitals, and 106,000 deaths per year due to "non-error, adverse effects of medication." The author further stated that "how cause of death and outpatient diagnoses are coded does not facilitate an understanding of the extent to which iatrogenic cause of death and ill health are operative" (Starfield 2000).

The pursuit of benign and effective nutritional approaches takes on enhanced importance if it is recognized that "harmful effects of health care interventions likely...account for a substantial proportion of the excess deaths" in the United States (Starfield 2000).

Without complicated analysis, it should be clear that the deaths due to unnecessary surgery would not have happened if unnecessary surgery were avoided. Similarly, deaths due to adverse effects of medication would not occur if medication became unnecessary due to success of a benign dietary intervention.

For clinicians, who see patients one at a time, the huge numbers presented above may seem unreal and far away. But, recall that in Dr. Esselstyn's study, in the group of 177 patients who adhered to the dietary protocol, 27 patients were able to avoid coronary artery stenting or bypass grafts which had previously been recommended (Esselstyn 2014). They therefore also avoided the risk of dying due to unnecessary surgery. What degree of risk would they have been facing? In a series of over 500,000 percutaneous coronary interventions (PCI) the in-hospital mortality risk was overall 1.27%, and ranged from 0.65% in elective PCI to 4.81% in ST-elevation myocardial infarction (Peterson et al. 2010). One may regard 0.65% as "low risk" equating to "only" a 1 in 154 risk of death for an elective PCI. At the lowest estimate, one in 154 patients undergoing elective PCI will die. If the elective surgery were avoided, that death would not occur. Since it has been shown that dietary intervention can make it possible for elective PCI to be avoided (Esselstyn 2014), it is truly imperative to present this option to patients.

The figure quoted above of 106,000 deaths due to "non-error adverse effects of medication" is a reminder that even the best intentioned and correctly prescribed medication may cause irreversible damage. Two of the studies cited in this chapter specifically address discontinuing of medication in the context of specific nutritional intervention for hypertension (Goldhamer et al. 2001, 2002). In Furhman's case series of autoimmune remissions, medications were discontinued (Fuhrman et al. 2002). Similarly, in the large outpatient series showing the effects of a plant-based, nutrient-dense diet on multiple parameters, many patients were able to discontinue prescribed medications (Fuhrman et al. 2015). Patients who take no medications are not exposed to the risks and adverse effects of medications, including death. Logically and ethically, if the use of diet can reduce or eliminate the need for medications, then diet should be offered and strongly encouraged as a first line treatment.

In Dr. Ornish's Lifestyle Heart Trial, patients in the control group were given treatment according to the prevailing "usual care," which offered the best standard of care at the time. That is, of course, the ethical way to do a randomized trial. The outcomes in the treatment group were significantly better than the outcomes of patients receiving "usual care." The results in Dr. Esselstyn's study similarly show that it is possible to achieve excellent results with dietary therapy. The same must be said of the work of Drs. Barnard, Kempner, Swank, Kjeldsden-Kragh, and Fuhrman, described in this chapter. And yet, the guidelines have not really changed.

Culturally and ethically, autonomy is a sacred right of patients. Patients depend on clinicians to inform them correctly so that they can make wise choices. While it may take time for official guidelines to change, the case can be made that conscientious clinicians have a duty to present dietary options to patients suffering from chronic diseases. Waiting for guidelines to catch up may be a case of "making the perfect into the enemy of the good," and while waiting, patients may be exposed to unnecessary iatrogenic harms.

CONCLUSION: "MIND THE GAP"

Nutrition is indeed a powerful force with respect to health, whether for the enhancement of health or its detriment. While most clinicians are aware of the causative role of nutrition with respect to chronic metabolic conditions such as coronary artery disease, hypertension, and diabetes, and many may acknowledge the possibility of prevention or attenuation of these conditions through a better diet, fewer are aware of the power of nutrition to reverse these conditions, and even fewer may be aware of the ability of nutrition to produce remission in inflammatory disease and reduce recurrence rates of malignancy.

Traditional medical education and many medical guidelines fail to consider the power of nutritional intervention. Some reasons for this have already been discussed in this chapter. There is a gap between the applied guidelines and published evidence which can be found in the medical literature. This phenomenon has been pointed out in several sections of this chapter.

A chapter of this length cannot pretend to treat in full such a vast subject as nutritional care of chronic diseases. It has been necessary to focus mainly on those conditions which cause the most morbidity and mortality, while presenting a sampling of other conditions which present clinical challenges, and for which drug toxicity is high.

It is hoped that, in addition to consulting relevant guidelines, conscientious clinicians will develop enough curiosity to search scientific databases such as PubMed for nutritional approaches to conditions that they treat, or at least read for themselves the main published studies presented here. It is hoped that clinicians will become more aware of the gap between guidelines and good evidence and become aware that guidelines, due to their very nature, may exclude good evidence. It is to be hoped that conscientious clinicians will understand the potential of nutrition in a way that will lead to emphasizing diet much more, and first offering chronic disease patients a chance to try benign, effective, non-toxic, and potentially more economic options, before moving on to conventional drug treatment. This approach has the potential for being a winner on many levels, improving patient outcomes, reducing costs, and improving clinician satisfaction.

REFERENCES

Academy of Nutrition and Dietetics. 2016. Position of the academy of nutrition and dietetics: Vegetarian diets. *J Acad Nutr Diet* 116:1970–1980.

Auterhoff H. 1967. *Nobel Lectures, Physiology or Medicine 1901–1921*. Amsterdam: Elsevier.

Barnard ND, Cohen J, Jenkins DJ et al. 2006. A low-fat vegan diet improves glycemic control and cardiovascular risk factors in a randomised clinical trial in individuals with type 2 diabetes. *Diabetes Care* 29(8):1777–1783.

Barnard ND, Cohen J, Jenkins DJ, Turner-McGrievy G, Gloede L, Green A, and Ferdowsian H. 2009. A low fat vegan diet and a conventional diabetes diet in the treatment of type 2 diabetes: A randomized, controlled, 74 week clinical trial. *Am J Clin Nutr* 89(suppl):1588S–1596S.

BNF (British National Formulary) 72. 2016. London: Pharmaceutical Press.

Brault MW, Hootman J, Helmick CG et al. 2009. Prevalence and most common causes of disability among adults—United States 2005. *MMWR* 58(16):421–426.

Campbell TC and Campbell TM. 2006. *The China Study*. Dallas: BenBella Books, Inc.

Campbell TC and Jacobson HJ. 2013. *Whole. Rethinking the Science of Nutrition*. Dallas: BenBella Books, Inc.

Campbell TM and Campbell TC. 2012a. The breadth of evidence favoring a whole foods, plant-based diet. Part I: Metabolic diseases and diseases of aging. *Primary Care Reports* 18(2). http://www.ahcmedia.com/articles/print/76976-the-breadth-of-evidence-favoring-a-whole-food-plant-based-diet

Campell TM and Campell TC. 2012b. The breadth of evidence favoring a whole foods, plant-based diet, Part II: Malignancy and inflammatory diseases. *Primary Care Reports* 18(3):25–36.

CDC. 2014. *Diabetes Report Card 2014*. Atlanta, GA: Centers for Disease Control and Prevention, U.S. Department of Health and Human Services.

Cohen PA. 2016. The supplement paradox. *JAMA* 316(14):1453–1454.

Cremer A, Amraoui F, Lip GyH et al. 2016. From malignant hypertension to hypertension-MOD: A modern definition for an old but still dangerous emergency. *J Hum Hypertens* 30:463–466.

Doll R, Peto R, Boreham J, and Sutherland I. 2004. Mortality in relation to smoking: 50 years' observations on male British doctors. *BMJ* 328:1519, doi: 10.1136/bmj.38142.AE

Donaldson M, Speight N, and Loomis S. 2001. Fibromyalga syndrome improved using a mostly raw vegetarian diet: An observational study. *BMC Complement Altern Med* 1:7.

Eckel RH, Jakicic JM, Ard JD et al. 2013. AHA/ACC guideline on lifestyle management to reduce cardiovascular risk: A report of the American College of Cardiology/American Heart Association Task Force on Practice Guidelines. *J Am Coll Cardiol* 63:2960–2984.

Esselstyn CB, Ellis SG, Medendorp, and Crowe TD. 1995. A strategy to arrest and reverse coronary artery disease: A 5-year longitudinal study of a single physician's practice. *J Fam Pract* 41(6):560–568.

Esselstyn CB, Gendy G, Doyle J, Golubic M, and Roizen M. 2014. A way to reverse CAD? *J Fam Pract* 63:7.

Fuhrman J, Sarter B, and Calabro D. 2002. Brief case reports of medically supervised water-only fasting associated with remission of autoimmune disease. *Alternative Therapies* 8(4):112, 140–1.

Fuhrman J and Singer M. 2015. Improved cardiovascular parameter with a nutrient dense plant-rich diet style: A patient survey with illustrative cases. *Am Journ Lifestyle Medicine* 11(3):264–273, doi 10.1177/1559827615611024

Giovannucci E, Harlan DM, Archer MC et al. 2010. Diabetes and cancer. *Diabetes Care* 33(7):1674–1685.

Goff LM, Bell JD, So BW, Dornhorst A, and Frost GS. 2005. Veganism and its relationship with insulin resistance and intramyocellular lipid. *Eur J Clin Nutr* 59:291–298.

Goldenberg D, Burckhard C, and Crofford L. 2004. Management of fibromyalgia syndrome. *JAMA* 292:2388–2394.

Goldhamer A, Helms S, and Salloum T. 2013. Fasting. In *Textbook of Natural Medicine*, eds Pizzorno J and Murray M, 296–305. St. Louis, MO: Elsevier Churchill Livingstone.

Goldhamer A, Lisle D, Parpia B, Anderson S, and Campbell TC. 2001. Medically supervised water-only fasting in the treatment of hypertension. *J Manipulative Physiol Ther* 24(5):335–339.

Goldhamer A, Lisle D, Sultana P, Anderson S, Parpia B, Hughes B, and Campbell TC. 2002. Medically supervised water-only fasting in the treatment of borderline hypertension. *J Altern Complement Med* 8(5):643–650.

Greger M and Stone G. 2015. *How Not to Die*. New York: Flatiron Books.

Harvinder D, Ravindra B, Sajja V et al. 2010. Effect of intensive lifestyle changes on endothelial function and on inflammatory markers of atherosclerosis. *J Cardiol* 105:362–367.

Haugen M, Fraser D, Forre O. 1999. Diet therapy for the patient with rheumatoid arthritis? *Rheumatology* 38(11):1039–1044.

Heron, M. 2016. Deaths, leading causes for 2014. *Natl Vital Stat Rep* 65(5):1–15.

Holton K. 2016. The role of diet in the treatment of fibromyalgia. *Pain Management* 6(4):317–320.

Hutchinson E. 2006. Milestone 8 (1950) Smoking and Cancer. Smoking Gun. http://www.nature.com/milestones/milecancer/full/milecancer08.html (accessed 30 Oct 2016)

Intersalt Cooperative Research Group. 1988. Intersalt: An international study of electrolyte excretion and blood pressure. Results for 24 hour urinary sodium and potassium excretion. *BMJ* 297:319–328.

James PA, Oparil S, Carter B et al. 2014. 2014 Evidence based guideline for the management of high blood pressure in adults. *Report from the Panel Members Appointed to the Eighth Joint National Committee (JNC 8) JAMA* 311(5):507–520.

Jelinek G. 2009. *Overcoming Multiple Sclerosis, an Evidence Based Guide to Recovery*. Crows Nest, NSW: Allen and Unwin.

Jelinek G and Hassed C. 2009. Managing multiple sclerosis in primary care. Are we forgetting something? *Quality in Primary Care* 17:55–61.

Kantor ED, Rehm CD, and Du, M. 2016. Trends in dietary supplement use among US adults from 1999–2012. *JAMA* 310(6):1464.

Kaplan N. 2015. Salt intake, salt restriction and primary (essential) hypertension. http://www.uptodate.com/contents/salt-intake-salt-restriction-and-primary-essential-hypertension

Kempner W. 1946. *Some effect of the rice diet treatment of kidney disease and hypertension*. The Bulletin. Durham, NC: Department of Medicine, Duke University School of Medicine. Lecture read Jan 15, 1946 before the Section of Medicine of the New York Academy of Medicine.

Kempner W. 1948. Treatment of hypertensive vascular disease with rice diet. *Am J Med* 4:545–577 reprinted in *Arch Int Med* 1974, 133(758–790).

Kitiyakara C and Guzman N. 1998. Malignant hypertension and hypertensive emergencies. *Journ Am Soc Neph* 9(1):133–14.

Kjeldsen-Kragh J. 1999. Rheumatoid arthritis treated with vegetarian diets. *Am J Clin Nutr* 70(suppl):594S–600S.

Kjeldsen-Kragh J, Haugen M, Borchgrevnick C et al. 1991. Controlled trial of fasting and one-year vegetarian diet in rheumatoid arthritis. *Lancet* 338:899–902.

Leishman AWD. 1959. Hypertension-treated and untreated, a study of 400 cases. *Br Med J* 1:1361–1368.

Lenders C, Gorman K, Milch H et al. 2013. A novel nutrition medicine education model: The Boston University experience. *Adv Nutr* 4(1):1–7.

Maisel M. 2015a. Eating for health: The whole food plant based diet. http://www.dr-maisel.co.il/en/health/eating-for-health-the-whole-food-plant-based-diet

Maisel M. 2015b. Vegetarian or vegan: Is it healthy? http://www.dr-maisel.co.il/en/health/vegetarian-vegan-healthy

Makary M, Joo S, Daniel M, and Xu T. 2016. Letter to CDC. https://assets.documentcloud.org/2822345/Hopkins-CDC-letter.pdf

Mayo Clinic. 2016. Is there a multiple sclerosis diet? https://www.mayoclinic.org/diseases-conditions/multiple-sclerosis/diagnosis-treatment/drc-20350274

McDougall J. 2013. Walter Kempner MD-Founder of the Rice Diet. *The McDougall Newsletter* 12(12):1–10.

McGuire M and Beerman K. 2013. *Nutritional Sciences, From Fundamentals to Food*. 3rd ed. Belmont, CA: Wadsworth.

McKay D, Oliver Chen C-Y, Salzman E, and Blumberg J. 2009. Hibiscus Sabdariffa L tea (Tisane) lowers blood pressure in pre-hypertensive and mildly hypertensive adults. *J Nutr* 140:298–303.

Murray CJL, Abraham, J, Ali, MK et al. 2013. The state of US Health 1990–2010, burden of diseases, injuries, and risk factors. *JAMA* 310(6):591–608.

National Collaborating Centre for Chronic Conditions. 2009. *Rheumatoid Arthritis: National Clinical Guideline for Management and Treatment in Adults*. London: Royal College of Physicians.

Newborg B and Nash F. 2011. *Walter Kempner and the Rice Diet*, Challenging Conventional Wisdom. Durham, NC: Carolina Academic Press.

NICE (National Institute for Health and Clinical Excellence). 2014. Multiple sclerosis in adults: Management. Clinical guideline. https://www.nice.org.uk/guidance/cg186

NIH (National Institutes of Health). 2003. Reference card from the Seventh Report of the Joint National Committee on Prevention, Detection. Evaluation and treatment of high blood pressure (JNC 7) NIH Publication No. 03-5231.

Novick J. 2013. Label reading. www.wholefoodplantbasedrd.com.wp-content/uploads/2013/08/LabelReading

Ornish D, Brown SE, Scherwitz LW et al. 1990. Can lifestyle changes reverse coronary heart disease? *The Lancet* 336:129–133.

Ornish, D. 1990. *Dr Dean Ornish's Program for Reversing Heart Disease*. New York: Random House.

Ornish D, Weidner G, Fair W et al. 2005. Intensive lifestyle changes may affect the progression of prostate cancer. *J Urol* 174:1065–1070.

Peterson ED, Dai D, DeLong ER et al. 2010. Contemporary mortality risk prediction for percutaneous coronary intervention. Results from 588,398 procedures in the National Cardiovascular Data Registry. *J Am Coll Cardio* 55:1923–32.

Rodriguez-Leyva D, Weighell W, Edel A et al. 2013. Potent anithypertensive action of dietary flaxseed in hypertensive patients. *Hypertension* 62:1081–1089.

Rueda-Clausen CF, Silva FA, Lindarte MA et al. 2007. Olive, soybean and palm oils have a similar acute detrimental effect of the endothelial function in healthy young adults. *Nutr Metab Cardiovasc Dis* 17(1):50–57.

Starfield B. 2000. Is US healthcare really the best in the world? *JAMA* 284(4):483–485.

Swank RL and Duggan BB. 1987. *The Multiple Sclerosis Diet Book*. New York: Doubleday.

Swank RL and Duggan BB. 1990. Effect of low saturated fat diet in early and late cases of multiple sclerosis. *Lancet* 336:37–39.

Velasquez M, Ramezani A, Manal A, and Raj DS. 2016. Trimethylamine-N-oxide: The good, the bad and the unknown. *Toxins* 8, 326, doi:10.3390/toxins8110326

Vogel R. 1999. Brachial artery ultrasound: A noninvasive tool in the assessment of triglyceride-rich lipoproteins. *Clin Cardiol* 22(suppl II):34–39.

Vogel R, Corretti M, and Plotnick G. 1997. Effect of a single high-fat meal on endothelial function in healthy subjects. *Am J Cardiol* 79:350–354.

Vogel R, Corretti M, and Plotnick G. 2000. The postprandial effect of components of the Mediterranean diet on endothelial function. *Journ Am Coll Cardiol* 36:1455–1460.

World Health Organization. 2013. *A Global Brief on Hypertension*. Geneva, Switzerland: WHO Press.

Yadav V, Marracci G, Kim E et al. 2016. Low-fat plant based diet in multiple sclerosis: A randomized controlled trial. *Multiple Sclerosis and Related Disorders* 9:80–90.

3 Orthomolecular Parenteral Nutrition Therapy

Arturo O'Byrne-Navia and Arturo O'Byrne-De Valdenebro

CONTENTS

Introduction..39
   Nutritional Deficiencies/Insufficiencies that Support Intravenous Supplementation.................40
   Injectable Solutions in the Clinical Practice 41
      Application Routes in Parenteral Nutrition 42
   Preparation of Mixtures for Parenteral Nutrition 43
      Special Care in the Preparation of Orthomolecular Mixtures 44
Specific Products for Use in Orthomolecular Intravenous Nutritional Therapy...........................47
   Historical Considerations..47
   Theoretical Basis for the Therapeutic use of Intravenous (IV) Nutrients 48
   Potential Side Effects Considerations 50
   Intravenous (IV) Orthomolecular Therapeutic Agents...51
      Antioxidant Agents...51
      Amino Acids...71
      Vitamins..78
      B Complex Vitamins 78
      Lipid-Soluble Vitamins 82
      Minerals and Trace Elements 82
      Electrolytes..95
      Multimineral Preparations..95
      Precursors of Antioxidant Enzymes 96
      Others 96
References...97

INTRODUCTION

Nutritional treatments by parenteral route can be considered as valuable tools in the integrative management when added to a conventional treatment set, both in acute and chronic diseases.

Its main objective is to recover quickly and regain stability in the internal environment (biological terrain). They are also directed to ensure the proper management of homeodynamic (Lloyd et al. 2001) mechanisms, and to maintain or recover the molecular chemical conditions that guarantee health. Their role is crucial in chronic degenerative diseases, which often oral supplementation of therapeutic nutrients does not elicit a proper response. One of the main limitations for the successful use of the oral route is the abnormal function of the gastrointestinal mucous membranes from toxic and proinflammatory dietary habits (Taira et al. 2015, Woting and Blaut 2016, Li et al. 2016). Along with the resulting disturbances of the microbiota, this usually causes abnormalities in the intestinal permeability and a compromised capacity in the absorption of nutrients, radically interfering factors involved in the absorption and utilization of nutrients.

During the last 30 years, orthomolecular nutrition has been developing a path in integrative medicine, based on the crucial role of basic nutrients in:

- The recovery of chronically ill patients,
- The optimization of therapeutic responses to conventional treatments,
- The strengthening of homeodynamic mechanisms (through the psycho-neuro-immuno-endocrine links).

All these possibilities allow the patients to return to normal daily life in a more physiological way, since many of the delays in the recovery processes are due to nutritional imbalances. Unfortunately, the lack of knowledge of many conventional colleagues regarding the therapeutic use of nutrients many times leads to criticism of a method of great value in daily clinical practice.

NUTRITIONAL DEFICIENCIES/INSUFFICIENCIES THAT SUPPORT INTRAVENOUS SUPPLEMENTATION

Nutrition and orthomolecular supplements are optimal aid measures for most medical treatments. A patient recovers easier when the immune, endocrine, and neural systems (as master regulator systems for the rest of the body) are well nourished. On the other hand, the patient with nutritional imbalances will experience more difficulties overcoming the tendency to biological deregulation.

Unfortunately, in the modern world, many circumstances combine to create an increasingly poor state of nutrients, especially because it is not easy to find the right way to ensure the maintenance of health and structural/functional remodeling.

Understanding the concepts of deficiency and insufficiency plays a pivotal role in understanding the importance of intravenous nutritional therapy. This fully justifies the use of this type of orthomolecular practice, when facing serious nutritional issues in many patients. An historical misconception in the therapeutic use of nutrients has been limiting them to the critical patient, ignoring that for several nutrients, deficiencies/insufficiencies are widespread in the general population.

For some clinical settings, dietary amounts of many nutrients or oral supplementation based on the Recommended Daily Allowance (RDA) can be considered unable to attain clinical responses. In other cases, clinical improvement will take months to appear, thus making intravenous supplementation an interesting method of treatment.

Nutritional foodstuff values' tables of the commonly consumed foods serve only as reference values. Nonetheless, these tables do not reflect necessarily the actual state of the nutrient contents. This has been explained by many factors, for example, the lack or deficiency of a specific nutrient in the soil where these foods have been grown (Joy et al. 2016, Li et al. 2016). There are many other influencing factors, like agrochemical exposure of the crops, environmental toxicity, conservation, manipulation, and transport conditions, refinement of many foods, cooking techniques (peeling, high temperatures, cooking time), and so on, which may significantly impair the nutritional quality of the foods we consume every day (Teixeira et al. 2012, Gemenet et al. 2016, Poblaciones and Rengel 2016). A sustained consumption of nutritionally poor foods, slowly but inexorably leads to nutrient deficiencies among the population.

Some examples of specific nutrient deficiencies in foods/others are

- Preservation and storage processes make vitamins E, C, and/or B1 significantly dwindle its biological potential.
- The consumption of refined grains increases the needs of B complex vitamins and chromium to maintain the glucolipidic balance.
- Inclusion of "fake foods" (artificial flavoring and coloring of foods) compromise the availability of other nutritional factors.

- The little exposure to sunlight promotes global epidemic of hypovitaminosis D.
- Tobacco components (active or passive) affect epithelial barrier and mucosal systems, increasing the need of antioxidants (e.g., vitamins C and E).

Alcohol, a known liver toxin, reduces the absorption and bioavailability of many micronutrients, like vitamin C, vitamin E, B complex vitamins (thiamin, niacin, pyridoxine, folic acid, cyanocobalamin), calcium, magnesium, zinc, vitamin A/carotenoids, and SAMe (Lieber 1990, Ghorbani et al. 2016).

- Modern world stressful way of life increases the requirement of nutrients like glutamic acid, L-glutamine, L-arginine, antioxidants, and/or B complex vitamins.

Significant imbalance of essential fatty acids favors a trend toward persistent low-grade inflammation as a consequence of the distortion from modern habits and our Paleolithic genome (Ruiz-Núñez et al. 2016).

- Drug interactions with nutrients can affect their metabolism. This can be seen especially in polypharmacy patients due to chronic and/or multiple diseases. In some cases, specific medications alter the dynamics of the gastrointestinal system, affecting the absorption of nutrients (e.g., azathioprine, many of the chemotherapeutics, antibiotic related diarrhea, etc.).

Processing, storing, and heating/cooling of food may cause a loss of 40% of vitamin A, 100% of vitamin C, 80% B complex vitamins, and 55% of vitamin E (Harris and Karmas 1975).

Cutting or crushing food during preparation of meals starts enzymatic oxidation reactions that destroy important nutrients. The average loss of minerals and other nutrients from vegetables can reach more than 30% (Saxena et al. 2009).

All these factors lead us to understand that there is a considerable possibility of requiring parenteral nutritional replacement in patients with chronic or degenerative diseases. In this particular situation, the orthomolecular treatment has to ensure a quick and effective recovery of the deficient/insufficient nutritional components. There are other contexts like the acute patient. In that case, some of the nutritional circumstances may be similar, but the intravenous supplementation regimes are usually used for short periods of time. After the cause of the acute problem has been detected and corrected, it can be expected that any resulting nutritional deficiency does not prolong after a supplementation period limited in time.

INJECTABLE SOLUTIONS IN THE CLINICAL PRACTICE

As in any other pharmaceutical specialty, orthomolecular medicine requires the knowledge of the respective methodology of preparation of the nutritional therapeutic solutions to prevent any avoidable risk for the patient. When prepared under the proper manufacturing conditions, the orthomolecular intravenous solutions can be applied safely by trained personnel (both in the outpatient and in the inpatient setting).

The supplements suitable for nutritional therapy should have either pharmaceutical grade or should be manufactured by specialty compound pharmacies with experience in the preparation of injectable medications (Remington 1995). On the other hand, the attending physician practicing parenteral nutrition therapy should know the legislation and regulatory issues according to the country of practice. This must be taken into account especially for those regulations pertaining to the use of parenteral solutions in patients.

There are some fundamental conditions that the nutritional solutions should fulfill. All injectable nutritional/functional supplements must be sterile, pyrogen-free, and meet the stability and physicochemical conditions to assure the medical objective sought with this methodology treatment, while avoiding any complication arising from manufacturing issues (Lawrence 2007).

The use of the injectable route for orthomolecular supplementation becomes even more important in some specific situations related to the patient's condition:

- When the oral route is not possible, or when the conditions of the gastrointestinal tract do not guarantee the proper absorption of nutrients (from widespread intestinal dysbiosis to precise pathologies like short intestine syndrome);
- When the chemical nature or characteristics of the drug impede a satisfactory absorption by the oral route (e.g., Glutathione);
- When a quick correction fluid or circulating electrolytes is needed, or when a particular nutritional correction is mandatory (e.g., hypokalemia);
- When a faster therapeutic effect is required, due to the clinical condition or urgency;
- When the attending physician prefers direct control over the components and dosage of a nutritional mixture, according to the therapeutic objective.

Similarly, one might consider some specific situations in which the parenteral route can be recognized as the best way to ensure safety in the patient's treatment:

- When the pharmacological/clinical effect needs to be guaranteed, since the plasmatic levels obtained by the intravenous route do not depend on the process of intestinal absorption;
- When the treatment schedule must be correctly complied within the scope of inpatient institutions, as well as home care services;
- When the osmolarity, pH, or tonicity of the supplements are factors to be considered in the context of the patient (e.g., renal, cardiac, or hepatic disorders).

It is important that the health professional is trained specifically in the methodology of orthomolecular parenteral therapy. That allows a correct diagnosis of a particular medical condition, a determination of the type of orthomolecular treatment. It also allows the suitable preparation and administration of injectable components, as well as the recognition and prevention of any possible complications. Although not commonly seen in routine practice, some examples of these are: phlebitis, thrombosis, tissue damage, stroke, and local or systemic infection. As in any injectable therapy, when mistakes in dosage, volumes, and combinations are avoided, the risk of complications is clearly decreased.

The orthomolecular parenteral therapy comprises both intravenous and intramuscular administration. The best pharmaceutical presentations for these therapeutic routes available in the market are

- Ready to use pharmaceutical aqueous solutions,
- Dry soluble products with specific solvents, and/or
- Concentrated pharmaceutical solutions, which can be diluted prior to their use.

Application Routes in Parenteral Nutrition

Aqueous solutions are employed for the intravenous application. A peripheral vein (in most cases from the upper limbs) is chosen and varying volumes ranging from 0.5 to 1000 mL are dripped intravenously.

In some cases, there is also the possibility to apply "boluses" with volumes up to 10 mL. In other cases, intermittent solution applications can be performed over time (e.g., once a week), with volumes ranging from 100 to 500 mL. If total infusion volume exceeds 1000 mL or in some specific contexts like chelation therapy, it is recommended to have an infusion pump to perform a more controlled drip.

As it was mentioned before, the intravenous route has the advantage of not depending on the enteral absorption since the orthomolecular mixture is injected directly into the bloodstream and from there to the interstitial compartment and to the cell. It must be taken into account that this is a faster route with more rapid clinical effects, but one should also be aware of possible dangers associated to this same reason. Adverse reactions may be related to:

- Inappropriate use of supplements (e.g., an excess of intravenous L-tryptophan or Zinc could cause headache in sensitive patients);
- Empirical or random combinations (e.g., including unbalanced proportions of antagonistic nutrients as copper/zinc or L-lysine/L-arginine in the same solution or mixes of multiple minerals with ascorbic acid);
- Negligence in preparing the mixture;
- Not considering physical parameters of the solutions, such as tonicity or pH.

All these previous factors can be clearly associated with the lack of knowledge regarding the proper methods of orthomolecular parenteral nutrition. In that sense, they can be prevented easily if simple measures are taken.

Nonetheless, there are some other plausible undesired effects related to idiosyncratic reactions, sometimes not adverted by the patient though his or her life. Some people can have individual sensitivity to any orthomolecular component, although some of them have produced this type of reaction more frequently than others (e.g., iodum, thiamine).

In their original presentation, most orthomolecular injectable solutions are hypertonic. If used in this form, they could generate hemolysis (Olszewer and Teruya 2009). Prior to the intravenous application, hypertonic presentations must be diluted in suitable physiological solutions, optimizing osmolarity. The final solution should be isotonic or slightly hypotonic, to be adequately tolerated by erythrocytes (Botella Dorta 2004).

Regarding the pH parameter, neutral solutions between pH 6 and 7.5 are recommended. It is important to mention that blood has a significant buffering capacity, mainly concerning acids.

The intramuscular route can also be considered for the supplementation of orthomolecular nutrients. In that case, liquid medications in aqueous solutions or aqueous/oily suspensions are preferred, with volumes ranging from 1 to 5 mL. For these applications, gluteal or deltoid muscles are ideal. Their striated muscle nature endows them with wide vascularity and few sensory innervations, allowing a better absorption accompanied with low pain (Botella Dorta 2011).

Intramuscular injection allows differential absorption times, depending on the nature of the applied solution. For aqueous solutions, rapid absorption will be seen, while oily solutions/suspensions can be considered a deposit form with slow absorption rates. The proportion between oil and water in these solutions will determine its absorption rate.

When the pH of intramuscularly injected products is close to the plasmatic one, the application shall be less painful. In another way, when the pH is too acidic or alkaline, this can generate secondary reactions. In most cases there could be a simple congestion, but in extreme cases there can be an inflammatory process and even tissue necrosis could occur (Lawrence 2007). A slight hypertonic solution could be more easily absorbed.

Some adverse reactions with intramuscular injection are related to the nature of the drug itself. It is widely known how vitamin B1 and B complex vitamins produce much more pain when injected through this route. This fact can be reduced in some degree when these types of orthomoleculars are injected deeply into the gluteal muscle.

PREPARATION OF MIXTURES FOR PARENTERAL NUTRITION

Due to the practical importance of this aspect, it will be also mentioned in this chapter.

Health professionals, who include orthomolecular parenteral nutrition among their practices, should be trained particularly in the preparation of nutrient mixtures. The development of an institutional "procedures manual" is strongly suggested (Sobotka et al. 2009). This type of manual should include: detailed instructions about all the processes related to the preparation of the mixtures (responsible personnel both for the preparation and application, proper facilities, available supplements, optimal quantities and number of supplements to be used, etc.).

The procedures manual is primarily a safety measure for the patient, the health staff, and the institution. It also plays an important role in the institutional qualification/habilitation processes with the local sanitary authorities granting the permissions required to perform such procedures.

The health personnel involved in parenteral orthomolecular therapy must include one coordinator (usually a registered nurse) skilled to conduct training to the rest of the team. This training should cover the following topics (Botella et al. 2002, World Health Organization 2003, Sobotka et al. 2009):

- Hygiene and aseptic techniques. This point is especially important due to the emergence of parenteral therapy-associated mycobacteriosis;
- Knowledge of possible physical or chemical incompatibilities between prescribed nutrients and/or between nutrients and diluents;
- Potential instability of intravenous mixture or nutrient diluent mixture;
- Hazards or risks of microbiological contamination during intravenous mixture preparation, during the time of peripheral access puncture, or during the mixture application;
- Restrictions on temperature, sunlight exposure, and other storage product requirements. Label-related issues (Kumar et al. 2013), such as passive errors due to lack of attention when reading the labels, poor quality labels (allowing deterioration of important data related to the supplement that makes them difficult to read), or even mislabel itself;
- Human errors like adding the same supplement more than once, or in excessive amounts;
- Lack of knowledge regarding a particular nutrient, particularly in the case of potential adverse reactions or adverse effect during its application.

Special Care in the Preparation of Orthomolecular Mixtures

Incompatibility

Incompatibility can result from physical or chemical interaction between components.

Attention must be called to the presence of physical incompatibility which is visually noticeable. It is characterized by a variety of possibilities as precipitation, clumping, cloudiness, frothiness, or changes in color of the mixture. Any of these abnormalities occurs when there is incompatibility between two or more components. Another option would be the incompatibility between any of the nutrients and the solvent vehicle. The physical changes can be evident in the solution bag even from the time of preparation of the mixture, but also during the application of it (Saldaña–Ambulódegui 2012).

Another potential incompatibility arises from the chemical interaction of orthomolecular mixture components. The possible responses to chemical incompatibilities include an affection of the purported therapeutic action of the supplementation (from partial to complete loss). It could also derive in the eventual augmentation of known potential toxicity of one component, or in the generation of toxic compounds with undesirable effects. The emergence of thrombophlebitis is not common but possible, mostly related to an incorrect management of the parenteral technique. As with any intravenous application, there exists the theoretical chance for developing embolisms, a rare complication not seen in more than 30 years of experience with orthomolecular injectable medications in our practice.

Usual potential factors affecting compatibility or stability of a parenteral nutrition solution are

- Problems with the pH of the mixture, which is considered the most critical factor (Olszewer and Teruya 2009).
  - Regarding the intravenous solutions, the closer the pH value is to 7, the less chance there is of having a painful or risky application. In physiologic conditions, blood has a pH of approximately 7.35, slightly alkaline. With the intramuscular injections, solutions with a pH between 4.4 and 8.5 are considered acceptable.

- Some components are known because of their very low pH: Thiamine, N-acetylcysteine, L-leucine, or Cyanocobalamin. In turn, there are others like DMSO, which tend to have alkaline pH (around 10).
- The sequence in which the components are added.
- Modifications of components by exposure to light and/or inadequate temperatures (previous or during the application; e.g., alpha lipoic acid, ascorbic acid).
- Difficulties or problems with dilution of any component of the mixture.
- Significant changes secondary to the time elapsed between preparation and application.
- Complications arising from the type of diluent used.
- Improper conditions of packaging, transporting, and storing.

The institutional procedures manual serves as a useful method to minimize the risk of incompatibilities, therefore preserving the integrity of patient care during orthomolecular injectable therapy. There are some specific recommendations to observe in that regard:

- The solutions to be injected must be prepared and then injected in the shortest possible time. Avoiding the preparation of orthomolecular mixtures in advance should be the general rule. The concept of mixture stocking should not have any role in orthomolecular nor in integrative medicine.
- The number of components of a nutritional mixture should be kept to the lowest, and should follow rational protocols established previously, according the therapeutic target(s).
- If the mixture includes components with different pH, a previous check of this pH in their labels is recommended, to mix and add them in descending pH order (from alkalines to acidics).
- There exist several incompatibilities between some injectable orthomoleculars. For example, ascorbic acid plus minerals in the form of sulfate salts, due to the precipitation possibility of the last ones. Incompatible medications should never be mixed. They should be prepared in different solution bags and attention should be paid to the order of intravenous application of these solutions.
- Many practitioners of integrative medicine perform orthomolecular infusions along with other types of therapeutic approaches. When using medications with bio-regulatory properties (antihomotoxics and/or homeopathics) simultaneously during the orthomolecular mixture, the intravenous catheter should be used. Ideally, a washout of the intravenous line with 10 mL of sterile water solution should be performed before and after the injection of the bio-regulatory medication. When using two or more bio-regulatory medications, a minimum of 5 minutes should be left between their application.
- In case of having any doubt, a consult with the pharmacist of the institution is highly recommended.

Instability

Instability of some orthomolecular nutrients arises from chemical reactions considered undesirable and preventable, but in most cases irreversible. These reactions occur either because of mixing incompatible components in the same solution or external influences. The result could be in the form of toxic compounds or as a compromise in the therapeutic effectiveness of the nutrients. The most known of these influences are

- Oxidation of antioxidants after exposure to light and/or heat (especially alpha lipoic acid, but attention must be paid also with ascorbic acid, glutathione (Yamamoto and Ishihara 1994, Fleming 2016), and vitamin B5);

- Destruction by the action of ultraviolet light (B complex vitamins, particularly riboflavin, thiamine, pyridoxine, Cyanocobalamin, and folic acid (www.helapet.co.uk/downloads/lightaffectingdrugs.pdf));
- Hydrolysis of amino acid (polypeptidic) chains can result from their inclusion in acidic solutions.

Sterility and Modifications Due to Contamination

The sterility of an injectable nutritional solution is a mandatory condition. Microbiological controls of injectable drugs must be carefully fulfilled. When handling solution bags, intravenous application equipment, catheters, and so on, sufficient precautions have to be taken care of.

Beyond the required quality of the used materials, contamination can occur during the preparation and/or the application procedure itself. This phenomenon can be related to inadequate staff hygiene when preparing and administrating the solutions, and also to inappropriate infrastructure institutional conditions (Akers and Larrimore 2003, Williams 2005, http://www.usp.org/sites/default/files/usp_pdf/EN/USPNF/generalChapterInjections.pdf).

Apyrogenicity

Nutritional products intended for parenteral use must be free of pyrogens. Defensive reactions against a variety of microorganisms (Gram-negative or Gram-positive bacteria, viruses, and fungi), or its endotoxins (lipopolysaccharides, LPS from Gram-negative bacteria) can be found in parenteral pharmaceuticals and medical. Endotoxins are large molecular weight complexes ($\sim$106 Da) associated with and expressed in the outer membranes of Gram-negative bacteria (Kluger 1990, Hartung and Wendel 1995, Henderson et al. 1996, Rosimar et al. 2004). This is a reason of concern to the pharmaceutical industry, and as such, all the necessary means to avoid this situation must be present.

In our system, the endotoxin/LPS binds to the specific toll-like receptor 4 (TLR4) complex on the monocyte membrane (Lu et al. 2008) initiating the signaling and transduction inflammatory pathway. This pathway comprises several reactions leading to the induction of endogenous pyrogens such as Interleukin-1β (IL-1β), Interleukin-6 (IL-6), and tumor necrosis factor-α (TNF-α). The endogenous pyrogens then cause a change in the thermoregulation in the hypothalamus toward a higher body temperature in order to optimize all the immune system responses. In the case of exogenous pyrogens, the Interleukin-8 (IL-8) is induced in the monocyte. This chemokine by nature has different functions than the previously mentioned ones.

Pyrogens are hyperthermia inducing substances. They can come from intact, dead, or disintegrated microorganisms, whether they are pathogenic or not. In the case of intact (living) microorganisms, they often result from their metabolic products such as denatured proteins. Gram-negative bacteria are particularly known due to their capacity of pyrogen production. In comparison to other pyrogens, LPS are more resistant to heat (Hartung et al. 2001, Roth and Blatteis 2014) inducing higher febrile reactions. In this context, it is mandatory that the sterilization process is performed with the correct temperatures and controls.

From the clinical point of view, regarding other types of microorganisms, pyrogens from fungi are considered less important since they tend to produce only a slight temperature elevation. As demonstrated in experiments with rabbits, fungal mannans can be considered pyrogens by themselves (Nagase et al. 1984). Its effect is independent from the one of LPS, but has a weaker intensity.

In cases of contaminated orthomolecular therapeutic mixtures administered intravenously, a febrile reaction occurs. This situation does not have any relationship with the nutritional agents included in the mixture, since none of the usual orthomoleculars is known to induce this type of reaction. This hyperthermical effect can go beyond 40°C (104°F) and have a duration ranging from 4 to 12 hours (Morimoto et al. 1988, Rosimar et al. 2004), if an antithermic measure is not taken. Other clinical features of the reaction against pyrogens include cold or chills, joint or lumbar pain, nausea and/or headache.

SPECIFIC PRODUCTS FOR USE IN ORTHOMOLECULAR INTRAVENOUS NUTRITIONAL THERAPY

HISTORICAL CONSIDERATIONS

The use of nutrition with therapeutic purposes has a long history in medicine, but it was only until the mid-twentieth century that the intravenous route was a feasible option. McCormick in Canada (McCormick 1959) was probably the first author to come up with the idea of the intravenous intervention in cancer, which according to his theories would arise from a defective collagen remodeling because of vitamin C deficiency.

During the 1970s, Linus Pauling and Ewan Cameron took back these interesting ideas (Cameron and Pauling 1973, 1974, Cameron et al. 1979). After encouraging clinical observations (Cameron et al. 1975), the group of Cameron later began their clinical research on terminal cancer patients, using high-dose intravenous Vitamin C. In their landmark publications (Cameron and Pauling 1976, 1978) they were able to show improvement in function and life expectancy in this oncologic group of patients. The patients receiving the high-dose vitamin C treatment had a median survival time of 300 days more compared to the non-treated patients (Cameron and Pauling 1978).

These claims were promptly scrutinized by researchers in the Mayo Clinic. They were not able to corroborate Pauling and Cameron's observations (Creagan et al. 1979, Moertel et al. 1985), thus disqualifying the treatment of oncologic disease with high-dose vitamin C. This publication closed the doors for the possibility of integrating vitamin C into conventional oncology treatment for many years.

It has already been clarified (González et al. 2005) that the trials from Pauling and Cameron and the ones from Moertel et al. are clearly different in their methodology. Pauling and Cameron used high-dose vitamin C delivered intravenously and the orally, in patients with moderately advanced disease. The Mayo Clinic trial used high-dose vitamin C delivered *only* orally in patients with severely advanced disease.

Additionally, at that time it was not known that the vitamin C pharmacokinetics differ clearly in the parenteral versus the oral use (Padayatty et al. 2004), rendering the studies by Cameron and Moertel incomparable. Prior observations of high-dose vitamin C researchers had already suggested such an effect, since the tumoral regression was possible only when the dose was maintained high enough (Cameron et al. 1975). Cameron did not have the pharmacokinetic data but emphasized the need of a continuous administration of high-dose vitamin C to achieve the expected results (Cameron 1991).

The following decades were characterized by the opposition of the two points of view. High-dose vitamin C advocates continued treating their patients with this approach, and conventional oncology continued rejecting this therapy. Hugh Riordan, MD in Wichita, Kansas contributed building a strong base of work from the practical therapeutic activity in complementary oncology. Dr. Riordan and his team have treated more than 40,000 cancer patients and have published research (Mikirova et al. 2008, 2016a,b, Riordan et al. 2005, Duconge et al. 2007, Padayatty et al. 2006) showing effectiveness for some cancers. The Riordan intravenous vitamin C (IVC) protocol for patients with oncologic disease (Riordan et al. 2003) involves the slow infusion of vitamin C at doses of 0.1–1.0 grams (g) of ascorbate per kilogram (kg) of body weight.

During the 1960s and the 1970s, John Myers, MD, an internist from Johns Hopkins Hospital in Baltimore, made particular remarks regarding the limitation of the oral route to provide an optimal nutrient intake (with therapeutic purposes). He concluded that since the average western world patient has a compromised capacity to absorb nutrients due to the lack of an optimal function of the digestive mucous membranes, the use of intravenous supplementation would be fully justified. Besides the absorptive limitation, there is also the inherent activity of detoxification systems (i.e., the "1st-pass effect"), turning the oral route into a suboptimal one. Hence, only a small fraction of the vitamins and minerals ingested by the average patient (either in food or in pills) are actually being successfully absorbed and then lead into the bloodstream. Dr. Myers started using a safe mixture of key nutritional supplements which were administered in a single intravenous infusion (directly providing these nutrients to each cell in the body).

Although the pioneering work of Dr. Myers has always been recognized in the orthomolecular medical community, the exact composition of the so-called "Myers' cocktail" was not precisely known. The information related to Myers' patients was incomplete and there weren't any official publications available about this orthomolecular treatment, beyond anecdotic material. According to the review made by Dr. Alan R. Gaby, MD (Gaby 2002) who took over Dr. Myers' practice in Baltimore after his passing, it seems that Myers used a 10-mL syringe to administer a combination of magnesium chloride, calcium gluconate, thiamine, pyridoxine, cyanocobalamin, calcium pantothenate, and vitamin C. The exact amounts of the individual components were unknown, but Myers apparently used a 2% solution of magnesium chloride, rather than the more widely available preparations containing 20% magnesium chloride or 50% magnesium sulfate.

Based on the alleged "Myers' cocktail" composition by Gaby, he administered such a mixture of magnesium, calcium, B complex vitamins, and vitamin C. This author along with a group of collaborators report (Ali et al. 2009) satisfactory clinical results in patients with migraine, fatigue (including chronic fatigue syndrome), fibromyalgia, acute muscle spasm, upper respiratory tract infections, chronic sinusitis, seasonal allergic rhinitis, acute asthma attacks, and other disorders. According to these authors, through the years they have administered more than 1500 Myers' cocktails to patients with various clinical conditions.

Other orthomolecular nutrients like Glutathione have also been reported to be useful when administered together with Myers' cocktail, particularly in the context of cardiovascular disease (Forman et al. 2009).

According to our experience, since 1975 in the Academia de Medicina Biológica de Los Robles (Los Robles Biological Medicine Academy) in Popayan, Colombia, Dr. Germán Duque, MD initiated the intravenous administration of the so-called Moros' mineral constellations. This combination of oligo and macroelements was developed by Dr. Gustavo Moros, a Venezuelan cardiologist some years before. Dr. Moros used fixed doses of various minerals in different salt forms. This supplementation allows the complete reposition of the relative circulating pool from the most important minerals, providing a basic nutritional load for the extracellular matrix and subsequently for the cells. This type of intravenous orthomolecular compound has been the basis of the parenteral nutritional approach in our clinic for the last 35 years. There are several commercial presentations available in South America, for example, MM–16 Forte (18 minerals) from HeilPro DKN® (Cali, Colombia), MinTraz (19 minerals) from OrthomoLab® (Cali, Colombia), and Nutri-MINS (16 minerals) from BioMolec® (Quito, Ecuador). All these multimineral compounds conserve the Moros' concept of including a myriad of mineral salts as the nutritional orthomolecular supplementation method in both chronic and acute patients.

THEORETICAL BASIS FOR THE THERAPEUTIC USE OF INTRAVENOUS (IV) NUTRIENTS

Therapeutic intravenous administration of nutrients has some advantages over other routes, and of course like any therapeutic measure, is not free of some disadvantages.

Regarding the advantages, this route can achieve serum concentrations which are not obtainable with oral or even intramuscular (IM) administration.

For example, as the oral dose of vitamin C is increased progressively, the serum concentration of ascorbate tends to approach an upper limit, because of both saturation of gastrointestinal absorption and a sharp increase in renal clearance of the vitamin (Blanchard et al. 1997).

When the daily intake of vitamin C is increased by 12-fold, from 200 mg/day to 2500 mg/day, the plasma concentration increases by only 25% (from 1.2 to 1.5 mg/dL). The highest serum vitamin C level reported after oral administration of pharmacological doses of ascorbate is 9.3 mg/dL (Harakeh et al. 1990). In contrast, the IV administration of 50 g/day of vitamin C resulted in a mean peak plasma level of 80 mg/dL (about 12 times higher).

Similarly, oral supplementation with magnesium results in little or no change in serum magnesium concentrations, whereas its IV administration can double or triple the serum magnesium levels (Okayama et al. 1987, Sydow et al. 1993).

Many nutrients have been shown to exert pharmacological effects, which are in many cases dependent on the concentration of the nutrient (so as in most medicinal substances).

For example, an antiviral effect of vitamin C has been demonstrated at a concentration of 10–15 mg/dL, a level achievable with IV but not oral therapy. In another context, at a concentration of 88 mg/dL in vitro, vitamin C was able to destroy 72% of the histamine present in the medium (Uchida et al. 1989).

Lower concentrations were not tested, but it is possible that serum levels of vitamin C attainable by giving several grams in an IV push would produce an antihistaminic effect in vivo. Such an effect would have implications for the treatment of various allergic conditions.

Magnesium ions promote relaxation of both vascular (Iseri and French 1984) and bronchial (Brunner et al. 1985) smooth muscles, specifically with higher doses. This effect might be useful in the acute treatment of vasospastic angina and bronchial asthma, respectively.

These are only a couple of examples, but it is likely that these and other nutrients exert additional pharmacological effects (currently unidentified) when used in high concentrations.

In addition to having direct pharmacological effects, IV nutrient therapy may be more effective than oral or IM treatment for the correction of intracellular nutritional deficits. Some nutrients are present at much higher concentrations in the cells than in the serum. For example, the average magnesium concentration in myocardial cells is 10 times higher than the extracellular concentration (Frustaci et al. 1987).

This ratio is maintained in healthy cells by an active-transport system that continually pumps magnesium ions into cells against the concentration gradient. In certain disease states, the capacity of membrane pumps to maintain normal concentration gradients may be compromised. In one study, the mean myocardial magnesium concentration was 65% lower in patients with cardiomyopathy than in healthy controls (Frustaci et al. 1987), implying a reduction in the intracellular-to-extracellular ratio to less than 4-to-1. Considering that magnesium plays a key role in mitochondrial energy production, intracellular magnesium deficiency may exacerbate heart failure and lead to a vicious cycle of further intracellular magnesium loss and more severe heart failure with potentially disastrous consequences.

Intravenous administration of magnesium, by producing a marked, though transient, increase in the serum concentration, provides an opportunity for ailing cells to take up magnesium against a smaller concentration gradient. Since these cells belong to a pathological context, the nutrients taken up by them after an IV orthomolecular infusion may eventually leak out again. Nonetheless there is always the aim of inducing repair and healing phases from the replenishment of nutrients, even before the leak out happens again. With time, if cells are repeatedly "flooded" with nutrients, this improvement may be cumulative.

In the author's clinical observation, some patients who receive a series of orthomolecular IV injections become progressively healthier, not only from their main cause of consultation, but also from other minor complaints in their clinical history. In these patients, the interval between treatments can be gradually increased, and eventually the injections might be no longer necessary.

This can be considered as one of the disadvantages of the IV route, since not all the patients are willing to receive injections. Of course, this is not limited to orthomoleculars, but extends to any injectable product/medication.

Other patients require regular injections for an indefinite period of time in order to control their medical problems. This prolonged necessity of orthomolecular IV injections could conceivably result from any of the following:

1. Chronic disease states which are hardly reversible (e.g., many oncologic patients).
2. Advanced age, since it is characterized among others by a difficulty in the normal intestinal absorption of nutrients and the secondary deficits.

A genetically determined impairment in the capacity to maintain normal intracellular concentrations of a specific nutrient (Henrotte 1980).

An inborn error of metabolism that can be controlled only by maintaining a higher than normal concentration of a particular nutrient (Camp et al. 2013).

3. A persistent renal leak of a nutrient (Booth and Johanson 1974) or several nutrients, like in CKD (Merrill 1956).

POTENTIAL SIDE EFFECTS CONSIDERATIONS

It is important to mention that the use of IV vitamin C must take into account a genetic defect called "Glucose-6-Phosphate Dehydrogenase Deficiency," or G6PD-deficiency, also known as "favism." This is a genetic mutation found in people of African or Mediterranean origin. If a patient with favism receives IV vitamin C, it can result in hemolysis (destruction of red blood cells, RBCs). This happens because without this critical enzyme, the RBC is not able to recycle Glutathione and thus is not able to handle oxidative stress/damage. Without Glutathione to protect it, the RBC will be destroyed, leading to anemia. This is a potentially very dangerous situation since it can end up in acute renal failure, and can even be fatal (although this is rare).

A genetic screening for G6PD-deficiency in patients programmed to receive IV vitamin C is thoroughly recommended. The practice of medicine and of orthomolecular supplementation is shaped by socioeconomical status. In that sense, we are aware of the screening being performed regularly in developed countries. On the other hand, in our experience in third world countries, where the test is expensive or simply not available, it is possible to begin IV vitamin C with low doses (e.g., 3–5 g) and tell the patient to pay attention to any change in the color of the first urination after the infusion. If there has been any low-level hemolysis (as evidenced by rose or light red color in the urine), the genetic test is indicated.

Although this genetic defect has been reported in the literature as a high incidence one (Minareci et al. 2006), in our particular Latin-American population we have not been able to see the first case in more than 30 years using low, medium, and high doses of IV vitamin C.

In any case, most patients with this mutation are already aware of their condition (given they were born with it) and the likelihood of red cell hemolysis/destruction with the ingestion of certain common foods, such as beans (especially fava beans). Any family history of favism reported by the patient obligates to the appropriate test before receiving IV vitamin C.

Another special group to consider is the chronic renal insufficiency (CKD) patient. In this case, some nutrients included in the orthomolecular infusions represent an increased risk of accumulation. This is due to the compromise in the blood filtering function of the kidneys, which helps maintain normal levels of fluid and ions in the bloodstream. If this process is impaired, receiving certain amounts of IV fluids possess an increased risk of "fluid overload" state. This applies also for patients with congestive heart failure and/or atrial fibrillation. Special precaution must be observed in patients taking Digoxin or other potassium-depleting drugs (e.g., some diuretics), since potential electrolyte imbalances in this group of patients can lead to heart arrhythmias in an easier way in comparison to the general population.

In any of these conditions, IV nutrients can be used but there are special cautions with volumes and duration of the infusions, to avoid a "fluid overload" state. Additionally, CKD can also impair the ability to filter and/or reabsorb specific minerals. Certain ions (K^+, Mg^+, Ca^{4+}) or mixes of them, with a higher osmolality, could eventually lead to accumulation of them and potential toxicity.

Intravenous magnesium is known to affect blood pressure (BP) and potentially lower its records. Magnesium influence in blood pressure is evident when it is used daily in hospitals around the world (particularly in the management of pregnancy-induced hypertension, or "toxemia gravidarum"). Patients with low blood pressure are advised to report any symptoms related to such conditions during and/or after an orthomolecular IV treatment. This phenomenon is usually counteracted with the total volume of the infusion, but it could persist if the tendency to hypotension is notorious and/or if the dose of magnesium is high. Thus, caution is recommended in patients with low BP.

A similar caution must be mentioned in patients with tendency to hypoglycemia. Some ortho-molecular nutrients have the capacity to influence the carbohydrate metabolism, such as chromium, zinc, manganese, vanadium, some B complex vitamins, among others (Sárközy et al. 2014). Glucose can bind to DMSO and be carried into cells. All these potential influences can lead to lower blood sugar levels. Patients with hypoglycemic tendencies are advised to report any symptom related to such condition during and/or after an orthomolecular IV treatment. In our institution, there is the universal recommendation of ingesting at least some food before any IV orthomolecular infusion.

Allergy is also a theoretical reason for concern, although the rarest of the potentially adverse reactions to occur. There is always of course the possibility of a patient with an unknown allergy. In that case, individual patients may have an allergy to a component of the IV combination and this can evoke an allergic response. Given the simple molecular characteristics of most of the orthomo-lecular nutrients used in IV infusions, it is not likely that an allergic reaction presents. Nonetheless, there are specific concerns about iodine, which in fact is recognized in medicine as a potentially strong allergen for some individuals. If there is any suspicion of a potential allergic sensitivity, the suspected substance should be avoided in the orthomolecular mixture. In the very infrequent case of an allergic reaction, the respective control treatment should be commenced quickly.

INTRAVENOUS (IV) ORTHOMOLECULAR THERAPEUTIC AGENTS

A wide range of substances that are part of the nutritional orthomolecular therapeutic approach can be injected through the veins into the bloodstream. Each nutrient has specific medical objec-tives, but since habitually a single nutrient is involved in several metabolic pathways and exerts actions in several tissues, it is common that the list of objectives/functions can rise to 5 or 6 per nutrient. When injected in conjunction with other nutrients with the same objective, a synergistic action can be expected, but this is more a theoretical concept given the difficulty to measure it. The nutrients in orthomolecular medicine can be grouped in several categories according either to their action or to their chemical structure. The most common ones will be reviewed in the next section of the chapter.

Antioxidant Agents

Vitamin C (Ascorbic Acid)

It is important to mention that vitamin C can act as an antioxidant or as a prooxidant depending on a variety of factors, like the dose administered and the physiologic or pathologic state of the recipient (Levine et al. 2011, Chakraborthy et al. 2014). Historically, lower doses up to 5 g have been consid-ered as antioxidants (Traber and Stevens 2011), while the higher doses from 15 g and above have been recognized as prooxidant (Chen et al. 2008, Mendes-da-Silva 2014). Although this concept can prevail most of the time, there have also been publications (Hininger et al. 2005) which challenge this postulate. Of course, oxidative stress is a complex phenomenon to study and drawing conclu-sions only from basic studies can not necessarily be applied to the clinical reality. In the clinical and therapeutic contexts (where type III complexity is the rule rather than the exception and thus they are better understood with a systems biology approach (Welsby 1999)) the dose concept cannot be static, as in the case for the use of IV vitamin C.

Different studies have been published suggesting beneficial results in many clinical situations. One of the most prominent fields for the use of IV vitamin C is the modulation of the tissues, result-ing in an aid to the healing process. This has been observed, for example, in a postsurgical set-ting, where the supraphysiologic supplementation of ascorbic acid resulted in improvements of the anastomosis healing. The authors attributed the effect to a better control of the local inflammatory process, and to a better quality and quantity of the collagen produced locally, resulting in a higher strength of the anastomosis (Cevikel et al. 2008).

Another possibility for the orthomolecular use of IV vitamin C is in the oncology field. In the clinical setting, doses of 10–75 g of vitamin C administered intravenously exhibited a cytotoxic effect upon entering cancer cells. According to their interesting results, the research team affiliated with the Bezmialem Vakif University Medical Faculty in Turkey encourages the use of IV vitamin C along with radiotherapy for the treatment of patients with bone metastases (Kiziltan et al. 2014).

The besought mechanism of action for the antitumoral effect of high dose IV vitamin C is the augmentation of hydrogen peroxide at the extracellular level (Riordan et al. 1995). Since the tumoral cells lack the proper antioxidative defenses (catalases, among others), they perish from the exposure to these type of doses (prooxidant) (Chen et al. 2007, Park 2013).

There are other possible additional mechanisms of action supporting the use of high dose IV vitamin C in cancer patients. In a basic study (Yeom et al. 2009) Korean authors found that the carcinostatic effect induced by high dose concentrations of ascorbic acid occurred through the inhibition of angiogenesis, according to several parameters of tumor evaluation (biopsy results, gene expression studies, and wound healing analysis, both in vivo and in vitro).

Several treatment protocols have been reported for high dose IV vitamin C as a therapeutic tool in patients with cancer. Most of them include the infusion of doses between 350 and 750 mg/kg every 3–5 days for a prolonged period of time. A thorough review of one of these protocols is provided by Mirikova et al from the Riordan clinic (Mikirova et al. 2013).

This, however, differs significantly from the original protocol used by Cameron et al. in the 1970s, and published in their landmark papers about the use of high dose IV vitamin C in cancer patients (Cameron and Campbell 1974, Cameron and Pauling 1976, 1978). In these observational studies, without the knowledge of vitamin C pharmacokinetics we have available nowadays, the most employed protocol combined the oral supplementation of several grams of vitamin C with daily IV infusions of 10 g of the agent for 10 days.

It is worth noting that despite the widespread use of high dose IV vitamin C in many integrative practices and clinics around the world, and of the interesting results that most of us constantly witness with the use of this measure in the oncologic patient, the available high-quality evidence on its effectiveness is still scant (Fritz et al. 2014). This precludes a definite and formal recommendation for this type of treatment, since to date there is only preliminary evidence which does not allow drawing strong conclusions about it. Nevertheless, according to this same evidence high dose IV vitamin C appears to have a good safety profile and a potential antitumor activity.

Regardless of the conceptual orientation of the consulted authors (Fritz et al. 2014, Jacobs et al. 2015), there seems to be much more agreement in the notion that high dose vitamin C infusions do play a role in the improvement of the quality of life and in the reduction of symptom severity in oncologic patients. We are optimistic that the years to come will bring substantial improvements in the quality of the evidence, through adequately designed and implemented controlled trials on the use of vitamin C in cancer treatment. This will be crucial not only for the growth and acceptance of the integrative oncology field, but also for the patients who will receive better medical care when infused with high dose vitamin C. Remaining questions dealing for instance with the most responsive tumors, or the optimal schemes of IV vitamin C (doses, rates of infusion, length of the treatment, etc.) still pose significant challenges even for the physician with years of experience in the field of orthomolecular medicine.

The clinical use of high dose IV vitamin C has another interesting chapter in the treatment of infectious diseases. Vitamin C has been used in many different aetiological contexts, but the viral infections are the ones that seem to exhibit a better response when this agent is utilized. Thanks to the laborious work of compilation of Robert McCracken (2004), it is possible to have access to many difficult to find publications in this area (e.g., articles from the 1930s to the 1970s, written by one of the most prominent pioneers in the clinical application of vitamin C, Dr. Fred R. Klenner).

In fact, many natural compounds have been tested in the search for the ability to suppress viral replication. IV vitamin C infusions produce a positive effect on disease duration and reduction of several viral antibody levels. Also from the group of the Riordan Clinic in Kansas (Mikirova and Hunninghake 2014), the publication of a clinical study of ascorbic acid and EBV infection showed a reduction in antibody titers of EBV EA IgG and EBV VCA IgM during the IV vitamin C treatment.

There are some other observations from the medical literature that serum vitamin C concentrations at the millimolar levels are able to hinder viral infection and replication in vitro. For example, suspensions of herpes simplex virus (HSV) types 1 and 2, cytomegalovirus (CMV), and parainfluenzavirus type 2 were inactivated within 24 hours of having been treated at 37°C with 1 mg (5.05 mM) of copper-catalyzed sodium ascorbate per mL. Ascorbate concentrations as high as 10 mg/mL (50.5 mM) demonstrated only a minimum increase in effect on viral inactivation. The loss of infectivity did not alter either the hemagglutination or complement fixation qualities of the antigens (White et al. 1986).

Vitamin C exerts plenty of influences in the immune system function, both from the quantitative and qualitative points of view. As reported by Sorice et al. in their broad review from 2014 covering this topic (Sorice et al. 2014), vitamin C enhances the cytokine production and the synthesis of immunoglobulins in response to infection (Stephensen et al. 2006); up-regulates the activity of NK cells (Ichim et al. 2011); impacts the lymphocytes proliferation in a dose-dependent fashion, with physiological concentrations increasing it and supraphysiological concentrations inhibiting it (Bruunsgaard et al. 2003, Furuya et al. 2008, Calder et al. 2009); polarizes the differentiation toward type 1 response (leading Th0 subset to differentiate to Th1 subset) (Holmannová et al. 2012); and affects both antimicrobial and NK cell activities, lymphocytic proliferation, chemotaxis, and delayed-type hypersensitivity (Zhang and Farthing 2000).

In the same instance but from an opposite direction, inflammation represents an obstacle for the action of vitamin C on endothelilal cells, due to an inhibition of its uptake due to proinflammatory cytokines like tumor necrosis factor-alpha and interleukin-1 beta (Seno et al. 2004). Vitamin C itself has the possibility to modulate inflammatory processes and it consequences (Zhang et al. 2000). For example, high doses of vitamin C may attenuate exercise-induced inflammatory reactions.

Our clinical experience in the use of intravenous vitamin C in the treatment of infectious diseases has led us to observe that the everyday infections in immunocompetent patients (e.g., cases of common cold, mild gastroenteritis, uncomplicated bronchitis) evolve faster and with much less symptoms derived from the infection. This results after a comparison with previous similar infectious episodes referred by the patient or with household contacts or close relatives with the same disease but who did not receive the vitamin C treatment for any reason. In these types of infections one or two vitamin C infusions of 5–10 g have been very useful.

In cases of complex or chronic infections treated in our institution, vitamin C infusions also have an important role. An important difference with the acute but trivial infection, in the chronic ones or the complex acute ones, usually the patient must be injected in a series of occasions during a more prolonged time. Two to five vitamin C infusions of 15–20 g, given every 3–5 days is the customary treatment for an uncomplicated pneumonia (along with other measures from the biological medicine and the proper antibiotic scheme).

In chronic infections like hepatitis C (HCV), a long course of weekly vitamin C infusions of 15–25 g for 6 months, followed by every other week infusions with similar amounts of vitamin C, have been helpful to manage symptoms referred by the patients as infection related (e.g., fatigue, appetite alterations, sensation of dullness in the right upper quadrant of the abdomen). From a small number of patients with chronic HVC infection treated in our institution, in some of them the viral load has responded favorably descending, while in most of them it has stabilized at the previous count for long periods of time, and in some cases (the least) the viral load has ascended.

In other chronic but less complicated infections like the ones produced by herpes virus (herpes simplex virus type 1 and 2), frequent relapses often represent a high burden in patients' daily activities and tend to impact negatively in their quality of life. Our patients with HSV1 or HSV2 related symptoms have had noticeable reductions in the frequency, intensity, and length of the relapses within the first 6 months of treatment with 4–6 weekly vitamin C IV infusions followed by every other week IV infusions for 2–4 months. The doses of vitamin C applied intravenously in these cases have been from 5 to 10 g per infusion.

Dengue fever is a relatively common reason of consultation in our area of Colombia, given the all-year-round warm weather (on average 26–33°C) with an altitude of 1000 m above sea level and the closeness to the Pacific shore where it is even hotter (on average 26–37°C), much more humid, and at the sea level. In addition to the occasional Dengue case from time to time as a routine scenario, during 2015 and 2016 in Colombia (as in most parts of the northern area of South America) there were pandemics of Chikungunya and Zika viral infections. Although our institution is not a reference center for the treatment of infectious diseases, some patients with these types of viral infections consulted, searching for additional measures others than the ones established by conventional physicians for symptom management. In Dengue, Chikungunya, or Zika cases (confirmed or clinically suspected) our typical IV vitamin C treatment included 2–5 every other day 15–20 g infusions followed by weekly applications for 4–8 weeks. As in other infections treated with biological medicine, patients referred an optimized and quicker evolution when compared to their same case before receiving the aforementioned scheme, or when compared to relatives, friends, or acquaintances of them who were not treated (for any reason).

At this point we consider of utmost importance to clarify that the practice of biological medicine goes far beyond the use of a single and isolated measure like IV vitamin C or even far beyond orthomolecular supplementation alone. In the biological medicine treatment of any viral infection, the vitamin C infusions are carried out in conjunction with other immune enhancing orthomolecular nutrients (for instance, oral vitamin C and oral/IV N-acetylcysteine, L-glutamine, and L-lysine) and also along with other measures from biological medicine like phytotherapeutics (Arena et al. 2008, Ciuman 2012, Lu et al. 2016), complex homeopathics to enhance Th1 antiviral response (Fimiani et al. 2000, Oberbaum et al. 2005, Enbergs 2006, Roeska and Seilheimer 2010), ozone therapy due to its immunostimulant and germicidal effects (Viebahn–Hänsler 2007), and/or neural therapy with procaine 0.5% both to ease the symptomatic burden and to modulate the inflammatory immune response.

In the story of vitamin C treatment in infectious disease, the episode of its use in the common cold is another one characterized by strong opinion struggles in the medical community. The current evidence regarding this issue points toward some already pretty well-established conclusions, but they are derived mostly from studies with oral vitamin C schemes.

According to the Cochrane review (Hemilä and Chalker 2013) on this issue (last updated by Hemilä and Chalker in 2013), there have been several clinical trials with different dosages of oral vitamin C which haven't been able to demonstrate a preventive/prophylactic effect of this supplement on the common cold. In that context 1 g per day of oral vitamin C was evaluated in several randomized and non-randomized trials, not resulting effective to reduce the incidence of the common cold when taken during the coldest months of winter. Although the general population may not achieve benefit from ingesting 1000 mg of vitamin C daily in terms of the common cold incidence reduction, specific populations subject to significant physical and/or thermal (cold) challenges (marathonists, skiers, and soldiers in six studies) may have an average of a 50% reduction in the incidence of this disease (Douglas and Hemilä 2005, Douglas et al. 2007).

Aside from the data on common cold incidence, a reduction of the intensity of symptoms and length of the infection has been seen consistently among those supplemented with oral vitamin C, both in therapeutic and prevention regimens. As a matter of fact, a 14% reduction in the length of colds was observed in children supplemented with vitamin C with a prophylactic intention, while the reduction in adults reached 8% (42). Larger doses have provided greater symptomatic benefit when compared to lower doses, when vitamin C was taken after the symptoms of the common cold had already started (Chambial et al. 2013, Hemilä and Chalker 2013).

In our clinical experience and taking into account the available information on vitamin C pharmacokinetics (Levine et al. 1996, Benke 1999, Levine et al. 1999, Duconge et al. 2008), small (in orthomolecular terms) but frequent doses of vitamin C have proved to be more useful in the case of an acute infection. This is important since due to the dynamic flow phenomenon in vitamin C kinetics (Hickey and Roberts 2005, Hickey et al. 2005) this type of dose will produce (for a short period of time) peak blood plasma concentrations well above the ones achieved by a consumption of the RDA for vitamin C. Another factor to observe here is a difference in the turnover of vitamin C in healthy subjects versus patients with acute diseases including infection and myocardial infarction, as evidenced in several leukocyte lines (Hume et al. 1972, Bergsten et al. 1990, Chambial et al. 2013, Ferrón-Celma et al. 2009).

The usual scheme we have employed in our clinical practice is 500 mg of vitamin C taken every half hour for the first 2 hours, followed by every hour doses for the next 4 hours, and then every 2 hours for rest of the day. The patient is emphatically instructed to begin taking vitamin C as soon as the first symptoms of the common cold appear (even the prodromal ones). The following 3–5 days the patient takes an average 4–8 doses of 500 mg vitamin C each day, distributed throughout the day. The number of doses per day depends on the symptomatic evolution of the cold, and it is adjusted over time, according to close medical supervision. In patients whose respiratory disease seems to progress despite the described scheme or in those at higher risk (elderly, immunocompromised, or those with chronic respiratory diseases), we have applied a series of 1–3 IV vitamin C infusions from 5 to 25 g (separated by 2–3 days between them). The IV route can also be implemented from the beginning of the disease (usually along with the oral scheme) at the discretion of the attending physician.

Our regimen has been useful to diminish considerably the symptoms of the common cold as referred by the patients, and in some cases the cold has been aborted after the first day or two days of the regimen. Although the described method is not the exactly the same as the one reported by Anderson et al. in an old but well-designed randomized controlled trial (Anderson et al. 1974), it also supports the notion that larger doses are more effective in terms of symptom reduction during the common cold when the disease has already started.

Modern societies have been struggling with vascular disease (both cardiovascular and cerebrovascular) for many decades. Since cholesterol levels and metabolic syndrome were declared as risk factors for the development of atherosclerosis, most of the attention was strongly diverted to pharmacological measures to diminish blood lipids. As shown by Thomas Levy in his controversial but thoroughly researched work (Levy 2006), lipids are an undeniable actor in the movie of cardiovascular disease (CVD) and atherosclerosis, but it is also true that long standing vitamin C deficiency also plays a key role in the process. Structural and functional consequences of chronic low levels of vitamin C influence the quality of connective tissue and thus prepare an ideal terrain for the atheromatous plaque to develop (Levy 2006). Today, the concept of a relationship between this particular nutritional deficiency and CVD has been gaining terrain into the predominant paradigm of lipid as exclusive culprit factor in CVD (Moser and Chun 2016).

On the other hand, taking these concepts from the bench to bedside has not been easy task. Conflicting results from different intervention trials with vitamin C supplements (most of them through the oral route) are without a doubt a considerable obstacle, precluding a universal therapeutic recommendation for the use of vitamin C in primary or secondary prevention in CVD (at least with the currently available data) (Cook et al. 2007, Sesso et al. 2008, Myung et al. 2013).

Anyhow, as pointed out by Tveden-Nyborg and Lykkesfeldt in their interesting review with a section devoted to this issue (Tveden-Nyborg and Lykkesfeldt 2013), the negative results in these clinical trials evaluating vitamin C in CVD could be related to a variety of factors. The factors range from the design of the study (e.g., biased population selection when not using poor vitamin C status as an inclusion criterion), to the potential authors' unawareness of vitamin C nonlinear kinetics (different in many ways to the usual kinetics of medications subject of evaluation in clinical trials), to the concurrent use of several supplements in the population evaluated (prior or during the study itself, resulting in a confounding factor), among others. We share the opinion that this plethora of failed characteristics should be considered before drawing a definite conclusion on this matter, and paraphrasing these Danish authors, "there is a critical need for well-designed large RCTs that select or offer the possibility to control for entry-level vitC status and also for the many potential co-deficiencies which may interfere with the interpretation of the results." The chapter of vitamin C in vascular disease is far from being closed.

In terms of mechanisms of action in vascular disease, it has long been recognized that due to the preponderant role of oxidative stress in endothelial dysfunction, the uptake of ascorbate and dehydroascorbate, so as the reduction of dehydroascorbate, and the release of ascorbate, may be of great importance in the regulation of local antioxidant capacity of the vascular bed, to preserve nitric oxide (NO) at physiological levels (Mendiratas et al. 1998). Vitamin C influences both on the NO synthase (eNOS) and on the cofactor tetrahydrobiopterin (BH4) are also significant in the NO activity and its potential impact on CVD and hypertension (61). Profound disturbances in NO bioavailability are a common feature observed in various cardiovascular pathologies including ischemic heart disease and hyperlipidemia (Mendiratas et al. 1998, Moser and Chun 2016).

Many other potential mechanisms of action have been put forward in the case of vitamin C in vascular disease according to results in experimental (animal and human) studies (Levy 2006, Tveden-Nyborg and Lykkesfeldt 2013, Moser and Chun 2016):

- Reduction in the monocyte adhesion to the endothelium;
- Limitation of the inflammation process, even at the intracellular signaling level due to reduction in the TNF-α-mediated NF-κβ activation;
- Prevention of LDL oxidation; enhancement of the activity of lipoprotein lipase (LPL) as a clearing factor for oxidized lipids in the bloodstream;
- Enhancement of vascular smooth muscle cells conditions, resulting in a delayed rate of apoptosis and a controlled rate of proliferation (both important when atherosclerosis has already developed);
- Decrease in blood pressure values.

L-Glutathione (GSH)

Glutathione is probably the most important antioxidant at the cellular level and has a direct participation in multiple specific detoxification pathways, which are essential to protect our cells and tissues against potential damages inflicted by an enormous variety of harmful substances. This antioxidant is ubiquitous, being present to variable extent in all the cells and organs of the human body. Glutathione has a high capacity as an electron donor and a high negative redox potential. These factors, combined with intracellular concentration at the millimolar levels (from 0.1 to 10 mM (Bremer et al. 1981)), give GSH a very efficient antioxidant profile. The usual plasma concentrations, on the other hand, are on the micromolar level.

From the chemical point of view, Glutathione is a linear tripeptide formed in our cells by the amino acids L-cysteine, L-glutamic, and Glycine (denominated technically γ-L-Glutamyl-L-cysteinylglycine). The result is a water-soluble compound with antioxidant properties (Murray 1996). After Glutathione has yielded the electron of the cysteinil portion of the sulfhydryl group, reduced Glutathione (GSH) turns into oxidized Glutathione (GSSG) through its disulfide bridges. This is a reversible and dynamic process. As long as the rereduction of GSSG takes place, a dynamic balance can be established between the synthesis of GSH, its utilization as an antioxidant and/or detoxifying agent, and its recycling from GSSG (Lomaestro and Malone 1995). A tight homeodynamic control of the GSH availability is established both in the intracellular and extracellular compartments (Kidd 1997). In physiological but also in pathological conditions, GSH:GSSG ratio has been considered a major determinant of the global oxidative stress load (Birben et al. 2012). Most of the intracellular Glutathione (>98%) exists in the thiol-reduced form (GSH), the rest being comprised by the oxidized form glutathione disulfide (GSSG), and other several minoritarian glutathione S-conjugates like thioether, mercaptide, or other thioester forms (Ballatori et al. 2009).

Glutathione results particularly important in the liver, where it is highly concentrated in the hepatocytes (up to 10 mM). Other tissues with high concentrations of Glutathione are the spleen, the kidneys, the crystalline, and blood cells like the erythrocytes and the leukocytes. Its conjugation is the primary mechanism to remove xenobiotics from the reactive oxygen species (ROS) type, some of which are carcinogens. Conjugation and reduction reactions require Glutathione as part of the process. The Glutathione S-transferase enzymes catalyze the metabolic pathways of Glutathione in the cytosol, microsomes, and mitochondria (Raza 2011). The family of glutathione S–transferase enzymes are responsible for quenching and detoxifying many environmental substances, including free radicals, peroxidized lipids, and xenobiotics (a wide variety of environmental toxins, but also medications like antibiotics, among others). The antioxidant responsive element (ARE) mediates the activation of many genes influenced by oxidative and chemical stress, whose promoter includes this particular element (Hayes and McLellan 1999).

GSH has also a role as "secondary antioxidant," given that it also interacts actively in the reduction of most antioxidants. GSH can turn these other antioxidants useful again after they had been oxidized, thus acting as a regeneration factor. Glutathione aids in the recycling of other antioxidants like ALA (Bast and Haenen 1988), and vitamins like ascorbic acid and alpha tocopherol (Birben et al. 2012). These antioxidants in turn help neutralize the free radical damage potentially inflicted to both cell organelles and also DNA.

Many chronic diseases have been linked to an augmented oxidative stress burden and to low glutathione levels (Ballatori et al. 2009). This includes neurodegenerative diseases (like, for instance, Amyotrophic Lateral Sclerosis, Parkinson's disease, Alzheimer's disease, Huntington's disease, and schizophrenia), also characterized by an affected GSH metabolism in the nervous system (Bains and Shaw 1997). Nonetheless, the ubiquity and pleiotropy of this tripeptide have made it difficult to establish strong links between its supplementation, a therapeutic potential, and specific diseases. From a theoretical perspective, neurodegenerative disease is one of the most prominent fields for GSH therapy (Bains and Shaw 1997, Zeevalk et al. 2008). A common feature in many of these ailments, including Alzheimer's disease and Parkinson's disease, is GSH deficiency at the neuronal and glial level. Neuronal survival depends on many factors, and GSH brain levels play a crucial role in the nervous system antioxidant defense. This has been postulated as the rationale for the development of therapeutic approaches using GSH replenishment in neurodegenerative diseases (Zeevalk et al. 2008).

The clinical studies about the efficacy of short experimental GSH IV supplementation schemes in Parkinson's disease patients have had mixed results. In 1996 Sechi et al. (1996) reported a 42% reduction in disability according to the modified Columbia University Rating Scale in their observational open-label study. The benefit lasted for 2–4 months, for the small sample (n = 9) of early stage, previously untreated Parkinson's disease patients, who received 600 mg of IV Glutathione twice daily for one month. Much closer to our days, a randomized placebo controlled trial was carried out in 2009 by Hauser and colleagues (Hauser et al. 2009) with 21 Parkinson's disease patients who were already in treatment. In this study, the treatment was well tolerated and consisted of 1400 mg IV Glutathion infusions, three times a week for a month. Also, there wasn't any difference in the unified Parkinson's disease rating scale (UPDRS) found between groups, but the authors make it clear that their main objective was not to assess the efficacy of the treatment but its tolerability and potential adverse effects.

As many other unconventional medical practices, IV Glutathione has also received strong criticism from the orthodox medical establishment. This was the type of reaction (Okun et al. 2010) after the publication of the trial from Hauser et al., with reasonable arguments dealing with discrepancies about the research methodology and the interpretation of the results. On the other hand, there were also very subjective arguments like considering the placement of an IV line as some kind of major challenge. It must be noted that thousands of IV lines are placed around the world every day to infuse all types of medications without any major complication. Even many complex conventional drugs can fill that category of "safe IV infusions" in the short term, regardless of their sometimes-disputable clinical effectiveness in the long term (Morgan et al. 2004). In fact, controversial facts and figures for effectiveness are far from being an unusual phenomenon, even for many of the most commonly used and prescribed medications (Leucht et al. 2015).

Also in this discussion (Okun et al. 2010), we consider some other arguments to be very debatable, like demonizing the fact of charging patients out of their own pocket for a medical practice (which in any case it was provided). This is an issue that usually will receive a more bitter criticism if the professional practices any form of unconventional medicine. On the other hand, regular critics of complementary medicine tend to ignore or understate the variety of scientific and medical behavior artifacts known for a long time in academic medicine. Prominent examples are: the influence of the pharmaceutical industry in the way research material is published as scientific articles in journals (Blumenthal et al. 1997, Bekelman et al. 2003, Landefeld and Steinman 2009, *PLoS Medicine* Editors 2009, Doshi et al. 2012); the ever-growing role of contract research organizations (CROs) and corporate sponsorship in clinical investigation (Davidoff et al. 2001, Smith 2005); the payments and fees made to doctors by the same pharmaceutical companies which economically support their research (McCarthy 2014); the overt or surreptitious commercial and economic ties established around the prescription of many conventional medications (Ornstein et al. 2017), a phenomenon not limited to high-cost drugs like biologics and oncologics, but it also includes many newly branded drugs in order to compete in crowded markets (Brodwin 2015).

It is true that most conventional colleagues will use a different mindset to judge the results from a clinical trial of any given medication, depending on the orientation it has (whether it comes from orthodox medicine or from complementary medicine). And so, the other reaction to Hauser and colleagues' study (Hauser et al. 2009) is a case report (Naito et al. 2010) of drug-induced hepatitis in a patient in Japan who received 1200 mg of IV Glutathione daily for 5 months. The alterations in transaminases remitted after 2 months of the suspension of IV Glutathione. Although it is very clear that this type of report is indeed important to construct a more complete safety profile of any medication, it must also be stressed that in our opinion, such an intensive scheme of IV Glutathione does not reflect the usual orthomolecular practice for this measure. The authors suggest that the doses of Hauser et al. study and the ones from their case report (16,800 mg vs. 24,000 mg IV Glutathione/month) are comparable. Not only do we not consider a 42% higher dose to be comparable, but we also emphasize that the length of the treatment in both scenarios is strikingly different: one month in the clinical trial versus 5 months in the case report. In any case, it turns very relevant to take additional control measures and foresights in any treatment scheme that could be considered experimental. If a patient would receive IV Glutathione for such a long period of time, it is strongly recommended to have a complete laboratory check up every month and any other evaluation pertinent to the liver function.

The arrival of a much clearer picture for the role of Glutathione in Parkinson's disease was only possible until recently, after new research was performed on this issue. The judicious work by Mischley and colleagues is proof that the constancy added to the proper conceptualization of a scientific investigation was able to yield interesting results in this matter (Mischley 2011, 31). The low molecular weight of Glutathione (around 307 Da) make this antioxidant an excellent candidate for the intranasal administration with therapeutic purposes (Mischley 2011).

Their first step was to investigate about any potential safety issues for the use of Glutathione in the intranasal presentation (Mischley et al. 2013). Among the thousands of registers in the database of the compound pharmacy which dispensed the intranasal Glutathione, 300 patients were randomly selected and the questionnaire was mailed to them. There were 70 respondents, whose majority had been prescribed intranasal Glutathione to treat three conditions: Multiple chemical sensitivity (MCS) (n = 22), chronic sinusitis/allergies (n = 21), or Parkinson's disease (n = 7). Adverse effects were common (with a lot of heterogeneity among groups), but all of them mild and mostly related to the route of administration of Glutathione (e.g., irritation of the nasal pathways, etc.). The authors highlight that most of the surveyed patients (78%) reported the overall experience with intranasal Glutathione as positive.

After this preliminary questionnaire-based evaluation of the safety of intranasal Glutathione, the next step by the group led by Mischley was to set up a double-blind, placebo controlled trial (Mischley et al. 2015) to gain further insight about the safety and tolerability of this measure in Parkinson's disease patients.

Thirty patients were unevenly allocated in 4 groups: two treatment groups with different intranasal Glutathione doses (300 and 600 mg/day) of 10 patients each, one placebo group (sterile saline was used) of 10 patients, and one watchful waiting group of 4 patients. The highest Glutathione dose of 4200 mg/week matched the one used in the study by Hauser et al. from 2009 (Hauser et al. 2009). During the 3 months of the intervention period, the patients were instructed to use the nasal spray with either Glutathione or placebo 3 times daily, and they should also keep a daily log of events in which they recorded a report on medication use and changes in symptoms (systemic and local) and general well-being according to validated scales (Monitoring of Side Effects Scale, MOSES and the SinoNasal Outcomes Test, SNOT-20). Laboratory evaluations including blood chemistry, complete blood count, and urianalysis were obtained at several points during and after the intervention (weeks 2, 4, 8, 12, 16). Besides the evaluation of the side effects (both positive and negative), the authors decided to include an assessment of the Parkinson's disease evolution during the study as well. For this purpose, UPDRS scores were used (also considered as a safety measure).

The treatment was well tolerated in both doses, without any statistically significant difference in comparison to the placebo group, both in the clinical and laboratory evaluations. This reflected the findings from previous studies (Hauser et al. 2009, Mischley et al. 2013) regarding the excellent profile of tolerability of Glutathione in Parkinson's disease patients. Aside from that, the authors report a slight clinical improvement according to the UPDRS symptoms scores in the two treatment groups over the placebo group. This trend persisted in the post hoc analysis of the results after the exclusion of the patients who changed medications throughout the study. According to their findings, which included a clinical response superior to placebo, without ignoring the fact of power limitations of this experimental design, Mischley et al. suggest the use of a delayed-start trial (or a similar) design in future investigations to determine a potential neuroprotective effect of intranasal Glutathione in Parkinson's disease. A compilation of the interesting works of Dr. Mischley can be found for further reading in her PhD thesis (Mischley et al. 2016).

Reproaches to the therapeutic use of Glutathione in the context of neurodegenerative diseases have been somehow repetitive (Schulz et al. 2000, Zeevalk et al. 2008, Okun et al. 2010). The controversy has revolved around the uncertainty about if the drug actually crosses the blood–brain barrier and if it does reach the central nervous system (CNS) in levels significant enough to generate any plausible biological or therapeutic activity. To address this problem, Mischley and colleagues carried out a proof-of-concept study using proton magnetic resonance spectroscopy (^{1}H-MRS) to measure the CNS uptake of Glutathione after intranasal delivery in a group of 15 mid-stage Parkinson's disease patients (Mischley et al. 2016). The results of this small pilot study consistently showed an augmentation of the GSH signal in ^{1}H-MRS brain after one single 200 mg intranasal dose. According to the authors, these preliminary findings warrant a more robust trial to evaluate the pharmacokinetic profile of intranasal Glutathione in a larger sample of patients with neurodegenerative diseases. Such a trial could provide information about the magnitude and duration of the increase of Glutathione in the CNS, and about the eventual repercussion of these variables in the efficacy of its use in Parkinson's disease. It could also allow optimizing Glutathione delivery techniques, dosing schedules, product stability, and intranasal formulations.

Glutathione supplementation has also been the subject of evaluation in other conditions outside the spectrum of the neurodegenerative diseases worsening with aging. In some clinical trials evaluating this antioxidant in chronic conditions characterized by a high load of oxidative stress (like cystic fibrosis, e.g. (Visca et al. 2015) or autism (Kern et al. 2011)), the use of oral Glutathione was able to induce changes in systemic oxidative stress biomarkers. It also showed benefits in particular aspects affected by the respective disease. Bear in mind that patients in these studies received Glutathione in oral high doses along with other routes of administration (e.g., intranasal or intradermal). Since there was a combined route of administration, the benefits observed cannot be attributed solely to oral Glutathione. In fact, given that the availability of GSH after the oral ingestion has produced conflicting results, and according to the aforementioned findings by Mischley and colleagues

(Mischley 2011, 2016, Mischley et al. 2013, 2015) about intranasal GSH, it is much more likely that the therapeutic action can be attributed to this way of administration.

Some important considerations must be noticed when supplementing Glutathione with a therapeutic perspective. First, many studies point out to the fact that achieving satisfactory blood levels after the ingestion of Glutathione is not reliable in the clinical practice (Witschi et al. 1992). Basic studies carried out in rodents in the early 1990s showed an increase in the concentrations of Glutathione after an oral load of the antioxidant, both in plasma (circulating free and protein-bound Glutathione) (Hagen et al. 1990) and in tissues (kidney, liver, brain, heart) (Aw et al. 1991).

In spite of these data, this situation does not seem to be replicable in humans and so it has long been known that Glutathione has a poor bioavailability after the oral supplementation (Hagen et al. 1990, Witschi et al. 1992), limiting its use as an oral therapeutic agent. The proteases in the small intestine carry out the protein digestion process, breaking down the Glutathione tripeptide into its basic constituents (just in the exact way it happens with all other peptide/protein chains). It has already been postulated that a possible explanation for the conflicting results about the eventual lack of effectiveness of GSH supplementation in clinical trials could rely on the lack of discrimination of individuals with high/poor antioxidant reserve among the sample of patients included in intervention studies to evaluate this measure.

In this regard, the limitation of an effective oral supplementation of GSH seems to be especially true for healthy adults. In this group, the alleged oxidative stress should not be high, at least from a theoretical point of view. For example, a 4-week protocol consisting of 500 mg of oral Glutathione taken twice a day, failed to induce any significant change in oxidative stress biomarkers in a randomized controlled trial including 40 healthy volunteers (Allen and Bradley 2011). In this study, the blood levels of GSH, GSSG, and the ratio of GSH to GSSG (as an indicator of oxidative stress) remained unchanged both in placebo of oral GSH group. In this same direction, Witschi and colleagues reported that during a 4.5-hour measurement period after the ingestion of a single high dose of Glutathione (3000 mg), it wasn't either capable of increasing blood concentration of glutathione, nor the one cysteine and glutamate as its primary constituents (Witschi et al. 1992).

The results of both these trials, however, have been found debatable by Richie Jr. and colleagues (Richie et al. 2013, 2015). Regarding Allen and Bradley clinical trial (Allen and Bradley 2011), they call the attention on how potential variations in red blood cells' volume and number can impact GSH levels. Furthermore, there is a disagreement in methodological aspects related to the moment of acidification of erythrocytes, which would eventually compromise the stability of both GSH and GSSG and thus could lead to erroneous measurements (Mills et al. 1994). Regarding Witschi and colleagues' publication (Witschi et al. 1992), they call on the attention about the short half-life of Glutathione (only 1–2 minutes), which makes it practically impossible to find an increase in its blood levels after a single oral dose (Kleinman and Richie 2000). Studying the pharmacokinetics of GSH (Aebi et al. 1991), other authors found a longer half-life for its high-dose IV infusion in healthy volunteers. Despite not having the enteric absorption as hindrance, and thus going directly through the blood stream and from there to the cells, IV high-dose Glutathione half-life remains always within the minutes' range (14.1 ± 9.2 min).

In contrast to these results there have been indeed some studies demonstrating an elevation of GSH levels after its oral supplementation. One example is the recent publication by the group of Richie Jr and colleagues (Richie et al. 2015) in which a much longer period of oral Glutathione supplementation (6 months) was able to demonstrate a significant rise in its plasmatic levels compared to placebo. In this clinical trial, 54 healthy adults were randomly divided into three groups: two treatment arms with differential doses of 250 mg/day and 1000 mg/day of Glutathione, and a placebo group. GSH was measured in several compartments and cell types at baseline and at 1, 3, 6, and 7 months (after 1 month of washout). Measurements included GSH in plasma and whole blood, lymphocytes, erythrocytes, and exfoliated buccal mucosal cells. Also, different immune response tests were performed. Phagocytosis and respiratory burst were assessed in neutrophils at baseline and at 3 and 6 months; NK cell cytotoxicity and lymphocyte proliferation was evaluated at baseline and at 3 months.

Both GSH doses produced changes in some of the parameters tested. For instance, regarding GSH levels in whole blood, low-dose and high-dose participants exhibited an increase at 1, 3, and 6 months of GSH supplementation. In other compartments (erythrocytes, plasma, and lymphocytes) mean GSH levels significantly augmented 30%–35% after 6 months of 1000 mg/day GSH. In exfoliated buccal mucosal cells obtained after a mouth rinse with distilled water and brushing of the cheeks and gums with a soft tooth brush, a significant 260% increase was present in the high-dose group. For the low-dose group (250 mg/day of oral GSH), whole blood GSH levels increased significantly (17%), a situation that was also evident in erythrocytes (29%). The authors also report a decrease in the oxidative stress of the supplemented participants, due to the significant reduction in the GSSG/GSH ratio induced in both low- and high-dose GSH dose groups. Moreover, after 3 months of oral GSH supplementation NK cell cytotoxicity increased in both dose groups, but only the high-dose GSH group reached a significant level of increase. In this immune parameter, the authors declare that larger sample sizes and longer evaluation times are necessary to generalize these findings. Except for the patients in the high-dose group, whose GSH levels remained significantly greater than baseline after the washout period, most of the evaluated parameters after GSH oral ingestion returned back toward baseline levels at the 7th month measurements. This would suggest the need for a permanent GSH supplementation if therapeutic/antioxidative action is desired.

In our experience, the use of IV Glutathione in the context of diseases characterized by an elevated oxidative stress burden has provided an interesting tool to enhance the potential antioxidant effects of IV infusions. This concept is applicable (at least from a theoretical perspective) when GSH is injected along with other orthomolecular medications sharing this profile, like vitamin C, ALA or Coenzyme Q10. In our patients, the doses have ranged from 200 mg to 1 g of IV Glutathione, 600 mg being the most common one. GSH is infused through a peripheral vein, diluted in saline solution (volumes of 200–400 mL), using a slow to moderate drip (40–60 drops per minute), and according to the individual tolerance (more on that below). Such antioxidant IV drips have resulted in faster recoveries from day to day infections. In other clinical situations, like chronic diseases, after the regular antioxidant drips including GSH some patients have referred a transient subjective sensation of better overall performance for their daily activities. This energy boost was felt both in the mental and the physical domains and lasts 2–5 days on average.

Although the concomitant use of vitamin C with GSH can be recommended in many pathological states, it has been discussed if this notion can be considered universal. Oncologic disease is one of the areas where this postulate has been put to debate. The Glutathione paradox in cancer has been exemplary described by Traverso and colleagues in their 2013 paper: "While GSH deficiency, or a decrease in the GSH/glutathione disulphide (GSSG) ratio, leads to an increased susceptibility to oxidative stress implicated in the progression of cancer, elevated GSH levels increase the antioxidant capacity and the resistance to oxidative stress as observed in many cancer cells" (Traverso et al. 2013). This poses interesting questionings about the role of GSH either as a potential treatment against cancer or as a cancer cell protector.

Based on years of clinical practice Dr. Harald Krebs, an experienced author from the field of complementary medicine, published protocols (Krebs 2010) using high-dose IV vitamin C (intended as a pro-oxidant) along with IV Glutathione, doses ranging from 1200 to 2400 mg (intended as an anti-oxidant). Even coming from the conventional medicine, there are several reports about the use of IV GSH for the enhancement of chemotherapy tolerability (Smyth et al. 1997). The concept of GSH as a protective agent against chemotherapy adverse effects in ovarian cancer patients treated with Cisplatin had already been propounded more than a decade before (Zunino et al. 1983, 1989, Oriana et al. 1987, Aebi et al. 1991). Initially GSH was conceptualized as a renal protective measure in tumoral rodent models (Zunino et al. 1983, Tedeschi et al. 1990), but the protection it provides against chemotherapy related neurotoxicity and ototoxicity was found out and investigated in the years afterward (Cascinu et al. 1995).

Intravenous GSH can also provide protection against damage inflicted by therapeutic radiation. This was assessed in a randomized pilot trial of patients who had been operated of endometrial tumors and were then scheduled to receive pelvic radiation therapy (DeMaria et al. 1992). The protocol included the intravenous administration of 200 mg of GSH or saline solution as placebo, performed 15 minutes before the pelvic radiotherapy sessions. Even though DeMaria and colleagues mention that their sample size does not allow to show significance, the patients who received IV GSH had less diarrhea (28% vs. 52% in the control group receiving chemotherapy alone), one of the most common adverse effects of pelvic radiation. Additionally, the IV GSH group had a greater chance to finish the complete cycle of Cisplatin-based chemotherapy (71% to 52%). As with many other chemotherapy schemes, failure to get complete cycles of Cisplatin has been associated with less partial/complete disease remission and/or more disease relapses. As in some other GSH-related publications in the field of oncology, the authors considered that it was unlikely for the antioxidant to interfere with Cisplatin (although this asseveration was not derived patient outcomes).

The issue of a direct potential role (whether inhibiting or promoting) for the simultaneous use of antioxidants with any of the conventional oncologic treatment options is probably one of the most controversial ones in unconventional medicine, and has been largely debated in medical and lay literature (Ladas and Kelly 2009). One of the papers cited as landmark by conventional oncologists who advise against the use of antioxidants by cancer patients is the one poorly done by Dr. Gabriella D'Andrea (2005). It appeared in *CA: A Cancer Journal for Clinicians*, a peer-reviewed journal published for the American Cancer Society, whose own Submission Guidelines acknowledge that "most CA articles are solicited reviews" (American Cancer Society 2017), raising doubts about the impartiality and objectivity of the editorial line of this journal. The particular D'Andrea paper led Ralph Moss to develop a thorough review on the issue in 2006 (Moss 2006), and probably influenced the posterior evaluations on this controversy published by Dr. Keith Block et al. (2007) and by Dr. Charles Simone et al. (2007a,b) in 2007.

This discussion is very complex indeed and goes far beyond reduced Glutathione; there are dozens of different antioxidants with a variety of chemical responses in the host. Besides, there have been interesting arguments both for and against the combination of antioxidants with conventional treatment schemes. In any case, as it has been consistently reported in the medical literature, most publications show that the groups of patients receiving chemotherapy and/or radiotherapy do not only have fewer complications derived from these conventional treatments, but also in many cases their survival time and disease-free time statistics have been longer than the patients who were under conventional management only. These concepts can also be applied to the utilization of IV GSH as a complementary measure in the oncologic patient.

Of course, some studies report a diminishment of the cytotoxic activity of chemotherapy when used in conjunction with GSH. These publications come mostly from the basic experiments in this issue (in vitro and in vivo). Chen and colleagues report their findings after supplementing ascorbic acid, GSH, or their combination in cancer experimental models. When GSH was added to ascorbic acid, cytotoxicity in cancer cells mediated by H_2O_2 production was reduced from 10% to 95% in comparison to the vitamin C alone. The authors conclude that GSH should not be co-administered with ascorbic acid in the context of oncologic treatments, since most cancer cells presented a cytotoxic response to pharmacologic ascorbic acid in concentrations easily achieved in human treatments (IC50 less than 4 mM) and this response could be affected by GSH when given together (Chen et al. 2011).

There are important considerations to take into account before considering Chen's et al. conclusions as fully valid. As noted by Dettman and colleagues in response to Chen's et al. work (Dettman et al. 2012), a closer analysis of their experimental model shows a clear disparity between the amount of GSH and vitamin C used in the in vitro part of the experiment and the one infused to the mice in the in vivo stage. For example, the quantity of GSH infused to the mice would be equivalent to 48 g of GSH if a proportional dose would be used in a 60-kg human. Extrapolation of basic studies' results to the clinical practice is never an easy task. But, when the infused GSH doses used in the in vivo experiments are equivalent to 20–40 times more GSH in comparison to the usual doses used in the orthomolecular clinical practice, this frankly impedes any extrapolation of these results to any real-world scenario. There are other reasons for criticism highlighted by Dettman et al., but they go beyond the purpose of this section of the chapter.

According to our clinical experience in the use of IV GSH (L Glutathione R 200 [200 mg/2 mL] and L Glutathione R 600 [600 mg/5 mL], HeilPro DKN, Cali, Colombia), we consider important to mention that when this antioxidant is added to an IV drip, it can be painful for some patients. This is a dose-dependent phenomenon, and the nuisance can be avoided or at least diminished using larger diluent volumes, slowing the velocity of the drip, or both. In some unusual but eventual cases, the aforementioned simple measures have not been effective enough. In these patients, the injection of a slow bolus of 2 mL of 1% procaine (not in the neuraltherapeutic sense but with local anesthetic purposes for the sensitive nerve endings in the vein wall) has been successful for the control of the local venous discomfort.

Taking into consideration the difficulties found with the GSH supplementation to obtain reliable elevations in GSH levels in humans, some authors began using N-acetylcysteine (NAC) as a way to induce GSH metabolic pathways and GSH raise as a consequence. While this has been tried successfully in diverse reports, a completely satisfactory definition of the profile for NAC as an antioxidant by itself is still lacking. Although at this time it is very clear that NAC acts as a precursor for building GSH (in fact, it is considered its limiting amino acid), its own activity as antioxidant should not be considered strong. Given the conflicting results of NAC supplementation in clinical settings, some authors (Rushworth and Megson 2014) have suggested that the success in the use of this orthomolecular medication will be relevant only in those cases of actual quantitative cellular deficits of GSH, being unlikely effective in cells with normal GSH repletion. A broader analysis of NAC as a potential antioxidant tool will be provided later in the specific section of this chapter devoted to this amino acid.

Alpha Lipoic Acid (ALA)

Alpha lipoic acid (ALA) is an endogenous antioxidant, also known as tioctic acid. It is synthetized at the mitochondria from cysteine and caprylic acid as precursors. From the chemical point of view, ALA is the 1,2-dithiolane-3-pentanoic acid. It can neutralize reactive oxygen species (ROS) both in aqueous and lipid cellular regions, since it can have lipophilic and/or hydrophilic affinities.

ALA represents an example of a substance that has been transiting the pathway from the orthomolecular field to a conventionally accepted medication for quite some time now. In fact, ALA has gained some recognition in diabetology (Papanas and Ziegler 2014) as a therapeutic measure with a level of evidence (several randomized controlled trials with positive results (Ziegler et al. 1999, Mijnhout et al. 2012)) for the treatment of diabetic peripheral neuropathy. The therapeutic effect of ALA has been linked more than anything to its antioxidant activity.

Studies have attributed four antioxidant properties to ALA (Biewenga et al. 1997):

- The capacity to chelate metals,
- The ability to scavenge reactive oxygen species (ROS),
- The capacity to regenerate/reduce antioxidants (endogenous or exogenous), and
- The role in oxidative damage reparation.

When applied systemically through the IV route, ALA accumulates in tissues and is converted to dihydrolipoic acid (DHLA) by the enzyme lipoamide dehydrogenase. Both forms (ALA and DHLA) are biologically active. There are important differences in the route of ALA supplementation. When ingested ALA rarely reaches tissue concentrations above the micromolar levels. In lower concentrations, it is considered unlikely that ALA can exert direct and primary antioxidant activities in the cells (Shay et al. 2009). This situation changes when ALA is injected directly to the blood stream, allowing higher concentrations. In that case, ALA can scavenge hydroxyl radical, subchloric acid, and singlet oxygen. Moreover, ALA can chelate transient ions. Due to these properties, ALA has been used with variable degrees of success in a variety of chronic diseases, like diabetic nephropathy, hepatic, cardiovascular, and neurodegenerative diseases according to the article by Huk-Kolega and Skibska (Huk-Kolega and Skibska 2011). Acute and potentially chronic situations, like fungal infections or metal intoxications are also interesting possibilities for the therapeutic utilization of ALA. The aforementioned review surveys the antioxidant ability of LA and its role in pathological states where increased concentration of ROS is observed.

As mentioned briefly in the introduction, diabetic neuropathy is one of the most prominent and investigated indications for the therapeutic use of ALA in the clinical practice. The earliest reports of its use in neuropathic conditions date as early as the last years of the 1950s (Bock and Schneeweiss 1959). According to Ziegler's meta-analysis from 2004 (Ziegler 2004), which included a large sample of diabetic patients (n = 1258) from several randomized controlled trials, a class Ia level of evidence can be granted to ALA for the treatment of this condition. The protocol of daily IV infusions with ALA at a dose of 600 mg/day over a 3-week period has been considered safe and effective to achieve a clinically meaningful reduction of peripheral neuropathic symptoms in diabetic patients (Bock and Schneeweiss 1959, Ziegler and Gries 1997). The favorable effect of IV ALA on neuropathic symptoms was associated with an improvement in neuropathic deficits. For the author of this meta-analysis, this clearly suggests a potential role in the enhancement of the underlying neuropathy. Diabetic neuropathy also affects the autonomic portion of the nervous system, causing cardiac dysfunction. Oral treatment with ALA at doses of 800 mg/day taken for a period of 4 months was able to improve this condition in non-insulin dependent diabetic patients (Bock and Schneeweiss 1959, Ziegler and Gries 1997), when evaluated through cardiac variability measures.

High blood pressure is another frequent component of metabolic disease. Some studies have been carried out to evaluate a potential usefulness of ALA in hypertension. With a hypothesis revolving around the role of the mitochondria and its derived oxidative stress in vascular disease, ALA was evaluated in combination with acetyl-L-carnitine in a double blind, crossover, placebo controlled trial (McMackin et al. 2007). In the group of 36 patients with previously known coronary artery disease, 8 weeks of the active treatment with this combination were able to induce a significant reduction in systolic blood pressure. This effect was more significant both in the subgroup of patients with blood pressure above the median and in the ones with metabolic syndrome. In addition to these functional changes, the active treatment also achieved a reduced arterial tone, interpreted from a significant increase in brachial artery diameter of 2.3%. The clinical utility of this preliminary finding, so as the confirmation of the effect in larger clinical trials is still awaited, according to the authors.

It is interesting how biological medicine can be integrated into conventional medical practice. Many diabetic patients have associated hypertension. This group of patients shows good response to angiotensin converting enzyme (ACE) inhibitors which have multiple advantageous characteristics. In them Quinalapril, for example, reduces blood pressure, proteinuria, and improves endothelial function. Although the addition of ALA to Quinalapril was not able to generate a further reduction in blood pressure levels (beyond the one produced by Quinalapril alone), it potentiated the decrease in the proteinuria and the endothelial-dependent flow-mediated dilation in a crossover, double blind study (Rahman et al. 2012). Rahman and colleagues from the Cardiology Division at Emory University School of Medicine consider that these results could represent a potential hamper for the usual deterioration of the vascular bed observed in hypertensive diabetic patients.

In experimental models of high blood pressure, long-term treatment with ALA decreased blood pressure in hypertensive animals, without significant changes in baseline heart rate. Baroreflex has sympathetic and parasympathetic components, whose sensitivity was increased after the ALA treatment. Normotensive animals were also treated with ALA, but did not experience changes in any of the parameters evaluated. Regarding their results, Queiroz et al. suggest that long-term supplementation of ALA exhibits an antihypertensive effect and improves baroreflex sensitivity in rats with renovascular hypertension (Queiroz et al. 2012).

Antioxidative properties have been proposed as the possible explanation for the ALA mechanism of action on the prevention of the development of hypertension and hyperglycemia. Midaoui et al.

(2003) assessed the effect of ALA supplementation on the prevention of an increase in heart mitochondrial superoxide anion production and in advanced glycation end-products (AGE) formation in the aorta of Sprague Dawley rats. The experimental rats had developed high blood pressure, hyperglycemia, hyperinsulinemia, and a 4-fold increase in an insulin resistance index after having been fed with a 10% D–glucose solution additional to their chow diet. The group of rats supplemented with ALA in conjunction with the hyperglycemic diet did not develop hypertension, nor was AGE accumulated in their aortas, nor augmented the production of superoxide in the mitochondrias of myocardial cells.

In the wide spectrum of possibilities of metabolic syndrome, some patients will express it also as non-alcoholic fatty liver disease (NAFLD). Long-term supplementation of ALA in rats resulted in prevention of NAFLD development, through a series of mechanisms. The effects include a reduction in hepatic alterations which characterize the disease, like steatosis, oxidative stress, immune activation, and local inflammation (Jung et al. 2012).

Alzheimer's disease is one of the most problematic degenerative diseases of the nervous system. In data from basic studies including cell cultures and animal models, it has been shown that a mixture of ALA with nutraceuticals like docosahexaenoic acid (from fish oil), curcumin (from Curcuma longa), and (-)-epigallocatechin gallate (from green tea) act synergistically to reduce generic aspects like oxidative stress and inflammation, but also specific aspects like amyloid beta levels and amyloid beta plaque load. An Australian group of authors led by Maczurek reviewed the diverse mechanisms of action of ALA in Alzheimer's disease, possible dosages and schemes derived from ALA pharmacokinetic data, and its possibilities as a treatment of this type of dementia (Maczurek et al. 2008).

In the complementary treatment of dementias, most beneficial effects have been linked to the use of the reduced form of lipoic acid, named dihydrolipoic acid (DHLA). Holmquist et al. (2007) inform about the possibility to use R-alpha lipoic acid instead of DHLA, as it is reduced by mitochondrial lipoamide dehydrogenase, a part of the PDH complex. They explore the therapeutic properties of lipoic acid, with particular emphasis on its R-alpha-enantiomer, to treat Alzheimer's disease and related dementia.

ALA can also be utilized in the field of clinical toxicology. ALA and other antioxidants have a role in the detoxification of heavy metal poisoning. One of the main problems with heavy metals is that they cause oxidative deterioration of many crucial bio-molecules, like nucleic acids (DNA and RNA), proteins and lipids through chain reactions mediated by free radicals. It has been proposed that ALA constitutes a preventive and also therapeutic measure in cases of cellular damage related to unsustainable loads of oxidative stress and derived from heavy metal intoxication (Veljkovic et al. 2012, Flora et al. 2013).

As reported by Xu and colleagues in a model of experimental cadmium exposure (Xu et al. 2015), ALA significantly protected cadmium-treated HepG2 cell cultures against cytotoxicity and lipid peroxidation, and it was able to reverse cellular GSH deficit ($p < 0.05$). The authors also reported an increase in the activity and the expressions of glutamate cysteine ligase (γ-GCL), a limiting critical first step enzyme in the glutathione metabolism.

We have experience with the use of injectable ALA in doses ranging from 30 to 300 mg, diluted in a solution bag and mixed with other orthomolecular nutrients and antioxidants. It is compatible with normal (0.9%) saline solution or with Ringer's lactate. We used to drip it along with vitamin C based IV infusions or along with mineral/trace element-based IV infusions. There are several presentations available in our countries:

- Ácido Alfa Lipóico (10 mL vials)
  30 mg/mL, for a total of 300 mg/vial, HeilPro DKN—Cali, Colombia
  2.5%, for a total of 250 mg/vial, Farmacia Milenium—Buenos Aires, Argentina
- Ácido Alfa Lipóico (2 mL ampoules)
  25 mg/mL, for a total of 50 mg/ampoule, MediBio—Bogotá, Colombia

- Ácido tióctico (10 mL vials)
  250 mg, Farmacia Francesa—Buenos Aires, Argentina
- A—Lipo R™ (24 mL vials)
  600 mg, Nutrabiotics—Bogotá, Colombia
- SAOX (50 mL vials)
  Includes 300 mg ALA + 1 gram of GSH + 9 grams of ascorbic acid, HeilPro DKN—
  Cali, Colombia

Normally IV ALA is well tolerated, but some precaution must be taken about the possibility of hypoglycemia during its infusion. This is a dose-dependent effect, rarely seen in doses below 120 mg. The glucometry values have been around 40–60 in these cases, and came accompanied by symptoms such as mild chills, blurred vision, or mental fogginess. It must be remembered that the use of glucometry to evaluate potential hypoglycemia in this context is limited in vitamin C-based infusions, since ascorbic acid can cause false positive alterations of this laboratory parameter. In that case, it should be the clinical picture that will guide the medical conduct with respect to the situation.

In any case, faster infusion rates, lower dilution solution volumes, and/or the concomitant use with the antioxidant DMSO or with medications like insulin or oral hypoglycemic agents could eventually act as potentiating factors. Simple measures are usually enough to prevent this phenomenon: the patient is instructed to ingest some food in the hour prior to any orthomolecular IV infusion. In the occurrence of hypoglycemia despite this measure (in sensitive patients), a slow bolus of 15–25 cc 5% dextrose has proven corrective of the symptoms associated with the disturbance of carbohydrate availability. Another recommendation to avoid IV ALA related hypoglycemia is to escalate the dose in a progressive manner, beginning with 100 mg and adding 100 mg every infusion (Nutrabiotics 2016), until reaching the objective of 600 mg of IV ALA in the case of neuropathy orthomolecular treatment.

Dimethyl Sulfoxide (DMSO)

Dimethyl sulfoxide (DMSO) is an amphipathic molecule, characterized by being a polar aprotic solvent miscible in water, but also in many different substances, both aqueous and organic. Besides water, DMSO is also soluble in acetone, ethanol, benzene, diethyl ether, and chloroform. It can act as a good solvent for unsaturated, nitrogen-containing, and aromatic compounds. Considering the hygroscopic properties of DMSO, it should be kept in sealed containers. DMSO has wide applications in the fields of biology and medicine (Walker 1993).

From the physico-chemical points of view, at room temperature DMSO can be found as a clear, colorless, and oily liquid, which distinctive characteristic is a more or less (depending on the concentration) noticeable bitter smell and taste, often referred to as garlic or vegetable-like (Wood and Wood 1975).

DMSO is a potent antioxidant/reactive oxygen species (ROS) scavenger and this is one of its main capabilities (Brayton 1986). It has been utilized for decades by unconventional medicine practitioners due to a variety of purported therapeutic actions. Dr. Stanley Jacobs, a surgeon affiliated with the Medical School at the Oregon Health Sciences University along with Dr. Robert Herschler, a chemist affiliated with Crown Zellerbach Corporation, were the pioneers for the introduction of DMSO in medicine as a therapeutic agent (Walker 1993). When searching for a better preservation agent in the context of transplant surgery, Jacobs came across this quite peculiar substance, which played an excellent role as a low-toxicity cryoprotectant for a variety of cells and tissues, thus allowing its prolonged storage at subzero temperatures.

Many of the properties of DMSO with a therapeutic potential made themselves evident even from the beginning (Wood and Wood 1975, Swanson 1985), in different biology experiments and basic sciences investigations. In the medical literature (Swanson 1985, Santos et al. 2003) DMSO is mentioned as an anti-inflammatory agent and topical analgesic, cell-differentiating inducer, cholinesterase inhibitor, hydroxyl radical scavenger and antioxidant, hydrogen-bound disrupter, topical analgesic, carrier for topical application of pharmaceuticals, cryoprotectant for tissues and cell conservation, and solubilizing agent used in sample preparation for electron microscopy, intracellular low-density lipoprotein-derived cholesterol mobilizer, intercellular electrical uncoupler, and also as an antidote to avoid the consequences of extravasating of vesicant oncologic medications (Kassner 2000).

During the first decades after the introduction of DMSO as a therapeutic tool, there were concerns about the potential toxicity it could bring when used for the treatment of humans. These concerns arose mainly from early observations in some animal studies reporting lenticular refractive changes in diverse species like dog, rabbit, swine (Rubin and Barnett 1967, Smith et al. 1969), and guinea pigs (Rengstorff et al. 1972). It results central to note that these ocular adverse effects are species-specific phenomena, and hence have not been able to be reproduced in primates nor in humans (Smith et al. 1969, de la Torre et al. 1981).

Moreover, the ocular safety of DMSO was specifically addressed in the study by Shirley et al. in 1989 (Shirley et al. 1989). In this randomized, double-blind trial, 84 patients with hand ulcers secondary to systemic progressive sclerosis (scleroderma) were divided into three groups to receive either topical 70% DMSO, topical 2% DMSO, or 0.85% normal saline solution as control. The treatment consisted in immersing the patients' hands into these solutions, three times per day for three months. For the results to be comparable to the doses previously used in animal studies, a theoretical maximum dose of 2.6 g DMSO/kg/day was considered. From the 55 patients who completed the study protocol, 46 went through a complete ophthalmologic evaluation before the immersions, and at 12 weeks after finishing the protocol. The ophthalmologist evaluated personal and familiar ocular history, past drug history, and performed pupillary examination, cycloplegic refraction, motility study, applanation tension, indirect dilated funduscopic examination, and slit-lamp examination. The ocular variables examined (e.g., visual acuity, lenticular changes, and cataract development) did not present any significant change among the three groups during the treatment period. None of the participants in this trial had any lenticular changes like the DMSO-related ones described in several animal studies (Shirley et al. 1989). Other reports in humans and primates (Brobyn 1975) have arrived at the same conclusions, and therefore DMSO is considered a safe drug for human use from the ophthalmic point of view.

We have deliberately decided to divide the description of our experience with the use of IV DMSO in two conceptual modes of use, according to the pursued therapeutic objective.

On the one hand, we used to apply IV DMSO in doses from 30 to 50 mg/kg/infusion as a theoretical carrier for many other nutrients, when dripped together in the same solution bag. The regular doses in this context range from 2 to 4 g of 99.9% DMSO into 200–250 mL of normal saline solution, along with other orthomolecular supplements. The final concentration of DMSO in this type of orthomolecular IV drip is 1%–2% on average. This can be infused every week to every 4 weeks, depending on the suspected or confirmed nutritional deficiencies, or according to the clinical necessities of the patient. Apart from the properties that DMSO can have on its own, it has also been largely known due to its ability to carry molecular from one compartment to another. In this sense, DMSO potentially binds to minerals, amino acids, and vitamins, and carries them from the intravascular compartment to the interstitial compartment, and from there to the intracellular space. In a reversible process, it has been shown how varying concentrations of DMSO are able to cross body membranes in animals (Wood and Wood 1975).

On the other hand, we have employed much larger doses mostly in the treatment of structural pain (joints, muscles, and bones). Such a medical use of DMSP has been described for many decades already (Demos et al. 1967). In our experience 200–250 mg/kg/infusion of IV DMSO works well and it is perfectly tolerated, but doses up to 1 gr/kg/infusion have been reported in the literature (Walker 1993, Olszewer et al. 2017). It must be noticed that the volume of physiologic saline to prepare the drip bag, so as the total infusion time both have to be augmented proportionally. A typical example of an orthomolecular treatment of this type would be to add 12 cc of 99.9% DMSO to 360 cc of normal saline solution for a 60-kg patient, to be dripped approximately in 2 hours (60 drops per minute). In this example, the final concentration of DMSO is 3.3%. Usually this is mixed with other orthomolecular supplements, depending on the clinical objective of the patient. In the search for a better aid in structural pain control, other orthomoleculars like magnesium chloride 20% (2–5 cc), cyanocobalamin 0.1% (2–4 cc) and/or L-phenylalanine 2.5% (1–3 cc) would be good examples.

Patients with diseases like rheumatoid arthritis, ankylosing spondylitis, and osteoarthritis (Eberhardt et al. 1995) quite often get a lot of symptomatic relief from serial IV DMSO infusions. This type of infusion is usually repeated much more often than the ones first described in the previous paragraph, every 3–7 days, depending on the clinical status of the patient. That is especially true at the beginning of the treatment (the first month to 3 months), when the proinflammatory spiral is still spinning its wheel fiercely. Afterward the rest of the measures of natural treatment gain strength in a progressive way. The patient also adopts a healthier way of living and the process tends to get easier, and then orthomolecular IV infusions can be performed less frequently. A healthy alkaline-based diet is one of the cornerstones of this approach, since it makes it difficult for the articular inflammation to thrive (Walker 1993). Analgesic properties of DMSO could rely on the induction of a concentration-dependent blockade of nerve fibers type C, as published by Evan et al. in 1993 (Evans et al. 1993).

Coenzyme Q10 (CoQ10)

Coenzyme Q10 (CoQ10) is an endogenous antioxidant molecule. It is also known as ubiquinone (oxidized) or ubiquinol (reduced). As these names suggest, it is present in all the organs and systems of the human body at the cellular (mitochondrial) level. Nevertheless, the concentration of CoQ10 is highly variable between organs, depending on their metabolic rate. In organs like the heart it is present in high amounts (114 ± 9.2 µg/gr tissue), while it is around half of the concentration in organs like the kidney or the liver (66.5 ± 6.6, and 54.9 ± 4.1 µg/g tissue, respectively) (Aberg et al. 1961, Turunen et al. 2004). Chemically CoQ10 is the trans 2, 3-dimethoxy-5-methyl-6-decaprenyl-1, 4-benzoquinone (in the reduced form). CoQ10 is a fat-soluble, vitamin-like compound, which has not been considered strictly essential since it does not necessarily have to be supplemented to be present in cells. Nonetheless, therapeutic action of CoQ10 is achievable mostly with pharmacologic supplemental doses.

The research in CoQ10 had an inflection point by the mid-twentieth century, when Dr. Frederick L. Crane and his team from the University of Wisconsin were able to isolate this antioxidant from cardiac muscle's mitochondria in 1957. One year later in 1958, Dr. Karl Folkers and colleagues of the University of Texas determined the chemical structure of CoQ10. This antioxidant has been used with various degrees of success and evidence in a series of clinical conditions (Garrido-Maraver et al. 2014), as reviewed by Garrido-Maraver and colleagues in 2014.

Considering that the heart is the tissue where CoQ10 is most concentrated in mammals including human beings, the cardiovascular system soon attracted the attention for a potential therapeutic use for this antioxidant. Conditions like high blood pressure (Rosenfeldt et al. 2007), cardiac failure (Belardinelli et al. 2006, Adarsh et al. 2008), ischemic heart disease (Celik and Iyisoy 2009, Ivanov et al. 2013b), and endothelial dysfunction (Belardinelli et al. 2006) (as a common denominator for the others) could be benefited from orthomolecular CoQ10 supplementation. It must be clarified that recent evidence of CoQ10 in hypertension shows that it is unable to lower blood pressure by itself, according to the Cochrane review on the topic by Ho and colleagues (Ho et al. 2016).

In the second half of the twentieth century, the abnormalities in blood lipid levels were characterized as a risk factor for cardiovascular disease. Statins emerged as the main treatment options, and with a wider portion of the population being treated with this type of drug, it became evident that patients on HMG-CoA reductase inhibitors due to blood lipid disorders have lower CoQ10 levels (Hargreaves et al. 2005). Some authors even refer to this situation as an acquired CoQ10 deficit disease (to differentiate it from the genetic inherited CoQ10 deficiencies).

Statins have a variety of adverse effects, myopathy being one of the most worrisome. Not only is muscle pain the most common side effect of statins (present in more than 1% of the patients) but in rare occasions, some patients can advance to severe stages even with rhabdomyolysis. To add confusion to the issue, in a randomized placebo-controlled trial with more than 20,000 subjects, the frequency of muscle pain in patients taking Simvastatin was the same as in those taking placebo (Heart Protection Study Collaborative Group 2002).

Some authors consider CoQ10 supplementation highly recommended in patients on statins in order to prevent the myopathy potentially induced by these medications (Garrido-Maraver et al. 2014), but without forgetting that the evidence regarding this indication for CoQ10 is not yet conclusive due to contradictory results in the trials analyzed (Mas and Mori 2010, Wyman et al. 2010). It has been suggested that some disturbances caused by this type of medication could be prevented or treated by supplementing CoQ10, at least to some extent according to the biochemical links between statins and CoQ10 deficit induction. In the orthomolecular sense, it would mean the reposition of a substance that is lacking in the patient's organism either due to the blockade in a metabolic pathway (like in this case) or due to insufficient cellular production or due to nutritional deficits from its precursors.

Some (conventional) sources even consider that implementing CoQ10 in statin treated patients with myalgia is feasible, mainly as a test and not as a routine measure. Marcoff and Thompson from Connecticut mention its use in myopathic statin-associated patients, given some anecdotal and preliminary evidence of an effect on muscle symptoms, and that there wouldn't be any risk associated with this antioxidant (Marcoff and Thompson 2007). In their opinion, some patients may respond to CoQ10, albeit they give chance only to a placebo effect in those cases.

Intravenous CoQ10 has been used with success limiting the extent of tissue damage in several experimental ischemia animal models. The group led by Prof. Oleg Medvedev from the Lomonosov Moscow State University in Russia has been dedicated to investigate the use of injectable CoQ10 in a variety of ischemic conditions, producing several interesting articles over the years. One of their initial investigations (Gorodetskaya et al. 2010) demonstrated a rapid rise in the plasma and tissue CoQ10 after an IV bolus in experimental rats. The plasma samples, and the cardiac, cerebral, and hepatic tissues showed important elevations of CoQ10, which were maintained in the plasma, heart, and liver after 48 hours, but not in the brain tissue. Some years later, Ivanov and colleagues (Ivanov et al. 2013a) reported significantly less cardiac structural and functional compromise after a single IV dose of CoQ10 in an animal model of myocardium infarction, with irreversible cardiac ischemia (Niibori et al. 1998, Verma et al. 2007). The cardioprotective effect of IV solubilized CoQ10 in a transient ischemia animal model after a single dose had beneficial repercussion on left ventricular lesion and after event function, but only if it was injected 1 hour after the experimentally induced ischemia and not when this measure was applied 3 hours after the event (Ivanov et al. 2014).

Also from this group and based on their previous findings (Gorodetskaya et al. 2010) Belousova and co-workers decided to investigate the action of CoQ10 in acute ischemic brain lesion. They performed an experiment injecting IV CoQ10 into laboratory rats after transient (6-hour arterial occlusion) focal brain ischemia and before reperfusion (Belousova et al. 2016a). The infarction area was reduced and the neurological impairment was milder in the treated animals in comparison with physiologic saline solution injected animals, demonstrating a robust neuroprotective role of CoQ10 in this induced ischemia model. CoQ10 was able to produce a lesser compromise of both functional and morphological markers of brain damage.

A similar neuroprotective capacity of Coq10 was found when the experimental ischemic lesion was irreversible (24-hour arterial occlusion) and the CoQ10 was injected IV in the first hour after the event began (Belousova et al. 2016b). The CoQ10 injected rats evidenced higher levels of the antioxidant in their brain tissue, presented less neurological deficit derived from the ischemia, and had an average of half the size of the infarction areas when compared to the control group (injected with normal saline solution).

CoQ10 also exerted a neuroprotective effect derived from its strong antioxidant and reactive oxygen species (ROS) scavenger properties. This orthomolecular nutrient was effective in the reduction of the biochemical and histological consequences of another type of experimental brain ischemia model, according to Ostrowski's publication (Ostrowski 2000).

Besides the cerebral ischemia models already detailed, there have been other experiments evidencing a positive role for CoQ10 supplementation in rats with brain ischemia after a head trauma. Kalayci and colleagues from the neurosurgery department at the Zonguldak Karaelmas University in Turkey developed an experimental traumatic brain injury model in laboratory rats and described their positive results after the use of CoQ10 in this context (Kalayci et al. 2011).

The aforementioned preliminary evidence strongly suggests the possibility of a therapeutic action from CoQ10 in acute cardiovascular/cerebral ischemic conditions (from different origins), but it still has to be subject to the proper review in clinical studies (human patients in real life conditions).

There are other systems and organs that can have benefits from a CoQ10 supplementation therapy. Among these, of the most prominent with several indications for its therapeutic use is the nervous system (Morris et al. 2013). As it was commented earlier in the glutathione section, the depletion of antioxidants has been linked to a variety of neurological disorders, mainly the neurodegenerative ones. This also applies to CoQ10, whose potential deficiency may have a role in the pathophysiology of morbid processes like depression, Parkinson's disease (Shults 2005), myalgic encephalomyelitis/chronic fatigue syndrome, and fibromyalgia.

A lot of disease-related aspects can ameliorate through a CoQ10 treatment in nervous system affection (Morris et al. 2013): enhancing the patient's quality of life in Parkinson's disease and fibromyalgia, decreasing depression intensity, reducing hyperalgesia and modulating inflammation hyperactivation in fibromyalgia (Cordero et al. 2014), delaying the progression in Parkinson's disease, improving the global energy levels in myalgic encepholamyletis/chronic fatigue syndrome. It has been postulated that most (if not all) of these effects can be explained by CoQ10 reduction of oxidative stress burden and by the protection to the mitochondria and its electron transport chain.

CoQ10 has been supplemented mostly by the oral route and injectable routes. Its typical absorption after oral intake is slow and limited, in relationship with physical characteristics like hydrophobicity and a relatively large molecular weight (Bhagavan and Chopra 2006, Nishimura et al. 2009). CoQ10 has a low absorption of 2%–3%, needing days to weeks of sustained supplementation to generate an impact in tissue CoQ10 levels. In experimental rats receiving oral CoQ10, some organs like the spleen or liver will show significant elevations of its CoQ10 levels, but in other organs like heart or kidney the levels were low to undetectable (Alessandri et al. 1988). All these limitations are more evident in the powder capsules of CoQ10. This can be partially enhanced when a solubilized form of CoQ10 is used, but the extent of the change is much more powerful (by many times) when CoQ10 is infused through an IV line in an injectable presentation.

The use of the IV route to supplement CoQ10 has some advantages, like the possibility to reach a much higher serum level, that correlates to a higher hepatic level. Due to the much longer period of time, the high levels remain in some organs, there have been some hypotheses about a reservoir for the antioxidant, probably at the hepatic level (Ivanov et al. 2013a) or at the intestinal level (through enterohepatic recirculation, anyway) (Yuzuriha et al. 1983). As mentioned by Bhagavan and Chopra (2006) in their article about CoQ10 pharmacokinetics, phenomena like a second plasma peak after both oral and IV administration led Yuzuriha et al. (1983) to propound a zero-order rate constant rather than first-order kinetics for CoQ10 supplementation (later came Tomono's research with radioactive labeled CoQ10 to expand this concept [Tomono et al. 1986]).

In our practice, we have experience with the use of injectable Coenzyme Q10 (2 mL ampoules with 40 mg, MediBio—Bogotá, Colombia; 0.1% vials of 10 mL, Farmacia Francesa—Buenos Aires, Argentina) at doses ranging from 10 to 80 mg. It is usually added to an antioxidant IV drip in conjunction with alpha lipoic acid and/or glutathione, amino acids, and a base of either multiple minerals or vitamin C. The main indications have been aiding in the recovery period of patients with recent ischemic events (either from coronary or cerebrovascular origin), neurodegenerative disorders (mostly Parkinson's disease), and fibromyalgia patients.

Regarding this last group of patients with fibromyalgia, we have had some whose response to the treatment with other biological medicine's interventions was not satisfactory, but changed radically after implementing the orthomolecular IV infusions (including CoQ10). Other groups have had interesting therapeutic experiences with the supplementation of CoQ10 in fibromyalgia patients (Cordero et al. 2011, 2012).

It is worth mentioning that in patients with fibromyalgia the usual response to a biological medicine treatment has been good to excellent. Most of them experience an important amelioration of their clinical picture 3–6 months after receiving a polymodal treatment including:

- Neural therapy according to Huneke (Dosch 1984) (local and segmental—metameric injections of a local anesthetic, preferably procaine 0.5%) and/or injected local anesthetics but not necessarily in the neural therapy context (e.g., IV drips, mainly lidocaine [Schafranski et al. 2009]),
- Bio-regulatory medicine (medications through the oral route + biopuncture [local and segmental—metameric injections]) (Goldman et al. 2015) (antihomotoxic medications through the oral route + biopuncture [local and segmental—metameric injections]) (Egocheaga and del Valle 2004, Präg 2004),
- Ozone therapy (ozone administered either with local injections, or systemically through an ozonated saline IV drip or through rectal insufflation) (Hidalgo-Tallón et al. 2013, Longas-Vélez 2014, Balestrero et al. 2017),
- Changes in alimentary patterns (toward a vegetarian diet [Arranz et al. 2010], an exclusion diet [Holton et al. 2009], an alkaline diet or a combination of several of these measures),
- An individually tailored exercise routine (Ortega 2016),
- And mind–body medicine techniques (like yoga or meditation) (Wahbeh et al. 2008, Theadom et al. 2015).

Nevertheless, for a few of them this approach was not able to produce an appropriate symptomatic relief, proving to be particularly challenging cases, and it was comforting to finally find relief with the orthomolecular aspect of the treatment. In some of these difficult cases the achieved clinical improvement through the addition of IV and oral orthomolecular supplementation schemes lasted for several months even after the discontinuation of the treatment.

Alterations in micronutrient levels are known to happen in fibromyalgia patients, although the information differs regarding the nutrient. According to the Joustra and co-workers, recent publication (Joustra et al. 2017), for example, while the status of manganese, vitamin B1, vitamin A (in the majority of studies), and vitamin E (studies with methodological issues) resulted consistently low in fibromyalgia patients, other nutrients' status was not statistically different when compared to healthy controls (folic acid, vitamin B12, iron, molybdenum, phosphorus, sodium, iodine, and the majority of studies about potassium and selenium). Some nutrients even showed important discrepancies (increased or decreased levels for the same nutrient) between the different studies analyzed, like it was the case for copper, ferritin, and zinc. Nutrients' role in pathophysiology of fibromyalgia is not completely understood and these deficiencies are not necessarily related to the clinical presentation of this condition (Arranz et al. 2010, Rosborg et al. 2007, Joustra et al. 2017). Within the scientific community, the notion of an orthomolecular origin of fibromyalgia or its use as a complementary measure treatment in fibromyalgia in order to aid in the patient health care is not free of controversy and some authors consider it unnecessary or lack merit (Rosborg et al. 2007, Joustra et al. 2017).

Amino Acids

Amino acids are organic molecules consisting of C, O, and N, and constitute the basic unit in the formation of proteins, one of the main components of the organic functions and structure. Proteins are among the most important substances in nature; in human health, they have notorious and variated roles, since enzymes, hormones, neurotransmitters, cytokines, albumin, collagen, and many others are proteins.

Although there is an undeniable importance of proteins, science and medicine have begun to appreciate the useful roles that have single amino acids or short dipeptidic/tripeptidic molecules. L-glutathione, which was covered earlier in this chapter, is a clear example of this. In this section, we will address single amino acids as therapeutic tools.

Amino acids are obtained from their ingestion and from their synthesis in the human organism. The liver must process and produce about 60% of the amino acids in our body. The remaining 40% depends on the diet protein content and the ability to degrade these proteins into smaller peptidic chains, tripeptides, dipeptides, and single amino acids. Afterward these must be absorbed in the digestive tract and then it can reach the blood stream, the hepatic metabolism, and the tissues.

N-Acetylcysteine (NAC)

Acetylcysteine is the N-acetylated form of the amino acid L-cysteine. As it has been extensively explained in the antioxidants section, it is the limiting precursor in the formation of the antioxidant glutathione in the tissues and cells. The thiol (sulfhydryl) group from L-cysteine confers NAC its antioxidant capacity, since this group has the possibility to reduce reactive oxygen species (ROS) (Mokhtari et al. 2017).

After an oral load of NAC it has an efficient and quick absorption, with a predominant first pass metabolism both in the small intestine cells and the liver. This facilitates the incorporation of this amino acid into proteins, and the excretion of its metabolites. After this broad hepatic metabolism (with a minor participation of CYP450), the arrival of intact NAC molecules to plasma and tissues/organs afterward, is thus very limited (albeit it occurs in a small percentage). Its urinary excretion is around 22%–30%, with a half-life of 5.6 hours in adults, and 11 hours in neonates (Kelly 1998).

Acetylcysteine serves as a prodrug to L-cysteine. L-cysteine is a precursor to the biologic antioxidant glutathione, and the limiting nutrient. Hence, administration of NAC is considered a good replenishment strategy of the glutathione stores (GA eBusiness Services 2013).

NAC also prevents tissue injury for its participation as a superoxide radical scavenger. Recent studies have established a link between oxidative stress and neurocognitive deficits in psychosis. As a glutathione precursor with glutamatergic properties, the administration of NAC has shown efficacy on negative symptoms in patients with schizophrenia, and in global functioning in patients with bipolar disorder. According to Rapado–Castro and Dodd, NAC may have an impact on cognitive performance in psychosis, as a significant improvement in working memory was observed in the NAC-treated group compared with placebo (Rapado-Castro and Dodd 2016). NAC is an antioxidant with direct and indirect antioxidant actions used in the clinical setting. NAC exerts a significant protective role in liver injury following intestinal ischemia reperfusion (IIR), which seems to be independent of any intestinal protective effect that this amino acid could have per se (Kalimeris and Briassoulis 2016).

NAC has the possibility to influence the effects of nitric oxide (NO). Shimada et al. performed a hemodynamic study demonstrating that the increased left ventricular mass produced by myocardial inflammation tended to be reduced in rats treated with NAC in the context of experimentally induced myocardium inflammation of autoimmune origin (Shimada and Uzui 2015). Taken together, nNO synthetase seems to be responsible for the increase of total NOS activity in the brain of SHR. SMTC inhibited 86% and 70% of NAC-induced increase of total NOS activity in the brainstem and cerebellum, respectively. Thus, nNOS is responsible not only for strain differences but also for NAC-induced increase of total NOS activity in the brain (Pechanova et al. 2009).

Nakagawa and co-workers investigated possible influences of NAC (also as a precursor of glutathione) on joint tissue, particularly in the cartilage. They were interested in a potential protective role of NAC in articular chondrocytes against nitric oxide (NO)-induced apoptosis and a potential prevention of the cartilage destruction in an experimental model of osteoarthritis (OA) in rats. One of their observations was that NAC was able to inhibit NO-induced apoptosis of chondrocytes through glutathione in vitro, and inhibits chondrocyte apoptosis and articular cartilage degeneration in vivo (Nakagawa et al. 2010).

NAC also plays important roles in respiratory/immune functions. Aliavi and Kurbanova analyzed 35 patients with community-acquired pneumonia. Studies of red blood cells and expired air condensate revealed significant nitric oxide metabolic disturbances in them. The established regularities in the balance change of nitric oxide metabolism in blood and expired air condensate at the height of the disease and positive changes during therapy including NAC suggest that nitric oxide plays an important role in the pathogenesis of community-acquired pneumonia (Aliavi and Kurbanova 2007). Other respiratory acute conditions are also susceptible to be treated complementarily with NAC, in relationship with an augmentation of glutathione levels after NAC supplementation in acute respiratory distress syndrome (Soltan-Sharifi et al. 2007).

One of the main and most investigated uses of NAC (even by conventional medicine) is the nephroprotection role. Intravenous and oral N-acetylcysteine may prevent contrast-medium–induced nephropathy with a dose-dependent effect in patients treated with primary angioplasty and may improve hospital outcome (Marenzi et al. 2006).

Glutathione precursor: NAC supplementation in diabetic patients is sufficient to increase intracellular GSH content in blood cells (Gamage et al. 2014). There are reports of a dose-dependent suppression of the insulin resistance phenomenon using some anti-oxidants, like NAC (Houstis et al. 2006).

The aim of this study was to investigate the effects of NAC on the levels of reactive oxygen species in sepsis. NAC treatment had beneficial effects on erythrocyte GSH, serum TNF-alpha, lung function, and kidney MDA levels in sepsis-induced rats. However, this beneficial effect was not confirmed as histopathological improvement (Gül et al. 2011). Oxidative stress and reduced brain levels of glutathione have been implicated in schizophrenia and bipolar disorder. N-acetylcysteine (NAC) is a precursor of glutathione and has additional effects on glutamate neurotransmission, neurogenesis, and inflammation. Glutathione depletion was reversed by NAC (1000 mg/kg) in saline-treated and amphetamine-treated (frontal cortex only) rats (Dean et al. 2011).

It has already been mentioned that the natural content of the thiol group confers NAC its antioxidant capacity. N-acetylcysteine is a natural thiol-containing antioxidant, a precursor for cysteine and glutathione, and a potential detoxifying agent for heavy metal ions (Sisombath and Jalilehvand 2015). Results show that Zn and NAC presented promising effects against the toxicity caused by $HgCl2$ (Oliveira et al. 2015). Cadmium (Cd) is known to cause severe damage to various organs including lung, liver, kidney, brain, and reproductive system. Several studies have reported the induction of oxidative stress pathways following Cd exposure. NAC can be used as a potential protective agent against Cd-induced testicular toxicity, especially with regard to oxidative stress-induced Leydig cell toxicity (Khanna et al. 2016). Cd is a well-known hepatotoxic environmental pollutant. Rat hepatocytes incubated with NAC and Cd simultaneously had significantly increased viability and decreased Cd-induced ROS generation. Our results suggested that Cd induces ROS generation that leads to oxidative stress. Moreover, NAC protects rat hepatocytes from cytotoxicity associated with Cd (Wang et al. 2014).

Stimulates Immune Function

NAC has also been hypothesized to exert beneficial effects through its modulation of glutamate and dopamine neurotransmission as well as its antioxidant properties.

Sulfur Amino Acids

Methionine, cysteine, homocysteine, and taurine are the four common sulfur-containing amino acids, but only the first two of these are actively incorporated into proteins. Cysteine, by its ability to form disulfide bonds, plays a crucial role in protein structure and in protein-folding pathways. Methionine metabolism begins with its activation to S-adenosylmethionine. Cysteine may be converted to such important products as glutathione and taurine (Brosnan and Brosnan 2006).

Antioxidant action due to the thiol groups of their molecules. Methionine residues constitute an important antioxidant defense mechanism. A variety of oxidants react readily with methionine to form methionine sulfoxide, and surface-exposed methionine residues create an extremely high concentration of reactant, available as an efficient oxidant scavenger (Levine et al. 1996, Di Buono et al. 2003, Moskovitz 2005).

5-Hydroxy tryptophan increases the production of serotonin in the nervous system (Jacobsen et al. 2016, Zhang and Zhao 2016). The amount of 5-HTP reaching the central nervous system (CNS) is affected by the extent to which 5-HTP is converted to serotonin in the periphery. This conversion is controlled by the enzyme amino acid decarboxylase, which, in the periphery, can be blocked by peripheral decarboxylase inhibitors (PDIs) such as carbidopa. Preclinical and clinical evidence for the efficacy of 5-HTP for depression is reviewed, with emphasis on double-blind, placebo-controlled (DB-PC) trials. Safety issues with 5-HTP are also reviewed, with emphasis on eosinophilia myalgia syndrome (EMS) and serotonin syndrome (Turner et al. 2006).

Branched Chain Amino Acids, Isoleucine, Leucine, Valine

AA mixture branched chain with direct stimulus to the nervous system and musculoskeletal system.

On the muscular mass, they exert an anabolic effect. Substantial evidence has been accumulated suggesting that branched-chain amino acid (BCAA) supplementation or BCAA-rich diets have a positive effect on the regulation of body weight, muscle protein synthesis, glucose homeostasis, the aging process, and extend healthspan (Bifari and Nisoli 2016).

Postinjury metabolism is characterized by breakdown of muscle protein as substrate for energy production and gluconeogenesis and by the resultant loss of lean body mass and weight loss. The results suggest that early nutritional support in the postoperative period will result in nitrogen equilibrium and that the infusion of the three BCAAs only in the postoperative state is as effective in preventing muscle catabolism as other more balanced amino acid solutions. In the postinjury state, balanced amino acid solutions rich in BCAA may prove beneficial (Freund et al. 1979).

Liver function optimization is another possible field for the use of BCAA supplements. These amino acids may also be useful in minimizing or reversing the catabolic state characteristic of patients with cirrhosis. A reduction of increased urinary 3-methylhistidine excretion by infusions of BCAAs in cirrhotic patients suggests an anticatabolic effect. These potential anticatabolic effects of BCAAs are interesting (Maddrey 1985).

L-Leucine

Optimizes hepatocyte function (Davuluri et al. 2016). Leucine supplementation has been reported to improve lipid metabolism. Chronic leucine supplementation reduced the body weight and improved the lipid profile of mice fed with a high-fat/cholesterol diet. This beneficial effect was ascribed to hepatic lipogenesis, adipocyte lipolysis, and white adipose tissue browning (Jiao et al. 2016) and neurons.

Besides its actions in lipid metabolism, leucine also promotes muscle mass gain, especially in the geriatric population (Murphy et al. 2016).

L-Carnitine

L-Carnitine has mitochondrial coenzyme functions (Valero 2014).

Useful in neurodegenerative diseases such as Alzheimer's disease (Lodeiro et al. 2014), review relevant experimental and clinical data on supplemental substances (i.e., curcuminoids, rosmarinic acid, resveratrol, acetyl-L-carnitine, and ω-3 (n-3) polyunsaturated fatty acids) that have demonstrated encouraging therapeutic effects on chronic diseases, such as Alzheimer's disease and neurodegeneration resulting from acute adverse events, such as traumatic brain injury (Gavrilova et al. 2011, Bigford and Del Rossi 2014).

Muscle degenerative diseases (La Guardia et al. 2013, D'Antona et al. 2014)

L-Carnitine is one of the usual orthomolecular supplements used in overweight patients, given some positive results regarding this indication. In a recent report, Pooyandjoo and colleagues published the results of their meta-regression analysis of the duration of the amino acid consumption (Pooyandjoo et al. 2016). They observed that although there was a weight reduction associated with carnitine supplementation, its magnitude significantly decreased over time (p = 0.002). In conclusion, the authors state that receiving the carnitine resulted in weight loss, and consider that a meta-analysis of the different medications to aid weight management and non-pharmacotherapy measures should be considered for future research.

L-Taurine

At the central nervous system level, taurine improves GABAergic neurotransmission and has neuroprotective activity (Hovsepyan et al. 2015, Qiao et al. 2015, Wang et al. 2016, Zhu et al. 2016).

Taurine also improves liver functions (Wu et al. 2015) after having a chelating activity on transition metals (Zhang et al. 2014).

L-Arginine

L-Arginine is a conditionally essential amino acid that is involved in protein synthesis, the detoxification of ammonia, and its conversion to glucose as well as being catabolized to produce energy. In addition to these physiological functions, arginine has been purported to have ergogenic potential. Athletes have taken arginine for three main reasons: (1) its role in the secretion of endogenous growth hormone; (2) its involvement in the synthesis of creatine; and (3) its role in augmenting nitric oxide. These aspects of arginine supplementation will be discussed as well as a review of clinical investigations involving exercise performance and arginine ingestion (Campbell et al. 2004).

Stimulating growth hormone; acute resistance exercise and L-arginine have both been shown to independently elevate plasma growth hormone (GH) concentrations (Forbes et al. 2014).

Arginine is one of the most important cofactors involved in the production of nitric oxide.

Glycine

Structurally speaking, glycine is the simplest amino acid. It also modulates GABAergic neurotransmission: GABA and glycine are major inhibitory neurotransmitters in the CNS and act on receptors coupled to chloride channels (Ito 2016).

It is used mainly in neurodegenerative diseases. Glycine receptors (GlyRs) are ligand-gated chloride ion channels that mediate fast inhibitory neurotransmission in the spinal cord and the brainstem. There these receptors are mainly involved in motor control and pain perception in the adult nervous system (Avila et al. 2013).

Glycine can also act as a brain protector. In cerebral hypoxia-ischemia (HI) experimental models, glycine was able to protect neonatal rat brains against HI, in part by inhibiting TNFα-induced inflammation and gliosis. Hence, systemic glycine infusions may have clinical utility for the treatment of HI injury in human newborns. The results of Mori et al. (2017) suggest that acute Gly treatment reduces ethanol-induced oxidative stress and neuronal cell loss in SH-SY5Y cells and in the developing rat brain. Therefore, Gly may be considered a potential treatment in ethanol-intoxicated newborns and infants (Amin et al. 2016). Glycine stabilizes energetics of brain mitochondria under conditions of brain hypoxia in vivo modeled by ligation of the common carotid artery in rats. It is concluded that both in the model of hypoxia in vivo and during in vitro modeling of hypoxia in cortical slices and mitochondria, glycine acts as a protector inhibiting generation of reactive oxygen species in mitochondria and preventing energetic disturbances in brain mitochondria (Selin et al. 2012).

Beta-Alanine (B-Ala)

B-Ala is a naturally occurring amino acid (a non-essential amino acid) that is not stored in the body as muscle tissue. Rather, research has shown that B-alanine works by increasing the muscle content of an important compound—carnosine. In fact, the production of carnosine is limited by the availability of B-alanine. B-Ala has some interesting scientific evidence about its possible performance enhancement.

This amino acid has an indirect antioxidant function, since it increases intracellular levels of carnitine, which serves to control free radicals.

Buffer agent for pH variations. Isokinetic average power/repetition was significantly increased post B-Ala supplementation compared with placebo. Beta-alanine may benefit short-duration, high-intensity exercise performance (IJSM 2013).

BA supplementation, by improving intracellular pH control, improves muscle endurance in the elderly. This, we believe, could have importance in the prevention of falls, and the maintenance of health and independent living in elderly men and women (Stout et al. 2007, 2008, Artioli et al. 2010, Derave et al. 2010, AIS 2011).

L-Tryptophan

L-Tryptophan (Trp) is a large neutral amino acid essential to human metabolism because it is the metabolic precursor of serotonin (a neurotransmitter), melatonin (a neurohormone), and niacin (vitamin B3) (Attenburrow et al. 2003).

Tryptophan's primary mechanism of action is its role as the metabolic precursor of the neurotransmitter serotonin. Other neurotransmitters and central nervous system (CNS) chemicals, such as melatonin, dopamine, norepinephrine, and beta-endorphin, have also been shown to increase following oral administration of tryptophan (van Praag and Lemus 1986).

Other neurotransmitters and central nervous system (CNS) chemicals, such as melatonin, dopamine, norepinephrine, and beta-endorphin, have also been shown to increase following oral administration of tryptophan (Guilleminault et al. 1973, Chadwick et al. 1975, den Boer and Westenberg 1990).

Through its intravenous administration, Trp stimulates the secretion of hormones like prolactin and growth hormone (Winokur et al. 1986).

L-Ornithine

L-Ornithine (ORN) is another amino acid that is not included in protein structures. ORN has its main function in the urea cycle (1), along with two other amino acids (arginine and citrulline) and five enzymes. The objective of the urea cycle is to regulate the body concentrations of urea and ammonia. As nitrogen is closely related, the urea cycle can also be understood as a nitrogen detoxifying pathway. Also, the urea cycle may be one of the pacemakers for the availability of protein/amino acids at the hepatic level, and then ORN can have an indirect anabolic effect (Sivashanmugam 2016).

Releasing growth hormone activity: A change magnitude of serum growth hormone was significantly larger in the L-ornithine hydrochloride condition than in the placebo condition (Demura et al. 2010).

L-Lysine

Immune humoral function: L-Lysine is classified as an essential amino acid; meaning the human body cannot synthesize lysine on its own and thus must rely on adequate dietary intake to function properly. Lysine is rapidly transported into muscle tissue (Longenecker and Hause 1959), within 5–7 hours after ingestion (Uhe et al. 1992), and is more concentrated in the intracellular space of muscle tissue compared to other essential amino acids (Flodin 1997). This suggests that muscle may serve as a reservoir for free lysine in the body.

Lysine is the most strongly conserved of the essential amino acids. Lysine is converted to acetyl CoA, a critical component in carbohydrate metabolism and the production of energy. Lysine is also the precursor of the amino acid carnitine, which aids in transporting long-chain fatty acids into the mitochondria for energy production and other metabolic functions. Once lysine is bound to a polypeptide structure, biosynthesis of carnitine is initiated by methylation of one of lysine's amine groups (Broquist 1982). Clinical indications are herpes, osteoporosis, and angina pectoris, where research is published (AMR 2007).

L-Phenylalanine

Phenylalanine (PHE) is a biologically essential aromatic amino acid that acts as a precursor to tyrosine and the catecholamines (epinephrine, norepinephrine, dopamine, and tyramine). It acts also as precursor of melanin and as a constituent of many central nervous system neuropeptides (Wurtman and Caballero 1988).

From the therapeutic perspective, PHE crosses easily the blood–brain barrier (easier than any other amino acid), making it able to exert a direct influence on brain biochemistry.

Phenylethylamine (PEA) is a metabolic end-product of phenylalanine. PEA is further metabolized by monoamine oxidase type B to phenylacetic acid (PAA) (Yang and Neff 1973).

PEA is believed to have amphetamine-like properties, and urine levels have been found to be reduced in patients with depression. Using it as a diagnostic tool, Sabelli found significantly lower levels of PEA in plasma and urine in depressed subjects, compared with normal controls. Treatment with phenylalanine improved mood in 78% of depressed subjects (Sabelli et al. 1986).

There are some precautions to consider before administering PHE. This amino acid is counter indicated in phenylketonuric patients since they are not able to metabolize it and it would worsen their symptoms of phenylketonuria. In some patients with schizophrenia there have been reports of aggravation of tardive dyskinesia with the use of PHE.

As a supplement, PHE is one of the few amino acids that can be administered in any of its isomeric presentations, D, L or DL (as with methionine). Liver enzymes take on the conversion to the useful form, L-phenylalanine.

We have experience with the use IV of L-phenylalanine in concentrations of 0.5% (HeilPro DKN, Cali, Colombia), 1% (Farmacia Francesa, Buenos Aires, Argentina), and 2.5% (Farmacia Milenium, Buenos Aires, Argentina). The average doses range from 15 to 75 mg diluted in IV drip solution, along with other orthomolecular nutrients. Habitual associations include other amino acids with neurotropic functions, like L-tryptophan and/or methionine.

Choline

Choline is required to make the phospholipids phosphatidylcholine, lysophosphatidyicholine, choline plasmalogen, and sphingomyelin—essential components of all membranes. It is a precursor for the biosynthesis of the neurotransmitter acetylcholine. Several lines of evidence suggest that choline might be an essential nutrient for humans. In many other mammals, including the monkey and rat, choline deficiency results in liver and renal dysfunction (Zeisel 1988).

The demand for choline as a methyl donor is probably the major factor that determines how rapidly a diet deficient in choline will induce pathology. As expected, humans ingesting a choline-deficient diet for 3 weeks had diminished plasma choline and phosphatidylcholine concentrations. Choline deficiency of longer duration would have resulted in more prominent evidence of liver dysfunction (Zeisel et al. 1991).

In another publication Zeisel also noted that choline consumed by the mother has a role in cerebral development, with potential protection against future cognitive dysfunction in the offspring (Zeisel 2004).

Amino Acid Complexes to Specific Conditions

In our practice, we use some amino acid combinations through the intravenous route, to treat specific conditions:

- Nutri-Detox® (Biomolec, Ecuador)
  - Cysteine, Cystine and Methionine combined
- Nutri-Brain® (Biomolec, Ecuador)
  - Glycine 25 mg, L Aspartic acid 5 mg, L-Asparagine 15 mg, L-Glutamic acid 25 mg, L-Glutamine 25 mg, L-Lysine 25 mg, L-Methionine 25 mg, L-Phenylalanine 25 mg, L-Tryptophan 10 mg, N-Acetyl L-Tyrosine 5 mg

- Nutri-AA-Pool (Biomolec, Ecuador)
  - Vial containing a series of important amino acids for the maintenance of protein synthesis and related metabolic activities. Also covers the possible indications related to the specific amino acids contained in the formula:
    - Arginine 58 mg, Lysine 97 mg, Proline 84 mg, Cysteine 3 mg, Histidine 46 mg, Aspartic acid 27 mg, Alanine 73 mg, Methionine 47 mg, Valine 43 mg, Tryptophan 18 mg, Ornithine 26 mg, and Serine 25 mg

Vitamins

Vitamins are one of the oldest orthomolecular nutrients that have been found useful from the therapeutic point of view. Their discovery had its highest points in the first 4 decades of the twentieth century. At that time, diseases like beriberi, rickets, or pellagra were much more common than today, and doctors and scientists were able to determine their biochemical origin only after investigating specific nutritional deficiencies. Vitamins can be grossly divided in two main groups, according to their solubility: those that are soluble in water and those that are soluble in lipids.

Vitamins can be divided according to their hydrophobic or hydrophilic properties. Water-soluble vitamins include vitamin C and a heterogenous group of vitamins called the B complex vitamins, which are grouped together mostly because they can be found in the same foods. Ascorbic acid (vitamin C) was covered sufficiently in the section devoted to antioxidants. Fat-soluble vitamins include vitamins A, D, E, and K.

B Complex Vitamins

B complex vitamins comprise 12 water-soluble vitamins, but only 8 of these are considered essential for humans, since they cannot be synthetized de novo and thus must be ingested with the diet (or taken as supplements). Usually B complex vitamins are not stored for any length of time in the human organism, and so they must be replenished on a daily basis. The eight essential B vitamins have both names and their corresponding numbers: vitamin B1 (thiamine), vitamin B2 (riboflavin), vitamin B3 (niacin), vitamin B5 (pantothenic acid), vitamin B6 (pyridoxine), vitamin B7 (biotin), vitamin 9 (folic acid), and vitamin B12 (cobalamin).

The B vitamins are widely required as coenzymes for different enzymes which are considered essential for many of the most determinant cell functions and metabolism. For example, B vitamins have an essential role on mitochondrial function maintenance. Energy production in the mitochondria can be compromised in the case of a maintained deficiency of any B vitamin.

B vitamins are found in whole unprocessed foods. Processed carbohydrates such as sugar and white flour tend to have lower B vitamins than their unprocessed counterparts. For this reason, it is required by law in many countries (including the United States, most European countries, Colombia and Argentina, among many others) that the B vitamins thiamine, riboflavin, niacin, and folic acid be added back to white flour after processing. Most of the times this practice is referred to as "Enriched Flour" on food labels. B vitamins are particularly concentrated in animal sources like some meats (e.g., in turkey, tuna, and liver) (Stipanuk 2006).

From the clinical point of view, B complex vitamins have had many different uses. Some of them have been more investigated than others. Neurodegenerative and psychiatric diseases, so as heart and cardiovascular diseases are among the most purported fields for its use.

They have been used as cofactors in some antioxidative protocols (e.g., the enzyme glutathione reductase is riboflavin-dependent, and it results essential to maintain intracellular concentrations of GSH). In our clinical practice we rarely use a single isolated nutrient, but rather a synergistic mix of them. B complex vitamins have also been utilized as pretreatment in some heavy metal chelation schemes.

Thiamine (Vitamin B1)

Thiamine is a vitamin B complex, also known as vitamin B1. Thiamine is a crucial nutrient in the correct functioning of the Krebs cycle for pyruvate decarboxylation (Frank et al. 2008). This

B complex vitamin also results essential for the oxidative decarboxylation of the multienzyme branched-chain ketoacid dehydrogenase complexes of the citric acid cycle (Depeint et al. 2006). The thiamine-dependent enzymes of the tricarboxylic acid (TCA) cycle are reduced following thiamine deficiency and in the brains of patients who died from multiple neurodegenerative disease. The results suggest that other TCA cycle enzymes should be measured in brains from patients that died from neurological disease in which thiamine-dependent enzymes are known to be reduced. The diminished activities of multiple TCA cycle enzymes may be important in our understanding of how metabolic lesions alter brain function in neurodegenerative disorders (Bubber et al. 2004). The observed increase in the excretion of pyruvate, lactate, 2-oxoglutarate (30-fold against control), and pentose phosphates (3-fold) with urine, depending on the degree of vitamin B1 deficiency, points to one of the essential mechanisms of cell metabolism stabilization under the given pathological condition (Gorbach et al. 1987).

Several groups of patients are at risk of thiamine deficiency, and the classic clinical picture of wet or dry beriberi is not always present, especially in cases of marginal deficiency (O'Keeffe et al. 1994).

Thiamine deficiency can be a cause of concern in groups with potentially low ingestion of this vitamin, like incarcerated prisoners, patients in drug rehabilitation, patients under prolonged parenteral nutrition, and institutionalized elders. Thiamine has also been found deficient in patients whose gastrointestinal absorption is compromised and/or the chronic nature of their disease suggests a possible increase in the output, like patients with hyperemesis gravidarum, anorexia nervosa, chronic kidney disease patients in hemodyalisis, oncologic disease, and AIDS (Hoffman 2011). Medications like furosemide and digoxine can hamper the pharmacokinetics and pharmacodynamics of thiamine, and thus the typical cardiologic patient receiving this type of drug for long periods of time can be at risk of deficiency (Zangen et al. 1998). Some regional risk of thiamine deficiency can be recognized in countries like Ireland or New Zealand, where it is not mandatory to supplement flour for human consumption with this vitamin (O'Keeffe et al. 1994).

Nevertheless, above all of these groups of thiamine deficient patients, alcoholics represent the most common and prototypical example for a variety of reasons. First, their main source of calories is alcohol, which also alters their judgment capacity and the proneness to consume a healthy and balanced diet. Second, ethanol by itself can diminish nutrient absorption at the gastrointestinal tract.

It is important to bear in mind that although adverse effects have been reported in the medical literature after the use of IV thiamine (Schiff 1941, Eisenstadt 1942, Leitner 1943, Stein and Morgenstern 1944, Reingold and Webb 1946, Assem 1973, Stephen et al. 1992, Leung et al. 1993, Morinville et al. 1998), this idiosyncratic reaction is exceedingly rare when compared to the hundreds of thousands of doses of IV thiamine that are given every year around the world.

Regarding this issue, Wrenn, Murphy, and Slovis carried out a prospective evaluation on the safety of thiamine hydrochloride (injected IV as a 100-mg bolus) (Wrenn et al. 1989). From a total of 1070 doses which had been given to 989 consecutive patients, they found an incidence of 0.093% for major reactions (one case of generalized pruritus) and 1.02% for minor reactions (11 cases of transient local irritation). Having a very low frequency of occurrence, the risk posed by this complication has been considered to be surpassed by the benefits of its supplementation in the case of thiamine deficiency and its consequences (mainly Wernicke encephalopathy).

In any case, as with any other potential adverse reaction with the use of any and all IV medication (Wrenn and Slovis 1992), staff should be prepared and trained in the proper treatment of allergic or adverse reactions.

Riboflavin (Vitamin B2)

Vitamin B2 plays an important role in enzymatic oxidoreduction systems. It also results in very important energy production via the respiratory chain.

In neurological diseases riboflavin has an antioxidant effect. The neuroprotective effects of riboflavin in motor disability of experimental autoimmune encephalomyelitis (EAE) as a model of multiple sclerosis. Riboflavin is capable of suppressing the neurological disability mediated by BDNF and proinflammatory cytokine IL-6 (Petrovski et al. 2015, Shashi et al. 2015, Naghashpour et al. 2016).

According to Song and colleagues, eight phenolic compounds including: p-coumaric acid, vainillic acid, caffeic acid, chlorogenic acid, trolox, quercetin, curcumin, and resveratrol were treated with riboflavin (RF) photosensitization, and in vitro antioxidant capacities of the mixtures. RF photosensitization may be a useful method to enhance antioxidant properties like ferric ion reducing abilities of some selected phenolic compounds (Song et al. 2016).

Pyridoxine (Vitamin B6)

Pyridoxine or vitamin B6 is part of the vitamin B group, and its active form, pyridoxal 5-phosphate (PLP) serves as a coenzyme in many enzyme reactions in amino acid, glucose, and lipid metabolic pathways.

Pyridoxal 5-phosphate is involved in reactions catalyzed by the coenzyme aminotransferase. It is involved in many aspects of macronutrient metabolism, neurotransmitter synthesis, histamine synthesis, hemoglobin synthesis and function, and overall gene expression. This vitamin generally serves as a coenzyme (cofactor) for many reactions, including (but not limited to) decarboxylation, racemization, transamination, replacement, beta-group interconversion, and elimination (Combs 2008).

In relationship with carbohydrates' metabolism, vitamin B6 is required as coenzyme for glycogen phosphorylase, which is the enzyme necessary for glycogenolysis to occur. It can catalyze transamination reactions that are essential for providing amino acids as a substrate for gluconeogenesis.

Pyridoxal 5-phosphate aids in the synthesis of hemoglobin, by serving as a coenzyme for the enzyme 5-aminolevulinic acid synthase (ALA-S), ALA-S is the first enzyme involved in the biosynthesis of the group heme (Erskine et al. 2003, Ajioka et al. 2006). For an enhanced binding of the oxygen to hemoglobin, PLP binds to two sites of this protein.

PLP also plays important indirect roles in the nervous system, since it acts as cofactor in the biosynthesis of the most important neurotransmitters: serotonin, norepinephrine, epinephrine, dopamine, and gamma-aminobutyric acid (GABA). Regarding the synthesis of histamine, PLP is also involved. Keep in mind that these neurotransmitters dynamically regulate neural and emotional aspects like mood, attention, and vigilance. Its deficiency or imbalance can lead to a variety of clinical symptoms associated with depression (Muss et al. 2016). Many of the most commonly used conventional antidepressant drugs in psychiatry exert their pharmacological action due to their role in the serotonin metabolism and aim the amelioration of symptoms of depression and mood disorders. The serotonergic pathways rely on nutritional cofactors such as pyridoxine together with essential mineral and trace elements.

In diabetic experimental models (alloxan-induced), intramuscular (IM) injections of the vitamin complex containing: thiamine chloride (B1), riboflavin (B2), lipoic acid (N), calcium pantothenate (B5), pyridoxine hydrochloride (B6), folic acid (B9), and ascorbic acid (C) can reduce the blood glucose level in serum of rats (Petrov et al. 2014). It also helped stabilizing the activity of some enzymes of energy metabolism, lactate dehydrogenase, and pyruvate dehydrogenase complex.

Niacin, Niacinamide (Vitamin B3)

Niacin, also known as vitamin B3 and nicotinic acid, is an organic compound, essential in humans. In the first half of the twentieth century, vitamin B3 deficiency was a major public health issue. Between 1906 and 1940, more than 3 million Americans were affected by pellagra and it was associated with more than 100,000 deaths. Nowadays niacin deficiency is sometimes seen in developed and developing countries. It can make itself evident in poor socioeconomic conditions with poverty, malnutrition, and chronic alcoholism (Pitsavas et al. 2004). There is also the possibility of a borderline or mild deficiency. In this case, vitamin B3 deficiency has been shown to slow metabolism, and also cause decreased performance of the immune response and hamper the tolerance to colds.

In animal models and in vitro, niacin produces marked anti-inflammatory effects in a variety of tissues—including the brain, gastrointestinal tract, skin, and vascular tissue (Offermanns and Schwaninger 2015).

Niacin can also act as an antioxidant that promotes reducing function.

Neuroprotection   Dietary intake and nutritional status of individuals are important factors affecting mental health and the development of psychiatric disorders. Lists of suggested nutritional components that may be beneficial for mental health are omega-3 fatty acids, phospholipids, cholesterol, niacin, folate, vitamin B6, and vitamin B12 (Lim et al. 2016). Niacin modulated the UPDRS scale, handwriting test, and quality of sleep parameters and showed the overall improvement without side effects (Wakade et al. 2015).

Cyanocobalamin (Vitamin B12)

Cyanocobalamin is a water-soluble vitamin that has a key role in the normal functioning of the brain and nervous system, and the formation of red blood cells. It is one of eight B vitamins involved in the metabolism of every cell of the human body, especially affecting DNA synthesis, fatty acid and amino acid metabolism (Yamada 2013).

No fungi, plants, or animals (including humans) are capable of producing vitamin B12.

Vitamin B12 deficiency is most commonly caused by low intakes, but can also result from malabsorption, certain intestinal disorders, low presence of binding proteins, and use of certain medications. Vitamin B12 is rare from plant sources, so vegetarians are most likely to suffer from vitamin B12 deficiency. Infants are at a higher risk of vitamin B12 deficiency if they were born to vegetarian mothers. The elderly who have diets with limited meat or animal products are vulnerable populations as well (Killen and Brenninger 2013).

Vitamin B12 deficiency can potentially cause severe and irreversible damage, especially to the brain and nervous system (van der Put et al. 2001). At levels only slightly lower than normal, a range of symptoms such as fatigue, depression, and poor memory may be experienced (National Institutes of Health—Office of Dietary Supplements 2016). Vitamin B12 deficiency can also cause symptoms of mania and psychosis (Sethi et al. 2005).

Vitamin B12 is a co-substrate of various cell reactions involved in methylation synthesis of nucleic acid and neurotransmitters (Bottiglieri et al. 2000).

Vitamin B12 also influences brain function. In animals, fortification of foods with vitamin B12 and omega-3 fatty acids improves brain development (Rathod et al. 2016). Vitamin B12 along with folate, and sulfur amino acid content may be modifiable risk factors for structural brain changes that precede clinical dementia. The study by Hooshmand and colleagues suggests that the acceleration of the aging process in the brain has relationships with both vitamin B12 and total homocysteine concentrations (Hooshmand et al. 2016). Folate-dependent enzyme methionine synthase and vitamin B12 intake have been crucially related to brain development and function. Zhang and colleagues report previously unrecognized low vitamin B12 cerebral levels across the lifespan in relation with an adaptation to an increase in the antioxidant demand, while accelerated deficits of this nutrient due to GSH deficiency may be a contribution factor to neurodevelopmental and neuropsychiatric diseases (Zhang et al. 2016). Brain's functional organization in health and disease states can be evaluated through the resting state functional MRI (rsfMRI). Using rsfMRI can be a useful tool to evaluate the consequences in brain derived from vitamin B12 deficiency. This vitamin plays an essential role in brain networks associated with cognition control, a process exhibiting compromise in vitamin B12 deficiency (Gupta et al. 2016).

Folic Acid

Folic acid, another form of which is known as folate, is one of the B vitamins. It may be taken by mouth or by injection. It is also used to treat anemia caused by folic acid deficiency. It is used as a supplement by women to prevent neural tube defects (NTDs) developing during pregnancy

(Drugs.com 2016). The National Health and Nutrition Examination Survey (NHANES III 1988–1991) and the Continuing Survey of Food Intakes by Individuals (1994–1996 CSFII) indicated most adults did not consume adequate folate (Alaimo et al. 1994).

Many drugs interfere with the biosynthesis of folic acid. Among them are the dihydrofolate reductase inhibitors such as trimethoprim, pyrimethamine, and methotrexate; the sulfonamides (competitive inhibitors of 4-aminobenzoic acid in the reactions of dihydropteroate synthetase). Valproic acid, one of the most commonly prescribed anticonvulsants that is also used to treat certain psychological conditions, is a known inhibitor of folic acid. All the patients taking any of these medications will have to supplement folic acid in order to avoid a medication-related deficiency and the clinical consequences derived from it.

More than 50 countries require fortification of certain foods with folic acid as a measure to decrease the rate of NTDs in the population (Bailey 2009, Obeid 2012).

There is growing concern worldwide that prenatal high folic acid in the presence of low vitamin B12 causes epigenetic changes in the unborn predisposing them to metabolic syndromes, central adiposity, and adult diseases such as Type 2 diabetes (Yajnik and Deshmukh 2008).

Recently, long-term supplementation of folic acid has been associated with small reductions in the risk of stroke and cardiovascular disease (Li et al. 2016).

Research at the University of York and Hull York Medical School has found a link between depression and low levels of folate (Gilbody 2007), because it is necessary for the increase of the production of neurotransmitters.

Lipid-Soluble Vitamins

Lipid-soluble vitamins include vitamin A (retinol), vitamin D (1, 25 dihydroxycholecalciferol), vitamin E (tocopherols), and vitamin K (phytomenadione). Due to their solubility in fats, they are not routinely used in the everyday intravenous orthomolecular supplementation. To be injected, lipid soluble vitamins have to be prepared in special forms (like the micellar ones).

Minerals and Trace Elements

Minerals are inorganic nutrients required in small amounts for the correct functioning of cells and tissues. Depending on the mineral, its requirements can range from less than 1 to 2500 mg per day. Their presence is necessary for most of the normal life processes, but also to respond properly in disease states (Hays and Swenson 1985, Ozcan 2003).

As with other essential food nutrients, mineral in humans and other vertebrates has been thoroughly recognized as indispensable for many body structures and functions (Underwood 1971, Darby 1976).

Minerals can be found in different quantities in the human body. They can be classified as macro (major) or micro (trace) elements, according to the amount of a particular mineral in the organism. A third category is the ultra-trace elements. The macro-minerals are required in amounts greater than 100 mg/dL and the micro-minerals are required in amounts less than 100 mg/dL (Murray et al. 2000).

The macro-minerals or macro-elements include: calcium (Ca), phosphorus (P), potassium (K), sodium (Na), and magnesium (Mg). Meanwhile the micro-elements include: iron (Fe), copper (Cu), cobalt (Co), chloride (Cl), iodine (I), zinc (Zn), manganese (Mn), molybdenum (Mo), fluoride (F), chromium (Cr), selenium (Se), and sulfur (S) (Eruvbetine 2003).

Ultra trace elements such as boron (B), silicon (Si), arsenic (As), and Nickel (Ni) have been found present in human tissues and are believed to be essential. Evidence for requirements and essentialness of other minerals like cadmium (Cd), lead (Pb), tin (Tn), lithium (Li), and vanadium (Va) is weak (Albion Research Notes 1996).

Human beings must acquire minerals from external sources, in order to allow biochemical and metabolic processes to occur normally. The most common source is (and will/should always be) feeding, but supplementation has gained a place mostly due to micronutrient deficiencies. These deficiencies lay upon many factors to develop, and currently represent a major public health problem. Traditionally it has been considered a problem affecting developing countries, with infants and pregnant women especially at risk, but the population from developed countries with highly westernized diets, and a significant load of antinutrient factors are also susceptible to have nutritional deficiencies (Batra and Seth 2002).

Infants need adequate micronutrients to maintain normal growth and development (Rush 2000).

When a trace element is deficient, a characteristic syndrome is produced which reflects the specific functions of the nutrient in the metabolism.

The trace elements are essential components of enzyme systems.

Simple or conditioned deficiencies of mineral elements therefore have profound effects on metabolism and tissue structure. To assess the dietary intake and adequacy of minerals, information needs to be collected on mineral element content of foods, diets, and water (Rao and Rao 1981, Simsek and Aykut 2007).

Mineral deficiencies or imbalances in soils and forages account partly for low animal production and reproductive problems. The uptake of minerals and other nutrients by plants is influenced by the concentration of these in soils, whose acidity and season of the year affect the availability of nutrients.

Plants use these minerals as structural components in carbohydrates and proteins; organic molecules in metabolism, such as magnesium in chlorophyll and phosphorus in ATP; enzyme activators like potassium, and for maintaining osmotic balance.

It has been reported to influence the mineral and trace element compositions of rice, wheat, oats, and barley, and these are mainly attributed to the altered soil conditions (Basargin and Peregudora 1969, Kavanek and Janicek 1969).

Uptake of copper, zinc, and manganese by plants is affected by the level of phosphate fertilizer (Mongia 1966, Baser and Deo 1967).

Cobalt, copper, iodine, and selenium deficiencies in the soil and flora in certain areas of the world have led to deficiencies of these minerals (Hays and Swenson 1985).

Antinutritional factors present in plants could also affect the absorption and availability of some minerals by humans and animals. Anti-nutritional factors reduce the nutrient utilization and/or food intake of plant foods (Osagie 1998).

Examples of antinutritional factors which could reduce the bioavailability of minerals are oxalates and phytates. Oxalic acid, like phytic acid, can bind some divalent metals such as calcium and magnesium thereby interfering with their metabolism. Phytic acid reduces the absorption of calcium from the gastrointestinal tract and consequently is implicated in the development of rickets when chicks are fed cereals such as sorghum (Blood and Radostits 1989).

Large amounts of calcium are required for the construction and maintenance of bone as well as for the normal function of nerves and muscles.

Phosphorus is an important constituent of adenosine triphosphate (ATP) as well as nucleic acid and essential for acid-base balance, bone and tooth formation.

Without iron, red blood cells cannot function properly. Iron is an important component of the cytochromes that function in the cellular respiration process.

Magnesium, copper, selenium, zinc, iron, manganese, and molybdenum are important co-factors found in the structure of certain enzymes and are indispensable in numerous biochemical pathways.

Vertebrates need iodine to make thyroid hormones.

Sodium, potassium, and chlorine are important in the maintenance of osmotic balance between cells and the interstitial fluid.

Magnesium is an important component of chlorophyll in plants.

The interactions between nutrition and diseases, nutrition and drug metabolism have been reported. The knowledge of the biochemistry of the mineral elements is also essential because individuals suffering from a chronic illness or taking medications that affect the body's use of specific nutrients need to be enlightened.

During two decades in our institution, we use macro- and micro-minerals in orthomolecular IV nutrition, with good results and excellent tolerance, as support in the treatment of many different pathologies, but at the same time as health support component, in sport practitioners and healthy people as functional boosters.

In the text below, we will address in detail the most important mineral elements we use in our daily practice.

Selenium

The trace mineral selenium (Se) is an essential nutrient of fundamental importance in human biology. As it is the case with many other mineral trace elements, Se performs its physiological functions not as an isolated ion, but in conjugation with other nutrients. For example, when it is bound to amino acids like cysteine in the form of selenocysteine, it plays important roles in many enzymatic reactions (Sunde 1997). Se is present as an integral component in more than 30 different selenoproteins (Mahima et al. 2012). Examples of Se-related enzymes are glutathione peroxidases, thioredoxin reductases, iodothyronine deiodinases, selenophosphate synthetase, among others (Arthur 2000, Rayman 2000). These enzymes are dependent on Se, with selenocysteine present at the active site. Rotruck and colleagues (Rotruck et al. 1973) had already suggested that selenium is a component of glutathione peroxidase more than 40 years ago.

Most of these selenoproteins wield fundamental roles both in general metabolic functions, for example, antioxidation in all the body systems and cells with glutathione reductases; organ-specific functions with influence on the whole system, for example, conversion of triiodothyronine (T_3) from its prohormone thyroxine (T_4) and regulation of its levels with thioredoxin reductases; and purely organ-specific functions, for example, potential protection of the developing sperm with spermatid selenoprotein 34 kDa (Rayman 2000). The detrimental consequences of Se deficiency in human and animal health can be easily understood after analyzing these enzymatic metabolic roles.

Se deficiency is recognized as a major health issue. By the beginning of the twentieth century it was estimated to affect from 0.5 to 1 billion people around the world (Combs 2001). Meanwhile, an even larger number of the world's population may be ingesting a lesser amount of selenium than the one required for the maintenance of optimal health (Haug et al. 2007). This deficiency has been identified in many parts of the world, like most of the European countries, China, and the South Island from New Zealand, just to provide some examples (Oldfield 2002, Rayman 2004). Volcanic regions for instance are noted for their low levels of Se in their soil. In many areas of Europe, aspects like the acidity of the soil, along with a higher soil complexity due to a high iron or aluminum content tend to reduce the uptake of Se by crops.

It should be mentioned that although there isn't any specific pathological condition in human beings associated exclusively to Se deficiency alone (Fordyce 2012), this mineral is nowadays considered essential and its deficiency has been implicated in a number of diseases (WHO 1996, Rayman 2012) affecting diverse organs and systems. Resembling a U-shaped dose/effect curve, the excessive intake of Se has also been linked to some diseases, known for centuries. Marco Polo and other chroniclers from antiquity described signs and symptoms compatible with what is recognized today as Se toxicity (selenosis) in pasture animals exposed to highly concentrated Se in forage grass or plants proceeding from soils later found to be excessive in Se (Fordyce 2012).

Human Se-deficiency diseases must be differentiated according to the severity of this deficiency. In some regions with extremely low intake of Se, particular clinical pictures may develop in severely depleted subjects. The two most iconic conditions derived from this extreme deficiency are (Reilly 1996, Fordyce 2012)

- Keshan disease, an endemic and potentially fatal dilated cardiomyopathy, whose name comes from an outbreak in Keshan County (northeast China) in 1935 but has been found in other regions of this country. There were several outbreaks during the rest of the twentieth century;

- Kashin-Beck disease, a deforming osteoarthropathy named after the Russian scientists who described it in the second half of the nineteenth century. It has been detected in several east countries (China, Siberia, North Korea, and possibly some parts of Africa).

These pathologies were first identified in areas of China where the soil is extremely low in selenium (Reilly 1996), and their incidence declined after compulsory Se supplementation (Reilly 1996, Rayman 2004), to the point that they are no longer considered public health problems in China. Nonetheless, in both cases other causative co-factors (dietary mycotoxins, chronic viral infection, iodine co-deficiency) besides Se severe deficiency are believed to play fundamental roles for the processes to develop (Rayman 2000).

Se has impact on several physiologic functions, including the balance in redox systems, the thyroid hormonal metabolism, and the immune system response, among others. Regarding the central role of the mineral in thyroid activity, Se is considered an essential micronutrient that is incorporated into iodothyronine deiodinases. These enzymes are directly involved in thyroid hormone metabolism (Köhrle 2015).

Se is a trace element that plays key roles in thyroid physiology, mediating in the conversion of T4 to its active form, T3. Se deficiency is associated with increased risk of thyroid disease. Some evidence suggests that Se supplementation may be beneficial in autoimmune thyroid disease (either hypo- or hyperthyroidism) (Negro et al. 2016). Se supplementation has been shown to decrease thyroid peroxidase antibodies (TPOAb) in autoimmune thyroiditis (van Zuuren 2013), although it is not completely clear yet if this decrease is protective or associated with less thyroid autoimmunity (Hegedüs et al. 2016).

Supplementation of (oral) Se has been considered quite safe, even after the long-term administration of 200 ug dosages in Se-deficient patients (Calissendorff et al. 2015) or 166 µg in Se-sufficient patients (Leo et al. 2017). Some mild to moderate adverse effects were reported in a small trial of chemoprevention for prostate cancer with a high-dose (1600 µg or 3200 µg), long-term (12 months in average) Se supplementation scheme was reported by Reid and colleagues (Reid et al. 2004). Most of these undesirable effects affected the skin and nails, and the authors emphasize that no serious adverse events occurred.

Se supplementation has been recommended by some authors in clinical situations with decreased antioxidant capacity, like hospitalization in the intensive care unit. Regarding this issue, there is still a great amount of debate over the utility of IV Se supplementation schemes in the critical patient. The recent publication of a critical review and meta-analysis by Manzanares and colleagues (2016) points out the lack of efficacy of Se as a monotherapy for the reduction of morbidity and/or mortality in the ICU.

Nonetheless there have also been reports of positive results with the simultaneous use of several antioxidants (Collier et al. 2008). The protocol published by Collier et al. consisted of the administration for 7 days of vitamin E (as alpha tocopherol, 1000 UI every 8 hours by naso or orogastric tube), vitamin C (as ascorbic acid, 1000 mg IV every 8 hours), and selenium (as selenious acid, 200 mcg IV daily in a 2-hour drip). Reductions in hospital mortality were statistically significant in this retrospective cohort study with 4294 trauma ICU patients (6.1% in the group of patients treated with antioxidants compared to 8.5% in the reference group of patients without the antioxidants; P = 0.001). This represented a 28% relative risk reduction in mortality.

The most complicated subgroup of the trauma patients (Trauma Revised Injury Severity Score [TRISS] 0.5) had a stronger reduction in the mortality rate. Other parameters (hospital/ICU length of stay, ventilator and ventilator-free days) did not change with the antioxidants scheme.

A later retrospective analysis of the trauma patients in the Collier study (Giladi et al. 2011) also revealed significant reductions in a variety of morbidity states associated with the critical patient. The group receiving the antioxidants had less respiratory failure rates (27.6% vs. 17.4%; P = 0.001), less abdominal wall complications (2.9% vs. 0.7%; P = 0.01), and less infections (both in the site of surgery [2.7% vs 1.3%; P = 0.002] and in the bloodstream originated in catheters [5.2% vs 4.9%; P = 0.02]). Other issues like renal failure and SIRS did not show significant differences between groups.

Traditionally Se has been linked to an antioxidant function, but it is important to note that it can also have a pro-oxidative role, depending on the compounds it incorporates into (Haygood et al. 2012).

Supplementation of Se in the clinical setting can be implemented through the oral and intravenous (IV) routes. As mentioned earlier in this chapter and in the same way it occurs with many other orthomolecular nutrients, each one of these routes has its own advantages and disadvantages. The oral route is safe, simple, and economically accessible, but needs weeks to months to achieve higher Se blood and plasmatic levels. As reported by Outzen et al., in the case of foods traditionally recognized as Se sources these levels did not raise so much as expected after the ingestion of 1 kg/week of fish and mussels for 26 weeks (~50 µg selenium/day) in a sample of healthy Danish men and women (Outzen et al. 2015).

Another potential oxidative stress rich situation where the use of Se has been considered potentially useful is malignant disease. Several tumor patients' populations have been found to have low Se serum levels in observational studies. This finding in cancer patients motivated further investigating supplemental oral Se to try to reduce the risk of developing malignant tumors. In this context, it is very important to consider that anticancer effect from Se was obtained from selenium-enriched yeast (SeEnY), but not from selenomethionine (SeMet) supplements. The NPC trial (Nutritional Prevention of Cancer trial) (Duffield-Lillico et al. 2003) was able to show a decrease in the prostate cancer incidence by 52%–65% with patients taking SeEnY, while the SELECT (Selenium and Vitamin E Cancer Prevention Trial) (Klein et al. 2011) patients did not achieve any benefit in prostate cancer risk reduction after 5.5 years taking different SeMet schemes (with or without vitamin E). The SELECT was ended prematurely due to lack of prevention in the antioxidant groups and, in fact, the vitamin E only group had a slight increase in the risk of developing prostate tumors in comparison to the placebo and other groups.

This phenomenon hasn't been clearly understood, while the information on Se biology is not yet complete and many questions remain unanswered about the cellular and genetic interactions of Se (Hatfield and Gladyshev 2009). Some have pointed to the very slight differences between the two forms of Se supplement. It is clear that both forms contain mainly selenomethionine, but SeEnY also contains little amounts of other sulfur compounds like gamma-glutamyl Se-methylselenocysteine and methylselenocysteine, which some have postulated as responsible for anticancer effects observed in the NPC trial. Apart from that, there are some discrete pro-oxidant properties of selenite, which is an Se species with potential contribution to ROS-mediated apoptosis. Malignant cells usually exist under mild oxidative conditions and many of them can be more vulnerable to oxidative stress than normal cells. There is some research toward the development of oncologic medications based on selenite that utilize oxidative damage as its main anticancer mechanism. These hypotheses were put to test in a recent trial that was able to demonstrate a different biochemical antioxidative profile derived from the use of SeEnY versus SeMet in a randomized trial with healthy volunteers (Richie et al. 2014).

In our orthomolecular experience, we use IV Se (as +4 selenite from HeilPro DKN, Cali, Colombia; oxide selenite from Farmacia Milenium, Farmacia Francesa, Buenos Aires, Argentina) in doses ranging from 60 to 120 µg added to other orthomolecular supplements, like high dose vitamin C and amino acids in the complementary treatment of malignant disease (as explained in the vitamin C section, every 4–6 days in average) or chronic infectious diseases (every 10–15 days on average). The treatment of acute infectious disease is another use we give to IV Se with high dose vitamin C drips (every 2–4 days for 2–5 infusions).

We've also used it in patients with autoimmune thyroid disease, but we tend to give preference to the oral route, long-term supplementation of Se in that situation. Another possibility we have put in practice is the combination of this permanent long-term oral Se supplementation dose with occasional Se IV drips (injected through IV drips along with multiple mineral preparations and amino acids).

Zinc (Zn)

Zinc is a micronutrient considered essential (since 1963 [Prasad 2013]) for the maintenance of health in humans and many animals. This trace element results in a wide range of organic functions

(Hambidge 2000). Some of these functions are related to cellular survival, proliferation, and development, even from the level of genetic expression (MacDonald 2000). Approximately 2 billion people around the world remain at risk of Zn deficiency, turning this into a public health issue which was underestimated for decades. Primary Zn deficiency syndromes may be due to diets poor in zinc (Hambidge 2000, Chatterjea and Rana 2012c).

Zn tissue contents vary depending on the organ (Chatterjea and Rana 2012a,b,c). It is high (70–86 mg/100 gm) in skin, and prostate. Zn is moderately concentrated (15–25 mg per 100 gm) in bones and teeth. Low Zn (2.3–5.5 mg/100 gm) can be found in most inner organs like kidneys, heart, pancreas, and spleen; also in muscles. The brain and the lungs have the lowest levels of tissue Zn (1.4–1.5 mg/100 gm).

There are cases in which the intake of Zn can be appropriate, but various conditions predispose to its inadequate handling or use by the organism. Secondary or conditioned zinc deficiency occurs in situations like malabsorption syndrome or total parenteral nutrition, many chronic diseases like sickle cell disease, diabetes, liver cirrhosis, chronic renal disease, several malignancies, and other chronic disorders (King and Cousins 2006). Some medications also interfere with adequate Zn storage and use, like in patients treated with ethambutol, penicillamine, and with some anticonvulsants.

Zn is found as a component of more than 300 enzymes and hormones, making it one of the most important trace elements (Riordan 1976). There are lots of metabolic reactions in which Zn is an indispensable co-factor. For example, it works on the synthesis and degradation of carbohydrates, lipids, proteins, and nucleic acids as well as in the metabolism of other micronutrients (King and Cousins 2006). Zn is crucial for enzymes like alkaline phosphatase, carnosinase, lactic dehydrogenase, alcohol dehydrogenase, and both RNA and DNA polymerase, for example, while it influences the activity of others like thymidine kinase and ribonuclease (Soetan 2010, Chatterjea and Rana 2012c). Zn is the only metal with presence in all enzyme classes (Osredkar and Sustar 2011).

Once absorbed in the gastrointestinal tract, most of Zn contained in plasma is transported bound to albumin, but 10% of this mineral is transported by α2-macroglobulin (Chatterjea and Rana 2012a,b,c). At the intracellular level, Zn is the most abundant metal ion found in cytosol, vesicles, organelles, and in the nucleus (Fleet 2000).

Given that Zn influences so many enzymatic and metabolic processes in the human organism, its deficiency can be found to affect a broad diversity of organs and systems, including the integumentary, gastrointestinal, central nervous system, immune, skeletal, and reproductive systems.

One of the roles of Zn is as adjuvant in carbohydrate metabolism. In this context, Zn is required for the crystallization of insulin. Although the Zn concentration is low when compared to other tissues, one of the organs where Zn can be found readily available is the pancreas. Within the pancreatic cells, Zn is also a constituent of stored insulin (Chatterjea and Rana 2012c).

Zn plays a vital role in the maintenance of immune functions, including cellular (Beck et al. 1997) and humoral immunity. Zn deficiency increases the susceptibility to infection since it affects multiple aspects of innate and adaptive immunity (Prasad et al. 1997). From the diverse subpopulations of T helper cells, the most sensitive to Zn deficiency is T helper subset 1 (Th1), whose response is essential to mount an effective defense against intracellular antigens (e.g., viral infections). In this regard, cytokines like IL–2 (as responsible for promoting lymphocyte proliferation in general), and IFN–γ (as the responsible for promoting Th1 proliferation in particular) showed important affection after the implementation of 8–12 weeks of experimental Zn-restricted diet (3–5 mg/d) in healthy human volunteers (Beck et al. 1997). It is to note that evident serum Zn deficit only appeared after 20–24 weeks of the institution of this experimental diet, much later than the impairment of the type 1 response cytokines' compromise. Th1 cells are indeed very sensitive to Zn depletion, while their main counterpart Th2 cells do not exhibit impairment in Zn-deficient diets in humans (Prasad 2000). An additional consequence of the limited IFN–γ production is the diminished monocytes/macrophages expansion. This certainly establishes a vicious circle, considering that these antigen presenting cells (APCs) both produce this cytokine (along with other proinflammatory molecules) and depend on it in order to get activated and to proliferate. Several interesting reviews have been published over the years covering the topic of the Zn role in immune function (Shankar and Prasad 1998, Maares and Haase 2016).

Immunosenescence is the progressive dysregulation of immune function capacity over the years, a condition especially noticeable in individuals after their sixth decade. The process's physiopathology is not fully understood yet, but factors like chronic infections through life (particularly cytomegalovirus infection), genetic predisposition to chronic low-grade inflammation (among others), and nutritional deficits have been postulated as predisposing elements to develop immunosenescence. Zn is one of the nutrients with most potential for the amelioration of age-dependent alterations on the immune system, along with other trace minerals like selenium, or vitamins like vitamin D and vitamin E. Recently Pae and Wu have provided a very complete review on this topic (Pae and Wu 2017), where they summarize the available intervention studies to date with Zn supplements in elderly patients. Besides playing a predominant supportive role in T-cell dependent immune response (in numbers and in function), Zn also induces augmentation of NK cell cytotoxicity and serves as a co-factor for thymulin, one of the thymus proteins declining with age. In Zn supplemented geriatric patients, additional immune achievements included an increase in delayed type hypersensitivity (DTH) response, and vaccination efficacy. The net result of this immune parameter enhancement was a reduction in morbimortality from infections in the Zn supplemented population (with doses ranging from 7 to 100 mg of Zn, and periods averaging several months). As with other indications, the authors emphasize that Zn supplements will have much more impact on the immune parameters in those elders with Zn deficiency, being less significant in those with normal Zn levels and healthy.

There are several infections (chronic and acute ones) in which Zn supplementation can be of potential benefit. For instance, Sharquie and Al-Nuaimy report on the successful local treatment of viral warts (especially the recalcitrant forms) with intralesional injection of 2% Zn sulfate (Sharquie and Al-Nuaimy 2002). Oral supplementation of Zn also proved effective in the treatment of this condition (Al-Gurairi et al. 2002).

Some recent publications (Maywald and Rink 2016, Rosenkranz et al. 2016) oblige us to consider also an immune tolerance induction role for Zn. From a general theoretical perspective, the immune system functioning is markedly complex: more frequently than not, a substance can have both immunopotentiating and immunomodulating behaviors. This will spin around the circumstances in which this substance acts (a nutrient, for instance). This could be the beginning of a possible role for Zn as an orthomolecular adjuvant measure in autoimmunity or transplantation tolerance induction, but the research is still young on this matter.

One of the subgroups of patients most expected to present a progressive deterioration of their immune function (including mucosal immunity/chronic diarrhea) is the one of those infected with HIV. In this case, Baum and colleagues performed a randomized controlled trial to evaluate oral long-term Zn supplementation (12–15 mg/day) as an adjuvant measure (Baum et al. 2010). They report a decrease in the likelihood of immunological failure and diarrhea in HIV+ patients with poor viral control. As with other essential nutrients, an increase in mortality and more advanced disease in HIV+ patients have been associated with persistently diminished Zn level in serum.

Diarrhea and enterocolitis have been areas of interest for the use of oral Zn supplements. The available evidence is not as strong as to recommend giving Zn to all patients with diarrhea, but it points to a beneficial effect on diarrhea in subjects belonging to populations with potential Zn deficiency. This has been observed mostly in developing countries with high rates of malnutrition and the usually associated Zn deficiency (Walker and Black 2010, Galvao et al. 2013). Some authors mention shorter diarrhea duration of 9%–23%, and a less severe disease in those children taking oral Zn when compared to control children with diarrhea but not taking the supplement (Black 1998).

The World Health Organization (WHO) and the United Nations Children's Fund (UNICEF) have recommended the use of Zn as part of the treatment of diarrhea since 2004 (WHO/UNICEF 2004), due to this positive influence in a disease with important mortality and morbidity around many areas of the world. Nonetheless, some authors from developed countries do not consider this recommendation necessary (Goldman 2013) in children who eat a regular diet, given their low prevalence of Zn deficiency. The opinion on the issue is far from being uniform, even between the medical community in the same country (Giles 2013), considering that (from the nutritional point of view) rural populations even in developed countries like Canada are very different from urban populations.

Concerning cutaneous issues, Zn facilitates wound healing, and helps maintain normal growth rates, and normal skin hydration. Zn-dependent matrix metalloproteinases augment autodebridement and keratinocyte migration during wound repair (Lansdown et al. 2007).

In the nervous system, Zn has several important roles. It intervenes in senses like taste and smell, and its deficiency has been linked to the clinical presentation of these symptoms. In the elderly population, when combined with frailty, memory disturbances, and the heavy use of medication, hypogeusia and hyposmia related to Zn deficiency can also represent another burden factor (Pisano and Hilas 2016).

Zn also has an interesting role in depression. Its supplementation can help optimize treatment results and lead to gain control of depressive symptoms in patients who were previously not responding to classic antidepressant medications. It should be clarified that Zn cannot be considered an antidepressant substance by itself. On the other hand, to date the results of the clinical intervention trials still yield conflicting results (Sarris et al. 2016). Being an antagonist of the glutamate N-methyl-D-aspartate (NMDA) receptor, Zn has a potential antidepressant-like activity in rodent tests/models of depression (Nowak et al. 2005). This trace mineral is also capable of inducing the gene expression of important neurotrophic factors like the brain derived neurotrophic factor (BDNF) (Szewczk et al. 2011).

The role of Zn in healthy aging is particularly important as it could help in the prevention of neoplastic cell growth. Zn is also involved in mitotic cell division, DNA and RNA repair (Tudor et al. 2005). It is involved in structural stabilization and activation of cytochrome P53 that appears to be an important component of the apoptotic process and also in activation of certain members of the caspase family of proteases (Dhawan and Chadha 2010), regulating the cell cycle.

As with many other orthomolecular supplements, like for example Se, N-acetylcysteine or vitamin C, Zn can also provide an antioxidative defense. From the conceptual point of view, the antioxidant mechanisms of Zn have been divided into two categories, depending on the duration of the Zn exposure (supplementation), whether it is acute or chronic. A detailed explanation of the mechanisms is provided by Powell in the review article about Zn antioxidant capacity (Powell 2000).

Diabetes mellitus is a chronic disease with a long list of complications, almost related entirely to the excess of oxidative stress. A role in the prevention of diabetes complications has been propounded recently by McCarty and DiNicolantonio for high dose Zn supplementation (McCarty and DiNicolantonio 2015). According to the authors, this action could be achieved not only due to the inherent capacity of this element to favorably influence the glycemic control in type 2 diabetics, and also to protect the pancreatic beta cells from oxidative stress thus reducing the risk for developing diabetes, but also due to the capacity of counteracting the copper effects through the induction of antioxidant protein metallothionein. Other measures reducing copper in experimental and clinical settings were able to reduce diabetic complications.

As any nutritional deficiency, Zn deficiency may arise from any alteration in one or more steps of the supply chain. Zn can be undersupplied, in cases of poor nutrition or anti-nutrient factors. But it could be ingested or supplemented in adequate amounts and not being properly absorbed. Even supposing a proper absorption, Zn could be handled deficiently and its transport in the body and/or its cell utilization could be impaired. Finally, Zn stores could be spent in a higher rate in most of the chronic diseases, being the issue an augmentation of its losses.

In some rare cases, Zn deficiency may result from a congenitally inherited defect of Zn absorption (deficiency of the Zn carrier protein ZIP4), called acrodermatitis enteropathica (AE). It is a severe Zn deficit syndrome, with an autosomal recessive genetic trait more common in families of Italian, Armenian, or Iranian origin. AE is usually lethal unless treated. It represents the most extreme of the consequences of Zn deficiency (Prasad 2013), with growth retardation, severe diarrhea, ophthalmic damage, skin and teguments compromise (with baldness or hair loss and skin rash localized most often around the genitalia and mouth), and immune impairment with thymic hypoplasia and recurrent infections due to a variety of pathogenic bacteria but also due to opportunistic germs like candida sp.

Much more commonly seen in the clinical practice, the Zn deficiency is mild to moderate in its presentation. It is acquired secondarily from a variety of factors affecting dietary Zn intake, absorption, or loss. An excellent example of a patient with limitation in the replenishment of Zn levels after oral supplementation was published recently by Vick and colleagues (Vick et al. 2015). In this clinical case, it is thought that the patient's original suboptimal response to oral supplementation of Zn and the improvement after receiving IV Zn were related to the prior surgical history of alteration of the gastroduodenal anatomy and bypass of the absorptive capacity at the duodenum and jejunum.

One of the conditions associated with Zn deficiency due to a combination of digestive factors including classical malabsorption syndrome is the one derived from Crohn's disease (Solomons et al. 1977, McClain et al. 1980a). In these patients, Zn deficiency is also frequently caused by low intake, besides the poor absorption of this and many other nutrients (Sturniolo et al. 1980). To make things even more complex, Crohn's disease patients also present with an excess of Zn fecal losses (Wolman et al. 1979).

Some patients with extensive Crohn's disease may need IV nutrition, which should include the replenishment of Zn along with many other nutrients (Driscoll and Rosenberg 1978). Zn deficiency in Crohn's disease patients is not only derived from the complex intestinal luminal phenomena characterizing this condition. A group of 10 patients with Crohn's disease who needed IV nutrition were supplemented with IV Zn through a period of 5 weeks, and their serum and urinary Zn status was evaluated by Main and colleagues in the early 1980s (Main et al. 1982). Presurgical orthopedic patients and healthy volunteers were used as controls. According to the serum/urine Zn dynamics observed during the trial, the authors suggest that IV Zn supplementation does not present an efficient tissue transport. Also, they considered that Zn supplementation might be partially excreted as small molecular weight chelates into urine, and provide recommendations to enhance Zn utilization during IV nutrition in this complex context.

Long-term IV nutrition can be complicated by the development of Zn deficiency (McClain et al. 1980b) unless this mineral is adequately supplemented. Actually, the development of many of the previously recognized moderate to severe Zn deficiency related symptoms in patients receiving total parenteral nutrition (TPN) before the recognition of the essentiality of Zn was one of the main reasons to grant this trace element its essential status by the FDA and medical authorities (AMA 1979). This consideration becomes even more important when the patient is affected by an anabolic state, when Zn deficiency is more prevalent due to a higher expenditure of the nutrient.

This is also the case in some pathologic states. Zn deficiency is also associated with acute and chronic liver disease. Zinc supplementation may protect against toxin-induced liver damage and it has been used as a therapeutic measure for hepatic encephalopathy in patients refractory to standard treatment (Takuma et al. 2010). Another example of organic disease with augmentation of Zn stores is type II diabetes mellitus (Kinlaw et al. 1983), whose patients also develop Zn deficiency with time.

The clinical picture of Zn deficiency varies according to the degree of deficit. In a 2004 article (Yanagisawa 2004), Yanagisawa has skillfully and succinctly summarized the relationship between a given symptomatology and the degree of Zn deficiency in the patient.

- In minor Zn deficiency, the patient may present with symptoms like a subjective reduction in the sense of taste, signs like non-fat weight loss, and laboratory findings like a reduction in serum testosterone levels with or without alteration in the sperm counts.
- When the Zn deficiency is moderate, some of the aforementioned features will aggravate, like in the case of reproductive health with signs of delayed gonadal development. The structural system can be affected and there could be also growth impairment and

retardation. Skin abnormalities are also usual, with delayed wound healing. The nervous system will manifest moderate Zn deficiency with anorexia, somnolence, reduced dark adaptation, and in the sensorial sphere, symptoms like hypogeusia and hyposmia can be present at this stage.

• Continuing with the intensification of the Zn deficiency, severe depletion of this micronutrient will cause more serious skin conditions with bullous or pustular dermatitis or premature balding; abnormalities in the mental/emotional sphere (mainly depression); mucosal manifestations like (chronic) diarrhea; and eventually also affected immune response with recurrent infections.

The pathological situations leading to each one of these deficiency degrees are obviously different (Yanagisawa 2004). Slight micronutrient deficiencies (including Zn) tend to be of the consequence of marginal dietary ingestion of the implicated trace element and/or presence of anti-nutrient factors. To develop a moderate Zn deficiency, a deeper compromise of the nutrient intake is necessary, usually accompanied by unbalanced nutrition (Yanagisawa 2004, Murthy 2010); but it can happen also in pathologic states like malabsorption syndromes or chronic liver/kidney disease. Severe Zn deficiencies are almost exclusively associated with specific Zn metabolism detrimental conditions, like, for example, acrodermatitis enteropathica, or prolonged ethambutol/penicillamine treatments, or prolonged high-calorie parenteral therapy (Prasad 1976).

Even though in the clinical practice plasma or serum Zn level measurements are the most commonly used tool to evaluate a potential Zn deficiency, the real cellular Zn status could not necessarily be reflected by these levels (Osredkar and Sustar 2011). The homeodynamic mechanisms involved in controlling plasma levels of most nutrients are tight, and hence there can be differences with the extracellular matrix and intracellular status of such nutrients. This reflects a situation that can be seen commonly when assessing the patient's status of many trace elements. There is always the possibility of having a patient with clinical effects of Zn (or other micronutrient) deficiency without the presence of abnormal laboratory measurements.

Already in a 1979 study published by Aamodt and colleagues in the *American Journal of Clinical Nutrition* (Aamodt et al. 1979), they were able to demonstrate that similar metabolic patterns were observed regardless of whether Zn was administered intravenously or orally, suggesting that these patterns were not affected by the route of administration for the cases studied.

As with many other orthomolecular nutrients, Zn supplementation is still a matter of continuous investigation. Ideal therapeutic dosing to effectively ameliorate Zn deficiency is not clear yet, but maximum plasmatic levels below 30 mmol of zinc/L (approximately 200 mg) are considered safe to avoid any potential detrimental effect on the immune system (Ibs and Rink 2003). A U-shaped effect has been observed for Zn and the immune system function, where low as high doses are detrimental for its optimal state.

The repetitive administration of Zn in the absence of copper (Cu) supplementation may cause a (progressive) decrease in serum Cu levels (Plum et al. 2010, Osredkar and Sustar 2011). Zn has a high safety profile; in fact, most of its potential toxic effects have been associated with the potential induction of Cu deficiency (anemia, neutropenia, among others) (Plum et al. 2010). Periodic determination of serum copper as well as Zn serum levels are suggested as a tool to guide the Zn supplemental administration. Zn is eliminated via the intestine and kidneys. The possibility of Zn retention must be taken into consideration in patients with significant alteration in excretory routes (e.g., chronic renal disease). In these cases, an adjustment of the Zn supplementation dose could be necessary according to a lesser capacity of renal clearance of the ion.

Oral Zn overdose is possible, although it is rare, since it would be required to ingest very large amounts of the mineral to cause toxicity (Plum et al. 2010). A large oral dose of more than 30–40 g of Zn sulfate has been reported fatal. Severe Zn intoxication symptoms include: nausea, vomiting, dehydration, electrolyte imbalances, dizziness, abdominal pain, lethargy, and incoordination. The administration of a single IV dose of 1–2 mg zinc/kg body weight has been reported to have been given to adult leukemic patients without any evident toxic manifestations. Normal plasma levels for zinc vary from approximately 88 to 112 mcg/100 mL. Plasma levels sufficient to produce symptoms of toxic manifestations in humans are not known. Calcium supplements could counteract Zn toxicity and may confer a protective effect.

In our clinic, we have experience with the use of zinc gluconate 1% solution (Farmacia Milenium, Buenos Aires, Argentina). The usual doses range from 20 to 80 mg, and it is added to the IV orthomolecular drip along with other nutrients according to the clinical picture and needs of the patient.

It is important to bear in mind that undiluted direct venous injections of Zn solutions should be avoided due to the potential risk of causing local irritation of the vessel (phlebitis), and there is a risk to induce a reflex augmentation of the Zn clearance at the renal level after a bolus injection of this mineral.

Copper (Cu)

Copper (Cu) is an essential trace element for humans and animals. It can be found in almost every cell of our organism, where Cu exists in the oxidized form. From the organs, the highest concentrations of copper are discovered in the brain and the liver; the central nervous system and the heart have high concentrations of copper as well (Gibson 2005). About 50% of total human body Cu content is stored in structural tissues, like bones and muscles (skeletal muscles alone contain about 25%). The other half of the Cu body content is distributed between the skin (15%), the bone marrow (15%), the brain (8%), and the liver (8%–15%).

Cu is a functional component of many essential enzymes, known as copper enzymes or cuproenzymes (Harris 1997). Some important examples are: cytochrome C oxidase, lysyl oxidase, feroxidase, 2-furoate-CoA dehydrogenase, amine oxidase, catechol oxidase, tyrosinase, dopamine beta-monooxygenase, D-galaktozo oxidase, D-hexozo oxidoreductase, indole 2,3-dioxygenase, L-ascorbatoxidase, nitratreductase, peptidylglycine monooxygenase, flavonol 2,4-dioxygenase, superoxide dismutase (SOD), PHM (peptidylglycine monooxygenase hydroxylation), and others. Some physiological functions are dependent on the presence of these enzymes in the organism (Rolff and Tuczek 2008).

Cu is absorbed mainly in the duodenum, but only about a third of Cu duodenal content coming from the diet can be absorbed. There are many factors limiting Cu absorption, like the presence of phytates, vitamins like ascorbic acid (but only in high amounts), and other minerals like zinc, molybdenum, cadmium, silver, and mercury (Chatterjea and Rana 2012).

The ability of copper to easily attach and accept electrons explains its importance in oxidative reduction processes and in disposing and removing free radicals from the organism (Uauy et al. 1998).

Changes in copper concentrations in body fluids and tissues are observed in different diseases and conditions. There are serious diseases, potentially caused by disorders in the metabolism of Cu in the organism. Low concentrations (abnormal) of Cu are found: Menkes syndrome (Kaler et al. 2008), Parkinson's disease, impaired intestinal resorption, parenteral nutrition (especially in the long term), excessive zinc supplementation, and diseases with protein loss (e.g., nephrotic syndrome, exudative enteropathy, and others). Meanwhile, other pathologic states exhibit increased Cu concentrations (Attri et al. 2006), like in pregnancy, cholestasis, malignant tumors and lymphomas, chronic degenerative liver disease (cirrhosis), increased ceruloplasmin—inflammation, myeloid leucosis, and Wilson's disease. Elevated circulating Cu concentration (hypercupremia) has been detected for decades in several situations, like acute and chronic infections and malignancies—leukemia, Hodgkin's disease, severe anemia hemochromatosis, myocardial infarction, hyperthyroidism, and so on (Lahey et al. 1953).

There is some controversy regarding the role of Cu in cardiovascular disease (Jones et al. 1997, Fox et al. 2000). While some scientists have suggested that elevated Cu levels can increase the risk of atherosclerosis (mainly through the oxidation of LDL), others mention how Cu deficiency (rather than Cu excess) would be associated with an increasing risk of cardiovascular disease. More recent evidence (Grammer et al. 2014) points out that both ceruloplasmin and Cu serum level are independent markers of all cause and cardiovascular disease associated mortality. Approximately 3253 persons were evaluated by coronary artery disease (CAD) angiography and mortality both from all causes and from cardiovascular disease. After the proper removal of several confounding factors, the authors declared that the association was reduced but remained statistically significant.

When the dietary intake of copper was low, adverse changes have been observed in blood cholesterol, including increased total and LDL cholesterol and decreased HDL-cholesterol (Klevay 1998). Nonetheless, Jones et al. (1997) show that high dose Cu supplements taken for 4–6 weeks did not lead to clinically significant changes in cholesterol levels.

Copper-containing enzyme lysyl oxidase is required for the development (cross-linking) of collagen, which is a key element in the consolidation of the organic bone extracellular matrix. Osteoporosis occurs in children and adults with severe Cu deficiency, while in healthy adult men and women studies showed that the use of Cu supplements is able to induce significant increases in bone density (Baker et al. 1999). In elderly patients with hip fractures the serum levels of Cu were found to be significantly lower than these of controls (Conlan et al. 1990).

In patients with poor metabolic control, the reduction in plasma Cu concentration is less strong in women than in men with diabetes (Ruiz et al. 1998).

Cu was related to the manifestation of type 2 diabetes and should be applied in the treatment of diabetic patients (Tanaka et al. 2009).

Studies in children with chronic diarrhea investigated Zn and Cu status. The level of both trace elements in serum was reduced. The authors have found deficit of serum Cu in chronic diarrhea (Rodriques et al. 1985, Sachdev et al. 1990).

Serum levels of copper are higher in patients who use contraceptives or estrogens.

Copper might have influence on iron metabolism. As reported by Turgut et al. the Cu blood content in anemic patients showed increased serum concentrations of Cu in some cases. In turn, high levels of Cu induced a reduction in the absorption of iron and adversely affected hematological indices (Turgut et al. 2007).

It is known that copper plays an important role in the development and maintenance of immune system function. For instance, although not a common cause, neutropenia can be a clinical sign of copper deficiency in the human organism. Adverse effects of copper deficiency on immune function are most pronounced in infants (Failla and Hopkins 1998).

Extracellular matrix structural defects: On the other hand, copper is involved in numerous physiological and metabolic processes critical for the appropriate functioning of almost all tissues in the human body. In the skin, copper is involved in the synthesis and stabilization of extracellular matrix skin proteins and angiogenesis (Borkow 2014).

Manganese (Mn)

Manganese (Mn) is distributed in tissues throughout the whole body, but the highest concentrations are present in the liver, thyroid, pituitary, pancreas, kidneys, and the bone. At the intracellular level, Mn is largely located in the mitochondria. The total manganese content of an average 70 kg man is approximately 12–20 mg. A minimum intake of 2.5–7 mg per day meets human needs (Hegsted 1976).

Many nutrients from different families have synergistic interactions with Mn. These include minerals like potassium, zinc, magnesium, iron, phosphorus, and vitamins like A, E, B1, B3, B5, and B6.

It activates numerous enzymes—such as hydrolases, transferases, kinases, and decarboxylases—and is a constituent of some enzymes; the most well-known manganese metalloenzyme is pyruvate carboxylase, which catalyzes the conversion of pyruvate to oxalo-acetate. Arginase is involved in the conversion of the amino acid arginine to urea as well as mitochondrial superoxide dismutase (SOD) (Scrutton et al. 1966).

Manganese activates enzymes associated with fatty acid metabolism and protein synthesis. Mn results are important in the fatty and carbohydrate metabolism. It is also involved in some vitamin metabolism (Wilson et al. 1979).

Manganese is required for normal thyroid function and is involved in the formation of thyroxin. Studies have revealed low manganese levels in hypothyroid patients (Pfeiffer 1975).

Absorption or utilization of manganese may be impaired when levels of insulin, parathyroid hormone (PTH), and estrogen are elevated, affecting thyroid function (Watts 1989).

Many similarities exist among species in manganese deficiency; including skeletal abnormalities, postural defects, impaired growth, impaired reproductive function, and disturbances in lipid and carbohydrate metabolism. Manganese deficiency has been associated with symptoms like fatigue, growth pains in children, irregular menses, nervous system functions alterations, and joint issues (Underwood 1977).

Mn can play a complementary role as a supportive measure in the diabetic patients, due to the protection that Mn superoxide dismutase has over the oxidative DNA damage (Madsen-Bouterse et al. 2010).

Mn participates in chondroitin and proteoglycan synthesis. As these are two of the main components in cartilage, Mn can represent an indirect cofactor in the treatment of joint diseases and osteoporosis. In the wide sense, Mn is involved in the biosynthesis of mucopolysaccharides (main components of any extracellular matrix). A deficiency in Mn can then play a role in cartilaginous and collagen disorders. Skeletal abnormalities include chondrodystrophy, or retarded bone growth with bowing. Perosis or "slipped tendon" is a widely recognized condition in chickens and ducks deficient in Mn (Davies 1972, Underwood 1977).

Mn also intervenes in sexual hormones synthesis. Reproductive function in manganese deficient patients (both male and female) is characterized by defective ovulation, ovarian and testicular degeneration, and increased infant mortality.

Although it is not one of the main therapeutic measures, Mn can provide some benefits in the complementary treatment of allergic patients.

Other abnormalities thought to be related to manganese deficiency have been reported. Epileptics were found to have lowered blood concentrations of manganese, thus hypothesized to be a possible cause of cerebral dysrhythmia (Papavasiliov 1979).

Chromium

Chromium is a trace mineral essential for many animals, including humans. It is an element with multiple valences, being the most common form of chromium the trivalent one (Cr^{3+}). In the oral presentations, chromium can be consumed as a supplement in the form of chromium chloride, chromium nicotinate, chromium picolinate, or high-chromium yeast. One of the main reasons to justify the use of this mineral via intravenous (IV) infusion is the difficult absorption when taken orally (only 1%–10% according to the source used to obtain it, and according to the chemical form administered). Albeit severe deficiency of chromium can be considered somehow a rare condition, since there are plenty of dietary sources. On the other hand, reaching an effective replenishment time in patients with marginal chromium levels can take months when supplementing it orally.

Although the role of chromium in the glucose tolerance factor (GTF) was described as early as 1957, this did not necessarily translate into a higher use of this mineral in the clinical practice. Actually, as with many other micronutrients (for instance, zinc or selenium), the clinical importance of chromium for human health was unveiled only after periods of shortage in ICU patients maintained with total parenteral nutrition (TPN) (Freund et al. 1979, Brown et al. 1986). It was observed in this setting that after the addition of chromium to TPN the patients without prior history of blood sugar issues had a better glycemic control, and those with a history of diabetes mellitus required less hypoglycemic medications and/or achieved better values after having had difficulties with their metabolic status while in the ICU (Jeejeebhoy et al. 1977).

Chromium aids in the control of insulin resistance, thus helping the organism to keep appropriate blood sugar levels (Suksomboon et al. 2014). This turns it into a useful tool in the pathologic states of the carbohydrate metabolism, like diabetes and hypoglycemia (Paiva et al. 2015).

In another component of the metabolic performance, chromium also has important results for the correct lipid metabolism. It has been proposed that it favors a better body weight control, while helping in the reduction of blood levels of LDL cholesterol and triglycerides.

Diabetes and obesity are diseases characterized by their increasing incidence every year. When comparing with healthy subjects, the serum levels of chromium (Cr) are lowered in these two diseases. Several studies conducted in laboratory animals with experimentally induced diabetes demonstrated that supplementation with chromium ions (III) decreased glucose concentration in the blood, reduced the probability of atherosclerosis and heart attack, and lowered the levels of cholesterol and low density lipoprotein (LDL) (Lewicki et al. 2014).

Utilizing the powerful technology of nutrigenomics to identify the genes regulated by chromium supplementation may shed some light on the underlying mechanisms of chromium-gene interactions, and thus provide strategies to mitigate and prevent insulin-resistance-related disorders (Lau et al. 2008).

Chromium deficiency can be related to clinical manifestations like tiredness, diabetes or hypoglicaemia, loss of hunger, or LDL augmentation.

Electrolytes

Magnesium

Magnesium (Mg) is one of the main minerals with a potential therapeutic spectrum in the structural system. As such, it has been used extensively as a muscle relaxant, and for the treatment of diverse painful conditions, like neuralgia among others.

It can also act as a mitochondrial antioxidant, where it is conveniently associated to Coenzyme Q10 and/or alpha lipoic acid (ALA).

In diabetic patients, Mg can be associated with amino acids like alanine, and minerals like chromium, zinc, and B complex vitamins, in order to facilitate a better carbohydrate metabolism.

We have used Mg intravenously as magnesium chloride 20% solution (HeilPro DKN, Cali, Colombia; Farmacia Milenium, Farmacia Francesa, Buenos Aires, Argentina) or magnesium sulfate 10% solution (Farmacia Milenium, Farmacia Francesa, Buenos Aires, Argentina). It is added to multiple mineral preparations, along with amino acids and antioxidants like DMSO. Our main experience has revolved around the utility of Mg as an aid in pain control, with interesting symptomatic results in bone, muscles, and joint complaints.

Calcium

Improves muscle contraction
Premenstrual syndrome
Replacement of calcium after EDTA chelation

Multimineral Preparations

In our clinical practice, we have been working for many years with multimineral complexes as the base for many of the orthomolecular IV drips. This type of orthomolecular presentation provides an easy way to supply the patient both with macro minerals and trace minerals in fixed doses. It is common that individual minerals are added to the IV drip solution on an individual basis. Also, amino acids and antioxidants are added, in accordance with the intended therapeutic objectives for the particular patient. The most used multimineral complexes we use are

- Mineral Complex Nutri–Min 16 (Biomolec, Quito, Ecuador);
- MM-16 Forte (HeilProDKN, Cali, Colombia);

- MinTraz (OrthomoLab, Jamundí, Colombia)
- MetaBas (Farmacia Milenium, Buenos Aires, Argentina);
- Gluco-Mins (Cr, Zn, Mn) complex for use in glucose metabolism alterations

Precursors of Antioxidant Enzymes

Zn, Cu, Mn in Complexation with SOD

This product can be added to a 250–500 cc volume of saline solution weekly during 4–8 infusions, and after that every 15 days for 2 or 3 months.

Others

Chelating Agents

- Disodium EDTA
  - Chelating calcium, magnesium, lead, cadmium, chromium
- EDTA or sodium-calcium
  - Chelating lead, chromium cadmium
- Deferoxamine
  - Trivalent metal chelator
- Lipoic acid
  - Chelating lead, arsenic, mercury

D-Ribose

D-ribose is a pentose, which utilizes the oxidative pathway of phophate pentoses (PPP). After its IV injection, D-ribose is captured quickly by the cells and it is phosphorylated to ribose 5 phosphate. D-ribose plays a fundamental role in all ischemic processes, even those occurring at the muscular level. Animal studies corroborated a role of D-ribose in the myocardium recovery after ischemic stages, with a positive influence on contractile function of this muscle.

This pentose enhances quality of life in patients with reduced coronary blood flow and myocardium affection. D-ribose allows a better tolerance of the heart to ischemia in patients with coronary artery disease.

D-ribose also acts as a cofactor for ATP resynthesis. It can help in muscle fatigue derived from the loss of intracellular phosphate, therefore augmenting the exercise tolerance.

From a theoretical point of view, D-ribose can enhance insulin and hypoglicemic agents' activity. It is a complementary nutrient in the treatment of disglycemic patients, but it must be potentially avoided in patients with a marked tendency to hypoglycemia.

Inositol

Inositol is used by the body to form cell membranes, and it allows for the proper functioning of cells. Inositol assists in the transmission of nerve signals, and helps to transport lipids within the body. This will help to contract muscles more efficiently and will help to use body fat as fuel.

Inositol is a simple polyol precursor in important brain second messenger systems. Cerebrospinal fluid inositol has been reported to be decreased in depressive patients. Inositol optimizes muscle metabolism.

Procaine

Procaine is not an orthomolecular supplement per se, but we chose to make a short reference to it, since it is used routinely in many biological medicine practices around the world in the context of neural therapy according to Huneke (NTH). NTH is used along with orthomolecular supplements and some other therapeutic tools of biological medicine. Procaine acts as a cell membrane resting potential regulator with special emphasis on the restoration of the proper function of the autonomic nervous system due to its role in disease (especially in the chronic ones) (Dosch 1984).

Apart from the neuratherapeutic use of procaine, many decades ago there were many reports by conventional colleagues about unexpected therapeutic effects after the application of local anesthetics. One interesting route is the IV procaine drip. Among other general regulatory actions, procaine is an inflammation modulator. Some bibliographic reports appeared in the 1940s by Graubard and colleagues. In the first one, the authors presented a method for the procaine IV drip and described 140 patients who received 608 intravenous procaine infusions for the management of pain in trauma and inflammation (Graubard et al. 1947). The next report was published the year after, including 448 cases with 1954 procaine infusions. In that one the authors wished to present further conclusions related to the safety of this method as a hospital procedure, and from the clinical point of view they mention that the average patient tolerated the procaine IV drip better when vitamin C is combined in solution (Graubard 1948). The same group continued working with IV procaine and producing reports about their advances (Graubard and Peterson 1949).

Considering the wide presence of the inflammatory process, the therapeutic action of local anesthetics holds a lot of promise for its clinical utility in many different areas and illnesses. Their noticeable effects on the inflammatory response and especially on several immune cells as promoters and effectors of the inflammatory response turns this class of drugs into modulating tools for a complex process. Some of the procaine and local anesthetics' effects have been evidenced mainly in polymorphonuclear granulocytes (PMNs), but macrophages and monocytes also exhibited changes. It is important to note that PMNs do not express Na channels, so the mechanisms of action must go beyond the classical one of the Na^+ channel blockade by local anesthetics (Krause et al. 1993).

From the point of view of biological medicine (and to some extent from conventional medicine [Cotran 1990, 1995]), the inflammatory cascade is essential for structural and functional repair of injured tissue. In some cases, however, inflammation can have a double-edged sword behavior. The uncontrolled and exaggerated generation of proinflammatory signals will lead invariably to a lesser or larger extent of tissue damage. This is what occurs in several disease states, and can be further aggravated due to tissue debris product from the same inflammatory process. Finding therapeutic tools that modulate rather than block the inflammatory response (e.g., procaine and local anesthetics) should eventually potentiate the favorable aspects of inflammation, while preventing excessive tissue damage. This postulate is in line with the principles of neural therapy.

Overactive inflammatory responses that destroy rather than protect are critical in the development of many perioperative disease states, such as postoperative pain, adult respiratory distress syndrome (ARDS), systemic inflammatory response syndrome (SIRS), and multiorgan failure. It accounts also as a big obstacle for the resolution in autoimmune diseases and many other chronic inflammatory conditions (e.g., COPD, neurodegenerative diseases, liver cirrhosis). Modulation of such responses is therefore a top priority from the point of view of any medical specialty that takes pride on practicing with a preventive orientation, like biological medicine.

Modern publications about the modulatory properties of local anesthetics in inflammatory diseases (Swanton and Shorten 2003, Pecher et al. 2004, Cassuto et al. 2006, Wright et al. 2008) echo the ones dating from more than a half century ago, but with a much broader view and fully equipped with many explanations about the molecular level interactions that these marvelous therapeutic agents have with effector proinflammatory cells.

REFERENCES

INTRODUCTION

A Guide to Parenteral Drugs Affected by Light. www.helapet.co.uk/downloads/lightaffectingdrugs.pdf, Accessed December 21, 2016.

Akers MJ, Larrimore DS. *Parenteral Quality Control. Sterility, Pyrogen, Particulate, and Package Integrity Testing.* 3rd Edition. Revised and Expanded. Bridgewater: New Jersey, 2003.

Botella Dorta C. Administración parenteral de medicamentos: la vía intravenosa (el goteo intravenoso). Actualizada el 12/11/2004. Servicio Canario de la Salud, España. https://www.fisterra.com/material/tecnicas/parenteral/viaiv.pdf, Accessed December 20, 2016.

Botella Dorta C. Administración parenteral de medicamentos: La vía intramuscular. Servicio Canario de la Salud, España, September 15, 2011. https://www.fisterra.com/material/tecnicas/parenteral/AdmonParentIM.pdf, Accessed December 20, 2016.

Botella M, Hernández OM, López ML et al. *Cuidados auxiliares de enfermería. Técnicas básicas de enfermería. Administración de medicamentos.* Gobierno de Canarias, Consejería de Educación, Cultura y Deportes: Santa Cruz de Tenerife, 2002, pp. 435–460.

Fleming A. Sigma–Aldrich Technical Service Letter on Glutathione stability. http://web.stanford.edu/~teruel1/Protocols/pdf/glutahione_stability.pdf, Accessed December 21, 2016.

Gemenet DC, Leiser WL, Beggi F et al. Overcoming phosphorus deficiency in West African Pearl Millet and sorghum production systems: Promising options for crop improvement. *Front Plant Sci* 2016 Sep 23; 7: 1389. https://www.ncbi.nlm.nih.gov/pubmed/27721815

General chapter injections corrections. http://www.uspnf.com/sites/default/files/usp_pdf/EN/USPNF/general-ChapterInjections.pdf

Ghorbani Z, Hajizadeh M, Hekmatdoost A. Dietary supplementation in patients with alcoholic liver disease: A review on current evidence. *Hepatobiliary Pancreat Dis Int* 2016 Aug; 15(4): 348–360. https://www.ncbi.nlm.nih.gov/pubmed/27498574

Harris RS, Karmas E. *Nutritional Evaluation of Food Processing.* AVI 2nd Edition. West Port, 1975. www.alceingenieria.net/nutricion/perdidas.pdf

Hartung T, Aaberge I, Berthold S et al. Novel pyrogen tests based on the human fever reaction. *ATLA* 2001; 29: 99–123. https://www.ncbi.nlm.nih.gov/pubmed/11262757

Hartung T, Wendel A. Detection of pyrogens using human whole blood. *ALTEX* 1995; 12(2): 70–75. https://www.ncbi.nlm.nih.gov/pubmed/11178418

Henderson B, Poole S, Wilson M. Bacterial modulins: A novel class of virulence factors which cause host tissue pathology by inducing cytokine synthesis. *Microbiol Res* 1996; 60: 316–341. https://www.ncbi.nlm.nih.gov/pubmed/8801436

Joy EJM, Ander L, Broadley MR et al. Elemental composition of malawian rice. *Environ Geochem Health* 2016; 39(4): 835–845. doi: 10.1007/s10653-016-9854-9. https://www.ncbi.nlm.nih.gov/pubmed/27438079

Kluger MJ. Fever: Role of pyrogens and cryogens. *Physiol Rev* 1990; 71: 93–127. https://www.ncbi.nlm.nih.gov/pubmed/1986393

Kumar K, Al Arebi A, Singh I. Accidental intravenous infusion of a large dose of magnesium sulphate during labor: A case report. *J Anaesthesiol Clin Pharmacol* 2013 Jul–Sep; 29(3): 377–379. https://www.ncbi.nlm.nih.gov/pmc/articles/PMC3788239/

Lawrence A. *Handbook of Injectable Drugs.* 14th Edition. Maryland: American Society of Health – System Pharmacists, 2007.

Li L, Yang T, Redden R et al. Soil fertility map for food legumes production areas in China. *Sci Rep* 2016; May 23(6): 26102. https://www.ncbi.nlm.nih.gov/pubmed/27212262

Lieber CS. Interaction of alcohol with other drugs and nutrients. Implication for the therapy of alcoholic liver disease. *Drugs* 1990; 40(Suppl. 3): 23–44. https://www.ncbi.nlm.nih.gov/pubmed/2081478

Lloyd D, Aon MA, Cortassa S. Why homeodynamics, not homeostasis? *Scientific World Journal* 2001; Apr 4(1): 133–145. https://www.ncbi.nlm.nih.gov/pubmed/12805697

Lu YC, Yeh WC, Ohashi PS. LPS/TLR4 signal transduction pathway. *Cytokine* 2008 May; 42(2): 145–151. https://www.ncbi.nlm.nih.gov/pubmed/18304834

Morimoto A, Nakamori T, Watanabe T et al. Pattern differences in experimental fevers induced by endotoxin, endogenous pyrogen, and prostaglandins. *Am J Physiol* 1988; 254(4 Pt 2): R633–R640. https://www.ncbi.nlm.nih.gov/pubmed/3258478

Nagase T, Mikami T, Suzuki S et al. Pyrogenicity of yeast mannans in rabbits. *Microbiol Immunol* 1984; 28(6): 651–657. https://www.ncbi.nlm.nih.gov/pubmed/6384740

Olszewer E, Teruya JR, eds. *Terapia Nutricional; Parenteral em Ortomolecular.* Sao Paulo, Brazil: Editora Apes, 2009, pp. 21–32.

Poblaciones MJ, Rengel Z. Soil and foliar zinc biofortification in field pea (Pisum sativum L.): Grain accumulation and bioavailability in raw and cooked grains. *Food Chem* 2016 Dec 1; 212: 427–433. https://www.ncbi.nlm.nih.gov/pubmed/27374552

Remington J. *The Science and Practice of Pharmacy.* 19th Edition. Volme 1. Pennsylvania: Mack Printing Co., 1995.

Rosimar L. Silveira, Simone S. Andrade, Schmidt CA et al. Comparative evaluation of pyrogens tests in pharmaceutical products. *Braz J Microbiol* 2004; 35: 48–53. http://www.scielo.br/scielo.php?script=sci_arttext&pid=S1517-83822004000100007

Roth J, Blatteis CM. Mechanisms of fever production and lysis: Lessons from experimental LPS fever. *Compr Physiol* 2014 Oct; 4(4): 1563–1604. https://www.ncbi.nlm.nih.gov/pubmed/25428854

Ruiz-Núñez B, Dijck-Brouwer DA, Muskiet FA. The relation of saturated fatty acids with low-grade inflammation and cardiovascular disease. *J Nutr Biochem* 2016 Oct; 36: 1–20. https://www.ncbi.nlm.nih.gov/pubmed/27692243

Saldaña–Ambulódegui E. *Manual de Inyectables y Venoclisis.* Trujillo: Perú, 2012. https://dokumen.tips/documents/manual-de-venoclisis-y-inyectables.html, Accessed April 10, 2018.

Saxena A, Bawa AS, Raju PS. Phytochemical changes in fresh-cut jackfruit (Artocarpus heterophyllus L) bulbs during modified atmosphere storage. *Food Chem* 2009; 115(4): 1443–1449. doi: 10.1016/j.foodchem.2009.01.080

Sobotka L, Schneider SM, Berner YN et al. ESPEN guidelines on parenteral nutrition: Geriatrics. *Clin Nutr* 2009; 28(4): 461–466. https://www.ncbi.nlm.nih.gov/pubmed/19464772

Taira T, Yamaguchi S, Takahashi A et al. Dietary polyphenols increase fecal mucin and immunoglobulin A and ameliorate the disturbance in gut microbiota caused by a high fat diet. *J Clin Biochem Nutr* 2015; Nov 57(3): 212–216. https://www.ncbi.nlm.nih.gov/pubmed/26566306

Teixeira TF, Collado MC, Ferreira CL et al. Potential mechanisms for the emerging link between obesity and increased intestinal permeability. *Nutr Res* 2012 Sep; 32(9): 637–647. https://www.ncbi.nlm.nih.gov/pubmed/23084636

Williams KL. *Microbial Contamination Control in Parenteral Manufacturing.* New Torl, NY: Marcel Dekker, 2005, p. 61.

World Health Organization (WHO). Aide-memoire for a national strategy for the safe and appropriate use of injections. Geneva, 2003. http://www.who.int/infection-prevention/tools/injections/AideMemoire-injection-safety.pdf, Accessed April 10, 2018.

Woting A, Blaut M. The Intestinal Microbiota in Metabolic Disease. *Nutrients* 2016 Apr 6; 8(4): 202. https://www.ncbi.nlm.nih.gov/pubmed/27058556

Yamamoto T, Ishihara K, eds. Stability of Glutathione in Solution. Developments in Food Engineering. *Proceedings of the 6th International Congress on Engineering and Food*, Springer, 1994, Chapter, pp. 209–211.

REFERENCES FOR PART II. A. SPECIFIC PRODUCTS FOR USE IN ORTHOMOLECULAR INTRAVENOUS NUTRITIONAL THERAPY

Ali A, Njike VY, Northrup V et al. Intravenous micronutrient therapy (Myers' Cocktail) for fibromyalgia: A placebo-controlled pilot study. *J Altern Complement Med* 2009; 15(3): 247–257.

Blanchard J, Tozer TN, Rowland M. Pharmacokinetic perspectives on megadoses of ascorbic acid. *Am J Clin Nutr* 1997; 66: 1165–1171.

Booth BE, Johanson A. Hypomagnesemia due to renal tubular defect in reabsorption of magnesium. *J Pediatr* 1974; 85: 350–354.

Brunner EH, Delabroise AM, Haddad ZH. Effect of parenteral magnesium on pulmonary function, plasma cAMP, and histamine in bronchial asthma. *J Asthma* 1985; 22: 3–11.

Cameron E. Protocol for the use of vitamin C in the treatment of cancer. *Med Hypotheses* 1991; 36(3): 190–194.

Cameron E, Campbell A, Jack T. The orthomolecular treatment of cancer. III. Reticulum cell sarcoma: Double complete regression induced by high-dose ascorbic acid therapy. *Chem Biol Interact* 1975; 11(5): 387–393.

Cameron E, Pauling L. Ascorbic acid and the glycosaminoglycans. An orthomolecular approach to cancer and other diseases. *Oncology* 1973; 27(2): 181–192.

Cameron E, Pauling L. The orthomolecular treatment of cancer. I. The role of ascorbic acid in host resistance. *Chem Biol Interact* 1974; 9(4): 273–283.

Cameron E, Pauling L. Supplemental ascorbate in the supportive treatment of cancer: Prolongation of survival times in terminal human cancer. *Proc Natl Acad Sci U S A* 1976; 73(10): 3685–3689.

Cameron E, Pauling L. Supplemental ascorbate in the supportive treatment of cancer: Reevaluation of prolongation of survival times in terminal human cancer. *Proc Natl Acad Sci U S A* 1978; 75(9): 4538–4542.

Cameron E, Pauling L, Leibovitz B. Ascorbic acid and cancer: A review. *Cancer Res* 1979 Mar; 39(3): 663–681.

Camp KM, Lloyd-Puryear MA, Yao L et al. Expanding research to provide an evidence base for nutritional interventions for the management of inborn errors of metabolism. *Mol Genet Metab* 2013 Aug; 109(4): 319–328. Epub 2013 May 23.

Creagan ET, Moertel CG, O'Fallon JR et al. Failure of high-dose vitamin C (ascorbic acid) therapy to benefit patients with advanced cancer. A controlled trial. *N Engl J Med* 1979; 301(13): 687–690.

Duconge J, Miranda-Massari JR, González MJ et al. Vitamin C pharmacokinetics after continuous infusion in a patient with prostate cancer. *Ann Pharmacother* 2007; 41(6): 1082–1083.

Forman HJ, Zhang H, Rinna A. Glutathione: Overview of its protective roles, measurement, and biosynthesis. *Mol Aspects Med* 2009; 30(1–2): 1–12.

Frustaci A, Caldarulo M, Schiavoni G et al. Myocardial magnesium content, histology, and antiarrhythmic response to magnesium infusion. *Lancet* 1987; 2: 1019.

Gaby AR. Intravenous nutrient therapy: The "Myers' cocktail". *Altern Med Rev* 2002; 7(5): 389–403.

González MJ, Miranda-Massari JR, Mora EM et al. Orthomolecular oncology review: Ascorbic acid and cancer 25 years later. *Integr Cancer Ther* 2005; 4(1): 32–44.

Harakeh S, Jariwalla RJ, Pauling L. Suppression of human immunodeficiency virus replication by ascorbate in chronically and acutely infected cells. *Proc Natl Acad Sci U S A* 1990; 87: 7245–7249.

Henrotte JG. The variability of human red blood cell magnesium level according to HLA groups. *Tissue Antigens* 1980; 15: 419–430.

Iseri LT, French JH. Magnesium: Nature's physiologic calcium blocker. *Am Heart J* 1984; 108: 188–193.

McCormick W. Cancer: A collagen disease, secondary to nutrition deficiency. *Arch Pediatr* 1959; 76: 166–171.

Merrill A. Nutrition in chronic renal failure. *Am J Clin Nutr* 1956; 4(5): 497–508.

Mikirova N, Hunnunghake R, Scimeca RC et al. High-dose intravenous vitamin C treatment of a child with neurofibromatosis type 1 and optic pathway glioma: A case report. *Am J Case Rep* 2016a; 17: 774–781.

Mikirova NA, Ichim TE, Riordan NH. Anti-angiogenic effect of high doses of ascorbic acid. *J Transl Med* 2008; 6: 50.

Mikirova N, Riordan N, Casciari J. Modulation of cytokines in cancer patients by intravenous ascorbate therapy. *Med Sci Monit* 2016b; 22: 14–25.

Minareci E, Uzunoğlu S, Minareci O. Incidence of severe glucose-6-phosphate dehydrogenase(G6PD) deficiency in countryside villages of the central city of Manisa, Turkey. *EJGM* 2006; 3(1): 5–10.

Moertel CG, Fleming TR, Creagan ET et al. High-dose vitamin C versus placebo in the treatment of patients with advanced cancer who have no prior chemotherapy: A randomized double-blind comparison. *NEJM* 1985; 312: 137–141.

Okayama H, Aikawa T, Okayama M et al. Bronchodilating effect of intravenous magnesium sulfate in bronchial asthma. *JAMA* 1987; 257: 1076–1078.

Padayatty SJ, Riordan HD, Hewitt SM, Katz A, Hoffer LJ, Levine M. Intravenously administered vitamin C as cancer therapy: Three cases. *CMAJ* 2006 Mar 28; 174(7): 937–942.

Padayatty SJ, Sun H, Wang Y et al. Vitamin C pharmacokinetics: Implications for oral and intravenous use. *Ann Intern Med* 2004; 140: 533–537.

Riordan H, Hunninghake RB, Riordan NH et al. Intravenous ascorbic acid: Protocol for its application and use. *P R Health Sci J* 2003; 22: 225–232.

Riordan HD, Casciari JJ, González MJ, Riordan NH, Miranda-Massari JR, Taylor P, Jackson JA. A pilot clinical study of continuous intravenous ascorbate in terminal cancer patients. *P R Health Sci J* 2005 Dec; 24(4): 269–276.

Sárközy M, Fekete V, Szűcs G et al. Anti-diabetic effect of a preparation of vitamins, minerals and trace elements in diabetic rats: A gender difference. *BMC Endocr Disord* 2014; 14: 72.

Sydow M, Crozier TA, Zielmann S et al. High-dose intravenous magnesium sulfate in the management of life-threatening status asthmaticus. *Intensive Care Med* 1993; 19: 467–471.

Uchida K, Mitsui M, Kawakishi S. Monooxygenation of N-acetylhistamine mediated by L-ascorbate. *Biochim Biophys Acta* 1989; 991: 377–379.

Vitamin C

Anderson TW, Suranyi G, Beaton GH. The effect on winter illness of large doses of vitamin C. *Canad Med Assoc J* 1974; 111(1): 31–36.

Arena A, Bisignano G, Pavone B et al. Antiviral and immunomodulatory effect of a lyophilized extract of Capparis spinosa L. buds. *Phytother Res* 2008; 22(3): 313–317.

Benke KK. Modelling ascorbic acid level in plasma and its dependence on absorbed dose. *J Aust Coll Nutr Environ Med* 1999; 18(1): 11–12.

Bergsten P, Amitai G, Kehrl J et al. Millimolar concentrations of ascorbic acid in purified human mononuclear leukocytes. Depletion and reaccumulation. *J Biol Chem* 1990; 265(5): 2584–2587.

Bruunsgaard H, Poulsen HE, Pedersen BK et al. Long-term combined supplementation with alpha-tocopherol and vitamin C have no detectable anti-inflammatory effects in healthy men. *J Nutr* 2003; 133(4): 1170–1173.

Calder PC, Albers R, Antoine JM et al. Inflammatory disease processes and interactions with nutrition. *Br J Nutr* 2009; 1: S1–S45.

Cameron E, Campbell A. The orthomolecular treatment of cancer: II. Clinical trial of high-dose ascorbic acid supplements in advanced human cancer. *Chem Biol Interact* 1974; 9: 285–315.

Cameron E, Pauling L. Supplemental ascorbate in the supportive treatment of cancer: Prolongation of survival times in terminalhumancancer. *Proc Natl Acad Sci USA* 1976; 73: 3685–3689.

Cameron E, Pauling L. Supplemental ascorbate in the supportive treatment of cancer: Reevaluation of prolongation of survival times in terminal human cancer. *Proc Natl Acad Sci USA* 1978; 75: 4538–4542.

Cevikel MH, Tuncyurek P, Ceylan F et al. Supplementation with high-dose ascorbic acid improves intestinal anastomotic healing. *Eur Surg Res* 2008; 40: 29–33.

Chakraborthy A, Ramani P, Sherlin HJ et al. Antioxidant and pro-oxidant activity of Vitamin C in oral environment. *Indian J of Dental Res* 2014; 25(4): 499–507.

Chambial S, Dwivedi S, Shukla KK et al. Vitamin C in disease prevention and cure: An overview. *Indian J Clin Biochem* 2013; 28(4): 314–328. https://www.ncbi.nlm.nih.gov/pmc/articles/PMC3783921/

Chen Q, Espey MG, Sun AY et al. Ascorbate in pharmacologic concentrations selectively generates ascorbate radical and hydrogen peroxide in extracellular fluid in vivo. *Proc Natl Acad Sci USA* 2007; 104: 8749–8754.

Chen Q, Espey MG, Sun AY et al. Pharmacologic doses of ascorbate act as a prooxidant and decrease growth of aggressive tumor xenografts in mice. *Proc Natl Acad Sci USA* 2008; 105: 11105–11109.

Ciuman RR. Phytotherapeutic and naturopathic adjuvant therapies in otorhinolaryngology. *Eur Arch Otorhinolaryngol* 2012; 269(2): 389–397.

Cook NR, Albert CM, Gaziano JM et al. A randomized factorial trial of vitamins C and E and betacarotene in the secondary prevention of cardiovascular events in women: Results from the Women's Antioxidant Cardiovascular Study. *Arch Intern Med* 2007; 167: 1610–1618.

Douglas RM, Hemilä H. Vitamin C for preventing and treating the common cold. *PLoS Med* 2005; 2(6): e168. doi: 10.1371/journal.pmed.0020168

Douglas RM, Hemilä H, Chalker E et al. Vitamin C for preventing and treating the common cold. *Cochrane Database Syst Rev* 2007; July 18(3): CD000980.

Duconge J, Miranda-Massari JR, Gonzalez MJ et al. Pharmacokinetics of vitamin C: Insights into the oral and intravenous administration of ascorbate. *P R Health Sci J* 2008; 27(1): 7–19.

Enbergs H. Effects of the homeopathic preparation Engystol on interferon-gamma production by human T-lymphocytes. *Immunol Invest* 2006; 35(1): 19–27.

Ferrón-Celma I, Mansilla A, Hassan L et al. Effect of vitamin C administration on neutrophil apoptosis in septic patients after abdominal surgery. *J Surg Res* 2009; 153(2): 224–230.

Fimiani V, Cavallaro A, Ainis O et al. Immunomodulatory effect of the homoeopathic drug Engystol-N on some activities of isolated human leukocytes and in whole blood. *Immunopharmacol Immunotoxicol* 2000; 22(1): 103–115.

Fritz H, Flower G, Weeks L et al. Intravenous vitamin C and cancer: A systematic review. *Integr Cancer Ther* 2014; 13(4): 280–300.

Furuya A, Uozaki M, Yamasaki H et al. H. Antiviral effects of ascorbic and dehydroascorbic acids in vitro. *Int J Mol Med* 2008; 22(4): 541–545.

Hemilä H, Chalker E. Vitamin C for preventing and treating the common cold. *Cochrane Database Syst Rev* 2013; 1: CD000980. doi: 10.1002/14651858.CD000980

Hickey S, Roberts H. Misleading Information on the Properties of Vitamin C. *PLoS Med* 2005; 2(9): e307. doi: 10.1371/journal.pmed.0020307

Hickey S, Roberts HJ, Cathcart RF. Dynamic flow: A new model for ascorbate. *J Orthomol Med* 2005; 20(4): 237–244.

Hininger I, Water R, Osman M et al. Acute prooxidant effects of vitamin C in EDTA chelation therapy and long-term antioxidant benefits of therapy. *Free Radic Biol Med* 2005; 38(12): 1565–1570.

Holmannová D, Koláčková M, Krejsek J. [Vitamin C and its physiological role with respect to the components of the immune system]. *Vnitr Lek* 2012; 58(10): 743–749.

Hume R, Weyers E, Rowan T et al. Leucocyte ascorbic acid levels after acute myocardial infarction. *Br Heart J* 1972; 34: 238–243.

Ichim TE, Minev B, Braciak T et al. Intravenous ascorbic acid to prevent and treat cancer-associated sepsis? *J Transl Med* 2011; 4: 9–25.

Jacobs C, Hutton B, NG T et al. Is there a role for oral or intravenous ascorbate (vitamin C) in treating patients with cancer? A systematic review. *Oncologist* 2015; 20: 210–223.

Kiziltan HS, Bayir AG, Demirtas M et al. Ascorbic-acid treatment for progressive bone metastases after radiotherapy: A pilot study. *Altern Ther Health Med* 2014; 20(Suppl. 2): 16–20.

Levine M, Conry-Cantilena C, Wang Y et al. Vitamin C pharmacokinetics in healthy volunteers: Evidence for a recommended dietary allowance. *Proc Nat Acad Scien USA* 1996; 93(8): 3704–3709.

Levine M, Padayatty SJ, Espey MG. Vitamin C: A concentration-function approach yields pharmacology and therapeutic discoveries. *Adv Nutr* 2011; 2: 78–88.

Levine M, Rumsey SC, Daruwala R et al. Criteria and recommendations for vitamin C intake. *JAMA* 1999; 281(15): 1415–1423.

Levy TE. *Stop America's # 1 Killer! Reversible Vitamin Deficiency Found to be Origin of All Coronary Heart Disease.* Henderson, NV: Livon Books, 2006.

Lu NT, Crespi CM, Liu NM et al. A phase I dose escalation study demonstrates quercetin safety and explores potential for bioflavonoid antivirals in patients with chronic hepatitis C. *Phytother Res* 2016; 30(1): 160–168.

McCracken RD. *Injectable Vitamin C and the Treatment of Viral and Other Diseases. A Compilation of Pioneering Literature.* 2nd Edition. Long Beach, CA: Hygea Publishing Co, 2004.

Mendes-da-Silva RF. Prooxidant versus antioxidant brain action of ascorbic acid in well-nourished and malnourished rats as a function of dose: A cortical spreading depression and malondialdehyde analysis. *Neuropharmacology* 2014; 86: 155–160.

Mendiratas S, Qu ZC, May JM. Erythrocyte ascorbate recycling: Antioxidant effects in blood. *Free Radic Biol Med* 1998; 24: 789–797.

Mikirova NA, Casciari JJ, Hunninghake RE et al. Intravenous ascorbic acid protocol for cancer patients: Scientific rationale, pharmacology, and clinical experience. *FFHD* 2013; 3(8): 344–366.

Mikirova NA, Hunninghake R. Effect of high dose vitamin C on Epstein-Barr viral infection. *Med Sci Monit* 2014; 20: 725–732.

Moser MA, Chun OK. Vitamin C and heart health: A review based on findings from epidemiologic studies. *Int J Mol Sci* 2016; 17(8): 1328.

Myung SK, Ju W, Cho B et al. Efficacy of vitamin and antioxidant supplements in prevention of cardiovascular disease: Systematic review and meta-analysis of randomised controlled trials. *BMJ* 2013; 346: f10.

Oberbaum M, Glatthaar-Saalmüller B, Stolt P et al. Antiviral activity of Engystol: An in vitro analysis. *J Altern Complement Med* 2005; 11(5): 855–862.

Park S. The effects of high concentrations of vitamin C on cancer cells. *Nutrients* 2013; 5(9): 3496–3505.

Riordan NH, Riordan HD, Meng X et al. Intravenous ascorbate as a tumor cytotoxic chemotherapeutic agent. *Med Hypotheses* 1995; 44: 207–213.

Roeska K, Seilheimer B. Antiviral activity of Engystol and Gripp-Heel: An in-vitro assessment. *J Immune Based Ther Vaccines* 2010; 8: 6.

Seno T, Inoue N, Matsui K et al. Functional expression of sodium-dependent vitamin C transporter 2 in human endothelial cells. *J Vasc Res* 2004; 41: 345–351.

Sesso HD, Buring JE, Christen WG et al. Vitamins E and C in the prevention of cardiovascular disease in men. *J Am Med Assoc* 2008; 300: 2123–2133.

Sorice A, Guerriero E, Capone F et al. Ascorbic acid: Its role in immune system and chronic inflammation diseases. *Mini Rev Med Chem* 2014; 14(5): 444–452.

Stephensen CB, Marquis GS, Jacob, RA et al. Vitamins C and E in adolescents and young adults with HIV infection. *Am J Clin Nutr* 2006; 83(4): 870–879.

Traber MG, Stevens JF. Vitamins C and E: Beneficial effects from a mechanistic perspective. *Free Radic Biol Med* 2011; 51(5): 1000–10013. doi: 10.1016/j.freeradbiomed.2011.05.017

Tveden-Nyborg P, Lykkesfeldt J. Does vitamin C deficiency increase lifestyle-associated vascular disease progression? Evidence based on experimental and clinical studies. *Antioxid Redox Signal* 2013; 19(17): 2084–2104.

Viebahn–Hänsler R. Chapter III – Indications for ozone therapy, section 4. Infections and virus caused disease. In: Viebahn–Hänsler R, ed. *The Use of Ozone in Medicine.* 5th English Edition. Iffezheim, Germany: Odrei Publishers, 2007, pp. 83–89.

Welsby PD. Reductionism in medicine: Some thoughts on medical education from the clinical front line. *J Eval Clin Prac* 1999; 5(2): 125–131.

White LA, Freeman CY, Forrester BD, Chappell WA. In vitro effect of ascorbic acid on infectivity of herpesviruses and paramyxoviruses. *J Clin Microbiol* 1986; 24(4): 527–531.

Yeom CH, Lee G, Park JH et al. High dose concentration administration of ascorbic acid inhibits tumor growth in BALB/C mice implanted with sarcoma 180 cancer cells via the restriction of angiogenesis. *J Transl Med* 2009; 7: 70.

Zhang ZW, Farthing MIG. Helicobacter Pylori and gastric malignancy: Importance of oxidants, antioxidants and other cofactors. In: Hunt RH, Tytgat GNJ, eds. *Helicobacter Pylor: Basic Mechanisms to Clinical Cure*. London: Kluwer Academic Publishers, 2000, pp. 513–524.

Zhang ZW, Patchett SE, Perrett D et al. Gastric alpha-tocopherol and beta-carotene concentrations in association with Helicobacter pylori infection. *Eur J Gastroenterol Hepatol* 2000; 12(5): 497–503.

L-Glutathione (GSH)

Aebi S, Assereto R, Lauterburg BH. High-dose intravenous glutathione in man. Pharmacokinetics and effects on cyst(e)ine in plasma and urine. *Eur J Clin Investig* 1991; 21: 103–110.

Allen J, Bradley RD. Effects of oral glutathione supplementation on systemic oxidative stress biomarkers in human volunteers. *J Altern Complement Med* 2011; 17(9): 827–833.

American Cancer Society. Editorial Board. CA: A Cancer Journal for Clinicians Author Guidelines'. *Submission Guidelines*. Available at: http://onlinelibrary.wiley.com/journal/10.3322/%28ISSN%291542-4863/homepage/CA_Author_Guidelines.pdf and http://onlinelibrary.wiley.com/journal/10.3322/%28ISSN%291542-4863/homepage/ForAuthors.html, Accessed May 22, 2017.

Aw TY, Wierzbicka G, Jones DP. Oral glutathione increases tissue glutathione in vivo. *Chem Biol Interact* 1991; 80(1): 89–97.

Bains JS, Shaw CA. Neurodegenerative disorders in humans: The role of glutathione in oxidative stress-mediated neuronal death. *Brain Res Brain Res Rev* 1997; 25: 335–358.

Ballatori N, Krance SM, Notenboom S et al. Glutathione dysregulation and the etiology and progression of human diseases. *Biol Chem* 2009; 390(3): 191–214.

Bast A, Haenen GR. Interplay between lipoic acid and glutathione in the protection against microsomal lipid peroxidation. *Biochim Biophys Acta* 1988; 963(3): 558–561.

Bekelman JE, Li Y, Gross CP. Scope and impact of financial conflicts of interest in biomedical research. *JAMA* 2003; 289: 454–465.

Birben E, Sahiner UM, Sackesen C et al. Oxidative stress and antioxidant defense. *World Allergy Organ J* 2012; 5(1): 9–19.

Block KI, Koch AC, Mead MN et al. Impact of antioxidant supplementation on chemotherapeutic efficacy: A systematic review of the evidence from randomized controlled trials. *Cancer Treat Rev* 2007; 33(5): 407–418.

Blumenthal D, Campbell EG, Anderson MS et al. Withholding research results in academic life science: Evidence from a national survey of faculty. *JAMA* 1997; 277: 1224–1228.

Bremer HJ, Duran M, Kameling JP. Glutathione. In: Bremer HJ, Duran M, Kamerling JP et al., eds. *Disturbances of Amino Acid Metabolism: Clinical Chemistry and Diagnosis*. Urban and Schwarzenberg: Baltimore-Munich, 1981, pp. 80–82.

Brodwin E. These Are The Drugs Doctors Get Paid The Most To Promote. *Bussiness Insider*, January 9, 2015. Available at: http://www.businessinsider.com/what-drugs-are-doctors-paid-the-most-to-promote-2015-1, Accessed April 8, 2017.

Cascinu S, Cordella L, Del Ferro E et al. Neuroprotective effect of reduced glutathione on cisplatin-based chemotherapy in advanced gastric cancer: A randomized double-blind placebo-controlled trial. *J Clin Oncol* 1995; 13(1): 26–32.

Chen P, Stone J, Sullivan G et al. Anti-cancer effect of pharmacologic ascorbate and its interaction with supplementary parenteral glutathione in preclinical cancer models. *Free Radic Biol Med* 2011; 51(3): 681–687.

D'Andrea G. Use of antioxidants during chemotherapy and radiotherapy should be avoided. *CA Cancer J Clin* 2005; 55: 319–321.

Davidoff F, DeAngelis CD, Drazen JM et al. Editorial: Sponsorship, authorship, and accountability. *N Engl J Med* 2001; 345: 825–826.

DeMaria D, Falchi AM, Venturino P. Adjuvant radiotherapy of the pelvis with or without reduced glutathione: A randomized trial in patients operated on for endometrial cancer. *Tumori* 1992; 78: 374–376.

Dettman I, Meakin C, Allen R. Co-infusing glutathione and vitamin C during cancer treatment—A reply. *ACNEM Journal* 2012; 31(1): 8–11. Available at: https://nutritioncollege.org/sites/default/files/Co-infusing%20glutathione%20and%20vitamin%20C%20during%20cancer%20treatment%20-%20a%20reply.pdf, Accessed May 26, 2017.

Doshi P, Jefferson T, Del Mar C. The imperative to share clinical study reports: Recommendations from the tamiflu experience. *PLoS Med* 2012; 9(4): e1001201. doi: 10.1371/journal.pmed.1001201

Hagen TM, Wierzbicka GT, Sillau AH et al. Bioavailability of dietary glutathione: Effect on plasma concentration. *Am J Physiol* 1990; 259(4 Pt 1): G524–G529.

Hauser RA, Lyons KE, McClain T et al. Randomized, double-blind, pilot evaluation of intravenous glutathione in Parkinson's disease. *Mov Disord* 2009; 24(7): 979–983.

Hayes JD, McLellan LI. Glutathione and glutathione-dependent enzymes represent a co-ordinately regulated defence against oxidative stress. *Free Radic Res* 1999; 31(4): 272–300.

Kern JK, Geier DA, Adams JB et al. A clinical trial of glutathione supplementation in autism spectrum disorders. *Med Sci Monit* 2011; 17(12): CR677–CR682.

Kidd PM. Glutathione: Systemic protectant against oxidative and free radical damage. *Altern Med Rev* 1997; 1: 155–176.

Kleinman WA, Richie JP Jr. Status of glutathione and other thiols and disulfides in human plasma. *Biochem Pharmacol* 2000; 60: 19–29.

Krebs H. 6. Kapitel: Onkologie. In: *Vitamin-C-Hochdosistherapie Leitfaden für die therapeutische Praxis*. Seiten 81–124. 2. Auflage. Elsevier Urban & Fischer Verlag, 2010.

Ladas E, Kelly KM. The antioxidant debate. Chapter 9. In: Abrams DI, Weil AT eds. *Integrative Oncology*. Oxford University Press: New York, 2009, pp. 195–214.

Landefeld CS, Steinman MA. The Neurontin legacy: Marketing through misinformation and manipulation. *New Engl J Med* 2009; 360: 103–106.

Leucht S, Helfer B, Gartlehner G, Davis JM. How effective are common medications: A perspective based on meta-analyses of major drugs. *BMC Med* 2015; 13: 253. doi: 10.1186/s12916-015-0494-1

Lomaestro BM, Malone M. Glutathione in health and disease: Pharmacotherapeutic issues. *Ann Pharmacother* 1995; 29: 1263–1273.

McCarthy M. US doctors earn speaking and consulting fees from drug companies that sponsor their research. *BMJ* 2014; 348: g2410; 348. Published March 27, 2014. doi: 10.1136/bmj.g2410

Mills BJ, Richie JP Jr, Lang CA. Glutathione disulfide variability in normal human blood. *Anal Biochem* 1994; 222: 95–101.

Mischley LK. Glutathione deficiency in Parkinson's disease: Intranasal administration as a method of augmentation. *J Orthomol Med* 2011; 26(1): 32–36.

Mischley LK. Glutathione in Parkinson's Disease. *A dissertation submitted in partial fulfillment of the requirements for the degree of Doctor of Philosophy*. University of Washington, 2016. Available at: https://digital. lib.washington.edu/researchworks/bitstream/handle/1773/36458/Mischley_washington_0250E_15659. pdf, Accessed March 25, 2017.

Mischley LK, Conley KE, Shankland EG et al. Central nervous system uptake of intranasal glutathione in Parkinson's disease. *NPJ* 2016; 2: 16002; 6 pages. doi: 10.1038/npjparkd.2016.2

Mischley LK, Leverenz JB, Lau RC et al. A randomized, double-blind phase I/IIa study of intranasal glutathione in Parkinson's disease. *Mov Disord* 2015; 30: 1696–1701.

Mischley LK, Vespignani MF, Finnell JS. Safety survey of intranasal glutathione. *J Altern Complement Med* 2013; 19(5): 459–463.

Morgan G, Ward R, Barton M. The contribution of cytotoxic chemotherapy to 5-year survival in adult malignancies. *Clin Oncol (R Coll Radiol)* 2004; 16(8): 549–560.

Moss RW. Should patients undergoing chemotherapy and radiotherapy be prescribed antioxidants? *Integr Cancer Ther* 2006; 5(1): 63–82.

Murray RK. Metabolism of xenobiotics. In: Murray RK, Granner DK, Mayes PA et al., eds. *Harper's Biochemistry*. 24th Edition. Stamford, CT: Appleton and Lange, 1996.

Naito Y, Matsuo K, Kokubo Y et al. Higher-dose glutathione therapy for Parkinson's disease in Japan: Is it really safe? *Mov Disord* 2010; 25(7): 962; author reply 962–963.

Okun MS, Lang A, Jankovic J. Reply: Based on the available randomized trial patients should say no to glutathione for Parkinson's disease. *Mov Disord* 2010; 25(7): 961–962; author reply 962–963.

Oriana S, Bohm S, Spatti G et al. A preliminary clinical experience with reduced glutathione as protector against cisplatin toxicity. *Tumori* 1987; 73: 337–340.

Ornstein C, Sagara E, Grochowski Jones R. As full disclosure nears, doctors' pay for drug talks plummets. In: *Dollars for Doctors. How Industry Money Reaches Physicians*. Available at: https://www. propublica.org/article/as-full-disclosure-nears-doctors-pay-for-drug-talks-plummets, Accessed April 10, 2017.

Raza H. Dual localization of glutathione S-transferase in the cytosol and mitochondria: Implications in oxidative stress, toxicity and disease. *FEBS J* 2011; 278(22): 4243–4251.

Richie JP, Nichenametla S, Calcagnotto A et al. Enhanced Glutathione Levels in Blood and Buccal Cells by Oral Glutathione Supplementation. *FASEB J* 2013; 27(Suppl. 1): 862.32.

Richie JP Jr, Nichenametla S, Neidig W et al. Randomized controlled trial of oral glutathione supplementation on body stores of glutathione. *Eur J Nutr* 2015; 54(2): 251–263.

Rushworth GF, Megson IL. Existing and potential therapeutic uses for N-acetylcysteine: The need for conversion to intracellular glutathione for antioxidant benefits. *Pharmacol Ther* 2014; 141(2): 150–159.

Schulz JB, Lindenau J, Seyfried J et al. Glutathione, oxidative stress and neurodegeneration. *Eur J Biochem* 2000; 267(16): 4904–4911.

Sechi G, Deledda MG, Bua G et al. Reduced intravenous glutathione in the treatment of early Parkinson's disease. *Prog Neuropsychopharmacol Biol Psychiatry* 1996; 20: 1159–1170.

Simone CB 2nd, Simone NL, Simone V et al. Antioxidants and other nutrients do not interfere with chemotherapy or radiation therapy and can increase kill and increase survival, Part 1. *Altern Ther Health Med* 2007a; 13(1): 22–28.

Simone CB 2nd, Simone NL, Simone V et al. Antioxidants and other nutrients do not interfere with chemotherapy or radiation therapy and can increase kill and increase survival, part 2. *Altern Ther Health Med* 2007b; 13(2): 40–47.

Smith R. Medical journals are an extension of the marketing arm of pharmaceutical companies. *PLoS Med* 2005; 2: e138.

Smyth JF, Bowman A, Perren T et al. Glutathione reduces the toxicity and improves quality of life of women diagnosed with ovarian cancer treated with cisplatin: Results of a double-blind, randomised trial. *Ann Oncol* 1997; 8(6): 569–573.

Tedeschi M, Bohm S, Di Re F et al. Glutathione and detoxification. *Cancer Treat Rev* 1990; 17(2–3): 203–208.

The PLoS Medicine Editors. An unbiased scientific record should be everyone's agenda. *PLoS Med* 2009; 6(2): e1000038. https://doi.org/10.1371/journal.pmed.1000038

Traverso N, Ricciarelli R, Nitti M et al. Role of glutathione in cancer progression and chemoresistance. *Oxid Med Cell Longev* 2013; 2013: 10, Article ID 972913, 10 pages, 2013. doi: 10.1155/2013/972913

Visca A, Bishop CT, Hilton S, Hudson VM. Oral reduced l-glutathione improves growth in pediatric cystic fibrosis patients: A randomized clinical trial. *J Pediatr Gastroenterol Nutr* 2015; 60(6): 802–810.

Witschi A, Reddy S, Stofer B, Lauterburg BH. The systemic availability of oral glutathione. *Eur J Clin Pharmacol* 1992; 43(6): 667–669.

Zeevalk GD, Razmpour R, Bernard LP. Glutathione and Parkinson's disease: Is this the elephant in the room? *Biomed Pharmacother* 2008; 62(4): 236–249.

Zunino F, Pratesi G, Micheloni A et al. Protective effect of reduced glutathione against cisplatin-induced renal and systemic toxicity and its influence on the therapeutic activity of the antitumor drug. *Chem Biol Interact* 1989; 70: 89–101.

Zunino F, Tofanetti O, Besati A et al. Protective effect of reduced glutathione against cis-dichlorodiammine platinum(II)-induced nephrotoxiclty and lethal toxicity. *Tumori* 1983; 69: 105–111.

Alpha Lipoic Acid (ALA)

Biewenga GP, Haenen GR, Bast A. The pharmacology of the antioxidant lipoic acid. *Gen Pharmacol* 1997; 29(3): 315–331.

Bock E, Schneeweiss J. Ein Beitrag zur Therapie der neuropathia diabetic. *Munchner Med Wochenschrift* 1959; 43: 1911–1912.

Flora SJ, Shrivastava R, Mittal M. Chemistry and pharmacological properties of some natural and synthetic antioxidants for heavy metal toxicity. *Curr Med Chem* 2013; 20(36): 4540–4574.

Holmquist L, Stuchbury G, Berbaum K. Lipoic acid as a novel treatment for Alzheimer's disease and related dementias. *Pharmacol Ther* 2007; 113(1): 154–164. https://www.ncbi.nlm.nih.gov/pubmed/16989905

Huk-Kolega H, Skibska B. Role of lipoic acid in health and disease. *Pol Merkur Lekarski* 2011; 31(183): 183–185.

Jung TS, Kim SK, Shin HJ et al. α-lipoic acid prevents non-alcoholic fatty liver disease in OLETF rats. *Liver Int* 2012; 32(10): 1565–1573.

Maczurek A, Hager K, Kenklies M et al. Lipoic acid as an anti-inflammatory and neuroprotective treatment for Alzheimer's disease. *Adv Drug Deliv Rev* 2008; 60(13–14): 1463–1470.

McMackin CJ, Widlansky ME, Hamburg NM et al. Effect of combined treatment with alpha lipoic acid and Acetyl-L-Carnitine on vascular function and blood pressure in coronary artery disease patients. *J Clin Hypertension (Greenwich, Conn)* 2007; 9(4): 249–255.

Midaoui AE, Elimadi A, Wu L et al. Lipoic acid prevents hypertension, hyperglycemia, and the increase in heart mitochondrial superoxide production. *Am J Hypertens* 2003; 16(3): 173–179.

Mijnhout GS, Kollen BJ, Alkhalaf A et al. Alpha lipoic acid for symptomatic peripheral neuropathy in patients with diabetes: A meta-analysis of randomized controlled trials. *Int J Endocrinol* 2012; 2012: 456279, Article ID 456279, 8 pages, 2012.

Nutrabiotics. NutraTips – Compendio de monografías 2016. Capítulo Ácido Alfa Lipóico en la regulación del metabolismo y de los sistemas enzimáticos mitocondriales. p. 67.

Papanas N, Ziegler D. Efficacy of α-lipoic acid in diabetic neuropathy. *Expert Opin Pharmacother* 2014; 15(18): 2721–2731.

Queiroz TM, Guimarães DD, Mendes-Junior LE et al. α-lipoic acid reduces hypertension and increases baroreflex sensitivity in renovascular hypertensive rats. *Molecules* 2012; 17(11): 13357–13367.

Rahman ST, Merchant N, Haque T et al. The impact of lipoic acid on endothelial function and proteinuria in quinapril-treated diabetic patients with stage I hypertension: Results from the QUALITY study. *J Cardiovasc Pharmacol Ther* 2012; 17(2): 139–145.

Shay KP, Moreau RF, Smith EJ et al. Alpha-lipoic acid as a dietary supplement: Molecular mechanisms and therapeutic potential. *Biochimica Biophysica Acta* 2009; 1790(10): 1149–1160. doi: 10.1016/j.bbagen.2009.07.026. Available at: www.ncbi.nlm.nih.gov/pubmed/19664690

Veljkovic AR, Nikolic RS, Kocic GM et al. Protective effects of glutathione and lipoic acid against cadmium-induced oxidative stress in rat's kidney. *Ren Fail* 2012; 34(10): 1281–1287.

Xu Y, Zhou X, Shi C et al. α-Lipoic acid protects against the oxidative stress and cytotoxicity induced by cadmium in HepG2 cells through regenerating glutathione regulated by glutamate-cysteine ligase. *Toxicol Mech Methods* 2015; 25(8): 596–603.

Ziegler D. Thioctic acid for patients with symptomatic diabetic polyneuropathy: A critical review. *Treat Endocrinol* 2004; 3(3): 173–189.

Ziegler D, Gries FA. Alpha-lipoic acid in the treatment of diabetic peripheral and cardiac autonomic neuropathy. *Diabetes* 1997; 46(Suppl. 2): S62–S66.

Ziegler D, Hanefeld M, Ruhnau KJ et al. Treatment of symptomatic diabetic polyneuropathy with the antioxidant alpha-lipoic acid. (ALADIN III Study). ALADIN III Study Group. *Diabetes Care* 1999; 22: 1296–1301.

Dimethyl Sulfoxide (DMSO)

Aberg F, Appelkvist EL, Dallner G et al. Distribution and redox state of ubiquinones in rat and human tissues. *Arch Biochem Biophys* 1961; 295(2): 230–234.

Adarsh K, Kaur H, Mohan V. Coenzyme Q10 (CoQ10) in isolated diastolic heart failure in hypertrophic cardiomyopathy (HCM). *Biofactors* 2008; 32(1–4): 145–149.

Alessandri MG, Scalori V, Giovannini L et al. Plasma and tissue concentrations of coenzyme Q10 in the rat after intravenous administration by a microsphere delivery system or in a new type of solution. *Int J Tiss React* 1988; 10: 99–102.

Arranz LI, Canela MA, Rafecas M. Fibromyalgia and nutrition, what do we know? *Rheumatol Int* 2010; 30(11): 1417–1427.

Balestrero R, Franzini M, Valdenassi L. Use of oxygen-ozone therapy in the treatment of fibromyalgia. *Ozone Therapy* 2017; 2: 6744.

Belardinelli R, Mucaj A, Lacalaprice F et al. Coenzyme Q10 and exercise training in chronic heart failure. *Eur Heart J* 2006; 27(22): 2675–2681.

Belousova M, Tokareva OG, Gorodetskaya E et al. Intravenous treatment with coenzyme Q10 improves neurological outcome and reduces infarct volume after transient focal brain ischemia in rats. *J Cardiovasc Pharmacol* 2016a; 67(2): 103–109.

Belousova MA, Tokareva OG, Gorodetskaya EA et al. Neuroprotective effectiveness of intravenous ubiquinone in rat model of irreversible cerebral ischemia. *Bull Exp Biol Med* 2016b; 161(2): 245–247.

Bhagavan HN, Chopra RK. Coenzyme Q10: Absorption, tissue uptake, metabolism and pharmacokinetics. *Free Radic Res* 2006; 40(5): 445–453.

Brayton CF. Dimethyl sulfoxide (DMSO): A review. *Cornell Vet* 1986; 76(1): 61–90.

Brobyn RD. The human toxicology of dimethyl sulfoxide. *Ann NY Acad Sci* 1975; 243: 497–506; Report of AD Hoc committee on dimethyl sulfoxide as a therapeutic agent. National Academy of Sciences, National Research Council, Division of Medical Sciences. Washington, DC, National Academy Press. 1973.

Celik T, Iyisoy A. Coenzyme Q10 and coronary artery bypass surgery: What we have learned from clinical trials. *J Cardiothorac Vasc Anesth* 2009; 23(6): 935–936.

Coenzyme Q10 (CoQ10)

Cordero MD, Alcocer-Gómez E, Culic O et al. NLRP3 inflammasome is activated in fibromyalgia: The effect of coenzyme Q10. *Antioxid Redox Signal* 2014; 20(8): 1169–1180.

Cordero MD, Alcocer-Gomez E, de Miguel M et al. Coenzyme Q10: A novel therapeutic approach for Fibromyalgia? Case series with 5 patients. *Mitochondrion* 2011; 11: 623–625.

Cordero MD, Cano-Garcia FJ, Alcocer-Gomez E et al. Oxidative stress correlates with headache symptoms in fibromyalgia: Coenzyme Q 10 effect on clinical improvement. *PLoS One* 2012; 7: e35677.

de la Torre JC, Sugeon JW, Ernest T et al. Subacute toxicity of intravenous dimethyl sulfoxide in rhesus monkeys. *J Toxicol Environ Health* 1981; 7: 49–57.

Demos CH, Beckloff GL, Donin MN, Oliver PM. Dimethyl sulfoxide in musculoskeletal disorders. *Ann NY Acad Sci* 1967; 141: 517–523.

Dosch P. *Manual of Neural Therapy According to Huneke.* 1st English Edition (translation of 11th German ed. Revised). Lindsay A, translator. Heidelberg, Germany: Karl F. Haug Publishers, 1984.

Eberhardt R, Zwingers T, Hoffman R. [DMSO in patients with active gonarthrosis. A double-blind, placebo-controlled phase III study.] [Article in German.]. *Fortschr Med* 1995; 113: 446–450.

Egocheaga J, del Valle M. Tratamiento con farmacología antihomotóxica de los síntomas asociados a fibromialgia. *Revista de la Sociedad Española del Dolor* 2004; 11(1): 4–8.

Evans MS, Reid KH, Sharp JB Jr. Dimethylsulfoxide (DMSO) blocks conduction in peripheral nerve C fibers: A possible mechanism of analgesia. *Neurosci Lett* 1993; 150(2): 145–148.

Garrido-Maraver J, Cordero MD, Oropesa-Ávila M et al. Coenzyme Q10 therapy. *Mol Syndromol* 2014; 5(3): 187–197.

Goldman AW, Burmeister Y, Cesnulevicius K et al. Bioregulatory systems medicine: An innovative approach to integrating the science of molecular networks, inflammation, and systems biology with the patient's autoregulatory capacity? *Front Physiol* 2015; 6: 225.

Gorodetskaya E, Kalenikova E, Medvedev O. PP.13.483 – Intravenous bolus of solubilized Coenzyme Q10 increased rapidly its myocardial and brain level. *J Hypertens* 2010; 28(e-Suppl. A): e196.

Hargreaves IP, Duncan AJ, Heales SJ et al. The effect of HMG-CoA reductase inhibitors on coenzyme Q10: Possible biochemical/clinical implications. *Drug Saf* 2005; 28(8): 659–676.

Heart Protection Study Collaborative Group. MRC/BHF Heart Protection Study of cholesterol lowering with simvastatin in 20,536 high-risk individuals: A randomised placebo-controlled trial. *Lancet* 2002; 360(9326): 7–22.

Hidalgo-Tallón J, Menéndez-Cepero S, Vilchez JS et al. Ozone therapy as add-on treatment in fibromyalgia management by rectal insufflation: An open-label pilot study. *J Altern Complement Med* 2013; 19(3): 238–242.

Ho MJ, Li ECK, Wright JM. Blood pressure lowering efficacy of coenzyme Q10 for primary hypertension. *Cochrane Database Syst Rev* 2016; Oct 7(3): CD007435. Art. No.: CD007435. doi: 10.1002/14651858. CD007435.pub3

Holton KF, Kindler LL, Jones KD. Potential dietary links to central sensitization in fibromyalgia: Past reports and future directions. *Rheum Dis Clin North Am* 2009; 35(2): 409–420.

Ivanov A, Gorodetskaya E, Kalenikova E et al. Single intravenous injection of CoQ10 reduces infarct size in a rat model of ischemia and reperfusion injury. *Bull Exp Biol Med* 2013a; 155(6): 771–778.

Ivanov AV, Gorodetskaya EA, Kalenikova EI et al. Single intravenous injection of coenzyme Q10 protects the myocardium after irreversible ischemia. *Bull Exp Biol Med* 2013b; 155(6): 771–774.

Ivanov A, Tokareva O, Gorodetskaya E et al. Cardioprotection with intravenous Injection of coenzyme Q10 is limited by time of administration after onset of myocardial infarction in rats. *Journal of Clinical and Experimental Cardiology* 2014; 5: 299.

Joustra ML, Minovic I, Janssens KA et al. Vitamin and mineral status in chronic fatigue syndrome and fibromyalgia syndrome: A systematic review and metaanalysis. *PLoS ONE* 2017; 12(4): e0176631. doi: 10.1371/journal.pone.0176631

Kalayci M, Unal MM, Gul S et al. Effect of Coenzyme Q10 on ischemia and neuronal damage in an experimental traumatic brain-injury model in rats. *BMC Neurosci* 2011; 12: 75 (7 pages).

Kassner E. Evaluation and treatment of chemotherapy extravasation injuries. *J Pediatr Oncol Nurs* 2000; 17(3): 135–148.

Longas-Vélez BP. Ozone therapy, a supplement for patients with fibromyalgia. *Revista Española de Ozonoterapia* 2014; 4(1): 39–49.

Marcoff L, Thompson PD. The role of Coenzyme Q10 in statin-associated myopathy. A Systematic Review. *J Am Coll Cardiol* 2007; 49: 2231–2237.

Mas E, Mori TA. Coenzyme Q(10) and statin myalgia: What is the evidence? *Curr Atheroscler Rep* 2010; 12(6): 407–413.

Morris G, Anderson G, Berk M et al. Coenzyme Q10 depletion in medical and neuropsychiatric disorders: Potential repercussions and therapeutic implications. *Mol Neurobiol* 2013; 48(3): 883–903.

Niibori K, Yokoyama H, Crestanello JA et al. Acute administration of liposomal coenzyme Q10 increases myocardial tissue levels and improves tolerance to ischemia reperfusion injury. *J Surg Res* 1998; 79: 141–145.

Nishimura A, Yanagawa H, Fujikawa N et al. Pharmacokinetic profiles of coenzyme Q 10: Absorption of three different oral formulations in rats. *J Health Sci* 2009; 55(4): 540–548.

Olszewer E, Sabbag FC, Zapata AR et al. DMSO (Dimethylsulfoxide) Treatments in Arthritis. *Supplement to The art of getting well.* Available at: http://arthritistrust.org/wp-content/uploads/2012/10/DMSO-Treatments-in-Arthritis.pdf. Accesed April 2, 2017.

Ortega E. The "bioregulatory effect of exercise" on the innate/inflammatory responses. *J Physiol Biochem* 2016; 72(2): 361–369.

Ostrowski RP. Effect of coenzyme Q(10) on biochemical and morphological changes in experimental ischemia in the rat brain. *Brain Res Bull* 2000; 53(4): 399–407.

Präg M. Traumeel-Injektion bei Ansatztendinosen der Muskulatur (Traumeel injections in the treatment of tendinosis). *Biologische Medizin* 2004; 33(3): 125–128.

Rengstorff RH, Petrali JP, Sim VM. Cataracts induced in guinea pigs by acetone, cyclohexanone and dimethyl sulfoxide. *Am J Optom* 1972; 49: 308–319.

Rosborg I, Hyllén E, Lidbeck J et al. Trace element pattern in patients with Fibromyalgia. *Sci Total Environ* 2007; 385: 20–27.

Rosenfeldt FL, Haas SJ, Krum H et al. Coenzyme Q10 in the treatment of hypertension: A meta-analysis of the clinical trials. *J Hum Hypertens* 2007; 21(4): 297–306.

Rubin LF, Barnett KC. Ocular effects of oral and dermal application of dimethyl sulfoxide in animals. *Ann N Y Acad Sci* 1967; 141: 333–345.

Santos NC, Figueira-Coelho J, Martins-Silva J et al. Multidisciplinary utilization of dimethyl sulfoxide: Pharmacological, cellular, and molecular aspects. *Biochem Pharmac* 2003; 65: 1035–1041.

Schafranski MD, Malucelli T, Machado F et al. Intravenous lidocaine for fibromyalgia syndrome: An open trial. *Clin Rheumatol* 2009; 28(7): 853–855.

Shirley HH, Lundergan MK, Williams HJ et al. Lack of ocular changes with dimethyl sulfoxide therapy of scleroderma. *Pharmacotherapy* 1989; 9(3): 165–168.

Shults CW. Therapeutic role of coenzyme Q10 in Parkinson's disease. *Pharmacol Ther* 2005; 107: 120–130.

Smith ER, Mason MM, Epstein E. The ocular effects of repeated dermal applications of dimethyl sulfoxide to dogs and monkeys. *J Pharmacol Exp Ther* 1969; 170(2): 364–370.

Swanson BN. Medical use of dimethyl sulfoxide (DMSO). *Rev Clin Basic Pharm* 1985; 5(1–2): 1–33.

Theadom A, Cropley M, Smith HE, Feigin VL, McPherson K. Mind and body therapy for fibromyalgia. *Cochrane Database Syst Rev* 2015; Apr 9(4): CD001980. Art. No.: CD001980. doi: 10.1002/14651858.CD001980.pub3

Tomono Y, Hasegawa J, Seki T et al. Pharmacokinetic study of deuterium-labelled coenzyme Q10 in man. *Int J Clin Pharmacol Ther Toxicol* 1986; 24: 536–541.

Turunen M, Olsson J, Dallner G. Metabolism and function of coenzyme Q. *Biochimica et Biophysica Acta (BBA) – Biomembranes* 2004; 1660(1–2): 171–199.

Verma DD, Hartner WC, Thakkar V et al. Protective effect of coenzyme Q10-loaded liposomes on the myocardium in rabbits with an acute experimental myocardial infarction. *Pharm Res* 2007; 24: 2131–2137.

Wahbeh H, Elsas SM, Oken BS. Mind–body interventions: Applications in neurology. *Neurology* 2008; 70(24): 2321–2328.

Walker M. Arthritis therapy and diet. Chapter 7. In: *DMSO—Nature's Healer.* Garden City Park, NY: Avery Publishing Group, Inc., 1993, pp. 103–124.

Walker M. *DMSO—Nature's Healer.* Garden City Park, NY: Avery Publishing Group, Inc., 1993.

Wood DC, Wood J. Pharmacologic and biochemical considerations of dimethyl sulfoxide. *Ann N Y Acad Sci* 1975; 243: 7–19.

Wyman M, Leonard M, Morledge T. Coenzyme Q10: A therapy for hypertension and statin-induced myalgia? *Clevel Clin J Med* 2010; 77(7): 435–442.

Yuzuriha T, Takada M, Katayama K. Transport of [14C] coenzyme Q10 from the liver to other tissues after intravenous administration to guinea pigs. *Biochimica Biophysica Acta* 1983; 759: 286–291.

N-Acetylcysteine (NAC)

Aliavi AL, Kurbanova GA. Nitric oxide metabolism in the inclusion of N-acetylcysteine into the complex therapy of patients with community-acquired pneumonia. *Probl Tuberk Bolezn Legk* 2007; (9): 20–24.

Dean OM, van den Buuse M et al. N-acetyl cysteine restores brain glutathione loss in combined 2-cyclohexene-1-one and d-amphetamine-treated rats: Relevance to schizophrenia and bipolar disorder. *Neurosci Lett* 2011 Jul 25; 499(3): 149–153.

GA eBusiness Services. Phebra Pty Ltd. January 16, 2013. Retrieved November 8, 2013.

Gamage AM, Lee KO, Gan YH. Effect of oral N-acetyl cysteine supplementation in type 2 diabetic patients on intracellular glutathione content and innate immune responses to Burkholderia pseudomallei. *Microbes Infect* 2014 Aug; 16(8): 661–671.

Gül M, Ayan M, Seydanoğlu A et al. The effect of N-acetyl cysteine on serum glutathione, TNF-alpha and tissue malondialdehyde levels in the treatment of sepsis. *Ulus Travma Acil Cerrahi Derg* 2011; 17(4): 293–297.

Houstis N, Rosen ED, Lander ES. Reactive oxygen species have a causal role in multiple forms of insulin resistance. *Nature* 2006; 440: 944–948.

Kalimeris K, Briassoulis P. N-acetylcysteine ameliorates liver injury in a rat model of intestinal ischemia reperfusion. *J Surg Res* 2016 Dec; 206(2): 263–272.

Kelly GS. Clinical applications of N-acetylcysteine. *Alt Med Rev* 1998; 3(2): 114–127.

Khanna S, Mitra S, Lakhera PC, Khandelwal S. N-acetylcysteine effectively mitigates cadmium-induced oxidative damage and cell death in Leydig cells in vitro. *Drug Chem Toxicol* 2016; 39(1): 74–80.

Marenzi G, Assanelli E, Marana I et al. N-acetylcysteine and contrast-induced nephropathy in primary angioplasty. *N Engl J Med* 2006; 354(26): 2773–2782.

Mokhtari V, Afsharian P, Shahhoseini M et al. A review on various uses of N-acetyl cysteine. *Cell Journal* 2017; 19(1): 11–17.

Nakagawa S, Arai Y, Mazda O et al. N-acetylcysteine prevents nitric oxide-induced chondrocyte apoptosis and cartilage degeneration in an experimental model of osteoarthritis. *J Orthop Res* 2010 Feb; 28(2): 156–163.

Oliveira VA, Oliveira CS, Mesquita M et al. Zinc and N-acetylcysteine modify mercury distribution and promote increase in hepatic metallothionein levels. *J Trace Elem Med Biol* 2015 Oct; 32: 183–188.

Pechanova O, Kunes J, Dobesova Z et al. Contribution of neuronal nitric oxide (NO) synthase to N-acetylcysteine-induced increase of NO synthase activity in the brain of normotensive and hypertensive rats. *J Physiol Pharmacol* 2009 Dec; 60(4): 21–25.

Rapado-Castro M, Dodd S. Cognitive effects of adjunctive N-acetyl cysteine in psychosis. *Psychol Med* 2016; Nov 29: 1–11.

Shimada K, Uzui H. N-acetylcysteine ameliorates experimental autoimmune myocarditis in rats via nitric oxide. *J Cardiovasc Pharmacol Ther* 2015; 20(2): 203–210.

Sisombath NS, Jalilehvand F. Similarities between N-Acetylcysteine and glutathione in binding to lead(II) ions. *Chem Res Toxicol* 2015 Dec 21; 28(12): 2313–2324.

Soltan-Sharifi MS, Mojtahedzadeh M, Najafi A et al. Improvement by N-acetylcysteine of acute respiratory distress syndrome through increasing intracellular glutathione, and extracellular thiol molecules and anti-oxidant power: Evidence for underlying toxicological mechanisms. *Hum Exp Toxicol* 2007; 26(9): 697–703.

Wang J, Zhu H, Liu X, Liu Z. N-acetylcysteine protects against cadmium-induced oxidative stress in rat hepatocytes. *J Vet Sci* 2014 Dec; 15(4): 485–493.

Sulfur Amino Acids

Brosnan JT, Brosnan ME. The sulfur-containing amino acids: An overview. *J Nutr* 2006; 136: 1636S–1640S.

Di Buono M, Wykes LJ, Cole DEC, Ball RO, Pencharz PB. Regulation of sulfur amino acid metabolism in men in response to changes in sulfur amino acid intakes. *J Nutr* 2003; 133: 733–739.

Jacobsen JP, Krystal AD, Krishnan KR, Caron MG. Adjunctive 5-hydroxytryptophan slow-release for treatment-resistant depression: Clinical and preclinical rationale. *Trends Pharmacol Sci* 2016 Nov; 37(11): 933–944.

Levine RL, Mosoni L, Berlett BS, Stadtman ER. Methionine residues as endogenous antioxidants in proteins. *Proc Natl Acad Sci USA* 1996; 93: 15036–15040.

Moskovitz J. Methionine sulfoxide reductases: Ubiquitous enzymes involved in antioxidant defense, protein regulation and prevention of aging-related diseases. *Biochim Biophys Acta* 2005; 1703: 213–219.

Turner EH, Loftis JM, Blackwell AD. Serotonin a la carte: Supplementation with the serotonin precursor 5-hydroxytryptophan. *Pharmacol Ther* 2006 Mar; 109(3): 325–338. Epub 2005 Jul 14.

Zhang H, Zhao H. 5-Hydroxytryptophan, a precursor for serotonin synthesis, reduces seizure-induced respiratory arrest. *Epilepsia* 2016 Aug; 57(8): 1228–1235.

Branched Chain Amino Acids, Isoleucine, Leucine, Valine

Bifari F, Nisoli E. Branched-chain amino acids differently modulate catabolic and anabolic states in mammals: A pharmacological point of view. *Br J Pharmacol* 2016 Sep 17; 174(11): 1366–1377.

Freund H, Hoover HC Jr, Atamian S, Fischer JE. Infusion of the branched chain amino acids in postoperative patients. Anticatabolic properties. *Ann Surg* 1979 Jul; 190(1): 18–23.

Maddrey WC. Branched chain amino acid therapy in liver disease. *J Am Coll Nutr* 1985; 4(6): 639–650.

L-Leucine

Davuluri G, Krokowski D, Guan BJ, Kumar A, Thapaliya S, Singh D, Hatzoglou M, Dasarathy S. Metabolic adaptation of skeletal muscle to hyperammonemia drives the beneficial effects of l-leucine in cirrhosis. *J Hepatol* 2016 Nov; 65(5): 929–937.

Jiao J, Han SF, Zhang W et al. Chronic leucine supplementation improves lipid metabolism in C57BL/6J mice fed with a high-fat/cholesterol diet. *Food Nutr Res* 2016 Sep 9; 60: 31304.

Murphy CH, Saddler NI, Devries MC, McGlory C, Baker SK, Phillips SM. Leucine supplementation enhances integrative myofibrillar protein synthesis in free-living older men consuming lower- and higher-protein diets: A parallel-group crossover study. *Am J Clin Nutr* 2016 Dec; 104(6): 1594–1606.

L-Carnitine

Bigford GE, Del Rossi G. Supplemental substances derived from foods as adjunctive therapeutic agents for treatment of neurodegenerative diseases and disorders. *Adv Nutr* 2014 Jul 14; 5(4): 394–403.

D'Antona G, Nabavi SM, Micheletti P, Di Lorenzo A, Aquilani R, Nisoli E, Rondanelli M, Daglia M. Creatine, L-carnitine, and ω3 polyunsaturated fatty acid supplementation from healthy to diseased skeletal muscle. *Biomed Res Int* 2014; 2014: 613890.

Gavrilova SI, Kalyn IaB, Kolykhalov IV, Roshchina IF, Selezneva ND. Acetyl-L-carnitine (carnicetine) in the treatment of early stages of Alzheimer's disease and vascular dementia. *Zh Nevrol Psikhiatr Im S S Korsakova* 2011; 111(9): 16–22.

La Guardia PG, Alberici LC, Ravagnani FG, Catharino RR, Vercesi AE. Protection of rat skeletal muscle fibers by either L-carnitine or coenzyme Q10 against statins toxicity mediated by mitochondrial reactive oxygen generation. *Front Physiol* 2013 May 15; 4: 103.

Lodeiro M, Ibáñez C, Cifuentes A, Simó C, Cedazo-Mínguez Á. Decreased cerebrospinal fluid levels of L-carnitine in non-apolipoprotein E4 carriers at early stages of Alzheimer's disease. *J Alzheimers Dis* 2014; 41(1): 223–232.

Pooyandjoo M, Nouhi M, Shab-Bidar S et al. The effect of (L-)carnitine on weight loss in adults: A systematic review and meta-analysis of randomized controlled trials. *Obes Rev* 2016; 17(10): 970–976.

Valero T. Mitochondrial biogenesis: Pharmacological approaches. *Curr Pharm Des* 2014; 20(35): 5507–5509.

L-Taurine

Hovsepyan LM, Zakaryan GV, Melkonyan MM, Zakaryan AV. The effects of taurine on oxidative processes in brain edema. *Zh Nevrol Psikhiatr Im S S Korsakova* 2015; 115(5): 64–67.

Qiao M, Liu P, Ren X, Feng T, Zhang Z. Potential protection of taurine on antioxidant system and ATPase in brain and blood of rats exposed to aluminum. *Biotechnol Lett* 2015 Aug; 37(8): 1579–1584.

Wang Q, Fan W, Cai Y, Wu Q, Mo L, Huang Z, Huang H. Protective effects of taurine in traumatic brain injury via mitochondria and cerebral blood flow. *Amino Acids* 2016 Sep; 48(9): 2169–2177.

Wu G, Tang R, Yang J et al. Taurine accelerates alcohol and fat metabolism of rats with alcoholic Fatty liver disease. *Adv Exp Med Biol* 2015; 803: 793–805.

Zhang Z, Liu D, Yi B, Liao Z et al. Taurine supplementation reduces oxidative stress and protects the liver in an iron-overload murine model. *Mol Med Rep* 2014; 10(5): 2255–2262.

Zhu XY, Ma PS, Wu W et al. Neuroprotective actions of taurine on hypoxic-ischemic brain damage in neonatal rats. *Brain Res Bull* 2016 Jun; 124: 295–305.

L-Arginine

Campbell BI, La Bounty PM, Roberts M. The ergogenic potential of arginine. *J Int Soc Sports Nutr* 2004; 1(2): 35–38.

Forbes SC, Harber V, Bell GJ. Oral L-arginine before resistance exercise blunts growth hormone in strength trained males. *Int J Sport Nutr Exerc Metab* 2014; 24(2): 236–244.

Glycine

Amin FU, Shah SA, Kim MO. Glycine inhibits ethanol-induced oxidative stress, neuroinflammation and apoptotic neurodegeneration in postnatal rat brain. *Neurochem Int* 2016 Jun; 96: 1–12.

Avila A, Nguyen L, Rigo JM. Glycine receptors and brain development. *Front Cell Neurosci* 2013 Oct 21; 7: 184.

Ito S. GABA and glycine in the developing brain. *J Physiol Sci* 2016; 66(5): 375–379.

Mori H, Momosaki K, Kido J et al. Amelioration of brain damage by glycine in neonatal rat brain following hypoxia-ischemia. *Pediatr Int* 2017 Mar; 59(3): 321–327. doi: 10.1111/ped.13164

Selin AA, Lobysheva NV, Vorontsova ON et al. Mechanism underlying the protective effect of glycine in energetic disturbances in brain tissues under hypoxic conditions. *Bull Exp Biol Med* 2012 May; 153(1): 44–47.

Beta-Alanine (B-Ala)

AIS Sports Nutrition. Australian Institute of Sport. B-alanine. Fact Sheets: Group B Supplements 2009. https://www.ausport.gov.au/ais/sports_nutrition/supplements/groupb, Accessed April 10, 2018.

Artioli GG, Gualano B, Smith A, Stout J et al. Role of beta-alanine supplementation on muscle carnosine and exercise performance. *Med Sci Sports Exerc* 2010; 42(6): 1162–1173.

Derave W, Everaert I, Beeckman S, Baguet A. Muscle carnosine metabolism and beta-alanine supplementation in relation to exercise and training. *Sports Med* 2010; 40(3): 247–263.

IJSM. The effect of beta-alanine supplementation on isokinetic force and cycling performance in highly trained cyclists. *Int J Sport Nutr Exerc Metab* 2013; 23: 562–570.

Stout JR, Graves BS, Smith AE et al. The effect of beta-alanine supplementation on neuromuscular fatigue in elderly (55-92 Years): A double-blind randomized study. *J Int Soc Sports Nutr* 2008; 5: 21. http://www.jissn.com/imedia/3329546222303903_article.pdf?random=19492

Stout JR, Cramer JT, Zoeller RF, Torok D et al. Effects of beta-alanine supplementation on the onset of neuromuscular fatigue and ventilatory threshold in women. *Amino Acids* 2007; 32(3): 381–386.

L-Tryptophan

Attenburrow MJ, Williams C, Odontiadis J et al. The effect of a nutritional source of tryptophan on dieting-induced changes in brain 5-HT function. *Psychol Med* 2003; 33: 1381–1386.

Chadwick D, Jenner P, Harris R et al. Manipulatio of brain serotonin in the treatment of myoclonus. *Lancet* 1975; 2: 434–435.

den Boer JA, Westenberg HG. Behavioral, neuroendocrine, and biochemical effects of 5-hydroxytryptophan administration in panic disorder. *Psychiatry Res* 1990; 31: 267–278.

Guilleminault C, Tharp BR, Cousin D. HVA and 5HIAA CSF measurements and 5HTP trials in some patients with involuntary movements. *J Neurol Sci* 1973; 18: 435–441.

van Praag HM, Lemus C. Monoamine precursors in the treatment of psychiatric disorders. In: Wurtman RJ, Wurtman JJ, eds. *Nutrition and the Brain.* New York, NY: Raven Press, 1986, pp. 89–139.

Winokur A, Lindberg ND, Lucki I et al. Hormonal and behavioral effects associated with intravenous L-tryptophan administration. *Psychopharmacology (Berl)* 1986; 88: 213–219.

L-Ornithine

Demura S, Yamada T, Yamaji S et al. The effect of L-ornithine hydrochloride ingestion on human growth hormone secretion after strength training. *Adv Biosci Biotechnol* 2010; 1: 7–11.
Sivashanmugam MJ. Ornithine and its role in metabolic diseases: An appraisal. *Biomed Pharmacother* 2016; 86: 185–194.

L-Lysine

AMR. *Alternative Medicine Review* Vol. 12, Number 2 2007.
Broquist HP. Carnitine biosynthesis and function. Introductory remarks. *Fed Proc* 1982;. 41: 2840–2842.
Flodin NW. The metabolic roles, pharmacology, and toxicology of lysine. *J Am Coll Nutr* 1997; 16: 7–21.
Longenecker JB, Hause NL. Relationship between plasma amino acids and composition of the ingested protein. *Arch Biochem Biophys* 1959; 84: 46–59.
Uhe AM, Collier GR, O'Dea K. A comparison of the effects of beef, chicken and fish protein on satiety and amino acid profiles in lean male subjects. *J Nutr* 1992; 122: 467–472.

L-Phenylalanine

Sabelli HC, Fawcett J, Gusovsky F et al. Clinical studies on the phenylethylamine hypothesis of affective disorder: Urine and blood phenylacetic acid and phenylalanine dietary supplements. *J Clin Psychiatry* 1986; 47: 66–70.
Wurtman RJ, Caballero B. Control of plasma phenylalanine levels. In: Wurtman RJ, Ritter-Walker E, eds. *Dietary Phenylalanine and Brain Function*. Birkhauser: Boston, MA, 1988, pp. 3–12.
Yang H, Neff NH. Monoamine oxidase: A natural substrate for type B enzyme. *Fed Proc* 1973; 32: 797.

Choline

Zeisel SH. "Vitamin-like" molecules: Choline. In: Shils M, Young V, eds. *Modern Nutrition in Health and Disease*. Lea & Febiger: Philadelphia, 1988, pp. 440–452.
Zeisel SH. Nutritional importance of choline for brain development. *J Am Coll Nutr* 2004; 23(6 suppl): 621S–626S.
Zeisel SH, Da Costa KA, Franklin PD et al. Choline, an essential nutrient for humans. *FASEB J* 1991; 5(7): 2093–2098.

B Complex Vitamins

Stipanuk MH. *Biochemical, Physiological, Molecular Aspects of Human Nutrition*. 2nd Edition. St Louis, MO: Saunders Elsevier, 2006, p. 667.

Thiamine (Vitamin B1)

Assem ESK. Anaphylactic reaction to thiamine. *Practitioner* 1973; 565.
Bubber P, Ke ZJ, Gibson GE. Tricarboxylic acid cycle enzymes following thiamine deficiency. *Neurochem Int* 2004; 45(7): 1021–1028.
Depeint F, Bruce WR, Shangari N et al. Mitochondrial function and toxicity: Role of the B vitamin family on mitochondrial energy metabolism. *Chem Biol Interact* 2006; 163(1–2): 94–112.
Eisenstadt WS. Hypersensitivity to thiamine hydrochloride. *Minn Med* 1942; 85: 861–863.
Frank RA, Kay CW, Hirst J et al. Off-pathway, oxygen-dependent thiamine radical in the Krebs cycle. *J Am Chem Soc* 2008; 130(5): 1662–1668.
Gorbach ZV, Maglysh SS, Nefedov LI et al. Characteristics of intracellular metabolism of carbohydrates and amino acids in animals with thiamine deficiency. *Biokhimiia* 1987; 52(1): 42–52.
Hoffman RS. Antidotes in depth (A25): Thiamine hydrochloride. In: Nelson L, Lewin N, Howland MA (authors) et al. *Goldfrank's Toxicologic Emergencies*. 9th Edition. McGraw–Hill Medical, 2011, pp. 1129–1133.
Leitner ZA. Untoward effects of vitamin B. *Lancet* 1943; 2: 474–475.
Leung R, Puy R, Czarny D. Thiamine anaphylaxis. *Med J Aust* 1993; 159: 355 (letter).

Morinville V, Jeannet-Peter N, Hauser C. Anaphylaxis to parenteral thiamine (vitamin B1). *Schweiz Med Wochenschr* 1998; 128(44): 1743–1744.

O'Keeffe ST, Tormey WP, Glasgow R et al. Thiamine deficiency in hospitalized elderly patients. *Gerontology* 1994; 40(1): 18–24.

Reingold IM, Webb FR. Sudden death following intravenous administration of thiamine hydrochloride. *JAMA* 1946; 130: 491–492.

Schiff L. Collapse following parenteral administration of solution of thiamine hydrochloride. *JAMA* 1941; 117: 609.

Stein W, Morgenstern M. Sensitization to thiamine hydrochloride: Report of another case. *Ann Intern Med* 1944; 70: 826–828.

Stephen JM, Grant R, Yeh CS. Anaphylaxis from administration of intravenous thiamine. *Am J Emerg Med* 1992; 10(1): 61–63.

Wrenn KD, Murphy F, Slovis CM. A toxicity study of parenteral thiamine hydrochloride. *Ann Emerg Med* 1989; 18(8): 867–870.

Wrenn KD, Slovis CM. Is intravenous thiamine safe? *Am J Emerg Med* 1992; 10(2): 165.

Zangen A, Botzer D, Zangen R et al. Furosemide and digoxin inhibit thiamine uptake in cardiac cells. *Eur J Pharmacol* 1998; 361(1): 151–155.

RIBOFLAVIN (VITAMIN B2)

Naghashpour M, Amani R, Sarkaki A et al. Brain-derived neurotrophic and immunologic factors: Beneficial effects of riboflavin on motor disability in murine model of multiple sclerosis. *Iran J Basic Med Sci* 2016 Apr; 19(4): 439–448.

Petrovski S, Shashi V, Petrou S et al. Exome sequencing results in successful riboflavin treatment of a rapidly progressive neurological condition. *Cold Spring Harb Mol Case Stud* 2015 Oct; 1(1): a000257.

Shashi V, Petrovski S, Schoch K et al. Sustained therapeutic response to riboflavin in a child with a progressive neurological condition, diagnosed by whole-exome sequencing. *Cold Spring Harb Mol Case Stud* 2015 Oct; 1(1): a000265.

Song J, Seol NG, Kim MJ, Lee J. Riboflavin phototransformation on the changes of antioxidant capacities in phenolic compounds. *J Food Sci* 2016 Aug; 81(8): C1914–C1920.

PYRIDOXINE (VITAMIN B6)

Ajioka RS, Phillips JD, Kushner JP. Biosynthesis of heme in mammals. *Biochim Biophys Acta* 2006; 1763(7): 723–736.

Combs GF, ed. *The Vitamins: Fundamental Aspects in Nutrition and Health*. 3rd Edition. San Diego, CA: Elsevier Academic Press, 2008, Table 4–12, page 90.

Erskine PT, Coates L, Butler D et al. X-ray structure of a putative reaction intermediate of 5-aminolaevulinic acid dehydratase. *Biochem J* 2003; 373: 733–738.

Muss C, Mosgoeller W, Endler T. Mood improving potential of a vitamin trace element composition—A randomized, double blind, placebo controlled clinical study with healthy volunteers. *Neuro Endocrinol Lett* 2016; 37(1): 18–28.

Petrov SA, Danilova AO, Karpov LM. The effect of a water-soluble vitamins on the activity of some enzymes in diabetes. *Biomed Khim* 2014 Nov–Dec; 60(6): 623–630.

NIACIN, NIACINAMIDE (VITAMIN B3)

Lim SY, Kim EJ, Kim A et al. Nutritional factors affecting mental health. *Clin Nutr Res* 2016 Jul; 5(3): 143–152.

Offermanns S, Schwaninger M. Nutritional or pharmacological activation of HCA(2) ameliorates neuroinflammation. *Trends Mol Med* 2015; 21(4): 245–255.

Pitsavas S, Andreou C, Bascialla F, Bozikas VP, Karavatos A. Pellagra encephalopathy following B-complex vitamin treatment without niacin. *Int J Psychiatry Med* 2004; 34(1): 91–95.

Wakade C, Chong R, Bradley E, Morgan JC. Low-dose niacin supplementation modulates GPR109A, niacin index and ameliorates Parkinson's disease symptoms without side effects. *Clin Case Rep* 2015 Jul; 3(7): 635–637.

CYANOCOBALAMIN (VITAMIN B12)

Bottiglieri T, Laundy M, Crellin R, Toone BK, Carney MW, Reynolds EH. Homocysteine, folate, methylation, and monoamine metabolism in depression. *Journal of Neurology, Neurosurgery & Psychiatry* 2000; 69(2): 228–232.

Gupta L, Gupta RK, Gupta PK et al. Assessment of brain cognitive functions in patients with vitamin B12 deficiency using resting state functional MRI: A longitudinal study. *Magn Reson Imaging* 2016 Feb; 34(2): 191–196.

Hooshmand B, Mangialasche F, Kalpouzos G et al. Resonance imaging measures in older adults: A longitudinal population-based study. *JAMA Psychiatry* 2016 Jun 1; 73(6): 606–613.

Killen JP, Brenninger VL. Vitamin B12 deficiency. *N Engl J Med* 2013; 368: 2040–2041.

National Institutes of Health—Office of Dietary Supplements. Dietary Supplement Fact Sheet: Vitamin B12. Fact Sheet for Health Professionals. Last update: February 11, 2016. Available at: https://ods.od.nih.gov/pdf/factsheets/VitaminB12-HealthProfessional.PDF

Rathod RS, Khaire AA, Kale AA, Joshi SR. Effect of vitamin B12 and omega-3 fatty acid supplementation on brain neurotrophins and cognition in rats: A multigeneration study. *Biochimie* 2016 Sep–Oct; 128–129: 201–208.

Sethi NK, Robilotti E, Sadan Y. Neurological manifestations of vitamin B-12 deficiency. *Internet J Nutr Wellness* 2005; 2(1).

van der Put NMJ, van Straaten HWM, Trijbels FJM, Blom HJ. Folate, homocysteine and neural tube defects: An overview. *Exp Biol Med* 2001; 226(4): 243–270.

Yamada K. Chapter 9. Cobalt: Its role in health and disease. In: Sigel A, Sigel H, Sigel R, eds. *Interrelations between Essential Metal Ions and Human Diseases. Metal Ions in Life Sciences.* Vol. 13. Dordrecht: Springer, 2013, pp. 295–320.

Zhang Y, Hodgson NW, Trivedi MS et al. Decreased brain levels of vitamin B12 in aging, autism and schizophrenia. *PLoS One* 2016 Jan 22; 11(1): e0146797.

FOLIC ACID

Alaimo K, McDowell MA, Briefel RR et al. Dietary intake of vitamins, minerals, and fiber of persons aged 2 months and over in the United States: Third National Health and Nutrition Examination Survey, Phase 1, 1988–91. *Adv Data from Vital and Health Statistics* 1994; Nov 14(258): 1–28.

Bailey LB. *Folate in Health and Disease.* 2nd Edition. Boca Raton, FL: CRC Press, p. 198. ISBN 9781420071252. Available at: https://www.crcpress.com/Folate-in-Health-and-Disease-Second-Edition/Bailey/p/book/9781138111882

Drugs.com. American Society of Health-System Pharmacists. January 1, 2010. Retrieved September 1, 2016.

Gilbody S, Lewis S, Lightfoot T. Methylenetetrahydrofolate reductase (MTHFR) genetic polymorphisms and psychiatric disorders: A HuGE review. *Am J Epidemiol* 2007; 165(1): 1–13.

Li Y, Huang T. Folic acid supplementation and the risk of cardiovascular diseases: A meta-analysis of randomized controlled trials. *J Am Heart Assoc* 2016 Aug; 5(8): e003768.

Obeid R, Herrmann W. The emerging role of unmetabolized folic acid in human diseases: Myth or reality? *Curr Drug Metab* 2012; 13(8): 1184–1195.

Yajnik CS, Deshmukh US. Maternal nutrition, intrauterine programming and consequential risks in the offspring. *Rev Endocr Metab Disord* 2008; 9(3): 203–211.

MINERALS AND TRACE ELEMENTS

Albion Research Notes. *A compilation of vital research updates on human nutrition*, 5: 2, Albion Laboratories, Inc. May, 1996.

Basargin NN, Peregudora LA. Zinc and molybdenum content of different varieties of spring and winter wheat. *Vop Pttan* 1969; 28: 65.

Baser BL, Deo R. Effect of superphosphate on the uptake of micronutrients by sorghum (jowar) and maize plants. *J Ind Soc Soil Sci* 1967; 15: 245. as cited by Kanwar JS, Randhawa NS. *Micronutrient Research in Soils and Plants in India (A Review).* 2nd Edition. New Delhi: Indian Council of Agricultural Research, 1974, pp. 41–78.

Batra J, Seth PK. Effect of iron deficiency on developing rat brain. *Indian J Clin Biochem* 2002; 17(2): 108–114.

Blood DC, Radostits OM. *Veterinary Medicine.* 7th Edition. London: Balliere Tindall, 1989, pp. 589–630.

Darby WJ. Deficiency of zinc in man and its toxicity. In: Prasad AS, Oberleas D, eds. *Trace Elements in Human Health and Disease.* Vol. 1. New York, San Francisco, London: Academic Press, 1976, p. 17.

Eruvbetine D. Canine Nutrition and Health. A paper presented at the seminar organized by Kensington Pharmaceuticals Nig. Ltd., Lagos on August 21, 2003.

Hays VW, Swenson MJ. Minerals and bones. In: *Dukes' Physiology of Domestic Animals.* 10th Edition. 1985, pp. 449–466.

Kavanek M, Janicek G. Effect of locality and variety on the content of some trace elements in oat grains. *Shorn Vys Skoly Chemtechnol Praze E* 1969; 24: 65.

Mongia AD. Phosphorus-zinc relationship in wheat as affected by sources and rates of applied phosphorus. MSc thesis, Punjab Agricultural University, Hissar, 1966.

Murray RK, Granner DK, Mayes PA, Rodwell VW. *Harper's Biochemistry.* 25th Edition. McGraw-Hill, Health Profession Division, 2000.

Osagie AU. Green leafy vegetables. In: Osagie AU, Eka OU, eds. *Nutritional Quality of Plant Foods.* Benin City, Nigeria: University of Benin, 1998, pp. 221–244.

Ozcan M. Mineral contents of some plants used as condiments in Turkey. *Food Chem* 2003; 84: 437–440.

Rao CN, Rao BSN. Trace element content of Indian foods and the dietaries. *Indian J Med Res* 1981; 73: 904–909.

Rush D. Nutrition and Maternal mortality in the developing world. *Am J Clin Nutr* 2000; 72(Suppl.): 2125–2405.

Simsek A, Aykut O. Evaluation of the microelement profile of Turkish hazelnut (Corylus avellana L) varieties for human nutrition and health. *Int J Food Sci Nutr* 2007; 58: 677–688.

Underwood EJ. *Trace Elements in Human and Animal Nutrition.* 3rd Edition. New York: Academic Press, 1971, p. 116.

SELENIUM

Arthur JR. The glutathione peroxidases. *Cell Mol Life Sci* 2000; 57(13–14): 1825–1835.

Calissendorff J, Mikulski E, Larsen EH et al. A Prospective investigation of Graves' disease and selenium: Thyroid hormones, autoantibodies and self-rated symptoms. *Eur Thyroid J* 2015; 2: 93–98.

Collier BR, Giladi A, Dossett LA et al. Impact of high-dose antioxidants on outcomes in acutely injured patients. *J Parenter Enteral Nutr* 2008; 32: 384–388.

Combs GF. Se in global food systems. *Br J Nutr* 2001; 85: 517–547.

Duffield-Lillico AJ, Dalkin BL, Reid ME et al. Selenium supplementation, baseline plasma selenium status and incidence of prostate cancer: An analysis of the complete treatment period of the Nutritional Prevention of Cancer Trial. *BJU Int* 2003; 91(7): 608–612.

Fordyce FM. Selenium deficiency and toxicity in the environment. In: Selinus O, ed. *Essentials of Medical Geology. Part II, Chapter 16.* Netherlands: Springer, 2012, pp. 375–416.

Giladi AM, Dossett LA, Fleming SB et al. High-dose antioxidant administration is associated with a reduction in post- injury complications in critically ill trauma patients. *Injury* 2011; 42: 78–82.

Hatfield DL, Gladyshev VN. The outcome of selenium and vitamin E cancer prevention trial (SELECT) reveals the need for better understanding of selenium biology. *Mol Interv* 2009; 9(1): 18–21.

Haug A, Graham RD, Christophersen OA et al. How to use the world's scarce selenium resources efficiently to increase the selenium concentration in food. *Microb Ecol Health Dis* 2007; 19(4): 209–228.

Haygood RJ, Dickerson RN, Brown RO. Review of intravenous selenium infusions for the critically Ill patient. *Hosp Pharm* 2012; 47(12): 933–938.

Hegedüs L, Bonnema SJ, Winther KH. Selenium in the treatment of thyroid diseases: An element in search of the relevant indications? *Eur Thyroid J* 2016; 5(3): 149–151.

Klein EA, Thompson IM Jr, Tangen CM et al. Vitamin E and the risk of prostate cancer: The selenium and vitamin E cancer prevention trial (SELECT). *JAMA* 2011; 306(14): 1549–1556.

Köhrle J. Selenium and the thyroid. *Curr Opin Endocrinol Diabetes Obes* 2015 Oct; 22(5): 392–401.

Leo M, Bartalena L, Rotondo Dottore G et al. Effects of selenium on short-term control of hyperthyroidism due to Graves' disease treated with methimazole: Results of a randomized clinical trial. *J Endocrinol Invest* 2017; 40(3): 281–287. Epub ahead of print.

Mahima, Verma AK, Kumar A et al. Inorganic versus organic selenium supplementation: A review. *Pak J Biol Sci* 2012; 15: 418–425.

Manzanares W, Lemieux M, Elke G et al. High-dose intravenous selenium does not improve clinical outcomes in the critically ill: A systematic review and meta-analysis. *Crit Care* 2016; 20: 356 (16 pages).

Negro R, Attanasio R, Colosimo E et al. A 2016 Italian survey about the clinical use of selenium in thyroid disease. *Eur Thyroid J* 2016; 5(3): 164–170.

Oldfield JE. *Selenium World Atlas*. 2nd Updated Edition. 2002. http://369.com.cn/En/Se%20Atlas%202002.pdf

Outzen, M, Tjønneland A, Larsen EH et al. The effect on selenium concentrations of a randomized intervention with fish and mussels in a population with relatively low habitual dietary selenium intake. *Nutrients* 2015; 7(1): 608–624.

Rayman MP. The importance of selenium to human health. *The Lancet* 2000; 356(9225): 233–241.

Rayman MP. The use of high-Se yeast to raise Se status: How does it measure up? *Br J Nutr* 2004; 92: 557–573.

Rayman MP. Selenium in human health. *The Lancet* 2012; 379(9822): 1256–1268.

Reid ME, Stratton MS, Lillico AJ et al. A report of high-dose selenium supplementation: Response and toxicities. *J Trace Elem Med Biol* 2004; 18(1): 69–74.

Reilly C. *Selenium in Food and Health*. 1st Edition. London, New York: Blackie Academic and Professional, 1996.

Richie JP, Das A, Calcagnotto AM et al. Comparative effects of two different forms of selenium on oxidative stress biomarkers in healthy men: A randomized clinical trial. *Cancer Prev Res (Phila)* 2014; 7(8): 796–804.

Rotruck JT, Pope AL, Ganther HE et al. Selenium: Biochemical role as a component of glutathione peroxidase. *Science* 1973; 179: 588–590.

Sunde RA. Selenium. In: O'Dell BL, Sunde RA, eds. *Handbook of Nutritionally Essential Mineral Elements*. Ch 18. New York: Marcel Dekker, Inc., 1997, pp. 493–556.

van Zuuren EJ. Selenium supplementation for Hashimoto's thyroiditis. *Cochrane Database Syst Rev* 2013; Jun 6(6): CD010223.

World Health Organization (WHO) – Food and Agriculture Organization (FAO), International Atomic Energy Agency expert group. *Trace Elements in Human Nutrition and Health*. Geneva: WHO, 1996.

ZINC (Zn)

Aamodt RL, Rumble WF, Johnston GS et al. Zinc metabolism in humans after oral and intravenous administration of Zn-69 m. *Am J Clin Nutr* 1979; 32(3): 559–569.

Al-Gurairi FT, Al-Waiz M, Sharquie KE. Oral zinc sulphate in the treatment of recalcitrant viral warts: Randomized placebo-controlled clinical trial. *Br J Dermatol* 2002; 146(3): 423–431.

AMA Department of Foods and Nutrition. Guidelines for essential trace element preparation for parenteral use. A statement by an expert panel. *JAMA* 1979; 241: 2051–2054.

Baum MK, Lai S, Sales S et al. Randomized, controlled clinical trial of zinc supplementation to prevent immunological failure in HIV-infected adults. *Clin Infect Dis* 2010; 50(12): 1653–1660.

Beck FW, Prasad AS, Kaplan J et al. Changes in cytokine production and T cell subpopulations in experimentally induced zinc deficient humans. *Am J Physiol Endocrinol Metab* 1997; 272: 1002–1007.

Black RE. Therapeutic and preventive effects of zinc on serious childhood infectious diseases in developing countries. *Am J Clin Nutr* 1998; 68(2 Suppl.): 476S–479S.

Chatterjea MN, Rana S. *Textbook of Medical Biochemistry*. 8th Edition. New Delhi, India: Jaypee Brothers Medical Publishers (P) Ltd, 2012a, p. 105.

Chatterjea MN, Rana S. *Textbook of Medical Biochemistry*. 8th Edition. New Delhi, India: Jaypee Brothers Medical Publishers (P) Ltd, 2012b, p. 581.

Chatterjea MN, Rana S. Zinc (Eds.). Section 4, Chapter 34 – Metabolism of minerals and trace elements. In: *Textbook of Medical Biochemistry*. 8th Edition. New Delhi, India: Jaypee Brothers Medical Publishers (P) Ltd, 2012c, pp. 626–628.

Dhawan DK, Chadha VD. Zinc: A promising agent in dietary chemoprevention of cancer. *Indian J Med Res* 2010; 132(6): 676–682.

Driscoll RH Jr, Rosenberg IH. Total parenteral nutrition in inflammatory bowel disease. *Med Clin North Am* 1978; 62: 185–201.

Fleet JC. Zinc, copper, and manganese. In: Stipanuk MH, ed. *Biochemical and Physiological aspects of Human Nutrition*. New York: Saunders, 2000, pp. 741–759.

Galvao TF, Thees MF, Pontes RF et al. Zinc supplementation for treating diarrhea in children: A systematic review and meta-analysis. *Revista Panamericana de Salud Pública* 2013; 33(5): 370–377.

Giles S. Do all Canadian children have enough zinc? *Can Fam Physician* 2013; 59(7): 726.

Goldman RD. Zinc supplementation for acute gastroenteritis. *Can Fam Physician* 2013; 59(4): 363–364.

Hambidge M. Human zinc deficiency. *J Nutr* 2000; 130(5S Suppl.): 1344S–1349S.

Ibs KH, Rink L. Zinc-altered immune function. *J Nutr* 2003; 133(5 Suppl. 1): 1452S–1456S.

King JC, Cousins RJ. Zinc. In: Shils ME, Shike M, Ross AC, Caballero B, Cousins RJ, eds. *Modern Nutrition in Health and Disease*. 10th Edition. Baltimore, MD: Lippincott Williams & Wilkins, 2006, pp. 271–285.

Kinlaw WB, Levine AS, Morley JE et al. Abnormal zinc metabolism in type II diabetes mellitus. *Am J Med* 1983; 75(2): 273–277.

Lansdown AB, Mirastschijski U, Stubbs N et al. Zinc in wound healing: Theoretical, experimental, and clinical aspects. *Wound Repair Regen* 2007; 15(1): 2–16.

Maares M, Haase H. Zinc and immunity: An essential interrelation. *Arch Biochem Biophys* 2016; 611: 58–65.

MacDonald RS. The role of zinc in growth and cell proliferation. *J Nutr* 2000; 130(5S Suppl.): 1500S–1508S.

Main ANH, Hall MJ, Russell RI et al. Clinical experience of Zn supplementation during IV nutrition in Crohn's disease—Value of serum and urine Zn measurements. *Gut* 1982; 23: 984–991.

Maywald M, Rink L. Zinc supplementation induces CD4+CD25+Foxp3+ antigen-specific regulatory T cells and suppresses IFN-γ production by upregulation of Foxp3 and KLF-10 and downregulation of IRF-1. *Eur J Nutr* 2016; 56: 1859; first online Jun 3. doi: 10.1007/s00394-016-1228-7

McCarty MF, DiNicolantonio JJ. The protection conferred by chelation therapy in post-MI diabetics might be replicated by high-dose zinc supplementation. *Med Hypotheses* 2015; 84(5): 451–455.

McClain C, Soutor C, Zieve L. Zinc deficiency: A complication of Crohn's disease. *Gastroenterology* 1980a; 78(2): 272–279.

McClain CJ, Soutor C, Steele N et al. Severe zinc deficiency presenting with acrodermatitis during hyperalimentation: Diagnosis, pathogenesis, and treatment. *J Clin Gastroenterol* 1980b; 2(2): 125–131.

Murthy SC, Udagani MM, Badakali AV et al. Symptomatic zinc deficiency in a full-term breast-fed infant. *Dermatol Online J* 2010; 16(6): 3.

Nowak G, Szewczyk B, Pilc A. Zinc and depression. An update. *Pharmacol Rep* 2005; 57(6): 713–718.

Osredkar J, Sustar N. Copper and zinc, biological role and significance of copper/zinc imbalance. *J Clinic Toxicol* 2011; S3: 001 (18 pages).

Pae M, Wu D. Nutritional modulation of age-related changes in the immune system and risk of infection. *Nutr Res* 2017; 41: 14–35.

Pisano M, Hilas O. Zinc and taste disturbances in older adults: A review of the literature. *Consult Pharm* 2016; 31(5): 267–270.

Plum LM, Rink L, Haase H. The essential toxin: Impact of zinc on human health. *Int J Environ Res Public Health* 2010; 7(4): 1342–1365.

Powell SR. The antioxidant properties of zinc. *J Nutr* 2000; 130(5S Suppl.): 1447S–1454S.

Prasad AS. Discovery of human zinc deficiency: Its impact on human health and disease. *Adv Nutr* 2013; 4(2): 176–190.

Prasad AS. Effects of zinc deficiency on Th1 and Th2 cytokine shifts. *J Infect Dis* 2000; 182(Suppl. 1): S62–S68.

Prasad AS. *Trace Elements in Human Health and Disease. Vol. 1. Zinc and Copper*. New York, London: Academic Press, 1976, pp. 107–113.

Prasad AS, Beck FW, Grabowski SM, Kaplan J, Mathog RH. Zinc deficiency: Changes in cytokine production and T-cell subpopulations in patients with head and neck cancer and in noncancer subjects. *Proc Assoc Am Physicians* 1997; 109: 68–77.

Riordan JF. Biochemistry of zinc. *Med Clin North Am* 1976; 60: 661–674.

Rosenkranz E, Maywald M, Hilgers RD et al. Induction of regulatory T cells in Th1-/Th17-driven experimental autoimmune encephalomyelitis by zinc administration. *J Nutr Biochem* 2016; 29: 116–123.

Sarris J, Murphy J, Mischoulon D et al. Adjunctive nutraceuticals for depression: A systematic review and meta-analyses. *Am J Psychiatry* 2016; 173(6): 575–587.

Shankar AH, Prasad AS. Zinc and immune function: The biological basis of altered resistance to infection. *Am J Clin Nutr* 1998; 68: 447S–463S.

Sharquie KA, Al-Nuaimy AA. Treatment of viral warts by intralesional injection of zinc sulphate. *Ann Saudi Med* 2002; 22(1–2): 26–28.

Soetan KO, Olaiya CO, Oyewole OE. The importance of mineral elements for humans, domestic animals and plants: A review. *AJFS* 2010; 4(5): 200–222.

Solomons NW, Rosenberg IH, Sandstead HH et al. Zinc deficiency in Crohn's disease. *Digestion* 1977; 16(1–2): 87–95.

Sturniolo GC, Molokhia MM, Shields R et al. Zinc absorption in Crohn's disease. *Gut* 1980; 21(5): 387–391.

Szewczk B, Kubera M, Nowak G. The role of zinc in neurodegenerative inflammatory pathways in depression. *Prog Neuropsychopharmacol Biol Psychiatry* 2011 Apr 29; 35(3): 693–701.

Takuma Y, Nouso K, Makino Y et al. Clinical trial: Oral zinc in hepatic encephalopathy. *Aliment Pharmacol Ther* 2010; 32(9): 1080–1090.

Tudor R, Zalewski PD, Ratnaike RN. Zinc in health and chronic disease. *J Nutr Health Aging* 2005; 9(1): 45–51.

Vick G, Mahmoudizad R, Fiala K. Intravenous zinc therapy for acquired zinc deficiency secondary to gastric bypass surgery: A case report. *Dermatol Ther* 2015; 28(4): 222–225.

Walker CL, Black RE. Zinc for the treatment of diarrhoea: Effect on diarrhoea morbidity, mortality and incidence of future episodes. *Int J Epidemiol* 2010; 39(Suppl. 1): i63–69.

WHO/UNICEF. *Joint Statement: Clinical Management of Acute Diarrhoea (WHO/FCH/CAH/04.07)*. Geneva and New York: World Health Organization, Department of Child and Adolescent Health and Development, and United Nations Children's Fund, Programme Division, 2004. Available at: https://www.unicef.org/nutrition/files/ENAcute_Diarrhoea_reprint.pdf, Accessed June 5, 2017.

Wolman SL, Anderson GH, Marliss EB et al. Zinc in total parenteral nutrition: Requirements and metabolic effects. *Gastroenterology* 1979; 76(3): 458–467.

Yanagisawa H. Zinc deficiency and clinical practice. *J Formos Med Assoc* 2004; 47(8): 359–364.

Copper (Cu)

Attri S, Sharma N, Jahagirdar S. Erythrocyte metabolism and antioxidant status of patients with Wilson disease with hemolytic anemia. *Pediatr Res* 2006; 59(4 Pt 1): 593–597.

Baker A, Harvey L, Majask-Newman G et al. Effect of dietary copper intakes on biochemical markers of bone metabolism in healthy adult males. *J Clin Nutr* 1999; 53(5): 408–412.

Borkow G. Using copper to improve the well-being of the skin. *Curr Chem Biol* 2014 Aug; 8(2): 89–102.

Chatterjea MN, Rana S. Copper (Eds.). Section 4, Chapter 34 – Metabolism of minerals and trace elements. In: *Textbook of Medical Biochemistry*. 8th Edition. New Delhi, India: Jaypee Brothers Medical Publishers (P) Ltd, 2012, p. 622.

Conlan D, Korula R, Tallentire D. Serum copper levels in elderly patients with femoral-neck fractures. *Age Ageing* 1990; 19(3): 212–214.

Failla ML, Hopkins RG. Is low copper status immunosuppressive? *Nutr Rev* 1998; 56: 59–64.

Fox PL, Mazumder B, Ehrenwald E et al. Ceruloplasmin and cardiovascular disease. *Free Radic Biol Med* 2000; 28(12): 1735–1744.

Gibson RS. *Principles of Nutritional Assessment*. 2nd Edition. New York: Oxford University, 2005, pp. 697–711.

Grammer TB, Kleber ME, Silbernagel G et al. Copper, ceruloplasmin, and long-term cardiovascular and total mortality (The Ludwigshafen Risk and Cardiovascular Health Study). *Free Radic Res* 2014; 48(6): 706–715.

Harris ED. Copper. In: O'Dell BL, Sunde RA, eds. *Handbook of Nutritionally Essential Minerals*. New York: Marcel Dekker, Inc., 1997, pp. 231–273.

Jones AA, DiSilvestro RA, Coleman M et al. Copper supplementation of adult men: Effects on blood copper enzyme activities and indicators of cardiovascular disease risk. *Metabolism* 1997; 46(12): 1380–1383.

Kaler SG, Holmes CS, Goldstein DS et al. Neonatal diagnosis and treatment of Menkes disease. *N Engl J Med* 2008; 358(6): 605–614.

Klevay LM. Lack of a recommended dietary allowance for copper may be hazardous to your health. *J Am Coll Nutr* 1998; 17(4): 322–326.

Lahey ME, Gubler CJ, Cartwright GE et al. Studies on Copper metabolism—VII. Blood Copper in pregnancy and various pathologic states. *J Clin Invest* 1953; 32(4): 329–339.

Rodriques A, Soto G, Torres S, Venegas G, Castillo-Duran C. Zinc and copper in hair and plasma of children with chronic diarrhea. *Acta Paediatr Scand* 1985; 74(5): 770–774.

Rolff M, Tuczek F. How do copper enzymes hydroxylate aliphatic substrates? Recent insights from the chemistry of model systems. *Angewandte Chemie International Edition* 2008; 47: 2344–2347.

Ruiz C, Alegria A, Barbera R et al. Selenium, zinc, and copper in plasma of patients with type I diabetes mellitus in different metabolic control states. *J Trace Elem Med Biol* 1998; 12: 91–95.

Sachdev HP, Mittal NK, Yadav HS. Serum rectal mucosal zinc levels in acute and chronic diarrhea. *Indian Pediatric* 1990; 27(2): 125–133.

Tanaka A, Kaneto H, Miyatsuka T et al. Role of copper ion in the pathogenesis of type 2 diabetes. *Endocr J* 2009; 56(5): 699–706.

Turgut S, Polat A, Inan M, Turgut G, Emmungil G, Bican M, Karakus TY, Genc O. Interaction between ane-mia and blood levels of iron, zinc,copper, cadmium and lead in children. *Indian J Pediatr* 2007; 74(9): 827–830.

Uauy, R., Olivares M., Gonzalez M. Essentiality of copper in humans. *J Clin Nutr* 1998; 67(5): 952–959.

MANGANESE (Mn)

Davies IJT. *The Clinical Significance of the Essential Biological Metals*. Illinois: Charles Thomas Pub., 1972.

Hegsted B. Food fortification. In: McLaren DS, ed. *Nutrition in the Community*. New York: John Wiley, 1976.

Madsen-Bouterse SA, Zhong Q, Mohammad G et al. Oxidative damage of mitochondrial DNA in diabetes and its protection by manganese superoxide dismutase. *Free Radic Res* 2010; 44(3): 313–321.

Papavasilious PS, Kutt H, Miller ST et al. Seizure disorders and trace metals: Manganese tissue levels in treated epileptics. *Neurology* 1979; 29(11): 1466–1473. https://www.ncbi.nlm.nih.gov/pubmed/574199

Pfeiffer CC. *Mental and Elemental Nutrients*. Connecticut: Keats Pub.: 1975.

Scrutton MC, Utter MF, Mildran AS. Pyruvate carboxylase VI. The presence of tightly bound manganese. *Biol Chem* 1966; 241(15): 3480–3487.

Underwood EJ. *Trace Elements in Human and Animal Nutrition*. 4th Edition. New York: Academic Press, 1977.

Watts DL. The nutritional relationships of the thyroid. *J Orthomol Med* 1989; 4(3): 165–169. Available at the web page: http://w3.traceelements.com/Docs/The%20Nutritional%20Relationships%20of%20Thyroid.pdf

Wilson ED, Fisher KH, Garcia PA. *Principles of Nutrition*. New York: John Wiley, 1979.

CHROMIUM

Brown RO, Forloines-Lynn S, Cross RE et al. Chromium deficiency after long-term total parenteral nutrition. *Dig Dis Sci* 1986; 31: 661–664.

Freund H, Atamian S, Fischer JE. Chromium deficiency during total parenteral nutrition. *JAMA* 1979; 241(5): 496–498.

Jeejeebhoy KN, Chu RC, Marliss EB et al. Chromium deficiency, glucose intolerance, and neuropathy reversed by chromium supplementation in a patient receiving long-term parenteral nutrition. *Am J Clin Nutr* 1977; 30: 531–538.

Lau FC, Bagchi M, Sen CK, Bagchi D. Nutrigenomic basis of beneficial effects of chromium(III) on obesity and diabetes. *Mol Cell Biochem* 2008 Oct; 317(1–2): 1–10.

Lewicki S, Zdanowski R, Krzyżowska M. The role of Chromium III in the organism and its possible use in diabetes and obesity treatment. *Ann Agric Environ Med* 2014; 21(2): 331–335.

Paiva AN, Lima JG, Medeiros AC. Beneficial effects of oral chromium picolinate supplementation on glyce-mic control in patients with type 2 diabetes: A randomized clinical study. *J Trace Elem Med Biol* 2015 Oct; 32: 66–72.

Suksomboon N, Poolsup N, Yuwanakorn A. Systematic review and meta-analysis of the efficacy and safety of chromium supplementation in diabetes. *J Clin Pharm Ther* 2014 Jun; 39(3): 292–306.

PROCAINE

Cassuto J, Sinclair R, Bonderovic M. Anti-inflammatory properties of local anesthetics and their present and potential clinical implications. *Acta Anaesthesiol Scand* 2006; 50(3): 265–282.

Cotran R, Kumar V, Robbins S. Inflamación y reparación. Chapter 2 in: Patología estructural y funcional. Cotran R, Kumar V, Robbins S (Eds.), 4th Edition, 1990. Editorial Interamericana McGraw-Hill, España; page 39.

Cotran R, Kumar V, Robbins S. Inflamación y reparación. Chapter 3 in: Patología estructural y funcional. Cotran R, Kumar V, Robbins S (Eds.), 5th Edition, 1995. Editorial Interamericana McGraw-Hill, España; page 57.

Dosch P. *Manual of Neural Therapy According to Huneke*. 1st English Edition (translation of 11th German ed., revised). Lindsay A, translator. Heidelberg, Germany: Karl F. Haug Publishers, 1984.

Graubard DJ, Robertazzi RW. One year's experience with intravenous procaine. *Anesth Analg* 1948; 27(4): 222–226.

Graubard DJ, Peterson MC. Intravenous use of procaine in the management of arthritis. *JAMA* 1949; 141(11): 756–761.

Graubard DJ, Robertazzi RW, Peterson MC. Intravenous procaine: A preliminary report. *N Y State J Med* 1947; 47: 2187.

Krause KH, Demaurex N, Jaconi M et al. Ion channels and receptor-mediated Ca21 influx in neutrophil granulocytes. *Blood Cells* 1993; 19: 165–173.

Pecher S, Böttiger BW, Graf B et al. ["Alternative" effects of local anesthetic agents]. *Anaesthesist* 2004; 53(4): 316–325.

Swanton BJ, Shorten GD. Anti-inflammatory effects of local anesthetic agents. *Int Anesthesiol Clin* 2003; 41(1): 1–19.

Wright JL, Durieux ME, Groves DS. A brief review of innovative uses for local anesthetics. *Curr Op Anaesthesiol* 2008; 21: 651–656.

4 Toxicology
Exploring the Concept of Exogenous and Endogenous Toxins

Stevan Cordas

CONTENTS

Importance of Dose...122
Endocrine Disruptors 122
Basics 123
    Pharmacokinetics 123
        Absorption..123
        Distribution..125
        Drug Metabolism...125
        Drug Excretion 126
    Pharmacodynamics 127
        Interference with Ion Passage through the Cell Membrane 128
        Enzyme Inhibition or Stimulation 128
        Incorporation into Macromolecules 128
        Interference with Metabolic Processes of Microorganisms 128
    Undesirable Responses to Drug Therapy 128
    Factors Affecting the Body's Response to a Drug 129
        Toxicity..130
        Synergism..130
        Susceptibility...130
    Subspecialties of Toxicology 131
    Medical Toxicology..131
    Chemical Toxicology 132
    Toxicology and Pharmacology...132
    Occupational Toxicology 134
    Regulatory Toxicology 137
    Toxic: Allergic Interaction 137
    Exogenous and Endogenous Toxins...137
        Tobacco 138
        Alcohol 141
    Endogenous Toxins 142
    Selective Toxic Metals 143
        Mercury 143
        Lead..144
    Toxicology and Psychoneuroimmunology...145
    Some Treatments and Measures to Reduce Individual Toxic Exposure 146
Summary..146
References..146

This chapter is written for various health-care providers, including physicians, nurse practitioners, nurses, pharmacists, and physician assistants. For that reason, portions may appear basic or simplistic but must be included to afford an appropriate overview of the subject.

Toxicology is the scientific study of adverse effects that occur in living organisms due to chemicals. These chemicals are referred to as "poisons." Thus, toxicology includes the investigation of the adverse effects of environmental agents and chemical compounds found in nature as well as those synthesized. It also includes pharmaceutical compounds. Some of these substances may be beneficial and even life-saving at a recommended dose but produce toxic effects in living organisms, including disturbance in growth patterns, disease and death at an abnormal amount and/or duration (concentration times the duration equals the dose).

IMPORTANCE OF DOSE

Virtually any substance can act as a "poison" and produce adverse effects. This even applies to water or the oxygen that we breathe. The key is the dose.

The dose of the substance is the most important factor in toxicology, as it has a significant relationship with the effects experienced by the individual. It is the primary means of classifying the toxicity of the chemical, as it measures the quantity of the chemical, or the exposure to the substance.

A conventional relationship between dose and toxicity has traditionally been accepted, in that greater exposure to a chemical leads to higher risk of toxicity. However, this concept has been challenged by a study of endocrine disruptors and may not be as straightforward as once thought.

ENDOCRINE DISRUPTORS

At a recent international conference the known evidence incriminating certain ubiquitous chemicals was emphasized. These chemicals have, in common, the ability to disrupt the endocrine system in living organisms, including humans. As an example, there has already been a correlation with fetal loss and elevated levels of phthalates in the occupational setting, however, recently a prospective cohort study by Dr. Masserlien on couples who received infertility treatment, not in the occupational setting, showed a significantly higher biochemical pregnancy loss in the group with the highest quartile of urinary phthalates than the lowest quartile. He measured four metabolites of d (ethylhexyl) phthalate (RR 3.4). This was presented at the American Society for Reproductive Medicine in 2015. Another study demonstrated an association between reduced female sexual desire and elevated phthalate urinary levels.[1]

A recent quote by the Endocrine Society published online September 2015 states *"This Executive Summary to the Endocrine Society's second Scientific Statement on environmental endocrine-disrupting chemicals (EDCs) provides a synthesis of the key points of the complete statement. The full Scientific Statement represents a comprehensive review of the literature on seven topics for which there is strong mechanistic, experimental, animal, and epidemiological evidence for endocrine disruption, namely: obesity and diabetes, female reproduction, male reproduction, hormone-sensitive cancers in females, prostate cancer, thyroid, and neurodevelopment and neuroendocrine systems. EDCs such as bisphenol A, phthalates, pesticides, persistent organic pollutants such as polychlorinated biphenyls, polybrominated diethyl ethers, and dioxins were emphasized because these chemicals had the greatest depth and breadth of available information. The Statement also included thorough coverage of studies of developmental exposures to EDCs, especially in the fetus and infant, because these are critical life stages during which perturbations of hormones can increase the probability of a disease or dysfunction later in life. A conclusion of the Statement is that publications over the past 5 years have led to a much fuller understanding of the endocrine principles by which EDCs act, including nonmonotonic dose-responses, low-dose effects, and developmental vulnerability. These findings will prove useful to researchers, physicians, and other healthcare providers in translating the science of endocrine disruption to improved public health."*[2]

BASICS

Most toxicological information is obtained from animal data, though human data are preferable. The data are then extrapolated to applications in humans. These data are evaluated and regulations are created by OSHA (Occupational Safety and Health Administration) for the workplace and the EPA (Environmental Protection Agency) outside the workplace. There are similar agencies that regulate chemicals in most developed countries. At the workplace, the toxicological information is found in the health hazard section of the Material Safety Data Sheet (MSDS). Such information is mandated to be available.

PHARMACOKINETICS

Pharmacokinetics considers the movement of drugs within the body and the way in which the body affects drugs with time. Once a drug has been administered, it will then undergo four basic processes:

- Absorption
- Distribution
- Metabolism
- Excretion

This applies to metals, synthetic compounds as well as natural substances, such as mushrooms, fish and snake toxins, and plants.

Absorption

In order for a substance to pose a threat it must be a small molecule that is either water or fat soluble. It may enter the body via the respiratory route (inhalation), transdermal route or the gastrointestinal route. In medicine, other routes exist which includes intravenous, sublingual, subcutaneous, transocular and transanal routes. This is termed absorption.

The process of absorption involves bringing the drug from the site of administration into the circulatory or lymphatic system. Almost all drugs, other than those administered intravenously or applied topically, must be absorbed before they can have an effect on the body. The term bioavailability is the proportion of the administered drug that has reached the circulation and that is available to have an effect. Drugs given intravenously may be considered to be 100% bioavailable as they are administered directly into the circulation and all of the drug may potentially cause an effect. Administration by other routes means that some of the drug molecules will be lost during absorption and distribution, and thus bioavailability is reduced.

Drugs administered orally are absorbed from the gastrointestinal tract, carried via the hepatic portal vein to the liver, and then undergo some metabolism by the liver before the drug has even had the opportunity to work. This removal of a drug by the liver, before the drug has become available for use, is called the first-pass effect. Some drugs, when swallowed and absorbed, will be almost totally inactivated by the first-pass effect (e.g., nitroglycerin). The first-pass effect can, however, be avoided if the drug is given by another route. Thus, nitroglycerin when administered sublingually or transdermally, avoids first-pass metabolism by the liver and is able to cause a therapeutic effect.

Factors Affecting Drug Absorption From the Gastrointestinal Tract

Since oral administration is the most common route, a number of variables exist that can influence absorption. These include:

- Gut motility: If motility is increased then transit time is increased, so there will be less time available for absorption of a drug. Hypomotility may increase the amount of drug absorbed if contact with the gut epithelium is prolonged.
- Gastric emptying: If increased, this will speed up drug absorption rate. If delayed, it will slow the delivery of drug to the intestine, therefore reducing the absorption rate.
- Surface area: The rate of drug absorption is greatest in the small intestine due to the large surface area provided by the villi.
- Gut pH: The pH of the gastrointestinal tract varies along its length. Different intestinal pHs will have different effects on medications and toxins. Optimal absorption of a drug may be dependent on a specific pH.
- Blood flow: The small intestine has a very good blood supply which is one reason why most absorption occurs in this part of the gut. Faster absorption rates will occur in areas where blood supply is ample.
- Luminal contents: Presence of food and fluid in the gastrointestinal tract: The presence of food in the gut may selectively increase or decrease drug absorption. For example, food increases the absorption of dicoumarol, while tetracycline absorption is reduced by the presence of dairy foods. Fluid taken with medication will aid dissolution of the drug and enhance its passage to the small intestine.
- Antacids: The presence of these in the gastrointestinal tract causes a change in environmental pH. They will increase absorption of basic drugs and decrease absorption of acidic ones.
- Drug composition: Various factors pertaining to the composition of the drug may affect the rate at which it is absorbed. For example, liquid preparations are more rapidly absorbed than solid ones, the presence of an enteric coating may slow absorption, and lipid-soluble drugs are rapidly absorbed.

Drugs may act locally or systemically. Locally implies that the effects of the drug are confined to a specific area. Systemically means that the drug has to enter the vascular and lymphatic systems for delivery to body tissues. The main route of administration to provide a local effect is topical, while oral or parenteral administration of drugs is the main route to provide a systemic effect. Some topical drugs can, however, have systemic effects, especially if given in large doses, in frequent doses or over a long period of time. For example, rhinitis medimatosa may occur from either prolonged use of intranasal or oral decongestants.

More specifically gastrointestinal absorption can occur through four processes:

- Passive diffusion is the most important and most common. If the drug is present in the gastrointestinal tract in a greater concentration than it is in the bloodstream, then a concentration gradient is said to exist. The presence of the concentration gradient will transport the drug to shift through the cell membrane and into the circulation. The drug will be shifted until the concentrations of drug are equal on either side of the cell membrane. No energy is expended during this process.
- Facilitated diffusion allows low lipid-soluble drugs to be transported across the cell membrane by combining with a carrier molecule. This also requires a concentration gradient and expends no energy.
- Active transport is only used by drugs which closely resemble natural body substances. This process works against a concentration gradient and requires a carrier protein and expended energy.

- Pinocytosis is not a common method for absorbing drugs. It requires energy and involves the cell membrane invaginating and engulfing a fluid-filled vesicle or sac.

Distribution

Once absorbed, each substance has its own pattern of distribution. Even though the discussion is predominately about drugs, the same principles apply to other chemical substances. During distribution, some drug molecules may be deposited at storage sites and others may be deposited and inactivated. Various factors influence how a drug is distributed.

- Blood flow: Distribution may depend on tissue perfusion. Organs that are highly vascular such as the heart, liver, and kidneys will rapidly acquire a drug. Levels of a drug in bone, fat, muscle, and skin may take some time to rise due to reduced vascularity. The patient's level of activity and local tissue temperature may also affect drug distribution to the skin and muscle.
- Plasma protein binding: In the circulation, a drug is either bound to circulating plasma proteins or is "free" in an un-bound state. The plasma protein usually involved in binding a drug is albumin. If a drug is bound, then it is said to be inactive and cannot have a pharmacological effect. Only the free drug molecules can cause an effect. As free molecules leave the circulation, drug molecules are released from plasma protein to re-establish a ratio between the bound and the free molecules. Binding tends to be non-specific and competitive. This means that plasma proteins will bind with many different drugs and these drugs will compete for binding sites on the plasma proteins. Displacement of one drug by another drug may have serious consequences. For example, warfarin can be displaced by tolbutamide producing a risk of hemorrhage, whereas tolbutamide can be displaced by salicylates producing a risk of hypoglycemia.
- Placental barrier: The chorionic villi enclose the fetal capillaries. These are separated from the maternal capillaries by a layer of trophoblastic cells. This barrier will permit the passage of lipid soluble, non-ionized compounds from mother to fetus but prevents entrance of those substances that are poorly lipid soluble.
- Blood–brain barrier: Capillaries of the central nervous system differ from those in most other parts of the body. They lack channels between endothelial cells through which substances in the blood normally gain access to the extracellular fluid. This barrier constrains the passage of substances from the blood to the brain and cerebrospinal fluid. Lipid-soluble drugs, for example, diazepam, will pass fairly readily into the central nervous system, whereas lipid-insoluble drugs will have little or no passage.
- Storage sites: Fat tissue is a storage site for lipid-soluble drugs, for example, anticoagulants, marijuana. Drugs that have accumulated in this tissue, may remain for some time, not being released until after administration of the drugs has ceased. Calcium-containing structures such as bone and teeth can accumulate drugs that are bound to calcium, for example, tetracycline.

Drug Metabolism

Drug metabolism or biotransformation refers to the process of modifying or altering the chemical composition of the drug. The pharmacological activity of the drug is usually removed though is some cases, hepatic transformation is required to activate the drug. Metabolites (products of metabolism) are produced which are more polar and less lipid soluble than the original drug, which ultimately promotes their excretion from the body. Most drug metabolism occurs in the liver, where hepatic enzymes catalyze various biochemical reactions. Metabolism of drugs may also occur in the kidneys, intestinal mucosa, lungs, plasma, and placenta.

Metabolism proceeds in two phases:

- Phase I. These reactions attempt to biotransform the drug to a more polar metabolite. The most common reactions are oxidations, catalysed by mixed function oxidase enzymes. Other phase I reactions include reduction and hydrolysis reactions.
- Phase II. Drugs or phase I metabolites which are not sufficiently polar for excretion by the kidneys, are made more hydrophilic by conjugation reactions with endogenous compounds provided by the liver. The resulting conjugates are then readily excreted by the kidneys.

With some drugs, given repeatedly, the metabolism of the drugs becomes more effective due to enzyme induction. Therefore, larger and larger doses of the drug become required in order to produce the same effect. This is referred to as drug tolerance (e.g., opiates).

Tolerance may also develop as a result of adaptive changes at cell receptors.

Various factors affect a client's ability to metabolize drugs. These include:

- Genetic differences: The enzyme systems which control drug metabolism are genetically determined. Some individuals show exaggerated and prolonged responses to drugs such as propranolol which undergo extensive hepatic metabolism. Also the new concepts of cancer chemotherapy utilize this concept.
- Age: In the elderly, first-pass metabolism may be reduced, resulting in increased bioavailability. In addition, the delayed production and elimination of active metabolites may prolong drug action. Reduced doses may, therefore, be necessary in the elderly. The enzyme systems responsible for conjugation are not fully effective in the neonate and this group of clients may be at an increased risk of toxic effects of drugs.
- Disease processes: Liver disease (acute or chronic) will affect metabolism if there is destruction of hepatocytes. Reduced hepatic blood flow as a result of cardiac failure or shock may also reduce the rate of metabolism of drugs.

Drug Excretion

Kidneys

Most drugs and metabolites are excreted by the kidneys. Small drug or metabolite molecules not bound to plasma proteins may be transported by glomerular filtration into the tubule. Active secretion of some drugs into the lumen of the nephron will also occur. This process, however, requires membrane carriers and energy.

Several factors may affect the rate at which a drug is excreted by the kidneys. These include:

- Presence of kidney disease, for example, renal failure.
- Altered renal blood flow.
- pH of urine.
- Concentration of the drug in plasma.
- Molecular weight of the drug.

Bile

Several drugs and metabolites are secreted by the liver into bile. These then enter the duodenum via the common bile duct, and move through the small intestine. Some drugs will be reabsorbed back into the bloodstream and return to the liver by the enterohepatic circulation. The drug then undergoes further metabolism or is secreted back into the bile. This is referred to as enterohepatic cycling and may extend the duration of action of a drug. Drugs secreted into bile, will ultimately pass through the large intestine and be excreted in the feces.

Lungs

Anesthetic gases, solvents, and small amounts of alcohol undergo pulmonary excretion.

Breast Milk

Milk-producing glands are surrounded by a network of capillaries, and drugs may pass from maternal blood into the breast milk. The amounts of drug may be very small, but may affect a suckling infant who has less ability to metabolize and excrete drugs.

Perspiration, Saliva, and Tears

Drugs may be excreted passively via these body secretions if the drugs are lipid soluble. Occasionally heavy solvent elimination is enhanced using an exercise-sauna methodology with controlled temperatures. This is termed controlled depuration.

The processes of drug metabolism, distribution, and drug excretion will ultimately determine the drug's half-life. This is the time taken for the concentration of drug in the blood to fall by half (50%) its original value. Standard dosage intervals are based on half-life calculations. This helps in the setting up of a dosage regime, which produces stable plasma drug concentrations, keeping the level of drug below toxic levels but above the minimum effective level.

There are occasions when an effective plasma level of drug must be reached quickly. This requires a dose of the drug which is larger than is normally given. This is called a loading dose. Once the required plasma level of drug has been reached, the normal recommended dose is given. This is then continued at regular intervals to maintain a stable plasma level and is called the maintenance dose.

Determining plasma levels of a drug at frequent intervals is undertaken when clients are prescribed drugs with a narrow therapeutic index such as digoxin, dilantin, or lithium. The therapeutic index is the ratio of the drug's toxic dose to its minimally effective dose. Usually, we measure this in terms of half-life of the drug or toxin. In order to completely eliminate a single dose of a substance, one must multiply the half-life by 5. The half-life may vary in different compartments. As an example, the half-life of inorganic mercury is 57 days in the blood but over 2 years in the brain. Pharmacologists measure drugs as having first-order kinetics or zero-order kinetics.

PHARMACODYNAMICS

While pharmacokinetics considers the way in which the body affects a drug by the processes of absorption, distribution, metabolism, and excretion, pharmacodynamics considers the effects of the drug on the body and the mode of drug action.

All body functions are mediated by control systems which depend on enzymes, receptors on cell surfaces, carrier molecules, and specific macromolecules such as the DNA. Most drugs act by interfering with these control systems at a molecular level. Once at their site of action, drugs may work in a very specific or non-specific manner. Specific mechanisms will be considered first.

Interaction with receptors on the cell membrane: A receptor is a protein molecule found on the surface of the cell or located intracellularly in the cytoplasm. Drugs frequently bind to receptors to form a drug–receptor complex. In order for a drug to interact with a receptor, it has to have a complementary structure in the same way that a key has a structure complementary to the lock in which it fits. Very few drugs are truly specific to a particular receptor and some drugs combine with more than one type of receptor. However, many drugs show selective activity on one particular receptor type.

A drug that has an affinity for a receptor, once bound to the receptor, can cause a specific response. Drugs that assist or boost a response are termed agonists whereas drugs that inhibit or antagonize a response are termed antagonists. Morphine is an opioid agonist that binds to mu receptors in the central nervous system to depress the perception of pain.

The action of the drug depends on whether it occupies the most receptors. For example, naloxone is a competitive antagonist for mu receptors and may be used to treat opioid overdose. It will compete with morphine for mu receptors and reverse the effects of an excessive dose of morphine. A non-competitive antagonist will inactivate a receptor so that an agonist cannot bind to the site.

Drug–receptor binding is usually reversible and the response to the drug is gradually reduced once the drug leaves the receptor site.

Interference with Ion Passage through the Cell Membrane

Ion channels are selective pores in the cell membrane that allow the movement of ions in and out of the cell. Some drugs will block these channels, which ultimately interferes with ion transport and causes an altered physiological response. Drugs working in this way include nifedipine, verapamil, and lidocaine.

Enzyme Inhibition or Stimulation

Enzymes are proteins and biological catalysts which speed up the rate of chemical reactions. Some drugs interact with enzymes in a manner similar to the drug–receptor complex mechanism already described. Drugs often resemble the structure of a natural substrate and compete for the binding site on the enzyme. A few examples of drugs interacting with enzymes include aspirin and angiotensin-converting enzyme (ACE) inhibitors such as enalapril.

Incorporation into Macromolecules

Some drugs may be taken up by a larger molecule and will interfere with the normal function of that molecule. For example, when the anticancer drug 5-fluorouracil is incorporated into messenger RNA, taking the place of the molecule uracil, transcription is affected.

Interference with Metabolic Processes of Microorganisms

Some drugs interfere with metabolic processes that are very specific or unique to microorganisms and thus kill or inhibit activity of the microorganism. Penicillin disrupts bacterial cell wall formation while trimethroprim inhibits bacterial folic acid synthesis.

Non-specific mechanisms involve:

- Chemical alteration of the extracellular environment. Drugs may not alter specific cell function, but because they alter the chemical environment around the cell, a cellular response or change occurs. Drugs which have this effect include osmotic diuretics (e.g., mannitol), osmotic laxatives (e.g., lactulose), and antacids (e.g., magnesium hydroxide).
- Physical alteration of the cellular environment. Drugs may not alter specific cell function, but because they alter the physical as opposed to the chemical environment around the cell, cellular responses or changes occur. Drugs which have this effect would include docusate sodium which lowers fecal surface tension and many of the barrier preparations available, which protect the skin.

UNDESIRABLE RESPONSES TO DRUG THERAPY

Most drugs are not entirely free of unwanted effects. However, drugs which are frequently prescribed, highly potent, or that have a narrow therapeutic index, are likely to increase the risk of unwanted effects.

Terms used to describe undesirable responses to drugs include:

- Adverse reaction. This refers to any undesirable drug effect.
- Side effect. This is used interchangeably with the term adverse reaction. It refers to unwanted but predictable responses to a drug.

- Toxic effect. This usually occurs when too much drug has accumulated in the body. It may be due to an acute high dose of a drug, chronic buildup over time or increased sensitivity to the standard dose of a drug.
- Drug allergy (hypersensitivity). The immune system recognizes the drug as an antigen and an immune response is mounted against the drug. This may be either an immediate or delayed response.

FACTORS AFFECTING THE BODY'S RESPONSE TO A DRUG

Many individual factors will determine an individual's clinical response to a drug. Some of these have already been identified but additional factors will also be considered here. The health-care provider should be fully aware of these factors and they should be incorporated into the patient's assessment before decisions are made about which drug to prescribe. In addition, they should be considered when monitoring drugs which are already being used by the patient, whether the drugs are prescribed or obtained "over-the-counter."

- Age. The very young and the elderly particularly have problems related to their ability to metabolize and excrete drugs. Neonatal hepatic enzyme systems are not fully effective, so drug metabolism will be reduced and there is an increased risk of toxicity. In the elderly, delayed metabolism by the liver and a decline in renal function means delayed excretion by the kidneys and drug action may be prolonged. Complicated drug regimens may be difficult for the elderly to follow which may mean inadequate or excessive doses of drugs are consumed.
- Body weight. The size of an individual will affect the amount of a drug that is distributed and available to act. The larger the individual, the larger the area for drug distribution. Lipid-soluble drugs may be sequestered in fat stores and not available for use. This is the reason that some drugs are given according to the client's body weight, that is, × milligrams per kilogram of body weight. All clients should have their weight recorded and this should be reassessed regularly if the client is receiving long-term drug treatment.
- Pregnancy and lactation. Lipid-soluble, non-ionized drugs in the free state will cross the placenta (e.g., opiates, warfarin). Some may be teratogenic and cause fetal malformation. Drugs can also be transferred to the suckling infant via breast milk and have adverse effects on the child (e.g., sedatives, anticonvulsants, and caffeine). A full drug history should be obtained pre-conception where possible or as soon as pregnancy has been diagnosed. Women must be educated not to take medication without consulting a health-care practitioner.
- Nutritional status. Patients who are malnourished may have altered drug distribution and metabolism. Inadequate dietary protein may affect enzyme activity and slow the metabolism of drugs. A reduction in plasma protein levels may mean that a more free drug is available for activity. A loss of body fat stores will mean less sequestering of the drug in fat and more drug available for activity. Normal doses in the severely malnourished may lead to toxicity. Nutritional assessment of clients is, therefore, essential and malnutrition should be managed accordingly.
- Food–drug interactions. The presence of food may enhance or inhibit the absorption of a drug. For example, orange juice (vitamin C) will enhance the absorption of iron sulfate, but dairy produce reduce the absorption of tetracycline. Monoamine oxidase inhibitors must not be taken with foods rich in tyramine, such as cheese, meat, yeast extracts, some types of alcoholic drinks and other products, due to risk of sudden hypertensive crisis. Health-care practitioners should have some knowledge of common food–drug interactions and drug administration may need timing in relation to mealtimes.

- Disease processes. Altered functioning of many body systems will affect a client's response to a drug. Only a few examples are therefore given:
  - Changes in gut motility and therefore transit time may affect absorption rates, for example, with diarrhea and vomiting absorption is reduced. Loss of absorptive surface in the small intestine, as occurs in Crohn's disease will affect absorption.
  - Hepatic disease (e.g., hepatitis, cirrhosis, and liver failure), will reduce metabolism of drugs and lead to a gradual accumulation of drugs and increase the risk of toxicity.
  - Renal disease (e.g., acute and chronic renal failure), will reduce excretion of drugs and drugs may accumulate.
  - Circulatory diseases (e.g., heart failure and peripheral vascular disease), will reduce distribution and transport of drugs.
- Mental and emotional factors. Many factors may affect a client's ability to comply with their drug regime. These include confusion, amnesia, identified mental illness, stress, bereavement, and many others. These types of problems may lead to inadequate or excessive use of medication resulting in unsuccessful treatment or serious adverse effects. The nurse must consider these issues during patient assessment.
- Genetic and racial factors. Enzyme systems controlling drug metabolism are genetically determined and therefore, genetic variation leads to differences in patient's abilities to metabolize drugs. For example, some individuals possess an atypical form of the enzyme pseudocholinesterase. When these individuals are given the muscle relaxant suxamethonium, prolonged paralysis occurs and recovery from the drug takes longer. Different races of people are also known to dispose of drugs at different rates.

The liver, kidney, and breath are our most important organs of elimination though sweating (controlled depuration) is sometimes helpful.

Toxicity

Those toxic substances that cannot be eliminated are then stored and can produce toxic effects. Some substances can be present without overt clinical effects. A good example is lead which is predominately stored in bones. Again, the dose is the key. Even subtle effects caused by toxic substances can easily be overlooked and can produce nonspecific signs. Many medical and osteopathic schools have improved their education regarding environmental and toxicological etiologies.

Synergism

Sometimes one can be exposed to more than one substance at the same time. Synergism when two compounds produce an adverse effect greater than that of either substance alone.

Drugs can also have an additive effect, which occurs when one drug effect is added to another.

Susceptibility

Another principle of toxicology is that some individuals are more susceptible to toxins than others. This is an area of intense investigation and genetic factors are often determined to be responsible.

A clinical example is a case of a school teacher supervising her class outdoors as they board a bus after school is dismissed. She was exposed to the exhaust from the bus for 10 minutes. When she returned to her classroom she became short of breath and began to cough. This led to a serious asthma attack that slowly responded to medical care, including high-dose steroids, over a three-week period. Her exposure time was brief (10 minutes). This case is atypical as the exposure was relatively brief but emphasizes the importance of bioindividuality and susceptibility. The same amount of exposure did not affect anyone else at that time. Historically she was atopic and an asthmatic though not on medications prior to the incident. Asthmatics often have low-grade eosinophilic and inflammatory responses with increased cytokines in their airways to begin with. Thus they are often hypersensitive to perfumes, colognes, fumes, and other vapors. Even OSHA acknowledges that there are sensitive individuals who may respond adversely in certain workplace areas in spite of measurements of concentration that meet Federal standards. In other words, Federal standards apply to a vast majority (~80%) of the workforce but not everyone in covered.

Another example of individual variability is demonstrated in patients with eczema. Such individuals are more prone to cutaneous aggravation after contact with a mild irritant in doses that would not affect normal skin.

Genetic susceptibility in processing different medications is well recognized. Over the past several years testing has become available at the physician's office to provide a genetic susceptibility overview.

There are some individuals who demonstrate multi-systemic manifestations when exposed to petroleum-based chemicals below levels considered at risk by OSHA or EPA. This condition is termed multiple chemical sensitivity. This syndrome is not uncommon. The cause of this condition is being investigated and is probably multifactorial. Phenotypic abnormalities in excretory pathways such as sulfation, glucuronidation, or with the numerous cytochrome P450 system members are suggested. Often there are psychological factors as well.[2-6]

SUBSPECIALTIES OF TOXICOLOGY

There are several subdisciplines of toxicology, which focus on particular aspects of toxicology. These include:

- Toxicogenomics
- Chemical toxicology
- Clinical toxicology
- Ecotoxicology
- Environmental toxicology
- Forensic toxicology
- Medical toxicology
- Occupational toxicology
- Regulatory toxicology

All these may interact. As an example, the Mine Safety Health Administration (MSHA) is a regulatory body created to lessen the morbidity and mortality rate among miners. Mine incidents were the most common cause of occupational-related death in past years. Working with the Occupational Safety and Health Administration, regulations were created to lessen the dangers in such an environment. The MSHA also depended on monitoring and research from the environmental toxicologist as well as the diagnosis and treatment of medical impairment from the clinical toxicologist and occupational physician. Teamwork is often essential when dealing with a toxicological event. Even a urinary test for illicit drugs involves both the physician and the toxicology laboratory, supervised by the clinical or laboratory toxicologist.

MEDICAL TOXICOLOGY

From a medical perspective, the physician usually perceives toxicology in the form of poisons and overdoses, best dealt with at a poison control center or more commonly, an emergency room.

In such centers, general principles apply while an effort to identify the poison is conducted.
First: ABCs

1. Establish and maintain an airway if needed
2. Ensure adequate oxygenation
3. Establish an intravenous route

4. Properly monitor vital signs
5. Assist ventilation and treat bronchoreactivity if present
6. Provide an antidote to the poison or toxin if known. Some toxins have specific antidotes
7. Remove or reduce the toxin (dialysis, diuresis, gastric lavage, etc.)
8. Monitor as some substances have a long half-life (e.g., methadone).

Certain substances produce characteristic clinical patterns which assist with decisions on proper treatment.

The best-known examples of these are:

1. Cholinergic syndrome which may have either a muscarinic or nicotinic pattern: Muscarinic pattern: Diarrhea (often with nausea and vomiting) excess urination, muscle fasciculation, miosis, bradycardia, bronchospasm, excessive lacrimation, excessive salivation—Mnemonic DUMBELS

   Nicotinic pattern: Weakness tachycardia, mydriasis, hyperglycemia, hypertension, muscle fasciculations, CNS excitation.

   The former can be found with organophosphates including nerve gases or certain pesticides. Certain mushrooms can also have this effect.
2. Anticholinergic syndrome: Flushing, dry skin and mucous membranes, mydriasis, loss of accommodation, and mental status changes, including convulsions, psychosis, delirium are classic manifestations. Fever, tachycardia, thirst, urinary retention are also seen. This pattern can be seen totally or partially with overdoses of atropine and similar anticholinergics. Mushrooms such as *Amanita muscarina*, plants like jimson weed, skeletal muscle relaxants, antipsychotics, antihistamines, or tricyclics can produce this effect.
3. Serotonin syndrome.
4. Extrapyramidal syndrome.
5. Excessive sympathetic syndrome.
6. Malignant hyperthermia.

A comprehensive review of medical toxicology is beyond the scope of this chapter, however, an excellent, no-cost app is available called PEPID.

Chemical Toxicology

Chemical toxicology is a subspecialty of toxicology that focuses on the structure of chemical agents and how it affects their mechanism of action on living organisms. It is a multidisciplinary field that includes computational and synthetic chemistry, in addition to people who specialize in the fields of proteomics, metabolomics, drug discovery, drug metabolism, bioinformatics, analytical chemistry, biological chemistry, and molecular epidemiology. It relies on technological advances to help understand the chemical components of toxicology more comprehensively. It is among the core sciences for the development of new drugs and consumer products. Such toxicologists are usually PhDs and may be educators of this subject, researchers, or advisors to pharmaceutical and consumer product companies.

Toxicology and Pharmacology

Toxicology and pharmacology are both studies that involve an understanding of chemical properties and their actions of these agents on the body, but differ considerably in other areas. They are like looking at two sides of the same coin.

Pharmacology primarily focuses on the therapeutic effects of pharmaceutical substances and how they can be used most effectively for medical purpose. On the contrary, toxicology is more closely related to the adverse effects of such substances that can occur in living organisms. Toxicologists are also more concerned with measuring the risk of certain substances with risk-assessment tools. Common terms used in this investigation are pharmacokinetics which is the study of what the body does to the drug and pharmacodynamics which is the study of what the drug does to the body.

As mentioned before, the toxic effects of a chemical frequently depend on the route of exposure (oral, intravenous, inhalation, or dermal) and the duration of exposure (subchronic, chronic, or lifetime). Thus, a full description of the toxic effects of a chemical includes a listing of what adverse health effects the chemical may cause and how the occurrence of these effects depends upon dose, route, and duration of exposure.

The toxicity assessment process is usually divided into two parts: the first characterizes and quantifies the non-cancer effects of the chemical, while the second addresses the cancer effects of the chemical. This two-part approach is employed because there are typically major differences in the time-course of action and the shape of the dose–response curve for cancer and non-cancer effects.

Essentially, all chemicals can cause non-cancer adverse health effects if given at a high enough dose. However, when the dose is sufficiently low, typically no adverse effect is observed. Thus, in characterizing the non-cancer effects of a chemical, the key parameter is the threshold dose at which an adverse effect first becomes evident. Doses below the threshold are considered to be safe, while doses above the threshold are likely to cause an effect.

Like any field of science, toxicology has its own abbreviations and phrases. LD50 is a useful term that refers to the dose of a substance that displays toxicity in that it kills 50% of a test population. In scientific research, rats or other surrogates are usually used to determine toxicity. The data are then extrapolated for humans.

The threshold dose is typically estimated from toxicological data (derived from studies of humans and/or animals) by determining the highest dose that does not produce an observable adverse effect and the lowest dose which does produce an effect. These are referred to as the "no-observed-adverse-effect-level" (NOAEL) and the "lowest-observed-adverse-effect-level" (LOAEL), respectively. The threshold is presumed to lie in the interval between the NOAEL and the LOAEL.

However, in order to be conservative (protective), non-cancer risk evaluations are not based directly on the threshold exposure level, but on a value referred to as the reference dose (RfD). The RfD is an estimate (with uncertainty spanning perhaps an order of magnitude) of a daily exposure to the human population (including sensitive subgroups) that is likely to be without an appreciable risk of deleterious effects during a lifetime.

The RfD is derived from the NOAEL (or the LOAEL if a reliable NOAEL is not available) by dividing by an "uncertainty factor." If the data are from studies in humans, and if the observations are considered to be very reliable, the uncertainty factor may be as small as 1.0. However, the uncertainty factor is normally at least 10 and can be much higher if data are limited. The purpose of dividing the NOAEL or the LOAEL by an uncertainty factor is to ensure that the RfD is not higher than the true threshold level for adverse effects. Thus, there is always a "margin of safety" built into an RfD, and doses equal to or less than the RfD are nearly certain to be without any risk of adverse effect. Doses higher than the RfD may carry some risk, but because of the margin of safety, a dose above the RfD does not mean that an effect will necessarily occur.

For cancer effects, the toxicity assessment process has two components. The first is a qualitative evaluation of the weight of evidence (WOE) that the chemical does or does not cause cancer in humans. For chemicals that are believed to be capable of causing cancer in humans, the second part of the toxicity assessment is to describe the carcinogenic potency of the chemical. This is done by quantifying how the number of cancers observed in exposed animals or humans increases as the dose increases. Typically, it is assumed that the dose–response curve for cancer has no threshold (i.e., there is no dose other than zero that does not increase the risk of cancer), arising from the origin and increasing linearly until high doses are reached. Thus, the most convenient descriptor of cancer potency is the slope of the dose–response curve at low doses (where the slope is still linear). This is referred to as the slope factor (SF), which has dimensions of risk of cancer per unit dose.

Estimating the cancer SF is often complicated by the fact that observable increases in cancer incidences usually occur only at relatively high doses, frequently in the part of the dose–response curve that is no longer linear. Thus, it is necessary to use mathematical models to extrapolate from the observed high-dose data to the desired (but unmeasurable) slope at low dose. In order to account for the uncertainty in this extrapolation process, the EPA typically chooses to employ the upper 95th confidence interval limit of the slope as the SF. That is, there is a 95% probability that the true cancer potency is lower than the value chosen for the SF. This approach ensures that there is a margin of safety in cancer as well as non-cancer risk estimates.

The International Agency for Research on Cancer (IARC) is part of the World Health Organization (WHO). Its major goal is to identify causes of cancer. The most widely used system for classifying carcinogens comes from the IARC. In the past 30 years, the IARC has evaluated the cancer-causing potential of more than 900 likely compounds, placing them into one of the following groups:

- Group 1: Carcinogenic to humans
- Group 2A: Probably carcinogenic to humans
- Group 2B: Possibly carcinogenic to humans
- Group 3: Unclassifiable as to carcinogenicity in humans
- Group 4: Probably not carcinogenic to humans

Thus far, the IARC has classified 117 substances as carcinogenic to humans, 74 as probably carcinogenic, 287 as possibly carcinogenic, 503 as unclassifiable, and 1 as probably not carcinogenic.[7]

The preferred source of toxicity data is EPA's **Integrated Risk Information System (IRIS)** database. Values in this database have been derived by expert toxicologists at EPA and most values have undergone thorough review and validation both within and outside EPA. If a toxicity value is available in IRIS, that value should be used in preference to any other value. If toxicity values for a contaminant of potential concern are not available in IRIS, the next source to consult is EPA's Provisional Peer Reviewed Toxicity Values (PPRTVs). This source includes toxicity values that have been developed by the Office of Research and Development/National Center for Environmental Assessment/Superfund Health Risk Technical Support Center (STSC).[8]

For those health-care professionals interested in expanding their knowledge of how to perform an environmental and occupational history as well as learning more about individual chemical agents, an excellent source is to contact the Agency for Toxic Substances and Disease Registry at 4770 Buford Hwy NE Atlanta, GA 30341, USA, Phone 800-CDC-INFO (800-232-4636), TTY: 888-232-6348.

Another source of toxicity seen commonly in clinical practice is from the effects of illicit drugs. Many cases of drug overdose flood our emergency rooms and cause significant mortality. Medical review officers are examined and certified by the Department of Transportation to evaluate mandated drug testing for interstate truck drivers in an effort to have safer highways.

OCCUPATIONAL TOXICOLOGY

Occupational toxicology involves the study of adverse effects of a large number of metals and chemicals found in the workplace. Single exposures can and do produce permanent impairment or even death. These are termed acute events and in such cases the concentration is usually high. At lower doses, insidious effects can occur with temporary or permanent damage. These are termed chronic effects. The toxicologist is involved with both of these patterns.

From a clinical perspective, physicians frequently encounter cases of occupational toxic exposure. Often these cases overlap with a consideration of potential allergic responses. The overlap can occur because some toxic substance can directly affect the immune system. These can cause both a toxic as well as an allergic response. Many cutaneous cases result in contact dermatitis and more rarely contact urticaria or photodermatitis.

Case 1: A 56-year-old male presented with severe pruritic dermatitis on his left forearm. It had been present for three weeks and was treated with topical steroids at the local clinic. He was referred to a specialist when he returned to work and his condition worsened and a second eruption occurred on the dorsal surface of his left hand.

Possible causes include industrial compounds, soaps, cosmetics, fragrances, jewelry, and plants, such as poison ivy or poison oak. Some people, such as this patient, are exposed to substances at work that may cause contact dermatitis. Due to different methods of treatment, especially with regard to engineering controls, it is important to identify if this problem is caused by an allergy or an irritant. It is important to obtain and properly interpret a standardized patch test to separate one from the other. This often requires the cooperation of an allergist or dermatologist.

In his case, the allergist and occupational specialist made an inventory of all the chemicals that he worked around. They then determined any chemical compounds that were new or altered in the weeks or months preceding the exposure as well as the type of personal protection that he utilized. (In a large facility, it is helpful to work with the industrial hygiene department as well as management.) By a process of elimination, the chemical involved was narrowed down to three possibilities. None of these were available in an FDA (Food and Drug Administration)-approved standard patch-test series (true test). The three chemicals are too toxic to be utilized as a prick test or subcutaneous test. They had to be custom made by a compounding pharmacist and were prepared as a patch test at an appropriate dilution in the pharmacy, utilizing a petroleum base. They were then applied to the patient's unshaven, clean skin, away from the area of dermatitis. A control was also utilized and read, and dermatographia of the skin is to be excluded initially. These reactions, if allergic, usually result in a delayed reaction and must be interpreted by the American Academy of Dermatology protocol at 24 and 48 hours and sometimes 72 hours. Irritant-type responses cause early irritant effects and pruritis. In his case, the product causing his skin allergy was an additive to a machine coolant. He reacted at the 48 hour evaluation.

There are four possible actions to take in a case of occupational allergy versus an irritant effect. If he is allergic, (a) engineering controls such as substitution of the compound for another one that he is not allergic to can solve the problem; (b) he may lose his symptoms by improving the work conditions, whereas his personal protection adequately prevents contact; (c) place him in another area of the plant (reasonable accommodation) or (d) terminate the employee. This patient had an allergy, so that even small amounts of contact with the substance potentially would cause problems.

With the more common irritant-type contact dermatitis, besides providing standard medical care, the key to prevention is education, improving personal protection, keeping a clean work area, and personal cleanliness. This patient's company would not provide a product substitution but provided him reasonable accommodation by placing him in another area of the plant where he only rarely is exposed to the product. He is treated approximately twice a year with steroids for a flare-up when exposed.

Case 2: A 28-year-old female presented with asthmatic symptoms. She had no prior history of allergy or asthma and did not appear clinically atopic at the time of her examination. Her pulmonary function testing revealed a normal diffusion capacity, slight increase in total lung and residual volume, slight reduction in vital capacity and moderate reduction in the forced expiratory volume during the first breath (FEV1). The forced vital capacity (FVC)/FEV1 ratio was 65%. There was a significant 23% increase in the FEV1 after a bronchodilator. The patient's history suggested that she may have been exposed to a product at work. She had been working in a paint manufacturing facility for 6 years and never had problems. She reports adequate ventilation and personal protection.

The problem here is to document whether she had adult asthma initiating independently of the work environment or was exposed to something different in the domiciliary (home) or work environment. In her case she noted that over the weekend, away from work, she improved and upon returning to work, she worsened. Furthermore she noticed that wearing her protective mask became increasing difficult due to shortness of breath. An investigation of her MSDSs and work environment eventually permitted us to establish a diisocyanate sensitivity. Many cases of diisocyanate allergy appear *de novo* in non-atopic individuals after working around this chemical for an extended time period. Unfortunately even small amounts of the agent will induce asthma once she is sensitized but her prognosis is favorable if she changes vocations. In this case, personal protection and engineering controls could not be reasonably provided.

About 15%–20% of individuals exposed to this product as auto-spray painters develop a sensitivity to this substance after performing this job for many years.

Occupational asthma is the most common type of occupational lung disease. About 15% of asthma in the United States is caused by occupational substances.

Statistically, the strongest evidence of association of occupational asthma with a worksite agent is with exposure to laboratory animals. Associations with moderate evidence level were obtained for alpha-amylase from *Aspergillus oryzae*, various enzymes from *Bacillus subtilis*, papain, bakeries, western red cedar, latex, psyllium, storage mites, rat, carmine, egg proteins, Atlantic salmon, fishmeal, Norway lobster, prawn, snow crab, seafood, trout and turbot, and reactive dyes. These reactions produce classic antibody responses and are relevant because exposure to even small amounts of the allergen (below OSHA PEL levels) will produce a bronchoreactive response.

Irritants can also trigger an asthma-type response. This was first described by Brooks et al., and is termed reactive airways disease or RADS.[9] The irritant agents at worksites that can produce RADS include numerous solvents, benzene-1,2,4-tricarboxylic acid, 1,2-anhydride (trimetallic anhydride), chlorine, platinum salts, cobalt, cement, environmental tobacco smoke, grain, welding fumes, construction work, as well as fumes from swine confinement. This condition is sometimes difficult in that the pulmonary function test at times does not look very abnormal and is disproportionate to the clinical manifestations. To verify, the patient may require a methacholine challenge test.

Over 40% of workers cleaning up after the World Trade Centre disaster in 2001 have persisting and sometimes disabling respiratory conditions. The persistent dust cloud with its airborne toxins as well as the longer duration of time working at the site significantly elevated the risk of respiratory problems. Many workers developed RADS. Post-traumatic stress disorder (PTSD) was also frequent among such workers, especially the non-police rescuers.

Another area of occupational toxicology is neurotoxicology. Solvents and heavy metals have clearly been associated with central nervous system dysfunction. Peripheral neuropathies also are well recognized. A list of agents that are neurotoxic are:

Acetone (1000 ppm)	Formaldehyde (3 ppm)
Alcohol	Glycerol
Aliphatic hydrocarbons	Hexane (500 ppm)
Alkanes	Isophorone (25 ppm)
Alkyl styrene polymers	Lead (0.05 mg/m³)
Ammonia (500 ppm)	Lithium grease
Amyl acetate (100 ppm)	Methanol (200 ppm)
Aniline (5 ppm)	Methyl acetate (200 ppm)
Antimony sulfide (0.5 mg/m³)	Nitrous oxide
Aromatic hydrocarbons	Oil, fuel no. 1
Asphalt	Oil, lube
Benzene (1 ppm)	Petroleum distillates
Butanol	Pine oil
Butyl acetate (150 ppm)	Polymethacrylate resin
Cadmium oxides (0.1 mg/m³)	Products of combustion
Carbon disulfide (20 ppm)	Propanol, 1-
Carbon tetrachloride (10 ppm)	Propylene glycol (200 ppm)
Chlorinated hydrocarbons	Shella
Chlorobenzene (75 ppm)	Sodium chloride

Continued

Chromium oxides	Solvents
Cresol (5 ppm)	Tetrachloroethylene 100 ppm
Cyclohexanol (50 ppm)	Toluene (200 ppm)
Cyclohexanone (50 ppm)	Trichlorobenzene
Degreaser	Trichloroethylene
Diacetone alcohol (50 ppm)	Trichlorofluromethane
Dichlorobenzene, ortho- (50 ppm)	Tricresyl phosphate
Dichlorotetrafluroethane	Tungsten oxides
Diphenylamine	Turpentine
Dyes	Vinyl chloride
Ethanol	Xylene (100 ppm)
Ethyl acetate (400 ppm)	Ethylene glycol (0.2 ppm)
Food additives	Mercury

REGULATORY TOXICOLOGY

Regulatory toxicology is of great importance as a component of State and Federal regulatory agencies. The National Institute of Safety and Health Administration (NIOSH) is the non-regulatory research arm of these regulatory bodies that compiles the data and analyzes the epidemiological and toxicological research to make decisions on safe thresholds levels (TLVs) and advise regulatory agencies. Engineering controls, NIOSH-approved respiratory protection, and appropriate personal protection are critical when working with toxic substances. Working in partnership with regulators and employers are important to prevent further morbidity and mortality in the workplace.

TOXIC: ALLERGIC INTERACTION

Toxic substances at the workplace, such as trimethyl anhydride (TMA), can activate the allergic response and can produce specific antibodies (often IgE), just as the case mentioned above did with diisocyanate. Cosmetics and personal care products have a lot of potential allergens. These include:

- Fragrances in soaps, colognes, deodorants, body creams, cosmetics, detergents, and tissues
- Preservatives and antibacterials, added to many liquids to keep them from becoming rancid or contaminated
- Substances added to thicken, color, or lubricate a product
- Chemicals in permanent hair dyes and other hair products
- Formaldehyde resin, an ingredient in many nail care products
- Sunscreens, often found in cosmetic moisturizers, lip balms, and foundations

Most of these sensitizing chemicals bind to a protein termed a haptene and the hypersensitivity reactions are to this chemical–protein complex. This is an example of another chemical response specifically creating allergic antibodies or responses. Some of these are type III or IV immune responses, though type I responses (IgE mediated) are also common.

Another area of concern is the concept of immunotoxicology. How is the immune system affected by the sum total of our chemical load? This field is gaining attention.[10]

EXOGENOUS AND ENDOGENOUS TOXINS

Many substances may act as toxins as described above that enter our bodies from outside. The most common are pharmaceuticals, environmental pollutants, and additives found in our home and work environment. These toxins are ubiquitous. You only have to live in a civilized society to acquire exogenous toxins. Also contributing, are our personal habits such as tobacco smoke (primary and second-hand) ethanol and recreational drugs such as heroin, marijuana, cocaine, phencyclidine (PCP), amphetamines, and numerous synthetics. Thus, we are exposed to a virtual sea of toxins.

Hydrocarbon-based compounds found at home and work environment are commonly encountered. These include solvents, strippers, cleaners, cutting oils, metals such as chromium, cadmium, lead, mercury, and less commonly, beryllium. Occupational texts tell us that there are over 60,000 different chemicals in the workplace, with new ones being produced all the time. Some are bioaccumulative, such as lead and mercury, other metals, and hydrocarbons, especially chlorinated pesticides. Many of these chemicals can cause disability and even death.

In a perfect world, we may be exposed to little or no external toxins and thus have a lower cancer rate and less functional impairment. Since none of us live in a truly perfect world, we are in a state of heterostasis where our body must continuously adapt and adjust to external and internal stressors, some of which are allergic, some are infectious, some are psychic, and some are toxic. This list is not inclusive. In fact, our bodies are designed to be in this state since the relative absence of stress, can cause stress.

Testing of our adipose tissue demonstrates a myriad of fat-soluble products that are accumulating. It is true that the kidney, liver, breathe, and sweat remove some toxins, but a wide variety of chemicals remain in all of us. Normally these remain silently within us but may contribute to carcinogenesis and other disorders, especially in genetically susceptible individuals.

Tobacco

What some of us do to ourselves contribute to the toxicological stress load in our bodies. Smoking is a good example. While many smokers look at smoking as a pleasurable experience, they are vaguely aware that it may cause cancer or chronic obstructive pulmonary disease (COPD). Many smokers tend to ignore this fact and often exhibit an immortality complex to indicate that such diseases affect "the other guy." After all, in the short term a cigarette may well be affiliated with a cup of coffee or a martini. The facts however are different.

The list of 599 additives approved by the US Government for use in the manufacture of cigarettes is something every smoker should be aware of. Submitted by the five major American cigarette companies to the Department of Health and Human Services in April of 1994, this list of ingredients had long been kept confidential.

Tobacco companies reporting this information were:

American Tobacco Company
Brown and Williamson
Liggett Group, Inc.
Philip Morris Inc.
R.J. Reynolds Tobacco Company

While these ingredients are approved as additives for foods, they were not tested by burning them, and it is the burning of many of these substances which changes their properties, often for the worse. Over 4000 chemical compounds are created by burning a cigarette—69 of those chemicals are known to cause cancer. Carbon monoxide, nitrogen oxides, hydrogen cyanides, and ammonia are all present in cigarette smoke. Manufacturers utilize various additives to enhance or change the "flavor" of the product. This includes grains. Here is a partial list:

• Acetic acid
• Acetone
• Acetophenone
• 6-Acetoxydihydrotheaspirane
• 2-Acetyl-3-ethylpyrazine

- 2-Acetyl-5-methylfuran
- Acetylpyrazine
- 2-Acetylpyridine
- 3-Acetylpyridine
- 2-Acetylthiazole
- Aconitic acid
- DL-Alanine
- Alfalfa extract
- Allspice extract, oleoresin, and oil
- Allyl hexanoate
- Allyl ionone
- Almond bitter oil
- Ambergris tincture
- Ammonia
- Ammonium bicarbonate
- Ammonium hydroxide
- Ammonium phosphate dibasic
- Ammonium sulfide
- Amyl alcohol
- Amyl butyrate
- Amyl formate
- Amyl octanoate
- α-Amylcinnamaldehyde
- Amyris oil
- *trans*-Anethole
- Angelica root extract, oil, and seed oil
- Anise
- Anise star, extract, and oils
- Anisyl acetate
- Anisyl alcohol
- Anisyl formate
- Anisyl phenylacetate
- Apple juice concentrate, extract, and skins
- Apricot extract and juice concentrate
- L-Arginine
- Asafetida fluid extract and oil
- Ascorbic acid
- L-Asparagine monohydrate
- L-Aspartic acid
- Balsam Peru and oil
- Basil oil
- Bay leaf, oil, and sweet oil
- Beeswax white
- Beet juice concentrate
- Benzaldehyde
- Benzaldehyde glyceryl acetal
- Benzoic acid, benzoin
- Benzoin resin
- Benzophenone
- Benzyl alcohol
- Benzyl benzoate

- Benzyl butyrate
- Benzyl cinnamate
- Benzyl propionate
- Benzyl salicylate
- Bergamot oil
- Bisabolene
- Black currant buds absolute
- Borneol
- Bornyl acetate
- Buchu leaf oil
- 1,3-Butanediol
- 2,3-Butanedione
- 1-Butanol
- 2-Butanone
- 4(2-Butenylidene)-3,5,5-trimethyl-2-cyclohexen-1-one
- Butter, butter esters, and butter oil
- Butyl acetate
- Butyl butyrate
- Butyl butyryl lactate
- Butyl isovalerate
- Butyl phenylacetate
- Butyl undecylenate
- 3-Butylidenephthalide
- Butyric acid
- Cadinene
- Caffeine
- Calcium carbonate
- Camphene
- Cananga oil
- Capsicum oleoresin
- Caramel color
- Caraway oil
- Carbon dioxide
- Cardamom oleoresin, extract, seed oil, and powder
- Carob bean and extract
- β-Carotene
- Carrot oil
- Carvacrol
- 4-Carvomenthenol
- 1-Carvone
- β-Caryophyllene
- β-Caryophyllene oxide
- Cascarilla oil and bark extract
- Cassia bark oil
- Cassia absolute and oil
- Castoreum extract, tincture, and absolute
- Cedar leaf oil
- Cedarwood oil terpenes and Virginiana
- Cedrol
- Celery seed extract, solid, oil, and oleoresin
- Cellulose fiber

- Chamomile flower oil and extract
- Chicory extract
- Chocolate
- Cinnamaldehyde
- Cinnamic acid
- Cinnamon leaf oil, bark oil, and extract
- Cinnamyl acetate
- Cinnamyl alcohol
- Cinnamyl cinnamate
- Cinnamyl isovalerate
- Cinnamyl propionate
- Citral
- Citric acid
- Citronella oil
- DL-Citronellol
- Citronellyl butyrate
- Citronellyl isobutyrate
- Civet absolute
- Clary oil
- Clover tops, red solid extract
- Cocoa
- Cocoa shells, extract, distillate and powder
- Coconut oil
- Coffee
- Cognac white and green oil
- Copaiba oil
- Coriander extract and oil
- Corn oil
- Corn silk
- Costus root oil
- Cubeb oil
- Cuminaldehyde
- *p*-Cymene
- L-Cysteine dandelion root solid extract
- Davana oil
- 2-*trans*, 4-*trans*-Decadienal
- δ-Decalactone

To complete this list go to: http://www.tricountycessation.org/tobaccofacts/Cigarette-Ingredients. html.

Alcohol

Since it is legal to consume alcohol and a majority of us have done so we recognize the effects of a higher dose of alcohol. Here are a few facts about alcohol. According to the National Institute of Alcohol Abuse and Alcoholism, in the United States, 17.6 million people—about one in every 12 adults—abuse alcohol or are alcohol dependent. Chronic alcohol-related neuroadaptations in key neural circuits of emotional and cognitive control play a critical role in the development of, and recovery from, alcoholism. Converging evidence in the neurobiological literature indicates that neuroplastic changes in the prefrontal–striatal–limbic circuit, which governs emotion regulation and decision-making and controls physiological responses in the autonomic nervous system and hypothalamic–pituitary–adrenal axis system, contribute to chronic alcoholism. These changes also are significant predictors of relapse and recovery. Alcohol is metabolized by alcohol dehydrogenase into acetaldehyde which can affect the microglia of the nervous system. The microglia are altered dendritic cells and a key component of the immune system in the brain. Alcoholics convert alcohol more rapidly than non–alcoholics, but not acetaldehyde. Thus, the latter can increase toxic levels leading to damage not only of the brain (microtubules, microglia, etc.) and peripheral nervous system, but other organs such as the heart and the digestive system.

Opiates: Heroin use is increasing in epidemic proportions in this country. As it does the drug-related mortality rate is increasing. There is a recent trend to add fentanyl to the heroin, causing almost instant overdosing, and sometimes death, in many users.

The White House has recently entered into the discussion by changing federal training and dispensing requirements for federal health-care providers.

Methadone is also a problem that must be mentioned. Methadone has a half-life of over 50 hours in the body yet its average analgesic effect is 6 hours. Since it is regarded as a safer alternate to many other narcotics when treating chronic pain patients, more methadone is being prescribed than previously. The patients are not properly informed of the dangers of methadone and especially are not aware of the differences in persistence (half-life) versus the relatively short time for this drug's pain suppressing duration so they take more than they should to control the pain. They are in danger of quietly dying in their sleep from respiratory arrest. Forty percent of opioid-related deaths are caused by methadone.

ENDOGENOUS TOXINS

In the uterus, the fetus is in a sterile environment. Shortly after birth it is introduced to *Candida* and various bacteria. There are estimated to be 50–100 of these organisms for every living cell in our body. This population of organisms usually adapts with each other as well as ourselves and becomes symbiotic. This population of organisms is termed the microbiome.

The micorbiome plays an important role in our digestive health but when it becomes imbalanced the bacteria may cause inflammation, affect the immune responses and produce systemic effects. Systemic candidiasis is not uncommon after aggressive antibiotic or steroid administration and in a patient with AIDS or other congenital conditions (mucocutaneous candidiasis, common variable immunodeficiency, selective immunoglobulin deficiencies, and T-cell regulation deficiencies) or acquired immune dysfunction (cancer chemotherapy, biologicals).

In some individuals without such obvious defects, low-grade polysystemic candidiasis responses can also be found. Sometimes they are aggravated by toxins, diabetes, inflammatory bowel disease, allergies, or other conditions. The microbiome can also be altered by hypochlorhydria or pancreatic insufficiency which permits increased fermentation, soponification, and putrefaction with a variety of end products.

Case 3: A 32-year-old female presented with a chief complaint of chronic urticaria. She had this problem for 11 months and steroids were provided repeatedly since antihistamines and H2 blockers were not particularly effective. Various causes were excluded including drugs, foods, infections, hereditary factors. A majority of these cases do not present with a specific cause. During the examination she smelled like "beer." Her tongue was whitish, she had intestinal bloating and excessive gas, and was fatigued. She also complained of brain fag. She was placed on a yeast-free, mold-free diet, fluconazole and probiotics with an initial worsening lasting 2 days (Jarish–Herxheimers reaction) and then her urticaria disappeared. It has remained in remission for 10 months thus far. The fluconazole was utilized for 40 days with hepatic monitoring. A digestive aid was also utilized. Is this a hypersensitive response or a toxic response or both to Candida albicans? Our testing suggested both. Both serial titration skin testing as well as IgG antibodies to Candida were abnormal. Three strains of Candida have demonstrated the production of alcohol-derived neurotoxins.

Besides the microbiome, most toxins were exogenous at one time. Some can remain in the body for many years and act as a component of our endogenous toxicity. Two examples are mercury and lead.

SELECTIVE TOXIC METALS

Mercury

Mercury is a silvery-white metal element that is liquid at ordinary room temperature; it has no taste or smell. It occurs as metallic mercury (Hg), as cinnabar (HgS), and in about 25 other organic mineral compounds. Mercury exists in three basic forms: the elemental (H0), inorganic salts (H2 and H3), and the organic state. The elemental state is a silver-gray liquid, which volatilizes slowly at room temperatures, and vaporizes more rapidly when heated. This form accounts for most occupational exposures. Inhalation of the elemental vapor is very hazardous and nearly 100% absorbed and 75% retained. Following vapor inhalation, only 7% is expelled through exhalation. Only about 0.01% is absorbed from the gastrointestinal tract when ingested. The fecal route is probably the primary route of excretion for elemental mercury with the urine also being an important route. The saliva and sweat are also potentially capable of excreting mercury.

This element has a short span in the body once inhaled and oxidizes to the mercuric ion at the cellular level, much of this prior to breaching the blood–brain barrier. Elemental mercury vapor readily crosses the placental and blood–brain barrier where further conversion to mercuric ion occurs. Elemental mercury accumulates in the brain, kidneys, liver, testes, adrenal glands, thyroid, ovaries, and the gastrointestinal tract. The highest concentration accumulates in the kidneys but the longest half- life occurs in the brain. The average half-life of elemental mercury is 58 days in man though 15% of a dose has a secondary half-life of over 2 years. The half-life of mercury can be prolonged by ethanol even in non-intoxicating dosages. The half-life of mercury in blood is 3 days so blood testing in whole blood is valuable only if continued exposure or acute exposure is occurring. A urine mercury concentration of over 20 μg/L or a blood level over 4 μg/dL is considered abnormal but often blood levels of 20 μg/dL are seen before symptoms appear with acute inorganic toxicity. If air monitoring indicates that the mercury level at the work area exceeds the TLV, an immediate 24 hour urine test and physical examination should be carried out.

Acute elemental mercurialism is characterized by chills, fever, shortness of breath, metallic taste in the mouth (these first four symptoms are characteristic of metal fume fever), confusion, chest pain, nausea, vomiting, and diarrhea, colitis, interstitial pneumonitis, necrotizing bronchiolitis, and pulmonary edema. Interstitial fibrosis, interstitial emphysema, pneumothorax, pneumatocele formation and mediastinal emphysema can result, especially in adults where an obstructive mechanism is more likely to result. Neuropsychological symptoms can also be present and permanent neurological damage can remain. The lung is the primary target for acute vapor exposure. Symptoms may resolve in 2–7 days or progress into more serious pulmonary involvement. Infants less than 30 months of age are especially likely to have a fatal outcome. Chronic manifestations from elemental mercury (usually as vapor) occur gradually and may take months or years to develop. Since mercury vapor is oxidized to and eventually excreted as the mercuric ion by the catalase system at the cellular level, this form of chronic elemental mercury accumulation eventually develops a form of intracerebral mercuric poisoning. The brain and the peripheral nervous system are the primary targets for chronic elemental mercurialism. Accordingly, neuropsychological symptoms, including autonomic nervous system symptoms result. Tremors occur, which may be of a fine type at rest. They characteristically become coarser on intention. Chronic subtoxic levels of this substance appear to produce "mild changes in short-term nonverbal recall and heightened distress generally, and particularly in categories of obsessive compulsion, anxiety, and psychoticism, without alterations in general intellectual functioning, attention, verbal recall, and motor skills. Erythrism (shyness, insomnia, and excessive irritability) occurs, as well as enhanced sensitivity to sounds and other stimuli, excessive salivation, and gingivostomatitis. In more severe cases, constriction of visual field, delayed peripheral neuritis (usually sensory), discoloration of the lens (a brown light reflex reflects from a brownish pigmentation of the anterior capsule of the lens), proteinuria, dermatitis, chronic pneumonia, kidney failure, and psychosis can occur. Conjunctivitis and a pruritic erythematous rash may occur from mild exposures to this element.

Mercury is found in trace amounts with every breath we take. Recent estimates of annual global mercury emissions from both natural and anthropogenic sources are in the range of 5000–8000 metric tons per year. These estimates include mercury that is re-emitted. Natural sources of mercury include volcanic eruptions and emissions from the ocean. Anthropogenic (human-caused) emissions include mercury that is released from fuels or raw materials, or from uses in products or industrial processes. It is a common contaminant in gold mining, coal mining, and oil-production industries. Other large sources of emissions are non-ferrous metals production and cement production.

Elevated mercury concentrations have been detected in about 25% of the groundwater and surface-water samples from 2783 hazardous waste sites tested by EPA.

Seafood consumption is a source with swordfish reported to contain the highest μg/gm content. Tuna contains less but is actually a greater per capita source due to its preferred consumption in our society. In fact, over 50% of a "silver" filling contains mercury and several groups have verified that large amounts may be emitted post mastication in some individuals.

Case 4: A 57-year-old male engineer presented with personality changes, fatigue, and tremor. His wife describes unusual mood swings and hostility not previously present, over the past 6 months. The physical examination confirmed an intention tremor. The tremor was not found at rest and there was no Parkinsonian-type tremor. A neurological evaluation included a urinary heavy metal screen, which indicated marked elevated urinary mercury levels. No source could be found in investigating his workplace as he worked from home whereas his wife worked outside the home. There were no children involved. Eventually, elevated mercury levels were found in his home water supply. Criminal investigation found that mercury was being purposely added by a neighbor and an arrest was made. He responded to chelation therapy over time, as well as modification to his water supply.

Lead

Lead can be found in all parts of our environment—the air, the soil, the water, and even inside our homes. Much of our exposure comes from human activities, including the use of fossil fuels including past use of lead and lead compounds, which have been used in a wide variety of products found in and around our homes, including paint, ceramics, pipes and plumbing materials, solders, gasoline, batteries, ammunition, and cosmetics. Leaded gasoline, some types of industrial facilities, and past use of lead-based paint in homes. Lead paint was often used before 1978. The EPA is responsible for monitoring and regulating the non-workplace environment. OSHA is responsible for the workplace environment. OSHA was originally initiated due to the use of lead-based undercoat paint in the auto industry and was the first to protect the workers' compensation while recovering from lead poisoning by mandate.

Lead can accumulate in our bodies over time, where it is stored in bones along with calcium. Lead can affect almost every organ and system in your body. Children six years old and younger are most susceptible to the effects of lead. Lead's effects, like mercury, are due to binding of lead with sulfhydryl groups on proteins, especially if these involve zinc-dependent enzyme systems. Primarily the brain, peripheral nervous system, bone marrow, liver, and kidneys are involved. Neurotransmitters are affected directly by lead.

Anemia results from interference of lead with several enzymes in heme synthesis, including δ-aminolevulinic acid as well as pyridimidine 5-nucleotidase, which is involved in the breakdown of RNA. This interference results in basophilic stippling in the red cell. 1-25-dihydroxy vitamin D production is blocked. Tubular renal function is altered and neurons and Schwann cells are affected. Inhibition of ferrochetalase results in an increase in uroporphorin in the urine and increase in protoporphorin in the blood. RBC protoporphorin levels in the adult will rise when the blood level is around 25–30 μg/dL.

Lead is absorbed only 10%–20% in the adult but up to 50% in the child. Recently, the lead level for children has changed to 5 μg/dL in the blood. The new, lower value means that more children are likely to be identified as having lead exposure allowing parents, doctors, public health officials, and communities to take action earlier to reduce the child's future exposure to lead. Organic lead but not the inorganic form can be absorbed through the intact skin. After absorption in the bloodstream, almost all of the lead is found in the RBC in a short term. With prolonged exposure, almost all of it ends up in the bone. Lead is substituted for calcium in the bone matrix. Lead crosses the blood–brain barrier and concentrates in the gray matter. It also crosses the placental barrier and may concentrate in the fetus.

Lead has a terminal half-life of 30 years. In workers with elevated blood levels, 50% reached 40 µg/dL in 180 days and 75% in 460 days. The sources of lead are paint, putty, folk remedies, contaminated clothing, dirt and air contamination, lead pipe or solder, glazed pots, bullets, indoor firing ranges and industrial sources with lead smelters, battery reclamation. Lead paint can be a hazard with workers who weld or use an acetylene torch on surfaces being heated.

Effects of Lead on Children

Even low levels of lead in the blood of children can result in:

- Behavior and learning problems
- Lower IQ and hyperactivity
- Slowed growth
- Hearing problems
- Anemia

In rare cases, ingestion of lead can cause seizures, coma, and even death.

During pregnancy, lead is released from bones as maternal calcium and is used to help form the bones of the fetus. This is particularly true if a woman does not have enough dietary calcium. This can result in serious effects to the mother and her developing fetus, including:

- Reduced growth of the fetus
- Premature birth

Adults working in a job or engaging in hobbies where lead is used, such as making stained glass, can increase exposure as can certain folk remedies containing lead. More subtle sources include leaded glass from foreign countries when acidic products such as vinegar or tomato sauce is added or stored. Lead contamination from neighboring communities with industrial runoff that contaminates the water supply (e.g., Flint, Michigan) can also be seen. Although encephalopathy is uncommon with excessive lead, motor loss such as wrist drop can be seen, as well as irritability, basophilic stippling, infertility, subtle personality changes, and fatigue. Abdominal pain, sometimes severe resulting in unnecessary surgery has been noted. Lead lines in the gums occur in about 15% of cases.

Although uncommon, other metals we encounter producing adverse responses include: chromium, barium, arsenic, cadmium, beryllium, antimony, cobalt, copper, nickel, selenium, gold, silver, thallium, tin, titanium, and zinc. Even essential elements can be toxic if taken in excess or through an unusual route of administration.

TOXICOLOGY AND PSYCHONEUROIMMUNOLOGY

Toxic substances and their effects act as physical stressors and can disrupt the nervous system, especially the hypothalamicopituitary axis (HPA) as well as the immune system. Both the brain and immune system are important adapting components of the body and a disruption of one can also lead to a disturbance of the other. The innate immune system is that part of the body's defenses that predominate to deal with internal and external threats for the first 72 hours. Not only bacteria or viruses but components of damaged tissue such as DNA and RNA fragments, uric acid and other exogenous and endogenous products including toxins have to be recognized as foreign and either be eliminated by this system or augmented by a specific and complementary system termed the adaptive immune system utilizing the T and B cells. Both of these systems are highly complex.

Toxic substances can provide specific clinical syndromes or can be subclinical and occult. When subclinical, the orchestra of toxins can assist in modulating adverse neuroendocrine and immunologic effects. This has been shown with certain endocrine disruptors and more research is required with other toxins.

SOME TREATMENTS AND MEASURES TO REDUCE INDIVIDUAL TOXIC EXPOSURE

Assure that your business is following OSHA regulations. PEL (personal exposure limits).

Consider measures to reduce heavy metals if that is found to be a problem. There are various chelating agents approved for different toxic metals.

If mold is contaminating the home or workplace, let a professional remediate the growth.

Ideally, choose foods with less pesticide exposure, such as organic fruits, vegetable, fish, and meat products.

Use gloves, glasses, and protective equipment when working with chemicals.

Avoid chemicals known to be toxic if you are actively trying to get pregnant (although this does not change past exposure). Also check with your doctor if considering taking any medication.

Reduce the amount of processed food and fast food you eat.

Eat lower amounts of deep-sea fish (swordfish, shark, king mackerel, and tilefish) to minimize mercury exposure, especially if you are trying to get pregnant or are pregnant.

Check for lead-based paint in your house to prevent exposure. Also you may wish to get your tap water tested (e.g., Flint, Michigan).

Natural methods commonly used for detoxification include homeopathy, supervised fasting, colon irrigations, "liver flushing," therapeutic clay and depuration. A detailed discussion of these is beyond the scope of this chapter.

SUMMARY

Thus, toxicology is more relevant today than ever before. Increased awareness, permits us to appreciate that the practicing toxicologist has many roles: working in poison control centers, Federal and State agencies that permit cleaner air, safer mines and workplaces, and provide safer food, well-studied pharmaceuticals and better consumer products. Toxicologists also investigate and treat the immediate and chronic effects of obvious poisons at home or at work. Finally, toxicologists confirm, forensically, the presence of illicit drugs as well as nefarious toxins that are sometimes used for criminal intent.

Dr. Cordas is certified in internal medicine as well as immunology/allergy. He is a clinical associate professor at the Texas College of Osteopathic Medicine UNTHSC. He also has earned a master's in public health in occupational medicine (toxicology).

REFERENCES

1. http://www.asrm.org/Phthalate_Exposure_May_Affect_Levels_of_Sexual_Interest_in_Premeno-pausal_Women/
2. http://press.endocrine.org/doi/10.1210/er.2015-1093
3. Doull J., Amdur M.O., Klaassen C.D. (Eds). *Casarett and Doull's Toxicology: The Basic Science of Poisons.* Fourth Edition, McGraw-Hill, New York, NY, 1991.
4. Massaro E.J. (Ed.). *Handbook of Human Toxicology*, CRC Press, Boca Raton, FL, 1997.
5. Gosselin R.E., Hodge H.C., Smith R.P. (Eds). *Clinical Toxicology of Commercial Products*, Fifth Edition, Williams and Wilkins, Baltimore, MD, 1984.

6. Haddad L.M., Winchester J.F. (Eds). *Clinical Management of Poisoning and Drug Overdose*, Second Edition, W.B. Saunders Company, Philadelphia, PA, 1990.
7. http://www.iarc.fr/en/cancertopics/index.php
8. http://www.epa.gov/iris/
9. Brooks S.M., Weiss M.A., Bernstein I.L. Reactive airways dysfunction syndrome (RADS): Persistent asthma syndrome after high level irritant exposures. *Chest*, 88, 1985, 376–384.
10. Burrell R., Flaherty D., Sauers L. (Eds). *Toxicology and the Immune System: A Human Approach*, Van Nostrand Reinhold, New York, NY, 1992.

5 Environmental Toxins and Chronic Illness

Clinical Management Using Traditional and Allostatic Load-Based Approaches

Jeffrey Moss

CONTENTS

Introduction: Bridging the Gap between Academic Publications on Environmental Toxicology and Clinical Application 150
Common Environmental Toxins and Their Impact on Health in High Amounts 152
Immunotoxicology 152
Neurotoxicity 152
Endocrine Toxicity 154
Other Published Research on Endocrine Toxicity 154
Mechanisms Involved in Creating the Impact of EDCs 155
Endocrine Disrupting Chemicals: Focus on Reproductive Health 155
Molecular Physiology of Environmental Toxins 156
Detoxification Pathways 156
Phases of Detoxification 157
Detoxification and Genetic Polymorphisms (SNPs) 159
Detoxification and Age 160
Detoxification and Gender 160
Detoxification and Dose 160
Detoxification and Route of Administration 160
Detoxification and Suboptimal Nutrient Intake 161
Detoxification and Medications 162
Detoxification of Environmental Toxins: Some Practical Considerations 162
    Assessment 162
    Assessment: History 164
    Assessment: Laboratory Analysis 164
    Assessment: Organic Chemicals 164
    Assessment: Heavy Metals 165
    Treatment: Traditional Approaches 165
Traditional Avoidance Treatments 166
Traditional Treatments that Improve the Ability of the Body to Metabolize and Eliminate 166
Traditional Treatments that May Assist in the Physical Removal of Toxins from the Body 167

Practical Concerns about Traditional Approaches to Environmental Toxicity Diagnosis and Treatment 167
When Detoxification Procedures Alone Do Not Reduce or Eliminate Chief Complaints in Patients Carrying a Significant Load of Environmental Toxins and Why 168
Allostatic Load, Environmental Toxins, and Detoxification Enzymes 170
Some Final Thoughts 172
References 173

INTRODUCTION: BRIDGING THE GAP BETWEEN ACADEMIC PUBLICATIONS ON ENVIRONMENTAL TOXICOLOGY AND CLINICAL APPLICATION

Over the last three to four decades, much has been published on the impact of the ever-increasing environmental load of toxic chemicals and metals on human health. Interestingly, many if not most of these publications have focused almost exclusively on identifying the chemical and metal toxins that pose the greatest threat and detailing the specific ways they create disease and affect biochemistry and physiology. In addition, they tend to focus on extreme levels of exposure (Lyon et al., 2005) that might occur in occupational settings, that is, chemical plant workers (Crinnion, 2013), or environmental disasters, that is, mercury in Minamata Bay, Japan (Crinnion, 2013) where ill-health can easily be traced back, almost exclusively, to the chemical or metal being addressed. Concerning treatment, little is often recommended other than avoidance of the offending agent plus, in the case of heavy metals, chelation therapy. A notable exception are papers and texts on the subject of environmental toxicity and detoxification written for the alternative medicine community that, in addition to avoidance procedures, recommend various diets, "cleanses," and nutritional supplements (Lyon et al., 2005; Crinnion, 2013). This approach to dealing with environmental toxins, not only from an efficacy standpoint but also from a cost-effectiveness, practicality, and patient compliance standpoint will be discussed later in this chapter.

Unfortunately, for the ever-increasing amount of health care practitioners whose practices are primarily composed of the rapidly growing amounts of chronically ill individuals of all ages, it is difficult, if not impossible to use the information in the more "mainstream" papers that address environmental toxins to create efficacious, cost-effective, and practical from a patient compliance standpoint treatment plans. Furthermore, even the more alternative medicine papers and texts that recommend dietary protocols, "cleanses," and nutritional supplements often yield less than optimal results for many clinicians from an efficacy, cost-effectiveness, and/or patient compliance standpoint. Why? One reason is that the vast majority of patients did not develop toxicity-related signs and symptoms due to singular, easy to define, and easy to eliminate or avoid sources. Rather, toxicity-related signs and symptoms developed due to chronic, long-term exposure to small amounts of sometimes dozens of different chemicals and heavy metals that are the reality of our modern-day society in industrialized nations (Liska et al., 2005; Crinnion, 2013). Because of this, avoidance may be impossible and, when possible, may be impractical from a patient compliance standpoint due to cost and the intrusive lifestyle changes involved to accomplish avoidance in meaningful amounts. However, there is one other extremely important reason that is rarely addressed in either mainstream or alternative medicine papers and texts that address environmental toxins.

Toxicity due to environmental toxin exposure is a state of being that is not only defined by often unavoidable levels of toxin exposure. Rather, it is a balance between exposure to toxins and the ability to metabolize and eliminate the toxins. Very often books such as this will suggest that the ability to metabolize and eliminate toxins is solely a function of the types of toxins involved, exposure levels, genetic strengths and weaknesses concerning detoxification enzymes, and nutritional status.

As will be discussed, the ability to metabolize and eliminate toxins is also affected by a whole host of environmental stressors which include:

- Suboptimal movement against gravity (exercise)
- Infection and/or microbial imbalance
- Psychological stress
- Electromagnetic stress

Furthermore, the whole-body or "allostatic" responses to these stressors can also have a profound impact on the ability to metabolize and eliminate environmental toxins. These allostatic responses include:

- Endocrine responses largely involving hyperinsulinemia, insulin resistance, elevated or depressed cortisol and/or glucocorticoid resistance
- Chronic inflammation

As suggested not only by the title of this chapter but also by the theme of this entire text, this chapter is not being written for academics. It is being written for clinicians desiring to assist chronically ill patients whose quality of life is being adversely impacted by environmental toxins in feeling better in an efficacious, cost-effective, and practical manner that is practical for both the practitioner and the patient. To do this, it certainly is important to address some of the basics of the science of toxicology both in terms of the precise nature of the chemicals and heavy metals that constitute environmental toxic load in modern, industrialized societies and the primary mechanisms of how they adversely affect human metabolism. Furthermore, it is important to address the basics of endogenous detoxification pathways, which includes genetic influences on detoxification enzyme function. This chapter, like so many other similar chapters in other texts of this type, will address these concerns. However, as was mentioned, in the opinion of this author, from a clinical standpoint, more is needed. Why? Years of clinical experience suggest that most clinicians treating the "usual" chronically ill patients are primarily interested in the following:

- The mechanisms of how small amounts of dozens, if not hundreds, of chemicals and heavy metal toxins to which everyone in industrialized societies are exposed everyday are contributing to the creation of signs and symptoms.
- Why, even though the vast majority of people in industrialized countries are exposed to similar amounts of the same chemicals and heavy metal toxins (Liska et al., 2005; Crinnion, 2013), these patients are experiencing signs and symptoms related to exposure to these substances while others are not.
- How to improve quality of life with the knowledge that long-term, meaningful avoidance is virtually impossible given the reality of ever-increasing opportunities for exposure in our polluted world (Liska et al., 2005; Crinnion, 2013).
- The bottom-line realities of what patients are willing to do and willing to pay for in terms of both avoidance and treatment.

To address these needs it is also the opinion of this author that, as was suggested above, more than the usual must be addressed. To fully understand the role of environmental toxins in the creation of chronic illness, it must be appreciated that many other environmental stressors such as those listed above are involved, not just the toxins themselves, poor diet, and genetic influences on detoxification capacity. Furthermore, it must be appreciated that the whole-body "allostatic" response to these other stressors that involve suboptimal insulin and cortisol metabolism plus chronic inflammation can have a profound effect on the ability to metabolize and eliminate environmental toxins and, when not addressed, reduce the efficacy of even the most detailed and aggressive avoidance, dietary, and supplemental protocols. Many of these other modifiers of detoxification capacity that are rarely addressed in books such as this will be discussed in this chapter.

COMMON ENVIRONMENTAL TOXINS AND THEIR IMPACT ON HEALTH IN HIGH AMOUNTS

As was mentioned above, most patients encountered in the typical integrative medicine practice have not suffered from massive exposure levels to any single environmental toxin. Instead they tend to suffer effects from long-term exposure to small amounts of often dozens of different environmental toxins. Nevertheless, because some extrapolation is possible to the low-dose, chronic scenario, there is much to be learned from the large volume of published research on the impact of large amounts of individual environmental toxins on health. One of the best reviews on this subject is the book chapter "Environmental Medicine" by Walter J. Crinnion (2013). In this chapter, Crinnion examines the basics of the impact of environmental toxin exposure in relation to their impact on health from three perspectives—immunotoxicology, neurotoxicology, and endocrine toxicology.

IMMUNOTOXICOLOGY

Crinnion begins with immunotoxicology because signs and symptoms relating to the immune system are often the first to occur with patients, specifically beginning with allergies (both food and airborne). What then often follows is sensitivity to various chemicals used in everyday life along with an increase in the incidence of chronic infections. Toxins that fall into this category include dichlorodiphenyldichloroethylene (DDE), which is the main metabolite of DDT (dichlorophenyl-trichloroethane). It has been found to compromise cellular immune responses. Another common environmental toxin that falls into this category is mercury. Mercury increases destruction of both monocytes and lymphocytes and reduces the phagocytic ability of monocytes. A family of chemical compounds that possess immunotoxic properties is polycyclic aromatic hydrocarbons (PAH), which can decrease T-cell dependent antibody response, splenic activity, T-cell effector function, T-cell cytotoxic induction, and natural killer cell activity. Organophosphorus pesticides (OP) have been found to decrease percentages of CD4 and CD5 cells, increase numbers and percentages of CD26 cells, and increase atopy, antibiotic sensitivity, and autoimmunity. Acute exposure to high levels of ozone has been found to exacerbate asthma and reduce lung function in hikers. Autoimmune responses have been reported with increased exposures to mercury compounds.

NEUROTOXICITY

OPs, even at levels of exposure that would not fall into the acute toxicity range, are well documented to cause symptoms of neurotoxicity such as depression, headache, fatigue, and cognitive dysfunction. In particular, this has been seen in greenhouse workers who are exposed to OPs who not only exhibited some of the above-mentioned symptoms but also tremors, parasthesias, longer reaction time, and reduced motor steadiness. Exposure to even low levels of chlorinated pesticides such as DDT has been reported to create a dimming of vision, a sense of fullness deep inside the skull, headache, slow thinking, concentration difficulty, and short-term memory loss. In addition, DDT exposure has been associated with muscle symptoms such as weakness, fatigue, dysphagia, and ataxia. Retired malaria control workers who worked with DDT were found, compared to a control group of retired persons, to have worse performance with cognitive, sensory, and motor testing. In particular, they demonstrated particularly poor performance with aspects of cognitive testing (verbal attention, visuomotor speed, and sequencing) and more psychiatric symptoms.

People living in an apartment complex where chlordane had been used, even after 7 years since application of the chlordane, demonstrated reduced reaction time, balance dysfunction, reduced cognitive function and perceptual motor speed, and reduced immediate and delayed verbal recall. Increased tension, depression, anger, and fatigue were also noted.

Solvent exposure has been documented to lead to chronic toxic encephalopathy (CTE). Interestingly, in agreement with the issue of decreased detoxification capacity mentioned above, Crinnion (2013) discusses research where individuals on antidepressants were four times more likely to demonstrate persistent CTE compared with those not on these medications. Crinnion (2013) suggests that one reason for this is the fact that many antidepressants inhibit phase I detoxification pathways in the liver. Other research has shown that workers with a genetic propensity for lower glutathione production demonstrated a significantly increased risk for development of CTE. Concerning specific solvents, toluene, which is often present in glues and paints, is highly linked with development of CTE. In one study on printers exposed to toluene, fatigue, impaired memory, impaired concentration, irritability, headaches, mood lability, and depression were often reported. In another study on shipyard painters, in addition to the some of the symptoms mentioned above, dizziness and insomnia were reported as well as a feeling of pressure in the chest and sweating with any work or movement. Finally, another study on female workers reported symptoms relating to manual dexterity, visual scanning, and verbal memory even though there was no overt evidence of classic toxicity.

Heavy metals such as lead and mercury have long been known to create neurotoxic effects. As demonstrated most recently in Flint, Michigan (Campbell et al., 2016), lead toxicity in particular can have devastating neurologic effects, particularly in children. Crinnion (2013) reports reduced IQ scores plus attention and behavioral problems. Both parents and teachers of children exposed to significant levels of lead have reported children having more somatic complaints, delinquency, aggressiveness, and internalizing and externalizing behavior. In a study on Yugoslavian children, perceptual-motor aspects of intelligence were most affected. On a more controversial note, lead exposure has been linked with autism and attention deficit hyperactivity disorder in several studies.

The impact of lead exposure has also been noted even when the exposure occurred several years earlier. In one study where people were exposed to lead as children 20 years earlier, significant issues with neurologic function were still present. Specifically, issues with comprehension, depression, insomnia, fatigue, and balance were noted. Also, older individuals who had no history of industrial exposure to lead still demonstrated a correlation between decreased cognitive function and total bone lead levels.

Mercury, as noted by Crinnion (2013) is a well-known neurotoxin that is neurotoxic in both organic and inorganic forms. It can inhibit uptake of dopamine, serotonin, and norepinephrine at synaptic sites. It also has a significant binding affinity for serotonin-binding sites. Concerning symptoms, it has been demonstrated for many years that mercury exposure can lead to irritability, excitability, temper outbursts, quarreling, fearfulness, restlessness, depression, and insomnia.

Methylmercury, an organic form of mercury that has been reported in many studies as a significant environmental pollutant often found in certain types of fish, accumulates in the brain, primarily in myelin sheaths, leading to demyelination. In terms of large-scale, overt methylmercury poisoning, probably the most famous case is pollution of Minamata Bay in Japan in the 1950s. Symptoms that were seen in those exposed to the polluted water in Minamata Bay primarily through ingestion of fish include ataxia, speech impairment, constriction of visual fields, hypoesthesia, dysarthria, hearing impairment, and sensory disturbances. What may be even more significant than the original occurrence is the fact 40 years after the spill and 30 years after a fishing ban was enacted symptoms of mercury neurotoxicity still persisted. Other studies, such as those performed on Amazonian children exposed to methylmercury as the result of local gold mining, demonstrated neurotoxic effects. In addition, more than 80% of the children had levels of hair mercury high enough to impact brain development. Neuropsychological testing in these children demonstrated deficits in motor function, attention, and visuospatial performance. In the United States, a study of patients in an internal medicine practice in San Francisco who ingested large fish regularly had blood levels of mercury above 5 mcg/L and demonstrated issues with fatigue, hair loss, troubled thinking, memory loss, muscle aches, and headaches. Furthermore, many of these patients reported a metallic taste in the mouth.

ENDOCRINE TOXICITY

During recent years endocrine toxicity and endocrine disrupting chemicals have received a tremendous amount of attention from the research community. First, consider information by Crinnion (2013) on the subject. He first points out the most common health issues that have been attributed to endocrine toxicity. These include:

1. Sleep disturbances or changes in energy level or mood
2. Alterations in weight, appetite, and bowel function
3. Sexual interest and function change; in females, and any menstrual change
4. Changes in temperature perception, sweating, or flushing
5. Alterations of hair growth and skin texture

Crinnion also states

The most common endocrine diagnoses associated with xenobiotic burden include:

1. Infertility
2. Hypothyroidism
3. Adult-onset diabetes and obesity

Crinnion (2013) next discusses several studies on endocrine disrupting chemicals based on three major clinical issues—infertility, hypothyroidism, and adult-onset diabetes. Concerning infertility, several studies have implicated herbicides and organophosphate and chlorinated pesticides, polychlorinated biphenyls (PCBs), that is, DDT, and solvents. Concerning hypothyroidism, a large volume of studies has implicated exposure to PCBs. One of the main reasons is that, structurally, PCBs closely resemble thyroxine. Both have two connected benzene rings with attached halogens. PCBs have chlorine molecules and thyroxine has iodine. Bisphenol-A is also similar in structure to thyroxin where each of the rings in bisphenol-A contains a bromine molecule. Because of this similarity, these endocrine disrupting chemicals can block utilization and transport of thyroxine. In addition, several studies have demonstrated an association between PCB exposure and elevated thyroid antibodies (antiperoxidase and antithyroglobulin). Concerning adult-onset diabetes, arsenic, chlorinated pesticides, dioxins, and PCBs have all been associated with increased incidence.

OTHER PUBLISHED RESEARCH ON ENDOCRINE TOXICITY

Due to increased incidence of endocrine-related disease as a function of endocrine disrupting chemicals (EDCs), many other researchers have been examining this relationship. In terms of increased incidence, Attina et al. (2016) pointed out that the disease cost of EDCs in the United States was much higher than in Europe ($340 billion vs. $217 billion). They also note that much of the difference was due to the impact of polybrominated diphenyl ethers on intelligence quotient (IQ). In the European Union, organophosphate pesticides were the biggest contributor to costs. Finally, they point out that disease due to EDC exposure in the United States has led to annual costs that take up more than 2% of the gross domestic product (GDP).

Compounding the problem is the immense number of chemicals used in daily life that have endocrine disrupting properties. According to Maqbool et al. (2016), this number is about 800. Furthermore, the authors point out that only some of them have been examined. What is known about these chemicals? Kabir et al. (2015) provide much more detail than what was presented above. First, what is the precise definition of an endocrine-disrupting compound? The authors answer this question by providing the U.S. Environmental Protection Agency (EPA) definition: "an agent that interferes with the synthesis, secretion, transport, binding, or elimination of natural hormones in the body that are responsible for the maintenance of homeostasis, reproduction, development and/or behavior." Kabir et al. (2015) then simplify this definition by stating: "this means that endocrine disruptors are chemicals, or chemical mixtures, that interfere with normal hormone function." Next, the authors divide EDCs into two categories. First, there are those that occur naturally such as natural chemicals found in human and animal food. These include phytoestrogens, genistein, and coumestrol. Second, there are those that are synthesized. These include industrial solvents and lubricants and their byproducts, for example, PCBs polybrominated biphenyls (PBBs), dioxins, plastics, bisphenol A (BPA), plasticizers, pesticides, fungicides, and some pharmaceuticals such as diethylstilbesterol (DES). Next, Kabir et al. (2015) group EDCs based on origin. First, there exists natural and artificial hormones such as phytoestrogens, omega-3 fatty acids, contraceptive pills, and thyroid medications. Second, there exists drugs with hormonal side effects such as naproxen, metoprolol, and clofibrate. Third, there exists industrial and household chemicals such as phthalates, alkylphenoltoxilate detergents, fire retardants, plasticizers, solvents, and PCBs. Finally, there exists side products of industrial and household processes such as polycyclic aromatic hydrocarbons (PAHs), dioxins, and pentachlorobenzene. Still another way of categorizing EDCs according to Kabir et al. (2015) is pesticides, chemicals in products used in everyday life which includes lead and brominated flame retardants, and food contact materials with BPA being the most common. Maqbool et al. (2016) provide additional information on the organ and systemic effects of EDCs. These include reproductive and developmental effects, carcinogenicity, obesity and diabetes, and effects on the thyroid, cardiovascular system and nervous system. Kabir et al. (2015) provide additional detail about reproductive effects, pointing out that EDCs have been linked with abnormal development during puberty, ovarian failure, menstrual irregularities, polycystic ovary syndrome, poor sperm quality, and male infertility.

MECHANISMS INVOLVED IN CREATING THE IMPACT OF EDCs

Maqbool et al. (2016) point out several mechanisms for the adverse impact EDCs have on health. These include oxidative stress, disruption of steroid hormone metabolism, disruption of optimal nuclear receptor activity, and disruption of hormone conduction pathways. Further detail concerning mechanisms of the adverse health impact of EDCs was provided by Kabir et al. (2015). These mechanisms include (1) acting as estrogen, androgen, and thyroid hormone analogs, potentially producing overstimulation of the respective organ systems, (2) acting as antagonists when binding to endogenous hormone receptors, thus preventing binding of endogenous hormones to these receptors, (3) altering liver metabolism of endogenous hormones, and (4) altering optimal function of transport proteins for endogenous hormones. It has also been suggested, according to Kabir et al. (2015), that EDCs can adversely affect health through their biotransformation to even more powerful disruption metabolites. Finally, the authors suggest that certain EDCs can accumulate in different parts of the body, mainly in fatty tissues, and then be slowly released over a period of years, potentially contributing to ill-health. Similarly, the authors suggest that certain EDCs can be passed from mothers to infants through breast milk, thus adversely affecting infant health.

ENDOCRINE DISRUPTING CHEMICALS: FOCUS ON REPRODUCTIVE HEALTH

Certainly, while EDCs have drawn attention due to their impact on numerous organ systems and physiologic processes, the impact that seems to have created the greatest concern over the last few years is that which deals with reproductive health. Fortunately, Zlatnik (2016) has recently published an excellent review of the literature on the subject, highlights of which will be presented here. As an introduction the author points out that a sampling of pregnant women in the United States showed that virtually every participant in the study had at least 43 different chemicals in her bloodstream. These chemicals included polychlorinated biphenyls, organochlorine pesticides, perfluorinated compounds, phenols, polybrominated diphenyl ethers, phthalates, polycystic aromatic hydrocarbons, and perchlorate. Next, to reiterate what was stated above about the realities of identification and management of environmental toxins in real-life clinical scenarios as opposed to the gross toxicity settings often discussed in published research on the subject consider the following quote:

> Environmental exposures and their outcomes can be hard to assess. This is multifactorial: exposure to chemicals is typically not documented outside of industrial settings, and different people have different levels of sensitivity (stemming from nutritional status, life stage, metabolism, or genetics). Additionally, the particular chemical involved may not be identifiable, even if an exposure was known to occur. The timing of exposure may be unclear or have occurred in the distant past.

Next, Zlatnik (2016) focuses on the major EDCs and their impact on reproductive health.

Bisphenol A—Bisphenol A (BPA) has phenyl groups that mimic estrogen and can bind to estrogen receptors. Because of this BPA can act as both an estrogen agonist and estrogen antagonist. In animal models BPA has been shown to contribute to obesity. However, the impact does not stop there as recent data suggest that BPA can have an adverse impact on normal fetal development. Still other research on occupational exposures suggests that BPA can also have an adverse impact on male reproductive health as reduced frequency of sexual intercourse, increased ejaculatory dysfunction, reduced satisfaction with sex life, reduced sex drive, and reduced ability to have an erection have been noted.

Phthalates—A large volume of research has reported that phthalates, often found in lotions and shampoos as a fragrance factor, and often used as plasticizers to change the physical characteristics of plastics found in flooring, shower curtains, packaging, and some medical equipment, can have an adverse impact on reproductive health in young and older males and females in addition to fetuses.

Flame retardants—Polybrominated diphenyl ethers (PBDEs) are often used as flame retardants in many consumer products. They have been suggested to adversely affect reproductive health by interacting with steroid hormone receptors and suppress normal thyroid hormone function.

Perfluorinated compounds—Perfluorinated compounds (PFCs) are used for waterproofing, stain resistance, and lubrication. They are found in many consumer products including food packaging and non-stick cookware. In animal and in vitro models, PFCs have been demonstrated to interact with estrogen and androgen receptors, thyroid hormones, and neurotransmitters. Alterations in thyroid function have also been demonstrated in humans.

Pesticides—It is well known that pesticides have far-reaching and numerous impacts on endocrine physiology and reproductive outcomes.

MOLECULAR PHYSIOLOGY OF ENVIRONMENTAL TOXINS

In addition to the research on the impact of environmental toxins on organ systems and physiologic pathways, other research has also focused on the impact on a molecular level, as reported by Lyon in the book chapter "Environmental Toxicology" (Lyon, 2013). The author states that (1) toxins can remove or impair the synthesis of specific molecules such as phospholipids, fatty acids, proteins, nucleotides, and glutathione, (2) toxins can alter structural entities such as mitochondria, cytoskeletons, plasma membranes, and nuclei, and (3) toxins can disturb cell signaling by adversely affecting cytokines, eicosanoids, hormones, calcium channels, and neurotransmitters.

DETOXIFICATION PATHWAYS

As has been demonstrated above, environmental toxins are both numerous and ubiquitous. Furthermore, identification and quantification of individual toxins in any particular patient is often difficult if not impossible. Finally, while, as suggested later in this chapter, avoidance and removal protocols can reduce toxic load to a certain extent, the realities of daily living in our toxic world make it clear that, for virtually all living beings on earth, a certain level of toxic burden is inevitable. Nevertheless, the impact on human health of this ongoing toxic load is never as great as data on exposure level and overall metabolic impact might suggest. Why is this? Environmental toxin exposure is not a new phenomenon that began with the industrial revolution approximately 200 years ago. Rather, exposure to many of the environmental toxins discussed above has been occurring for thousands, if not millions, of years via volcanos and outgassing from the earth's crust (Mahaffey, 1999; Crinnion, 2000). Therefore, evolutionary processes have placed a high priority on the development of endogenous detoxification pathways which, as will be demonstrated later in this chapter, are highly developed and function quite well in reasonably healthy, well-nourished individuals who are not subject to environmental stressors that lead to chronically elevated levels of inflammation. What follows next is an overview of endogenous detoxification pathways. This will be followed by a discussion of various factors that can adversely impact functionality of detoxification enzyme systems. These include:

- Genetics/single nucleotide polymorphisms (SNPs)
- Age
- Gender
- Dose
- Route of administration
- Suboptimal nutrient intake
- Medications
- Allostatic responses that include chronic inflammation

PHASES OF DETOXIFICATION

As noted by Croom (2012), metabolism of xenobiotics can be divided into three major steps or phases. Phase I reactions are the first step and are largely designed to convert highly lipophilic compounds into more hydrophilic metabolites (Liska et al., 2005; Croom, 2012). They are found most abundantly in the liver but can also be found in the gastrointestinal tract, lung, brain, and kidney and virtually every other tissue in the body (Xu et al., 2005; Croom, 2012). There exist several different families or subfamilies of phase I enzymes, all of which are based on amino acid sequence identities or similarities (Xu et al., 2005). Phase I enzymes are often designated as "cytochrome P450" enzymes because they are hemoproteins that absorb light at 450 nm after the heme is reduced and bound by carbon monoxide (Croom, 2012). In the vast majority of phase I reactions a toxic lipophilic compound is rendered less toxic. However, it is not rare for phase I reaction to yield a more toxic metabolite (Lyon, 2013). Hence, there is a need for phase II reactions (also called conjugation reactions), which enhance the detoxification effect by increasing hydrophilicity and excretion in the bile and/or urine (Xu et al., 2005). As with phase I reactions, while most of the phase II reactions yield a less toxic metabolite, under certain conditions phase II reactions will result in a more active metabolite, thereby increasing toxicity (Xu et al., 2005). Phase III, which involves transporter proteins such as P-glycoprotein and multidrug resistance-associated protein, are expressed in tissues such as the liver, intestine, kidney, and brain and have the role of transporting conjugated metabolites out of the body via the urine or bile (Xu et al., 2005; Croom, 2012). Other organs that contain phase III transporter proteins are the testes, prostate, breast, adrenal glands, heart, and skeletal muscle (Croom, 2012). Figure 5.1 shows the relationship between the first two phases of the detoxification process.

Most of the phase I conversions involve oxidative processes. However, they can involve demethylation, hydroxylation, or dehalogenation (Lyon, 2013). Phase II reactions primarily result in conjugation of a xenobiotic or metal ion with a carrier molecule such as glutathione, cysteine, sulfate, glycine, glucuronic acid, thiosulfate, and glutamine (Croom, 2012; Lyon, 2013). However, another important phase II family of enzymes is the methyltransferase enzymes that add a methyl group to a

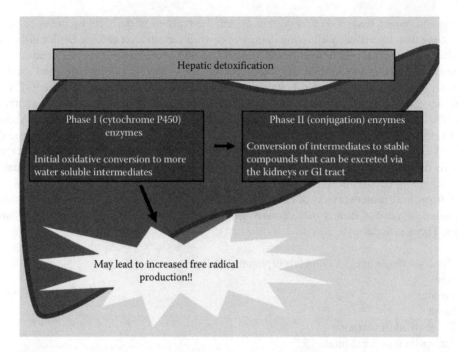

FIGURE 5.1   Hepatic detoxification: Relationship between phase I and phase II.

compound. For almost all methylation reactions S-adenosylmethionine (SAM) is the methyl donor (Croom, 2012).

One phase II methylation enzyme, in particular, has received much attention in the research and clinical communities because of its involvement in metabolism of estrogen metabolites that may promote breast cancer formation. During phase I metabolism estradiol (E2) is metabolized to the strongly procarcinogenic compound 4-hydroxy-estradiol (4-OH-E$_2$) (Zhu, 2003). Fortunately, the adverse impact on health of this metabolite is greatly minimized by the phase II methylation enzyme catechol-O-methyltransferase (COMT), which converts 4-OH-E$_2$ to the relatively inert O-methylated metabolite 4-methoxyestradiol (4-MeO-E$_2$) (Zhu, 2003). However, the anticarcinogenic properties of COMT do not end here. COMT also converts 2-hydroxyestradiol (2-OH-E$_2$) to 2-methoxyestradiol (2-MeO-E$_2$) (Zhu, 2003). 2-MeO-E$_2$ is associated with reduced cancer formation in several ways. First, it has little or no estrogen receptor-binding activity. Next, it may actually prevent cancer formation due to its antiproliferative, cytotoxic, and apoptotic actions (Zhu, 2002).

Because of the importance of COMT in reducing accumulation of potentially procarcinogenic estradiol metabolites, attention has also been focused on environmental toxins or endogenous metabolites that may interfere with its activity. Garner et al. point out that PCBs are not only substrates for COMT but can inhibit its activity, potentially leading to increased accumulation of carcinogenic estradiol metabolites (Garner et al., 2000). Concerning endogenous metabolites, Zhu points out that accumulation of S-adenosyl-L-homocysteine (SAH), which often occurs in association with elevated homocysteine, can act as a strong noncompetitive inhibitor of COMT-mediated methylation of both 2-OH-E$_2$ and 4-OH-E$_2$ (Zhu, 2003).

Of course, no current discussion on xenobiotic metabolism would be complete without mentioning the role of gut microflora. In most cases, microfloral reactions with xenobiotics yield a less toxic metabolite but not always. One notable exception where microfloral metabolism can increase toxicity is where gut organisms can act upon metabolites that have gone through phase II conjugation metabolism and remove the conjugating factor, that is, glutathione, sulfate, methyl group, and so on. This can lead to the release of a more toxic metabolite in the intestine that can be reabsorbed through a process called enterohepatic recirculation (Croom, 2012).

Additional ways that gut microflora can affect detoxification were discussed by Swanson (2015). Gut microbiota can affect expression of phase I and II enzymes in ways that either metabolically activate or inactivate drugs through processes that involve reduction, hydrolysis, dihydroxylation, acetylation, deacetylation, proteolysis, deconjugation, and deglycosylation. An example of this has been seen with sulfalzine, which is used to treat gut inflammation. Microbial enzymes in the gut will convert it to its pharmacologically active form, 5-amino 5-salicyclic acid. Concerning xenobiotics, the organism *Desulfovibrio desulfuricans* has been reported to participate in the metabolism of arsenic by producing hydrogen sulfide (H_2S) that converts monomethylarsonic acid to monomethyl monothioarsonate, a more toxic form of arsenic. Finally, another xenobiotic example is hydrazine, which has been used, along with its derivatives, as a rocket propellant and as a constituent of several industrial processes and agricultural chemicals. Gut microflora can significantly reduce the toxicity of this substance.

DETOXIFICATION AND GENETIC POLYMORPHISMS (SNPs)

It has now been firmly established that virtually all phase I and II detoxification enzymes can demonstrate a whole variety of genetic polymorphisms that vary from person to person which can profoundly affect the ability to detoxify xenobiotic compounds. As pointed out by Sim et al., these polymorphisms involve a gene copy number variation which can include amplification and deletion. However, the polymorphism that has received the most attention in the clinical and functional medicine community is the single-nucleotide polymorphism (SNP) (Sim et al., 2013). As noted by Croom (2012), phase I polymorphisms generally result in decreased activity of the enzymes rather than complete loss of function. In contrast, polymorphisms of phase II enzymes can result in complete loss of activity. A notable example that was pointed out by Croom (2012) is glutathione-S-transferase M1 (GSTM1), which has a null frequency of about 40%. Most polymorphisms yield a decrease in activity. However, some result in no change or even an increase in activity (Croom, 2012).

One of the most well-documented phase I enzyme polymorphisms is one that involves the phase I enzyme CYP2D6. Liska et al. (2005) point out that 5%–10% of the Caucasian population have low activity of this enzyme, which is an important metabolizer of more than 25 therapeutic drugs including antiarrhythmics, antidepressants, and antipsychotics plus a wide range of xenobiotics. Interestingly, this polymorphism can be expressed in two forms, with one gene that encodes the wild type (yielding average activity) and another that possesses an SNP that yields lower activity. Persons in this category are classified as poor metabolizers and may require lower dosages than usual of certain drugs in order to avoid adverse reactions. Interestingly, some individuals possess polymorphisms that increase activity of CYP2D6. They are known as extensive metabolizers and will need higher doses of certain drugs to achieve certain therapeutic effects. Another key point about extensive metabolizers is that they will tend to have the ability to handle higher loads of environmental toxins before demonstrating adverse effects.

Of course, given its high prevalence worldwide, including the United States (Levin and Varga, 2016), the C677 T methylenetetrahydrofolate reductase (MTHFR) polymorphism, of all polymorphisms, has probably attracted the most attention over the last few years. Given that this polymorphism can lead to significantly decreased enzyme function (Rai, 2016), which is to facilitate methylation reactions, could the activity of the phase II detoxification enzyme COMT, which acts by facilitating methylation of environmental toxins and, as mentioned above, endogenous estrogen metabolites, be adversely affected? This question has been examined by several studies on behavioral disorders where it has been found that individuals with certain behavioral disorders not only demonstrated the MTHFR C677 T polymorphism but COMT polymorphisms such as COMT Val158Met and COMT324AA (Muntjewerff et al., 2008; Peerbooms et al., 2012; Kontis et al., 2013; Wang et al., 2015; Rahimi et al., 2016). However, this author could not find studies linking MTHFR and COMT polymorphisms in relation to the role of COMT in detoxification reactions.

Nevertheless, research does exist that makes it clear that COMT polymorphisms alone can have an adverse impact on detoxification reactions. For example, it was found that estrogen levels in women were significantly correlated with COMT genotype (Worda et al., 2003). Conversely, it has also been found estrogen can down-regulate COMT gene transcription (Shu-Leong and Ramsden, 1999). Could COMT polymorphisms be clinically significant in terms of breast cancer risk? This is indeed true as demonstrated by Goodman et al. (2001). Still another fascinating and clinically significant relationship between estrogen metabolism and COMT activity was reported by Li et al., who noted that equine estrogens, which are a major constituent of many hormone replacement drugs, can inhibit the activity of variant forms of COMT. According to the authors, this impact of hormone replacement therapies containing equine estrogens could reduce the ability of COMT to clear endogenous and exogenous estrogens from cells, "...thus prolonging their ability to cause toxicity" (Li et al., 2004).

DETOXIFICATION AND AGE

According to Croom (2012), age can play a significant role in the activity of detoxification enzymes. For example, neonates and fetuses usually have a lower detoxification enzyme capacity than children or adults. However, after age 45 this trend reverses with a decline in detoxification ability with age.

DETOXIFICATION AND GENDER

According to Liska et al. (2005), the phase I family of enzymes, CYP3A, is particularly sensitive to hormones, being regulated, at least in part, by progesterone or the ratio of progesterone and estrogen. Evidence of this demonstrated by the fact that premenopausal women often show 30%–40% more activity of CYP3A4 compared to men or postmenopausal women. CYP3A activity also appears to be higher during pregnancy. However, overall xenobiotic metabolism during pregnancy, according to Croom (2012), is decreased. The author theorizes that this is a protective mechanism to reduce the formation of toxic metabolites.

DETOXIFICATION AND DOSE

As stated by Paracelsus several hundred years ago, "All things are poison and nothing is without poison, only the dose permits something not to be poisonous" (Mattson and Calabrese, 2010). In more modern terms, according to Croom (2012), "The dose makes the poison." The author goes on to point out that, as the dose shifts from low to high of any particular substance, there is a change in the relative importance of various detoxification enzymes involved in metabolism of the substance. Croon (2012) then presents an example of this. For acetaminophen, lower therapeutic doses go through the phase II pathways glururonidation and sulfotransferase conjugation. However, higher doses overwhelm the cofactors available for phase II conjugation, leaving the phase I pathway CYP2E1 to become predominant. Unfortunately, CYP2E1 activity leads to the formation of the highly reactive metabolite N-acetyl-p-benzoquinoneimine (NAPQI). According to Liska et al. (2005), NAPQI is a highly neurotoxic substance that, if not cleared by glutathione conjugation, can lead to severe toxicity.

DETOXIFICATION AND ROUTE OF ADMINISTRATION

Generally, toxins taken in orally go through first-pass metabolism where the toxin goes directly from the GI tract to the liver for detoxification. The advantage of this is that much less of the toxin is available to travel to key organs such as the brain or bladder (Croom, 2012). However, if the exposure is through significant inhalation or dermal absorption, much more of the toxin is available to the general circulation, which can greatly increase the overall damaging effect of the toxin. Fortunately, given that the nasal epithelium has a higher phase I activity than any other extrahepatic tissue, the potential overall metabolic impact of an inhaled toxin may be reduced (Parkinson, 1996).

DETOXIFICATION AND SUBOPTIMAL NUTRIENT INTAKE

The role of various nutrients in detoxification pathways has been extensively discussed, primarily in the functional medicine literature. These nutrients can be broadly subdivided into two categories. First, there are the essential nutrients that act as true co-factors in various detoxification reactions. Second, there are the nutrients, largely plant derived and generally named "phytonutrients" which, even though they may not be categorized as essential, have been found, when administered supplementally, to enhance and/or optimize various detoxification pathways. According to Liska et al. (2005), the following essential nutrients are required for optimal phase I and II activity:

- Vitamin A (phase II)
- Riboflavin (phase I)
- Niacin (phase I)
- Pyridoxine (phase I)
- Folate (phase I)
- Cobalamin (phase I)
- Branched-chain amino acids (phase I)
- Methionine (phase II)

According to the authors, phase I and II activity can be enhanced or optimized by the following non-essential nutrients:

- Glutathione (phase I)
- Flavonoids (phase I)
- Phospholipids (phase I)
- Glycine (phase II)
- Taurine (phase II)
- Glutamine (phase II)
- N-acetylcysteine (phase II)
- Cysteine (phase II)

Lyon et al. (2005) also point out that inorganic sulfate and selenium are important to support phase II activity. Concerning phytonutrients, the authors suggest grapefruit will reduce both phase I and II activity and St. John's wort will accelerate it. Furthermore, foods such as onions, garlic, and cruciferous vegetables can act in many and sometimes complex ways to optimize function of both detoxification phases. They go on to note that food constituents and herbals such as chlorophyll, terpenoids (e.g., citrus, *Ginkgo biloba*, menthol, camphor), and bioflavonoids (e.g., citrus, pine bark, grape seed, and green tea) can have similar beneficial activities.

Croom (2012) provides further detail on the impact of nutrition on detoxification. For example, food in general can affect the amount of xenobiotic available for metabolism by impacting its solubility and altering gastric emptying and bioavailability. In addition, polycyclic aromatic hydrocarbons found in grilled meats and vegetables can induce the expression of the phase I enzyme CYP1A.

Lyon (2013) notes that moderately high-protein diets can upregulate P450 enzymes in a way that decreases susceptibility to pesticides and other xenobiotics, where low-protein diets can do the opposite. Similarly, high carbohydrate diets can down regulate P450 enzymes in a way that promotes an undesirable reduction in the metabolism of several drugs and hormones. Of course, for some populations, lack of food in general, either due to circumstance or by choice (fasting) needs to be considered because of its impact on detoxification pathways. As pointed out by Lyon (2013), phase I enzymes are, for the most part, resistant to depletion due to suboptimal food intake and may even be induced by products of fasting metabolism such as ketones and xenobiotics released from stored fat. On the other hand, complete fasts, juice fasts, and other nutritionally marginal fasting regimens will lead to significant decreases in phase II enzyme function. The net result of suboptimal food intake has been described as "unbalanced detoxification" where phase I enzymes are often induced and phase II enzymes are decreased. This can lead to significant increases in oxidative stress and what has been described as "detox reactions." Therefore, according to Lyon (2013), traditional methods of detoxification that involve different fasting regimens may be ill-advised, especially for long periods of time.

One essential nutrient that has recently attracted great interest in relation to detoxification processes is vitamin D. As noted by Wang et al. (2013), of all the phase I enzymes, CYP3A4 is the most important in relation to drug metabolism since it is involved in clearance of almost half of all the orally ingested therapeutic agents that undergo metabolic transformation. The fully activated form of vitamin D, $1\alpha,25$ $(OH)_2D_3$, induces transcription of CYP3A4 though its relationship with vitamin D receptors (VDR). In particular, VDR helps regulate CYP3A4 enzyme content in the liver and small intestine mucosa.

Wang et al. (2013) also point out that phase I enzymes play a vital role in the metabolism of vitamin D. For example, the conversion in the liver of vitamin D_3 to 25-hydroxy D_3 ($25OHD_3$) involves 1α-hydroxylation, which is catalyzed primarily by CYP27B1. Furthermore, CYP3A4 in the intestine and liver may contribute to the metabolic clearance of fully activated vitamin D ($1\alpha,25(OH)_2C_3$) as well as $25OHD_3$, particularly when expression of CYP3A4 has been induced.

More recent research on vitamin D suggests phthalates and bisphenol A may alter circulating levels of total 25(OH)D in adults due to inhibition and/or induction of the cytochrome P450 family of enzymes that are involved in the conversion of vitamin D to 25(OH)D (Johns et al., 2016).

DETOXIFICATION AND MEDICATIONS

As pointed out by Liska et al. (2005), certain medications can impact on phase I detoxification enzymes in such a way that adversely affects the metabolism of both endogenous and exogenous toxins, thus allowing more of these toxins to remain in the body in an untransformed state, causing toxic reactions. Examples of this are medications such as SSRIs, macrolide antibiotics, and H2 blockers such as cimetidine that can inhibit one or more phase I enzyme systems.

DETOXIFICATION OF ENVIRONMENTAL TOXINS: SOME PRACTICAL CONSIDERATIONS

Assessment

Given that, from the patient's standpoint, resolution of chief complaints is the primary objective and elimination of toxins is only important insofar as it leads to resolution of chief complaints, assessment must incorporate two objectives:

1. The determination of not only which toxins are present but in what quantity
2. The determination of whether the toxins determined to be present are actually contributing to the creation of chief complaints

As will be demonstrated, most of the information on toxicity assessment only focuses on objective #1 with little or no specific determination of whether what was found is actually related to the clinical symptom presentation. Why is this a problem? Certainly clinical experience suggests that, most of the time, reduction in the body burden chemical and metal toxins will lead to reduction in chief complaints. However, as will also be demonstrated, this is not the case for many patients. Why is this? One theory that will be greatly expanded upon shortly revolves around the concept of what is known as "allostatic load." One of the main precepts of this theory is that chief complaints occur as the result of the cumulative effect of many different stressors in patients' lives. Certainly there is no question, as has been discussed above, that virtually everyone in the industrialized world, including patients, carries a certain level of environmental toxin burden. However, not everyone will experience clinically significant symptomatic profiles. Could the difference for the symptomatic patient not be just the presence of toxins per se, but the presence of toxins plus the additive effect of other life stressors such as poor diet, too much or too little exercise, chronic infections, lack of sleep, worry, and so on? This is what is suggested by allostatic load principles. Furthermore, if cumulative stress load, which includes but is not limited to environmental toxins, is the true cause of patient symptoms, it would stand to reason that, even if the clinical presentation is similar from one patient to the next, the patient for whom, for example, environmental toxicity is 80% of the total cumulative stress load, would be expected to respond favorably from a symptomatic standpoint to detoxification procedures alone. On the other hand, if environmental toxicity only accounts for 10% of the total cumulative stress load, it would also seem likely that there would be minimal symptomatic improvement with detoxification procedures alone. Therefore, it is not only important to determine the presence of environmental toxins, it is also important to determine if a primary focus on environmental toxins both from a diagnostic and treatment standpoint will predictably lead to improvements in chief complaints for any particular patient. This point was emphasized by Lyon et al. (2005) in a chapter subsection by Crinnion who points out that the important question to address in today's patient is not whether the patient is toxic given that the average number of toxins per person has been found to be 91. Instead, we need to ask the following:

- Is this patient's toxic burden a causative factor in his or her illness?
- If so, is it an obstacle to cure?
- If yes, what can be done to help the patient?

Crinnion goes on to point out, as suggested above, that the answers to these questions can be hard to come by since the subject has not been adequately researched even in small clinical trials:

"Connecting the toxic burden directly to the patient's illness is very difficult and sometimes impossible."

A good example of this is the study by Levy et al. (2004) where it was found that even though there was a direct correlation between the amount of mercury amalgam restorations in children and urinary mercury levels, no conclusions could be made concerning possible adverse health effects.

It is the opinion of this author that an understanding of allostatic load concepts will greatly enhance the ability of the clinician to determine more precisely if toxic burden is actually related to patient illness.

Before leaving this topic, practical, patient compliance issues should be addressed as to why it is so important to determine, as best as possible, if the toxins found to be present are key factors creating symptoms. Many, if not most, of the laboratory tests and treatment interventions to be discussed in this section often involve significant cost. In addition, many may entail significant changes and disruption of daily routines. Finally, some treatment modalities and laboratory tests that involve what is known as "challenge testing" carry with them sometimes significant risk of unpleasant side effects. It is certainly not difficult to imagine the patient dissatisfaction that would be incurred when, after going through significant costs, inconvenience, and side effects, substantial improvements in chief complaints are not realized. Yes, many lectures, papers, and textbooks have tended to focus on the many success stories. However, as will demonstrated, the frequency of lack of clinical improvement after going through extensive testing and treatment is often enough that it is the opinion of this author that no discussion of clinical management of the patient exposed to environmental toxins is complete without a discussion of how to identify the patient whose symptoms are not primarily related to the presence of these toxins alone, no matter how high the amount.

ASSESSMENT: HISTORY

Certainly, one of the best ways of accomplishing both objectives mentioned above is a thorough patient history. Liska et al. (2005) suggest evaluation of the following warning signs that would suggest a relationship between toxicity and patient chief complaints:

- A history of increasing sensitivity to exogenous exposures (toxic xenobiotics)
- Abundant use of medications
- Significant use of potentially toxic chemicals in the home or work environment
- Sensitivity to odors
- Musculoskeletal symptoms (similar to fibromyalgia)
- Cognitive dysfunction
- Unilateral paresthesia
- Autonomic dysfunction and recurrent patterns of edema
- Worsening of symptoms after anesthesia or pregnancy
- Paradoxical responses or sensitivity to medications or supplements

Lyon et al. (2005) suggest the following mnemonic, C(H2) OP(D4), that can act as a guide to determine whether various lifestyle and environmental issues may be contributing to toxic load and/ or symptomatology. This mnemonic stands for community, home, hobbies, occupation, personal habits, diet, drugs, dental, and development. The authors emphasize the importance of using this mnemonic as guideline in questioning patients as patients will often not be aware or will forget important sources of toxic exposure.

ASSESSMENT: LABORATORY ANALYSIS

What follows is an overview of some of the most popular and time-tested laboratory tests used to determine the presence of environmental toxins. For a more detailed description of these tests plus others such as organic acids and routine blood chemistry that have been used to assess environmental toxin levels, please consult *Laboratory Evaluations for Integrative and Functional Medicine, Revised Second Edition* by Lord and Bralley (2012).

ASSESSMENT: ORGANIC CHEMICALS

As noted by Lyon et al. (2005) while it is possible to assess blood, urine, and adipose tissue for levels of organic toxins such as PCBs, organochlorine pesticides, PBDE fire retardants, furans, and dioxins, the sheer numbers of these toxins that may be present in any patient makes testing impractical from a financial standpoint. However, given that chemical toxicity results from an interaction between chemical exposure and the ability to detoxify chemicals (Liska et al., 2005), assessment of phase I and II detoxification enzyme function via challenge testing that employs probe substances known to be eliminated by specific phase I and/or phase II enzymes has gained in popularity. Because caffeine is metabolized through the phase I CYP1A2 pathway, a caffeine challenge test has been used to assess phase I enzyme capacity. Concerning phase II enzymes, acetaminophen has been used as a probe substance to assess glucuronidation and sulfation and sodium benzoate has been used to assess phase II glycine conjugation (Liska et al., 2005). In addition, salicylic acid (aspirin) has been used as a probe substance to assess phase II glucuronidation and glycination (Lord and Bralley, 2012).

Given that detoxification capacity, as mentioned above, can be affected by SNPs, laboratory assessment tools are also available to determine the presence of SNPs for certain phase I enzymes and phase II enzymes such as glutathione-S-transferase (Lyon, 2013).

Assessment: Heavy Metals

Certainly, the most commonly used laboratory assessment tool over the years for heavy metals is trace mineral analysis using hair. On the positive side, as pointed out by Lyon (2013), the test is simple, inexpensive, and provides reasonably useful information on lead and methylmercury from seafood. On the negative side, Lyon et al. (2005) point out that interpretation of the findings on hair analysis can be challenging. For example, it has been suggested that low levels of mercury in autistic children may be a sign of poor excretion rather than a healthy finding and high hair mercury levels may indicate a healthy excretion pattern. Another negative is that the precision of this technology is limited, making findings about metals other than lead and mercury, which may be toxic at extremely low levels, of questionable use clinically.

One time or "spot" urine or blood tests for heavy metals such as lead are of limited use for most patients who are experiencing ongoing, low-grade exposure due to the fact that spot urine and blood tests only reflect current exposure and may have little relationship to actual tissue levels (Lyon, 2013). Because of this, Lyon (2013) advocates evaluating metals such as lead and mercury via urine after ingestion of a chelating agent such as dimercapto-propane sulfonate (DMPS). This type of challenge testing has also employed another oral chelator, dimercaptosuccinic acid (DMSA). Interestingly, there is a difference of opinion on the value of DMSA in terms of providing clinically useful information on heavy metal status. Lyon (2013) suggests that the DMSA postprovocative challenge test does not accurately reflect mercury body burden. In contrast, Lord and Bralley (2012) indicate that both DMPS and DMSA can provide useful information.

An endogenous detoxification factor that is specific for heavy metals is metallothionein (MT) (Lyon, 2013). While MT is involved in the transport and short-term storage of zinc and copper, it is involved in both the protection against and elimination of heavy metals, particularly cadmium and mercury. While there does not appear to be a commercially available laboratory test for MT, assays are available that will assess SNPs of MT (Lyon, 2013).

Of course, considering what was discussed above, none of these assessment modalities for heavy metals can reliably predict a close correlation between the presence of heavy metals and chief complaints in any particular patient. Because of this, a relatively new functional medicine assessment has been developed, urinary porphyrin profiling, which can reliably suggest that the presence of heavy metals is not just associated with chief complaints but represents true cause and effect (Lord and Bralley, 2012). Porphyrins are actually enzymatically produced metabolites that are intermediates in the production of heme. Heavy metal toxins such as arsenic, lead, and mercury can interfere with the various enzymes involved in the porphyrin pathway. Furthermore, each of these heavy metals will often present a unique enzyme-inhibition "signature" that suggests not only is the heavy metal present in significant quantities, but also it is having an adverse effect on key metabolic pathways that could very well be involved with patient chief complaints. In turn, as suggested by Lord and Bralley (2012):

"Elevated porphyrins in urine serve as biomarkers to verify the clinical observations of symptomatic effects of toxicity."

Treatment: Traditional Approaches

It is well documented that heavy metals such as lead, cadmium, and mercury can be actively removed using chelators such as DMSA and DMPS (Lyon, 2013). Can other toxins be removed from the body via use of therapeutic agents which physically remove toxins from the body? This controversial question will be addressed in the text that follows. However, for the most part, traditional treatment of environmental toxicity involves modalities that either reduce exposure levels or improve the ability of the body to metabolize and eliminate.

TRADITIONAL AVOIDANCE TREATMENTS

Crinnion (2013) first advocates for the chemically sensitive patient the creation of a chemically safe dwelling. To do this, the following specific procedures are recommended:

- No wearing of shoes indoors
- Replace furnace filters every 6 weeks with a high efficiency filter
- Air out dry-cleaning clothing outside the house for one week
- No indoor smoking
- Replace carpeting with tile or stone flooring
- Use non-scented laundry soap and fabric softeners
- Obtain a high-quality air purifier that has a large enough capacity to clear the air in the bedroom at least once every 30 minutes

Of course, Crinnion (2013) also points out that these steps may be difficult for many to accomplish. Therefore, while these interventions may be optimal, given the very real compliance issues that they may elicit because of the significant time and cost commitments involved, is there more that can be done in terms of avoidance? As will be discussed in detail in the section on allostatic load, avoidance of virtually any environmental stressor such as excessive use of computers, too little exercise, lack of sleep, and excessive worry can be just as effective in dealing with the impact of environmental toxins on patient chief complaints.

Concerning dietary avoidance procedures, Crinnion (2013) recommends avoiding foods that may elicit allergic reactions and certain fruits and vegetables that are known to be treated with herbicides and/or pesticides. In addition, avoidance of farmed salmon, high mercury fish, and nonorganic dairy products is recommended to reduce toxin exposures from food. Similar to what was stated above, though, a legitimate concern about these dietary recommendations for many patients is their practicality from both compliance and financial standpoints. Can clinical success with chief complaints be attained with a more relaxed, patient-friendly approach to diet? Applying allostatic load concepts to care of the toxic patients, as will be discussed, suggests that the answer to this question is yes.

TRADITIONAL TREATMENTS THAT IMPROVE THE ABILITY OF THE BODY TO METABOLIZE AND ELIMINATE

Crinnion (2013) recommends that macro- and micronutrient deficiencies that may compromise function of phase I and II enzymes be addressed. Specific nutrients that might be of concern are protein, folate, and choline. Liska et al. (2005) expand upon this theme by advocating optimal hydration to promote elimination and the supplementation of nutrients that function as cofactors or are otherwise involved in optimal functioning of phase I and II enzymes. (See the section above on detoxification enzymes and nutrition.) They also advocate supplementation of food factors that support optimal phase I and II enzyme activity such as flavonoids, monoterpenoids, curcumin, forskolin, and indole-3-carbinol. Lyon et al. (2005) suggest the utilization of a whole foods diet that is high in alkalizing foods, fiber, cruciferous vegetables, olive oil, onions, and garlic. They also recommend supplementation of the herb milk thistle, alkalizing minerals (Ca, Mg, K, Zn), a multivitamin/trace element supplement, DHA/EPA, N-acetylcysteine, lipoic acid, and antioxidants (vitamins C and E, grape seed extract, green tea extract). Finally, they advocate use of detoxification medical food products (research on the efficacy of these products will be addressed later).

TRADITIONAL TREATMENTS THAT MAY ASSIST IN THE PHYSICAL REMOVAL OF TOXINS FROM THE BODY

It is well recognized that heavy metals such as cadmium, lead, and mercury can be successfully chelated using chelating agents such as 2,3-dimercapto-1-propanesulfonic acid (DMPS), meso-2,3-dimercaptosuccinic acid (DMSA), and ethylenediamine tetraacetic acid (EDTA). Specifically, according to Fitzgerald et al. (2012), cadmium can be chelated with EDTA and DMSA, lead can be chelated with EDTA, and mercury can be chelated with DMSA and DMPS. It should be noted, though, side effects have been reported with all chelating agents. For example, treatment with both DMSA and DMPS have led to transient skin reactions, mild neutropenia, and moderately elevated liver enzymes (Aaseth et al., 2015).

There are many "detoxification" remedies and procedures that have been recommended over the years to remove toxins, many of which are quite controversial in terms of efficacy. Some of these are rice bran fiber (Crinnion, 2013), chlorophyll (Crinnion, 2013), "cleanses" that employ saunas (Crinnion, 2013) (Lyon et al., 2005), hydrotherapy (Crinnion, 2013) (Lyon et al., 2005), colonic irrigation (Crinnion, 2013), constitutional homeopathy (Crinnion, 2013), body therapies (Crinnion, 2013), counseling (Crinnion, 2013), fasting (Lyon, 2013), exercise (Lyon et al., 2005), and sleep and relaxation (Lyon et al., 2005).

PRACTICAL CONCERNS ABOUT TRADITIONAL APPROACHES TO ENVIRONMENTAL TOXICITY DIAGNOSIS AND TREATMENT

There is no question, based on both published and anecdotal evidence, that the diagnostic and treatment modalities just described have yielded success in terms of reduction or elimination of chief complaints in a great many patients. However, does this very direct approach that heavily focuses on identification, metabolism, and elimination of toxins ever yield less than optimal results? Published research that will be described shortly suggests that the answer to this question is in the affirmative. While there may be many reasons for this lack of efficacy, there is one very important reason that revolves around patient lifestyle issues. Of course, the overall tone of the literature I have just reviewed is that, if patients experiencing environmental toxicity want to reduce or eliminate chief complaints, there must be fairly rigid adherence to diagnostic and treatment regimens. Unfortunately, practicalities involving cost, side effects, and general lifestyle demands revolving around family, job, and key social interactions can very often render rigid compliance difficult if not impossible. Furthermore, the metabolic and psychological stress that can accompany the above-mentioned diagnostic treatment protocols due to cost, side effects, and inconvenience in terms of job, family, and social connections can actually create metabolic imbalances that can significantly negate even the most comprehensive detoxification program. In what way? Allostatic load principles, which will be described shortly, tell us that any stressor or set of stressors which may include toxicologic stress, dietary stress, or psychological stress will upregulate production of inflammatory mediators and lead to a state of chronic inflammation. Chronic inflammation, in turn, can powerfully down regulate activity of both phase I and II detoxification enzymes, as has been demonstrated in numerous studies (Cheng and Morgan, 2001; Morgan, 2001; Jover et al., 2002; Rivory et al., 2002; Haas et al., 2003; Kim et al., 2004; Renton, 2004; Mimche et al., 2014). One of the most powerful inducers of chronic inflammation may be a detoxification program that requires rigid adherence to diet that is not only very different from what the patient typically ingests but what spouses, family, and friends typically ingest. Why? With this scenario, it is not unusual that patient adherence to the detoxification diet and lifestyle can lead to social isolation, as noted by Bratman in his book *Health Food Junkies* (Bratman, 2000). In turn, social isolation can lead to significant increases in production of inflammatory mediators (Hackett et al., 2012). Because of the significant impact of inflammation on phase I and II detoxification enzyme function that will be described shortly, an ironic situation ensues where the psychological stress induced by rigid adherence to a detoxification program that involves significant cost and radical changes in lifestyle can highly compromise any positive impact the detoxification program may theoretically have on overall detoxification efficacy.

WHEN DETOXIFICATION PROCEDURES ALONE DO NOT REDUCE OR ELIMINATE CHIEF COMPLAINTS IN PATIENTS CARRYING A SIGNIFICANT LOAD OF ENVIRONMENTAL TOXINS AND WHY

All the references discussed above make mention through case reports and other data that detoxification procedures clearly assist in reduction of chief complaints in many patients carrying a significant load of environmental toxins. Unfortunately, some of the statements made in these references also suggest that, with optimal compliance, success is assured. A landmark study published in 2003 that examined clinical efficacy of virtually all the treatment modalities discussed above in patients with multiple chemical sensitivity suggests this is indeed not true. In "Perceived Treatment Efficacy for Conventional and Alternative Therapies Reported by Persons with Multiple Chemical Sensitivity" by Gibson et al. (2003), 917 individuals were evaluated. About 82% were women and 95% were Caucasian. Ages ranged from 20 to 82 years with a mean age of 53 years. There were 7% that identified the severity of their multiple chemical sensitivity (MCS) as mild, 32% as moderate, 45% as severe, and 13% as totally disabling. Patient evaluations of 108 different treatments were categorized by percentage in terms of the following:

- Very helpful
- Somewhat helpful
- No noticeable effect
- Somewhat harmful
- Very harmful

In addition, treatments were rated in terms of which had the best help/harm ratio. As will be described below, detoxification procedures were far from 100% successful in terms of patient satisfaction. Furthermore, these procedures elicited an alarmingly high level of adverse reactions.

Which therapies performed best in terms of help/harm ratio? It should come as no surprise that "chemical-free living space" and "chemical avoidance" performed the best. But what about detoxification procedures like many of those described above?

- Chelation—46% felt it was helpful, 27% felt there was no change, and 23% felt it was harmful. Given the popularity of this procedure, clinicians should seriously consider the implications of the possibility that over 20% of a clinician's patients who are chelated may complain about feeling worse after therapy.
- Removal of amalgam fillings—44% felt it was helpful, 47% felt there was no change, and 9% felt it was harmful. Given the cost and inconvenience of amalgam removal, the latter two percentages are both sobering and significant when considering treatment options.
- Milk thistle—49% felt it was helpful, 42% felt there was no change, and 9% felt it was harmful.

Other detoxification procedures performed similarly in that none were reported to be helpful more than 60% of the time. Equally significant from a practice management standpoint is that virtually all the detoxification procedures evaluated elicited harmful ratings well into the double digits from a percentage standpoint.

Concerning therapeutic interventions, what were the top three that performed best based on help/harm ratio? As you will see, none of the following were mentioned in the research discussed above and none would be considered "detox remedies" in the traditional sense:

- Prayer—64% felt it was helpful, 34% felt there was no change, and, most importantly, only 1% felt it was harmful.
- Meditation—54% felt it was helpful, 43% felt there was no change, and only 2.8% felt it was harmful.
- Acupressure—67% felt it was helpful, 38% felt there was no change, and 4.5% felt it was harmful.

Concerning diet, which intervention worked best based on help/harm ratio? Was it the type of regimented, restrictive diet mentioned above? Not even close. A rotation diet, which does not emphasize absolute restrictions as much as it emphasizes variety and reduction in certain offending foods, making it much more practical, was reported to be helpful by 72% of the respondents. About 22% felt there was no change, and 5.7% felt it was harmful.

Which supplements delivered the best help/harm ratio? Again, none that would be traditionally regarded as "detox" supplements:

- Acidophilus—52% felt it was helpful, 44% felt there was no change, and 4% felt it was harmful.
- Magnesium—52% felt it was helpful, 41% felt there was no change, and 6% felt it was harmful.

Another very interesting and telling list presented by Gibson et al. (2003) was the treatments that were rated as much more harmful than helpful. Not surprisingly, the majority on this list were medications such as antidepressants and Valium. However, there was one popular nutritional supplement on the list—a leading detoxification medical food. For this product 34% felt it was helpful, 30% felt there was no change, and, most importantly, close to 36% felt it was harmful.

In the opinion of this author, what are the important conclusions that can be taken away from this study? First, as noted by the authors, the highest rated therapies were fairly non-invasive and low risk. In addition, except for "chemical-free living space" and "chemical avoidance," they tended to be low cost and involved minimal to moderate disruption of daily activities and social interactions. How important is cost according to Gibson et al. (2003)? The authors state:

> "It is important to find efficacious treatments that minimize the financial depletion of a population that has difficulty remaining in gainful employment."

Second, the references in many of the studies reviewed above suggest that emphasis should primarily be placed on biochemical optimization of toxic load and detoxification pathways based on laboratory testing and this emphasis alone will lead to predictably good patient outcomes. They also suggest that, as long as biochemical optimization of toxic load and detoxification pathways is attained, issues of cost, convenience, and practicality need not be prioritized to maximize patient outcomes. The data from the Gibson et al. (2003) suggest just the opposite. In fact, probably the most important determinant of a successful practice that addresses the needs of toxic patients, patient satisfaction, which is based not only on reduction of chief complaints but focuses on cost, convenience, and practicality, is not going to be based solely on the ability to remove toxins and optimize detoxification pathways by the traditional methods discussed above. Rather success will involve avoidance, removal, and procedures that improve detoxification capacity in ways that are balanced with considerations of cost, convenience, and practicality.

Of course, I would suspect that many readers may be thinking by now that an "unscientific" approach to the toxic patient is being advocated that deemphasizes removal and avoidance of toxins and optimization of detoxification pathways in favor of interventions that do little more than create patient satisfaction via a placebo effect. Furthermore, I would suspect that many readers may be of the opinion, in contrast to what has been just stated, that successful detoxification and optimization of patient satisfaction can only be accomplished by the modalities discussed above that emphasize a somewhat rigid, regimented, "all or none" approach to interventions. In short, "How can the job be done effectively if so many compromises based on cost, convenience, and patient oriented lifestyle practicalities are instituted?"

In the opinion of this author, the answer to this question is "allostatic load."

ALLOSTATIC LOAD, ENVIRONMENTAL TOXINS, AND DETOXIFICATION ENZYMES

As was suggested in the text above, traditional functional medicine approaches to toxicology would regard many of the most effective modalities in the Gibson et al. (2003) study, even though they delivered impressive results in reducing chief complaints in MCS patients, as having little to do with the actual metabolism and elimination of environmental toxins. This line of thought, though, is seriously flawed. As will be demonstrated, there is every reason to believe that prayer, meditation, rotation diets, magnesium supplementation, and all the other most clinically effective interventions in the Gibson et al. (2003) paper did more than just help patients "feel better." Research about to be presented makes a strong case that they acted as powerful optimizers of detoxification enzyme function. In what way? The short answer can be summed up in one word: *Inflammation.* As was pointed out above, inflammation can powerfully suppress activity of both phase I and phase II enzymes. Could interventions such as prayer, meditation, rotation diets, magnesium supplementation, and so on have a major impact in reducing inflammation in the participants in the Gibson et al. (2003) study? To answer this question, the principles of allostasis and allostatic load need to be considered.

As noted by Danese and McEwen (2012), human biochemistry and physiology is constantly adapting to changes in the external and internal environment to maintain homeostatic indicators such as blood pressure, pulse, body temperature, and so on. Of course, these adaptations to a constantly changing environment do not happen randomly. In contrast, they act in an organized and predictable manner. This organized collection of responsive processes has been give the title of *allostasis.* The biological systems involved in allostasis include the hypothalamic–pituitary–adrenocortical (HPA) axis, the autonomic nervous system, and the metabolic and immune systems (Steptoe et al., 2014). Thus, as noted by Steptoe et al. (2014), allostasis is essential for maintaining homeostasis. What types of environmental changes elicit activity of allostatic mechanisms? As noted by Beckie (2012), virtual psychological or environmental stressors. These would include childhood adversity, infection, poor diet, lack of sleep, genetic polymorphisms, lack of optimal exercise, and environmental toxins. Furthermore, perceptions or expectations of any of these stressors through worry or fear can upregulate activity of allostatic mechanisms without actually encountering the specific stressor being feared. Unfortunately, as noted by Steptoe et al. (2014), these allostatic mechanisms have a limited capacity to respond to real and perceived stressors and maintain optimal homeostatic balance. Therefore, with repeated and sustained cumulative real and perceived stress levels, the very mechanisms involved in allostatic processes that are health-promoting with short-term, acute stress will, because of constant and prolonged activity, promote ill-health and loss of homeostasis with long-term, chronic stress. This overactivity of allostatic mechanisms during long-term, chronic stress has been termed *allostatic load.* What specifically happens with allostatic load to create ill-health? As noted by Steptoe et al. (2014), the cortisol production that is beneficial in the short term becomes dysregulated in the long term leading to numerous metabolic imbalances. The insulin production that is beneficial in the short term leads to blood sugar dysregulation in the long term. Of course, what is most pertinent to this discussion is that the production of inflammatory mediators that is beneficial in the short term leads to elevation of inflammatory, acute phase reactants such as interleukin-6 (IL-6) and C-reactive protein (CRP), which can cause numerous alterations in optimal metabolic function (Beckie, 2012; Steptoe et al., 2014). Most notably, as was reported above, increased production of acute phase reactants such as IL-6 and CRP can lead to profound decreases in phase I and II detoxification enzyme activity. An overview of the impact of allostatic load on detoxification pathways can be seen in Figure 5.2.

Before leaving this overview discussion of allostasis and allostatic load, please note again the phrase "sustained cumulative real and perceived stress levels" from the previous paragraph. Stressors act cumulatively to create allostatic load, which includes increased inflammation and subsequent decreases in phase I and II detoxification enzyme activity. Because of this, *any* stressor or combination of stressors, which may or may not include environmental toxins, can powerfully down regulate the ability of the body to detoxify. This would include common stressors found in many chronically ill patients such as too much or too little exercise, infection, poor diet, too much time in front of computers (electromagnetic stress), lack of sleep, and, what is, in the opinion of this author, a major source of allostatic load inducing, pro-inflammatory stress that is often unrecognized and under-appreciated in patients experiencing high levels of environmental toxins, perceived stress (worry and fear).

Of course, the fact that any combination of real or perceived stressors that is present in high enough levels for a sustained period of time can contribute to toxicity promoting inflammation and thereby down-regulating detoxification capacity also presents detoxification options not usually considered in references such as those discussed above. Certainly, as suggested above, detoxification can be enhanced through diet and key nutritional, herbal, and nutraceutical supplements that directly enhance and support phase I and II enzyme activity. However, detoxification can also be enhanced by any modality that reduces allostatic load and inflammation such as optimum exercise, ideal sleep habits, elimination of chronic infections and dysbiosis, and, most especially, activities that reduce fear and worry. In addition, it could be hypothesized that since so many interventions outside of those that have a direct impact on toxin levels and detoxification enzymes can have a positive impact on toxicity, a more relaxed, low cost, and patient friendly approach can be implemented where small changes are made with a large variety of lifestyle issues. Because this approach is not only effective in reducing inflammation and thereby optimizing phase I and II enzyme activity but

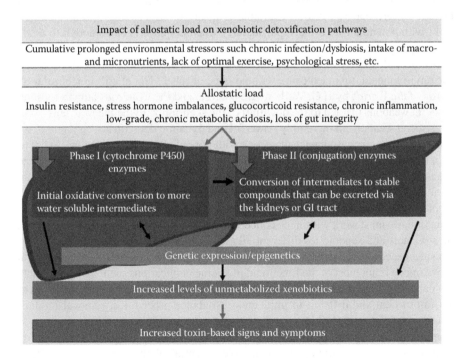

FIGURE 5.2   Impact of allostatic load on xenobiotic detoxification pathways.

also can maximize both short-term and long-term compliance, there is every reason to believe that it may be just as effective, if not more so, than an aggressive, sometimes costly and inconvenient, regimented, all-or-none approach that focuses solely on avoidance, diet, and supplements.

With the above in mind, the results seen in Gibson et al. (2003) should be easier to understand. For example, could the cost and inconvenience involved with the detoxification measures that had limited efficacy and created significant side effects have led to pro-inflammatory fear and worry that sabotaged possible beneficial impacts of these modalities? The fact that the most effective interventions were "fairly noninvasive and low risk" suggests that the answer to this question is yes. In addition, because it could be suggested that, based on the allostatic load principles discussed above, interventions such as rotation diets, prayer, meditation, and so on are highly effective at reducing inflammation both directly and indirectly due to their ability to reduce perceived fear and worry, they may be extremely effective detoxification modalities even though they do not have a direct, conventionally understood impact on environmental toxins and detoxification enzymes.

SOME FINAL THOUGHTS

As much as we wish it were otherwise, the world we live in, due largely but not exclusively to the industrial revolution that began approximately 200 years ago, is a dirty place that has left its mark on virtually every living being on Earth. In addition, despite our protests and best efforts, this situation will not radically change anytime soon. Therefore, it is no longer a question of whether we, our patients, or anyone else we encounter will be carrying a load of sometimes dozens of chemical and metal toxins. The only question is how much, and will it lead to clinically relevant signs and symptoms.

When we encounter someone who appears to have signs and symptoms related to environmental toxin load, it is logical to think first in terms of avoidance and removal. Unfortunately, from a practical standpoint, avoidance is difficult in the short term and virtually impossible in the long term, unless an individual is well off financially, totally free of commitments that limit life choice options, and incredibly committed and determined. Removal is certainly an option, particularly for heavy metals. Unfortunately, the tools available to us are often difficult to implement, expensive, and fraught with potential side effects, particularly when employed often enough to deal with the realities of ongoing, somewhat inevitable exposure.

Does this mean that many of us are doomed to a lifetime of suffering due to the ongoing ravages of chronic environmental toxin exposure with no hope of relief? Not at all!! For, similar to the scenario in *War of the Worlds* by H.G. Wells where bacteria and the wondrous human immune system were the secret weapons that led to the downfall of the seemingly invincible Martians, we also have a wondrous secret weapon, an incredibly powerful and dynamic detoxification system that has been honed and perfected as a consequence of coping with not only 200 years of the industrial revolution but eons of dealing with natural exposures from sources such as volcanos, forest fires, and natural earth outgassing.

William Rea, MD, one of the world's greatest clinical toxicologists, has pointed out, as stated in the chapter by Liska et al. (2005), that when considering the relationship between chemicals and human function, we must work within the concept of total load, which states that the central question as to how toxicants and xenobiotics differentially affect humans is the assessment of both sources of foreign substances and the patient's ability to deal with and process these foreign substances. As stated above, much if not most of the functional medicine publications seem to suggest that our ability to help patients deal with and process these foreign substances is limited to sometimes expensive and often impractical and difficult to implement avoidance procedures, removal modalities, and herbal, dietary, and supplemental interventions that are designed to optimize processing.

It is the opinion of this author that, while often effective, these approaches are only the beginning in terms of truly maximizing the incredible potential of the amazingly wondrous human detoxification system. While this chapter was certainly intended to share previous, somewhat well-known writings on these ways of dealing with environmental toxins, the primary intent was to show what this author feels is much less well-known. Allostatic load principles tell us that detoxification is not just a function of genetics and a few macro- and micronutrients, herbals, and phytonutrients. Rather, it is a whole-body phenomenon that is affected not only by everything we eat, but everything we do and every thought we think. If we can start thinking in terms of the detoxification lifestyle which includes our every thought and action, instead of merely detoxification diets and supplements, then we will truly release the awesome and incredible power of the human detoxification system. Furthermore, we will accomplish this in a cost-effective manner that respects not only the unique personal needs and desires that make life enjoyable and worth living for each patient, but also, to paraphrase the words of George Goodheart, the father of applied kinesiology, the need "to have a beer and a hot dog once in a while." For many if not most individuals, even in the face of ongoing environmental toxin onslaught, this will be more than enough to maintain and even optimize quality of life for many years to come.

REFERENCES

Aaseth J et al. 2015. Chelation in metal intoxication—Principles and paradigms. *J Trace Elements Med Biol* 31: 260–266.

Attina TM et al. 2016. Exposure to endocrine-disruptins chemicals in the USA: A population-based disease burden and cost analysis. *Lancet Diabetes Endocrinol* 4(12): 996–1003.

Beckie TM. 2012. A systematic review of allostatic load, health, and health disparities. *Biol Res Nursing* 14(4): 311–346.

Bratman S. 2000. *Health Food Junkies*. Broadway Books: New York.

Campbell C et al. 2016. A case study of environmental injustice: The failure in Flint. *Int J Environ Res Public Health* 13(10): 1–11.

Cheng PY and Morgan ET. 2001. Hepatic cytochrome P450 regulation in disease states. *Curr Drug Metab* 2: 165–183.

Crinnion WJ. 2000. Environmental medicine, part three: Long-term effects of chronic low-dose mercury exposure. *Alt Med Rev* 5(3): 209–233.

Crinnion WJ. 2013. Environmental medicine. In: *Textbook of Natural Medicine*, 4th ed., Pizzorno JE and Murray MT (Eds.). Elsevier: St. Louis, MO; pp. 266–279.

Croom E. 2012. Metabolism of xenobiotics of human environments. In: *Progress in Molecular Biology and Translational Science: Toxicology and Human Environments*, Hodgson, E (Ed.) Academic Press: Oxford, UK; Volume 112, pp. 31–88.

Danese A and McEwen B. 2012. Adverse childhood experiences, allostasis, allostatic load, and age-related disease. *Physiology & Behavior* 106: 29–39.

Fitzgerald KN et al. 2012. Nutrient and toxic elements. In: *Laboratory Evaluations for Integrative and Functional Medicine*, Revised Second Edition, Lord RS and Bralley JA (Eds.) Genova Diagnostics: Duluth, GA; pp. 63–172.

Garner CE et al. 2000. Catechol metabolites of polychlorinated biphenyls inhibit the catechol-O-methyltrans-ferase-mediated metabolism of catechol estrogens. *Toxicol Appl Pharmacol* 162(2): 115–123.

Gibson, PR, Elms, AN-M, and Ruding, LA. 2003. Perceived treatment efficacy for conventional and alternative therapies reported by persons with multiple chemical sensitivity. *Environmental Health Perspectives* 111(12): 1498–1504.

Goodman JE et al. 2001. COMT genotype, micronutrients in the folate metabolic pathway and breast cancer risk. *Carcinogenesis* 22(10): 1661–1665.

Haas CE et al. 2003. Cytochrome P450 activity after surgical stress. *Crit Care Med* 31(5): 1338–1346.

Hackett RA et al. 2012. Loneliness and stress-related inflammatory and neuroendocrine responses in older men and women. *Psychoneuroendocrinology* Published online ahead of print.

Johns LE et al. 2016. Relationships between urinary phthalate metabolite and bisphenol A concentrations and vitamin D levels in U.S. adults: National Health and Nutrition Examination Survey (NHANES), 1005–2010. *J Clin Endocrinol Metab* 101(11): 4062–4069.

Jover R et al. 2002. Down-regulation of human CYP3A4 by the inflammatory signal interleukin 6: Molecular mechanism and transcription factors involved. *FASEB J* Published Online September 19, 2002.

Kabir ER et al. 2015. A review on endocrine disruptors and their possible targets on human health. *Environ Toxicol Pharmacol* 40: 241–258.

Kim MS et al. 2004. Suppression of DHEA sulfotransferase (Sult2A1) during the acute phase response. *Am J Physiol* 287: 731–738.

Kontis D et al. 2013. COMT and MTHFR polymorphisms interaction on cognition in schizophrenia: an exploratory study. *Neurosci Lett* 537: 17–22.

Levin BL and Varga E. 2016. MTHFR: Addressing genetic counseling dilemmas using evidence-based literature. *J Genet Counsel* 25: 901–911.

Levy M et al. 2004. Childhood urine mercury excretion: dental amalgam and fish consumption as exposure factors. *Environ Res* 94(3): 283–290.

Li Y et al. 2004. Equine catechol estrogen 4-hydroxyequilenin is a more potent inhibitor of the variant form of catechol-O-methyltransferase. *Chem Res Toxicol* 17(4): 512–520.

Liska D et al. 2005. Detoxification and biotransformational imbalances. In: *Textbook of Functional Medicine*, Jones DS (Ed.). Institute for Functional Medicine: Gig Harbor, WA; pp. 275–298.

Lord RS and Bralley JA 2012. *Laboratory Evaluations for Integrative and Functional Medicine*. Metametrix Institute, Duluth, GA.

Lyon M. 2013. Functional toxicology. In: *Textbook of Natural Medicine*, 4th ed., Pizzorno JE and Murray MT (Eds.). Elsevier, St Louis, MO; pp. 475–487.

Lyon M et al. 2005. Clinical approaches to detoxification and biotransformation. In: *Textbook of Functional Medicine*, Jones DS (Ed.). Institute for Functional Medicine: Gig Harbar, WA; pp. 543–580.

Mahaffey, KR. 1999. Methylmercury: A new look at the risks. *Public Health Reports* 114(5): 397–415.

Maqbool F et al. 2016. Review of endocrine disorders associated with environmental toxicants and possible involved mechanisms. *Life Sciences* 145: 265–273.

Mattson MP and Calabrese EJ (Eds.). 2010. Hormesis: What it is and why it matters. In: *Hormesis: A Revolution in Biology, Toxicology, and Medicine*. Springer: New York; pp. 1–13.

Mimche SM et al. 2014. Hepatic cytochrome P450 s, phase II enzymes and nuclear receptors are down regulated in a Th2 environment during Schistosoma mansoni infection. *Drug Metab Dispos* 42: 134–140.

Morgan ET. 2001. Regulation of cytochrome P450 by inflammatory mediators: Why and how? *Drug Metab Dispos* 29(3): 2007–2212.

Muntjewerff JW et al. 2008. Polymorphisms in catechol-O-methyltransferase and methyltransferase reductase in relation to the risk of schizophrenia. *Eur Neuropsychopharmacol* 18(2): 99–106.

Parkinson A. 1996. Biotransformation of xenobiotics. In: *Casarett & Doull's Toxicology: The Basic Science of Poisons*, Fifth Edition, Klaassen CD et al. (Eds.). McGraw-Hill: New York; pp. 113–186.

Peerbooms O et al. 2012. Evidence that interactive effects of COMT and MTHFR moderate psychotic response to environmental stress. *Acta Psychiatr Scand* 125(3): 247–256.

Rahimi Z et al. 2016. The T allele of MTHFR c.C677 T and its synergism with G (Val 158) allele of COMT c.G472A polymorphism are associated with the risk of bipolar I disorder. *Genet Test Mol Biomarkers* 20(9): 510–515.

Rai V. 2016. Association of methylenetetrahydrofolate reductase (MTHFR) gene C677 T polymorphism with autism: evidence of genetic susceptiblity. *Metab Brain Dis* 31: 727–735.

Renton KW. 2004. Cytochrome P450 regulation and drug biotransformation during inflammation and infection. *Curr Drug Metab* 5(3): 235–243.

Rivory LP et al. 2002. Hepatic cytochrome P450 3A drug metabolism is reduced in cancer patients who have an acute-phase response. *Br J Cancer* 87(3): 277–280.

Shu-Leong TX and Ramsden D. 1999. Characterization and implications of estrogenic down-regulation of human catechol-O-methyltransferase gene transcription. *Mol Pharm* 56: 31–38.

Sim SC et al. 2013. Pharmacogenomics of drug-metabolizing enzymes: A recent update on clinical implications and endogenous effects. *Pharmacogenomics J* 13: 1–11.

Steptoe A et al. 2014. Disruption of multisystem responses to stress in type 2 diabetes: Investigating the dynamics of allostatic load. *PNAS* 111(44): 15693–15698.

Swanson HI. 2015. Drug metabolism by the host and gut microflora: A partnership or rivalry? *Drug Metab Dispos* 43: 1499–1504.

Wang LJ et al. 2015. A potential interaction between COMT and MTHFR genetic variants in Han Chinese patients with bipolar II disorder. *Scientific Reports*.

Wang Z et al. 2013. Interplay between vitamin D and the drug metabolizing enzyme CYP3A4. *J Steroid Biochem Mol Biol* 136(July): 54–58.

Worda C et al. 2003. Influence of the catechol-O-methyltransferase (COMT) codon 158 polymorphism on estrogen levels in women. *Hum Reprod* 18(2): 262–266.

Xu C et al. 2005. Induction of phase I, II and III drug metabolism/transport by xenobiotics. *Arch Pharm Res* 28(3): 249–268.

Zhu BT. 2002. Catechol-O-methyltransferase (COMT)-mediated methylation metabolism of endogenous bioactive catechols and modulation by endobiotics and xenobiotics: Importance to pathophysiology and pathogenesis. *Curr Drug Metab* 3: 321–349.

Zhu BT. 2003. Medical hypothesis: hyperhomocysteinemia is a risk factor for estrogen-induced hormonal cancer. *Int J Oncol* 22(3): 499–508.

Zlatnik MG. 2016. Endocrine-disrupting chemicals and reproductive health. *J Midwifery Women's Health* 61(4): 442–455.

6 Neuroprotection, Aging, and the Gut–Brain Axis

Translating Traditional Wisdom from the Mediterranean Diet into Evidence-Based Clinical Applications

Miguel A. Toribio-Mateas

CONTENTS

Introduction 177
What is Genomic Instability? 178
    Why is this Important? Plus, Some Important Considerations 181
        The Alzheimer's—Diabetes Type 2—Cardiovascular—Inflammation Link 183
Key Nutritional Therapeutic Agents—A Rationale in Support of Multi-Supplementation 183
    The Mediterranean Diet: A Naturally Occurring Model for Multi-Nutrient
    Supplementation 184
    Emulating the Nutrient Synergies in the Mediterranean Diet Model 186
Other Key Nutrients in a "Neuroprotective Supplementary Prescription" 188
    Vitamin A 188
    Methyl Donor B Vitamins: B6, B9 (Folate), and B12 188
The "MediterrAsian Diet" 188
Calorie Restriction Mimetics 189
The Microbiota: Gut–Brain Axis 189
A Complex Communication System 190
    From Eubiosys to Dysbiosis 192
    Assessing Function—Laboratory Testing and n = 1 Trials 193
    Dietary Neuroprotection, from the Gut Up 194
Conclusion 196
References 196

INTRODUCTION

Why do we age? Is aging pre-programmed or is it accidental? Is there a "biological clock" that sets the appropriate times for the various changes that characterize older age to take place? Is aging mainly the consequence of the accumulation of oxidative damage to tissues caused to body systems by free radicals? Is aging the result of the sheer accumulation of molecular damage that individuals gather throughout their life trajectory, becoming symptomatic and manifesting itself as diseases like Alzheimer's, cardiovascular disease, or cancer? Clear-cut answers to these questions aren't forthcoming, but what recent literature is unequivocal about is the fact that aging sits within a multifactorial network of physiopathological changes stemming from both genetic and stochastic factors that result in an altered metabolic homeostatic state (Barzilai et al. 2017), and that genomic instability is both a trigger and a mediator of these changes (Wu and Roks 2014; Edifizi and Schumacher 2015). Current research is also explicit about the fact that the role of diet in human health goes far beyond mere nutrition and the provision of macro- and micro-nutrients in the right quantities that avoid deficiencies. Nutrients, including those provided as food supplements, exhibit a range of additional, non-strictly nutritive functions that help preserve genome integrity, lowering DNA damage and thereby supporting successful aging (Bhullar and Rupasinghe 2013; Garcia-Calzon et al. 2015; Lee et al. 2015; Meramat et al. 2015; Sharif et al. 2015). A growing body of evidence documents the supporting role of nutritional supplements, such as vitamins, minerals, and compounds of plant origin—as well as other natural therapeutic agents such as pro- and prebiotics—in the prevention and clinical management of age-related disorders.

However, there is inconsistent evidence as to the efficacy of nutritional supplements in general (Balk et al. 2006; Huang et al. 2006; Fortmann et al. 2013; Schwingshackl et al. 2015), and while some studies report the many benefits of supplementation to the quality of life of aging individuals who use them regularly (van der Meij et al. 2012; Figueroa-Mendez and Rivas-Arancibia 2015; Xu et al. 2015), some show no significant statistical correlation between all individual nutrient deficiencies and the pathogenesis of age-related disorders (Arlt et al. 2012; Farina et al. 2012; Loef et al. 2012).

Additionally, although nutritional supplements are generally regarded as safe, some—mostly high dose antioxidant nutrients, and chiefly beta-carotene for smokers could even prove to have potentially harmful effects (Bjelakovic et al. 2008; Druesne-Pecollo et al. 2010; Bjelakovic et al. 2014). What seems clear is that supplementation with single nutrients is most often ineffective, with some exceptions that will be explored more fully as part of this chapter, which the author limits to the context of age-related disorders with a specific focus on brain aging, the author's doctoral research subject. That multi-supplementation may be more appropriate than mono-supplementation fits well with the fact that aging is a complex process and that attempting to modulate the many pathways involved in it by means of one single nutrient may just be too much of a simplistic approach.

WHAT IS GENOMIC INSTABILITY?

Post-mitotic neurons suffer from an innate deficiency in the repair of nuclear and mitochondrial DNA that makes them particularly prone to accumulation of the type of molecular damage seen in several neurodegenerative disorders, including Alzheimer's disease (AD), Parkinson's disease (PD), Huntington's Disease (HD), and amyotrophic lateral sclerosis (ALS) (Jeppesen et al. 2011). Much of this damage is stochastic and is triggered by well-known stressors such reactive oxygen species (ROS) (Wang et al. 2006), although a number of contributing factors such as protein modifications and aggregation, as well as metabolic stress and cytokine-mediated damage by microglial activation during the maturation process also play an important part in the process (Brettschneider et al. 2012; Nakanishi et al. 2011) that see differentiated neurons "continuously subjected to the genomic stress of different protein modifications, oxidation, metabolic stress, transcriptional and neuronal activities" (Chow and Herrup 2015), as seen in Figure 6.1.

Genomic stress is a key factor in neurodegeneration that mediates the progressive loss of fidelity in DNA repair (Tsutakawa et al. 2014). Environmental and lifestyle factors, including toxic exposure, physical activity, and nutrition, also play an important role in determining gene expression, thus influencing the likelihood that accumulated DNA damage translates into the misfolding of proteins (Golde et al. 2013; Wang and Ding 2014; Ciechanover and Kwon 2015), and neuroinflammation leading to loss of synapses (Lauritzen et al. 2010; Bazan 2012), as seen in Figure 6.2.

In simpler terms, Figure 6.2 illustrates the means whereby the aging exposes neurons to a number of insults that result in the accumulation of increasing amounts of irreparable damage to DNA.

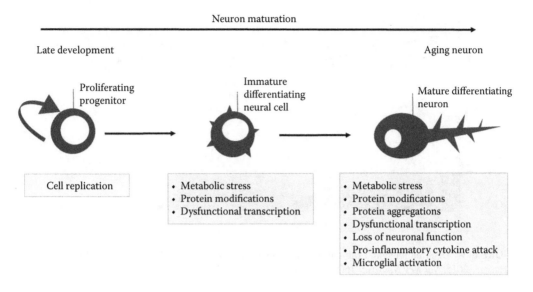

FIGURE 6.1 Causes of DNA damage in the developing, mature, and aging nervous system. (Adapted from Chow, H. M., and K. Herrup. 2015. *Nat Rev Neurosci* 16(11): 672–684.)

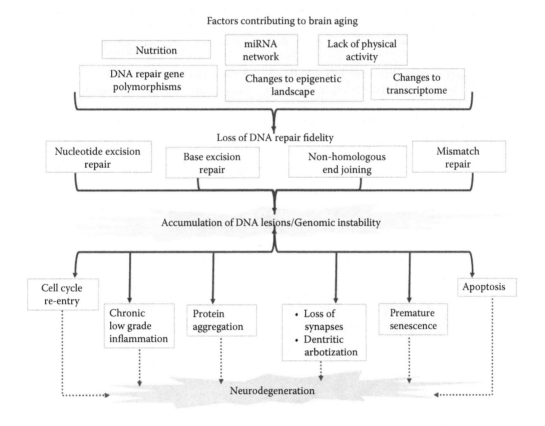

FIGURE 6.2 Factors contributing to the neurodegenerative process in aging neurons, with the resulting reduction of DNA integrity and increased genomic instability. (Adapted from Chow, H. M., and K. Herrup. 2015. *Nat Rev Neurosci* 16(11): 672–684.)

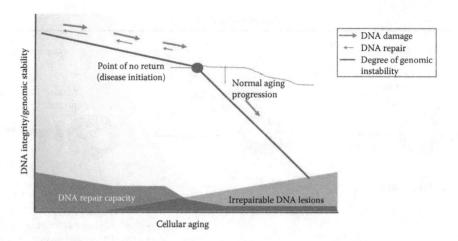

FIGURE 6.3   DNA damage and the onset of neurodegenerative disease. (Adapted from Chow, H. M., and K. Herrup. 2015. *Nat Rev Neurosci* 16(11): 672–684.)

Molecular, cellular, and organismal mechanisms of repair are influenced by nutrition (or lack thereof) as part of a wider set of factors contributing to the loss of repair efficiency, ultimately leading to the accumulation of lesions that characterizes neurodegenerative diseases. Seen in a timeline, there is a "point of no return" where the system is unable to withstand the pressure exerted by all the factors contributing to the lack of repair efficiency, thereby perpetuating a situation where the damage exceeds the system's ability to repair, thus resulting in its degeneration, as seen clearly in Figure 6.3.

Mitochondria possess their own DNA (mtDNA), which is also exposed to the same insults as nuclear DNA, with the added exposure to increased oxidative stress that mitochondrial tissue withstands throughout its lifespan. As mitochondria progressively decay, exposure to the ongoing oxidative burst leads to increased inflammation, which translates into loss of biomass, lower ATP production and, ultimately, low cellular function, as seen in Figure 6.4.

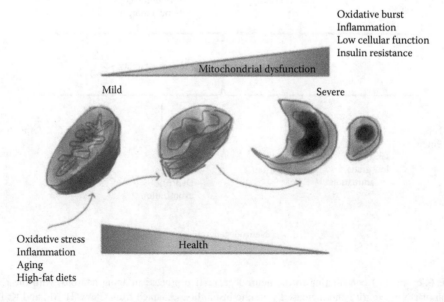

FIGURE 6.4   Mutations in mitochondrial DNA accompanied by different disease-suggestive phenotypes. (Reproduced from Hernandez-Aguilera, A. et al. 2013. *Mediators Inflamm* 2013: 135698. With permission.)

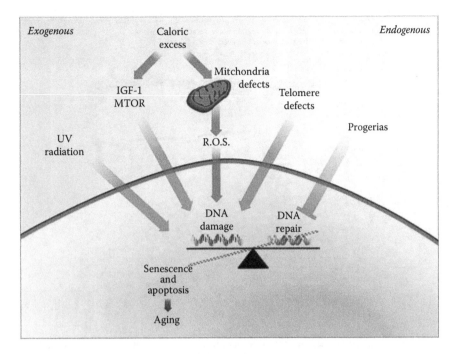

FIGURE 6.5 A variety of theories on aging converge on accumulated DNA damage. (Reproduced from St Laurent, G. 3rd, N. Hammell, and T. A. McCaffrey. 2010. *Mech Ageing Dev* 131(5): 299–305. With permission.)

Some common dietary factors such as caloric excess, a common occurrence in the Western diet, are also known to accelerate mitochondrial dysfunction and decay, perpetuating elevated levels of ROS and ultimately contributing to increased nuclear DNA damage (St Laurent et al. 2010), as seen in Figure 6.5. Additionally, deficiencies in vitamins B5 (pantothenic acid) and biotin are also known to increase mitochondrial oxidants through oxidant leakage resulting from selectively dysfunctional heme metabolism through diminished complex IV function (Ames et al. 2005). Some other factors such as radiation and smoking have an effect on DNA damage and aging (Soares et al. 2014).

WHY IS THIS IMPORTANT? PLUS, SOME IMPORTANT CONSIDERATIONS

Having defined genomic instability, a driving factor in neurodegeneration and nutrition, as a key modulator in DNA repair fidelity, the context is set to explore strategies that allow for nutritional interventions to be applied in the clinical management of neurodegenerative disease and in the promotion of a healthy lifespan in humans.

But before embarking on the review of the various agents that impact DNA repair capacity, an important consideration must be made. As seen in the appropriately humorous Figure 6.6, animal research models that aim to understand the physiopathology of neurodegenerative diseases abound, but often their outcomes do not translate into strategies that can be successfully implemented in the clinical management of the conditions in humans. The amount of positive results in human studies can fill researchers with somewhat false hope that the same results will replicate in humans, but there are a number of issues to influence clinical outcomes. Some are as simple as the bioavailability of nutrients used, or whether they can cross the blood brain barrier in order to exert their beneficial activity where it is most needed. Some are behavioral. For example, expecting an individual suffering from even mild cognitive decline to remember to take several tablets/capsules everyday (or indeed several times a day everyday) can also be unrealistic.

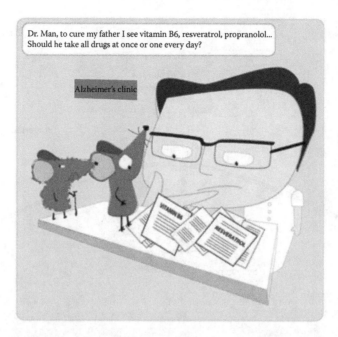

FIGURE 6.6 There is a distinct deficit in translational research in nutritional neuroscience. The success of individual nutrients or even nutrient combinations that work in mice fails to translate to human neuroprotection. (Reproduced from Franco, R., and Cedazo-Minguez, A. 2014. *Front Pharmacol* 5: 146. With permission.)

So, treatment compliance issues are also paramount when considering the overall efficacy of nutritional interventions. Plus, there is also a monetary aspect. Most nutritional supplements are not covered by insurers or national health services. Some are on prescription, but even the prescription charge can be prohibitive for some, unless these are issued for free, as is the case for chronic patients in some countries. Most times dosages prescribed are conservative in comparison studies that have reported good clinical outcomes.

This means that engaging in a preventive strategy based on nutritional supplements is largely a self-funding exercise, which makes the subject of choosing the right product, dose, purity, and so on even more of a minefield for most people. Nutrition health professionals—such as clinical nutritionists, nutritional therapists, and registered dietitians with a functional approach—play the key role of translating benefits into practice, educating patients to make better dietary and supplement choices with healthy aging in mind (Ruxton et al. 2016).

Another important aspect to consider when reviewing literature on nutrient-based interventions of vitamins, minerals and natural agents is the lack of funding necessary for these studies to take place. Funding from government agencies and charitable foundations for these types of studies is hard to come by (Zachwieja et al. 2013), and food supplements cannot be patented and sold following a model that resembles that used by pharmaceutical companies which constitutes an additional hurdle for securing industry funding for both single-nutrient and multi-supplementation intervention studies, making it an increasingly difficult task, particularly for double-blind randomized controlled trials of sufficient duration and with large enough samples to endow them with credible statistical power and significance.

Some pharmaceutical companies have adapted natural products used traditionally for the management of age-related diseases, for example, Glaxo's Lovaza, a lipid-regulating agent consisting of ethyl esters of omega-3 fatty acids sourced from fish oils (Weintraub 2014), contributing to the body of evidence to promote the use of the natural alternative by proxy, that is, a "regular" fish oil supplement as opposed to its prescription equivalent.

However, some critics have raised their concerns about the potential bias of industry funded studies that can influence public health guidelines (Aveyard et al. 2016). In any event, the relevance of this point is around the fact that the sample of studies reporting the effects of both single and multiple supplementation may not be fully representative because of the very small size and the generalized lower methodological quality compared with pharmacological interventions.

The Alzheimer's—Diabetes Type 2—Cardiovascular—Inflammation Link

Although the causal relationship remains poorly understood, there's an ample body of evidence documenting the fact that individuals with type 2 diabetes have an increased risk for developing Alzheimer's disease (AD) (Stanley et al. 2016). The postulated mechanism of action is likely to consist of alterations in insulin signaling (IS) in the AD brain. Additionally, it appears that amyloid-β (Aβ) deposits can lead to neuronal insulin resistance and intranasal insulin is being explored as a potential therapy for AD (Claxton et al. 2015). Conversely, elevated insulin levels are found in AD patients and high insulin has been reported to increase Aβ levels and tau phosphorylation (Freude et al. 2005), which could exacerbate AD pathology.

Dysglycemias rarely occur as isolated conditions and are frequently seen alongside dysregulation of cardiovascular function. In fact, there is mounting evidence that middle-aged men and women at risk for heart disease may also face a higher chance of dementia later in life, and that risk factors such as smoking, high blood pressure, and diabetes might increase the odds of dementia are comparable to genetically raise the risk of developing Alzheimer's disease by APOE3/4 or APOE4/4 carriers (Chatterjee et al. 2016). Moreover, APOE4 is only present in ∼50%–60% of individuals with AD, suggesting that other factors are involved in AD pathogenesis (Holtzman et al. 2011).

The popular belief among clinicians and the general public that dietary saturated fat clogs arteries as though they were pipes furred with greasy slime might be evocative, but is starting to be disproven (Rothberg 2013). Instead, a high total cholesterol to high-density lipoprotein (HDL) ratio is starting to surface as the best predictor of cardiovascular risk, as well as a surrogate marker for insulin resistance (Malhotra et al. 2017). A recent systematic review published in the British Medical Journal by a multinational team of cardiovascular experts (Ravnskov et al. 2016) concluded that "LDL cholesterol is not associated with cardiovascular disease and is inversely associated with all-cause mortality." In the author's own clinical experience, a high total cholesterol to HDL ratio drops rapidly when introducing dietary changes that follow the principles of a lower-carbohydrate, higher fat Mediterranean diet, and the supplementary nutrients that are discussed in the following sections of this chapter all help modulate the inflammatory processes that underline neurodegenerative, cardiovascular, and metabolic diseases alike. As illustrated in Figure 6.7, management of these dysfunctional processes requires transdisciplinary novel approaches that hold much promise for understanding and intervening in human chronic disease, complete lifestyle medicine approaches that combine a healthful diet and regular movement with stress reduction as a means to improve quality of life, and reduce cardiovascular and all-cause mortality (Epel and Lithgow 2014).

KEY NUTRITIONAL THERAPEUTIC AGENTS—A RATIONALE IN SUPPORT OF MULTI-SUPPLEMENTATION

A recent systematic review and meta-analysis by Lopes da Silva et al. (2014) provides a comprehensive correlation between the adequacy of various nutrients and brain function in Alzheimer's patients. The review featured a number of nutrients essential for brain function, including vitamins A, C, D, and E, as well as the methyl donors B12 (cobalamin), B6 (pyridoxine), and folate, plus B1 (thiamin), and the minerals manganese, calcium, copper, iron, magnesium, selenium, and zinc, and the essential fatty acids DHA (docosahexaenoic acid) and EPA (eicosapentaenoic acid), and concluded that lower plasma nutrient levels in patients with AD are indicative of their impaired systemic availability, which puts these individuals at further risk of neurodegeneration.

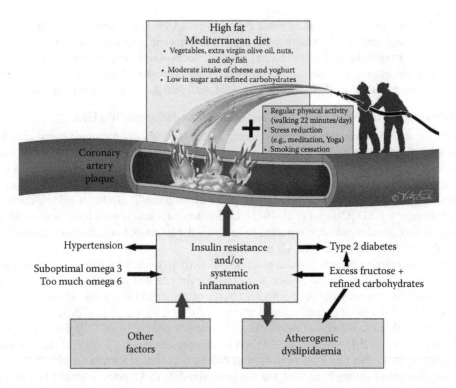

FIGURE 6.7 Lifestyle interventions for the prevention and treatment of coronary disease with the Mediterranean Diet at the core of them. (Reproduced from Malhotra, A., R. F. Redberg and P. Meier. 2017. *Br J Sports Med* 51(15): 1111–1112. With permission.)

THE MEDITERRANEAN DIET: A NATURALLY OCCURRING MODEL
FOR MULTI-NUTRIENT SUPPLEMENTATION

So why is the above systematic review relevant? The author finds that the multi-supplementation model investigated as part of the meta-analysis features all of the nutrients that are naturally occurring in the Mediterranean diet, a broad dietary umbrella describing the dietary practices of inhabitants in regions around the Mediterranean Sea, for example, Italy, Spain, Greece, and Turkey, and that is characterized by the presence of high levels of fresh vegetables, fruits, nuts, seeds and whole grains, as well as fresh fish (including oily fish like sardines, anchovies, mackerel, etc.) and reduced amounts of meat compared to other Western diet types.

Other typical features of the Mediterranean diet include the regular consumption of pulses (e.g., lentils, chickpeas, beans), fresh dairy produce, and moderate red wine consumption. The Mediterranean diet is naturally rich in vitamins with antioxidant properties such as vitamins A, K, C, E, and D, as well as in methyl donors such as folate and vitamins B6 and B12 (Feart et al. 2012; Balci et al. 2014). Additionally, the Mediterranean diet is also one of the richest dietary patterns in polyunsaturated omega-3 (ω-3) fatty acids (PUFAs) (Widmer et al. 2015) and polyphenolic compounds (Bonaccio et al. 2017). Of particular relevance are a myriad of antioxidant compounds in olive oil, which are well documented to possess anti-inflammatory effects (Bonaccio et al. 2015; Scoditti et al. 2015) and to aid with the clinical management of a variety of conditions (Buckland and Gonzalez 2015).

A Mediterranean dietary pattern has long been correlated with lower levels of pro-inflammatory proteins such as CRP and cytokines such as TNF-α and IL-10, as well as with lower levels of lipid peroxidation (measured by means of malondialdehyde) and of DNA damage, assessed by means of 8-hydroxy-2'-deoxyguanosine (8-OHGH). It is believed that the high amount of naturally occurring

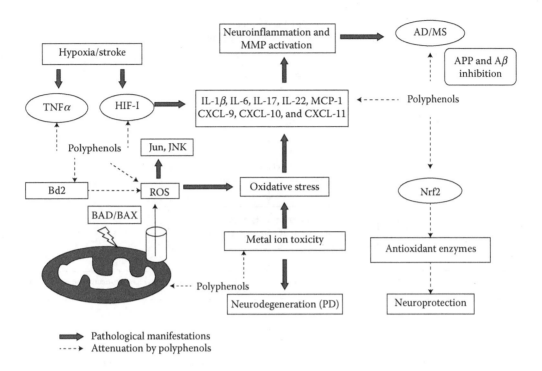

FIGURE 6.8 A diagram illustrating some of the neuroprotective pathways modulated by dietary polyphenols. (Reproduced from Bhullar, K. S. and H. P. Rupasinghe. 2013. *Oxid Med Cell Longev* 2013: 891748. With permission.)

polyphenols in this type of diet accounts for the improvement of DNA repair capacity (Pedret et al. 2012), as illustrated in Figure 6.8.

Perhaps more interesting is the emerging evidence of the synergy among the various molecules, including the ω-3 PUFAs, the oleic acid (a monounsaturated ω-9 fatty acid), and neuroprotective phenolic compounds such as hydroxytyrosol and oleocanthal (Abuznait et al. 2013; de la Torre-Robles et al. 2014) which seem to work better together than as individual agents (Scoditti et al. 2014). Hydroxytirosol has been shown to enhance mitochondrial biogenesis and to improve cellular repair and defense mechanisms (Hao et al. 2010), thereby improving genomic integrity. Melatonin is also known for its ability to reduce genomic instability (Belancio 2015) and has recently been discovered in grape products typically included in the Mediterranean diet (Iriti and Varoni 2015). It is therefore quite possible that the rich, complex nutritional matrix provided by a typical Mediterranean diet is the reason explaining the reduction in the risk of cardiovascular disease, cancer, AD, and PD seen reported by large recent studies (Toledo et al. 2015; Tuttolomondo et al. 2015). The reduced cardiovascular risk is associated with an improved lipid profile reporting protective high-density lipoprotein (HDL) cholesterol levels at higher concentrations than their low-density (LDL) counterpart (Penalvo et al. 2015).

The polyphenols in a typical Mediterranean-style diet have an additional mode of action. They regulate the deacetylation of DNA by means of activation of Sirtuin (SIRT) enzymes. Sirtuin activation is correlated with enhanced mitochondrial biogenesis and function, as well as with improved neurogenesis and reduced oxidative stress and inflammation, all consistent with improved genomic integrity (Chatzianagnostou et al. 2015), as seen in Figure 6.9.

On that basis, for individuals who do not follow a Mediterranean eating pattern, it would be advisable to include a supplement containing a variety of polyphenols such as those that would be featured in a Mediterranean region, like quercetin, resveratrol, and grape seed extract, in a dose that resembles that of a typical dietary exposure for an inhabitant of the area. It is likely

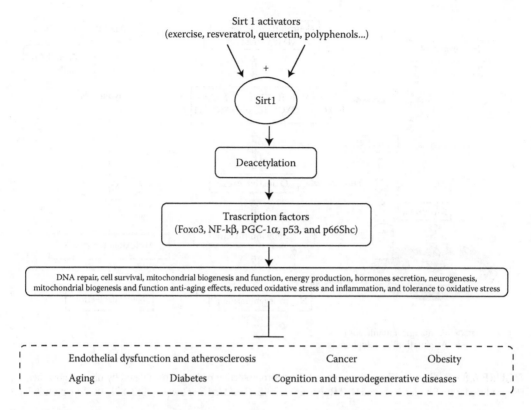

FIGURE 6.9   A schematic representation of the mechanisms of action whereby the Mediterranean diet exerts its protective effects. (From Chatzianagnostou, K. et al. 2015. *Antioxidants (Basel)* 4(4): 719–736. With permission.)

that the benefits of these phenolic compounds are driven not only by dose but by continuity of exposure, as well as by compound synergy which means that doses should be low in order to be safe.

Additionally, some further considerations need to be taken into account. Although the benefits of resveratrol and red wine as a source thereof are well documented, alcohol in itself adds a risk factor for the development of AD for individuals with single nucleotide polymorphisms (SNPs) to their methylenetetrahydrofolate reductase (MTHFR) gene, particularly MTHFR 677CT (Fowler et al. 2012). This may sound counterintuitive and it proves that nutritional and dietary advice must be individualized in order to obtain the most favorable clinical outcomes. Some of the pathways modulated by resveratrol are illustrated in Figure 6.10.

EMULATING THE NUTRIENT SYNERGIES IN THE MEDITERRANEAN DIET MODEL

A recent systematic review by Shah (2013) found that those adhering to a Mediterranean-type diet appeared at less risk of developing AD. Incidentally, the same review compared the results of adherence to the Mediterranean diet with the supplementation with a commercially available product that contains 300 mg EPA, 1200 mg DHA, 106 mg phospholipids, 400 mg choline, 600 mg uridine monophosphate, 40 mg vitamin E, 80 mg vitamin C, 60 μg selenium, 3 μg vitamin B12, 1 mg vitamin B6, and 400 μg folic acid. This patented formula has been shown to have "beneficial effects on functional ability, behaviour, or global clinical change, including improvements in verbal recall in patients at early stages of AD" (Onakpoya and Heneghan 2017), demonstrating that a multinutrient supplement can be used to promote successful aging, with measurable endpoints.

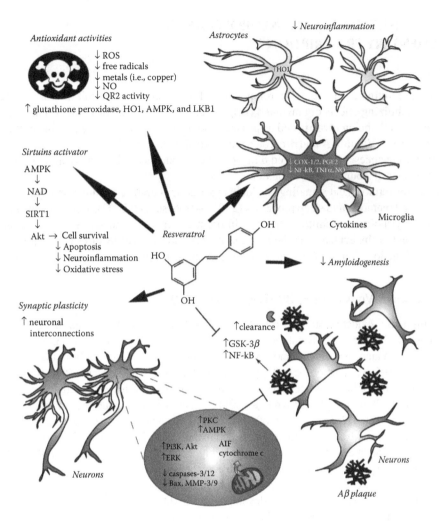

FIGURE 6.10 Some of the pathways modulated by resveratrol. (Reproduced from Bastianetto, S., C. Menard, and R. Quirion. 2015. *Biochim Biophys Acta* 1852(6): 1195–1201. With permission.)

Another recent study by Gutierrez-Mariscal et al. (2012) also compared the Mediterranean diet with a "bolt-on" supplement, in this case, coenzyme Q10 (CoQ10), and found that the supplementation group presented with reduced postprandial oxidative DNA damage in elderly subjects, measured by means of plasma 8-OHdG. As oxidative stress is one of the drivers of genomic instability and DNA damage, the findings of this study appear to suggest CoQ10 supplemented at a dose of 200 mg/ day provided prevention of oxidative processes associated with the aging process. Conversely, a large interventional study (n = 600) published in the *Journal of the American Medical Association* in 2014 by Beal et al. found no clinical benefit of supplementing with CoQ10.

Participants were either allocated to a placebo, a 1200 mg/day, and a 1600 mg/d of CoQ10, a much larger dose than that used in the study by Gutierrez-Mariscal (2012) and reported no statistical difference between groups (Beal et al. 2014), which reinforces the hypothesis that the synergy among the various bioactive components characteristic of the Mediterranean diet may make the whole more than the sum of its individual parts. It also poses the question about the unmeasured effects of other factors such as exercise and conviviality, which are part of the "Mediterranean lifestyle" diet and that aren't accounted for or replicated as part of the study design of most studies, thereby adding bias to the statistical significance of the results.

OTHER KEY NUTRIENTS IN A "NEUROPROTECTIVE SUPPLEMENTARY PRESCRIPTION"

Vitamin A

Retinol, retinal, retinoic acid, and β-carotene have all been shown to inhibit the formation, extension, and destabilizing effects of amyloid β (Aβ) proteins in *in vitro* studies of AD. These inhibitory effects are currently being investigated as possible therapeutic targets for the treatment of AD (Ono and Yamada 2012). Vitamin A and β-carotene are also abundant in a Mediterranean-type diet, from sources including cheese and fermented dairy products (sources of vitamin A), and carrots, melon, and summer squash (sources of β-carotene).

Additionally, retinoic acid signaling is widely reported in literature documenting synaptic plasticity, learning and memory, and sleep processes (Tafti and Ghyselinck 2007), appearing to enhance the effects on acetylcholine transmitter functions in brain cholinergic neurons (Szutowicz et al. 2015). Given the extent of the evidence on the amount of neurobiochemical features that require retinoids for optimum function, vitamin A is warranted a spot on the supplementary prescription list.

Methyl Donor B Vitamins: B6, B9 (Folate), and B12

Neuroinflammatory oxidative stress is a hallmark of AD pathology. A common biomarker for that, which allows healthcare professionals to assess the severity of this inflammation, is homocysteine (HCY). HCY is an auto-oxidative amino acid (Cook and Hess 2005) resulting from the metabolism of its homologue cysteine as part of the methylation cycle. High (HCY) levels are often seen in individuals whose serum and/or blood red cell levels of methyl donor B-vitamins, for example, folate (B9), B6, and cobalamin (B12) are low (De Bruyn et al. 2014). This biochemical picture is more prevalent after the age of 60 (Risch et al. 2015) and very often seen in AD patients (Chen et al. 2015). In fact, a recent comprehensive meta-analysis of 68 studies published in the *Journal of Alzheimer's Disorders* (Shen and Ji 2015) not only confirmed the correlations between higher HCY and lower folate and B12 levels in AD patients, it also showed a statistically significant difference with controls.

The authors also went further to say that high HCY combined with low folic acid levels may themselves constitute risk factors for the development of AD.

Methyl donor B vitamins are provided in ample amounts by a Mediterranean-type diet, by means of readily available foods such as spinach, cabbages, wholegrains, and fresh meats, as well as organ meats. Not all individuals are able to process dietary folate and B12 appropriately due to unfavorable genetic variations to their MTHFR gene. This means that there are genetic considerations to take into account, particularly those around MTHFR SNPs. While some SNPs seem to be negatively associated with the development of AD, for example, MTHFR 776CG in individuals with the MTHFR 1298AA genotype (Cascalheira et al. 2015), others, for example, MTHFR C677 T, show a significant association with susceptibility to the development of the disease (Rai 2017). A simple saliva swab test carried out by a licensed healthcare provider can help determine the MTHFR status of the individual, providing further support for the clinical decision to include supplementary folate as part of their prescription. As with other genetic risk factors for the development of AD, for example, apolipoprotein E (APOE) ε4 status, environmental/epigenetic factors are as important or possibly more than those of a genetic nature, meaning clinical management must pivot around the individual with their own idiosyncrasies, and that healthcare providers should not be tempted to "treat the SNPs."

THE "MEDITERRASIAN DIET"

The myriad of protective benefits attributed to a Mediterranean-type diet have been discussed in detail. However, there are other dietary patterns from around the world that also deserve some attention, particularly what could be widely defined as an "Asian" or "Oriental"-style diet, that is, such as a typical Japanese diet, or perhaps a hybrid between a Japanese, Chinese, and Indian diet. The bioactive components of a Mediterranean diet can be complemented and enhanced by adding some of those characteristics of Asian diets, for example, soybean isoflavones shown to improve cognition by means of modulation of estrogen receptors (Soni et al. 2014) and epigallocatechin gallate (EGCG) phenolic compounds from green tea which exhibit a number of beneficial properties, from radical scavenging to transition metal (e.g., iron and copper) chelating, thereby providing neuroprotective activity (Weinreb et al. 2004). Another interesting compound is curcumin, which is known to improve (Aβ) destabilization in mouse models (Zhang et al. 2010) and has a well-documented anti-inflammatory activity in humans (Hu et al. 2015). Soy isoflavones, green tea extracts, and curcumin can all be supplemented, but the author proposes that, in order to improve compliance and limit the amount of supplements to be taken daily, these are supplemented by means of inclusion of these "functional foods" in the patient's daily diet, for example, by adding half a teaspoon of turmeric powder to cooking a few times a week. This may not normally form part of a typically British or Western diet, so the supplementation model proposed for these bioactive substances is to see the foods providing them as supplements themselves.

CALORIE RESTRICTION MIMETICS

Perhaps one of the best documented interventions in aging science is caloric restriction. The number of human studies carried out is small compared with those that use animal models. The evidence of efficacy of this single intervention in animal studies is unequivocal, with some promising recent evidence in humans (Stein et al. 2012; Ravussin et al. 2015). Fasting is known to reprogram metabolic and cellular resilience/stress endurance pathways, thereby promoting longevity. Polyphenols can mimic this reprogramming effect by interacting directly with nuclear transcription factors such as FoxO1 (Barbato et al. 2015). Indeed, some of the key antioxidant molecules in the Mediterranean diet, for example, resveratrol and the most recently discovered dietary melatonin, also activate the same molecular pathways as caloric restriction, which are modulated by the SIRT enzymes discussed previously (Ramis et al. 2015). A combination of the Mediterranean and the Asian foods can therefore promote SIRT activation and caloric restriction mimicry, and a MediterrAsian diet (term coined by Pallauf et al. (2013)) and/or supplementation with the foods providing the bioactive components that characterize this dietary style are seen as additional tools to enhance neuroprotection.

THE MICROBIOTA: GUT–BRAIN AXIS

A growing body of preclinical and clinical evidence supports the concept of bidirectional brain–gut microbiome interactions. The complexity of this intricate communication system is such, and the amount of studies published every week is so large that this section only attempts to provide the integrative clinician with an overview of the matter, focusing on the most salient aspects with regard to the implications for practice of the current literature.

The microbe population living in our gastrointestinal (GI) tract, collectively known as "gut microbiota" (and traditionally referred to as "gut flora"), interacts with the human host through immune, neuroendocrine, and neural pathways. Bacteroidetes and Firmicutes are the two main phyla in the GI tract (Sekirov et al. 2010; Belkaid and Naik 2013), with quantity and diversity increasing from stomach to small intestine to colon (Sekirov et al. 2010; Brown et al. 2013). The human microbiota can cast local as well as systemic effects on host biology, both in health and disease. For example, gastrointestinal dysbiosis—an alteration in normal commensal gut microbiota with an increase in pathogenic microbes which deranges homeostasis—has been consistently reported as a key contributory factor to the development of metabolic disease. A recent review by Martinez et al. (2017) highlights the effects of a "typical Western diet" on the gut microbiota and how changes mediated by the latter then become key contributory factors to the development of metabolic disease. We know that the gut microbiota are capable of regulating host fat deposition, metabolism, and immune function and that environmental influences such as diet, exercise, and early life exposures can significantly impact the composition of the microbiota (Nehra et al. 2016). In turn, increased gastrointestinal permeability (traditionally referred to by integrative medicine practitioners as "leaky gut") induced by microbial dysbiosis is seen alongside increased blood–brain barrier permeability, and mediate or affect the pathogenesis of neurodegenerative disorders associated with aging, for example, Alzheimer's disease (AD) (Jiang et al. 2017). Though the primary risk factor for AD is advancing age, other factors such as diabetes type 2, hyperlipidemia, obesity, vascular factors, and depression play a role in its pathogenesis. Indeed, the specific role of gut microbiota in modulating neuro-immune functions well beyond the gastrointestinal tract may constitute an important influence on the process of neurodegeneration (Kohler et al. 2016). In Parkinson's disease (PD) antibiotic treatment ameliorates, while microbial recolonization promotes pathophysiology in adult animals, suggesting that postnatal signaling between the gut and the brain modulates disease and that alterations in the human microbiome represent a risk factor for the development of the condition (Sampson et al. 2016; Erny and Prinz 2017).

A COMPLEX COMMUNICATION SYSTEM

Emerging data from human studies suggests that the function and health of the central nervous system, and the brain as the key organ in it, is modulated by the complex interaction among a number of factors. Multiple routes of communication between the gut and brain have been established and these include the vagus nerve, the immune system, short chain fatty acids, and tryptophan (Dinan and Cryan 2015). According to Sundman et al. (2017) these channels can be summarized as follows:

1. The composition of the gut microbiota
2. Neurotransmitters, hormones, and immune- and neuropeptides produced in the gut and communication between these and gut microbes
3. The integrity of the intestinal wall serving as the physical barrier to the external environment

The influence of the gut microbiota on the function of the central nervous system (CNS) is manifested in both normal and disease conditions. In disease states, the basic mechanism of action is mediated by inflammation triggered by loss of the natural eubiotic state of the GI tract and its progression toward dysbiosis. For example, the low-grade, often chronic inflammation and/or immune activation that underlies the etiology of IBS is seen as an increased risk factor in mood disorders such as depression (O'Malley et al. 2011), obsessive compulsive disorder (OCD) (Turna et al. 2016), and autism (Mangiola et al. 2016). Additionally, this type of abnormality in the gut–brain axis affecting individuals with IBS and IBS-like symptoms is seen to be associated with several chronic non-communicable disorders including, but not limited to, chronic fatigue syndrome (CFS)/fibromyalgia (Galland 2014), obesity (Beaumont et al. 2016; Pallister and Spector 2016), cardiovascular disease (Tang et al. 2017), and type 2 diabetes mellitus (T2DM) (Ali et al. 2006). With the amount of patients with IBS-like symptoms who seek the support of integrative clinicians, this illustrates how the gut–brain axis involves communication among a number of interconnected systems, including the central nervous system (CNS), the autonomic nervous system (ANS), the hypothalamic–pituitary–adrenal (HPA) axis or "stress system," as well as the (gastrointestinal) corticotropin-releasing factor system, and the intestinal immune response system, featuring the intestinal mucosal barrier and the luminal microbiota (Bonaz and Bernstein 2013). Taking these components into account one can see how regulation of the CNS by the gut microbiota is achieved not only through neural, but through endocrine, metabolic, and immunological pathways.

Neural communication pathways lay within the enteric nervous system (ENS), a main division of the ANS that governs GI function and vagal afferent nerves (VAN) that transmit sensory information from the visceral organs to the CNS. Receptors expressed on VAN are able to sense regulatory gut peptides such as leptin and ghrelin (de Lartigue et al. 2011) as well as information contained in nutrients such as carbohydrates or fat (Hamilton and Raybould 2016), relaying these signals to the CNS (de Lartigue et al. 2011).

Apart from being mediated via stress factors, the microbiota-gut-brain axis has the ability to alter intestinal permeability and motility through the release of mucus rich in immune molecules such as secretory IgA and neurotransmitters, for example, serotonin, melatonin, gamma-aminobutyric acid, histamines and acetylcholine (Wells et al. 2017). Gut microbiota also synthesize nutrients that are essential for optimum human health span. As an example of the metabolic activity of some human gut bacteria, folate and vitamin B12 (cobalamin) are produced by Lactobacillus reuteri (Spinler et al. 2014). Both are important for development of the nervous system during the early years (Marques et al. 2010) as well as for healthy brain aging later in life (Lim et al. 2016). Some of these pathways are summarized in Figures 6.11 and 6.12.

Practitioners with a whole-person clinical approach are only too aware of how psychosocial stress can affect gut function. This stress normally manifests itself as changes in bowel motion regularity and/or stool consistency, most likely triggered by secondary changes in intestinal microbiota composition. In long-term cases of exposure to stress, these changes can contribute to low-grade inflammation, causing ultrastructural epithelial abnormalities, and altering bacterial-host interactions allowing greater microbial translocation (Gareau et al. 2008).

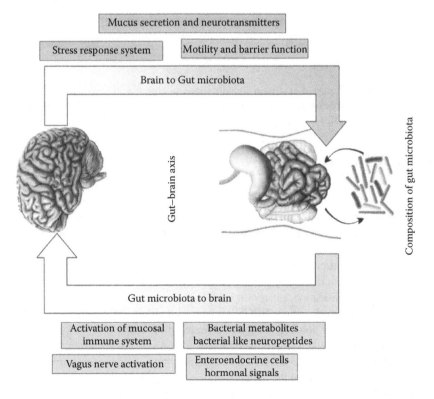

FIGURE 6.11 Bidirectional communication between the gut microbiota and the central nervous system (CNS). (Reproduced with permission from Al-Asmakh, M. et al. 2012. *Gut Microbes* 3(4): 366–373.)

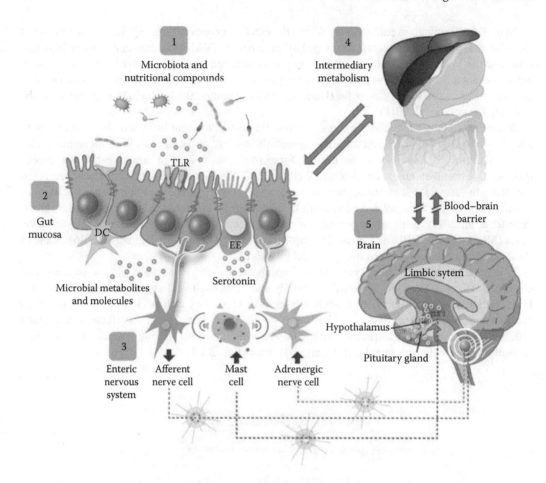

FIGURE 6.12 Schematic model of gut–brain signaling representing five components, with a central role of host-microbe interaction and intestinal barrier function. (Reproduced from Wells, J. M., R. J. Brummer, M. Derrien et al. 2017. *Am J Physiol Gastrointest Liver Physiol* 312(3): G171–G193.)

FROM EUBIOSYS TO DYSBIOSIS

Overgrowth of pathogenic bacteria results in an increase in lipopolysaccharide (LPS) levels which triggers the production of pro-inflammatory cytokines in the gut axis (Tremlett et al. 2017). For example, in irritable bowel syndrome (IBS), gut-related inflammation is pivotal in promoting endo-toxemia, systemic inflammation, and neuroinflammation, all of which lead to cognitive impairment (Daulatzai 2014). Similarly, in non-celiac gluten sensitivity (NCGS) patients, dysbiosis causes gut inflammation, diarrhea and/or constipation, visceral hypersensitivity, abdominal pain, a dysfunc-tional metabolic state characterized by enhanced energy harvest, and deranged peripheral immune and neuro-immune communication, a pathologic cascade that may promote oxidative stress, neuroin-flammation, and cognitive dysfunction. NCGS is a newly identified pathological entity that describes the symptoms experienced by non-celiac subjects. They experience celiac-like symptoms because of gluten intake, including IBS-like symptoms as well as abdominal pain, nausea, bloating, flatulence, diarrhea, or constipation (Czaja-Bulsa 2015) with gluten as the confirmed causative factor. Although it's tempting to assume that many of the patients who seek the advice of integrative clinicians may be suffering from NCGS, in a recent small-scale study by Bardella et al. (2016) only 8% of 37 patients were diagnosed with NCGS. The rest of the participants were affected by Fermentable, Oligo-, Di-, Mono-saccharides and Polyols (FODMAPS) in wheat and not by gluten itself.

ASSESSING FUNCTION—LABORATORY TESTING AND n = 1 TRIALS

We share one-third of our gut microbiota with most people, while two-thirds are specific to each one of us. This means that the peculiarities in our gut microbiota can provide scientists and clinicians with information about our health and susceptibility to the development of various diseases. The last 5 years has seen an explosion of research in the gut microbiome brought about by gene testing of the microbes using a small stool sample to assess the thousands of different species (Shankar 2017). Thanks to this latest generation sequencing based on 16S rRNA technology, we know that in a small human stool sample we're likely to find tens of trillions of microorganisms, including at least 1000 different species of known bacteria with more than 3 million genes. That's 150 times more than human genes (Backhed et al. 2005). In fact, based on current findings, a single microbiome test can provide more reliable information about a person's health than a genome screen and major disruptions are easier to see in the results of a stool test than in results of genetic sequencing. While treating every patient as a research subject, health professionals should see every meal as an opportunity, and every food as a potential drug (Toribio-Mateas and Spector 2017). These stool tests—available from a range of functional or integrative medicine laboratories—provide a holistic snapshot of gut health and diversity which is not diagnostic in nature, as the results can vary from one day to another day. Reports and accuracy continue to improve with time and with the use of larger datasets for benchmarking patients against healthy and diseased populations, but the most interesting property of functional stool testing is the increase in patient compliance reported by integrative practitioners. The demanding twenty-first century patient who seeks the support of an integrative medicine practitioner looks for individualized advice that moves away from the concept of "the average person" promoted by large-scale trials. These patients expect their clinicians to take personalization to the next level making care participative by involving them in the process, accounting for differences in their gut, their genes, their environment, and their lifestyle. This type of patient doesn't want their clinician to wait for years so that science can make it from bench to bedside and are happy to engage in n = 1-style trials, the basis of personalized medicine (Schork 2015). In the words of Tim Spector, Professor of Genetic Epidemiology at King's College London, "while treating every patient as a research subject, health professionals should see every meal as an opportunity, and every food as a potential drug." Stool testing can help motivate the patient to comply with the recommendations issued by clinicians, so even if the science is not absolutely there yet, based on the fact that the interventions are likely to be very safe for most and the results likely to be positive, one can be a little adventurous in the clinical application of emerging findings.

The most reliable biomarkers for clinicians to assess gut–brain function are as follows:

- *Microbial diversity*—Gut microbiota profiles in a variety of conditions including autism, major depression, and Parkinson's disease show that individuals suffering from ill-health tend to show narrowing in microbial diversity (Dinan and Cryan 2015), rendering the host more susceptible to infection and consequently negatively affecting innate immune function (Patterson et al. 2014). Additionally, recent studies have identified that subject biological age but not chronological age correlate with a decrease in stool microbial diversity (Maffei et al. 2017), that is, pathological aging is associated with a narrowing in microbial diversity while healthy aging correlates with a more diverse microbiota (Dinan and Cryan 2017).
- *Fecal calprotectin*—A recent study carried out on 22 Alzheimer's patients by Leblhuber et al. (2015) showed that almost three-quarters of AD patients presented fecal calprotectin concentrations higher than normal (>50 mg/kg). This is interpreted to be a sign of gastrointestinal permeability/leaky gut, where fecal calprotectin would have translocated from the gut into the circulation via disturbed intestinal barrier function. Calprotectin is heterodimer formed by pro-inflammatory proteins S100A8 and S100A9. The latter has been established as a biomarker for the diagnosis and progression of AD and dementia (Horvath et al. 2016).

- *Zonulin and nutrient status*—Zonulin is a physiological modulator of intercellular tight junction function and thus a regulator of gut permeability (Fasano 2012). Exposure to air pollution (Calderon-Garciduenas et al. 2015) as well as microbial dysbiosis, high-fructose and high-fat dietary patterns, and nutritional deficiencies, for example, vitamin D, vitamin A, and zinc, are also factors known to affect gastrointestinal permeability (Teixeira et al. 2012).

DIETARY NEUROPROTECTION, FROM THE GUT UP

Working on neuroprotection from the gut is not difficult and can be a very satisfying job for the integrative clinician. The two main interventions will consist of the use of pre- and probiotics, both of which have been used traditionally for gastrointestinal health. With advancing knowledge on the communication system that connects the gut and the brain, integrative practitioners can now tackle neuroprotection from the gut upward.

So what are probiotics and prebiotics? How do we define them? How these natural substances are defined is important not only for the scientific community, but also for regulatory agencies, the food industry, consumers, and healthcare professionals (Hutkins et al. 2016). They provide practitioners with the possibility to regulate their patient's microbiota, restoring gastrointestinal homeostasis, and thereby influencing mucosal and systemic immune function that helps dampen down neuroinflammation.

According to Valcheva and Dieleman (2016) dietary prebiotics are defined as "selectively fermented ingredients that result in specific changes in the composition and/or activity of the gastrointestinal microbiota, thus conferring benefit(s) upon host health." According to an expert consensus statement issued recently by The International Scientific Association for Probiotics and Prebiotics (ISAPP), the definition and scope of prebiotics is "currently established prebiotics are carbohydrate-based, but other substances such as polyphenols and polyunsaturated fatty acids converted to respective conjugated fatty acids might fit the updated definition assuming convincing weight of evidence in the target host" (Gibson et al. 2017). The reason this updated definition is relevant for clinicians is the fact that dietary plant polyphenols such as catechins (in tea and cocoa), anthocyanins (in berries), resveratrol (in red grapes and wine), quercetin (in apples, onions, and other bulbs like leeks), and epigallocatechin gallate (in green tea) constitute a class of nutrients that aren't absorbed in the small intestine. Instead, they reach the colon where they undergo extensive biotransformation by the microbiota (Clifford 2004). With the amount of evidence available, it is safe to say that considering polyphenols as mere antioxidant agents is now somewhat outdated. Instead, the new way to see these compounds is as providers of health benefits resulting from microbial metabolism. Thus, integrative clinicians should regard dietary polyphenols as contributors to the maintenance of gastrointestinal health "by preserving microbial balance through the stimulation of the growth of beneficial bacteria (i.e., lactobacilli and bifidobacteria) and the inhibition of pathogenic bacteria, exerting prebiotic-like effects" (Duenas et al. 2015). There is also evidence that the metabolism of polyphenols by gut microbiota increases their bioavailability to the host (Fernandes et al. 2017).

As a word of caution, it is important to remember that research into the modulation of the gut–brain axis via the gastrointestinal microbiota is still-emerging frontier science and that most evidence is based on basic science and animal models that may lack translatability into measurably effective human interventions. Therefore, the highly sophisticated, individualized prescriptions of specific prebiotic compounds and probiotic strains that would constitute the ideal of personalization for integrative practitioners still remains utopian. While the risk of harm to the patient when experimenting with prebiotics and probiotics is most likely to be minimal, if any, it is advised that practitioners use their clinical judgement and weigh the likely benefits against any potential disadvantages.

Manipulating gut bacteria through the use of prebiotics and probiotics doesn't have to be complicated. Given the lack of extensive human clinical data, using simple strategies such as increasing dietary diversity are easy to implement in patients' busy lifestyles and have been found to have an influence on both gut health and emotional wellbeing. In fact, in a recent retrospective, non-controlled assessment of nutritional therapy work, carried out in the United Kingdom by a team featuring a nutrition practitioner and a health psychologist it was found that a simple intervention consisting of increasing the diversity of the participants' diets to aim to include up to 50 different food ingredients per week, with a focus on brightly colored fruits and vegetables, had a statistically significant positive effect on digestion, cognition, and physical and emotional wellbeing (Lawrence and Hyde 2017). The results of this study resonate with those of another human experiment where 45 participants were given a prebiotic fiber supplement or placebo for 3 weeks and cortisol levels were measured to assess emotional processing. Participants receiving the prebiotic supplements showed increased attentional vigilance to positive versus negative stimuli similar to those seen following administration of pharmacological agents such as the selective serotonin reuptake inhibitor citalopram or the benzodiazepine diazepam in healthy individuals (Schmidt et al. 2015). These results are very interesting because they show that certain saccharides such as the fiber inulin—present in Jerusalem artichokes, leeks, and onions—and other fructo-oligosaccharides, galacto-oligosaccharides, and polydextrose, all of which have been widely used to improve gastrointestinal outcomes, also appear to influence distant sites, including improvements in neural and cognitive processes, immune functioning, and serum lipid profiles (Collins and Reid 2016). Sources of prebiotic fiber often provide other interesting nutrients that are useful neuroprotective agents. For example, the pseudo-grain buckwheat has been reported to possess prebiotic and antioxidant activities. In vitro and animal studies suggest that some of its bioactive compounds, such as D-chiro-inositol and the flavonoids rutin and quercetin, may be partially responsible for the observed neuroprotective effects (Giménez-Bastida and Zieliński 2015). Equally, resistant starch from beans, lentils, green bananas, and cooked and cooled potatoes and rice is known to have a positive effect on the gut microbiota, increasing the concentration of short-chain fatty acids such as butyrate, increasing insulin sensitivity, and improving cardiovascular and kidney health (Yang et al. 2017).

Fermented foods, both dairy-based and non-dairy also provide an effective way to modulate the patient's gut microbiota (Jandhyala et al. 2015), thereby influencing brain health via the many pathways that connect the GI tract with the CNS. In a recent randomized, double-blind, placebo-controlled trial involving 75 petrochemical workers conducted by nutrition researchers at the University of Tehran, addition of a daily probiotic yoghurt containing two strains of *Lactobacillus acidophilus* LA5 and *Bifidobacterium lactis* BB12 with a total of min 1×10^7 colony forming units (CFU) to the participants' diet resulted in similar improvements to mental health to supplementation with a multi-species probiotic capsule containing seven probiotic bacteria species (*Actobacillus casei* 3×10^3, *L. acidophilus* 3×10^7, *L. rhamnosus* 7×10^9, *L. bulgaricus* 5×10^8, *Bifidobacterium breve* 2×10^{10}, *B. longum* 1×10^9, and *S. thermophilus* 3×10^8 CFU/g) with 100 mg fructo-oligosaccharide and lactose as carrier substances. The control group was given a conventional yoghurt containing the starter cultures of *Streptococcus thermophilus* and *Lactobacillus bulgaricus* and experienced no statistically significant improvement in mental health markers, which included changes to experience of depression, anxiety, and stress based on validated scales. The comparable effectiveness of the interventions reported in this study supports the use of live probiotic bacteria from whole foods as opposed to the obligatory use of probiotics supplements. There are advantages to using a whole food approach, including lower cost and improved patience compliance.

Another widely available food is milk fermented by kefir grains, or simply known as "kefir." Drinking this probiotic food daily has been shown to increase secretory IgA in feces while reducing the expression of pro-inflammatory cytokines in the gastrointestinal tract (Carasi et al. 2015). As discussed previously, inflammation mediates dysbiosis, and the subsequent bacterial translocation that contributes to cognitive decline. On that basis, downregulating inflammation in the gut is assumed to have similar systemic effects. Kefir is the author's favorite source of probiotic microbes not least because of its symbiotic nature, being a combination of bacteria and yeast—at least 30 different types for most grain types—but also because of the many health properties that patients can achieve with regular consumption, including immunomodulation, antimicrobial and anticarcinogenic activity, as well as control of serum glucose and cholesterol and control of lactose intolerance (Ahmed et al. 2013; Nielsen et al. 2014). While there are non-dairy varieties of kefir available in health food shops, and some dairy-sensitive patients even ferment their own non-dairy milk alternatives with kefir grains at home, there is a definite benefit in including dairy products in the diets of patients seeking to enhance neuroprotection.

A recent study published in the *American Journal of Clinical Nutrition* found that individuals who consumed cheese daily had better circulating levels of the endogenous antioxidant glutathione (Choi et al. 2015). Glutathione is used by brain cells to fight free radical formation, while cheese and other fermented dairy produce such as yoghurt is a source of probiotic bacteria—particularly if made with unpasteurized/raw milk. Therefore, unless patients express a concern about dairy, it is advisable that they include it as part of their daily diets. For vegan patients or those who cannot tolerate dairy at all, either because of extreme lactose intolerance or because of sensitivity to milk proteins, for example, casein, soy, coconut, oat and almond "milks" can be fermented successfully by kefir grains, with soy being particularly suitable in terms of the consistency achieved (Bau et al. 2013, 2015). There are also many other alternative non-dairy substrates, such as fruit and vegetable juices, as well as plain sugared water (using cane sugar or molasses), that can be fermented by kefir grains for the production of probiotic drinks with distinct sensory characteristics that engage patients with specific dietary preferences.

Another slightly more exotic fermented food reported in the literature is fermented papaya, which has been used in humans as a wholefood supplement that elicits significant reductions in urinary 8-OHdG, a guanine byproduct of DNA breakdown used as a biomarker of genomic instability (Aruoma et al. 2010; Barbagallo et al. 2015).

Discussing supplementation with different strains of probiotic bacteria in detail is outside of the scope of this chapter. However, it is important for integrative practitioners to remind themselves that there's an argument for the use of a multistrain probiotic supplement over single-strain products, even if these claim to be "high potency."

CONCLUSION

Given the multifactorial nature and the complexity of the aging processes, it would be simplistic to assume that the consumption of high levels of single nutrients or specific food items would be able to modulate the many pathways involved therein. Instead a diverse and naturally occurring dietary pattern, such as the Mediterranean diet, provides practitioners with a model that's well documented for its range of beneficial actions on gut, brain, and systemic health. It is hoped that this chapter has provided integrative practitioners with an insight as to how this model is a much better fit for ongoing neuroprotection primarily mediated by means of ongoing minimization of genomic instability and sustained protection of genomic integrity, mostly by means of wholefoods and with the use of targeted nutraceuticals, prescribed on the basis of individual requirements.

REFERENCES

Abuznait, A. H., H. Qosa, B. A. Busnena, K. A. El Sayed, and A. Kaddoumi. 2013. Olive-oil-derived oleocanthal enhances beta-amyloid clearance as a potential neuroprotective mechanism against Alzheimer's disease: In vitro and *in vivo* studies. *ACS Chem Neurosci* 4(6): 973–982.

Ahmed, Z., Y. Wang, A. Ahmad, S. T. Khan, M. Nisa, H. Ahmad, and A. Afreen. 2013. Kefir and health: A contemporary perspective. *Crit Rev Food Sci Nutr* 53(5): 422–434.

Al-Asmakh, M., F. Anuar, F. Zadjali, J. Rafter, and S. Pettersson. 2012. Gut microbial communities modulating brain development and function. *Gut Microbes* 3(4): 366–373.

Ali, S., M. A. Stone, J. L. Peters, M. J. Davies, and K. Khunti. 2006. The prevalence of co-morbid depression in adults with Type 2 diabetes: A systematic review and meta-analysis. *Diabet Med* 23(11): 1165–1173.

Ames, B. N., H. Atamna, and D. W. Killilea. 2005. Mineral and vitamin deficiencies can accelerate the mitochondrial decay of aging. *Mol Aspects Med* 26(4–5): 363–378.

Arlt, S., T. Muller-Thomsen, U. Beisiegel, and A. Kontush. 2012. Effect of one-year vitamin C- and E-supplementation on cerebrospinal fluid oxidation parameters and clinical course in Alzheimer's disease. *Neurochem Res* 37(12): 2706–2714.

Aruoma, O. I., Y. Hayashi, F. Marotta, P. Mantello, E. Rachmilewitz, and L. Montagnier. 2010. Applications and bioefficacy of the functional food supplement fermented papaya preparation. *Toxicology* 278(1):6–16.

Aveyard, P., D. Yach, A. B. Gilmore, and S. Capewell. 2016. Should we welcome food industry funding of public health research? *BMJ* 353: i2161.

Backhed, F., R. E. Ley, J. L. Sonnenburg, D. A. Peterson, and J. I. Gordon. 2005. Host-bacterial mutualism in the human intestine. *Science* 307(5717): 1915–1920.

Balci, Y. I., A. Ergin, A. Karabulut, A. Polat, M. Dogan, and K. Kucuktasci. 2014. Serum vitamin B12 and folate concentrations and the effect of the Mediterranean diet on vulnerable populations. *Pediatr Hematol Oncol* 31(1): 62–67.

Balk, E., M. Chung, G. Raman, A. Tatsioni, P. Chew, S. Ip, D. DeVine, and J. Lau. 2006. B vitamins and berries and age-related neurodegenerative disorders. *Evid Rep Technol Assess (Full Rep)* (134): 1–161.

Barbagallo, M., F. Marotta, and L. J. Dominguez. 2015. Oxidative stress in patients with Alzheimer's disease: Effect of extracts of fermented papaya powder. *Mediators Inflamm* 2015: 6.

Barbato, D. L., G. Tatulli, K. Aquilano, and M. R. Ciriolo. 2015. Mitochondrial Hormesis links nutrient restriction to improved metabolism in fat cell. *Aging (Albany NY)* 7(10): 869–881.

Bardella, M. T., L. Elli, and F. Ferretti. 2016. Non celiac gluten sensitivity. *Curr Gastroenterol Rep* 18(12): 63.

Barzilai, A., B. Schumacher, and Y. Shiloh. 2017. Genome instability: Linking ageing and brain degeneration. *Mech Ageing Dev* 161(Pt A): 4–18.

Bastianetto, S., C. Menard, and R. Quirion. 2015. Neuroprotective action of resveratrol. *Biochim Biophys Acta* 1852(6): 1195–1201.

Bau, T. R., S. Garcia, and E. I. Ida. 2013. Optimization of a fermented soy product formulation with a kefir culture and fiber using a simplex-centroid mixture design. *Int J Food Sci Nutr* 64(8): 929–935.

Bau, T. R., S. Garcia, and E. I. Ida. 2015. Changes in soymilk during fermentation with kefir culture: Oligosaccharides hydrolysis and isoflavone aglycone production. *Int J Food Sci Nutr* 66(8): 845–850.

Bazan, N. G. 2012. Neuroinflammation and proteostasis are modulated by endogenously biosynthesized neuroprotectin D1. *Mol Neurobiol* 46(1): 221–226.

Beal, M. F., D. Oakes, I. Shoulson et al. 2014. A randomized clinical trial of high-dosage coenzyme Q10 in early Parkinson disease: No evidence of benefit. *JAMA Neurol* 71(5): 543–552.

Beaumont, M., J. K. Goodrich, M. A. Jackson et al. 2016. Heritable components of the human fecal microbiome are associated with visceral fat. *Genome Biol* 17(1): 189.

Belancio, V. P. 2015. LINE-1 activity as molecular basis for genomic instability associated with light exposure at night. *Mob Genet Elements* 5(3): 1–5.

Belkaid, Y. and S. Naik. 2013. Compartmentalized and systemic control of tissue immunity by commensals. *Nat Immunol* 14(7): 646–653.

Bhullar, K. S. and H. P. Rupasinghe. 2013. Polyphenols: Multipotent therapeutic agents in neurodegenerative diseases. *Oxid Med Cell Longev* 2013: 891748.

Bjelakovic, G., D. Nikolova, and C. Gluud. 2014. Antioxidant supplements and mortality. *Curr Opin Clin Nutr Metab Care* 17(1): 40–44.

Bjelakovic, G., D. Nikolova, L. L. Gluud, R. G. Simonetti, and C. Gluud. 2008. Antioxidant supplements for prevention of mortality in healthy participants and patients with various diseases. *Cochrane Database Syst Rev* 2: Cd007176.

Bonaccio, M., C. Cerletti, L. Iacoviello, and G. de Gaetano. 2015. Mediterranean diet and low-grade subclinical inflammation: The Moli-sani study. *Endocr Metab Immune Disord Drug Targets* 15(1): 18–24.

Bonaccio, M., G. Pounis, C. Cerletti, M. B. Donati, L. Iacoviello, and G. de Gaetano. 2017. Mediterranean diet, dietary polyphenols and low-grade inflammation: Results from the MOLI-SANI study. *Br J Clin Pharmacol* 83(1): 107–113.

Bonaz, B. L. and C. N. Bernstein. 2013. Brain-gut interactions in inflammatory bowel disease. *Gastroenterology* 144(1): 36–49.

Brettschneider, J., J. B. Toledo, V. M. Van Deerlin, L. Elman, L. McCluskey, V. M. Lee, and J. Q. Trojanowski. 2012. Microglial activation correlates with disease progression and upper motor neuron clinical symptoms in amyotrophic lateral sclerosis. *PLoS One* 7(6): e39216.

Brown, E. M., M. Sadarangani, and B. B. Finlay. 2013. The role of the immune system in governing host-microbe interactions in the intestine. *Nat Immunol* 14(7): 660–667.

Buckland, G., and C. A. Gonzalez. 2015. The role of olive oil in disease prevention: A focus on the recent epidemiological evidence from cohort studies and dietary intervention trials. *Br J Nutr* 113(Suppl 2): S94–101.

Calderon-Garciduenas, L., A. Vojdani, E. Blaurock-Busch et al. 2015. Air pollution and children: Neural and tight junction antibodies and combustion metals, the role of barrier breakdown and brain immunity in neurodegeneration. *J Alzheimers Dis* 43(3): 1039–1058.

Carasi, P., S. M. Racedo, C. Jacquot, D. E. Romanin, M. A. Serradell, and M. C. Urdaci. 2015. Impact of kefir derived Lactobacillus kefiri on the mucosal immune response and gut microbiota. *J Immunol Res* 2015: 361604.

Cascalheira, J. F., M. Goncalves, M. Barroso, R. Castro, M. Palmeira, A. Serpa, A. C. Dias-Cabral, F. C. Domingues, and S. Almeida. 2015. Association of the transcobalamin II gene 776C → G polymorphism with Alzheimer's type dementia: Dependence on the 5, 10-methylenetetrahydrofolate reductase 1298A → C polymorphism genotype. *Ann Clin Biochem* 52(Pt 4): 448–455.

Chatterjee, S., S. A. E. Peters, M. Woodward et al. 2016. Type 2 diabetes as a risk factor for dementia in women compared with men: A pooled analysis of 2.3 million people comprising more than 100,000 cases of dementia. *Diabetes Care* 39(2): 300–307.

Chatzianagnostou, K., S. Del Turco, A. Pingitore, L. Sabatino, and C. Vassalle. 2015. The mediterranean lifestyle as a non-pharmacological and natural antioxidant for healthy aging. *Antioxidants (Basel)* 4(4): 719–736.

Chen, H., S. Liu, L. Ji, T. Wu, F. Ma, Y. Ji, Y. Zhou, M. Zheng, M. Zhang, and G. Huang. 2015. Associations between Alzheimer's disease and blood homocysteine, vitamin B12, and folate: A case-control study. *Curr Alzheimer Res* 12(1): 88–94.

Choi, I. Y., P. Lee, D. R. Denney, K. Spaeth, O. Nast, L. Ptomey, A. K. Roth, J. A. Lierman, and D. K. Sullivan. 2015. Dairy intake is associated with brain glutathione concentration in older adults. *Am J Clin Nutr* 101(2): 287–293.

Chow, H. M., and K. Herrup. 2015. Genomic integrity and the ageing brain. *Nat Rev Neurosci* 16(11): 672–684.

Ciechanover, A., and Y. T. Kwon. 2015. Degradation of misfolded proteins in neurodegenerative diseases: Therapeutic targets and strategies. *Exp Mol Med* 47: e147.

Claxton, A., L. D. Baker, A. Hanson, E. H. Trittschuh, B. Cholerton, A. Morgan, M. Callaghan, M. Arbuckle, C. Behl, and S. Craft. 2015. Long acting intranasal insulin detemir improves cognition for adults with mild cognitive impairment or early-stage Alzheimer's disease dementia. *J Alzheimers Dis* 45(4): 1269–1270.

Clifford, M. N. 2004. Diet-derived phenols in plasma and tissues and their implications for health. *Planta Med* 70(12): 1103–1114.

Collins, S., and G. Reid. 2016. Distant site effects of ingested prebiotics. *Nutrients* 8(9).

Cook, S., and O. M. Hess. 2005. Homocysteine and B vitamins. In von Eckardstein, A. (ed.), *Atherosclerosis: Diet and Drugs*. Berlin, Heidelberg: Springer, pp. 325–338.

Czaja-Bulsa, G. 2015. Non coeliac gluten sensitivity—A new disease with gluten intolerance. *Clin Nutr* 34(2): 189–194.

Daulatzai, M. A. 2014. Chronic functional bowel syndrome enhances gut-brain axis dysfunction, neuroinflammation, cognitive impairment, and vulnerability to dementia. *Neurochem Res* 39(4): 624–644.

De Bruyn, E., B. Gulbis, and F. Cotton. 2014. Serum and red blood cell folate testing for folate deficiency: New features?"*Eur J Haematol* 92(4): 354–359.

de la Torre-Robles, A., A. Rivas, M. L. Lorenzo-Tovar, C. Monteagudo, M. Mariscal-Arcas, and F. Olea-Serrano. 2014. Estimation of the intake of phenol compounds from virgin olive oil of a population from southern Spain. *Food Addit Contam Part A Chem Anal Control Expo Risk Assess* 31(9): 1460–1469.

de Lartigue, G., C. B. de La Serre, and H. E. Raybould. 2011. Vagal afferent neurons in high fat diet-induced besity; intestinal microflora, gut inflammation and cholecystokinin. *Physiol Behav* 105(1): 100–105.

Dinan, T. G., and J. F. Cryan. 2015. The impact of gut microbiota on brain and behaviour: Implications for psychiatry. *Curr Opin Clin Nutr Metab Care* 18(6): 552–558.

Dinan, T. G., and J. F. Cryan. 2017. Gut instincts: Microbiota as a key regulator of brain development, ageing and neurodegeneration. *J Physiol* 595(2): 489–503.

Druesne-Pecollo, N., P. Latino-Martel, T. Norat, E. Barrandon, S. Bertrais, P. Galan, and S. Hercberg. 2010. Beta-carotene supplementation and cancer risk: A systematic review and metaanalysis of randomized controlled trials. *Int J Cancer* 127(1): 172–184.

Duenas, M., I. Munoz-Gonzalez, C. Cueva, A. Jimenez-Giron, F. Sanchez-Patan, C. Santos-Buelga, M. V. Moreno-Arribas, and B. Bartolome. 2015. A survey of modulation of gut microbiota by dietary polyphenols. *Biomed Res Int* 2015: 850902.

Edifizi, D., and B. Schumacher. 2015. Genome instability in development and aging: Insights from nucleotide excision repair in humans, mice, and worms. *Biomolecules* 5(3): 1855–1869.

Epel, E. S., and G. J. Lithgow. 2014. Stress biology and aging mechanisms: Toward understanding the deep connection between adaptation to stress and longevity. *J Gerontol A Biol Sci Med Sci* 69(Suppl 1): S10–16.

Erny, D., and M. Prinz. 2017. Microbiology: Gut microbes augment neurodegeneration. *Nature* 544(7650): 304–305.

Farina, N., M. G. Isaac, A. R. Clark, J. Rusted, and N. Tabet. 2012. Vitamin E for Alzheimer's dementia and mild cognitive impairment. *Cochrane Database Syst Rev* 11: Cd002854.

Fasano, A. 2012. Intestinal permeability and its regulation by zonulin: Diagnostic and therapeutic implications. *Clin Gastroenterol Hepatol* 10(10): 1096–1100.

Feart, C., B. Alles, B. Merle, C. Samieri, and P. Barberger-Gateau. 2012. Adherence to a mediterranean diet and energy, macro-, and micronutrient intakes in older persons. *J Physiol Biochem* 68(4): 691–700.

Fernandes, I., R. Pérez-Gregorio, S. Soares, N. Mateus, and V. de Freitas. 2017. Wine flavonoids in health and disease prevention. *Molecules* 22(2).

Figueroa-Mendez, R., and S. Rivas-Arancibia. 2015. Vitamin C in health and disease: Its role in the metabolism of cells and redox state in the brain. *Front Physiol* 6: 397.

Fortmann, S. P., B. U. Burda, C. A. Senger, J. S. Lin, and E. P. Whitlock. 2013. Vitamin and mineral supplements in the primary prevention of cardiovascular disease and cancer: An updated systematic evidence review for the U.S. Preventive Services Task Force. *Ann Intern Med* 159(12): 824–834.

Fowler, A. K., A. Hewetson, R. G. Agrawal et al. 2012. Alcohol-induced one-carbon metabolism impairment promotes dysfunction of DNA base excision repair in adult brain. *J Biol Chem* 287(52): 43533–43542.

Franco, R., and Cedazo-Minguez, A. 2014. Successful therapies for Alzheimer's disease: Why so many in animal models and none in humans? *Front Pharmacol* 5: 146.

Freude, S., L. Plum, J. Schnitker, U. Leeser, M. Udelhoven, W. Krone, J. C. Bruning, and M. Schubert. 2005. Peripheral hyperinsulinemia promotes tau phosphorylation *in vivo*. *Diabetes* 54(12): 3343–3348.

Galland, L. 2014. The gut microbiome and the brain. *J Med Food* 17(12): 1261–1272.

Garcia-Calzon, S., G. Zalba, M. Ruiz-Canela et al. 2015. Dietary inflammatory index and telomere length in subjects with a high cardiovascular disease risk from the PREDIMED-NAVARRA study: Cross-sectional and longitudinal analyses over 5 y. *Am J Clin Nutr* 102(4): 897–904.

Gareau, M. G., M. A. Silva, and M. H. Perdue. 2008. Pathophysiological mechanisms of stress-induced intestinal damage. *Curr Mol Med* 8(4): 274–281.

Gibson, G. R., R. Hutkins, M. E. Sanders et al. 2017. Expert consensus document: The International Scientific Association for Probiotics and Prebiotics (ISAPP) consensus statement on the definition and scope of prebiotics. *Nat Rev Gastroenterol Hepatol* 14(8): 491–502.

Giménez-Bastida, J. A., and H. Zieliński. 2015. Buckwheat as a functional food and its effects on health. *Journal of Agricultural and Food Chemistry* 63(36): 7896–7913.

Golde, T. E., D. R. Borchelt, B. I. Giasson, and J. Lewis. 2013. Thinking laterally about neurodegenerative proteinopathies. *J Clin Invest* 123(5): 1847–1855.

Gutierrez-Mariscal, F. M., P. Perez-Martinez, J. Delgado-Lista et al. 2012. Mediterranean diet supplemented with coenzyme Q10 induces postprandial changes in p53 in response to oxidative DNA damage in elderly subjects. *Age (Dordr)* 34(2): 389–403.

Hamilton, M. K., and H. E. Raybould. 2016. Bugs, guts and brains, and the regulation of food intake and body weight. *Int J Obes Suppl* 6(Suppl 1): S8–S14.

Hao, J., W. Shen, G. Yu, H. Jia, X. Li, Z. Feng, Y. Wang, P. Weber, K. Wertz, E. Sharman, and J. Liu. 2010. Hydroxytyrosol promotes mitochondrial biogenesis and mitochondrial function in 3T3-L1 adipocytes. *J Nutr Biochem* 21(7): 634–644.

Hernandez-Aguilera, A., A. Rull, E. Rodriguez-Gallego, M. Riera-Borrull, F. Luciano-Mateo, J. Camps, J. A. Menendez, and J. Joven. 2013. Mitochondrial dysfunction: A basic mechanism in inflammation-related non-communicable diseases and therapeutic opportunities. *Mediators Inflamm* 2013: 135698.

Holtzman, D. M., J. C. Morris, and A. M. Goate. 2011. Alzheimer's disease: The challenge of the second century. *Sci Transl Med* 3(77): 77sr1.

Horvath, I., X. Jia, P. Johansson et al. 2016. Pro-inflammatory S100A9 Protein as a robust biomarker differentiating early stages of cognitive impairment in Alzheimer's disease. *ACS Chem Neurosci* 7(1): 34–39.

Hu, S., P. Maiti, Q. Ma, X. Zuo, M. R. Jones, G. M. Cole, and S. A. Frautschy. 2015. Clinical development of curcumin in neurodegenerative disease. *Expert Rev Neurother* 15(6): 629–637.

Huang, H. Y., B. Caballero, S. Chang et al. 2006. The efficacy and safety of multivitamin and mineral supplement use to prevent cancer and chronic disease in adults: A systematic review for a National Institutes of Health state-of-the-science conference. *Ann Intern Med* 145(5): 372–385.

Hutkins, R. W., J. A. Krumbeck, L. B. Bindels et al. 2016. Prebiotics: Why definitions matter. *Curr Opin Biotechnol* 37: 1–7.

Iriti, M., and E. M. Varoni. 2015. Melatonin in Mediterranean diet, a new perspective. *J Sci Food Agric* 95(12): 2355–2359.

Jandhyala, S. M., R. Talukdar, C. Subramanyam, H. Vuyyuru, M. Sasikala, and D. Nageshwar Reddy. 2015. Role of the normal gut microbiota. *World J Gastroenterol* 21(29): 8787–8803.

Jeppesen, D. K., V. A. Bohr, and T. Stevnsner. 2011. DNA repair deficiency in neurodegeneration. *Prog Neurobiol* 94(2): 166–200.

Jiang, C., G. Li, P. Huang, Z. Liu, and B. Zhao. 2017. The Gut Microbiota and Alzheimer's Disease. *J Alzheimers Dis* 58(1): 1–15.

Kohler, C. A., M. Maes, A. Slyepchenko, M. Berk, M. Solmi, K. L. Lanctot, and A. F. Carvalho. 2016. The Gut-Brain Axis, Including the Microbiome, Leaky Gut and Bacterial Translocation: Mechanisms and Pathophysiological Role in Alzheimer's Disease. *Curr Pharm Des* 22(40): 6152–6166.

Lauritzen, K. H., O. Moldestad, L. Eide, H. Carlsen, G. Nesse, J. F. Storm, I. M. Mansuy, L. H. Bergersen, and A. Klungland. 2010. Mitochondrial DNA toxicity in forebrain neurons causes apoptosis, neurodegeneration, and impaired behavior. *Mol Cell Biol* 30(6): 1357–1367.

Lawrence, K., and J. Hyde. 2017. Microbiome restoration diet improves digestion, cognition and physical and emotional wellbeing. *PLoS ONE* 12(6): e0179017.

Leblhuber, F., S. Geisler, K. Steiner, D. Fuchs, and B. Schütz. 2015. Elevated fecal calprotectin in patients with Alzheimer's dementia indicates leaky gut. *J Neural Transm* 122(9): 1319–1322.

Lee, S. L., P. Thomas, and M. Fenech. 2015. Genome instability biomarkers and blood micronutrient risk profiles associated with mild cognitive impairment and Alzheimer's disease. *Mutat Res* 776: 54–83.

Lim, S. Y., E. J. Kim, A. Kim, H. J. Lee, H. J. Choi, and S. J. Yang. 2016. Nutritional factors affecting mental health. *Clin Nutr Res* 5(3): 143–152.

Loef, M., N. von Stillfried, and H. Walach. 2012. Zinc diet and Alzheimer's disease: A systematic review. *Nutr Neurosci* 15(5): 2–12.

Lopes da Silva, S., B. Vellas, S. Elemans, J. Luchsinger, P. Kamphuis, K. Yaffe, J. Sijben, M. Groenendijk, and T. Stijnen. 2014. Plasma nutrient status of patients with Alzheimer's disease: Systematic review and meta-analysis. *Alzheimers Dement* 10(4): 485–502.

Maffei, V. J., S. Kim, E. t. Blanchard, M. Luo, S. M. Jazwinski, C. M. Taylor, and D. A. Welsh. 2017. Biological aging and the human gut microbiota. *J Gerontol A Biol Sci Med Sci* 72(11): 1474–1482.

Malhotra, A., R. F. Redberg, and P. Meier. 2017. Saturated fat does not clog the arteries: Coronary heart disease is a chronic inflammatory condition, the risk of which can be effectively reduced from healthy lifestyle interventions. *Br J Sports Med* 51(15): 1111–1112.

Mangiola, F., G. Ianiro, F. Franceschi, S. Fagiuoli, G. Gasbarrini, and A. Gasbarrini. 2016. Gut microbiota in autism and mood disorders. *World J Gastroenterol* 22(1): 361–368.

Marques, T. M., R. Wall, R. P. Ross, G. F. Fitzgerald, C. A. Ryan, and C. Stanton. 2010. Programming infant gut microbiota: Influence of dietary and environmental factors. *Curr Opin Biotechnol* 21(2): 149–156.

Martinez, K. B., V. Leone, and E. B. Chang. 2017. Western diets, gut dysbiosis, and metabolic diseases: Are they linked? *Gut Microbes* 8(2): 130–142.

Meramat, A., N. F. Rajab, S. Shahar, and R. Sharif. 2015. Cognitive impairment, genomic instability and trace elements. *J Nutr Health Aging* 19(1): 48–57.

Nakanishi, H., Y. Hayashi, and Z. Wu. 2011. The role of microglial mtDNA damage in age-dependent prolonged LPS-induced sickness behavior. *Neuron Glia Biol* 7(1): 17–23.

Nehra, V., J. M. Allen, L. J. Mailing, P. C. Kashyap, and J. A. Woods. 2016. Gut Microbiota: Modulation of Host Physiology in Obesity. *Physiology (Bethesda)* 31(5): 327–335.

Nielsen, B., G. C. Gurakan, and G. Unlu. 2014. Kefir: A multifaceted fermented dairy product. *Probiotics Antimicrob Proteins* 6(3–4): 123–135.

O'Malley, D., E. M. Quigley, T. G. Dinan, and J. F. Cryan. 2011. Do interactions between stress and immune responses lead to symptom exacerbations in irritable bowel syndrome? *Brain Behav Immun* 25(7): 1333–1341.

Onakpoya, I. J., and C. J. Heneghan. 2017. The efficacy of supplementation with the novel medical food, Souvenaid, in patients with Alzheimer's disease: A systematic review and meta-analysis of randomized clinical trials. *Nutr Neurosci* 20(4): 219–227.

Ono, K., and M. Yamada. 2012. Vitamin A and Alzheimer's disease. *Geriatr Gerontol Int* 12(2): 180–188.

Pallauf, K., K. Giller, P. Huebbe, and G. Rimbach. 2013. Nutrition and healthy ageing: Calorie restriction or polyphenol-rich "MediterrAsian" diet? *Oxid Med Cell Longev* 2013: 707421.

Pallister, T., and T. D. Spector. 2016. Food: A new form of personalised (gut microbiome) medicine for chronic diseases? *J R Soc Med* 109(9): 331–336.

Patterson, E., J. F. Cryan, G. F. Fitzgerald, R. P. Ross, T. G. Dinan, and C. Stanton. 2014. Gut microbiota, the pharmabiotics they produce and host health. *Proc Nutr Soc* 73(4): 477–489.

Pedret, A., R. M. Valls, S. Fernandez-Castillejo et al. 2012. Polyphenol-rich foods exhibit DNA antioxidative properties and protect the glutathione system in healthy subjects. *Mol Nutr Food Res* 56(7): 1025–1033.

Penalvo, J. L., B. Oliva, M. Sotos-Prieto, I. Uzhova, B. Moreno-Franco, M. Leon-Latre, and J. M. Ordovas. 2015. Greater adherence to a Mediterranean dietary pattern is associated with improved plasma lipid profile: The Aragon Health Workers Study cohort. *Rev Esp Cardiol (Engl Ed)* 68(4): 290–297.

Rai, V. 2017. Methylenetetrahydrofolate reductase (MTHFR) C677 T polymorphism and Alzheimer disease risk: A meta-analysis. *Mol Neurobiol* 54(2): 1173–1186.

Ramis, M. R., S. Esteban, A. Miralles, D. X. Tan, and R. J. Reiter. 2015. Caloric restriction, resveratrol and melatonin: Role of SIRT1 and implications for aging and related-diseases. *Mech Ageing Dev* 146–148: 28–41.

Ravnskov, U., D. M. Diamond, R. Hama et al. 2016. Lack of an association or an inverse association between low-density-lipoprotein cholesterol and mortality in the elderly: A systematic review. *BMJ Open* 6(6): e010401.

Ravussin, E., L. M. Redman, J. Rochon et al. 2015. A 2-year randomized controlled trial of human caloric restriction: Feasibility and effects on predictors of health span and longevity. *J Gerontol A Biol Sci Med Sci* 70(9): 1097–1104.

Risch, M., D. W. Meier, B. Sakem, P. Medina Escobar, C. Risch, U. Nydegger, and L. Risch. 2015. Vitamin B12 and folate levels in healthy Swiss senior citizens: A prospective study evaluating reference intervals and decision limits. *BMC Geriatr* 15: 82.

Rothberg, M. B. 2013. Coronary artery disease as clogged pipes. *A Misconceptual Model* 6(1): 129–132.

Ruxton, C. H., E. Derbyshire, and M. Toribio-Mateas. 2016. Role of fatty acids and micronutrients in healthy ageing: A systematic review of randomised controlled trials set in the context of European dietary surveys of older adults. *J Hum Nutr Diet* 29(3): 308–324.

Sampson, T. R., J. W. Debelius, T. Thron et al. 2016. Gut microbiota regulate motor deficits and neuroinflammation in a model of Parkinson's disease. *Cell* 167(6): 1469–1480.e1412.

Schmidt, K., P. J. Cowen, C. J. Harmer, G. Tzortzis, S. Errington, and P. W. Burnet. 2015. Prebiotic intake reduces the waking cortisol response and alters emotional bias in healthy volunteers. *Psychopharmacology (Berl)* 232(10): 1793–1801.

Schork, N. J. 2015. Personalized medicine: Time for one-person trials. *Nature* 520(7549): 609–611.

Schwingshackl, L., G. Hoffmann, B. Buijsse et al. 2015. Dietary supplements and risk of cause-specific death, cardiovascular disease, and cancer: A protocol for a systematic review and network meta-analysis of primary prevention trials. *Syst Rev* 4: 34.

Scoditti, E., C. Capurso, A. Capurso, and M. Massaro. 2014. Vascular effects of the Mediterranean diet-part II: Role of omega-3 fatty acids and olive oil polyphenols. *Vascul Pharmacol* 63(3): 127–134.

Scoditti, E., M. Massaro, M. A. Carluccio, M. Pellegrino, M. Wabitsch, N. Calabriso, C. Storelli, and R. De Caterina. 2015. Additive regulation of adiponectin expression by the mediterranean diet olive oil components oleic Acid and hydroxytyrosol in human adipocytes. *PLoS One* 10(6): e0128218.

Sekirov, I., S. L. Russell, L. C. Antunes, and B. B. Finlay. 2010. Gut microbiota in health and disease. *Physiol Rev* 90(3): 859–904.

Shah, R. 2013. The role of nutrition and diet in Alzheimer disease: A systematic review. *J Am Med Dir Assoc* 14(6): 398–402.

Shankar, V. 2017. Gut microbiome profiling tests propelled by customer demand. *Nat Biotechnol* 35(1): 9.

Sharif, R., P. Thomas, P. Zalewski, and M. Fenech. 2015. Zinc supplementation influences genomic stability biomarkers, antioxidant activity, and zinc transporter genes in an elderly Australian population with low zinc status. *Mol Nutr Food Res* 59(6): 1200–1212.

Shen, L., and H. F. Ji. 2015. Associations between homocysteine, folic acid, Vitamin B12 and Alzheimer's disease: Insights from meta-analyses. *J Alzheimers Dis* 46(3): 777–790.

Soares, J. P., A. Cortinhas, T. Bento, J. C. Leitao, A. R. Collins, I. Gaivao, and M. P. Mota. 2014. Aging and DNA damage in humans: A meta-analysis study. *Aging (Albany NY)* 6(6): 432–439.

Soni, M., T. B. Rahardjo, R. Soekardi, Y. Sulistyowati, Lestariningsih, A. Yesufu-Udechuku, A. Irsan, and E. Hogervorst. 2014. Phytoestrogens and cognitive function: A review. *Maturitas* 77(3): 209–220.

Spinler, J. K., A. Sontakke, E. B. Hollister et al. 2014. From prediction to function using evolutionary genomics: Human-specific ecotypes of Lactobacillus reuteri have diverse probiotic functions. *Genome Biol Evol* 6(7): 1772–1789.

St Laurent, G. 3rd, N. Hammell, and T. A. McCaffrey. 2010. A LINE-1 component to human aging: Do LINE elements exact a longevity cost for evolutionary advantage? *Mech Ageing Dev* 131(5): 299–305.

Stanley, M., S. L. Macauley, and D. M. Holtzman. 2016. Changes in insulin and insulin signaling in Alzheimer's disease: Cause or consequence? *J Exp Med* 213(8): 1375–1385.

Stein, P. K., A. Soare, T. E. Meyer, R. Cangemi, J. O. Holloszy, and L. Fontana. 2012. Caloric restriction may reverse age-related autonomic decline in humans. *Aging Cell* 11(4): 644–650.

Sundman, M. H., N. K. Chen, V. Subbian, and Y. H. Chou. 2017. The bidirectional gut-brain-microbiota axis as a potential nexus between traumatic brain injury, inflammation, and disease. *Brain Behav Immun* 66: 31–44.

Szutowicz, A., H. Bielarczyk, A. Jankowska-Kulawy, A. Ronowska, and T. Pawelczyk. 2015. Retinoic acid as a therapeutic option in Alzheimer's disease: A focus on cholinergic restoration. *Expert Rev Neurother* 15(3): 239–249.

Tafti, M., and N. B. Ghyselinck. 2007. Functional implication of the vitamin A signaling pathway in the brain. *Arch Neurol* 64(12): 1706–1711.

Tang, W. H., T. Kitai, and S. L. Hazen. 2017. Gut microbiota in cardiovascular health and disease. *Circ Res* 120(7): 1183–1196.

Teixeira, T. F., M. C. Collado, C. L. Ferreira, J. Bressan, and C. Peluzio Mdo. 2012. Potential mechanisms for the emerging link between obesity and increased intestinal permeability. *Nutr Res* 32(9): 637–647.

Toledo, E., J. Salas-Salvado, C. Donat-Vargas et al. 2015. Mediterranean diet and invasive breast cancer risk among women at high cardiovascular risk in the PREDIMED trial: A randomized clinical trial. *JAMA Intern Med* 175(11): 1752–1760.

Toribio-Mateas, M. A., and T. Spector. 2017. Could food act as personalized medicine for chronic disease? *Personalized Medicine* 14(3): 193–196.

Tremlett, H., K. C. Bauer, S. Appel-Cresswell, B. B. Finlay, and E. Waubant. 2017. The gut microbiome in human neurological disease: A review. *Ann Neurol* 81(3): 369–382.

Tsutakawa, S. E., J. Lafrance-Vanasse, and J. A. Tainer. 2014. The cutting edges in DNA repair, licensing, and fidelity: DNA and RNA repair nucleases sculpt DNA to measure twice, cut once. *DNA Repair (Amst)* 19: 95–107.

Turna, J., K. Grosman Kaplan, R. Anglin, and M. Van Ameringen. 2016. What's bugging the gut in ocd? A review of the gut microbiome in obsessive-compulsive disorder. *Depress Anxiety* 33(3): 171–178.

Tuttolomondo, A., A. Casuccio, C. Butta et al. 2015. Mediterranean Diet in patients with acute ischemic stroke: Relationships between Mediterranean Diet score, diagnostic subtype, and stroke severity index. *Atherosclerosis* 243(1): 260–267.

Valcheva, R., and L. A. Dieleman. 2016. Prebiotics: Definition and protective mechanisms. *Best Pract Res Clin Gastroenterol* 30(1): 27–37.

van der Meij, B. S., J. A. Langius, M. D. Spreeuwenberg, S. M. Slootmaker, M. A. Paul, E. F. Smit, and P. A. van Leeuwen. 2012. Oral nutritional supplements containing n-3 polyunsaturated fatty acids affect quality of life and functional status in lung cancer patients during multimodality treatment: An RCT. *Eur J Clin Nutr* 66(3): 399–404.

Wang, J., W. R. Markesbery, and M. A. Lovell. 2006. Increased oxidative damage in nuclear and mitochondrial DNA in mild cognitive impairment. *J Neurochem* 96(3): 825–832.

Wang, P., and K. Ding 2014. Proteoglycans and glycosaminoglycans in misfolded proteins formation in Alzheimer's disease. *Protein Pept Lett* 21(10): 1048–1056.

Weinreb, O., S. Mandel, T. Amit, and M. B. Youdim. 2004. Neurological mechanisms of green tea polyphenols in Alzheimer's and Parkinson's diseases. *J Nutr Biochem* 15(9): 506–516.

Weintraub, H. S. 2014. Overview of prescription omega-3 fatty acid products for hypertriglyceridemia. *Postgrad Med* 126(7): 7–18.

Wells, J. M., R. J. Brummer, M. Derrien et al. 2017. Homeostasis of the gut barrier and potential biomarkers. *Am J Physiol Gastrointest Liver Physiol* 312(3): G171–G193.

Widmer, R. J., A. J. Flammer, L. O. Lerman, and A. Lerman. 2015. The Mediterranean diet, its components, and cardiovascular disease. *Am J Med* 128(3): 229–238.

Wu, H., and A. J. Roks. 2014. Genomic instability and vascular aging: A focus on nucleotide excision repair. *Trends Cardiovasc Med* 24(2): 61–68.

Xu, J., L. L. Wang, E. B. Dammer, C. B. Li, G. Xu, S. D. Chen, and G. Wang. 2015. Melatonin for sleep disorders and cognition in dementia: A meta-analysis of randomized controlled trials. *Am J Alzheimers Dis Other Demen* 30(5): 439–447.

Yang, X., K. O. Darko, Y. Huang, C. He, H. Yang, S. He, J. Li, J. Li, B. Hocher, and Y. Yin. 2017. Resistant starch regulates gut microbiota: Structure, biochemistry and cell signalling. *Cell Physiol Biochem* 42(1): 306–318.

Zachwieja, J., E. Hentges, J. O. Hill, R. Black, and M. Vassileva. 2013. Public-private partnerships: The evolving role of industry funding in nutrition research. *Adv Nutr* 4(5): 570–572.

Zhang, C., A. Browne, D. Child, and R. E. Tanzi. 2010. Curcumin decreases amyloid-beta peptide levels by attenuating the maturation of amyloid-beta precursor protein. *J Biol Chem* 285(37): 28472–28480.

7 The Dental Connection to Health

Dental and Gingival Health and Its Relation to Chronic Illness

Alyse Shockey, Lisa Marie Samaha, and Dawn Ewing

CONTENTS

Understanding Dentinal Fluid Transfer 208
What Influences the Reversal of the Dentinal Fluid Flow? 210
Characteristics of a Caries-Prone Patient... 210
    Fluid Reversal 210
Periodontal Disease and the Oral Systemic Connection.. 211
Some Thoughts about Materials Used in Dentistry 214
    Tooth/Body Connection 216
    Root Canal—Understanding the Implications 216
        Evidence.. 217
        The Tooth and Organ Connection 218
    Oral Home Care 221
        Fluoride 222
        Propylene Glycol...222
        FD&C Color Pigments 222
        Artificial Sweeteners 222
        Ethanol (Ethyl Alcohol)...222
        Triclosan 222
        Trisodium Phosphate (TSP) 222
        Glycerin..222
        Calcium 222
        Flavoring...222
        Detergents and Surfactants...222
        Carrageenan..222
        Hydrated Silica 223
        Carbomer..223
    A Holistic Approach to Dental Care 223
References..223

Dentistry is on the "cusp" of understanding that there is a relationship between the oral cavity and the metabolism of the rest of the body. Modern dental research has revealed many breakthroughs by discovering the importance of the oral-systemic connection in overall health. As time passes, this connection can help save lives and shift dentistry into a collaborative effort with the medical community.

We have been taught that tooth decay prevention is done by brushing twice a day, flossing, and regular dental checkups, yet the staggering number of cavities, crowns, root canals, and extracted teeth confirm that we have missed the mark in our oral care. Even with the dawn of fluoride treatments, fluoridated toothpastes, and medicated mouth rinses, there has been more dental decay in the past 100 years than in any other century. Successful oral care goes far beyond brushing and flossing. Teeth are alive, and given the right environment, they can regenerate; and therefore the internal factors that nourish the teeth are of the utmost importance. Eating whole plant-based foods, maintaining hormonal balance, absorbing minerals, and proper fluid exchange in and out of the teeth are essentials for good oral health.

We think of our teeth as separate from our bodies and this has stuck with the general population. In addition, the theory of how we get cavities in the mouth has been adopted from less than desirable politics. Through the 1930s there were two tracks of investigations: the *dominant track* favored the Acidogenic Theory and the *lesser track* examined the possible role of systemic factors. The Acidogenic Theory is the perception of dentists and dental schools that sugar and acids sitting on the teeth are the cause of decay. This theory grew from Willoughby D. Miller in 1890, who stated that nonspecific bacteria in the plaque would ferment refined carbohydrates to produce acid that demineralized tooth enamel.[1]

This quote from the Colgate website is evidence of the continuity of the theory:

> *Everyone develops plaque because bacteria are constantly forming in our mouths. These bacteria use ingredients found in our diet and saliva to grow. Plaque causes cavities when the acids from plaque attack teeth after eating. With repeated acid attacks, the tooth enamel can break down and a cavity may form. Plaque that is not removed can also irritate the gums around your teeth, leading to gingivitis (red, swollen, bleeding gums), periodontal disease and tooth loss.*[2]

This theory makes the teeth pretend like they are "inert appendages" or "not alive" and ignores the possibility of them being capable of resistance. Teeth are more than just bone. The enamel is alive. The dentin is alive. So are the pulp, the blood vessels, the saliva, the nerves, and the gums. They are living things with the ability to heal and regenerate.

In the 1940s the Acidogenic Theory was adopted by the American Association of Dental Research by committee vote, rather than science (Erosion vs. Systemic). The investigators of the *lesser track*, who emphasized the possible existence of a dentinal fluid flow system that begins with the odontoblasts and extends through the dentin, were effectively ignored thereafter.

Dr. Ralph Steinman was a dentist in the 1950s. He suffered with chronic asthma and every summer he had to shut down his practice for a few weeks because he would get so sick from his asthma.

He studied information on diet and eating, which lead him to cure his asthma thus concluding the link between health and diet. This was not much of a topic in the 1950s. He was also interested in dental textbooks and articles that were from the 1800s, theorizing that if someone were to get a cavity that it was due to systemic reasons. These textbooks also suggested that there must be some sort of fluid that is connecting the teeth with the rest of the body and histological morphology of teeth clearly indicates that they are designed for maintaining fluid flow through the dentin and enamel. This also indicates that there must be some mechanism to control fluid flow.

Plus, in spite of a destructive oral environment, there are physiological mechanisms that are linked to the teeth that allow them to withstand the assault of a hostile environment (Figure 7.1).

In Dr. Steinman's private dental practice, his confidence in the acidogenic theory began to diminish because what he observed in his patients' mouths did not always follow the "theory." The theory ignored the potential defensive role of the host. He stopped practicing dentistry in 1958 and went fully into dental research with Dr. Webster Price who helped establish the School of Dentistry at Loma Linda.

Many of his faculty associates didn't share his ideas and criticized him severely, even to the point of putting a sign on his laboratory door which said, "Searching for a systemic explanation for cariogenesis is akin to looking for the 'holy grail'."

For the next 40 years, he continually proved that there is "dentinal fluid transport" in the teeth that is similar to the lymphatic system, a system that connects the teeth to the rest of the body.

Dr. Steinman discovered that there are approximately 3 miles of microscopic dentinal tubules leading from the teeth to glands in our brain, like the hypothalamus and pituitary.

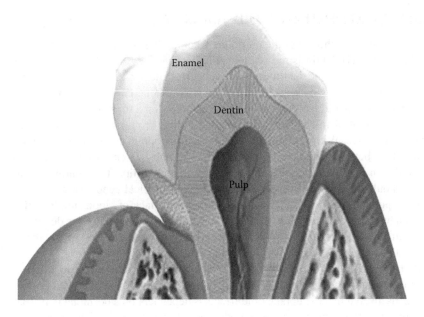

FIGURE 7.1 Anatomy of a tooth.

Steinman did an experiment by injecting fluorescent dye,[3] acriflavine hydrochloride, near the stomach of rats to see if he could observe the dentinal fluid flow that he questioned. He was astonished to find out that the dye was visible in the pulp of the tooth within 6 minutes and eventually visible in the enamel in 1 hour. He proved this theory over and over again. Steinman wanted to know how the teeth could become decayed if the fluid was flowing correctly and where did this fluid come from. When he studied the morphology of the tooth, he noted that it is designed to maintain a fluid flow through its structure (Figure 7.2).

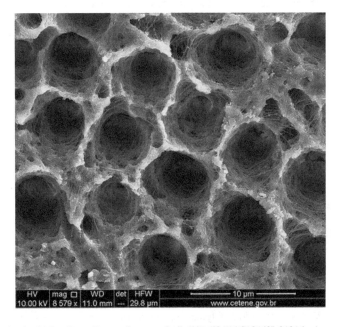

FIGURE 7.2 Dentinal tubules (http://www.forp.usp.br/bdj/Bdj9(1)/t0191/f5t0191.jpg).

UNDERSTANDING DENTINAL FLUID TRANSFER

It is necessary to identify three significant points when understanding the significance of dentinal fluid transfer (DFT):[4] (1) dentin is morphologically designed for fluid flow through a multitude of canaliculi that extends from the dentin-pulp interface to the dentin-enamel interface; also, enamel is porous to facilitate fluid flow onto its surface, (2) teeth are noncompliant structures, and (3) dentin has no vascular supply but like all living tissue is dependent on a transport mechanism for survival.

Dentin is composed of microscopic tubules that radiate from the dentin-pulp interface to the dentin-enamel interface. Within the dentin is a layer of odontoblast and preodontoblast cells that form the interface between the dentin and pulp. Functionally, odontoblasts secrete dentin matrix and because dentin is a living tissue, they maintain dentin vitality. The dentin, despite it being a living tissue, should have a blood supply to maintain physiological needs. However, the blood supply ends in the pulp chamber. In order to compensate for the lack of blood supply in the dentin, the odontoblasts have a dentinal fluid flow transport mechanism that inundates the dentin with essential nutrients obtained from the blood. The dental lymph is comprised of blood minus the large protein molecules and its purpose is to give vitality to the dentin.

The pulp has capillaries that are fenestrated (have windows) to allow these nutrients to diffuse out of the circulation into the pulp chamber in a lymph-like fluid which is taken up by the odontoblasts. It was discovered that the uptake of nutrients is dependent on a hormone in the parotid gland. This hormone alters the permeability of the odontoblast membranes which enables the transfer of nutrient-containing fluid into the odontoblasts. Another attribute of the odontoblasts is that they have cytoplasmic myofibrils that allow them to function as pumps (Figure 7.3).

Physiologically, the dentinal fluid always moves in a centrifugal direction[5] and eventually appears on the surface of the enamel as a fluid layer. This could have a protective role by preventing inward diffusion of oral cytotoxic bacterial products.[6,7] If any cracks are in the enamel, the dentinal fluid flow is increased because the hydrostatic pressure within the tooth is greater than oral pressure and so harmful bacteria outside of the teeth cannot penetrate the tooth. For this reason, the teeth remain caries-free[8] (Figures 7.4 and 7.5).

He demonstrated that the composition of a diet (cariogenic vs. noncariogenic) affected the dynamics of this dentinal fluid flow.[9] The rats that were on a noncariogenic diet showed the dye moved quickly from the pulp-dentin interface to the dentin-enamel interface compared to the suppressed flow in the rats on the cariogenic diet. This information did not explain the mechanism that regulated the dentinal flow so in the mid-1960s he collaborated with Dr. John Leonora, PhD,

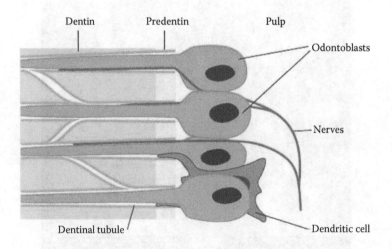

FIGURE 7.3 Fish EW. The circulation of lymph in the dentinal tubules with some observations on the metabolism of the dentin. (From *Proc R. Soc. Med.* 1926;19:59–72. With permission.)

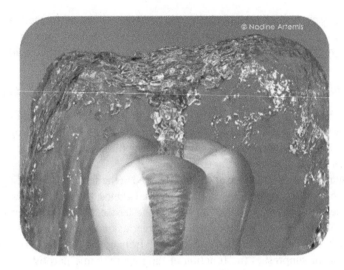

FIGURE 7.4 Centrifugal action of dentinal fluid illustrated. (From Artemis N., *Holistic Dental Care: The Complete Guide to Healthy Teeth and Gums (Kindle Locations 205)*. North Atlantic Books, 2013-10-08. With permission.)

an endocrinologist, and together they concluded that this is possible because of the hypothalamus which is our "endocrine/hormonal" system.[10]

The system begins with chewing, which communicates to neural endings in the oral mucosa and tongue to detect nutritive substrates. These substrates activate nerves that signal the hypothalamus. The hypothalamus responds by telling the parotid gland to release a hormonal secretion (parotid hormone).

The parotid gland is the only salivary gland that secretes a hormone which forms the dentin and regulates the flow and can "switch" the flow of the dentinal fluid. Dr. Steinman's research also showed there was a low incidence of caries when the dentinal fluid flow was high and the inverse when the dentinal fluid flow was low because it acts like a buffer. The pH of the fluid is similar to blood, 7.4, and can neutralize bacterial acids both within the tooth and on the surface of the teeth. The dental fluid, also known as dental lymph, contains nutrients essential for maintaining the vitality of dentin: amino acids for synthesizing dentinal collagen, glucose for metabolism, and minerals to mineralize the dentinal collagen.

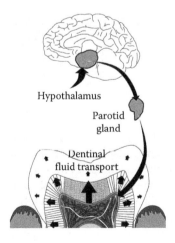

FIGURE 7.5 Diagram explaining the human hypothalamus-parotid gland endocrine axis. (From Roggenkamp C. *Dentinal Fluid Transport*, ix. Loma Linda, CA: Loma Linda University Press, 2004. With permission.)

Once the fluid passes through the enamel it will coat the surface of the teeth and form a barrier against the pathogens in the mouth by acting as a buffer. If any cracks in the enamel are present, the fluid flow will be greater there to prevent bacterial invasion and to neutralize acids.

WHAT INFLUENCES THE REVERSAL OF THE DENTINAL FLUID FLOW?

Deficiency in minerals signals the body to rob minerals from the teeth and bones. The first indication of this is a drop in the pH of the first morning urine from a normal reading of 6.4–7.0 to the 5.0–5.8 range. A deficiency of vitamins C, D, and A during the calcification process (when the teeth are forming) leaves the teeth less resistant to decay.[11]

Calcium is drawn from the bone tissue and is then carried in the serum calcium. Sugar is also disruptive to the endocrine system, the hypothalamus, the adrenal glands, the pituitary glands, and the pineal glands as well as the hormonal secretions of cortisol, progesterone, DHEA, testosterone, and estrogen.

Like the bones, the teeth react to deficiencies of minerals and trace elements imposed by either a direct deficiency in the diet or by a relative deficiency from an excess of sucrose and other refined foods in the diet. Sugar suppresses the function of the hypothalamic-parotid gland endocrine axis which leads to a decrease in the parotid hormone secretion.[12] There are three preconditions required for caries to occur: bacteria, fermentable carbohydrates, and susceptibility of the tooth (plus time). When sugar in the diet is replaced by polysaccharides such as a starch, the rate of caries is reduced. Conversely, when sugar was injected intraperitoneally, the rate of caries increased and for this reason slowly absorbed sugars would be more advisable. Monitoring the effects of dietary carbohydrates is important such as the quantity in the diet, the rate of absorption, availability of phosphate, endocrine stability, and the nutrients necessary for metabolism.[13]

CHARACTERISTICS OF A CARIES-PRONE PATIENT

1. Consuming "enriched" white flour versus natural whole wheat flour.[14] Enriched flour has less pyridoxine, pantothenic acid, zinc, chromium, molybdenum, fluoride, and phosphate.
2. Large amounts of added nutritive diluting sucrose in the diet or draining cooking water from vegetables.
3. Consumption of low nutritive foods like sugary foods between meals that are typically deprived of vitamins, minerals, and trace elements.
4. Endocrine system imbalances.

Caries susceptibility can be predicted by "caries-activity tests" that provide valuable information about the bacterial population in the mouth; however, they tell nothing about the response of the tooth to this environment. Classifying caries potential was done through the study of acid produced by various food-saliva mixtures and the rate of decay. Unfortunately this data was not verified and all of the studies failed to consider the response of the tooth because it was thought to be an inert object in a destructive environment.[15]

FLUID REVERSAL

The primary reason for fluid reversal is insulin imbalance that originates from refined carbohydrates and sugar. Sugar inhibits the hypothalamus from functioning properly, which suppresses the hypothalamus-parotid gland endocrine system and odontoblasts from pumping the fluid.[16]

The tooth will draw bacteria and acid inward (centripetal)[4] from the mouth like a straw. This fluid contains microbes, bacteria, acid, and fungi. They cause inflammation in the pulp chamber and allow the tooth to experience oxidative damage which postures the tooth for demineralization and decay begins to show on the enamel. The salivary enzymes begin to digest tooth structure and bacteria increase in response to dying tissue (Figure 7.6).

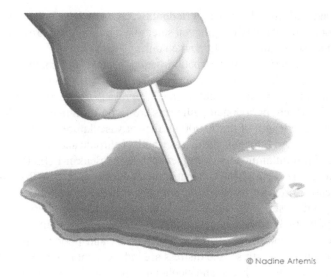

© Nadine Artemis

FIGURE 7.6 Centripetal action of dentinal fluid illustrated. (From Artemis N., *Holistic Dental Care: The Complete Guide to Healthy Teeth and Gums (Kindle Locations 205)*. North Atlantic Books, 2013-10-08. With permission.)

Every effort should be given to other influences to the parotid gland and how it functions. Lack of exercise contributes to lymph stagnation, and radiation can contribute to parotid gland tumors.

The teeth are alive, they can create new tissue, and the vitality of the teeth comes from the core of the tooth. Eating foods that are plant-based seems to provide a variety of nutrients versus eating the Standard American Diet (SAD) that is loaded with processed sugar, boxed and canned food, and fast food. Resistance to decay depends on normal dentinal fluid transport and decay can be arrested when the malfunction is corrected by the nutritional value of the diet. Normal functioning teeth are caries resistant. Everything that affects the health and welfare of our bodies may affect the health of the teeth. Increasing micronutrients in the diet and reducing sucrose are essential for the teeth.[17]

PERIODONTAL DISEASE AND THE ORAL SYSTEMIC CONNECTION

Periodontal disease is an aggressive and insidious disease of the oral cavity, affecting the tissues that support the teeth, known as the periodontium. The periodontium consists of gingival tissue, cementum, periodontal ligament, and alveolar bone.[18] In health, the tissue is firm, non-ulcerative, and robustly supportive of the teeth. In disease, the gingival tissues are swollen, inflamed, and often receding while the bone is deteriorating around the necks of the teeth. In all of its stages, from gingivitis to periodontitis, periodontal disease has the potential to negatively impact the overall health of the host.[19]

Periodontal disease is the leading cause of tooth loss in the adult population worldwide and one of the body's most abundant sources of chronic, low-grade inflammation.[20,21]

Both inflammatory and infectious, periodontal disease is typically present as a chronic condition and destruction often occurs in a silent (i.e., asymptomatic) manner until it becomes well established. Typically, people with mild and moderate stages of periodontal disease are unaware of their condition because they may have no pain until the disease reaches a severe stage. At times, and given the right host environment, periodontal disease can manifest episodes of acute exacerbation. An acute lesion is known as a "periodontal abscess." Such an acute response is typically painful and more aggressive from both oral and systemic perspectives. Individuals with more advanced periodontal disease may present with multiple periodontal abscesses at any given time. In the early stages of gingivitis, the tissue lining the gingival sulcus is ulcerated. Since this area lies against the root of the tooth, the infection is not visible. If left untreated, gingivitis may transition into the more destructive periodontal infection known as periodontitis, characterized by loss of gum tissue attachment and alveolar bone. Bleeding of the gingival sulcus becomes more aggressive during evaluation and initial treatment, and purulence is often noted during examination.

The initial process of periodontal destruction begins silently and characteristically leads to a breech in the sulcular epithelium, even in its early stage, known as gingivitis. This early stage may be devoid of clinical signs or symptoms, although it is representative of an open wound (Figure 7.7).

As a result of this breech, periodontal pathogens are free to migrate throughout the rest of the body, traversing the entire length of the 70,000+ miles of vasculature, resulting in widespread systemic health effects.[20,22–24] Additionally, the disease, both in chronic and acute periods, stimulates the activity and release of pro-inflammatory cytokines such as interleukin-1 (IL-1), interleukin-6 (IL-6), tumor necrosis factor alpha (TNF alpha) and matrixmetalproteinases (MMPs) into the circulation.[25]

Periodontal disease primarily results from a highly complex, anaerobic and dysbiotic biofilm that breeds in the gingival sulcus.[19] The disease is exacerbated by a variety of issues: host immunity, genetic susceptibility, hormonal changes, and a vast array of systemic disease states, including obesity, diabetes, osteoporosis, nutritional deficiencies, and poor dietary and sleep habits.[26] Emotional states of depression, stress, and distress are independent risk factors for periodontal disease.[26] Lifestyle choices such as tobacco and alcohol use, poor oral hygiene and lack of professional care also contribute to the inflammatory response and eventual degradation of the periodontal tissues. Localized oral factors contributing to periodontal disease include decayed teeth, defective

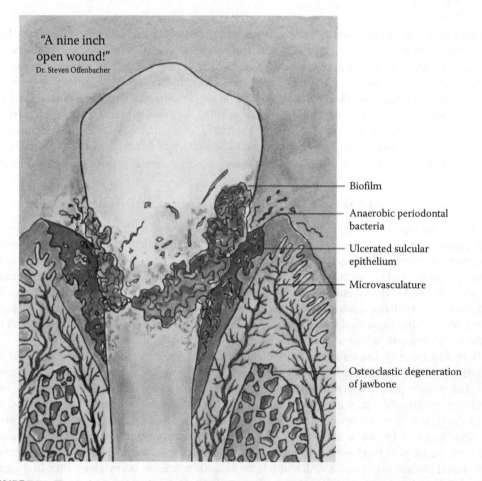

FIGURE 7.7   The oral dynamics of periodontal disease. (Illustration by Lisa Marie Samaha, DDS, Perio Arts Institute, © 2017.)

restorations, fractured teeth, occlusal imbalances, ill-fitting fixed and removable prostheses, habitual grinding and clenching, xerostomia, and infectious contact.[26,27]

Periodontal disease is generally preventable, yet according to the U.S. Centers for Disease Control, it afflicts 80% of the American population. With the United States' reputation for its relative obsession with oral hygiene in comparison to the rest of the world, we might assume the percentage of periodontal disease is even more dramatic elsewhere.[27]

Periodontics became an approved specialty of dentistry in the United States in 1947.[28] Regrettably, the standard-of-care for the diagnosis and treatment of periodontal disease has remained mostly unchanged, focusing on a traditional therapeutic technique known as "scaling and root planing."[29] The traditional technique has consisted of mechanical removal of the soft, sticky biofilm known as "plaque," and the hard, calcified concretions that result from mineral deposition within plaque, known as "calculus" via a mechanical process known as scaling and root planing. It is noteworthy that when such a procedure is performed, bacteria is mobilized into the bloodstream creating a systemic bacteremia, which can result in untoward medical issues elsewhere in the body. Salivary bacterial DNA testing to properly identify the pathogens involved in the individual's periodontal disease before clinical care is instituted can help protect the patient, as DNA testing will allow for the prescribing of the appropriate, targeted systemic or oral antibiotic rinses to help prevent negative sequelae in the rest of the body and allow for improved therapeutic results of periodontal therapy. Historically, diagnostics have only consisted of clinical signs and symptoms of bleeding upon probing, increased probing depth, evidence of radiographic bone loss, gingival recession, mobility, and clinical attachment loss.

While advanced diagnostic and treatment methodology is used by a small cadre of forward-thinking dental health professionals, the development and generally accepted implementation of a standard protocol in clinical practice has, for the most part, been lacking.[27] Therefore, traditional means remain the standard-of-care, as evidenced in a study funded by the American Dental Association and released in the *Journal of the American Dental Association*, 2015.[29]

Based on salivary DNA microbial testing, periodontal disease appears to be a subclinical disease in its initial stages, that is, one that has taken hold well before any of the traditional means of diagnosis are manifest, such as increased probing depth, bleeding upon probing, gingival recession, clinical attachment loss, mobility, and radiographic evidence of bone loss. DNA testing can also identify those with a genetic predisposition to periodontal disease.[30,31]

By the mid-1990s, scientific research had begun to establish a link between periodontal disease and systemic disease. Connections documented in the scientific literature are found at differing levels with some weakly linked, others bordering on causative and some bi-directionally related in cause or exacerbation of adverse systemic conditions.

Periodontal disease is linked to cardiovascular disease,[32–36] cerebrovascular disease,[37] diabetes,[38–41] Alzheimer's disease and dementia,[41–45] rheumatoid arthritis,[46–48] adverse pregnancy outcome for mother and baby,[49–51] infertility and erectile dysfunction,[52] kidney disease and lung diseases,[53–55] brain abscesses[56,57] and a myriad of cancers throughout the body, to include oral cancer, breast cancer, colon cancer, lung and kidney cancers, multiple myeloma, Hodgkin's lymphoma, and prostate and pancreatic cancers.[58]

By the early part of the twenty-first century, challenges to the status quo were surfacing due to a small number of progressive dental professionals. These individuals had come to believe that dentistry must play an integral role in the establishment of total body health and focus its collective efforts on establishing interprofessional communications and collaboration with our colleagues throughout the field of medicine.[27,59,60]

Although scientific research had established a bona fide connection between periodontal disease and a myriad of untoward systemic conditions, the science, for all intents and purposes, remained locked within academic and research institutions with no universally accepted clinical protocol developed to move the oral-systemic agenda forward.

Over the past two decades, researchers, academicians, and clinicians within the medical/dental communities have engaged in lengthy conversation over dentistry's role in this emerging dynamic.

Knowledge was present, yet patients were suffering. Unacceptable to a relatively small but leading-edge cadre of dental health professionals who were willing to push the envelope, a variety of methods for improved diagnosis and treatment were sought out and integrated into their clinical practices.

The phase contrast microscope is being used with increasing frequency in the general dental office to screen for pathogenic bacterial activity. By 2006, salivary DNA testing for assessing periodontal pathogens and genetic risk was available in the United States.[27]

New piezo ultrasonic technologies and patient oral hygiene aids are utilized. Pharmaceutical grade nutritional supplements, oral probiotics, essential oils, and antioxidant rinses have been developed and integrated into use.[27,59,60] Blood testing has been added as a screening tool for systemic disease and conversations about inflammation, gut health, and whole body genomics became relevant within clinical practice.[27,59,61-65]

The use of various lasers (such as CO_2, NdYag, diode) and medical ozone therapies (gaseous injections, gas insufflation, and oils) became a part of this groundbreaking movement and are all successfully used to treat periodontal and other dental diseases.[27,59,66,67]

Approximately 70% of the United States' population visits a dentist once a year; twice the number who visit their medical doctors annually.[68] According to the U.S. Surgeon General's report "Oral Health in America, 2000," an oral examination can reveal signs and symptoms of more than 90% of systemic diseases.[20] Dental health professionals, responsible for healing the mouth, clearly have a profound opportunity for an integral role in assisting in the healing of the entire body.[27,63,64]

With many options available to them, a relatively small number of astute dental professionals ushered in a bold new era in dentistry, transforming the manner by which they help people heal.[27] As a result, they have fostered an increased level of communication and collaboration with medical colleagues of all disciplines, both within clinical practice as well as academia.

As of this writing, ozone therapy remains one of the least understood and utilized of the implemented modalities previously referenced. In dentistry, ozone therapeutics can be used as a stand-alone therapeutic agent or in combination with any or all of the above treatment options. In addition to its use in periodontal therapy, ozone is effective in the treatment of a vast array of soft and hard tissue oral lesions: caries control, wound healing from trauma, oral surgical procedures, and endodontic therapies.[27,66]

Due to the complex nature of periodontal disease, there exists a high rate of recurrence subsequent to traditional scaling and root planning therapy and surgical periodontal therapy.[69]

Through scientific research and clinical observation, it is apparent that a multifaceted protocol for diagnosing and treating periodontal disease will best serve our patients—one that includes the structured implementation of the techniques and technology described above, in a predictable and objectively measurable manner.

The dental profession is transitioning into a profession that requires consideration of systemic issues in every patient interaction just as the medical profession is transitioning into a profession that requires consideration of oral disease in every patient interaction.[70-72]

Without a collective focus through the lens of total body health, the healing professions cannot achieve long-term periodontal or systemic health.

SOME THOUGHTS ABOUT MATERIALS USED IN DENTISTRY

Products with heavy metals are often disastrous in terms of long-range tissue acquisition and tissue/organ interference and toxicity. Products with metals in the noble category are relatively safe although they could pose problems for some people.

Mercury amalgams are often misrepresented as a "silver filling." Although they are silver in color and they do contain a small amount of silver, they are 50% mercury. Mercury is a toxic substance. It was long thought that once mixed with the silver it would not leech out of the filling. We now know that is not true. The "mer" in thimerosal stands for mercury.

The most dangerous and absorbable form of mercury is in a vapor form. When a dentist removes an amalgam with a drill it creates a cloud of invisible vapor. A mercury-safe office will follow a very strict protocol to protect the patient, the staff, and the environment. This protocol is available at The International Academy of Biological Dentistry and Medicine (www.IABDM.org). The protocol is ever-changing as they gather new data so it is up to date.

Therefore, if we are going to steer clear of the mercury amalgams, what do we use? Through the years, dental materials have become stronger, better, and more aesthetic. But to be clear, there is nothing as good as what you were born with. Manufactured materials are chemicals and many people are sensitive to chemicals. Why certain people are sensitive to certain chemicals whereas others are not is an entire subject in itself. This is why most biological dentists will have their patients get tested for reactivity so that they are not placing something in their mouth that they are reactive to.

Dental materials used for white fillings can be composed of ceramic, plastics, and even glass materials. Each of those different materials will require different glue or bonding agents to create a tight seal with the tooth. Denture materials can range from vinyl to acrylic; there are different sutures and anesthetics as well.

How dental work is done can alter a person's bite (the way the teeth fit together). Changing that bite could create headaches, neck stiffness, or even make a person snore at night. This means that a person's teeth have always played a bigger role in their quality of life than most people have ever imagined.

Another factor regarding the use of composite resins, white filling materials, is the dentist must expose the materials of the adhesives and resins with a proper light source. The light acts as a catalyst and causes the materials to set. Each time the light is used it should be on for a minimum of 20 seconds. If these materials not properly cured, they will "out gas" and can be harmful to the patient's health. These materials are layered because multiple materials are used to make up a filling and the light has limitations in its ability to penetrate more than 4–6 mm. These are the steps taken to fill a prepared site; at each step, the material must be cured for approximately 20 seconds.

1. An etchant is used to prepare the surface of the tooth.
2. An adhesive is applied to fill in the rough surface and mechanically attach to the root's surface.
3. A flowable composite is placed for its ability to seal the margins.
4. A filler or thicker material is placed to "shape the filling" and make it take the tooth's form.

Taking shortcuts while placing composite resin materials may save the dentist time but could hurt the patient. Regarding the idea that wearing out of composites might stress the biochemical system of the body may have merit. However, the symptoms that have been described (to a "T") are that of myofascial pain dysfunction that results from the loss of what is known as posterior support. The composites wear out leaving a less than optimal structural platform for function to occur. When this happens, the muscles try harder and harder to work with the poorly balanced structures (teeth). The muscles then are in dysfunction and cause pain syndromes with the symptoms that have been described.

As for the other characteristics: It is true that everything wears. An underlying issue to answer is why are they wearing. Natural teeth, in a well-balanced system, do not exhibit wear. The problems then come in when people have some other mitigating condition. For example, TMJ problems, neurological problems, or airway problems can and do lead to horrendous issues of health and tooth destruction. Dentists are very good at repairing a tooth but all too often it is simply restored into the dysfunction that caused the problem to begin with.

Think of teeth as circuit breakers. In this context, when there is an overload in the system "upstream" the downstream weak link, the tooth/teeth, pop. This can be seen as a vertical fracture of the whole tooth, an oblique fracture of the tooth, a notch at the gum line, the death of the pulp, vertical bone loss, and so on. It is imperative to get a proper diagnosis of these upstream problems to truly help the patient rather than just looking to the teeth and the materials of restoration as the inciting problem. It is rather most often the resultant obvious problem that even a casual observer can detect.

TOOTH/BODY CONNECTION

Remember the children's song "the shin bone's connected to the knee bone"?[66] Well, what if you knew your wisdom teeth have an energetic connection to your heart? Have you heard of eye teeth? The cuspids are called the eye teeth and actually lie on the meridian associated with the eye.

Thousands of years ago, the Chinese discovered the human body was flowing with an invisible energy. They called the energy Qi (also spelled Chi) pronounced "Chee." The Chinese found ways to measure the amount of chi and discovered a network of pathways on which the energy flowed. These pathways are called meridians.

The flow of the Chi is essential to good health. When the body is in good health, the chi flows smoothly. Any disturbance in the ease of flow may result in disease. Think of breathing—when healthy, the air goes in and out smoothly. When there is a disturbance in that flow, the results cause either disease or death.

The meridians connect particular organs together to create balance. Every Yin (female) organ is paired with a Yang (male) organ. Examples are liver with the gallbladder, lungs with large intestine, kidney with bladder, stomach with spleen, and heart with small intestine. Each of these meridians have designated teeth to specific organs.

Our bodies are electric! The flow of energy through the body on these meridians is invisible to the naked eye, it is not imaginary! We use EKGs and EEGs to measure the electricity in our heart tissue and brains. If energy is flowing through these meridians and a disturbance occurs it would be like you blowing a circuit breaker and having a lamp not work in the bedroom and yet, two rooms away the washer now does not work and neither does the dishwasher. They are all on the same circuit breaker in that home. Would you go out and buy a new lamp, dishwasher, or washing machine to fix the problem? No, you would correct the flow of electricity on that circuit.

Dr. Voll was a German physician who found a way to measure the flow of the energy on the meridians in the 1940s. He felt that 80% of the disturbances in the flow of chi were found in the oral cavity.

Forty years of electrodermal screening research by Dr. Reinhard Voll demonstrated that about 80% of all illness is related to decay in the mouth.[73] His research shows that since the teeth are connected to every organ and gland via the blood stream, any infection that the mouth harbors affects the body's overall health.

Dr. Voll developed equipment to measure the burdens of dead teeth, extraction sites, and dental restorations on the body. I had a patient with a gold crown placed on a lower molar who experienced an elevation of blood pressure. Your traditional physician rarely asks what dental work you have recently had done before writing a prescription. Those lower molars are on the energetic pathway for arteries and veins. The gold can stimulate an increase in blood pressure. In that case, changing the crowns to a different material solved the issue.

Implants are often titanium. Titanium placed into a jaw can short out the meridian and thus create a problem for the organs related to that area. A patient with a compromised immune system might react to the material, not just react like an allergy but react by reducing T-cells.

ROOT CANAL—UNDERSTANDING THE IMPLICATIONS

Most people think of their teeth as just a piece of nonliving bone. They think it is solid and not porous. Truth is, a tooth is a living organ. It has a blood supply, a nerve, and a lymphatic supply. It is made of microscopic tubes. When a tooth is healthy a flow of fluid goes from the inside through the tubules to the outside. Think of it as if the tooth is detoxing. It pushes the waste away through those tubules to the outside of the tooth. When a root canal is done, the dentist attempts to remove the blood supply, nerve, and lymphatic tissues.

Over 50,000,000 (50 million) teeth are "saved" in the United States alone every year by having a "root canal" done on them. This common name for this treatment is really a misnomer. The root canal in a tooth is the portion in the center of the tooth that goes down into the roots (usually two roots—sometimes three or even four). When a "root canal" is done by the dentist, he or she removes the nerve in the center of the tooth and the pulp which surrounds it. This nerve and pulp go all the way down from under the "crown" of the tooth to the end of the roots in the jaw. This is usually done because the decay has penetrated the center of the tooth and a "normal" filling is impossible because it would press on the nerve and be incredibly painful. The "root canal" process itself has a reputation for being quite painful.

When the nerve and pulp of the tooth are removed by this procedure, they are replaced with an inert substance—usually the rubber-like "gutta percha." The dentist attempts to sterilize the tooth before the gutta percha is inserted in the "root canal." The object is to cut off the normal circulation of bacteria through the tooth and make it permanently sterile.

Unfortunately, this never works and it has been proven that this is impossible. The tooth becomes a dead piece of bone in the jaw. The bacteria that were in the millions of tiny "tubules" in the dentin of the tooth (the portion between the enamel and the root canal) mutate into "anaerobic" bacteria. The one thing that is impossible for a dentist to remove is the flesh inside those small tubules that make up the tooth. In some teeth that can be 3 miles of tubules. These are bacteria that do not require oxygen. Every root canal-filled tooth has them. No exceptions. They occur because of the structure of the root canal filling. It is impossible to eliminate them and they are 1000 times more toxic than any other bacteria. In fact, the toxins they put out are in the form of a gas called "thio-ethers" which can easily migrate through the enamel of the tooth and down through the roots into the bloodstream. These toxins travel throughout the body, as do many of the bacteria themselves. These are responsible for most chronic degenerative conditions…not just cancer, but rheumatoid arthritis, heart disease, multiple sclerosis, lupus, ALS, and diabetes. Think of it as botulism in a tooth, but actually it is more toxic than botulism. Once a root canal is done, a crown is placed because the tooth becomes brittle and can fracture at the gum. Even if a root canal is lasered or ozonated to reduce the bacteria, that procedure will not last long at all because the flesh inside those tubules starts to rot. Where else in medicine do we taxidermy an organ and leave it in the living body and then tell the patient you will be fine? For a diabetic, this chronic low grade infection can and usually does make their blood sugars unmanageable. For a person with a compromised immune system we see things like rheumatoid arthritis, elevated ANA (antinuclear antigen) and, of course, cancer.

Evidence

Dr. Weston Price, beginning in 1903, led a study by 60 prominent dentists. Their mission was to find a safe way to perform a root canal filling. In 1923, they submitted their 1174 pages of research to the American Dental Association (ADA). The team's conclusion: there is no safe way to do a root canal filling. Why, you ask, are 50 million of these done every year in the United States 87 years later? And why are they done exactly the same way they were in Dr. Price's time? A key assumption of Dr. Weston Price's team was something called "focal infection." This just means that an infection somewhere in your body (your mouth, for example) can affect organs distant from it. This concept is taught in all medical schools now and has been for many years. At the time, however, it was controversial. The conservatives at that time rejected Dr. Price's team's conclusions because they did not believe in the "focal infection" concept. You'll find Dr. Price's research summarized in a book called *Root Canal Cover-Up* by Dr. George Meinig, D.D.S., F.A.C.D. Dr. Meinig passed away in 2008. He was a prominent endodontist (root canal specialist). After he retired in 1993 from 50 years of practice, he discovered Dr. Price's 1923 research report. He was horrified when he considered the thousands of people whose health he had ruined in his 50 years of practice by doing root canal fillings. As a "*mea culpa,*" Dr. Meinig wrote the *Root Canal Cover-Up* and spent the last 15 years of his life trying to get his message out to people about how deadly root canal-filled teeth are. Here's what Dr. Hal Huggins says about Dr. Weston Price's research: "*Dr. Weston Price and Mayo Clinic of 1910 to 1920 described finding bacterial growth in root canals that could be transferred into animals and create the same diseases the donor human had in from 80 to 100% of the animals. Heart disease, in particular, could be transferred 100% of the time. His research has since been suppressed by the various Dental Associations in the United States.*"

A root canal can create a total blockage in the flow of energy to the organs on that meridian which could result in disease. Sometimes the disturbance in the flow of energy is with an organ on that meridian which can cause a toothache or, even worse, a spontaneous abscess.

If the patient is not responding to conventional therapy, start looking for a root cause. Often this involves looking at the patient's dental charting and using a dental meridian chart to find the link between the tooth and the organ. There are ways to test the burdens of the individual teeth and extraction sites.

Many people postpone getting their jaw evaluated by one of these competent dentists. It is common to procrastinate on dental work. It is costly, usually not covered by insurance, and often painful. This procrastination or ignorance has cost millions of people their lives (Figure 7.8).

The Tooth and Organ Connection

The teeth are connected to the rest of the body and are aligned with the circuitry of many meridians of energy (Figure 7.8). This is helpful information in determining why a tooth may display decay or discomfort.[75]

Tooth #1 Upper right third molar (wisdom tooth): Anterior lobe of the pituitary gland, internal ear on the right side, part of the tongue on the right, ulnar side of the right shoulder, plantar side of the right foot, right toes, ulnar side of the right elbow, ulnar side of the right hand, sacro-iliac joint on the right, segments of spinal marrow and dermatomes (SC1, SC2, SC8, STH1, STH5, STH6, STH7, SS1, SS2), vertebrae (C1, C2, C7, TH1, TH5, TH6, TH7, S1, S2), right side of the heart, duodenum, terminal ileum on the right, central nervous system, limbic system, the mid trapezius muscle.

Tooth #2 Upper right second molar: Shares with #3. *The right side of parathyroid gland and the right side of abdominal muscle relate to #2 only.*

Tooth #3 Upper right first molar: Tongue on right, maxillary sinus, oropharynx, larynx, jaw on right side, right anterior hip, right anterior knee, right medial ankle joint, spinal marrow and dermatomes (SC1, SC2, STH11, STH12, SL1), vertebrae (C1, C2, TH11, TH12, L1), pancreas, esophagus, right side of the stomach, right breast. *The right latissimus dorsi and the right side of the thyroid relate to #3 only.*

Tooth #4 Upper right second bicuspid: Shares with #5. *The thymus gland, right breast, and the right side of the diaphragm muscle relate to tooth #4 only.*

Tooth #5 Upper right first bicuspid: Nose on the right side, ethmoid sinus, radial side of shoulder on the right, radial side of elbow on the right, radial side of hand on the right, right foot, big toe on the right foot, spinal marrow and dermatomes (SC1, SC2, SC5, SC6, SC7, STH2, STH3, STH4, SL4, SL5), vertebrae (C1, C2, C5, C6, C7, TH2, TH3, TH4, L4, L5), right lung, bronchi, large intestine on the right side. The pectoralis major clavicular relates to both tooth #4 and #5. *The right coracobrachialis popliteus and posterior lobe of the pituitary gland relate to #5 only.*

Tooth #6 Upper right cuspid: Intermediate lobe of the pituitary gland, hypothalamus, posterior portion of the right eye, sphenoidal sinus, tonsilla palate, posterior portion of the right knee, right hip, lateral side of the right ankle, spinal marrow and dermatomes (SC1, SC2, STH8, STH9, STH10), vertebrae (C1, C2, TH8, TH9, TH10), right side of the liver, gall bladder, biliary ducts on the right side. The right deltoid and right anterior serratus.

Tooth #7 Upper right lateral incisor: Same meridian as #8. *The right subscapularis relates to tooth #7 only.*

Tooth #8 Upper right central incisor: Pineal gland, the nose, sphenoidal sinus and frontal sinus on the right side, posterior right knee, right sacro-coccygeal joint, posterior right ankle joint, spinal

Upper arch (teeth 1–16)

Tooth	Traditional Chinese meridian organs	Associated western medicine joints, organs and glands
1	Heart, small int., circulation/sex, triple warmer	Right: shoulder, elbow, hand (ulnar) sacroiliac, foot, toes, middle Ear. Right heart, Rt. duodenum, terminal ileum. CNS. Ant pituitary
2, 3	Stomach pancreas	Right: TMJ, anterior hip/knee, medial ankle. Sinus: maxillary. oropharynx, larynx, esophagus, Rt. side of stomach. #2 parathyroid; #3 Thyroid Right breast
4, 5	Lung large intestine	Right: shoulder, elbow, hand (radial), foot, big toe. Sinus: paranasal and ethmoid. Bronchus, nose. Right lung. Right side of large intestine #4 Right breast
6	Liver gallbladder	Right: post. knee, hip, lateral ankle. Sinus: sphenoid. palatine tonsil. Eye. Hypothal. Rt. liver, gallbladder.
7, 8	Kidney bladder	Right: Post. knee. Sacroiliac joint. Post. ankle. Sinus: frontal pharyngeal tonsil. Pineal. Right kidney, bladder, ovary, uterus, prostate, testicle, rectum
9, 10	Kidney bladder	Left: Post. knee. Sacroiliac joint. Post. ankle. Sinus: frontal pharyngeal tonsil. pineal. left kidney, bladder, ovary, uterus, prostate, testicle, rectum
11	Liver gallbladder	Left: post. knee, hip. lateral ankle. Sinus: sphenoid. Palatine tonsil. Eye. Hypothal. Left liver, biliary ducts.
12, 13	Lung large intestine	Left: shoulder, elbow, hand (radial), foot, big toe. Sinus: paranasal and ethmoid. bronchus, Nose. Left lung. Left side large intestine #13 Left Breast
14, 15	Stomach spleen	Left: TMJ, anterior hip/knee, medial ankle. Sinus: Maxillary. Oropharynx, Larynx, esophagus, Left Side of stomach. #14: Thyroid #15: Parathyroid Left breast
16, 17	Heart, small int., circulation/sex, triple warmer	Left: Shoulder, elbow, hand (ulnar) sacroiliac, foot, toes, middle ear. Left heart, Jejunum, Ileum. CNS. Ant pituitary

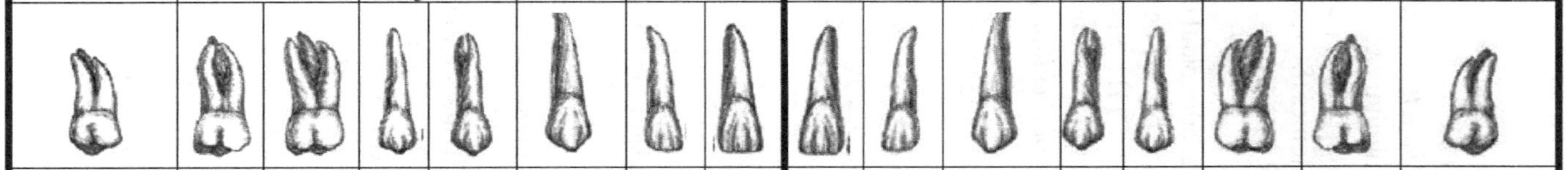

Lower arch (teeth 17–32)

Tooth	Traditional Chinese meridian organs	Associated western medicine joints, organs and glands
32	Heart, small int., circulation/sex, triple warmer	Right: shoulder, elbow, hand (ulnar) sacroiliac, foot, toes, middle Ear. Right heart, Rt. duodenum, terminal ileum. CNS.
31, 30	Lung large intestine	Right: shoulder, elbow, hand (radial) Sinus: paranasal and ethmoid. Bronchus, nose. Right lung. Right side of large intestine
29, 28	Stomach pancreas	Right: TMJ, anterior hip/knee, medial ankle. Sinus: maxillary. Oropharynx, larynx, esophagus, Rt. side of stomach. #28: ovaries, Testes right breast
27	Liver gallbladder	Right: Post. knee, hip, lateral ankle Sinus: sphenoid Palat. Tonsil. Eye ovaries testes Rt. liver, gallbladder.
26, 25	Kidney bladder	Right: post. knee. Sacroiliac joint. Post. ankle. Sinus: frontal Pharyngeal tonsil. Adrenal. Right kidney, bladder, ovary, uterus, prostate, testicle, rectum
24, 23	Kidney bladder	Left: post. knee. Sacroiliac joint. Post. ankle. Sinus: frontal Pharyngeal tonsil. Adrenal. Left kidney, bladder, ovary, uterus, prostate, testicle, rectum
22	Liver gallbladder	Left: post. knee, hip, lateral ankle. Sinus: sphenoid Palat. Tonsil. Eye. Ovaries, testes. Left liver, biliary ducts.
21, 20	Spleen stomach	Left: TMJ, anterior hip/knee, medial ankle. Sinus: Maxillary. Oropharynx, larynx, esophagus, left Side of stomach. #21: ovaries, Testes left breast
19, 18	Lung large intestine	Left: shoulder, elbow, hand (radial), foot, big toe. Sinus: paranasal and ethmoid. Bronchus, nose. Left lung. Left side large intestine
17	Heart, small int., circulation/sex, triple warmer	Left: shoulder, elbow, hand (ulnar) sacroiliac, foot, toes, middle ear. Left heart, Jejunum, Ileum. CNS. Ant pituitary

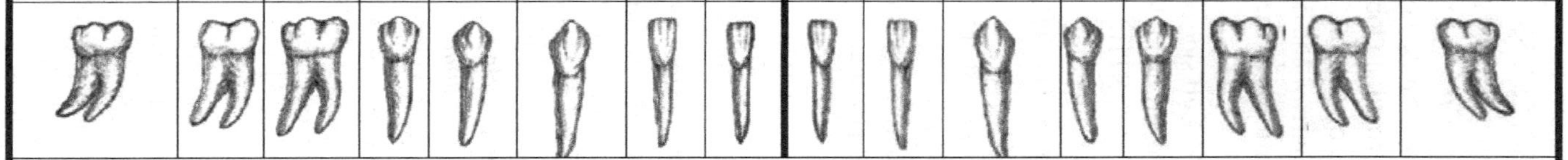

FIGURE 7.8 A traditional Chinese tooth organ chart.

marrow and dermatomes (SC1, SC2, SL2, SL3, SS3, SS4, SS5, SCo), vertebrae (C1, C2, L2, L3, S3, S4, S5, SCo), right kidney, right side of the bladder, ovary, testicle, prostate, uterus, rectum, and anal canal. *The right side neck flexors and extensors relate to #8 only.*

Tooth #9 Upper left central incisor: Pineal gland, the nose, sphenoidal sinus and frontal sinus on the left side, posterior left knee, left sacro-coccygeal joint, posterior left ankle joint, spinal marrow and dermatomes (SC1, SC2, SL2, SL3, SS3, SS4, SS5, SCo), vertebrae (C1, C2, L2, L3, S3, S4, S5, SCo), left kidney, urinary bladder left side, ovary, testicle, prostate, uterus, rectum, and anal canal. *The left side neck flexors and extensors relate to tooth #9.*

Tooth #10 Upper left lateral incisor: Same as #9. *The left subscapularis relates to #10 only.*

Tooth #11 Upper left cuspid: Intermediate lobe of pituitary gland, hypothalamus, posterior portion of the left eye, sphenoidal sinus on the left, tonsilla palate, posterior of the left knee, left hip, lateral side of the left ankle, spinal marrow and dermatomes (SC1, SC2, STH8, STH9, STH10), vertebrae (C1, C2, TH8, TH9, TH10), left side of the liver, bilary ducts on the left side. The left deltoid and left anterior serratus.

Tooth #12 Upper left first bicuspid: Left side of nose, ethmoidal cells, radial side of left shoulder, radial side of left elbow, radial side of left hand, left foot, big toe on the left foot, spinal marrow and dermatomes (SC1, SC2, SC5, SC6, SC7, STH2, STH3, STH4, SL4, SL5), vertebrae, (C1, C2, C5, C6, C7, TH2, TH3, TH4, L4, L5), left lung, bronchi, large intestine on the left side. The pectoralis major clavicular relates to #12 and #13. *The left coracobrachialis popliteus and posterior lobe of the pituitary gland relates to #12 only.*

Tooth #13 Upper left second bicuspid: Shares the meridian with #12. *The thymus gland, breast, and the left diaphragm relate to #13 only.*

Tooth #14 Upper left first molar: *Thyroid gland relates to #14 only.* Tongue on the left, maxillary sinus, orapharynx, larynx, left side of jaw, anterior left hip, anterior left knee, left medial ankle joint, spinal marrow and dermatomes (SC1, SC2, STH11, STH12, SL1), vertebrae (C1, C2, TH11, TH12, L1), spleen, esophagus, left side stomach, left breast. *Tooth #14 is related to the left latissimus dorsi.*

Tooth #15 Upper left second molar: Shares meridian with #14. *The parathyroid gland and the left abdominal muscle relate to #15 only.*

Tooth #16 Upper left third molar (wisdom tooth): Anterior lobe of pituitary gland, internal ear on left side, part of the tongue on the left side, ulnar side of the left shoulder, plantar side of the left foot, left toes, ulnar side of the left elbow, ulnar side of the left hand, sacro-iliac joint on left, spinal marrow and dermatomes (SC1, SC2, SC8, STH1, STH5, STH6, STH7, SS1, SS2), vertebrae (C1, C2, C7, TH1, TH5, TH6, TH7, S1, S2), left side of heart, duodenum, ileum, jejunum, central nervous system, limbic system, mid-trapezius muscle.

Tooth #17 Lower left third molar (wisdom tooth): Tongue, middle external ear, sacro-iliac joint on left side, ulnar side of left hand, plantar side of left foot, toes, left shoulder, left elbow, spinal marrow and dermatomes (SC1, SC2, SC8, STH1, STH5, STH6, STH7, SS1, SS2), vertebrae (C1, C2, C7, TH1, TH5, TH6, TH7, S1, S2), left side of the heart, left side of jejunum, left side of ileum, peripheral nerves, energy exchange, psoas muscle.

Tooth #18 Lower left second molar: Shares the meridian with #19. *The arteries and the left quadriceps relate to tooth #18 only.*

Tooth #19 Lower left first molar: Nose, ethmoid cells, radial side of left hand, foot, big toe, left shoulder, left elbow, spinal marrow and dermatomes (SC1, SC2, SC5, SC6, SC7, STH2, STH3, STH4, SL4, SL5), vertebrae (C1, C2, C5, C6, C7, TH2, TH3, TH4, L4, L5), left lung, left side of large intestine. *The veins and the left muscles gracilis and sartorius relate to #19 only.*

Tooth #20 Lower left second bicuspid: Shares the meridian with #21. *The lymph vessels, and the left pect. maj. sternal relate to tooth #20 only.*

Tooth #21 Lower left first bicuspid: Tongue, left maxillary sinus, left jaw, left medial ankle joint, left anterior hip, left anterior knee, spinal marrow and dermatomes (SC1, SC2, STH11, STH12, SL1), vertebrae (C1, C2, TH11, TH12, L1), spleen, esophagus, stomach on the left side, left mammary glands, hamstrings. *The left gonads and left quadratus lumborum relate to #21 only.*

Tooth #22 Lower left cuspid: Gonads, anterior portion of the left eye, sphenoidal sinus, lateral left ankle joint, left hip, posterior left knee, spinal marrow and dermatomes (SC1, SC2, STH8, STH9, STH10), vertebrae (C1, C2, TH8, TH9, TH10), left side of the liver, left biliary ducts, gluteus maximus.

Tooth #23 Lower left lateral incisor: Shares the meridian with #24. *The left tensor fasciae latae and left pyriformis are related to #23 only.*

Tooth #24 Lower left central incisor: Adrenal gland, sphenoidal sinus, frontal sinus, posterior of left ankle joint, left sacro-coccygeal joint, posterior of left knee, spinal marrow and dermatomes (SC1, SC2, SL2, SL3, SS3, SS4, SS5, SCo), vertebrae (C1, C2, L2, L3, S3, S4, S5, Co), left kidney, rectum, anal canal, urinary bladder, left ovary/testicle, prostate/uterus. *The gluteus medius on the left side relates to #24 only.*

Tooth #25 Lower right central incisor: Shares meridian with #26. *The gluteus medius on the right side relates to #25 only.*

Tooth #26 Lower right lateral incisor: Adrenal gland, sphenoidal sinus, frontal sinus, posterior of right ankle, right sacro-coccygeal joint, posterior of right knee, spinal marrow and dermatomes (SC1, SC2, SL2, SL3, SS4, SS5, SCo), vertebrae (C1, C2, L2, L3, S3, S4, S5, Co), right kidney, rectum, anal canal, urinary bladder, right ovary/testicle, prostate/uterus. *The right tensor fasciae latae and right pyriformis relate to #26 only.*

Tooth #27 Lower right cuspid: Gonads, anterior portion of the right eye, sphenoidal sinus, lateral of right ankle joint, right hip, posterior of right knee, spinal marrow and dermatomes (SC1, SC2, STH8, STH9, STH10), vertebrae (C1, C2, TH8, TH9, TH10), right side of the liver, biliary ducts right side, gallbladder, right gluteus maximus.

Tooth #28 Lower right first bicuspid: Shares the meridian with #29. *The right gonads and right quadratus lumborum relate to #28 only.*

Tooth #29 Lower right second bicuspid: Tongue, right maxillary sinus, right jaw, medial of right ankle, right anterior hip, anterior of right knee, spinal marrow and dermatomes (SC1, SC2, STH11, STH12, SL1), vertebrae (C1, C2,TH11, TH12, L1), pancreas, esophagus, right side of stomach, right mammary glands, hamstrings. *The lymph vessels and the right pect. maj. sternal relate to #29 only.*

Tooth #30 Lower right first molar: Shares the meridian with #31. *The veins and the right muscles gracilis and sartorius relate to #30 only.*

Tooth #31 Lower right second molar: Nose, ethmoidal cells, radial side of the right hand, right foot, big toe, right shoulder, right elbow, spinal marrow and dermatomes (SC1, SC2, SC5, SC6, SC7, STH2, STH3, STH4, SL4, SL5), vertebrae (C1, C2, C5, C6, C7, TH2, TH3, TH4. L4, L5), lung on the right side, large intestine on the right side, ileo-cecal area. *The arteries and the right quadriceps relate to #31 only.*

Tooth #32 Lower right third molar (wisdom tooth): Tongue, middle external ear, sacro-iliac joint on right side, ulnar side of the right hand, plantar side of the right foot, toes, right shoulder, right elbow, spinal marrow and dermatomes (SC1, SC2, SC8, STH1, STH5, STH6, STH7, SS1, SS2), vertebrae (C1, C2, C7, TH1, TH5, TH6, TH7, S1, S2), right side of the heart, terminal ileum, peripheral nerves, energy exchange, psoas muscle.

ORAL HOME CARE

Traditional oral hygiene care can be effective; however, many toothpastes, mouthwashes, whitening products, and fluoride contain chemicals that can alter the health of the body. Special attention should be given to reading labels and understanding the efficacy of the ingredients especially in the "harmful if swallowed" aisle of the store. The true health of the teeth comes from within and external products have their limitations. The multitude of chemicals that are used in commercial toothpastes are not ideal for the delicate tissue in the body because they are absorbed through the mucous membranes. This is especially true when bleeding gums are evident because anything in the mouth will have direct access to the bloodstream. The following synthetic ingredients are commonly found in most toothpaste.

Fluoride

Tooth decay is not from a fluoride deficiency. Fluoride accumulates in the body and can lower IQ, form as deposits in the brain related to Alzheimer's, promotes early onset of puberty, and so on.[74]

Propylene Glycol

This is frequently used as antifreeze and to deice airplanes. It is produced from fossil fuels during the oil-refining process and can irritate the skin and mucous membranes and increase overall acidity of the body, leading to metabolic acidosis. Although it is present in toothpaste in small amounts, daily use makes it potentially harmful.

FD&C Color Pigments

Many of the food, drug and cosmetic (FD&C) coloring additives approved by the U.S. Food and Drug Administration are tainted with heavy metals that can accumulate in the body.

Artificial Sweeteners

Ethanol (Ethyl Alcohol)

A drying agent that facilitates the entry of other toothpaste ingredients into the gums.

Triclosan

A biopersistent chemical, triclosan is registered as a pesticide that destroys fragile aquatic ecosystems.

Trisodium Phosphate (TSP)

TSP is widely used in household cleaners and detergents as a powerful cleaner and degreaser. When consumed, it can reduce lactic acid buildup, which may be important since artificial sweeteners in toothpastes are metabolized into lactic acid. Overtime, TSP can cause tumor lesions, gum bleeding, and nerve inflammation.

Glycerin

A clear, slick gel is an inexpensive filler and carrier for the low-concentration substances that are highlighted as active ingredients. It is made up of dried vegetables that are repeatedly bleached and deodorized. When it coats the teeth, it also blocks the saliva's ability to remineralize the enamel.

Calcium

Calcium carbonate is an abrasive cleaning agent added to toothpaste to remove calculus and plaque plus help with tooth sensitivity. It is found in eggshells, seashells, limestone, chalk, marble, and other kinds of stones; however, it is not water soluble or readily bioavailable.

Flavoring

Flavoring is typically added to mask the unpleasant taste of the detergents in toothpaste. These synthetic flavors are made in a beaker rather than from a plant such as menthol and cinnamaldehyde.

Detergents and Surfactants

These create the foaming action of toothpaste using sodium laureth sulfate (SLES), ammonium laureth sulfate (ALES), sodium lauryl sulfate (SLS), and ammonium lauryl sulfate (ALS). They are known as skin irritants, hormone and endocrine disruptors, and suspected gene mutagens and carcinogens.

Carrageenan

A gummy, gel-like substance that is extracted from red seaweed. These can potentially upset the gastrointestinal system and immune system.

Hydrated Silica

This is added to create an abrasiveness for polishing and scrubbing the surface of the teeth in gel toothpastes. Pollutants and toxins are usually added to this natural product in the manufacturing and refining process.

Carbomer

This is an airy, white powder carbomer that absorbs water and thickens liquid ingredients into a paste and stabilizes the paste so it doesn't separate. This is a polymer of acrylic acid, one of the by-products of gasoline production. These polymers are acid so another chemical is necessary to neutralize it enough to prevent burning in the mouth. They can include sodium hydroxide, tetra sodium EDTA, or triethanolamine (TEA).

A HOLISTIC APPROACH TO DENTAL CARE

Incorporating natural products is generally safer, gentler, and more potent. All botanical oils are antibacterial, antiviral, antifungal, and can remove harmful oral microbes. They can rejuvenate the gum tissue and increase blood circulation to the gums and blood vessels in the mouth. As a result, they can prevent the immune system from becoming compromised. They reduce bacteria, viral loads, chronic inflammation, and a congested lymph system. Essential oils and extracts are highly concentrated lipophilic liquids. Some botanical oils will require an entire plant to create a single drop of oil. Due to the fact that essential oils are lipid-soluble, they can penetrate the lipid layer of the skin and gums and reach the immune system quickly. Bacteria will not develop resistance to essential oils yet they can become resistant to antibiotics.

REFERENCES

1. Larmas M. Dental caries seen from the pulpal side: A nontraditional approach. *J Dent Res* 2003;82:253. Miller WD. The human mouth as a focus of infection. *Dent Cosmos* 1891;33:689, 789, 913.
2. Colgate quote from website. http://www.colgate.com/en/us/oc/oral-health/conditions/plaque-and-tartar/article/what-is-plaque.
3. Steinman RR, O'Day P. Intraperitoneal injected carbohydrate on the incidence of caries, dentinal circulation related to diet. 1958.
4. Roggenkamp C. *Dentinal Fluid Transport*, xiii. Loma Linda, CA: Loma Linda University Press, 2004.
5. Leonora J, Steinmann RR. DFT, its cariostatic effect. Teaching syllabus, ca. 1981.
6. Steinman RR, Smith LV. The physiological basis for caries susceptibility and resistance. *J South Calif Dent Assn* 1961;29(7):221–224.
7. Tièche JM, Leonora J. Acute secretion of immunoreactive parotid hormone in response to different diets in the pig. *Arch Oral Biol* 1995;40(6):559–565.
8. Roggenkamp C. *Dentinal Fluid Transport*, ix. Loma Linda, CA: Loma Linda University Press, 2004.
9. Steinman RR, Leonora J. Relationship of fluid transport through the dentin to the incidence of dental caries. *J Dent Res* 1971;50(6) Part 2:1536–1543.
10. Steinman RR. The control of dental caries by manipulating dentinal fluid movement. *J Missouri Dent Assn* 1977;57(7):15–18.
11. Sanchez A, Steinman RR, Leonora J. Effect of diet on dentinal fluid movement in germfree and non-germfree rats. *Am J Clin Nutr* 1970;23:686–690.
12. Huggins HA. *Why Raise Ugly Kids? How You Can Fulfill Your Child's Health and Happiness Potential.* Westport, CT: Arlington House, 1981, 145–146.
13. Steinman RR. Can dental caries susceptibility be affected by the ingestion of carbohydrates? *J Indiana State Dent Assoc* 1960;39:130–134.
14. Steinman RR. The clinical significance of the physiologic approach to the control of dental caries. *J Missouri Dental Assn* 1977;57(7):15–18.
15. Steinman RR, Leonora J. Susceptibility to dental caries. *Austral Dent J* 1979;24:222–224.
16. Artemis N. *Holistic Dental Care: The Complete Guide to Healthy Teeth and Gums (Kindle Location 375).* Berkeley, CA: North Atlantic Books, 2013-10-08.

17. Steinman RR. The physiologic nature of caries susceptibility. Part III. Physiologic aspects of resistance to dental caries. *J Alabama Dent Assn* 1983;67:46–49.
18. Zijnge V et al. Oral biofilm architecture on natural teeth. *PLoSOne* 2010;5(2):e9321.
19. Sbordone L, Bortolaia C. Oral microbial biofilms and plaque-related disease: Microbial communities and their shift from oral health to disease. *Clin Oral Investig.* 2003;7(4):181–188.
20. Evans CA, Kleinman DV. Oral health in America: A report of the surgeon general. The surgeon general's report on America's oral heath: Opportunities for the dental professional. *JADA* 2000;131:1728. US Dept. of Health and Human Services National Institute of Health.
21. El-Shinnawi U, Soory M. Associations between periodontitis and systemic inflammatory diseases: Response to treatment. *Recent Pat Endocr Metab Immune Drug Discov.* 2013;7(3):169–188.
22. Ambooken M et al. Periodontal infections and atherosclerosis: Mechanisms of association. *Oral Maxilloac Pathol J* 2015;6(2):615–620.
23. Pessi T et al. Bacterial signatures in thrombus aspirates of patients with myocardial infarction. *Circulation* Mar 2013 19;127(11):1219–1228.
24. Gurenlian J. Inflammation: The relationship between oral health and systemic disease. Access. April 2006.
25. Beck J et al. Periodontal disease and cardiovascular disease. *J Periodontol* 1996;67:1123–1137.
26. Genco RJ, Borgnakke WS. Risk factors for periodontal disease. *Periodontol 2000* 2013;62:59–94.
27. www.perioartsinstitute.com
28. Palcanis K. Executive Director, American Board of Periodontology. 2015.
29. Smiley C et al. Evidence based clinical practice guideline on the nonsurgical treatment of chronic periodontitis by means of scaling and root planning with or without adjuncts. *JADA* 2015;146(7):525–535.
30. Scannapieco FA. The oral microbiome: Its role in health and in oral and systemic infections. *Clinical Micorbiology Newsletter* 2013;35:163–169.
31. Giannobile WV. Salivary diagnostics for periodontal diseases. *J Am Dent Assoc* 2012;143(Suppl 10):6S–11S.
32. Mattila KJ et al. Association between dental health and acute myocardial infarction. *BMJ* 1989;298:779–781.
33. Axel S et al. Role of periodontal bacteria and importance of total pathogen burden in coronary artery event and periodontal disease (CORODENT) study. *Arch Intern Med* 2006;166(5):554–559.
34. Beck JD et al. Oral health and systemic disease: Periodontitis and cardiovascular disease. *J Dent Educ* 1998;62:859–870.
35. Mantyla P et al. Subgingival aggregatibacter actinomycetemcomitans associates with the risk of coronary artery disease. *J Clin Periodontol* 2013;40:583–590.
36. Bahekar AA et al. The prevalence and incidence of coronary heart disease is significantly increased in periodontitis: A meta-analysis. *American Heart Journal (AHJ)* 2007;154(5):830–837.
37. Bale B et al. High-risk periodontal pathogens contribute to the pathogenesis of atherosclerosis. *Postgrad Med J* 2016;0:1–6. doi:10.1136/postgradmedj-2016-134279
38. Mealey BL, Rose LF. Diabetes mellitus and inflammatory periodontal diseases. *Curr Opin Endocrinol Diabetes Obes* 2008;15:135–141.
39. Llambes F et al. Relationship between diabetes and periodontal infection. *World J Diabetes* 2015;6(7):927–935 and Preshaw PM et al. Periodontitis and diabetes: A two-way relationship. *Diabetologia* 2012 Jan;55(1):21–31.
40. Soorya KV et al. The effect of scaling and root planing on glycaemic control, periodontal status and gingival crevicular fluid TNF-α levels in an Indian population—To Reveal the Ambivalent Link. *J Clin Diagn Res* 2014;8(11):ZC22–ZC26.
41. Lamster IB et al. The relationship between oral health and diabetes mellitus. *J Am Dent Assoc* 2008;139(Suppl):19–24.
42. Van der Putten C et al. Hot topic in geriatric medicine: The importance of oral health in (frail) elderly people—a review. *European Geriatric Medicine* 2013;4:339–344.
43. Miklossy J. Alzheimer's Disease—a neurospirochetosis: Analysis of the evidence following Koch's and Hill's criteria. *J Neuroinflammation* 2011;8:90.
44. Singhrao S et al. Porphyromonas gingivalis: Periodontal infection and its putative links with Alzheimer's disease. Mediators of Inflammation. http://dx.doi.org/10.115/2015/137357
45. Watts A et al. Inflammation as a potent mediator for the association between periodontal disease and Alzheimer's disease. *Neuropsychiatr Dis Treat* 2008;4(5):865–876.
46. Ogrendik M. Rheumatoid arthritis is an autoimmune disease caused by periodontal pathogens. *Int J Gen Med* 2013;6:383–386.

47. Kobayashi T et al. Host Response in the link between periodontitis and rheumatoid arthritis. *Curr Oral Health Rep* 2015;2:1–8.
48. Smolik I et al. Periodontitis and rheumatoid arthritis: Epidemiological, clinical and immunological associations. *Compend Contin Educ Dent* 2009;30(4):188–192.
49. Han Y. Fusobacterium nucleatum: A commensal-turned pathogen. *Current Opinion in Microbiology* 2015;23:141–147.
50. Nwhator SO et al. Could periodontitis affect time to conception? *Ann Med Health Sci Res* 2014;4(5):817–822.
51. Hart R et al. Periodontal disease: A potential modifiable risk factor limiting conception. *Hum Reprod* 2012;27(5):1332–1334.
52. Goepfert A et al. Periodontal disease and upper genital tract inflammation in early spontaneous pre-term birth. *Obstetrics & Gynecology* 2004;100(4):777–783 and Xiong X, et al. Periodontal disease and adverse pregnancy outcomes: A systematic review. *BJOG An International Journal of Obstetrics and Gynaecology* 2006;113:135–143.
53. Usher A, Stockley R. The link between chronic periodontitis and COPD: A common role for the neutrophil? *BMC Medicine* 2013;11:241.
54. Peter KP et al. Association between periodontal disease and chronic obstructive pulmonary disease: A reality or just a dogma? *J Periodontol* 2013;84(12):1717–1723.
55. Scannapieco FA, Genco RJ. Association of periodontal infections with atherosclerotic and pulmonary diseases. *J Perio Research.* 1999;7(34):340–345.
56. Marks PV et al. Multiple brain abscesses secondary to dental caries and severe periodontal disease. *Br J Oral Maxillofac Surg.* 1988;26(3):244–247 and Mylonas AI et al. Cerebral abscess of odontogenic origin. *J Craniomaxillofac Surg* 2007 Jan;35(1):63–7.
57. Martin BF et al. Brain abscess due to actinobacillus actinomycetemcomitans. *Neurology* 1967;17:833–837.
58. Tezal M et al. Chronic periodontitis and the incidence of head and neck squamous cell carcinoma. *Cancer Epidemiol Biomarkers Prev* 2009;18:2306–2412.
59. www.Centersfordentalmedicine.com
60. Garcia MN et al. One-year Effects of vitamin D and calcium supplementation on chronic Periodontitis. *J Periodontol* 2011;82(1):25–32.
61. Barasch A et al. Random blood glucose testing in dental practice: A community-based feasibility study from The Dental Practice Based Research Network. *J Am Dental Assoc* 2012;143:262–269.
62. Rosedale M, Strauss S. Diabetes screening at the periodontal visit; patient and provider experiences with two screening approaches. *Int J Dent Hyg* 2012;10:250–258.
63. Sun WL et al. Inflammatory cytokines, adinopectin, insulin resistance, and metabolic control after periodontal intervention in patients with type 2 diabetes and chronic periodontitis. *Intern Med* 2011;50:1569–1574.
64. Shetty S et al. Gingival blood glucose estimation with reagent test strips: A method to detect diabetes in a periodontal population. *J Periodontol* 2011;82(11):1548–1555.
65. Lopez NJ et al. Effects of periodontal therapy on systemic markers of inflammation in patients with metabolic syndrome: A controlled clinical trial. *J Periodontol* Mar. 2012;267–271.
66. www.AAOSH.org
67. www.IAOH.org
68. Igari K et al. Association between periodontitis and the development of systemic diseases. *Oral Biol Dent* 2014;2:4.
69. Manife E et al. Prevalence of periodontitis in adults in the United States: 2009–2010. *J Dent Res* 2012;91(10):914–920.
70. Quijano A et al. Knowledge and orientation of internal medicine trainees towards periodontal disease. *J Periodontol* 2010;81(3):359–363.
71. Whitney, C. It is time to bridge the cosmetic-systemic gap. *Journal of Cosmetic Dentistry.* Summer 2014;30(2):88–89/144.
72. Bell KP et al. Incorporating oral-systemic evidence into patient care: practice behaviors and barriers of North Carolina Dental Hygienists. M.Sc thesis, University of North Carolina, Chapel Hill.
73. Breiner MA. *Whole-Body Dentistry: A Complete Guide to Understanding the Impact of Dentistry on Total Health.* Fairfield, CT: Quantum Health Press, 2011, 22.
74. Padilla SJ. Building a database of developmental neurotoxicant: Evidence from human and animal studies, *presented at the Society of Toxicology Annual Meeting*, Baltimore, MD, March 15–19, 2009.
75. Ewing D. *Let the Tooth be Known*, Holistic Health Alternative, 3rd edition, June 2002, pp. 115–121.

8 The Crucial Role of Craniofacial Growth on Airway, Sleep, and the Temporomandibular Joint

Mayoor Patel and Julia Worrall

CONTENTS

Introduction 228
Craniofacial Growth and Development 228
    Effect of Mouth Breathing on Facial Growth 231
    Effect of Tongue Function on Facial Growth and Airway 232
    Effect of Airway on Sleep 233
        NREM (Non-Rapid Eye Movement) Stage 1 233
        NREM Stage 2 234
        NREM Stage 3 (Has Been Merged with Stage 4 and Is Also Called Slow-Wave Sleep) 234
        REM Sleep 234
    Obstructive-Sleep Disordered Breathing (Sleep Apnea) 234
    Effect of Airway and Sleep during Infancy and Childhood 235
    Effect of Airway on Posture 237
    Effect of Posture on Cerebrospinal Fluid and Energy Flow 238
    Effect of Airway on Neurological System 240
    Effect of Airway on Cardiovascular System 240
    Effect of Airway on Endocrine System 242
    Craniofacial Pain 242
    Odontogenic Pain 243
    Oral Mucous Membrane Disorders 244
    Salivary Gland Disorder 244
    Nose and Paranasal Sinus Disorders 244
    Maxilla and Mandibular Disorders 244
    Eye and Ear Disorder 244
    Tumors 246
    Temporomandibular Joint Disorders 246
    Epidemiology of TMDs 247
    Etiology of TMD 247
    TMJ Symptoms 249
    Clinical Evaluation 249
Management 252
    Effects of TMD 253
References 255

INTRODUCTION

The human brain is the source of our thoughts, emotions, perceptions, and memories. It is what makes us uniquely us. Much time and attention has been spent trying to understand this most complicated of all biological structures. Advances have been made in the field of neuroscience to create deep brain stimulation therapies for Parkinson's patients which can restore motor circuit function for up to several years. There is extensive research into brain circuits for mood and emotion which will no doubt lead to advances in psychiatric treatment in similar ways (http://www.braininitiative. nih.gov).

As we begin to gain deeper knowledge into how our brains work, we will begin to understand ourselves differently, treat our patients more decisively, educate our children more effectively, challenge laws with greater insight and develop understanding of others whose brains have been molded through different circumstances.

To achieve this vision, we must train and support a new generation of multidisciplinary practitioners to assimilate the rapid expansion of technology and the knowledge that is being provided. For example, we know so much more about the brain and its function during sleep than ever before in history, and yet, many providers are still practicing with the body of knowledge they gained many, many years ago. To this point, the study of the brain and the current BRAIN initiative program is sure to yield tremendous results for the field of medicine, similar to the advances made through the GENOME project. We could hardly imagine practicing medicine today without a firm grasp of DNA and gene mapping. Similarly, one day we will not be able to imagine a complete history and physical that does not include a full craniofacial, airway, and sleep assessment. It only stands to reason that no study of the brain would be complete without due attention given to the bony structures that contain it...and so follows a brief consideration of craniofacial development, and its effect on our airway overall health.

CRANIOFACIAL GROWTH AND DEVELOPMENT

Our society is obsessed with appearances. The effect of this idealization of the perfect man or woman on our young ones has been well documented. Add to this the stigma of either a genetic anomaly or a developing defect in the facial structures of a child and one can hardly ignore the self-concept, dysmorphic disruption that is bound to occur. Figure 8.1 shows that attractiveness is associated with optimum physiological function, whereas unattractiveness is often linked to structural defects.

Are there any deformities of the face and cranium that don't interfere with physical and mental well-being? Unlikely. And yet, we have come to look at a person's face and make a stereotypical judgement about their attractiveness, intellectual abilities, their worth as a person and value to society as opposed to seeing the facial-cranial abnormality as a sign that the patient needs intervention to minimize long-term damage to the brain, the mind, and self-image (Singh and Moss 2015).

Their facial appearance interferes with personal life, employability, and social interaction. Many investigations have shown that these disfiguring conditions can lead to various psychosocial problems such as a high level of social anxiety and social avoidance, and poorer quality of life.

Studies have further shown that the earlier the intervention (Pertschuk and Whitaker 1982), the greater the improvement in psychosocial adjustment. Many of this group also require extensive orthodontic work and occlusal realignment. Therefore, an integrative approach is the best practice for managing this population. Good facial and dental aesthetics have a profound effect on behavior and self-esteem and should no longer be considered "cosmetic" or "elective." This is a departure from the current norm. Most practitioners find this area of facial growth overwhelming and thus merely observe and accept the clinical outcomes of atypical growth without considering the long-term consequences.

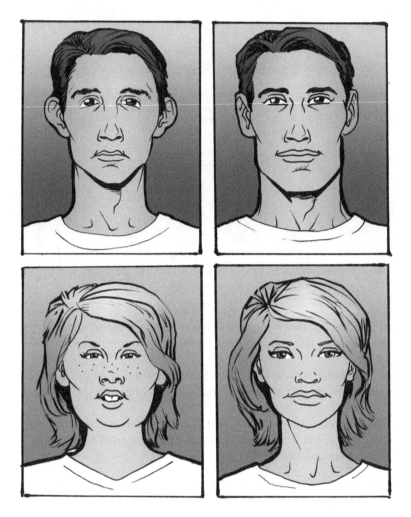

FIGURE 8.1 Attractiveness is associated with optimum physiological function, whereas unattractiveness is often linked to structural defects.

Such consequences include functional problems, temporomandibular disorders (TMD), breathing problems, sleep apnea along with other health issues. Although multiple factors may affect the pattern of growth and development of facial bones, it is fairly understood to be strongly associated with genetic factors (Enlow and Hans 1996), with environment factors affecting this process (Legović and Ostrić 1990). Facial growth and developmental process is strictly under the control of a biological process that is ongoing. Atypical growth begins when a disruption occurs with this biological balance. Bone growth itself is not predetermined within the bone itself but relies on multiple growth-related signals derived from the function of the surrounding soft tissue. The blueprint for facial bone growth lies within the muscles, tongue, cheeks, lips, mucous, connective tissue, nerves, blood vessels, airway, pharynx, tonsils, adenoids, and various other organ masses (Enlow and Hans 1996, Rubin 1987). Movement of bone growth includes physical movement of a facial bone while it simultaneously remodels. Understand that the expansion force of all growing soft tissues that surround and attach to it by anchoring fibers regulates this physical displacement of facial bones. There are three principal regions of facial and neurocranial development that ultimately guide facial growth and act together to maintain equilibrium of function and stability.

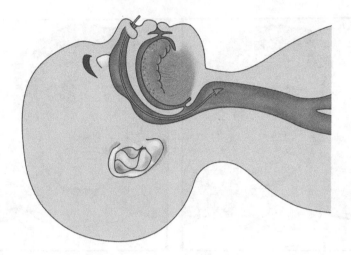

FIGURE 8.2 Obligate nose breathing allows the milk to accumulate at the back of the mouth without aspirating. The flap then opens to swallow, occluding the windpipe.

1. Brain and associated sensory organs and basicranium—Determine head form type and topographic features that characterize a facial type (brachycephalic, dolichocephalic, mesocephalic).
2. Facial and pharyngeal airway—Being a keystone for the face, regulates the arch form of the orbits, nasal and oral sides of the palate, maxillary arch, sinuses, zygomatic arch, and other arched structures of the face.
3. Oral complex—Reflects the stability of the facial and pharyngeal airway and any asymmetry of the basicranium. The nasomaxillary complex and mandible serves as an indicator of normal or atypical growth.

During the first months of life, mammalian infants are considered to be "obligate nose breathers" (Moss 1965) although the qualifying term "preferred nose breathers" was proposed subsequently (Rodenstein et al. 1986). Figure 8.2. shows an obligate nose breathing child. The fact is that newborn and very young mammals depend on nasal breathing to adapt their behavior competently, especially in relation to ingestion and, in newborns, to sucking (breastfeeding).

There are so many reasons why "Breast is Best," and the breast milk is just *one* of those. As critical to the development of the baby, its airway and future overall health, is the unique mechanical coordination of the facial muscles, the jaw, and the tongue. The process is much different from what is required for a baby to drink from a bottle, and this can affect craniofacial development. Figure 8.3 shows the difference of bottle feeding versus breastfeeding.

Satisfactory maternal breastfeeding has been associated with growth and development of the maxillomandibular complex (Neiva et al. 2003, Pierotti 2001, Carrascoza et al. 2006, Sánchez-Molins et al. 2010). This association can be neuromuscular stimuli resulting from the act of sucking the nipple, which increases perioral tonus and favors the correct arrangement of the structures responsible for mastication, swallowing, nose breathing, and phonation (Enlow and Hans 1996, Moss 1997). It has been speculated that such stimuli, when produced abnormally, could generate bone reactions with possible changes in the inadequate growth of the maxillary (Benkert 1996). Affecting the growth of the maxilla in return will affect the mandible and other bony structures within the craniofacial bones. These changes in pattern of growth and development can in turn lead to poor relationships between the dental elements, also resulting in dental malocclusions. There is much evidence on the effect of the parafunctional oral habits in malocclusion. Time and again, the type of "sucking" done in infancy is linked to better or worse dental health later in life (Neville

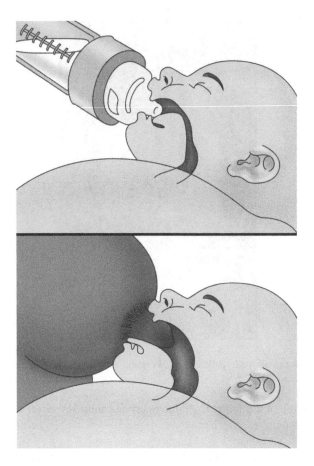

FIGURE 8.3 Bottle feeding develops the muscles at the front of the tongue and cheeks, breastfeeding encourages development of the pharyngeal muscles and temporomandibular joint.

2001). Those children who had been breastfed as a baby are much less likely to have problems with the alignment of their teeth or an overcrowded mouth later. Sleep apnea becomes much more common when someone has a high palate and narrow dental arch—conditions that are more likely to develop with bottle-feeding and other forms of artificial nipples; pacifiers, thumb or finger sucking, mouth breathing, and bruxism have been associated with alterations on the shape and size of the jaws and to higher prevalence of malocclusion (Greven 2011, Jabbar et al. 2011).

EFFECT OF MOUTH BREATHING ON FACIAL GROWTH

According to Moss's theory of functional matrix, nasal breathing allows proper growth and development of craniofacial and dentofacial complex (Moss and Salentijn 1969). We are normally nasal breathers (warming, filtration, and humidification of inhaled air); which optimizes both pulmonary exchanges and chemosensory reception (Churchill et al. 2004). However, when the nasal airway integrity is compromised, the tendency toward oral (mouth) breathing occurs. This disrupts the balance discussed above, leading to aberrant growth patterns including retrognathism and downward growth of the nasomaxillary complex (midface), underdevelopment of the lateral orbital rims, narrow deep palate, malocclusion, and excess vertical growth of the face. Figure 8.4 shows a typical appearance of a child with improper nasal patency. Other compensatory compensation may involve the ramus of the mandible, variation in maxillary size and shape, anterior teeth crowding, gonial angle remodeling, occlusal plane rotations, and other such variations that are seen clinically.

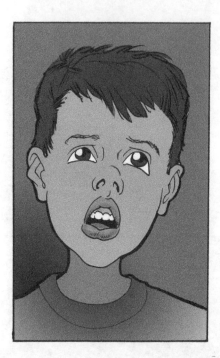

FIGURE 8.4 Before assuming your patient has allergies, ensure proper craniofacial development and nasal patency.

Additionally, one or more of the following three neuromuscular responses to the change of mouth breathing will be observed:

1. Altered mandibular posture—Mandible rotates down and backward
2. Altered tongue posture—Tongue moves inferiorly and anteriorly
3. Extended head posture—Mandible is held in position while the cranium and maxilla rotate upward to assist in increasing the size of the airway

Although mouth-breathing etiology is multifactorial, the most common causes are anatomical obstruction, such as palatine and pharyngeal tonsil hypertrophy, allergic rhinitis, nasal septal deviation, nasal polyps, and nasal turbinate hypertrophy (Harari et al. 2010). In particular, allergic rhinitis, a chronic respiratory problem with a high prevalence, results from a complex, allergen-driven mucosal inflammatory process that can result in nasal obstruction with consequent transition from nasal to mouth breathing (Settipane and Schwindt 2013). Linder-Aronson (1970) looked at 81 children who had severe nasal obstruction and open mouth breathing and were matched age and gender to nasal breathers. The findings demonstrated that children with obstructed nasal breathing were characterized by increased lower face height, increased total facial height, and more retrognathic mandibles compared to the control group.

EFFECT OF TONGUE FUNCTION ON FACIAL GROWTH AND AIRWAY

To swallow is the most complex reflex activity the human nervous system performs, and it is done without conscious effort. The ideal head balance is nasal breathing, lips sealed, the teeth slightly apart at rest, and the tongue positioned in the roof of the mouth. With each swallow, the teeth are brought into maximum occlusion (contact) by the masticatory muscles, the lips continue to be sealed, and the tongue pushes the bolus of food posteriorly against the palate. At the end of the swallow, the tongue returns to its resting position. A normal swallow provides maximum bracing for the head on the spinal column. Ideally, the tongue is in contact with the roof of the mouth at rest during subconscious swallowing and during nasal breathing. During the swallowing process, the tongue exerts an outward and forward force, which is compensated for by the inward force of the cheeks and lips. When the tongue is positioned in the roof of the mouth, it functions ideally and produces healthy palatal and dental development (Enlow and Hans 1996).

Constriction of the oral pharyngeal space may be caused by grossly enlarged tonsils or adenoids, which may lead to a forward placement of the tongue and an inferior displacement of the hyoid bone. Even though these changes may be reversed after a tonsillectomy or adenoidectomy, reinitiation of a normal swallow may not necessarily follow. In such cases, the child's swallow pattern must be retrained to produce a normal swallow.

EFFECT OF AIRWAY ON SLEEP

First, what is healthy sleep? Many theories have prevailed regarding the value of sleep. Until recently, most people thought of sleep as a passive, dormant part of our daily lives. New research highlights an active role for sleep in protecting mental health, physical health, quality of life, and safety. The quality and quantity of sleep has a profound effect on learning and memory (Rasch and Born 2013). Figure 8.5 demonstrates normal sleep breathing through a patent nasopharyngeal airway.

No practitioner can optimize their patient's health without seriously addressing issues arising from the one-third of their life while they are completely unaware and unconscious. To that end, let's review the normal, healthy stages of sleep and the purpose of each.

NREM (Non-Rapid Eye Movement) Stage 1

- Normal sleep begins and ends with Stage 1 sleep. This is the stage between wakefulness and sleep, which lasts around 5 to 10 minutes, and accounts for about 5% of total sleep time. During this stage, we drift in and out and can be awakened easily. Our body begins to relax, our eyes move very slowly, and overall muscle activity slows, sudden twitches or jerks often accompanied by a falling sensation may occur. A person may be aware of sounds and conversations but unwilling to respond.
- Stage 1 sleep is about 5% of total sleep time and those who are awakened during this period often believe they have never slept at all and may experience sleep inertia for a few minutes and up to 4 hours after waking. In fact, people have been observed to be driving

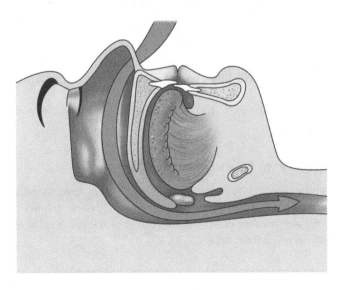

FIGURE 8.5   Normal sleep breathing through patent nasopharyngeal airway.

while in stage 1 sleep. Reaction time in those with sleep inertia can be comparable to those of drunk people.
- Motor learning seems to depend on the amount of lighter stages of sleep.

NREM Stage 2

- Stage 2 is the true onset of sleep where the person becomes disengaged from their surroundings. Stage 2 lasts about 20 minutes each cycle and accounts for about 50% of total sleep time.
- Eye movements stop and brain activity becomes slower with occasional bursts of rapid waves called sleep spindles. Body temperature falls, heart rate and breathing slows as you begin to reach a state of total relaxation in preparation for deeper sleep.

NREM Stage 3 (Has Been Merged with Stage 4 and Is Also Called Slow-Wave Sleep)

- Stage 3 has an average onset of 35–45 minutes after falling asleep and can last anywhere from 5–15 minutes. The first deep sleep of the night is more likely to last an hour or so. This is the time when the body does most of its repair work, tissue growth, and regeneration. Growth hormone is released during this stage.
- Slow wave sleep (SWS) and extremely slow brain waves called delta waves begin to appear. This is the start of the deepest, most restorative stage of sleep. There is no eye movement or muscle activity. It is very difficult to wake someone up and this is when a person is most likely to sleep through noise and movements without showing any reaction.
- SWS plays a significant role in declarative memory by processing and consolidating newly acquired information. Visual learning is also dependent upon the amount and timing of SWS and REM sleep.

REM Sleep

- The first period of REM sleep usually begins about 90 minutes after you start drifting off and lasts for about 10 minutes. As the night progresses, the periods of REM sleep become longer with the final episode lasting an hour or so.
- Babies spend as much as half of their sleep time in REM. Healthy adults spend about 20%–25% of their sleep in REM. REM sleep diminishes with age.
- Rapid eye movement (REM) sleep describes the stage of sleep where our breathing becomes more rapid, irregular, and shallow, our eyes jerk rapidly in various directions, and our limb muscles become temporarily paralyzed.
- Our brain activity and blood flow increases, our blood pressure rises, males develop penile erections. During REM sleep your brain is about as active as it is when you are awake. This is when people dream and your limbs go through periods of paralysis to prevent you from acting out those dreams.
- REM sleep plays a crucial role in the consolidation of procedural memory, remembering "how" to do something.

OBSTRUCTIVE-SLEEP DISORDERED BREATHING (SLEEP APNEA)

Sleep apnea is a condition marked by pauses in breathing during sleep. A pause, called an apnea, can last between 10 seconds to minutes. Pauses can occur 5 to 30 or more times per hour. Figure 8.6. shows an obstructed airway because of lax muscular tone of the pharyngeal airway as well as an edematous tongue and narrow palatal arch.

- *Obstructive sleep apnea* occurs when a physical barrier blocks or collapses the air passageway.

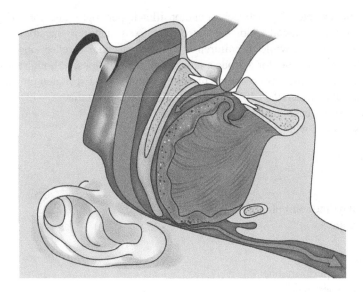

FIGURE 8.6 Obstructed airway results from lax muscular tone of the pharyngeal airway as well as an edematous tongue and narrow palatal arch.

- *Central sleep apnea* occurs when the brain fails to send signals to muscles that control breathing.
- *Complex or mixed sleep apnea* is a combination of both obstructive and central sleep apnea.

Obstructive sleep apnea is the most common, making up 84% of cases of sleep apnea.

In cases of obstructive sleep apnea, a pause in breath is often followed by a choking, gasping, or snoring sound as air passes through a narrowed or blocked airway.

More than 12 million Americans have sleep apnea, per the National Institutes of Health. More than half of those with obstructive sleep apnea are overweight. Daytime signs of sleep apnea include sleepiness, morning headaches, morning dry throat, as well as irritability, depression, and difficulty concentrating due to lack of quality sleep. Untreated sleep apnea can increase risks of an irregular heartbeat and heart disease, stroke, high blood pressure, and diabetes.

The risk of sleep apnea is higher among males, increases with age, and is more common in African Americans, Latinos, and Pacific Islanders than Caucasians.

All too often, sleep apnea goes undiagnosed because the person with the condition remains unaware that irregular breathing occurred during the night. However, a bed partner, or family member, is able to observe snoring and can encourage that person to see his or her doctor. A physician, through family history, medical examination, and sleep studies, can diagnose sleep issues.

These days there are a variety of treatment options available to someone with sleep apnea. A doctor can determine if lifestyle changes, mindful breathing, positional therapy, dental appliances, a continuous positive airway pressure (CPAP) breathing device, or surgery would most effectively treat the causes of sleep apnea.

EFFECT OF AIRWAY AND SLEEP DURING INFANCY AND CHILDHOOD

Obstructive sleep-disordered breathing (SDB) is commonly characterized by central hypoventilation and disorders of respiratory muscles in children (Hersi 2010). Children with other comorbid conditions, such as genetic syndromes that may alter craniofacial airway anatomy, central control of breathing, or respiratory muscle function represent a large percentage of pediatric patients presenting with obstructive sleep apnea (OSA).

There is a complex interplay between adenotonsillar hypertrophy and loss of neuromuscular tone. Children with craniofacial syndromes also have fixed anatomic variations that predispose them to airway obstruction, while in children with neuromuscular disease, obstruction is caused by hypotonia. Obesity accounts for a modest number of presentations, although these numbers are growing. Snoring is by far the most common presenting complaint. Estimated prevalence of snoring is 3%–12%, while OSA affects 1%–10%. Recent studies have shown that 4%–13% of Sudden Infant Death Syndrome (SIDS) cases had a history of apnea.

Conditions associated with sleep disordered breathing:

- Cor pulmonale
- Cyanosis
- Enuresis
- Excessive daytime somnolence
- Gasping for air
- Irritability
- Night-time awakening
- Poor academic performance
- Pulmonary hypertension
- Snoring
- Unusual daytime behavior
- Physical examination
  - Craniofacial abnormalities
  - Adenotonsillar hypertrophy
  - Lingual tonsils
  - Laryngeal pathology
- Growth disturbances
  - Failure to thrive
  - Obesity

Neurobiologically, closely linked modulatory systems appear to regulate sleep, alertness, and attention span. Therefore, the practitioner should include a full facial development and airway assessment in the medical differential when evaluating for signs and symptoms of the following:

- Attention deficit hyperactivity disorder (ADHD)
- Gastroesophageal reflux disease (GERD)
- Pervasive developmental disorders
- Mental retardation
- Down syndrome
- Prader–Willi syndrome
- Smith–Magenis syndrome
- Tourette disorder
- Nocturnal asthma
- Depressive disorders
- Anxiety disorders
- Mania
- Neuromuscular disorders
- Nocturnal seizures
- Kleine–Levin syndrome
- Chronic fatigue syndrome
- Headaches
- Blindness with associated sleep disorder

The best medical practice is to facilitate the recognition of these issues as potentially related to facial development, airway or sleep problems and refer for further evaluation.

EFFECT OF AIRWAY ON POSTURE

"Natural head posture (NHP) is the upright position of the head of a standing or sitting subject, while it is balanced by the post-cervical and masticatory-suprahyoid-infrahyoid muscle groups, with the eyes directed forward so that the visual axis is parallel to the floor" (Özbek et al. 1998).

Enlarged tonsils, adenoids, and chronic respiratory problems have been associated with compensatory adaptations of natural head posture (NHP) in children. Adult patients with OSA also tend to exhibit a craniocervical extension (CCE) with a forward head posture (FHP). The CCE and FHP in OSA patients is associated with a higher disease severity, longer and larger tongue, a lower hyoid bone position in relation to the mandibular plane, a smaller nasopharyngeal and larger hypopharyngeal cross-section area, and a higher body mass index. Figure 8.7 shows posture change due to compensatory adaptations.

Experimental studies demonstrated an immediate head extension and changes in postural EMG activity in the craniofacial muscles following the obstruction of the nasal airways. Correspondingly, the studies in children emphasized the role of enlarged tonsils and adenoids and chronic respiratory problems such as asthma and perennial rhinitis, in increased craniocervical extension.

Certain physiological and anatomical factors that cause the nocturnal respiratory problems persist when the patients are awake. Studies have determined significant differences in craniofacial, upper airway, and related structures between awake OSA patients and controls. Furthermore, several studies have demonstrated that the neuromuscular properties of pharyngeal and genioglossus muscles are also compromised in awake OSA patients when compared with controls. These anatomical and physiological characteristics of the upper airway and related structures in OSA patients may trigger the chain of interactions between the muscles of the craniomandibular complex (including the pharyngeal and post-cervical muscles) resulting in a CCE and FHP.

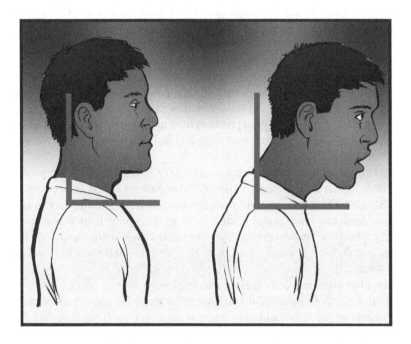

FIGURE 8.7　A chronic obstructive airway, whether naso or oropharynx, results in an unnatural protrusion of the head to artificially open the airway.

The most significant set of correlations in this study was observed between tongue size and shape and the NHP measurements. A longer and thinner tongue with an increased cross-sectional area was related to an increased CCE and FHP. The present findings also suggest that certain facial characteristics, such as an increased lower anterior facial height with a posterior rotation pattern of the mandible, and a tendency for a sagittal skeletal Class II relationship that have been observed in subjects with CCE and FHP may be due to a larger and longer tongue, which has also been suggested to be related to similar facial patterns.

EFFECT OF POSTURE ON CEREBROSPINAL FLUID AND ENERGY FLOW

Optimal health depends on correct postural alignment so that there is no impedance to cerebrospinal fluid (CSF). CSF has powerful vitalistic properties. From the base of the spine to the crown of the head, energy is said to flow up the spinal pathway while it maintains the electrolytic environment of the entire central nervous system (CNS). CSF influences systemic acid-base balance, serves as a medium for the supply of nutrients to neuronal and glial cells, functions as a lymphatic system for the CNS by removing the waste products of cellular metabolism, and transports hormones, neurotransmitters, releasing factors, and other neuropeptides throughout the CNS (Whedon and Glassey 2009).

CSF comes from arterial blood that has been filtered through the blood–brain barrier to the point where it is mostly water. CSF then leaves the brain through the venous system. Most of the CSF produced by the brain eventually makes its way up to the superior sagittal sinus where it empties into the venous system, the rest follows routes along cranial nerves, spinal nerves, and the lymphatic system. The CSF that leaves the brain on its way down to the cord must first pass through the tight neural (spinal) canal of the upper cervical spine. Likewise, on its return trip back to the brain, it must again pass through the neural canal of the upper cervical spine. Therefore, the upper cervical spine is a critical link in the flow of CSF between the subarachnoid space of the brain and the cord. It is vital to maintain the correct volume and flow of CSF in order to provide sufficient brain support and protection. Vertebral arteries supply the brain, and vertebral veins drain the brain. Any mechanical backups in this venous drainage system will invariably affect CSF pulsations, energy flow, and lymphatic drainage (Flanagan 2011). Figure 8.8 shows that energy flow is dependent on unimpeded flow of CSF.

Recently, the University of Virginia Department of Neuroscience discovered that the brain has a series of lymphatic vessels directly linking the brain to the immune system. This changes entirely the way we perceive the neuroimmune interaction. It appears the lymphatic system functions as a second step in the drainage of fluid from the brain after plasma proteins and other cellular debris are drained into the CSF through the glymphatic system and then back into the bloodstream along deep cervical lymph nodes. This new discovery directly links the brain's lymphatic system with the peripheral immune system.

Forward head posture, mouth breathing, craniofacial anomalies, trauma, genetic defects, and degenerative conditions may all cause rotational misalignment of the upper cervical spine and restrict vital CSF flow. Diseases like multiple sclerosis, Alzheimer's and autism suddenly make sense if, in fact, there are mechanical obstructions to the removal of wastes and proteins in the brain by alterations of these vessels. New research is warranted and will fundamentally change the way people look at postural alignment, CSF flow, and the CNS's relationship with the immune system.

Therapies aimed at affecting CSF, lymph, and improving overall energy flow include: maxillofacial orthodontics, temporomandibular realignment, osteopathic care, craniosacral therapy, chiropractic adjustments of the spine and cranium, massage therapy (including lymphatic drainage techniques), yoga, therapeutic breathwork, and CSF technique. Figure 8.9 explains that with new understanding of the role of the lymphatic system in the head, neck, and around the brain will change the way we treat neurological symptoms.

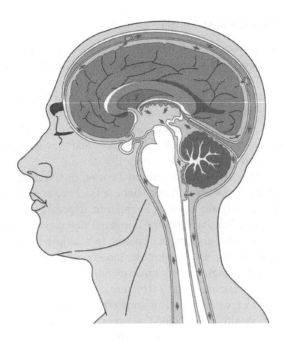

FIGURE 8.8 Energy flow is dependent on unimpeded flow of cerebrospinal fluid. Conversely, neurocognitive and physical decline is clear with CSF stasis.

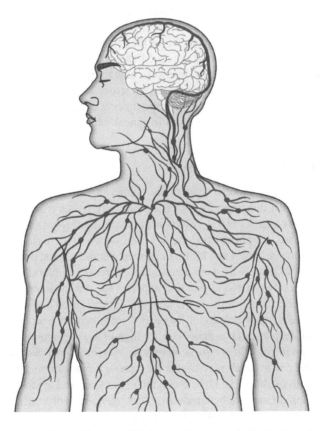

FIGURE 8.9 New understanding of the role of the lymphatic system in the head, neck, and around the brain will change the way we treat neurological symptoms.

EFFECT OF AIRWAY ON NEUROLOGICAL SYSTEM

Sleep helps your brain work properly. While you're sleeping, your brain is preparing for the next day. Studies show that a good night's sleep improves learning, enhances problem-solving skills, helps you pay attention, make decisions, and be creative.

Sleep deficiency alters activity in the brain and has been linked with depression, suicide, and risk-taking behavior. Children and teens who are sleep deficient may have problems getting along with others. They may feel angry and impulsive, have mood swings, feel sad or depressed, or lack motivation. They may also have problems paying attention, and they may get lower grades and feel stressed (Watson, Ceriana, and Fanfulla 2012, Leiter 1996).

Obstructive sleep apnea (OSA) leads to impaired daytime functioning in various neuropsychological and affective domains. The most common abnormalities are executive dysfunction, impaired vigilance, depression, and possibly anxiety and, in children, hyperactivity.

Neuroimaging shows that patients with severe, untreated sleep apnea had a significant reduction in white matter fiber integrity and gray matter volume in multiple brain areas. This brain damage was accompanied by impairments to cognition, mood, and daytime alertness. Three months of CPAP therapy produced improvements in white matter integrity and gray matter volume, but only limited improvements to damaged brain structures. Twelve months of CPAP therapy led to an almost complete reversal of white matter abnormalities. Treatment also produced significant improvements in nearly all cognitive tests, mood, alertness, and quality of life.

Some patients have persistent deficits despite effective treatment. This raises the possibility of a remaining subtle structural brain damage; such damage has been demonstrated through the use of sensitive functional and other neuroimaging techniques. Prefrontal cortical damage may underlie the cognitive dysfunction in OSA. Early recognition and treatment may prevent this untoward effect of OSA (El-Ad and Lavie 2005).

OSA and stroke are frequent, multifactorial entities that share several risk factors. Stroke of respiratory centers can lead to apnea. Snoring preceding stroke, documentation of apneas immediately prior to transient ischemic attacks, the results of autonomic studies, and the circadian pattern of stroke suggest that untreated OSA can contribute to stroke (Dyken and Im 2009). There is also evidence that lesions or impingement to the 5th cranial nerve at the base of the mouth or nose may lead to failure of automatic respiration and result in apneas which lead to stroke.

EFFECT OF AIRWAY ON CARDIOVASCULAR SYSTEM

OSA is responsible for repeated blood oxygen desaturations and accompanying increases in arterial carbon dioxide levels. When this happens your brain partially wakes from sleep and sends signals to the nervous system to constrict blood vessels to increase the flow of oxygen to your heart and brain. A persistent increase in sympathetic tone has been shown to increase blood pressure at night to keep oxygen flowing to your heart and brain. In general, people's blood pressure drops 10%–20% during sleep, but many patients with sleep apnea show increases in blood pressure of 10%–20%. Unfortunately, these increases in blood pressure experienced during sleep often begin to overlap into periods of wakefulness. This results in the potential for increased blood pressure always.

High blood pressure is a major risk factor for heart disease, stroke, heart attack, and many other medical problems, and sleep apnea is a major risk for high blood pressure.

Sleep apnea causes an increase in sympathetic nervous system activity associated with respiratory event-related hypoxemia and arousals may trigger the fight or flight response. These changes include elevations in heart rate to facilitate the rapid circulation of oxygen and glucose to muscles that need fuel to flee or flight, pupil dilation for better vision, water retention to minimize loss in fluid volume, and increases in the clotting of blood that minimize blood loss in the event of wounding.

In the case of potentially life-threatening events, such as apneas during sleep, our brains are geared to respond rapidly, since fast responses improve chances of survival. The hypothalamus promotes this function, raising a body-wide alarm response within minutes, followed at a slightly slower pace by an even broader "stress response." The stress response, described by Hans Szabo (Szabo, Tache, and Somogyi 2012) is elicited through stimulation of the hypothalamic–pituitary–adrenocortical (HPA) axis, which results in secretion of cortisol. The adrenal cortex facilitates conversion of norepinephrine to epinephrine. Together, the effects of cortisol, epinephrine, and norepinephrine engage system-wide defense mechanisms, fostering mobilization through processes such as secretion and distribution of glucose and stored energy, in part through inhibition of insulin secretion and promotion of insulin resistance (Leung and Douglas Bradley 2001).

OSA is an independent risk factor for ischemic stroke that is not included in the usual cardioembolic risk assessments for patients with atrial fibrillation (AF). The severity of OSA is independently associated with elevated markers of systemic inflammation, including C-reactive protein which is directly associated with an increased AF burden. Sleep apnea has been associated with left atrial enlargement (Yaranov et al. 2015).

In contrast, bradyarrhythmias are probably related to the prolonged apnea and hypoxemia in OSA that elicit the cardiac vagal activation reflex, with simultaneous sympathetic activation to the peripheral blood vessels, including muscle, renal, and splanchnic but not cerebral vasculature. Although the vagal response will often elicit a discernible bradycardia, in a minority of OSA patients (approximately 10%), bradyarrhythmias such as atrioventricular block and asystole may develop even in the absence of cardiac conduction disease. These are most likely to occur during REM sleep and with a decrease in oxygen saturation of at least 4%. Re-entry mechanisms may occur through the vagal stimulation that results from respiration against a partially occluded airway, which may lead to bradycardia-dependent increased dispersion of atrial repolarization predisposed to intra-atrial entry. Additionally, OSA/SDB-related mechanical effects of negative intrathoracic pressure on the atrial and ventricular free walls promote cardiac stretching, which may predispose one to arrhythmias by way of mechanical electrical feedback mechanisms. Figure 8.10 shows the arterial supply to the head. Of all patients having myocardial infarction (MI) between 12 AM and 6 AM, 91% had OSA. Additionally, cerebral vascular accidents (CVA) correlate 71.9% with OSA.

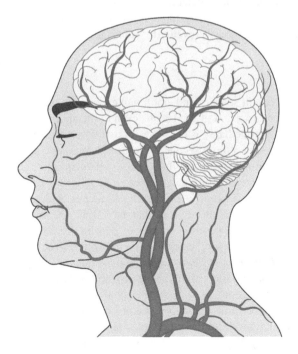

FIGURE 8.10 Of all patients having myocardial infarction (MI) between 12 AM and 6 AM, 91% have obstructive sleep apnea. Additionally, cerebral vascular accidents (CVA) correlate 71.9% with OSA.

EFFECT OF AIRWAY ON ENDOCRINE SYSTEM

OSA is associated with increased cardiovascular and cerebrovascular morbidity as discussed above. In addition, many subjects with OSA have central obesity and other features of metabolic syndrome, comprising of hyperinsulinemia, glucose intolerance, dyslipidemia, central obesity, and hypertension. These features are otherwise known as "insulin resistance syndrome" (Ip et al. 2002).

In support of all the increases in metabolic demand, epinephrine and cortisol increase the production and release of glucose, and inhibit insulin activity and secretion. During fight/flight, digestion and other activities such as energy storage are also inhibited. In effect, during fight/flight "we stop digesting the food in our stomachs and intestines and begin digesting ourselves," as stored glucose, proteins, and fats are utilized for energy.

Interestingly, the presence of OSA in nonobese individuals is significantly associated with impaired glucose metabolism, which can be responsible for future risk for diabetes and cardiovascular disease (Kim et al. 2013). It becomes imperative then, that practitioners determine if sleep apnea has any effect on insulin resistance and implement early, preventative interventions in their patients.

Other endocrine disorders correlated to OSA include:

- Hypothyroidism
- Polycystic ovarian syndrome
- Acromegaly
- Hypogonadism
- Growth hormone (GH) deficiency

In rare instances, OSA may be improved or even cured by treatment of underlying endocrine disorders: this is the case of hypothyroidism and acromegaly, situations in which OSA is mainly related to UA narrowing due to reversible thickening of the pharyngeal walls.

However, when irreversible skeletal defects and/or obesity are present, OSA may persist despite treatment of endocrine disorders and may thus require complementary therapy. This is also frequently the case in patients with obesity, even after substantial weight reduction.

CRANIOFACIAL PAIN

Pain is defined as an unpleasant sensory and emotional experience that is associated with actual or potential tissue damage, or described in such terms even in the absence of any obvious tissue damage. Nociceptive pain, on the one hand, is caused by actual tissue injury and inflammation, such as seen with pulpal involvement of a tooth secondary to dental decay.

Craniofacial pain is a common symptom that causes significant morbidity. Diagnosis requires a detailed history and examination. As the trigeminal nerve supplies a great deal of sensory and motor innervation to the face and jaw, it is not surprising that branches of this nerve are most commonly responsible for orofacial pain conditions. Cranial nerves VII, IX, X, and XII can also be involved. Although there are many different potential causes of pain in the head and neck region, the vast majority of cases fall into the following categories based on the structures affected: *odontogenic, myofascial, temporomandibular joint, neuropathic,* and *headache.*

An individual's perception of pain is highly subjective and is influenced by the underlying cause, which may not be clinically evident, as well as emotional and psychological factors. Key components of the history include: the timing, duration, quality, and intensity of pain; modifiers that make the pain better or worse; other sites of pain; previous pain history; social history (including major life events); and sleep history. Psychiatric history is also important; specifically regarding treatment for anxiety, depression, and panic attacks, all of which can be associated with chronic pain conditions. A pain score using a 0–10 numerical scale with descriptors should be obtained consistently at each visit.

A careful history accompanied by a comprehensive examination in most cases is sufficient to determine the correct diagnosis, although laboratory tests and imaging studies may be indicated on occasion.

Craniofacial pain deserves special consideration, given the complex anatomy and specialized sensory innervation of the head and neck. Many craniofacial pain syndromes also are unique, and represent a clinical diagnostic challenge. This chapter presents an introduction to practical issues regarding assessment and treatment of common craniofacial pain disorders and discusses the role of the oropharynx and airway.

The structures of the face have a rich, sensory innervation supplied by the trigeminal system. As such, pain is one of the most prominent symptoms of disease in this general area. In many cases, the acute pain symptoms closely correlate with other signs and symptoms of disease. However, correlation between pain and symptoms may not be evident in several more complex, chronic pain problems, particularly those involving the masticatory system. The diverse potential for pain arising from the vast area of the trigeminal innervation accounts for the need for interdisciplinary collaboration in the evaluation and treatment of these complex patients.

ODONTOGENIC PAIN

Dental infections are common; these must always be included in the differential diagnosis for orofacial pain. Hot or cold sensitivity that quickly resolves when the stimulus is removed is characteristic of reversible pulpal inflammation. Spontaneous, pounding pain often occurs once the pulp has become severely inflamed or necrotic. Formation of a periapical abscess may cause pain with chewing and when the tooth is *percussed* (tapped gently with a dental instrument).

Dental pain is usually well localized and the quality of pain can range from a dull ache to severe electric shocks, depending on the specific etiology and extent of disease. Dental pain is typically provoked by thermal or mechanical stimulation of the damaged tooth. Clinical and radiographic findings of dental decay, tooth fracture, or abscess drainage may confirm the source of dental pain.

Periodontitis is generally not a chronically painful disorder. Typically, patients may notice gingival sensitivity and tenderness, or gingival enlargement caused by inflammation and bleeding with brushing or probing examination. There is loss of gingival attachment around the necks of and soft tissue pocketing around the roots of the tooth with loss of bone support, which may result in tooth sensitivity, tenderness, and mobility. Pain secondary to periodontal disease is typically dull, generalized to a larger area, and more constant. In the presence of an acute infection in the periodontal tissues, tenderness to the touch, erythema, and bleeding may be evident. An acute periodontal abscess may cause swelling and purulence. When inflammation or infection occurs in the soft tissue or bone around an erupting or partially erupted tooth (particularly third molars), similar signs and symptoms may be seen with pain as a primary complaint.

An acute abscess also may have to be locally incised and drained. Areas of generalized periodontitis may be treated with tooth scaling and curettage of the gingival pocketing and possibly local or systemic antibiotic therapy.

Acute dental pain and periodontal disorders generally respond to nonsteroidal anti-inflammatory drugs (NSAIDs). Opioid analgesics also are occasionally indicated, depending on the extent of objective pathology.

Odontogenic pain unrelated to infection can be caused by a small crack in a tooth or maladjustment of the occlusion. If there is any concern regarding an odontogenic etiology, patients should be referred to a dentist for evaluation.

Tooth pulp has a specialized and possibly exclusively nociceptive innervation. In contrast, periodontal tissues are innervated by a wide variety of sensory afferents.

ORAL MUCOUS MEMBRANE DISORDERS

Diseases of the oral mucosa are numerous and caused by a variety of local and systemic etiologies. Pain often accompanies acute, recurrent, or persistent primary disease process, secondary to an associated process (i.e., infection), or related to damaged oral mucosa (i.e., cheek biting, tongue biting, chewing foods, thermal, chemical). Typically, these diseases produce pain and oral mucosal lesions. Lesions include vesicles, bullae, erosions, erythema, or red and white patches. Reduction in pain is often achieved by palliative care using analgesic medication or treatment of the underlying disorder using local and systemic analgesic agents.

SALIVARY GLAND DISORDER

Disorders of the three major pairs of salivary glands (parotid, submandibular, and sublingual) and many hundreds of minor salivary glands within the oral cavity also may produce pain as a primary or associated complaint. Pain originating in the salivary glands is typically of inflammatory, infectious, traumatic, or neoplastic origin. These disorders often are not difficult to diagnose due to accompanied signs and symptoms, such as pain occurring on eating, swelling, firmness, drainage, or tenderness of the affected gland. Disorders of the parotid gland can locally extend to produce otologic symptoms, or cranial nerve (V, VII, or IX) involvement. Disorders of the submandibular gland may result in symptoms of impaired swallowing or impairment of cranial nerves V, IX, or XII.

NOSE AND PARANASAL SINUS DISORDERS

These disorders are grouped together because of the intimate relationship between the nose and paranasal sinuses (maxillary, ethmoid, frontal, and sphenoid sinuses) as these sinuses communicate with the nasal passages through the small ostia. When the ostia become blocked due to inflammation or obstruction (anatomic variation, tumors), fluid and bacteria accumulate, leading to signs and symptoms of sinusitis. Patients frequently would experience nasal discharge, nasal purulence, postnasal drip, facial pressure and pain, alteration in sense of smell, cough, fever, halitosis, fatigue, dental pain, otalgia, and headache. Often patients describe their facial pain problem as a "sinus headache." However, sinus disorders do not cause chronic headaches, and the clinician should look for a more specific etiology for pain symptoms in such cases (Tepper 2004). Diseases of the nose and paranasal sinuses typically cause acute pain associated with multiple other symptoms that are generally related to the specific nasal or sinus disease (i.e., allergic, inflammatory, infections). Acute dentoalveolar pathology of the maxillary posterior teeth (dental abscess) often has signs and symptoms consistent with sinus disease. This process can cause secondary maxillary sinus inflammation or infection. These are typically acute in nature, but can become chronic. This condition is often confused with other facial pain and headache disorders. Palpation of the maxillary sinuses for tenderness, Valsalva Maneuver, and bending forward are helpful diagnostic methods of detecting pain from sinusitis.

MAXILLA AND MANDIBULAR DISORDERS

Numerous disorders of the bony substrate of the jaws can produce pain. These disorders are generally classified as being of odontogenic or nonodontogenic origin, cystic, cystic-like or tumor, or benign or malignant (either primary or metastatic disease). Often additional historical or examination findings warrant further evaluation (i.e., swelling, mass, discoloration, numbness, weakness, bleeding, drainage, tooth loss, or mobility).

EYE AND EAR DISORDER

Pain in and around the eye is a common complaint that may be either primary or referred as listed in Table 8.1. Most patients with eye pain often have obvious ocular symptoms, signs, or history

TABLE 8.1
Pain Arising from the Eyes

Primary Pain	Referred Pain
Corneal disease	Orbital apex syndrome
Glaucoma	Saccular aneurysms
Ocular inflammation	Cavernous sinus inflammation
Superior orbital fissure syndrome	Carotid artery dissection
Orbital tumors	Myofascial Pain
Convergence disorders (heterophoria or heterotropia)	Parasellar syndrome
Painful ophthalmoplegia	Temporal tendonitis
	Sinus
	Temporomandibular Joint
	Supraorbital neuritis/neuralgia
	Lesser occipital neuralgia

that implicates the eye as the origin of pain. Most ocular diseases are not painful, however. The retina and optic nerve are not capable of nociception; however, the cornea, conjunctiva, and iris have an abundant supply of nociceptors. Pain may be perceived as originating in the orbit when the optic nerve is stimulated at any point along its path to the cortex (intracranial tumors, tumors of the orbit or paranasal sinuses, cavernous sinus inflammation, carotid aneurysms) (Rosenblatt and Sakol 1989).

Ear aches are due to structural lesions of the external or middle ear 50% of the time (Göbel and Baloh 1999). Primary otalgia is pain with an etiology in the ear and usually it can be diagnosed by examination of the pinna, auditory canal, and tympanic membrane. Referred otalgia does not have a distinct otologic etiology and has also been termed secondary or nonotogenic otalgia. Referred pain may be a result from pathological factors involving the sensory supply of the V, IX, X cranial nerves and the spinal nerves C2 and C3 (Mehta et al. 2011). Primary otalgia listed in Table 8.2 may

TABLE 8.2
Pain Arising from the Ears

Primary Pain	Referred Pain
Infections of the auricle, external auditory canal, tympanic membrane and middle ear	Temporomandibular disorders
	Myofasical pain
Cholesteatoma	Toothache
Mastoiditis	Auriculotemporal syndrome
Herpes simplex virus	Carotid artery dissection
Herpes zoster virus	Red ear syndrome
Tumors	Hypopharynx pain
	Larynx pain
	Nasopharynx pain
	Oromucosal pain
	Sinus pain
	Tongue pain
	Ramsay hunt syndrome
	Hyoid bone syndrome
	Hamular bursitis
	Temporal arteritis
	Eagles syndrome

TABLE 8.3

Syndromes with Eye and Ear Pain

- Cluster headache and cluster-tic syndrome
- Paroxysmal hemicrania
- SUNCT syndrome (short-lasting unilateral neuralgiform headache with conjunctival injection and tearing)
- Trigeminal neuralgia
- Sphenopalatine neuralgia (Sluder's neuralgia)
- Icepick headache
- Ice cream headache
- Hypnic headache
- Nonorganic pain and headache (psychosomatic and psychiatric disorders)
- Ernest syndrome
- Occipital (greater/lesser) neuralgia

---

be accompanied by symptoms such as vertigo, deafness, or tinnitus (Loeser and Bonica 2001). Often pain in and around these structures is also associated with a variety of other craniofacial and headache syndromes as listed in Table 8.3.

TUMORS

Numerous intra- and extracranial tumors can cause oropharyngeal, facial, and head pain as a primary symptom. Cancers of the upper digestive tract, jaws, base of the skull, and neck may demonstrate pain along with other associated signs and symptoms. In addition, numerous intracranial tumors and lesions (i.e., vascular malformations) can exhibit facial pain and headache. Headache and facial pain of unknown origin should warrant a careful evaluation for an underlying occult tumor (Nguyen et al. 1986, Cheng, Cascino, and Onofrio 1993, Mathews and Scrivani 2000).

Oral cancer accounts for about 2% of all malignant tumors. Over 90% of malignant cancers of the mouth are squamous cell carcinomas arising from mucosal epithelium. The remainder are adenocarcinomas of minor salivary glands or metastases (Cawson and Odell 2008).

Patients presenting with facial pain or headache should undergo a comprehensive medical history and careful physical examination with particular attention to the cranial neurologic examination. Consideration should be given to obtaining appropriate imaging studies including computed tomography (CT), magnetic resonance imaging (MRI), and magnetic resonance angiography (MRA).

TEMPOROMANDIBULAR JOINT DISORDERS

Temporomandibular disorder (TMD) is yet another prominent orofacial pain disorder with various signs and symptoms associated with it. The temporomandibular joint (TMJ) and muscles of mastication function together as a unit that is one of the most heavily utilized structures in the human body. TMD is a collective term that encompasses a number of clinical problems involved in the masticatory muscles, TMJ, and its associated structures (Johansson et al. 2003).

Pain in and around the TMJ may arise from structural abnormalities of the bony joint, disk (meniscal) problems, or muscular dysfunction. Trauma, degenerative changes, disc displacement, and inflammatory arthritis may also affect the joint. Tumors, infections, and growth or congenital abnormalities are rarely involved.

In addition to pain, TMD may include additional complaints including the following: headache, face pain, eye pain, ear symptoms, temporomandibular joint symptoms, neck pain, and arm and back symptoms (Magnusson, Egermark, and Carlsson 2000, Carlsson, Egermark, and Magnusson 2002).

The most common diagnosis in patients suffering from TMD is pain in the muscles of mastication (myofascial pain) accounting for 55% of TMD cases (Mehta et al. 2011). Muscle pain usually is accompanied by restriction of functional movement. Chewing or other jaw activities aggravate the patient's pain experience. Other common complaints include jaw pain, earache, headache, and facial pain.

Non-painful masticatory muscle hypertrophy and abnormal tooth wear associated with oral parafunctional such as bruxism (jaw clenching and/or teeth grinding) may be related problems.

EPIDEMIOLOGY OF TMDS

Cross-sectional epidemiologic studies of selected nonpatient populations (adult) show that 40%–70% have at least one sign of joint dysfunction, that is, movement abnormalities, joint noise, and tenderness on palpation. Approximately 33% have at least one symptom, that is, face pain or jaw pain (Rugh and Solberg 1985, Schiffman and Fricton 1988, Schiffman et al. 1990, Dworkin et al. 1990).

Demographically, TMD in individuals who exhibit pain is experienced more often by females than males in reported ranges 3:1 to 9:1 in patients seeking care.

Prevalence of TMD in children and adolescents varies widely in the literature. Prevalence increased during developmental stages and girls in general were more affected than boys. A study investigating TMD in over 1000 preschool and school children (age 3–7 years) showed an incidence of TMD in approximately 14% males and 18% females also demonstrating a statistical difference strongly suggestive of early gender preference (Thilander et al. 2002). Overall signs and symptoms observed in children and adolescents show a lower prevalence than in adults (Motegi et al. 1992, Keeling et al. 1994).

ETIOLOGY OF TMD

Historically, in 1934, James Costen, an otolaryngologist, evaluated 13 patients who presented with pain in or near the ear, tinnitus, dizziness, a sensation of ear fullness, and difficulty swallowing (Costen 1934). He observed that these patients had many missing teeth and, as a result, their jaws were over-closed. The symptoms seemed to diminish when their missing teeth were replaced and the proper vertical dimension (height) of the occlusion was restored. Costen believed that the malocclusion and improper jaw position were the cause of both "disturbed function of the temporomandibular joint" and the associated facial pain. Thereafter, the emphasis of treatment for this condition focused on altering the affected patient's dental occlusion. Figure 8.11 illustrates the complex interplay of CSF, blood, lymph, nerves, muscle, and bones and highlights the need to take any complaint of craniofacial pain seriously. An asymmetry in one area creates a cascade of responses sure to impact structural integrity and optimal function.

More recently, advances in the understanding of joint biomechanics, neuromuscular physiology, autoimmune and musculoskeletal disorders, and pain mechanisms have led to changes in our understanding of the cause of temporomandibular disorders (De Leeuw and Klasser 2008). It can be said that it may be understood at different levels, utilizing different paradigms. It has been accepted that through careful analysis TMD can be broken down into three categories.

1. Structural/anatomical component is based primarily on jaw position which is determined by the relationship of the maxilla and mandibular dentition, which is also influenced by the position of the head and neck. Muscles, nerves, ligaments, joints, blood vessels, and lymphatics are all involved to maintain this relationship (Dawson 1989, Simons, Travell, and Simons 1999, Milani et al. 2000, Makofsky 2000). Any condition that affects these components can result in a structural or chemical discrepancy resulting in a temporomandibular disorder. Take, for example, dehydration, excess water retention, lack of good nutrition, mineral balance, heavy metal toxicity, infection, and macro- or micro-trauma.

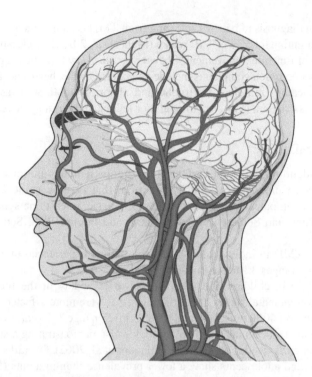

FIGURE 8.11 The complex interplay of CSF, blood, lymph, nerves, muscle, and bones highlights the need to take any complaint of craniofacial pain seriously. An asymmetry in one area creates a cascade of responses sure to impact structural integrity and optimal function.

2. Biochemical components frequently underlie the pathophysiological factors responsible for TMDs. These factors can be far-reaching and may include nutritional deficiencies, inflammatory or infectious process, drug and neurotoxic exposures, as well as genetic and metabolic disorders. Within this category the relationship of TMDs to the autonomic nervous system as described by Klinghardt have become an important consideration. He reports that toxicity of the autonomic ganglia associated with head and neck can occur by way of infectious agents, nutritional deficiencies, trauma, heavy metals, and so on. Unresolved emotional issues through the limbic-hypothalmic axis have also been explained by him (Klinghardt and Willis 1993).

3. Emotional or psychosocial components include stress and emotional or psychological issues which can be current or past (e.g., loss of loved one, job loss, work or domestic stress, emotional issues, childhood abuse, etc.) (Pert 1997, Sarno 2001). Reactions as such as well as other stressors may result in production of catecholamines and other neurotransmitters, which start a chain of events leading to effects such as muscle tightness, pain, insomnia, and other such effects. The impact of such a process may also have a direct or indirect effect on the immune system making the body more susceptible to infections (Yap et al. 2002, Korszun et al. 1998, Auerbach et al. 2001).

Trauma, whether it is micro (teeth grinding) or macro, direct or indirect, is an underlying dynamic force affecting TMJs. Clinically teeth wear or cervical abractions are seen due to such forces (Grippo, Simring, and Schreiner 2004). Pathomechanics in the knee and TMJ are numerous, the majority being macrotrauma through impact or hyperextension of the joint (Bertolucci 1990).

It is widely accepted that acute macrotrauma is probably the most common cause of an internal derangement of the TMJ. Examples of events contributing to it are blows to the jaw, endotracheal intubations, cervical traction, and iatrogenic stretching of the mouth during dental or oral surgery procedures (Huang and Rue 2006, Kaplan and Assael 1991). Trauma to the TMJ structures can affect ligaments, articular cartilage, articular disk, and bone which can lead to intra-articular bio-chemical alterations that have been shown to produce oxidative stress and to generate free radicals. Subsequent inflammatory changes in synovial fluid with the production of a variety of inflamma-tory cytokines can then lead to alteration in the functioning of normal tissues and degenerative disease in the TMJ (Milam and Schmitz 1995, Zardeneta, Milam, and Schmitz 1997, Israel et al. 2006, Ratcliffe et al. 1998).

Genetic marker studies of genes involved with catecholamine metabolism and adrenergic recep-tors suggest that certain polymorphisms (e.g., in the catechol O-methyltransferase [$COMT$] gene) might be associated with changes in pain responsiveness and pain processing in patients with chronic temporomandibular disorders (Diatchenko, Nackley et al. 2006, Diatchenko, Anderson et al. 2006). Differences in pain modulation have been shown between women and men with these disorders, with women showing decreased thresholds to noxious stimuli and more hyperalgesia. In addition, some studies suggest that the affective component of pain in women with temporoman-dibular disorders may be enhanced during the low-estrogen phase of the menstrual cycle (Bhalang et al. 2005, Diatchenko et al. 2005, Bragdon et al. 2002, de Leeuw et al. 2006).

TMJ Symptoms

Pain and sounds are very common with TMJ disorders (Egermark, Carlsson, and Magnusson 2001, Matsumoto, Matsumoto, and Bolognese 2002). Signs and symptoms associated with TMD are a common source of chronic pain complaints in the head and orofacial structures. The primary signs and symptoms associated with TMD originate from the masticatory structures and, therefore, are associated with jaw function. Patients often report pain unilaterally in the preauricular areas, face, or temples. It is important to appreciate that pain associated with most TMD is increased with jaw function. When a patient's pain complaint is not influenced by jaw function, other sources of (oro-facial) pain should be suspected. TMJ sounds are also frequent complaints and may be described as clicking, popping, grating, or crepitus in nature. In many instances, the joint sounds are not accom-panied by pain or dysfunction, and are merely a nuisance to the patient. However, on occasion, joint sounds may be associated with locking of the jaw during opening or closing, or with pain. Patients may even report a sudden change in their bite coincident with the onset of the painful condition. Figure 8.12 illustrates the location of symptoms a patient may experience that is suffering from a TMJ disorder.

TMD can be subdivided into two broad categories related to their primary source of pain and dysfunction: masticatory muscle disorders and intracapsular (TMJ) disorders.

Clinical Evaluation

When a patient presents with craniofacial pain, the first challenge one has to meet is to make a diag-nosis. The clinician must decide if the patient's chief complaint is a TMD issue, or if they show signs of a non-TMD problem such as migraine, neuralgia, intracranial lesion, neoplasm, radiculopathy, tooth pulpalgia, third molar pericoronitis, and so on that may require referral to a different medical or dental specialty. Figure 8.13 demonstrates normal position of the condyle relative to the meniscus within the fossa.

The most common symptom reported by patients with temporomandibular disorders is unilat-eral facial pain. Pain may radiate into the ears, temporal and periorbital region, to the angle of the mandible, and frequently to the posterior neck. The pain is usually reported as a dull, con-stant ache that is worse at certain times of the day. There can be bouts of more severe, sharp pain typically triggered by movements of the mandible. The pain may be present daily or intermittently, but many patients have pain-free intervals. Mandibular motion is usually limited, and attempts at active motion, such as chewing, talking, or yawning, increase the pain. Patients frequently describe

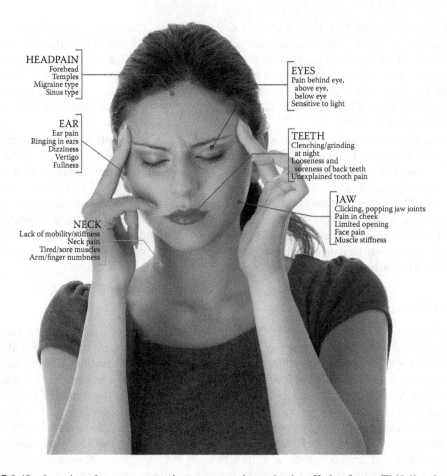

HEADPAIN
Forehead
Temples
Migraine type
Sinus type

EYES
Pain behind eye,
above eye,
below eye
Sensitive to light

EAR
Ear pain
Ringing in ears
Dizziness
Vertigo
Fullness

TEETH
Clenching/grinding
at night
Looseness and
soreness of back teeth
Unexplained tooth pain

JAW
Clicking, popping jaw joints
Pain in cheek
Limited opening
Face pain
Muscle stiffness

NECK
Lack of mobility/stiffness
Neck pain
Tired/sore muscles
Arm/finger numbness

FIGURE 8.12 Location of symptoms a patient may experience that is suffering from a TMJ disorder.

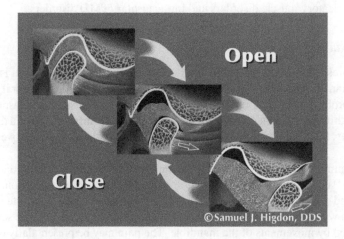

FIGURE 8.13 Normal position of the condyle relative to the meniscus within the fossa. Normal movement of condyle on opening and closing.

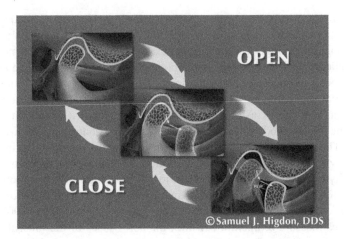

FIGURE 8.14 Meniscus positioned anterior to the condyle, on opening a joint sound is heard suggesting that the meniscus has reduced back into place. On closing the meniscus slips out anterior to the condyle.

"locking" of the jaw, either in the closed-mouth position, with inability to open (most common), or in the open-mouth position, with inability to close the jaw. These symptoms are often worse in the morning, particularly in patients who exhibit parafunctional habits (clenching, grinding, involuntary mandibular movements). Along with limitation of motion there is often deviation to the affected side of the mandible on opening and a "clicking" or "popping" (reducing disc) noise in the joint. This is suggestive of the disc reducing as the jaw opens. Figure 8.14 demonstrates an abnormal position of the meniscus within the fossa. In chronic conditions a clicking jaw may go quiet (nonreducing disc), which shows the jaw on opening deflection to the affected side accompanied with some degree of limited mouth opening. Figure 8.15 demonstrates a meniscus positioned anterior to the condyle within the fossa. On opening the meniscus does not reduce back into place.

Physical examination should include observation and measurement of mandibular motion (maximal interincisal opening, lateral movements, and protrusion), palpation of the muscles of mastication (masseter, temporalis, medial and lateral pterygoid muscles) and the cervical musculature, palpation, or auscultation of the TMJ, and examination of the oral cavity, dentition, occlusion, and salivary glands and inspection and palpation of the anterior and posterior neck. Examination of the cranial nerves, with special attention to the trigeminal system, should also be part of the physical examination.

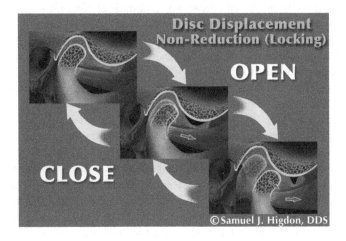

FIGURE 8.15 Meniscus positioned anterior to the condyle, on opening no change in meniscus position suggests that the meniscus has not reduced back into place.

Diagnostic studies are designed to rule out other disorders. They may include the use of blood and serum inflammatory markers to rule out autoimmune disorders and vasculitis. Imaging such as panoramic radiograph (a single-cut tomogram of the entire jaw) remains the most useful screening tool. Plain radiographs have been almost completely replaced by computed tomography (CT) for evaluation of bony morphology and pathology of the joint, mandibular ramus, and condyle. Cone-beam maxillofacial CT is a newer and faster technique, with a lower radiation dose, than conventional whole-body CT (Hashimoto et al. 2014). Magnetic resonance imaging (MRI) has replaced other imaging methods for evaluation of soft-tissue abnormalities of the joint and surrounding region. The anatomy of the joint and the position and structure of the intra-articular disk can be accurately visualized both at rest and in motion. MRI allows for analysis of the blood supply and vascularity of the condyle and for detection of pathologic accumulations of fluid within and around the joint. Diagnostic nerve blocks and muscle trigger point injections may in certain cases provide the only method to identify the true genesis of pain (Bell 1990). Thermography imaging techniques measure temperature within the soft tissues of the musculoskeletal system. Temperature changes on the surface of the skin may correlate with underlying pathosis (Biagioni et al. 1996). This method of imaging does not produce ionizing radiation and therefore is extremely safe with no known side effects.

MANAGEMENT

Treatment often includes a combination of dental, medical, and physical medicine (Simmons III and Gibbs 2005), and stress management through biofeedback relaxation (Johansson et al. 2003). The ultimate management goals mimic those of other orthopedic principles or those for rheumatologic disorders. In the craniofacial and cervical patient population, the reduction of occlusal loading (biting forces), stabilization of the TMJ, and relaxation of muscles allow for easier function of the joint. The majority of patients with temporomandibular disorders present with a chronic pain history of the head and neck, multidisciplinary management tends to be more successful than individual treatments. Conservative management techniques aimed at behavioral modification, supportive medication, physical medicine, and intraoral occlusal guards tend to be successful in 85%–90% of patients. The key to successful management is accurate diagnosis of the precipitating and perpetuating factors for the individual.

Nonsteroidal anti-inflammatory agents are often of value in the acute stage (Dionne 1997, Schütz, Andersen, and Tufik 2007, Ta and Dionne 2004). Treatment is usually administered for 10–14 days, at which time the patient should be reevaluated. Muscle relaxants are frequently used for episodes of acute pain but have not been proven efficacious in chronic conditions. Long-term use of opioid analgesics should be avoided, if at all possible (Dionne 1997). Antidepressants have a long history of effectiveness for the treatment of chronic pain. Their use is often justified, especially when the pain and dysfunction are part of the complex of generalized muscle pain with signs and symptoms of depression (Onghena and Van Houdenhove 1992, Max et al. 1992, Rowbotham et al. 2004).

Tricyclic antidepressants are the most widely used, and a bedtime-only schedule of 10 to 50 mg of nortriptyline, desipramine, or doxepin can be expected to alleviate symptoms in 2–4 weeks (Onghena and Van Houdenhove 1992). If treatment is successful then maintained for 2–4 months, then tapering to a low dose is recommended. Selective serotonin-reuptake inhibitors have also been used as part of the treatment regimen (Dionne 1997). However, some of these agents (fluoxetine and paroxetine) have been implicated in producing increased masticatory muscle activity (bruxism), especially during sleep, and are generally not recommended (Kishi 2007, Lobbezoo et al. 2001).

It is well documented that chronic pain and disability have a strong psychological component and most patients require some form of treatment ranging from simple home health tips (moist heat application, soft diet) and cognitive behavioral intervention to structured psychological and psychiatric intervention, which may include a comprehensive stress management program (sleep management, electromyography [EMG] biofeedback, and progressive relaxation), and lifestyle changes.

Counseling, relaxation techniques, stress management, work pacing, guided imaging, biofeedback, cognitive therapy, and other behavioral approaches to treatment have all been reported as helpful (Dworkin 1996, Raphael et al. 2003, Crider, Glaros, and Gevirtz 2005).

A 1996 National Institutes of Health Consensus Conference on Behavioral Medicine in the Management of Chronic Pain outlined techniques that are considered effective and indications for using them (Health 1995).

Physical medicine treatments address the structural aspects of temporomandibular and craniocervical disorders and may include myofascial (dry needling) and craniosacral physical therapy, orthopedic correction for the cervical spine, muscle education, and TMJ pain relief therapies. Manual manipulation, massage, ultrasonography, and iontophoresis are helpful in reconditioning and retraining the masticatory and the other craniocervical muscles that are usually involved in temporomandibular disorders (Medlicott and Harris 2006). Passive motion has also been reported as effective in rehabilitating some of the biochemical and biomechanical changes that occur in injured synovial joints, muscles, and periarticular tissues (Israel and Syrop 1997). Modification of the patient's nutritional factors, daily activities, and posture is important to the overall effectiveness of the treatment program.

Patients who present with craniocervical and mandibular dysfunctions and a history of trauma often have chronic headaches and neck pain in addition to the specific TMD. In these patients, it is beneficial to add orthopedic intraoral appliances, referred to as night guards, bite plates, bite splints, or bruxism guards, which are effective in relaxing jaw muscles, relieving jaw and joint pain, and stabilizing the maxillomandibular bite relationship. They are designed to improve function of the TMJ by altering joint mechanics and increasing potential mobility, to improve the function of the masticatory motor system while reducing abnormal muscle function, and also to protect the teeth from jaw clenching and potential tooth fracture or attrition. It has been hypothesized that these devices may make patients more conscious of their oral parafunctional habits, altering proprioceptive input and central motor system areas that initiate and regulate masticatory function (Dao and Lavigne 1998, Fricton 2007, 2006).

The aim of these devices should be used as a short-term treatment until symptoms subside. Dental corrections of the bite should not be attempted until the pain and dysfunction have subsided. Surgery of the TMJ is usually not initially recommended unless there is an acute injury or a specific joint-related problem that has not been resolved with nonsurgical management.

EFFECTS OF TMD

From our understanding of the impact of a temporomandibular joint condition and its relationship with the trigeminal nerve a vast series of symptoms can be treated or more effectively managed.

Simmons and Gibbs demonstrated that treating patients with an anterior repositioning appliance for temporomandibular disorders provided significant relief for most symptoms in their patient population. Most frequent symptoms management were frontal cephalalgia, temporal cephalalgia, occipital cephalalgia, otalgia, TMJ pain, painful and difficult mastication, back of neck pain, and pain on opening/closing of the mouth (Simmons III and Gibbs 2005). The association of sleep bruxism and painful TMD also greatly increases the risk for episodic migraine, episodic tension type headache, and chronic migraine (Graff-Radford and Bassiur 2014, Fernandes et al. 2013, Ciancaglini and Radaelli 2001, Franco et al. 2010).

Studies have shown that a TMJ disorder has some effect on head and body posture (Kritsineli and Shim 1991, Lee, Okeson, and Lindroth 1995, Zonnenberg et al. 1996, Cuccia and Caradonna 2009, Ciancaglini, Testa, and Radaelli 1999, Ayub, Glasheen-Wray, and Kraus 1984, Kaplan and Assael 1991). Figure 8.16 shows posture changes in patients with malocclusions, asymmetries, and forward head posture. These can create kyphosis and lordosis postures with resulting pain syndromes. It stands to reason that whole-body wellness is dependent on a treatment plan that focuses on realignment of this crucial system.

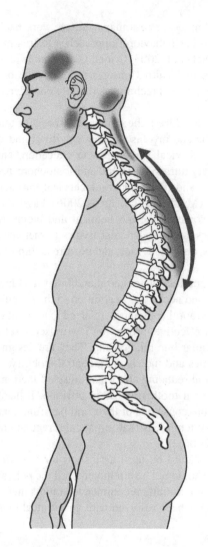

FIGURE 8.16 Malocclusions, asymmetries, and forward head posture create kyphosis and lordosis with resulting pain syndromes. It stands to reason that whole-body wellness is dependent on a treatment plan that focuses on realignment of this crucial system.

Olmos et al. showed that improvement in the condyle fossa relationship was related to decreased forward head posture. Their study suggests that optimizing mandibular condyle position should be considered in the management of forward head posture (adaptive posture) (Olmos et al. 2005). As also mentioned early in this chapter, the effect of airway on posture can also be reflective of the point that the position of the mandible affects both airway and TMD symptoms in some patients.

While the medical community understands this concept when it comes to the insertion of orthotics by a podiatrist, effectively realigning the knees, hips, and spine from the bottom up, we believe that the evolving science of postural neurology will demonstrate that temporomandibular occlusal therapy supports the complex interplay between the cranial nerves, cervical spine, and shoulders, effectively realigning the spine from the top down.

Simms and Stack have also demonstrated in a pilot study that by addressing a TMJ disorders, an internal derangement condition such as Tourette's syndrome, which is termed a structural-reflex disorder, can be quite effectively managed by using a neurocranio vertical distractor (NCVD) (Stack 2012, Sims and Stack 2009, 2010).

Clinical work suggests that the auriculotemporal (AT) nerve, a branch of the mandibular nerve, the largest of the three divisions of the trigeminal nerve, plays a critical role in TMD sequelae. The AT nerve provides the somatosensory fibers that supply the joint, the middle ear, and the temporal region. By projecting fibers toward the otic ganglion, the AT nerve establishes an important bridge to the sympathetic system. As it courses posteriorly to the condylar head of the TMJ, compression, injury, or irritation of the AT nerve can lead to significant neurologic and neuro-muscular disorders, including Tourette's syndrome, torticollis, gait or balance disorders, and Parkinson's disease (Demerjian, Sims, and Stack 2011).

Future research is needed to determine whether the suppression of dystonic and nondystonic movement disorders by jaw realignment arises from the decompression of injured AT nerves in the TMJs, the action of altered sensory-motor feedback loops within trigeminal-brainstem-supra brainstem interactions, a combination of these, or other mechanisms (Sims, Clark, and Cooper 2012).

This glimpse into the importance of enhancing health by starting with the correct development of one's face and cranium, understanding how these affect cranial innervation and ultimately their airway, will no doubt lead to an increased effort to collaborate with dental specialists and integrate these concepts into your current practice.

REFERENCES

http://www.braininitiative.nih.gov/.

Auerbach SM, DM Laskin, LME Frantsve, and T Orr. 2001. Depression, pain, exposure to stressful life events, and long-term outcomes in temporomandibular disorder patients. *Journal of Oral and Maxillofacial Surgery* 59 (6):628–633.

Ayub E, M Glasheen-Wray, and S Kraus. 1984. Head posture: A case study of the effects on the rest position of the mandible*. *Journal of Orthopaedic & Sports Physical Therapy* 5 (4):179–183.

Bell WE. 1990. *Temporomandibular Disorders: Classification, Diagnosis, Management.* Chicago: Year Book Medical Pub.

Benkert KK. 1996. The effectiveness of orofacial myofunctional therapy in improving dental occlusion. *The International Journal of Orofacial Myology: Official Publication of the International Association of Orofacial Myology* 23:35–46.

Bertolucci LE. 1990. Trilogy of the Triad of O'Donoghue in the knee and its analogy to the TMJ derangement. *Cranio: The Journal of Craniomandibular Practice* 8 (3):264–270.

Bhalang K, A Sigurdsson, GD Slade, and W Maixner. 2005. Associations among four modalities of experimental pain in women. *The Journal of Pain* 6 (9):604–611.

Biagioni PA, RB Longmore, JG McGimpsey, and PJ Lamey. 1996. Infrared thermography. Its role in dental research with particular reference to craniomandibular disorders. *Dentomaxillofacial Radiology* 25 (3):119–124.

Bragdon EE, KC Light, NL Costello, A Sigurdsson, S Bunting, K Bhalang, and W Maixner. 2002. Group differences in pain modulation: Pain-free women compared to pain-free men and to women with TMD. *Pain* 96 (3):227–237.

Carlsson GE, I Egermark, and T Magnusson. 2002. Predictors of signs and symptoms of temporomandibular disorders: A 20-year follow-up study from childhood to adulthood. *Acta Odontologica Scandinavica* 60 (3):180–185.

Carrascoza KC, R de Fátima Possobon, LM Tomita, and AB Alves de Moraes. 2006. Consequences of bottle-feeding to the oral facial development of initially breastfed children. *Jornal de pediatria* 82 (5):395–397.

Cawson RA and EW Odell. 2008. *Cawson's Essentials of Oral Pathology and Oral Medicine.* London, UK: Elsevier Health Sciences.

Cheng TMW, TL Cascino, and BM Onofrio. 1993. Comprehensive study of diagnosis and treatment of trigeminal neuralgia secondary to tumors. *Neurology* 43 (11):2298–2298.

Churchill SE, LL Shackelford, JN Georgi, and MT Black. 2004. Morphological variation and airflow dynamics in the human nose. *American Journal of Human Biology* 16 (6):625–638.

Ciancaglini R and G Radaelli. 2001. The relationship between headache and symptoms of temporomandibular disorder in the general population. *Journal of Dentistry* 29 (2):93–98.

Ciancaglini R, M Testa, and G Radaelli. 1999. Association of neck pain with symptoms of temporomandibular dysfunction in the general adult population. *Scandinavian Journal of Rehabilitation Medicine* 31 (1):17–22.

Costen JB. 1934. A syndrome of ear and sinus symptoms dependent upon disturbed function of the temporo-mandibular joint. *Annals of Otology, Rhinology & Laryngology* 43:1–15.

Crider A, AG Glaros, and RN Gevirtz. 2005. Efficacy of biofeedback-based treatments for temporomandibular disorders. *Applied Psychophysiology and Biofeedback* 30 (4):333–345.

Cuccia A and C Caradonna. 2009. The relationship between the stomatognathic system and body posture. *Clinics* 64 (1):61–66.

Dao TT and GJ Lavigne. 1998. Oral splints: The crutches for temporomandibular disorders and bruxism? *Critical Reviews in Oral Biology & Medicine* 9 (3):345–361.

Dawson PE. 1989. *Evaluation, Diagnosis, and Treatment of Occlusal Problems*. St. Louis: Mosby Inc.

de Leeuw R, RJC Albuquerque, AH Andersen, and CR Carlson. 2006. Influence of estrogen on brain activa-tion during stimulation with painful heat. *Journal of Oral and Maxillofacial Surgery* 64 (2):158–166.

De Leeuw R and GD Klasser. 2008. Orofacial pain: Guidelines for assessment, diagnosis, and management.

Demerjian GG, AB Sims, and BC Stack. 2011. Proteomic signature of Temporomandibular Joint Disorders (TMD): Toward diagnostically predictive biomarkers. *Bioinformation* 5 (7):282–284.

Diatchenko L, AD Anderson, GD Slade, RB Fillingim, SA Shabalina, TJ Higgins, S Sama et al., 2006. Three major haplotypes of the β2 adrenergic receptor define psychological profile, blood pressure, and the risk for development of a common musculoskeletal pain disorder. *American Journal of Medical Genetics Part B: Neuropsychiatric Genetics* 141 (5):449–462.

Diatchenko L, AG Nackley, GD Slade, K Bhalang, I Belfer, MB Max, D Goldman, and W Maixner. 2006. Catechol-O-methyltransferase gene polymorphisms are associated with multiple pain-evoking stimuli. *Pain* 125 (3):216–224.

Diatchenko L, GD Slade, AG Nackley, K Bhalang, A Sigurdsson, I Belfer, D Goldman et al., 2005. Genetic basis for individual variations in pain perception and the development of a chronic pain condition. *Human Molecular Genetics* 14 (1):135–143.

Dionne RA. 1997. Pharmacologic treatments for temporomandibular disorders. *Oral Surgery, Oral Medicine, Oral Pathology, Oral Radiology, and Endodontology* 83 (1):134–142.

Dworkin SF. 1996. The case for incorporating biobehavioral treatment into TMD management. *The Journal of the American Dental Association* 127 (11):1607–1610.

Dworkin SF, KH Huggins, L LeResche, M Korff, J Howard, E Truelove, and E Sommers. 1990. Epidemiology of signs and symptoms in temporomandibular disorders: Clinical signs in cases and controls. *The Journal of the American Dental Association* 120 (3):273–281.

Dyken ME and KB Im. 2009. Obstructive sleep apnea and stroke. *CHEST Journal* 136 (6):1668–1677.

Egermark I, GE Carlsson, and T Magnusson. 2001. A 20-year longitudinal study of subjective symptoms of temporomandibular disorders from childhood to adulthood. *Acta Odontologica Scandinavica* 59 (1):40–48.

El-Ad B and P Lavie. 2005. Effect of sleep apnea on cognition and mood. *International Review of Psychiatry* 17 (4):277–282.

Enlow DH and MG Hans. 1996. *Essentials of facial growth*. Philadelphia, PA: WB Saunders Company.

Fernandes G, Franco AL, Gonçalves DA, Speciali JG, Bigal ME, and CM Camparis. 2013. Head Pain, TMJ Pain. *J Orofac Pain* 27 (1):14–20.

Flanagan M. 2011. https://uprightdoctor.wordpress.com/2011/02/06/c1-c2-and-csf-flow/. Accessed September 2.

Franco AL, DAG Goncalves, SM Castanharo, JG Speciali, ME Bigal, and CM Camparis. 2010. Migraine is the most prevalent primary headache in individuals with temporomandibular disorders. *Journal of Orofacial Pain* 24 (3):287.

Fricton J. 2006. Current evidence providing clarity in management of temporomandibular disorders: Summary of a systematic review of randomized clinical trials for intra-oral appliances and occlusal therapies. *Journal of Evidence Based Dental Practice* 6 (1):48–52.

Fricton J. 2007. Myogenous temporomandibular disorders: Diagnostic and management considerations. *Dental Clinics of North America* 51 (1):61–83.

Göbel H and RW Baloh. 1999. Disorders of ear, nose, and sinus. In: *The Headaches*, 2nd ed., Olesen J, Tfelt-Hansen P, and Welch KMA (Eds.) Philadelphia, PA: Lippincott Williams & Wilkins: 908–912.

Graff-Radford SB and JP Bassiur. 2014. Temporomandibular disorders and headaches. *Neurologic Clinics* 32 (2):525–537.

Greven M. 2011. TMD, bruxism, and occlusion. *American Journal of Orthodontics and Dentofacial Orthopedics* 139 (4):424.

Grippo JO, M Simring, and S Schreiner. 2004. Attrition, abrasion, corrosion and abfraction revisited: A new perspective on tooth surface lesions. *The Journal of the American Dental Association* 135 (8):1109–1118.

Harari D, M Redlich, S Miri, T Hamud, and M Gross. 2010. The effect of mouth breathing versus nasal breathing on dentofacial and craniofacial development in orthodontic patients. *The Laryngoscope* 120 (10):2089–2093.

Hashimoto K, S Kawashima, S Kameoka, Y Akiyama, T Honjoya, K Ejima, and K Sawada. 2014. Comparison of image validity between cone beam computed tomography for dental use and multidetector row helical computed tomography. *Dentomaxillofacial Radiology* 36 (8):465–471.

Health, US National Institutes of. 1995. Integration of behavioral and relaxation approaches into the treatment of chronic pain and insomnia. *Technology Assessment Conference Statement* 313–318.

Hersi AS. 2010. Obstructive sleep apnea and cardiac arrhythmias. *Annals of Thoracic Medicine* 5 (1):10.

Huang GJ and TC Rue. 2006. Third-molar extraction as a risk factor for temporomandibular disorder. *The Journal of the American Dental Association* 137 (11):1547–1554.

Ip MSM, B Lam, MMT Ng, WK Lam, KWT Tsang, and KSL Lam. 2002. Obstructive sleep apnea is independently associated with insulin resistance. *American Journal of Respiratory and Critical Care Medicine* 165 (5):670–676.

Israel HA, C-J Langevin, MD Singer, and DA Behrman. 2006. The relationship between temporomandibular joint synovitis and adhesions: Pathogenic mechanisms and clinical implications for surgical management. *Journal of Oral and Maxillofacial Surgery* 64 (7):1066–1074.

Israel HA and SB Syrop. 1997. The important role of motion in the rehabilitation of patients with mandibular hypomobility: A review of the literature. *Cranio-Journal of Craniomandibular Practice* 15 (1):74–83.

Jabbar NSA, AB Miguel Bueno, PE da Silva, H Scavone-Junior, and RI Ferreira. 2011. Bottle feeding, increased overjet and Class 2 primary canine relationship: Is there any association? *Brazilian Oral Research* 25 (4):331–337.

Johansson A, L Unell, GE Carlsson, B Söderfeldt, and A Halling. 2003. Gender difference in symptoms related to temporomandibular disorders in a population of 50-year-old subjects. *Journal of Orofacial Pain* 17 (1):29–35.

Kaplan AS and LA Assael. 1991. *Temporomandibular Disorders: Diagnosis and Treatment*. Philadelphia: WB Saunders Company.

Keeling SD, S McGorray, TT Wheeler, and GJ King. 1994. Risk factors associated with temporomandibular joint sounds in children 6 to 12 years of age. *American Journal of Orthodontics and Dentofacial Orthopedics* 105 (3):279–287.

Kim NH, NH Cho, C-H Yun, SK Lee, DW Yoon, HJ Cho, JH Ahn, JA Seo, SG Kim, and KM Choi. 2013. Association of obstructive sleep apnea and glucose metabolism in subjects with or without obesity. *Diabetes Care* 36 (12):3909–3915.

Kishi Y. 2007. Paroxetine-induced bruxism effectively treated with tandospirone. *The Journal of Neuropsychiatry and Clinical Neurosciences* 19 (1):90–91.

Klinghardt D and T Willis. 1993. The autonomic nervous system and it's relationship to headache. *The Journal of Neurological and Orthopaedic Medicine and Surgery* (14):109–109.

Korszun A, E Papadopoulos, M Demitrack, C Engleberg, and L Crofford. 1998. The relationship between temporomandibular disorders and stress-associated syndromes. *Oral Surgery, Oral Medicine, Oral Pathology, Oral Radiology, and Endodontology* 86 (4):416–420.

Kritsineli M and YS Shim. 1991. Malocclusion, body posture, and temporomandibular disorder in children with primary and mixed dentition. *The Journal of Clinical Pediatric Dentistry* 16 (2):86–93.

Lee W-Y, JP Okeson, and J Lindroth. 1995. The relationship between forward head posture and temporomandibular disorders. *Journal of Orofacial Pain* 9 (2):161–167.

Legović, M and L Ostrić. 1990. The effects of feeding methods on the growth of the jaws in infants. *ASDC Journal of Dentistry for Children* 58 (3):253–255.

Leiter JC. 1996. Upper airway shape: Is it important in the pathogenesis of obstructive sleep apnea? *American Journal of Respiratory and Critical Care Medicine* 153 (3):894–898.

Leung RST and T Douglas Bradley. 2001. Sleep apnea and cardiovascular disease. *American Journal of Respiratory and Critical Care Medicine* 164 (12):2147–2165.

Linder-Aronson S. 1970. Adenoids. Their effect on mode of breathing and nasal airflow and their relationship to characteristics of the facial skeleton and the denition. A biometric, rhino-manometric and cephalometro-radiographic study on children with and without adenoids. *Acta oto-laryngologica. Supplementum* 265:1.

Lobbezoo F, RJA van Denderen, JGC Verheij, and M Naeije. 2001. Reports of SSRI-associated bruxism in the family physician's office. *Journal of Orofacial Pain* 15 (4):340–346.

Loeser JD and JJ Bonica. 2001. *Bonica's Management of Pain*. Philadelphia: Lippincott Williams & Wilkins.

Magnusson, T, I Egermark, and GE Carlsson. 2000. A longitudinal epidemiologic study of signs and symptoms of temporomandibular disorders from 15 to 35 years of age. *Journal of Orofacial Pain* 14 (4):310–319.

Makofsky HW. 2000. The influence of forward head posture on dental occlusion. *Cranio: The Journal of Craniomandibular Practice* 18 (1):30–39.

Mathews ES and SJ Scrivani. 2000. Percutaneous stereotactic radiofrequency thermal rhizotomy for the treatment of trigeminal neuralgia. *The Mount Sinai Journal of Medicine, New York* 67 (4):288–299.

Matsumoto MA, W Matsumoto, and AM Bolognese. 2002. Study of the signs and symptoms of temporomandibular dysfunction in individuals with normal occlusion and malocclusion. *Cranio: The Journal of Craniomandibular Practice* 20 (4):274–281.

Max MB, SA Lynch, J Muir, SE Shoaf, B Smoller, and R Dubner. 1992. Effects of desipramine, amitriptyline, and fluoxetine on pain in diabetic neuropathy. *New England Journal of Medicine* 326 (19): 1250–1256.

Medlicott MS and SR Harris. 2006. A systematic review of the effectiveness of exercise, manual therapy, electrotherapy, relaxation training, and biofeedback in the management of temporomandibular disorder. *Physical Therapy* 86 (7):955–973.

Mehta N, GE Maloney, DS Bana, and SJ Scrivani. 2011. *Head, Face, and Neck Pain Science, Evaluation, and Management: An Interdisciplinary Approach.* New Jersey: John Wiley & Sons.

Milam SB and JP Schmitz. 1995. Molecular biology of temporomandibular joint disorders: Proposed mechanisms of disease. *Journal of Oral and Maxillofacial Surgery* 53 (12):1448–1454.

Milani RS, DD De Periere, L Lapeyre, and L Pourreyron. 2000. Relationship between dental occlusion and posture. *Cranio: The Journal of Craniomandibular Practice* 18 (2):127–134.

Moss ML. 1965. The veloepiglottic sphincter and obligate. Nose breathing in the neonate. *The Journal of Pediatrics* 67 (2):330–331.

Moss ML. 1997. The functional matrix hypothesis revisited. 2. The role of an osseous connected cellular network. *American Journal of Orthodontics and Dentofacial Orthopedics* 112 (2):221–226.

Moss ML and L Salentijn. 1969. The primary role of functional matrices in facial growth. *American Journal of Orthodontics* 55 (6):566–577.

Motegi E, H Miyazaki, I Ogura, H Konishi, and M Sebata. 1992. An orthodontic study of temporomandibular joint disorders Part 1: Epidemiological research in Japanese 6–18 year olds. *The Angle Orthodontist* 62 (4):249–256.

Neiva FCB, DM Cattoni, JL de A Ramos, and H Issler. 2003. Desmame precoce: Implicações para o desenvolvimento motor-oral. *J Pediatr* 79 (1):7–12.

Neville MC. 2001. Anatomy and physiology of lactation. *Pediatric Clinics of North America* 48 (1):13–34.

Nguyen M, Raymond M, Anthony B, Charles P, and Robert O. 1986. Facial pain symptoms in patients with cerebellopontine angle tumors: A report of 44 cases of cerebellopontine angle meningioma and a review of the literature. *The Clinical Journal of Pain* 2 (1):3–9.

Olmos SR, D Kritz-Silverstein, W Halligan, ST Silverstein. 2005. The effect of condyle fossa relationships on head posture. *CRANIO* 23 (1):48–52.

Onghena P and B Van Houdenhove. 1992. Antidepressant-induced analgesia in chronic non-malignant pain: A meta-analysis of 39 placebo-controlled studies. *Pain* 49 (2):205–219.

Özbek MM, K Miyamoto, AA Lowe, and JA Fleetham. 1998. Natural head posture, upper airway morphology and obstructive sleep apnoea severity in adults. *The European Journal of Orthodontics* 20 (2):133–143.

Pert CB. 1997. *Molecules of Emotion*, 1st ed., New York, NY: Simon & Scribner.

Pertschuk MJ and LA Whitaker. 1982. Social and psychological effects of craniofacial deformity and surgical reconstruction. *Clinics in Plastic Surgery* 9 (3):297–306.

Pierotti SR. 2001. Breastfeeding: Influence on occlusion, oral habits and functions. *Rev Dent Press Orthodon Ortop Facial* 6:91–98.

Raphael KG, JJ Klausner, S Nayak, and JJ Marbach. 2003. Complementary and alternative therapy use by patients with myofascial temporomandibular disorders. *Journal of Orofacial Pain* 17 (1):36–41.

Rasch B and J Born. 2013. About sleep's role in memory. *Physiol Rev* 93 (2):681–766.

Ratcliffe A, HA Israel, F Saed-Nejad, and B Diamond. 1998. Proteoglycans in the synovial fluid of the temporomandibular joint as an indicator of changes in cartilage metabolism during primary and secondary osteoarthritis. *Journal of Oral and Maxillofacial Surgery* 56 (2):204–208.

Rodenstein DO, A Kahn, D Blum, and DC Stănescu. 1986. Nasal occlusion during sleep in normal and near-miss for sudden death syndrome infants. *Bulletin européen de physiopathologie respiratoire* 23 (3):223–226.

Rosenblatt MA and PJ Sakol. 1989. Ocular and periocular pain. *Otolaryngologic Clinics of North America* 22 (6):1173–1203.

Rowbotham MC, V Goli, NR Kunz, and D Lei. 2004. Venlafaxine extended release in the treatment of painful diabetic neuropathy: A double-blind, placebo-controlled study. *Pain* 110 (3):697–706.

Rubin RM. 1987. Effects of nasal airway obstruction on facial growth. *Ear, Nose, & Throat Journal* 66 (5): 212.

Rugh JD and WK Solberg. 1985. Oral health status in the United States: Temporomandibular disorders. *Journal of Dental Education* 49 (6):398–406.

Sánchez-Molins M, CJ Grau, GC Lischeid, and TJM Ustrell. 2010. Comparative study of the craniofacial growth depending on the type of lactation received. *European Journal of Paediatric Dentistry: Official Journal of European Academy of Paediatric Dentistry* 11 (2):87–92.

Sarno JE. 2001. *Healing back pain: The mind-body connection*, New York: Grand Central Publishing.

Schiffman E and JR Fricton. 1988. Epidemiology of TMJ and craniofacial pain. *TMJ and Craniofacial Pain: Diagnosis and Management*, St. Louis, MO: Ishiaku Euro American: 1–10.

Schiffman EL, JR Fricton, DP Haley, and BL Shapiro. 1990. The prevalence and treatment needs of subjects with temporomandibular disorders. *The Journal of the American Dental Association* 120 (3):295–303.

Schütz TCB, ML Andersen, and S Tufik. 2007. Effects of COX-2 inhibitor in temporomandibular joint acute inflammation. *Journal of Dental Research* 86 (5):475–479.

Settipane RA and C Schwindt. 2013. Chapter 15: Allergic rhinitis. *American Journal of Rhinology and Allergy* 27 (3):S52–S55.

Simmons III, H Clifton, and S Julian Gibbs. 2005. Anterior repositioning appliance therapy for TMJ disorders: Specific symptoms relieved and relationship to disk status on MRI. *CRANIO®* 23 (2):89–99.

Simons DG, JG Travell, and LS Simons. 1999. *Travell & Simons' myofascial pain and dysfunction: Upper half of body*, Vol. 1, Baltimore, MD: Lippincott Williams & Wilkins.

Sims AB, VP Clark, and MS Cooper. 2012. Suppression of movement disorders by jaw realignment. *Pain Medicine* 13 (5):731–732.

Sims A and B Stack. 2009. Tourette's syndrome: A pilot study for the discontinuance of a movement disorder. *Cranio* 27 (1):11–18.

Sims AB and BC Stack. 2010. An intraoral neurocranial vertical distractor appliance provides unique treatment for Tourette's syndrome and resolves comorbid neurobehavioral problems of obsessive compulsive disorder. *Medical Hypotheses* 75 (2):179–184.

Singh VP and TP Moss. 2015. Psychological impact of visible differences in patients with congenital craniofacial anomalies. *Progress in Orthodontics* 16 (1):1.

Stack BC. 2012. My journey from orthodontics to craniofacial pain and TMJ to movement disorders. *CRANIO®* 30 (3):156–158.

Szabo S, Y Tache, and A Somogyi. 2012. The legacy of Hans Selye and the origins of stress research: A retrospective 75 years after his landmark brief 'letter' to the editor of nature. *Stress* 15 (5):472–478.

Ta LE and RA Dionne. 2004. Treatment of painful temporomandibular joints with a cyclooxygenase-2 inhibitor: A randomized placebo-controlled comparison of celecoxib to naproxen. *Pain* 111 (1):13–21.

Tepper SJ. 2004. New thoughts on sinus headache. *Allergy and Asthma Proceedings* 25 (2):95–96.

Thilander B, G Rubio, L Pena, and C de Mayorga. 2002. Prevalence of temporomandibular dysfunction and its association with malocclusion in children and adolescents: An epidemiologic study related to specified stages of dental development. *The Angle Orthodontist* 72 (2):146–154.

Watson PL, P Ceriana, and F Fanfulla. 2012. Delirium: Is sleep important? *Best Practice & Research Clinical Anaesthesiology* 26 (3):355–366.

Whedon JM and D Glassey. 2009. Cerebrospinal fluid stasis and its clinical significance. *Alternative Therapies in Health and Medicine* 15 (3):54.

Yap AUJ, EK Chua, SF Dworkin, HH Tan, and KBC Tan. 2002. Multiple pains and psychosocial functioning/psychologic distress in TMD patients. *International Journal of Prosthodontics* 15 (5):461–466.

Yaranov DM, A Smyrlis, N Usatii, A Butler, JR Petrini, J Mendez, and MK Warshofsky. 2015. Effect of obstructive sleep apnea on frequency of stroke in patients with atrial fibrillation. *The American Journal of Cardiology* 115 (4):461–465.

Zardeneta G, SB Milam, and JP Schmitz. 1997. Presence of denatured hemoglobin deposits in diseased temporomandibular joints. *Journal of Oral and Maxillofacial Surgery* 55 (11):1242–1248.

Zonnenberg AJ, CJ Van Maanen, RA Oostendorp, and JW Elvers. 1996. Body posture photographs as a diagnostic aid for musculoskeletal disorders related to temporomandibular disorders (TMD). *Cranio: The Journal of Craniomandibular Practice* 14 (3):225–232.

9 The Role of the Clinical Laboratory in Nutritional Assessment

Harvey W. Kaufman

CONTENTS

Traditional Laboratory Tests that Assess Nutritional Status: Protein-Calorie Deficits.................263
   Nitrogen Balance...264
   Amino Acids..264
   Vegetarian and Other Diets 265
   Environmental Respiratory Factors and Nutrition 265
      Tobacco: Cigarettes 265
      Air Pollution 265
      Environmental Allergies and Asthma 266
   Exposure to Lead, Mercury, and Other Heavy Metals..266
Our Bodies and Nutrition..267
   Genes...267
   Alcohol..267
   ABO Blood Groups...268
   APO E Gene 268
   Physiology...269
      Menstrual Cycle 269
      Hydration...269
Medical Conditions 270
   Anorexia Nervosa and Bulimia and Other Eating Disorders 270
   Kidney Stones 270
Body Mass Index 270
   Post-Bariatric Surgery 271
   Cardiovascular Disease 271
   Hormones 272
      Diabetes...272
      Thyroid Disease...272
   The Hunger Games: Hormones...273
   Malabsorption 273
   Inflammatory Bowel Disease 275
   Sweat Chloride (Cystic Fibrosis) 275
   Celiac Disease 275
   Lactose and Soy Intolerance 276
   Food Allergy...276
Diet and Supplements and Herbal Medicine 277
   Vitamins and Minerals 277
      Iron Deficiency 277

Folic Acid (Vitamin B9) 278
Vitamin B12 (Cobalamin) 279
Vitamin D 279
Fat-Soluble Vitamins 280
Vitamin E (Tocopherol) 280
Water-Soluble Vitamins and Micronutrients 280
Other Micronutrients and Trace Elements 281
Infections 281
Foreign Bodies 281
Helicobacter pylori (*H. pylori*) 282
Gut Flora (Microbiota) 282
Closing 283
References 283

Nutrition is essential for our well-being. We can readily observe the effects of some forms of nutritional imbalance, such as kwashiorkor (severe protein-energy malnutrition) and overeating. We can see the bone deformation of rickets and observe the spots associated with scurvy. However, evidence for less extreme nutritional deficiencies and suboptimal levels and excesses of nutrients is best provided by clinical laboratory assessment. Laboratory tests can also identify latent disease and guide nutritional choices. In short, the clinical laboratory can provide insight into what is occurring within our organs and our cells, invisible to the human eye and out of reach from the gentle hands and stethoscope of the physician.

The U.S. Department of Health and Human Services and Department of Agriculture created guidelines for healthy eating but not for nutritional assessment.[1] There are, at best, limited medical professional guidelines on laboratory assessment of nutritional status in terms of whom should be tested, the indications for testing, and which tests to employ. This near vacuum contributes to the great variability in testing among healthcare providers and, most likely, to gross underutilization of the clinical laboratory to support medical decision-making and patient management for nutritional assessment. Exceptions include the Endocrine Society guidance for vitamin D testing and other medical organizations that provide guidance for patients with specific medical conditions such as diabetes.

This brief chapter describes the essential role the clinical laboratory can play in understanding human nutrition and in evaluating our well-being. A premise in this chapter is that too little or too much of anything can contribute to health impairment and, when severe, to death. There is a point or a range when the concentration of nutrients is "optimal," meaning we can perform at our peak capacity. Suboptimal or excessive levels of nutrients can dampen our function or interfere with achieving our peak capacity. Figure 9.1 is a conceptual portrayal of the need to stay in balance and the impact of deficiencies and excessive amounts of nutrients. This balance of our nutritional needs changes as we grow, as we place demands on our bodies, and in complex interactions among systems and medical conditions.

The x-axis represents the range of nutritional status with ideal in the center and gross deficiency and excess at each end. The y-axis represents an arbitrary scale of physiological states from optimal health (100) to overt disease (20) at each periphery.

This chapter takes a wide view on "nutrition" and includes what we put into our bodies including the air we breathe. What we put into our body can be intended, for example, our diets, or unintended, for example, contaminants and toxins. This chapter will *not* address medications, illicit drugs, vaccines, or over-the-counter herbs and supplements that affect our health and well-being. There are clinical laboratory tests that address many of these topics, but they fall outside of the broad definition of "nutrition."

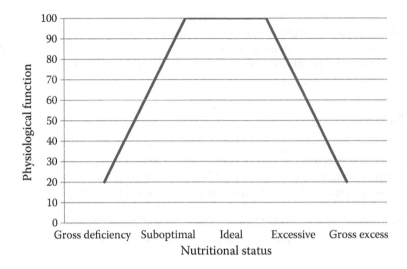

FIGURE 9.1 Physiological function relative to nutritional status.

TRADITIONAL LABORATORY TESTS THAT ASSESS NUTRITIONAL STATUS: PROTEIN-CALORIE DEFICITS

Protein-calorie deficits are common in countries with insufficient food supplies. But even in countries with apparently adequate food supplies, protein-calorie deficits can be common in poor communities, in households with poor diets, and among patients who are unable to eat without pain. People who are alcoholic or have protein-losing enteropathies or malabsorption may also have protein-calorie deficits.

Core laboratory testing for nutritional status includes assessment of four serum proteins (albumin, transthyretin [prealbumin], retinol-binding protein, transferrin), iron status, and vitamin D (25-hydroxyvitamin D). The four protein tests are usually reserved for patients with eating disorders, diets that restrict protein, calories, or essential nutrients, or medical conditions that compromise healthy eating, absorption, and utilization of nutrients. Because these proteins are produced in the liver, levels may be suppressed in liver disease. Also, malnutrition, renal loss (e.g., nephrotic syndrome), hormone therapy, and pregnancy may account for low levels. The four proteins are also considered "negative acute phase reactant" proteins; in the presence of inflammation, levels of these four proteins are suppressed. Thus, interpreting low protein levels associated with malnutrition requires ruling out inflammation and liver disease. The half-lives of the proteins help to understand when protein levels decline and when they recover. Transthyretin levels are sensitive to short-term changes in protein-calorie deficits and recovery (Table 9.1).

TABLE 9.1
Protein Assessment of Protein-Calorie Deficits

Protein	Function	Half-Life (Days)
Albumin	Primary serum protein; primary carrier protein for many substances and hormones; provides plasma oncotic pressure	14–21
Transthyretin (Prealbumin)	Carrier for retinol-binding protein; binds to thyroxine	2–3
Retinol-binding protein	Vitamin A transport protein	12–24
Transferrin	Involved in iron transport	8–10

The four serum protein tests are used to assess protein-calorie malnutrition and to monitor parental nutrition. Levels of ceruloplasmin, alpha-2-macroglobulin, and haptoglobin are decreased in malnutrition but increased as acute-phase reactants. C-reactive protein is also useful to assess inflammation. Testing of healthy people, including athletes, has no value.[2] Testing should be reserved for patients suspected of protein-calorie malnutrition.

NITROGEN BALANCE

The classic approach to assessing protein balance is measuring nitrogen balance. Approximately 16% of protein is nitrogen, and our body's balance of nitrogen is close to zero. We lose only small amounts through sweat, hair, and skin loss. Children and adolescents are in positive nitrogen balance, whereas starvation induces negative nitrogen balance (Table 9.2).

$$\text{Nitrogen balance} = \text{Nitrogen intake (grams of protein/24 hours)/6.25}$$
$$- (\text{urinary nitrogen (grams per 24 hours)} + 2 \text{ g/24 hours})$$

The most direct measures of calorie excess and deficiency are changes in body weight and body fat composition. Although both are components of wellness programs provided by laboratories, neither assessment fits the definition of a clinical laboratory assessment. Later in the chapter, causes of weight change, such as infection and hormonal imbalances, will be addressed.

AMINO ACIDS

Classically, amino acid analysis was limited to evaluating children with suspected inborn errors of metabolism. With the growth of protein and amino acid supplements, there is growing interest in the role that amino acid analysis and supplementation may play in our well-being and, especially, athletic performance. Diets that are very low in protein or very restrictive in the types of protein consumed (e.g., vegetarian diets) may not provide sufficient amounts of each of the required amino acids.

Compared to the general population, athletes require greater daily intakes of protein (in the range of 1.3–1.8 g/kg per day) to maximize muscle protein synthesis.[3] Evaluation of the essential amino acids can reveal information about skeletal muscle status. For example, the branched-chain amino acids (BCAA) leucine, isoleucine, and valine increase the rates of protein synthesis and degradation in resting human muscle.[4] BCAA levels may be informative about whether BCAA supplementation is affecting skeletal muscle protein synthesis signaling[5] though there is no consensus that BCAA supplementation is effective.[6] BCAA levels may also suggest if diet, stress, or disease states are affecting an athlete's skeletal muscles. There are a few other examples in which specific amino acids may indicate muscle status based on their roles in skeletal muscle. Other amino acids patterns

---

TABLE 9.2
Examples of Nitrogen Balance

	Intake Grams of Protein/24 Hours	Urinary Urea Nitrogen Grams/24 Hours	Balance
Person 1 (typical)	75	10	0 (balanced)
Person 2	60	15	−7.4 grams of nitrogen or 46 grams of protein

(e.g., elevated tryptophan, decreased glutamine) have been associated with fatigue and suboptimal training capacity in athletes and suggest specific amino acids that may serve as biomarkers of muscle quality/status.[7,8]

VEGETARIAN AND OTHER DIETS

Vegetarian diets have been associated with a lower risk of death from ischemic heart disease and lower overall cancer rates. Compared to nonvegetarian, vegetarians also appear to have lower LDL cholesterol levels, lower blood pressure, and lower rates of hypertension and diabetes. However, some vegetarian diets may be deficient in protein, iron, zinc, calcium, vitamin D, and vitamin B12, along with other nutrients. The need for these nutrients varies individually and when needs change, for example, pregnancy, change in physical activity, and development of chronic diseases.[9] With a well-balanced diet, routine laboratory assessment is not recommended unless there are specific indications. There are numerous other diets that focus on restricting certain types of foods, that similar to vegetarian diets may cause unanticipated nutritional deficiencies if the body's needs are unmet.

ENVIRONMENTAL RESPIRATORY FACTORS AND NUTRITION

Environmental respiratory factors may seem like an unlikely topic in a discussion of nutrition. We typically think of nutrition in terms of what we eat and drink. What we inhale affects our bodies just as what we ingest. We can influence our body's health and well-being by avoiding noxious air and fumes and by breathing clean air.

Tobacco: Cigarettes

Use of cigarettes and other tobacco products is a leading cause of death worldwide. Smoking tobacco suppresses appetite, impairs the sense of smell, and impacts the ability to absorb calcium, vitamins C and D, and other nutrients. Many companies, organizations, and governments restrict smoking. Because insurers and employers may provide financial incentives not to smoke, employees who do use tobacco products may misrepresent their use. Cotinine, a metabolite of nicotine, has a longer plasma half-life and is more amenable to testing than nicotine. Thus, companies may use cotinine testing to validate self-reported tobacco status. Many of us tend to overestimate our height, underestimate our weight and waist circumference, and falsely claim tobacco abstinence. Accordingly, physicians can validate their patients' assertions about tobacco abstinence through cotinine testing.

Air Pollution

Air pollution affects the respiratory system. The effects of inhaling noxious substances may be insidious and not easily detectable. In contrast, contaminated air may be obvious and the impact immediate. For example, four days of heavy London smog in December 1952 were associated with four thousand deaths.[10] Air pollution in developing countries with poor regulatory oversight affects children and adults alike. In a study of rats, those exposed to polluted air gained more weight, had higher levels of respiratory inflammation, exhibited more oxidative stress, and had higher levels of total cholesterol than the control rats who breathed filtered air.[11] Indoor pollution involves gases and particles that can be irritants and harmful. These include radon and formaldehyde. Air pollutants can also affect crops and therefore the availability of foods we consume. A study published in 1925 described a 70% reduction in crop yield of the most polluted compared to the least polluted crops in the northern English city of Leeds.[12] Crop yield affects crop prices and the food locally available which influences the choices we make in our diets.

Environmental laboratories, not clinical laboratories, test for radon, formaldehyde, and other noxious substances that can be in our homes, offices, buildings, and external environment. These air contaminants are not directly measured in our bodily fluids.

Environmental Allergies and Asthma

Allergies and asthma can make those affected feel terrible, both directly and through medications used to treat them. Asthma is often an allergic-based lung disorder in which spasms and inflammation of the bronchial passages restrict the flow of air in and out of the lungs. Difficulty breathing can affect appetite, which can in turn have negative effects on diet, mood, and general well-being.

Leukotrienes contribute to the allergic and inflammatory reactions in asthma. Because leukotrienes are derived from arachidonic acid, which is unique to animal products, a vegetarian diet is often helpful by reducing leukotriene formation.[13] When such a diet was followed for 1 year in conjunction with many specific dietary changes (such as avoidance of caffeine, sugar, salt, and chlorinated tap water) and combined with a variety of herbs and supplements, significant improvements were reported in one group of asthmatics.[13]

Magnesium, vitamin B6, and omega-3 fatty acids also play a role in asthma. Magnesium levels are often low in patients with asthma. Small studies suggest short-term benefit with magnesium supplements.[14,15] Likewise, vitamin B6 levels are often low in patients with asthma. This deficiency may relate to the asthma itself or to certain asthma drugs (such as theophylline and aminophylline) that deplete vitamin B6.[16] Clinical studies suggest patients taking supplements of vitamin B6 have fewer and less severe asthmatic attacks.[17] Finally, fish oils contain the essential fatty acids eicosapentaenoic acid (EPA) and docosahexaenoic acid (DHA), which block the production of leukotrienes. Research shows that fish oil supplements reduce reactions to allergens that can trigger attacks in some patients with asthma.[18]

Clinical laboratories can assess environmental or respiratory allergens, including mold, dust mites, animal hair and dander, and plant (e.g., ragweed, grass, weed, and tree) allergens. The blood-based tests are objective and quantitative, with increasing levels somewhat correlated with symptoms.[19] Skin tests are also commonly available to assess allergen sensitization.

EXPOSURE TO LEAD, MERCURY, AND OTHER HEAVY METALS

Lead and mercury are two metals that can affect child development and diet. Lead can be found in drinking water, contaminated soil, and paint chips and paint dust in older homes built when lead was used in paints. Nutrition can play a pivotal role in reducing childhood lead poisoning. Good nutrition can help minimize the amount of lead that is absorbed and stored in the bones.[20] When calcium and iron are deficient in the body, lead absorption is increased. Children with diets deficient in these minerals retain more of the lead than they would otherwise.

Mercury accumulates in tissues, in both fish and humans. Larger and older fish have eaten more, so they accumulate more. Farmed fish tend to have lower methylmercury levels because they have a shorter life span and enhanced growth rates (thus, bioaccumulation is lessened). Mercury is eliminated from our bodies in a few days or a few months, depending on the organ of deposition and the form of mercury. The half-life (time required for the concentration to fall to half of its initial value) is approximately 45–70 days in the human body. The nutrients we consume can interact with toxic metals at various points in the body, including absorption, excretion, transport, binding, metabolism, and oxidation. Many vegetables and fruits, in particular, along with omega-3s and mineral-rich protein sources, can support mercury detoxification and elimination. Fetuses can be exposed to methylmercury when their mothers eat fish and shellfish that contain methylmercury. This exposure can adversely affect fetal brains and nervous systems development. These systems may be more vulnerable to methylmercury than the brains and nervous systems of adults are.

Other heavy metals also affect our health.[21] Toxicity is uncommon. Arsenic, a naturally occurring element, is found throughout the environment; for most people, food is the major source of exposure. Inorganic arsenic is a deadly poison, but its organic form is an essential trace element; the necessary intake may be as low as 0.01 mg/day. Among foods, some of the highest levels are found in fish and shellfish; however, this arsenic exists primarily as organic compounds, which are essentially nontoxic.[22]

Aluminum, although not technically a heavy metal, is often considered one when it comes to health. Aluminum is one of the most abundant minerals, representing about 12% of the Earth's crust. More so than arsenic, aluminum is found in large biological quantities in every plant and animal. At higher levels, and in an inorganic form, aluminum is considered toxic and is associated with cognitive disorders such as dementia. At trace levels, organic or bound aluminum is essential to life through its action on a small number of enzymes such as succinic dehydrogenase and d-aminolevulinate dehydratase.

Aluminum is eliminated through action of the kidneys. Patients on hemodialysis can accumulate aluminum and if undetected can develop bone disease, microcytic anemia, and encephalopathy. Baseline blood levels should be <20 µg/L and in dialysate fluids, <0.01 mg/L.[23]

Reference toxicology laboratories may measure heavy metals in hair and body fluids and assist in detoxification. Clinical laboratories focus on detecting toxic levels as defined by the U.S. Environmental Protection Agency (EPA) and Occupational Safety and Health Administration (OSHA).[24]

OUR BODIES AND NUTRITION

GENES

The best-known example of the influence of genetics on nutrition is classic phenylketonuria (PKU) caused by rare inherited (autosomal recessive) mutations in the phenylalanine hydroxylase gene. Affected newborns cannot metabolize the amino acid phenylalanine. Blood testing, typically performed from a heel-stick specimen collected 24 hours after birth, is required throughout the country. Implementing a low phenylalanine diet shortly after birth ameliorates the phenotype of severe cognitive impairment and a host of medical problems.

Beyond our ability to metabolize the amino acid phenylalanine, our genes affect our ability to metabolize alcohol, certain foods, and drugs, and also affect our risk for medical conditions such as diabetes and celiac disease. Gene expression profiles could become important in understanding an individual's responses to specific nutrients. Different responses to nutrients could be used to design diets. Given that many vitamins and nutrients are involved in DNA stabilization and repair, it is possible that diets could be designed to optimize gene stability and thereby decrease the risk of cancer and other medical conditions.

Genetic and epigenetic elements may play a role in our size or over-size. These genetic and epigenetic elements may have complex interactions with our environment and diet that lead to excessive weight. Approximately two-thirds of American adults are overweight or obese. The high percentage of teenagers who are overweight or obese is also ominous. Yet, some obese individuals have lipid levels (total, LDL, and HDL cholesterol and triglycerides) and glucose and hemoglobin A1c levels (markers of prediabetes and diabetes) in the optimal range or display only slightly elevated insulin resistance. It is possible that these healthier obese individuals have altered gene expression.[25] The point is not to assess genes to see if it is healthy to be overweight or obese, but to underscore the important role that genes play in our susceptibility to disease.[26] Further studies will elucidate the complex role of genes that affect our metabolism and risk for chronic disease.

This discussion about the interplay of genetics and nutrition raises many interesting areas for research. At this time, outside of newborn testing, nutritional genetic testing is limited to research. The Academy of Nutrition and Dietetics concluded that this is an emerging science; testing is not advised for routine clinical use.[27]

ALCOHOL

In this chapter, what enters our bodies is considered nutrition and thus the important inclusion of alcohol. Alcohol is a source of calories and affects the gastrointestinal system. Further, excessive acute alcohol intake and alcoholism can have profound effects on our health. The National Institute on Alcohol and Alcoholism reported that 7.2% or approximately 17 million American adults suffer from alcohol use disorders.[28] Alcohol is a leading cause of automobile crashes and deaths.

Alcohol affects our mood, inhibitions, visual perception, and decision-making. Chronic alcoholism can lead to liver damage, cirrhosis, and liver failure. Approximately 10%–15% of people with alcohol use disorders develop cirrhosis in their lifetimes.[29] There is evidence that modest alcohol intake may confer cardiac protection that may in itself be associated with higher HDL cholesterol levels.[30] No randomized controlled study has been conducted to confirm or refute these observed associations.

Upon absorption, alcohol is oxidized to acetaldehyde, mainly by the enzyme alcohol dehydrogenase, and acetaldehyde is oxidized by the enzyme aldehyde dehydrogenase to acetate. The gene for aldehyde dehydrogenase is *ALDH2*. Half of the Japanese population are either heterozygous or homozygous for a null variant of this gene. Consequently, peak alcohol levels are 5 or 18 times higher in individuals who are heterozygotes or homozygotes for this gene relative to people with the wild type of the gene.[31] Thus, many Japanese people and others who are affected generally avoid alcohol because the consequences include flushing, heart palpitations, and drowsiness. This common genotype among Japanese, especially men, appears to be associated with much lower rates of hypertension compared to men with wild type *ALDH2*.

Testing of *ALDH2* and other genes associated with alcohol metabolism has only research interest. However, clinical laboratory testing for certain liver enzymes can provide evidence of alcohol-associated liver impairment. Such testing is often performed on behalf of life insurance companies to help guide premium decisions: higher insurance premiums can be assigned to applicants with evidence of alcohol-associated liver damage, because such applicants are likely to have shorter life expectancies than those without evidence of liver impairment by alcohol.

The two primary biomarkers of alcoholism are gamma glutamyl transferase (GGT) and carbohydrate-deficient transferrin (CDT).[32] Phosphatidylethanol is another biomarker of regular alcohol consumption. In a 1989 study, 19 of 22 (86%) self-reported alcoholics had elevated CDT levels, versus none of 47 patients with non-alcoholic liver disease.[33] In a more current study, of the various biomarkers for alcoholism, CDT had the highest area under the curve (0.77), followed by GGT (0.68).[34] The percentage of excessive drinkers with aspartate aminotransferase:alanine aminotransferase ratio (AST:ALT) >2 was only 2%, a very low sensitivity. CDT typically normalizes within weeks of abstinence. Importantly, there are other causes of elevated CDT levels, including congenital disorders of glycosylation (e.g., hereditary fructosamine and galactosemia) and other genetic and nongenetic causes of liver disease.

ABO Blood Groups

People with certain blood types can have a higher or lower risk of some diseases.[35] Conjecture is that ABO blood groups affect our diet or that we should modify our diet based on our ABO blood group. For example, people with type O have a lower risk of cardiovascular disease, but a higher risk of gastric ulcers.[36] However, there are no studies showing this to have *anything* to do with diet. In a large observational study of 1455 young adults, eating a type A diet (lots of fruits and vegetables) was associated with better health markers. But this effect was seen in everyone following the type A diet, not just individuals with type A blood.[37] In a 2013 review study where researchers reviewed over 1000 studies, they did not find a single well-designed study looking at the health effects of the blood type diet.[38]

APO E Gene

There are some interesting studies that examine the impact of genes beyond the ABO blood group genes on our nutritional status.[39] The studies are outside of the mainstream of traditional nutrition and medicine. Yet, they raise interesting perspectives that may guide additional research. One of the most interesting relationships is between lipid metabolism and the APO E gene. There are three common isoforms of the APO E (E2, E3, and E4) and, because we have two copies of each gene, these three isoforms code for six genotypes (E2/E2, E2/E3, E2/E4, E3/E3, E3/E4, and E4/E4). Approximately 60% of the U.S. population have genotype E3/E3. E2 is associated with lower levels of cholesterol while E4 is associated with higher levels. E4 carriers benefit most from low fat, high-carb diets while E2 carriers benefit most from high-fat, low-carb diets.[40] APO E4 is associated with increased risk for Alzheimer's disease and cardiovascular disease and shortened life expectancy.[41] Thus, testing for APO E provides much more information than just cholesterol levels.

PHYSIOLOGY

This section on physiology refers to how our bodies respond as we age, based on the menstrual cycle for women, and hydration.

As we age, the nutritional needs of our bodies change, from birth to senior living. For example, older adults tend to be less active and have decreased caloric needs. Aside from studies on children and adolescents, there is a paucity of data on changes in laboratory test interpretation as it pertains to nutrition in aging. Likewise, there is little research on the nutritional needs of older adults with cancer.[42] It may be that nutritional assessment is fundamentally unaltered in the aging adult.

Menstrual Cycle

Some research has shown that fluctuations in ovarian hormones, that is, estradiol and progesterone, predict the changes in binge eating and emotional eating across the menstrual cycle. Fluctuations in weight preoccupation across the menstrual cycle appear to be influenced primarily by emotional eating rather than ovarian hormones.[43] There is no role for clinical laboratory testing to assess nutritional needs associated with the menstrual cycle. However, premenopausal women have a high prevalence of iron deficiency related in large part to blood loss.

Hydration

Hydration refers to our water balance. Too little water leads to dehydration and too much water leads to over-hydration. With dehydration, there is a shift in fluid to our extracellular compartment from interstitial tissues. Dehydration caused by volume loss can be due to blood loss, vomiting, diarrhea, excessive sweating, and fluid shifts (e.g., fluid shifts into the abdominal cavity). Dehydration can also be caused by insufficient fluid intake. In contrast, hypervolemia can result from renal failure, excessive fluid or salt intake, liver cirrhosis, hyperaldosteronism, and congestive heart failure.

Correction of hydration imbalances starts with real-time measurement of hydration status. This is of strong interest for professional and everyday athletes and their athletic trainers who seek to maximize athletic performance.[44] Fluid imbalance may impact athletic performance, especially distance and endurance events including baseball, soccer, basketball, lacrosse, hockey, and football. Some marathoners become severely dehydrated at the end of the race. Other runners overcompensate and drink too much.[45] There is a range in fluid loss and salt loss among marathoners. Knowing our hydration status during an event may help us correct imbalances and last longer and perform better.[46]

Laboratory testing has a role in assessing hydration status. The simplest laboratory test for hydration status, one we can all perform, is simply looking at urinary color. Dr. Larry Armstrong developed an 8-point urine color scale with 1 being the lightest and 8 the darkest color. The threshold of dehydration is color 4 and colors of 5–8 are consistent with dehydration.[47] The classic laboratory tests used to assess hydration include tests of renal function: urea nitrogen (BUN) and creatinine, electrolytes—especially serum sodium—and urinary specific gravity. Serum sodium and urinary specific gravity are useful measurements in patients on diuretics or suspected of having an altered hydration status. In the future, assessment of sweat during athletic events and physical exercise may be useful to guide fluid replacement. This research is ongoing and may lead to improved performance by both professional athletes and those of us who have more pedestrian athletic ambitions.

People vary dramatically in the quantity and salt content of sweat during strenuous physical exercise. Estimations of the volume and salt content of sweat often vary from actual loss during athletic events. Laboratory analysis of sweat could be used to identify low-, medium-, and high-volume sweaters and those who sweat low, medium, and high concentrations of salt in our sweat. Further, during endurance events, real-time sweat analysis may be useful to guide fluid replacement. The science of sweat analysis for athletes is in development.[48,49]

MEDICAL CONDITIONS

ANOREXIA NERVOSA AND BULIMIA AND OTHER EATING DISORDERS

The position of the American Dietetic Association is that nutritional intervention, including nutritional counseling, by a registered dietician is an essential component during assessment and treatment across the continuum of care for patients with anorexia nervosa, bulimia nervosa, and other eating disorders. Patients need a complete nutritional assessment (generally by a dietician or clinical expert) with support of clinical laboratory tests to identify deficiencies and assess protein and liver function status. More than one-half of the patients with anorexia nervosa fail to meet the recommended dietary allowance for vitamin D, calcium, folate, vitamin B12, zinc, magnesium, and copper.[50]

KIDNEY STONES

Kidney stones are relatively common, affecting 1 in 11 people.[51] Twenty-four hour urine specimens are useful in evaluating minerals associated with stone development. Clinical laboratories evaluate kidney stones. Different types of stones have different etiologies and recommendations for reducing the risk of reoccurrence. Healthcare providers and dieticians can design diets that reduce the likelihood of recurrences. Typically, diets low in animal-protein may reduce the likelihood of developing kidney stones.

Calcium oxalate kidney stones are the leading type of kidney stones. Oxalate is naturally found in many foods, including fruits and vegetables, nuts and seeds, grains, legumes, and even chocolate and tea. Some examples of foods that contain high levels of oxalate include peanuts, rhubarb, spinach, beets, chocolate, and sweet potatoes. Another common type of kidney stone is a uric acid stone. Red meat and shellfish have high concentrations of a natural chemical compound known as a purine. High purine intake leads to a higher production of uric acid, which then accumulates as crystals in the joints or as stones in the kidneys. Again, based on the type of kidney stone, different diets and medication are prescribed. Monitoring 24-hour urine is often used in patient management to reduce reoccurrence.[52]

BODY MASS INDEX

Hippocrates said, "Let food be thy medicine and medicine be thy food." Some of us have overdosed. More than one-third of adults are obese, and black non-Hispanic and Hispanic populations have age-adjusted obesity rates of 48.4% and 42.6%, respectively. The nutritional needs of people who are obese are challenging. While some may initiate diets, or alternate between programs, they may neglect their basic nutritional needs. People who are obese are more likely to have iron, folate, and vitamin D deficiencies.[53] Likewise, nutritional assessment is essential after surgical procedures intended to reduce weight (see section on post-bariatric surgery).

People who are underweight also need special attention because they may be restricting their diets and have unsuspected nutrient deficiencies.

POST-BARIATRIC SURGERY

Bariatric surgery is growing in the United States, with approximately 100,000 operations in 2011. The U.S. National Institutes of Health recommends bariatric surgery for patients who are morbidly obese (BMI $\geq$40 kg/m²) or have a BMI of $\geq$35 kg/m² with coexisting medical conditions such as diabetes.[54] Medical guidelines suggest even lower BMI thresholds for surgical consideration.

Different surgical procedures are performed to aid people who are obese. Nutrient deficiencies are common, and malabsorption may develop following surgery with some dependence on procedure and post-surgical diet.[55,56] The Endocrine Society has provided clinical practice guidelines to address nutritional needs post-surgery.[57] Laboratory tests to consider before and after surgery include complete blood count, liver function tests, electrolytes, glucose, creatinine, vitamin B12, folate, iron studies, calcium, vitamin D, and possibly zinc, and vitamin B1 (thiamine).

CARDIOVASCULAR DISEASE

The primary nutrition-related test for cardiovascular disease is the lipid panel highly sensitive C-Reactive Protein, and advanced cardiovascular testing including cholesterol sub-particle analysis. These tests are the cornerstone of the laboratory assessment of cardiovascular disease risk. For more than half a century, the relationship between dietary intake of cholesterol and cardiovascular disease was perpetuated. The 2015 Dietary Guidelines Advisory Committee of the U.S. Department of Agriculture has recommended limits on dietary cholesterol be removed from the "Dietary Guidelines for Americans."[58]

An emerging test of cardiovascular disease risk related to nutrition is omega-3 fatty acids. Omega-3 fatty acids, also called n-3 polyunsaturated fatty acids (n-3 PUFAs), are involved in multiple biological pathways, including coagulation, muscle function, cellular transport, and cell division and growth. The three major omega-3 fatty acids are eicosapentaenoic acid (EPA), docosahexaenoic acid (DHA), and alpha-linolenic acid. Fish oil and fatty fish such as salmon, mackerel, herring, and tuna are the primary dietary sources of EPA and DHA. Alpha-linolenic acid is found in plant-based foods such as green leafy vegetables, beans, and vegetable oils; it is metabolized to EPA and then, though very inefficiently, to DHA after being ingested.[59,60]

A diet rich in omega-3 fatty acids is associated with a decreased risk of cardiovascular events, including sudden cardiac death; studies are summarized by De Caterina.[61] The American Heart Association[62] and the European Society for Cardiology[63] recommend dietary intake of omega-3 fatty acids to reduce cardiovascular disease risk. Up to 4 g/d of purified omega-3 fatty acids is considered safe,[64] but higher levels have not been thoroughly tested in clinical trials.

Although intake of omega-3 fatty acids is related to cardiovascular risk, EPA and DHA measurements can provide a more accurate prediction of clinical events.[65] The sum of EPA and DHA, expressed as a percentage of total phospholipid fatty acids, is called the omega-3 index.[66] The index can be used as an indicator of risk for sudden cardiac death and nonfatal cardiovascular events and as a therapeutic target.[64] It can also be used to assess adherence to omega-3 therapy and/or success or failure of such therapy.

In contrast to omega-3 fatty acids, omega-6 fatty acids (e.g., arachidonic acid [AA]) and their metabolites are more pro-inflammatory than anti-inflammatory. Two proposed markers of cardiovascular risk incorporate both omega-3 and omega-6 fatty acids: the omega-6/omega-3 ratio and the EPA/AA ratio. The omega-6/omega-3 ratio is still used by some physicians, but the clinical utility of the ratio has been called into question.[67] One drawback of the ratio is that it does not differentiate fatty acids that have different physiologic properties (e.g., effect on platelet function and lowering triglycerides).[66] Recent data indicate that the EPA/AA ratio, which includes specific types of omega-3 and omega-6 fatty acids, can be a useful alternative.[65,68] Higher EPA/AA ratios are associated with lower cardiac risk.[67]

HORMONES

There are many endocrine disorders associated with weight gain or weight loss. Many hormones affect our nutrition, notably insulin. The inability to produce insulin causes type 1 diabetes and the inability to have sufficient insulin receptors causes type 2 diabetes. Diabetes is a common medical condition associated with altered metabolism.

Diabetes

There are different types of diabetes. Type 1 diabetes is associated with insulin deficiency whereas type 2 is associated with insulin resistance. Clinical laboratory testing is essential for diagnosis of diabetes and of pre-diabetes. In addition, long-term trends may pre-stage development of pre-diabetes and diabetes. Just as we tend to slowly gain weight as we age, our glucose levels tend to creep higher. Further, patients with glucose results in the upper portion of the "normal" range are more likely to develop diabetes later in life than people with glucose levels in the lower portion of the normal range. An interesting theory is that type 2 diabetes may be a consequence of poor fetal and post-natal nutrition.[69]

Patients with diabetes need to continually monitor glycemic control. Laboratory tests include glucose (short-term), fructosamine (intermediate-term), and hemoglobin A1c (long-term). Urinary albumin creatinine ratio (formerly known as "microalbumin"), urinary protein, and urinary ketones are also useful to monitor glycemic control. Hyperglycemic excursions describe the length of accumulated time that glucose levels are elevated.[70] Higher amounts of hyperglycemic excursions are associated with poorer clinical outcomes.[71] Hyperglycemic excursions can be monitored with 1,5-anhydroglucitol (GlycoMark®).[72]

Patients with diabetes should consult with a nutritional expert about food selection.[73] Evidence does not support omega-3 fatty acid and anti-oxidant supplementation or monitoring. Assessment of nutritional status, especially vitamin D and lipids, is appropriate. However, evidence on the role of vitamin D supplementation in improving glycemic control is conflicting.

Other endocrine conditions associated with weight gain that are far less common or rare include:

Cortisol excess (endogenous Cushing or iatrogenic)
Hyperinsulinemia
Hypothyroidism
Leptin deficiency
MC4R receptor defects

In contrast, weight loss is associated with the following endocrine conditions:

Adrenal cortisol insufficiency
Hyperthyroidism
Gastrinomas
Type 1 diabetes and other autoimmune endocrine diseases

Thyroid Disease

Severe iodine deficiency is associated with thyroid goiter and hypothyroidism. Such deficiencies are rare in the United States except among recent immigrants who may have come from countries without salt iodination. In 1990, the United Nations World Summit for Children established the goal of eliminating iodine deficiency worldwide. Considerable progress has since been achieved, largely through programs of universal salt iodization. Variations in population iodine intake do not affect risk for hyperthyroid autoimmune thyroiditis, that is, Graves' disease, or thyroid cancer.

Adequate nutritional supply of selenium, together with the two other essential trace elements iodine and iron, is required for a healthy thyroid during development and adolescence, as well as in the adult and aging populations. Selenium administration in both autoimmune thyroiditis (Hashimoto) and mild Graves' disease improves clinical scores and well-being of patients and reduces autoimmune antibody titers in several prospective, placebo-controlled supplementation studies.[74] None of these analytes should be measured unless there is specific cause to suspect deficiencies.

THE HUNGER GAMES: HORMONES

Some of the hormones that affect our hunger and metabolism include adiponectin, cholecystokinin, peptin, gherelin, and leptin. Measuring these hormones is of interest for research but is not part of a routine clinical laboratory assessment.

Adiponnectin modulates glucose regulation and fatty acid oxidation.[75] It enhances the ability of muscles to use carbohydrates for energy and acts to curb appetite. Adiponectin is produced in adipose tissue, and levels correlate with body fat in adults.[76] Adiponectin levels are higher after weight reduction and during statin use.[77,78]

Cholecystokinin is a hormone released by intestinal cells in response to ingestion of fat and proteins. Cholecystokinin acts to slow the rate of digestion and activates our sense of satiety.

Leptin, like adiponectin, is a hormone produced in adipose tissues. It helps to regulate energy balance by inhibiting hunger. Its action opposes that of another hormone, ghrelin, that is referred to as the "hunger hormone." Ghrelin is a hormone produced in the stomach and signals hunger. Research shows that ghrelin levels stay above the upper limit of the reference range even after 12 months of a reduced-calorie diet.[79] In people who are obese, decreased sensitivity to leptin results in a decreased ability to detect satiety despite high energy stores.[80] Leptin deficiency is associated with weight gain.[81]

MALABSORPTION

Malabsorption may be caused by:

- Acquired immunodeficiency syndrome (AIDS)
- Biliary atresia (bile ducts do not develop normally)
- Celiac disease
- Chronic liver disease
  - Common causes include alcoholism, chronic hepatitis B or C, biliary obstruction, and biliary cirrhosis.[82] Non-alcohol fatty liver disease is also a common cause that may be secondary to obesity or post-jejunoileal bypass.
- Cholestasis of pregnancy (bile flow from the liver is slowed or blocked)
- Crohn's disease (inflammatory disease affecting the distal end of the small intestine and beginning of the large intestine)
- Milk intolerance
- Whipple's disease (caused by infection with a form of bacteria called *Tropheryma whippelii*)
- Medications such as cholestyramine, tetracycline, some antacids, colchicine, acarbose, and phenytoin
- Following gastrointestinal surgery, that is, gastrectomy or removal of portions of the gastrointestinal tract

A few of these conditions are discussed here. What is essential is that malabsorption can lead to protein-calorie deficits and specific nutritional deficits of minerals and vitamins such as iron, fat-soluble vitamins, calcium, and vitamin B12. There are specific clinical laboratory and pathology tests for the diagnosis and management of these conditions. Fecal fat can be measured to reflect malabsorption (Table 9.3).

TABLE 9.3

Laboratory Tests for Common Malabsorption Conditions

Condition	Laboratory Tests
Human Immunodeficiency Virus/AIDS	HIV-1/2 antigen and antibodies, fourth generation, with reflex to western blot confirmation.
Biliary atresia	• Total and direct (conjugated) bilirubin with direct bilirubin levels often >2 mg/dL or 20% of total bilirubin. • Liver function tests such as Alkaline phosphatase, 5′ nucleotidase, Gamma-glutamyl transpeptidase (GGT), Alanine aminotransferase (ALT), Aspartate aminotransferase (AST). • Serum alpha-1-antitrysin with Pi typing and Sweat chloride (for cystic fibrosis) can assist if suspected.
Celiac disease	• IgA (to detect low or deficient levels). • If IgA is not low then tissue Transglutaminase (tTG) antibodies, IgA. • If tTG, antibodies, IgA is detected then Endomysial antibodies, IgA is used as additional screening. • If IgA is low then tTG, antibodies, IgG. • Unless tTG antibody titers are extremely high, then diagnosis is dependent upon small bowel biopsies which reveal decreased size or absence of villi.
Chronic liver disease	• Chronic liver disease often means having elevated aminotransferase levels two-times or greater than the upper limit of the reference range for at least six months. • Prothrombin time (PT-INR), complete blood count (CBC), and liver function tests often reflect the impact of chronic liver disease. • Liver fibrosis panels. • Liver biopsy. • Specific tests such as for hepatitis B virus, hepatitis C virus, hemochromatosis, and alcoholism are appropriate when clinically indicated.
Cholestasis of pregnancy	• Serum bile acids are typically >10 μg/L. • Aspartate aminotransferase (AST) and Alanine aminotransferase (ALT) may be slightly to greatly elevated. • Total bilirubin may be elevated and generally after the onset of pruritus. • Other liver function tests may be useful but must be interpreted in the context of pregnancy and production from the placenta.
Crohn's disease	• Inflammatory markers such as Sedimentation rate (sed rate) and C-reactive protein (CRP) are generally elevated. • Complete blood count is used to detect anemia and to evaluate for macrocytosis (high Mean corpuscular volume (MCV). • Fecal calprotectin levels correlate with intestinal inflammation. • *Saccharomyces cerevisisae* antibodies (ASCA) are more commonly found in patients with Crohn's disease than ulcerative colitis whereas Perinuclear antineutrophil cytoplasmic antibody (p-ANCA, a myeloperoxidase antigen, is found more commonly in patients with ulcerative colitis than with Crohn's disease.
Milk intolerance	• Often diagnosed based on clinical history. Lactose tolerance test involves administration of 50 g of lactose. Glucose is measured at baseline and at 1 and 2 h. An increase of glucose of <9 mg/dL is supportive of lactose intolerance.
Whipple's disease	• Tissue biopsy of the small intestine. • *Tropheryma whippleii* DNA, real-time polymerase chain reaction testing detects the causative organism.

INFLAMMATORY BOWEL DISEASE

Nutritional deficiencies, especially of micronutrients, are common in patients with inflammatory bowel disease (IBD). Protein-calorie malnutrition is of concern.[83] Vitamin A, vitamin D, and zinc deficiency are common in patients newly diagnosed with IBD.[84] Diet is known to have a major role in the expression of IBD. Specifically, high dietary intakes of total fats, polyunsaturated fatty acids, omega-6 fatty acids, and meat are associated with an increased risk of Crohn's disease and ulcerative colitis. The role of dietary interventions and enteral nutrition in the management of IBD remains an active area of research.

Patients with irritable bowel disease often present with symptoms similar to those of IBD. Fecal calprotectin can be a highly sensitive way of detecting inflammatory bowel disease; generally, a calprotectin result in the reference range rules out IBD, thereby sparing most people with irritable bowel syndrome from having to undergo invasive investigations such as a colonoscopy.[85]

SWEAT CHLORIDE (CYSTIC FIBROSIS)

An important clinical laboratory test to aid in the diagnosis of cystic fibrosis is sweat chloride. The test measures the amount of chloride in sweat. Pilocarpine and electrical stimulation encourage sweating. A patch collects the sweat for analysis. Many patients with cystic fibrosis have pancreatic insufficiency, which imposes special nutritional needs. The Cystic Fibrosis Foundation published a guideline for nutrition-related management.[86]

CELIAC DISEASE

Celiac disease is an autoimmune disorder in which people cannot tolerate gluten because it damages the inner lining of the small intestine and prevents the absorption of many nutrients. In response to gluten found in wheat, rye, and barley, the immune system responds by damaging or destroying villi lining of the small intestine. Consequences include malnutrition and deficiencies of fat-soluble vitamins, iron, zinc, and other micronutrients, and potentially vitamin B12 and folic acid. Although many patients experience gastrointestinal symptoms, some patients have a specific skin disease, dermatitis herpetiformis. Many patients have no symptoms but suffer from malabsorption. Long-term consequences, when untreated, include growth retardation in children, osteoporosis, infertility and miscarriage, and neurological conditions such as migraines and epilepsy.

As many as 1 in 141 Americans has celiac disease, although most patients remain undiagnosed.[87] Celiac disease is genetic. One in 22 first-degree relatives (parent, sibling, child) tested will be diagnosed with celiac disease. Half of those affected have one or more family members who, when screened, will be identified as having celiac disease.[88]

Diagnosis starts with a thorough medical history and physical exam.[89] IgA antibodies to tissue transglutaminase (tTG, IgA) are generally elevated. Endomysial antibodies are used as additional support for identifying patients who should proceed to a more definitive, diagnostic small bowel biopsy. (In children under two years of age, IgG-deaminated gliadin peptide antibodies should also be tested.) The definitive diagnosis is based on small bowel biopsies in which the villi are greatly diminished in height. If testing is negative, and among family members who are at risk, genetic testing is often provided.[90] Those who are negative for the human leukocyte antigens HLA D2 and D8 (70% of the population) need not worry about future development of celiac disease.[91] Those who test positive for either or both HLA markers should be tested for antibodies if symptoms develop or periodically retested in the absence of symptoms.[92]

In addition to celiac disease and allergies to wheat, rye, or barley, there are many people who have non-celiac gluten sensitivity (NCGS). Symptoms are similar to those of celiac disease. There are no diagnostic tests for NCGS. Patients with NCGS have no hereditary predisposition, do not experience nutrient deficiencies that are associated with celiac disease, and are not at risk for conditions associated with celiac disease. Patients with NCGS do respond positively to a gluten-free diet.

LACTOSE AND SOY INTOLERANCE

Lactose, a disaccharide that comprises the monosaccharides glucose and galactose, is the primary carbohydrate found exclusively in mammalian milk. Absorption requires the enzyme lactase that is found in the small intestine. Approximately 70% of the world's population has primary lactase deficiency.[93] In populations with a predominance of dairy foods in the diet, particularly northern European people, as few as 2% of the population has primary lactase deficiency. In contrast, the prevalence of primary lactase deficiency is 50%–80% in Hispanic people, 60%–80% in black and Ashkenazi Jewish people, and almost universal in Asian and American Indian people.

Diagnosis often begins with a good medical history that associates lactose ingestion with symptoms. An approach once widely used is the lactose challenge test, in which an absolute lactose-free diet for two weeks is followed by reintroduction of lactose to determine if symptoms dissipate and then recur. In recent years this has been replaced by the hydrogen breath test. For some patients with symptoms similar to those of lactose tolerance, the cause may be parasitic infections affecting the small intestine (e.g., *Giardia lamblia* and *Cryptosporidia* species).[94]

Soy intolerance and allergy among children are reported but often not confirmed. The U.S. Food and Drug Administration estimates that 0.2% of the population have soy allergies, though clinically confirmed diagnoses are uncommon. A survey of pediatric allergists estimated prevalence at 1.1%.[95] The American Academy of Asthma, Allergy, and Immunology includes soy as one of the eight most common causes of food allergy. The risk of soy intolerance is highest in the first year of life and then decreases. Double-blind placebo controlled challenge testing and IgE-specific soy antibody testing provide a foundation for diagnosis.[96]

FOOD ALLERGY

More than 50 million Americans have an allergy. Food allergies affect 4%–6% of children and 4% of adults, according to the American College of Allergy, Asthma, and Immunology.[97] Approximately eight food allergens account for 90% of all allergic sensitizations: eggs, milk, peanuts, tree nuts, fish, shellfish, wheat, and soy. Young infants in particular are susceptible to food protein-induced enterocolitis syndrome (FPIES), typically 2–6 hours after ingestion of milk, soy, and grains. Infants with FPIES often have repetitive vomiting and dehydration.

Typical allergy symptoms include vomiting or stomach cramps, tight, horse throat and trouble swallowing, shortness of breath, and wheezing. Anaphylaxis is uncommon but of great concern. The severity of symptoms varies by person, and there is some correlation between the level of IgE sensitization and symptoms. Allergic sensitization can be a trigger for asthma, and patients with asthma should be evaluated for allergies.[98] The National Institutes of Health (NIH) guidelines on asthma shed light on the clear connection between allergic rhinitis and asthma, and how asthma may be difficult or impossible to control without concurrent diagnosis and treatment of hay fever.

Diagnosis starts with a good history of food exposure and symptoms. Three diagnostic tests are food challenge, skin-prick tests, and blood tests. Blood tests employ IgEs specific to food components. These tests are quantitative, reproducible, and safe and easy to perform. Hundreds of different standardized food allergens are available for evaluation through blood tests.

Appropriate allergy testing can help identify allergies that, undiagnosed, might lead to suboptimal performance of daily activities. Conversely, allergy testing can also help avoid unnecessary dietary restrictions that could cause nutritional imbalances and create undue stress. Many food allergies are outgrown, especially those identified in childhood. Appropriate testing and retesting thus provides information to guide healthy nutritional choices.

DIET AND SUPPLEMENTS AND HERBAL MEDICINE

The diet and supplement business is a multi-billion dollar business that continues to grow. More than half of all adults take dietary supplements, especially multivitamins, vitamin D, calcium, and folic acid.[99] Blindly taking supplements without knowledge of the body's concentrations leads many people to take too little or too much. The clinical laboratory provides quantitative assessment to guide dosage and assurance that deficiencies and overdoses are avoided. A prime example is vitamin D where dosing can be adjusted based on laboratory measurement of 25-hydroxyvitamin D, season, skin pigmentation, and sun exposure.

The U.S. Food and Drug Administration (FDA) regulates dietary supplements under a different set of regulations than those covering "conventional" foods and drug products. The manufacturers are responsible for the safety of their products. Manufacturers are not required to test new ingredients or supplements in clinical trials. Fortunately, most such products, such as daily multivitamins, are consumed by millions of people without adverse effects. Unfortunately, some supplements are not what is claimed and may contain fillers and contaminants. There are environmental laboratories that can authenticate the claimed ingredients; however, these services are usually employed by the manufacturers or researchers. In contrast, clinical laboratories test patient specimens for drug and nutrient levels. Toxin levels, such as heavy metals, could be assessed but such testing is usually reserved when there is a high index of suspicion of toxicity, not in the context of dietary supplements and herbal medicine use.

VITAMINS AND MINERALS

The easiest approach to vitamins and micronutrients is to sort them by where they are absorbed. The fat-soluble vitamins are vitamins A, D, E, and K. Anything that interferes with fat absorption should decrease absorption of these vitamins. The water-soluble vitamins and micronutrients include: biotin, folic acid, pantothenic acid, vitamins B1 (thiamine), B2 (riboflavin), B3 (niacin), B6 (pyridoxine), B12, and vitamin C. Our body stores for thiamine are typically only approximately 18 days versus a decade or longer for vitamin B12. Finally, there are other micronutrients and trace elements, such as calcium, chromium, iodine, iron, magnesium, manganese, selenium, and zinc that can be grouped together.

This discussion starts with a focus on the most commonly ordered tests for vitamin and mineral deficiencies: iron, folate, vitamin B12, and vitamin D.

Iron Deficiency

Iron deficiency is one of the most common nutritional deficiencies. Iron deficiency anemia develops when iron storage falls below the hematopoietic needs for erythrocyte (red blood cell) production to replace red blood cell loss. Iron deficiency anemia affects approximately 1 billion people worldwide.[100]

An adult body typically contains approximately 4 g of iron. Approximately 60%–65%, or 2500 mg, is within erythrocytes; 25%–30%, or 1000 mg, is within the bone marrow, liver, spleen, and other body stores; 300 mg is contained within myoglobin and respiratory enzymes; and only 4 mg (0.1% of the body iron) is within the plasma. Each day we lose approximately 1–2 mg, and this must be replaced to stay in balance. Foods high in iron include cashews, spinach, lentils, chickpeas, and bread and cereals fortified with iron. Transferrin, produced in the liver, is essential for iron transport throughout the body.

A common cause of iron deficiency in older adults is colorectal polyps and cancer. Fecal immunochemical tests (FIT) are used to identify blood in the lower gastrointestinal tract that requires further evaluation including potentially a colonoscopy. Often there is a benign colonic polyp or cancer that is bleeding into the colon. With sufficient bleeding, the body's ability to produce enough new red blood cells falls behind the loss of blood and iron deficiency anemia may develop.

Often the first clues of iron deficiency and iron deficiency anemia are found in the complete blood count (CBC) and iron studies, specifically iron, total iron binding capacity (TIBC), and ferritin. Other laboratory tests may include urinary hemoglobin, hemoglobin electrophoresis, sickle cell screen, reticulocyte count, and bone marrow examination. Although iron staining of the bone marrow is the definitive test, practically, the diagnosis is based on clinical laboratory tests. Many of the other tests, including bone marrow evaluation, are reserved for the differential diagnosis of iron deficiency to allow the primary cause to be identified and addressed. Often a trial or iron supplementation is provided prior to additional expensive and invasive testing. Of note, iron staining of the bone marrow may provide misleading interpretation after a trial of iron supplementation.[101]

The CBC is useful in iron deficiency because hemoglobin and the hematocrit are low. The mean corpuscular volume (MCV) is low in pure iron deficiency but may be in range in combined deficiencies with vitamin B12 or folate deficiencies. The red cell distribution width (RDW) often is increased with anemia, reflecting increased variability in the size of the red blood cells. An elevated RDW may be among the first signs of iron deficiency. The platelet count may be slightly elevated due to cross-reactivity of erythropoietin or in response to anemia, with thrombopoietin that stimulates platelet production. On the peripheral blood smear, the erythrocytes are microcytic and hypochromatic. In contrast to thalassemias, target cells are not observed in iron deficiency.

Ferritin is an excellent test for assessing body iron stores. Unfortunately, ferritin is elevated in response to chronic inflammation. Thus, only low concentrations can be viewed as supportive of a diagnosis of iron deficiency. Generally, iron levels should be interpreted in conjunction with TIBC and ferritin. Many individuals take iron supplements alone or as part of daily multivitamins. For an accurate assessment of iron, no iron supplements should be consumed within 24 hours before testing. Likely, iron-rich foods such as liver should be avoided as well prior to testing. In iron deficiency, TIBC is elevated. TIBC is also used to calculate the percent saturation. This is the percent of iron divided by TIBC. The ratio is also referred to as iron saturation and transferrin saturation. Very low levels of percent saturation are highly correlated with iron deficiency. Factors that influence iron and TIBC must be considered, too.

Folic Acid (Vitamin B9)

Folic acid (vitamin B9), as with all the eight B vitamins, is involved in converting carbohydrates into glucose. This vitamin is important in mental health and emotional well-being. It has a role in DNA and RNA production and is essential in periods of rapid body growth. Folic acid is a required vitamin, yet we cannot produce it; we need to consume folic acid in foods or supplements. All of the B vitamins are water-soluble, so we have no body stores.

Folic acid deficiency is associated with increased fetal risk of open neural tube defects.[102] Women who are planning on becoming pregnant are urged to take prenatal folic acid supplementation. Among women ages 20–39 years, approximately one in three take folic acid supplements. The rate is 41% among non-Hispanic white women, 24% among non-Hispanic black women, and only 19% among Mexican Americans.[98] Measuring folate levels is used to determine adequate levels and potential dosage for supplementation. Folate levels are commonly measured in the presence of macrocytic anemia.

Folate storage in the body is limited so levels can fall in the absence of intake of foods such as green vegetables, beans and legumes, and citrus fruits. Most grains are fortified with folate. Interestingly, increased excretion of folate can occur after vitamin B12 deficiency. During the development of vitamin B12 deficiency, methylenetetrahydrofolate reductase accumulates. In turn, large amounts of folate filter through the glomerulus, and urine excretion increases (referred to as the "folate trap phenomenon").

Macrocytic anemia is a late consequence of folate deficiency. Folate may become deficient secondarily to celiac disease, Crohn's disease, alcoholism, or certain medications such as phenytoin and sulfasalazine or secondary to lack of adequate intake of fruits and vegetables.

Vitamin B12 (Cobalamin)

Vitamin B12 (cobalamin) is one of the eight water-soluble B vitamins. It is found naturally in animal proteins including meats, eggs, and milk. Vitamin B12 is important in DNA and RNA production. It has an important role in metabolism and brain function. Body stores of vitamin B12 typically last a decade or more.

Deficiencies of vitamin B12 and folate are common causes of macrocytic anemia.[103] Pernicious anemia, a type of vitamin B12 anemia, is caused by insufficient production of intrinsic factor. Pernicious anemia typically occurs at 60 years of age or older.[104] The etiology of vitamin B12 deficiency is diverse and includes lack of intrinsic factor, altered pH in the small intestine, and lack of absorption of B12 complexes in the terminal ileum. As with folate deficiency, poor intake of leafy vegetables can cause vitamin B12 deficiency. Other foods rich in vitamin B12 include eggs, dairy products, fortified cereal or soy beverages, tempeh, and miso (tempeh and miso are foods made from soybeans). Atrophy or loss of the gastric mucosa can prevent vitamin B12 absorption. Bacterial overgrowth in the intestine can lead to bacteria competing for cobalamin. Bowel resection and tapeworm infections, such as with *Diphyllobothrium latum*, also can lead to vitamin B12 deficiency.

Vitamin B12 testing is common when macrocytic anemia and when certain neurologic conditions or malabsorption are suspected or diagnosed. The evaluation of vitamin B12 deficiency starts with a thorough medical history and examination. The complete blood count is the starting place for clinical laboratory testing. Vitamin B12 and folate levels can be followed with measurement of homocysteine and methylmalonic acid.[105] Using both homocysteine and methylmalonic acid to define vitamin B12 deficiency improves sensitivity. Accordingly, the prevalence of vitamin B12 deficiency in the elderly may be 15%–20%. Levels of intrinsic factor are detectable in approximately 85% of all patients with pernicious anemia. Parietal cell antibodies are present in approximately 90% of patients with pernicious anemia but they are less specific than intrinsic factor antibodies. Often the two types of antibodies are interpreted together to provide a better assessment.[106]

Vitamin D

Of all the laboratory tests of nutrients, none has grown to be as popular as vitamin D. Vitamin D is a hormone with receptors on most cells. We understand its role in bone disease. In addition, vitamin D plays a role in a wide host of functions, many still under investigation. Although there is a tremendous focus on the role of vitamin D in bone status, the other roles may prove to be as vital. The Institute of Medicine and others state that levels of 25-hydroxyvitamin D <20 ng/mL are deficient.[107] With this definition, approximately one in three Americans is deficient; the percent is significantly higher among people with pigmented skin, including non-white Hispanics and African Americans. Insufficiency is commonly defined as levels of 25-hydroxyvitamin D of 20–29 ng/mL.[108] It may be that the optimal level for other functions is lower or higher. There is controversy as to the optimal level of 25-hydroxyvitamin D. A recent meta-analysis suggests the optimal level of 25-hydroxyvitamin D is greater than 30 ng/mL.[109] The Endocrine Society suggests the optimal target of 25-hydroxyvitamin D may be 40 ng/mL or higher.[110]

Vitamin D is found in foods such as milk, soy, and other fortified foods. Diet may be inadequate to achieve and maintain healthy levels. We can also manufacture vitamin D within our skin with a mix of sunlight (UV exposure) that converts cholesterol to an inactive form that is then activated through hepatic and renal enzymes. However, few of us, especially in northern latitudes, obtain sufficient amounts of vitamin D through sunlight exposure or dietary vitamin D; thus, prescription or over-the-counter supplements may be appropriate for most people.[111] Laboratory evaluation provides quantitative assessment of 25-hydroxyvitamin D levels. Based on this data, the appropriate dose can be recommended. Monitoring response to therapy can guide the need for continuing supplementation and dosage adjustments.

Often overlooked is that there is considerable seasonal variation in 25-hydroxyvitamin levels, with a difference from peak to trough levels of approximately 7 ng/mL.[110] This requires interpretation in the context of seasons. In the Northern hemisphere, a peak 25-hydroxyvitamin D level that is optimal in March will likely be optimal throughout the year whereas a peak level that is just optimal in September is likely to be suboptimal throughout the remainder of the year.

Although observational studies support a potential role of vitamin D in endocrine disease, high quality evidence from clinical trials does not exist to establish a place for vitamin D supplementation in optimizing endocrine health. Testing is suggested for populations with the following:

- Obesity
- Chronic kidney disease
- Nephrotic syndrome
- Osteomalacia
- Fat malabsorption disorders, short bowel syndrome
- Hypercalcemia of cancer
- Hyperparathyroidism, primary and secondary
- Lymphoma and granulomatous disorders
- Medications that increase vitamin D metabolism, for example, anticonvulsants, antiretovirals, and glucocorticoids
- Rickets

FAT-SOLUBLE VITAMINS

The fat-soluble vitamins are vitamins A, D, E, and K. Vitamin D was previously discussed. Vitamins A and K are rarely measured. There is no basis for the routine measurement of either vitamin A or vitamin K. Toxicity of vitamin A results from ingesting too much preformed vitamin A from foods (e.g., fish or animal liver, supplements, or prescription medications). In the 1913 Far Eastern Party exploration of Antarctica, two explorers had vitamin A toxicity and one may have died after eating the livers of their sled dogs. Serum levels of vitamin A are relatively constant, despite wide ranges of vitamin A intake, and are a poor indicator of liver reserves. Measurement of retinyl esters may be more reliable as a marker of chronic hypervitaminosis A.[112]

Vitamin E (Tocopherol)

Vitamin E is a fat-soluble vitamin that acts as an anti-oxidant, protecting the body from free-radicals that harm the body. Vitamin E is involved in the immune system, production of red blood cells, and prevention of blood clots, among its many functions. Two large observational studies, both published in the prestigious *New England Journal of Medicine* in 1993, reported an association between short-term vitamin E supplementation and lower risk of coronary heart disease.[113,114] Yet, a well-controlled randomized study found no benefit to vitamin E supplementation.[115] Like vitamins A and K, there is no basis for the routine measurement of vitamin E.

WATER-SOLUBLE VITAMINS AND MICRONUTRIENTS

Vitamins B1 (thiamine), B3 (niacin), B6 (pyridoxine), and C (ascorbic acid) are vital for energy, carbohydrate, lipid, and amino acid metabolism and in the regulation of the cellular redox state.

Severe vitamin B1 (thiamine) deficiency may lead to serious complications involving the nervous, skeletal, and gastrointestinal systems and heart. Thiamine deficiency is associated with alcoholism, poor nutrition, cancer, vomiting associated with pregnancy, bariatric surgery, and hemodialysis.

Severe vitamin B3 (niacin) deficiency causes pellagra with skin, gastrointestinal, and nervous system manifestations. The most common cause of low levels of niacin is alcoholism.

Overt vitamin B6 deficiency is rare, but insufficient levels may be common. Insufficient levels may be associated with cardiovascular disease risk; supplementation does not appear to lower cardiovascular disease risk.

Just as with vitamin E, an initial observation found an inverse association between vitamin C (ascorbic acid) levels and coronary heart disease that was not confirmed in a well-controlled randomized study.[116,117] Vitamin C deficiency causes scurvy, associated with brown spots on the skin, spongy gums, and mucosal bleeding. Deficiency is extremely rare in the United States because of extensive fortification of foods. Serum levels reflect recent dietary intake.

None of these vitamins is routinely measured.

OTHER MICRONUTRIENTS AND TRACE ELEMENTS

Other micronutrients and minerals include:

- Calcium
- Chromium
- Copper
- Iodine
- Magnesium
- Manganese
- Selenium
- Zinc

Generally, none of these is measured as part of a nutritional assessment except for people with unusual diets such as having no fruits or vegetables, premature babies, patients on enteral therapy, and patients who are alcoholics or who have liver or kidney disease or malabsorption. A typical diet provides sufficient levels of these micronutrients and trace elements. Toxicity is occasionally observed in people who take excessive amounts of supplements. Although there are a few interesting studies that examined selenium supplementation, the consensus is there is insufficient evidence to support its control of disease.[118]

Another concern is contaminants in our drinking water as the unfortunate situation in Flint, Michigan drew our attention to lead poisoning from municipal-supplied drinking water.[119] Fluoride has been added to drinking water in many municipalities to reduce dental cavities. Some municipalities have not taken this public health measure in fear of fluoride toxicity despite many decades of safety throughout the country. Environmental laboratories are available to test environmental specimens including air, water, and soil.

INFECTIONS

From tapeworms to salmonella, shigella, and giardia, there are numerous infections of our gastrointestinal tract that can cause malabsorption and massive loss of fluids. For example, tapeworms of the *Diphyllobothrium* genus absorb a large amount of vitamin B12 and interfere with vitamin B12 absorption from the ileum, resulting in vitamin B12 deficiency (see Vitamin B12 [cobalamin]). Proper diagnosis of lower gastrointestinal tract infection starts with a complete physical history and examination. Clinical laboratory tests include stool culture.

FOREIGN BODIES

In the broad sense used in this chapter, "nutrition" includes what goes into our bodies. Infections can occur when our skin or mucosal surfaces are penetrated by foreign bodies. Another example is toxic shock syndrome, a potentially fatal bacterial infection caused by the entertoxin type B or TSST-1 and *Streptococcus pyogenes*. Toxic shock syndrome is associated with the use of tampons, menstrual sponges, diaphragms, and cervical caps.[120] These foreign bodies are not transmitters of infection; they provide the mechanism for infection to take root. Staphylococcal toxic shock syndrome has an estimated risk of 3–4/100,000 tampon users per year.[121]

Other examples of infections due to insertion of foreign bodies include blood-borne pathogens, for example, HIV and hepatitis C virus, associated with contaminated needles including needles used for tattooing and infections with contact lenses due to improper cleaning, disinfection, and storage.[122]

HELICOBACTER PYLORI (H. PYLORI)

Upper gastrointestinal disease can cause post-prandial distress and affect diet and nutrition. A common culprit is *Helicobacter pylori* (*H. pylori*), a Gram-negative spiral-shaped bacterium that specifically colonizes the gastric epithelium. It causes one of the most common infections worldwide, affecting about half of the world's population. *H. pylori* is the primary cause of gastric and duodenal ulcers and infection can lead to gastric cancer. *H. pylori* is a harmful human pathogen responsible for serious and sometimes lethal diseases. Thus, the proper goal is to eradicate *H. pylori* infection.[123]

However, *H. pylori* may play a protective role in our health. Whereas it infected up to 80% of the population before antibiotics, only 5% of children now carry the bacteria. The prevalence of *H. pylori*, particularly in the Western world, has significantly decreased coinciding with an increase of some autoimmune and allergic diseases, such as asthma. *H. pylori* appears to bolster the immune system. Children who lack the bacteria are 60% more likely to develop asthma.[124] Various epidemiological studies have also documented a negative association between *H. pylori* colonization and the presence of gastroesophageal reflux disease and risk of esophageal cancer.[125] Additionally, an upward trend of obesity raises a question about the relationship between *H. pylori* infection and body mass index (BMI).

H. pylori infection leads to chronic active gastritis in all infected individuals and thereby interferes with the release of gastric hormones, which are involved in the regulation of appetite and food intake.[126] *H. pylori* infection leads to a decrease in circulating ghrelin, through a reduction in ghrelin-producing cells in the gastric mucosa, and to an increase in gastric leptin.[127] As noted above, ghrelin and leptin are important factors in appetite and satiety regulation. After successful eradication of *H. pylori*, the number of ghrelin-positive cells in the gastric mucosa returns to normal. Based on these observations, weight gain caused by increased appetite after *H. pylori* eradication has been suggested.[128]

GUT FLORA (MICROBIOTA)

This is the appropriate way to end a discussion of the role of the clinical laboratory in nutritional assessment. The microbial composition of our gastrointestinal system varies along the digestive tract. These microorganisms are essential to metabolize food for our survival. The microorganisms are involved in absorption of nutrients, fermenting unused energy substrates, and synthesizing biotin and vitamin K. The colon has up to a trillion microorganisms per gram of intestinal content. Although there may be 1000 different species, 30–40 species account for 99% of the microorganisms in our intestines.[129] Approximately 60% of the dry weight of our stool is bacteria. The predominance of different species relates to our diet. Altering the diet changes the microbiota.[130]

Bacterial colonization may play a role in IBD.[131] A relatively new treatment approach is fecal microbiota transplant, whereby fecal material from a healthy donor is provided to a recipient to restore the gut microbiota. This treatment has been used on patients with *Clostridium difficile* infection that is unresponsive to antibiotics.[132] Fecal microbiota transplant is being studied in other medical conditions. Entrepreneurs from the Massachusetts Institute of Technology established the first stool bank in the United States to provide healthy stool for treatment and research.[133] We will see what role the clinical laboratory plays in evaluating our gut microbiota.

CLOSING

In closing, the clinical laboratory provides insights into our health and well-being that guide us in identifying disease and disease risk including those that are beyond the ability of our external senses. Laboratory results can guide our diet and need for supplements. Laboratory testing may be useful to assess allergen sensitization to what we breathe and infections secondary to foreign bodies. In the future, the clinical laboratory will provide new clues and new evidence as we explore ways to improve the quality of our lives, advance our ability to perform at optimal levels throughout our lifespans, and extend our life expectancy.

REFERENCES

1. U.S. Department of Health and Human Services and U.S. Department of Agriculture. *2015–2020 Dietary Guidelines for Americans.* 8th ed. December 2015. Available at http://health.gov/dietaryguidelines/2015/guidelines/. Accessed October 31, 2016.
2. Crespo R, Relea P, Lozano D, Macarro-Sanchez M, Usabiaga J, Villa LF, Rico H. Biochemical markers of nutrition in elite-marathon runners. *J Sports Med Phys Fitness.* 1995;35(4):268–72.
3. Phillips SM, Van Loon LJ. Dietary protein for athletes: From requirements to optimum adaptation. *J Sports Sci.* 2011;29:S29–38.
4. Blomstrand E, Eliasson J, Karlsson HK, Köhnke R. Branched-chain amino acids activate key enzymes in protein synthesis after physical exercise. *J Nutr.* 2006;136:269S–73S.
5. Apro W, Blomstrand E. Influence of supplementation with branched-chain amino acids in combination with resistance exercise on p70S6 kinase phosphorylation in resting and exercising human skeletal muscle. *Acta Physiol (Oxf).* 2010;200:237–48.
6. Mattick JSA, Kamisoglu K, Ierapetritou MG, Androulakis IP, Berthiaume F. Branched chain amino acid supplementation: Impact on signaling and relevance to critical illness. *Rev Syst Biol Med.* 2013;5:449–60.
7. Kingsbury KJ, Kay L, Hjelm M. Contrasting plasma free amino acid patterns in elite athletes: Association with fatigue and infection. *Br J Sports Med.* 1998;32:25–33.
8. Smith DJ, Norris SR. Changes in glutamine and glutamate concentrations for tracking training tolerance. *Med Sci Sports Exerc.* 2000;32:684–9.
9. Craig WJ, Mangels AR. Position of the American Dietetic Association: Vegetarian diets. *J Am Diet Assoc.* 2009;109:1266–82.
10. Bell ML, Davis DL, Fletcher T. A retrospective assessment of mortality from the London smog episode of 1952: The role of influenza and pollution. *Environ Health Perspect.* 2004;112:6–8.
11. Wei Y, Zhang J, Li Z et al. Chronic exposure to air pollution particles increases the risk of obesity and metabolic syndrome: Findings from a natural experiment in Beijing. *FASEB.* 2016;30(6):2115–22, *FASEB J* fj.201500142; published ahead of print February 18, 2016, doi: 10.1096/fj.201500142
12. Cohen JB, Ruston AG. *A Study of Town Air.* Edward Arnold, London, England. 1925.
13. Lindahl O, Lindwall L, Spångberg A, Stenram Å, Öckerman PA. Vegan regimen with reduced medication in the treatment of bronchial asthma. *J Asthma.* 1985;22:45–55.
14. Gaur SN, Dogra V. Editorial: Nutritional considerations in bronchial asthma. *J Allergy Asthma Immunol.* 2014;28:61–2.
15. Hill J, Micklewright A, Lewis S, Britton J. Investigation of the effect of short-term change in dietary magnesium intake in asthma. *Eur Respir J.* 1997;10:2225–9.
16. Weir MR, Keniston RC, Enriquez JI, McNamee GA. Depression of vitamin B6 levels due to theophylline. *Ann Allergy.* 1990;65:59–62.
17. Reynolds RD, Natta CL. Depressed plasma pyridoxal phosphate concentrations in adult asthmatics. *Am J Clin Nutr.* 1985;41:684–8.
18. Nagakura T, Matsuda S, Shichijyo K, Sugimoto H, Hata K. Dietary supplementation with fish oil rich in omega-3 polyunsaturated fatty acids in children with bronchial asthma. *Eur Respir J.* 2000;16:861–5.
19. Dolen WK. IgE antibody in the serum—Detection and diagnostic significance. *Allergy.* 2003;58:717–23.
20. U.S. Environmental Protection Agency. https://www.epa.gov/sites/production/files/documents/nutrition.pdf. Accessed on May 6, 2016.
21. Levander OA. Nutritional factors in relation to heavy metal toxicants. *Fed Proc.* 1977;36:1683–7.
22. Agency for Toxic Substances and Disease Registry (ATSDR). Toxicological Profile for Arsenic (Update). U.S. Public Health Service, U.S. Department of Health and Human Services, Atlanta, GA. 2007.

23. National Kidney Foundation. K/DOQI clinical practice guidelines for bone metabolism and disease in children with chronic kidney disease. *Am J Kidney Dis* 2005;46(4 Suppl 1):S1–121.

24. National Institute for Occupational Safety and Health (NIOSH). Pockey guide to chemical hazards. U.S. Department of Health and Human Services, Public Health Service, Centers for Disease Control and Prevention. Cincinnati, OH. 2007.

25. Telle-Hansen VH, Halvoresen B, Dalen KT, Narverud I, Wesseloft-Rao N, Granlund L, Ulven U, Holven KB. Altered expression of genes involved in lipid metabolism in obese subjects with favorable phenotype. *Genes Nutr.* 2013;8:425–34.

26. Paoloni-Giacobino A, Grimble R, Pichard C. Genetics and nutrition. *Clin Nutrition.* 2003;22:429–35.

27. Camp KM, Trujillo E. Position of the Academy of Nutrition and Dietetics: Nutritional genomics. *J Acad Nutrition and Dietetics.* 2014;114:299–312.

28. NIAAA.NIH.gov. Accessed May 3, 2016.

29. Jinjuvadia R, Liangpunsakul S. Trends in alcoholic hepatitis-related hospitalizations, financial burden, and mortality in the United States. *J Clin Gastroenterol.* 2015;49:506–11.

30. Rimm E. Commentary: Alcohol and coronary heart disease—Laying the foundation for future work. *Int J Epidemiol.* 2001;30:738–9.

31. Enomoto N, Takase S, Yasuhara M, Takada A. Acetaldehyde metabolism in different aldehyde dehydrogenase-2 genotypes. *Alcohol Clin Exp Res.* 1991;15:141–4.

32. Bell H, Tallaksen C, Sjahelm T, Weberg R, Raknerud N, Orjasaeter H, Try K, Haug E. Serum carbohydrate-deficient transferrin as a marker of alcohol consumption in patients with chronic liver diseases. *Alcohol Clin Exp Res.* 1993;17(2):246.

33. Kapur A, Wild G, Milford-Ward A, Triger DR. Carbohydrate deficient transferrin: A marker for alcohol abuse. *BMJ.* 1989;299:427–31.

34. Gough G, Heathers L, Puckett D, Westerhold C, Ren X, Yu Z, Crabb DW, Liangpunsakul S. The utility of commonly used laboratory tests to screen for excessive alcohol use in clinical practice. *Alcohol Clin Exp Res.* 2015;39:1493–500.

35. Yamamoto F, Cid E, Yamamoto M, Blancher A. ABO research in the modern era of genomics. *Transfu Med Rev.* 2012;26:103–18.

36. He M, Wolpin B, Rexrode K, Manson JE, Rimm E, Hu FB, Qi L. ABO blood group and risk of coronary heart disease in two prospective cohort studies. *Atherosclerosis.* 2012;32:2314–20.

37. Wang J, García-Bailo B, Nielsen DE, El-Sohemy A. ABO genotype, "Blood-Type" diet and cardiometabolic risk factors. *PLoS ONE.* 2014;9(1):e84749.

38. Cusack L, De Buck E, Compernolle V, Vandkerckhove P. Blood type diets lack supporting evidence: A systematic review. *Am J Clin Nutr.* 2013;98:99–104.

39. Lucock MD, Martin CE, Yates ZR, Veysey M. Diet and our genetic legacy in the recent Anthropocene: A Darwinian perspective to nutritional health. *J Evidence-Based Complimentary & Alternative Med.* 2014;19:68–83.

40. McDonald P. *The Apo E Diet.* Penscott Medical Corporation, Danville, CA. 2007.

41. Raichlen DA, Alexander GE. Exercise, APOE genotype, and the evolution of human lifespan. *Aging and Metabolism.* 2014;37:247–55.

42. Presley CJ, Dotan E, Soto-Perez-de-Celis E et al. Gaps in nutritional research among older adults with cancer. *J Geriatr Oncol.* 2016;7(4):281–92.

43. Hildebrandt BA, Racine SE, Keel PK, Burt A, Neale M, Boker S, Sisk CL, Klump KL. The effects of ovarian hormones and emotional eating on changes in weight preoccupation across the menstrual cycle. *Int J Eating Disorders.* 2015;48:477–86.

44. Casa DJ, Armstrong LE, Hillman SK, Montain SJ, Reiff RV, Rich BSE, Roberts WO, Stone JA. National Athletic Trainers' Association position statement: Fluid replacement for athletes. *J Athletic Training.* 2000;35:212–24.

45. Almond SD, Shin AY, Fortescue EB, Mannix RC, Wypij D, Binstadt BA, Duncan CN, Olson DP, Selerno AE, Newburger JW, Greenes DS. Hyponatremia among Runners in the Boston Marathon. *NEJM.* 2005;352:1550–6.

46. Bergeron MF, Harvreaves M, Haymes EM et al. ACSM position stand: Exercise and fluid replacement. *Med Sci Sports Exerc.* 2007;39:377–90.

47. McKenzie AL, Munoz CX, Armstrong LE. Accuracy of urine color to detect equal to or greater than 2% body mass loss in men. *J Athl Train.* 2015;50(12):1306–9.

48. Ring M, Lohmueller C, Raul M, Eskofier BM. On sweat analysis for quantitative estimation of dehydration during physical exercise. *37th Annual International Conference of the IEEE Engineering in Medicine and Biology Society*, Milan, Italy, August 25–29, 2015, pp. 7011–4.

49. Deignan J, Florea L, Coyle S, Diamond D. Wearable chemical sensing—Optimizing fluidics for real-time sweat analysis. In: Conference on Analytical Sciences Ireland 2016, April 14–15, 2016, Dublin City University, Dublin, Ireland.

50. Hadigan CM, Anderson EJ, Miller KK, Hubbard JL, Herzog DB, Klibanski A, Grinspoon SK. Assessment of macronutrient and micronutrient intake in women with anorexia nervosa. *Int J Eat Disord.* 2000;28:284–92.

51. Scales Jr CD, Smith AC, Hanley JM, Saigal CS. Prevalence of kidney stones in the United States. *Eur Urol.* 2012;62:160–5.

52. Mardis HK, Parks JH, Muller G, Ganzel K, Coe FL. Outcome of metabolic evaluation and medical treatment for calcium nephrolithiasis in a private urological practice. *J Urol.* 2004;171:85–8.

53. Van Rutte PWJ, Aarts EO, Smulders JF. Nienhuijs. Nutrient deficiencies before and after sleeve gastrectomy. *Obes Surg.* 2014;24:1639–46.

54. Robinson MK. Surgical treatment of obesity-weighing the facts. Editorial. *New Eng J Med.* 2009;361:520–1.

55. Bal BS, Finelli FC, Shope TR, Koch TR. Nutritional deficiencies after bariatric surgery. *Nat Rev Endocrinol.* 2012;8:544–56.

56. Koch TR, Finelli FC. Postoperative metabolic and nutritional complications of bariatric surgery. *Gastroenterol Clin North Am.* 2010;39:109–24.

57. Heber D, Greenway FL, Kaplan LM, Livingston E, Salvador J, Still C. The Endocrine Society: Endocrine and nutritional management of the post-bariatric surgery patient: An Endocrine Society clinical practice guideline. *J Clin Endocrinol Metab.* 2010;95:4823–43.

58. Scientific Report of the 2015 Dietary Advisory Committee. Unites States Department of Agriculture. 2015.

59. Brenna JT, Salem N Jr, Sinclair AJ, Cunnane SC. alpha-Linolenic acid supplementation and conversion to n-3 long-chain polyunsaturated fatty acids in humans. *Prostaglandins Leukot Essent Fatty Acids.* 2009;80:85–91.

60. Kris-Etherton PM, Taylor DS, Yu-Poth S, Huth P, Moriarty K, Fishell V, Hargrove RL, Zhao G, Etherton TD. Polyunsaturated fatty acids in the food chain in the United States. *Am J Clin Nutr.* 2000;71:179S–88S.

61. De Caterina R. n-3 fatty acids in cardiovascular disease. *N Engl J Med.* 2011;364:2439–50.

62. Smith SC Jr, Benjamin EJ, Bonow RO et al. AHA/ACCF secondary prevention and risk reduction therapy for patients with coronary and other atherosclerotic vascular disease: 2011 update: A guideline from the American Heart Association and American College of Cardiology Foundation. *Circulation.* 2011;124:2458–73.

63. Perk J, De Backer G, Gohlke H et al.; European Association for Cardiovascular Prevention & Rehabilitation (EACPR); ESC Committee for Practice Guidelines (CPG). European guidelines on cardiovascular disease prevention in clinical practice (version 2012). The Fifth Joint Task Force of the European Society of Cardiology and Other Societies on Cardiovascular Disease Prevention in Clinical Practice (constituted by representatives of nine societies and by invited experts). *Eur Heart J.* 2012;33:1635–701.

64. Lovaza [package insert]. Research Triangle Park, NC: GlaxoSmithKline; 2014. Accessed September 30, 2016.

65. von Schacky C. Omega-3 fatty acids vs. cardiac disease—The contribution of the omega-3 index. *Cell Mol Biol (Noisy-Le-Grand).* 2010;56:93–101.

66. Superko HR, Superko SM, Nasir K et al. Omega-3 fatty acid blood levels: Clinical significance and controversy. *Circulation.* 2013;128:2154–61.

67. Harris WS. The omega-6/omega-3 ratio and cardiovascular disease risk: Uses and abuses. *Curr Atheroscler Rep.* 2006;8:453–9.

68. Itakura H, Yokoyama M, Matsuzaki M et al. Relationships between plasma fatty acid composition and coronary artery disease. *J Atheroscler Thromb.* 2011;18:99–107.

69. Hales CN, Barker DJP. Type 2 (non-insulin-dependent) diabetes mellitus: The thrifty phenotype hypothesis. *Int J Epidemilogy.* 2013;42:1215–22.

70. Monnier L, Colette C, Rabasa-Lhoret R, Lapinski H, Caubel C, Avignon A. Morning hyperglycemic excursions. *Diabetes.* 2002;25:737–41.

71. Selvin E, Rawlings A, Lutsey P, Maruthur N, Pankow JS, Steffes M, Coresh J. Association of 1,5-anhydroglucitol with cardiovascular disease and mortality. *Diabetes.* 2016;65:201–8.

72. Dąbrowska AM, Tarach JS, Kurowska M. 1,5-Anhydroglucitol (1,5-Ag) and its usefulness in clinical practice. *Med Biol Sci.* 2012;26:11–7.

73. Evert AB, Boucher JL, Cypress M et al. Nutrition therapy recommendations for the management of adults with diabetes. *Diabetes Care.* 2014;37(S1):S120–43.

74. Köhrle J. Selenium and the thyroid. *Curr Opin Endocrinol Diabetes Obes.* 2013;20:441–8.

75. Díez JJ, Iglesias P. The role of the novel adipocyte-derived hormone adiponectin in human disease. *Eur J Endocrinol.* 2003;148:293–300.

76. Ukkola O, Santaniemi M. Adiponectin: A link between excess adiposity and associated comorbidities? *J Mol Med.* 2002;80:696–702.

77. Coppola A, Marfella R, Coppola L, Tagliamonte E, Fontana D, Liguori E, Cirillo T, Cafiero M, Natale S, Astarita C. Effect of weight loss on coronary circulation and adiponectin levels in obese women. *Int J Cardiol.* 2009;134:414–6.

78. Lim S, Quon MJ, Koh KK. Modulation of adiponectin as a potential therapeutic strategy. *Atherosclerosis* 2014;233(2):721–8.

79. Rossow LM, Fukuda DH, Fahs CA, Loenneke JP, Stout JR. Natural bodybuilding competition preparation and recovery: A 12-month case study. *Int J Sports Physiol Perform.* 2013;8:582–92.

80. Pan H, Guo J, Su Z. Advances in understanding the interrelations between leptin resistance and obesity. *Physiol Behav.* 2014;130:157–69.

81. Singh P, Peterson TE, Sert-Kuniyoshi FH, Glenn JA, Davison DE, Romero-Corral A, Pusalavidyasagar S, Jensen MD, Somers VK. Leptin signaling in adipose tissue: Role in lipid accumulation and weight gain. *Circ Res.* 2012;111:599–603.

82. Heidelbaugh JJ, Bruderly M. Cirrhosis and chronic liver failure: Part I. diagnosis and evaluation. *Am Fam Physician.* 2006;74:756–62.

83. Massironi S, Rossi RE, Cavalcoli FA, Valle SD, Fraquelli M, Conte D. Nutritional deficiencies in inflammatory bowel disease: Therapeutic approaches. *Clin Nutrition.* 2013;32:904–10.

84. Alkhouri A, Humaira H, Baker RD, Gelfond D, Baker SS. Vitamin and mineral status in patients with inflammatory bowel disease. *J Ped Gastroenterology & Nutrition.* 2013;56:89–92.

85. Waugh N, Cummins E, Royale P, Kandala N-B, Shyangdan D, Arasaradnam R, Clar C, Johnston R. Faecal calprotectin testing for differentiating amongst inflammatory and non-inflammatory bowel diseases: Systematic review and economic evaluation. *Health Technol Assess.* 2013;55:xv–xix.

86. Stallings VA, Stark LJ, Robinson KA, Feranchak AP, Quinton H. Clinical Practice Guidelines on Growth and Nutrition Subcommittee, Ad Hoc Working Group. Evidence-based practice recommendations for nutrition-related management of children and adults with cystic fibrosis and pancreatic insufficiency: Results of a systematic review. *J Am Diet Assoc.* 2008;108(5):832–9.

87. Rubio-Tapia A, Ludvigsson JF, Brantner TL, Murray JA, Everhart JE. The prevalence of celiac disease in the United States. *Am J Gastroenterol.* 2012;107:1538–44.

88. Fasano A, Berti I, Gerarduzzi T et al. A multicenter study on the sero-prevalence of coeliac disease in the United States among both at risk and not at risk groups. *Arch Int Med.* 2003;163:286–92.

89. Rubio-Tapia A, Hill ID, Kelly CP, Calderwood AH, Murray JA. ACG clinical guidelines: Diagnosis and management of celiac disease. *Am J Gastroenterol.* 2013;108:656–76.

90. Karinen H, Kärkkäinen P, Pihlajamäki J et al. HLA genotyping is useful in the evaluation of the risk for coeliac disease in the 1st-degree relatives of patients with coeliac disease. *Scand J Gastroenterol.* 2006;41:1299–304.

91. Rostom A, Murray JA, Kagnoff MF. American Gastroenterological Association (AGA) Institute technical review on the diagnosis and management of celiac disease. *Gastroenterology.* 2006;131:1981–2002.

92. Celiac Disease Foundation. www.celiac.org. Accessed May 13, 2016.

93. Kretchmer N. Lactose and lactase: A historical perspective. *Gastroenterology.* 1971;61:805–13.

94. Heymann MB for the Committee on Nutrition. Lactose intolerance in infants, children, and adolescents. *Pediatrics.* 2006;118:1279–86.

95. Johnstone DE, Roghmann KJ. Recommendations for soy infant formula: A review of the literature and a survey of pediatric allergists. *Pediatr Asthma Allergy Immunol.* 1993;7:77–88.

96. Savage JH, Kaeding AJ, Matsui EC, Wood RA. The natural history of soy allergy. *J Allergy Clin Immunol.* 2010;125:683–6.

97. ACAAI.org. Accessed on May 3, 2016.

98. Expert Panel 3 Report: Guidelines for the Diagnosis and Management of Asthma; National Heart Lung & Blood Institute, National Institutes of Health. 2007.

99. Gahche J, Bailey R, Burt V, Hughes J, Yetley E, Dwyer J, Picciano MF, McDowell M, Sempos C. Dietary supplement use among U.S. adults has increased since NHANES III (1988–1994). NCHS Data Brief No. 61, Centers for Disease Control and Prevention. April 2011.

100. Vos T, Flaxman AD, Naghavi M et al. Years lived with disability (YLDs) for 1160 sequelae of 289 diseases and injuries 1990–2010: A systematic analysis for the global burden of disease study 2010. *Lancet.* 2012;380(9859):2163–96.

101. Thomason RW, Almiski MS. Evidence that stainable bone marrow iron following parental iron therapy does not correlate with serum iron studies and may not represent readily available storage iron. *Am J Clin Pathol.* 2009;131:580–5.

102. Czeizel AE, Dudás I, Vereczkey A, Bánhidy F. Folate deficiency and folic acid supplementation: The prevention of neural-tube defects and congenital heart defects. *Nutrients.* 2013;5:4760–75.

103. Stabler SP. Clinical practice. Vitamin B12 deficiency. *N Engl J Med.* 2013;368:149–60.

104. Bizzaro N, Antico A. Diagnosis and classification of pernicious anemia. *Autoimmun Rev.* 2014;13:565–8.

105. Berg R, Shaw GR. Laboratory evaluation for vitamin B_{12} deficiency: The case for cascade testing. *Clin Med Res.* 2013;11:7–15.

106. Consensus guidelines on anti-intrinsic factor antibody testing. Prepared by Australasian Society of Clinical Immunology and Asthma in conjunction with the Royal Australasian College of Pathologists. November 2004 revision. http://allergy.org.au/images/stories/pospapers/ASCIA_Guidelines_IFA_1-%20 Nov04.pdf. Accessed May 31, 2016.

107. Ross AC, Manson JE, Abrams SA et al. The 2011 report on dietary reference intakes for calcium and vitamin D from the Institute of Medicine: what clinicians need to know. *J Clin Endocrinol Metab.* 2011;96:53–8.

108. Rosen CJ. Vitamin D insufficiency. *N Engl J Med.* 2011;364:248–54.

109. Bischoff-Ferrari HA. Optimal serum 25-hydroxyvitamin D levels for multiple health outcomes. *Adv Exp Med Biol (Review).* 2014;810:500–25.

110. Holick MF, Binkley NC, Bischoff-Ferrari HA, Gordon CM, Hanley DA, Heaney RP, Murad MH, Weaver CM. Evaluation, treatment, and prevention of vitamin D deficiency: An Endocrine Society clinical practice guideline. *J Clin Endocrinol Metab.* 2011;96:1911–30.

111. Kroll MH, Bi C, Garber CC et al. Temporal Relationship between Vitamin D Status and Parathyroid Hormone in the United States. *PLoSONE.* 2015;10(3):e0118108.

112. Penniston KL, Tanumihardjo SA. The acute and chronic effects of vitamin A. *Am J Clin Nutr.* 2006;83:191–201.

113. Rimm EB, Stampfer MJ, Ascherio A, Giovannucci E, Colitz GA, Willett WC. Vitamin E consumption and the risk of coronary heart disease in men. *New Eng J Med.* 1993;328:1450–6.

114. Stampfer MJ, Hennekens CH, Manson JE, Colditz GA, Rosner B, Willet WC. Vitamin E consumption and the risk of coronary heart disease in women. *New Eng J Med.* 1993;328:1444–9.

115. Eidelman RS, Hollar D, Hebert PR, Lamas GA, Hennekens CH. Randomized trials of vitamin E in the treatment and prevention of cardiovascular disease. *Arch Intern Med.* 2004;164:1552–6.

116. Khaw K-T, Bingham S, Welch A, Luben R, Wareham N, Oakes S, Day N. Relation between plasma ascorbic acid and mortality in men and women in EPIC- Norfolk prospective study: A prospective population study. *Lancet.* 2001;357:657–63.

117. Heart Protection Study Collaborative Group. MRC/BHF Heart Protection Study of antioxidant vitamin supplementation in 20536 high-risk individuals: A randomised placebo-controlled trial. *Lancet.* 2002;360:7–22.

118. Bjelakovic G, Nikolova D, Gluud LL, Simonetti RG, Gluud C. Antioxidant supplements for prevention of mortality in healthy participants and patients with various diseases. *Cochrane Database Syst Rev.* 2012;3(3):CD007176.

119. Hanna-Attisha M, LaChance J, Sadler RC, Champney Schnepp A. Elevated blood lead levels in children associated with the flint drinking water crisis: A spatial analysis of risk and public health response. *Am J Public Health.* 2015;106:283–90.

120. Toxic Shock Syndrome (Other Than Streptococcal) (TSS). 2011 Case Definition. Centers for Disease Control and Prevention. https://wwwn.cdc.gov/nndss/conditions/toxic-shock-syndrome-other-than-streptococcal/case-definition/2011/. Accessed January 17, 2017.

121. Lyons JS. A new generation faces toxic shock syndrome. The Seattle Times. Knight Ridder Newspapers. First published as "Lingering Risk." *San Jose Mercury News,* December 13, 2004.

122. Cope JR, Collier SA, Rao MM et al. Contact lens wearer demographics and risk for contact lens-related eye infections – United States, 2014. *Morbidly and Mortality Weekly Report.* 2015;64:865–70.

123. Kusters JG, van Vliet AHM, Kuipers EJ. Pathogenesis of *Helicobacter pylori* infection. *Clin Microbiol Rev.* 2006;19:449–90.

124. Arnold IC, Dehzad N, Reuter S, Martin H, Becher B, Taube C, Müller A. Helicobacter pylori infection prevents allergic asthma in mouse models through the induction of regulatory T-cells. *J Clin Investig.* 2011;121:3088–93.

125. Bocian KM, Jagusztyn-Krynicka EK. The controversy over anti-Helicobacter pylori therapy. *Pol J Microbiol.* 2012;61:239–46.
126. Weigt J, Malfertheiner P. Influence of *Helicobacter pylori* on gastric regulation of food intake. *Curr Opin Clin Nutr Metab Care.* 2009;12:522–5.
127. Tatsuguchi A, Miyake K, Gudis K, Futagami S, Tsukui T, Wada K, Kishida T, Fukuda Y, Sugisaki Y, Sakamoto C. Effect of *Helicobacter pylori* infection on ghrelin expression in human gastric mucosa. *Am J Gastroenterol.* 2004;99:2121–7.
128. Malfertheiner P, Selgrad M. *Helicobacter pylori* infection and current clinical areas of contention. *Curr Opin Gastroenterol.* 2010;26:618–23.
129. Beaugerie L, Petit JC. Antibiotic-associated diarrhoea. *Best Practice & Research Clinical Gastroenterology* 2004;18:337–52.
130. Wu GD, Chen J, Hoffmann C et al. Linking long-term dietary patterns with gut microbial enterotypes. *Science.* 2011;334(6052):105–8.
131. Hugot J-P. Inflammatory bowel disease: A complex group of genetic disorders. *Best Pract Res Clin Gastroenterol* 2004;18:451–62.
132. Drekonja D, Reich J, Gezahegn S, Greer N, Shaukat A, MacDonald R, Rutks I, Wilt TJ. Fecal microbiota transplantation for *Clostridium difficile* Infection: A systematic review. *Ann Intern Med.* 2015;162:630–8.
133. Smith PA. A new kind of transplant bank. February 17, 2014. *The New York Times.* Accessed May 13, 2016.

Section II

Integrative Medicine

10 Revisioning Cellular Bioenergetics

Food as Information and the Light-Driven Body

Sayer Ji and Ali Le Vere

CONTENTS

How We Got Here 292
The Cerebral Aspects of Nutrition 292
The Sociocultural Meaning of Food 293
Back to the "Food Itself" 293
The Old Story of Food as a Thing 294
    Food as Matter 294
    Food as Energy 294
The New Story: Food as Information 295
    The Microbiome of Food 297
    Food Timing and Quality 297
    Powerful Implications for the Future of Food 299
Biophotons: The Human Body Emits, Communicates with, and Is Made from Light 299
    The Physical and "Mental" Eye Emits Light 300
    Our Cells and DNA Use Biophotons to Store and Communicate Information 301
    The Body's Circadian Biophoton Output 301
    Medical Applications of Biophoton Emissions 302
    Meditation and Herbs Affect Biophoton Output 303
    The Electromagnetic Body and Consciousness 303
    Human Skin May Capture Energy and Information from Sunlight 304
    The Body's Biophoton Outputs Are Governed by Solar and Lunar Forces 306
Water as an Alternative Cellular Fuel Source 307
    Implications of EZ Water for Circulatory Flow 308
    Implications of EZ Water for Skeletal Muscle Structure 308
    Consequences of EZ Water for Human Health 309
    Can Human Cells Exploit Photosynthesis? 309
Intention is a Living Force of Physiology 310
The Bioelectromagnetic Body 310
    Biofields and Energetic Medicine 311
    The "Life Energy" and Holistic Health 312
References 312

Food, while being a prerequisite for the possibility of all life itself, is rarely appreciated for its true power. We are all hardwired to be deeply concerned with food when hungry, an interest that rapidly extinguishes the moment we are sated. But as an object of everyday interest and scientific inquiry, food often makes for a bland topic. This is all the more apparent when juxtaposed against its traditional status in ancient cultures as literally the sacred substrate of our lives, the very divine clay from which we are fashioned.

HOW WE GOT HERE

The modern Western conception of food is a byproduct of a centuries old process of intense materialism, reductionism, and secularization (Owen, 1996). Food is conceived largely in terms of its economic value as a commodity and its nutritional value as a source of physical sustenance. Regarding the latter, its value is quantified through the presence and molecular weight of macro- and micronutrients. In the process of reducing food's value to these quantities, only to what is measurable, it has lost its soul. Food is no longer believed to possess a vital life force, much less a sacred one, lest those claiming such to be the case be accused of "magical thinking."

Despite these reductionistic prejudices, consider how Nature designed our first experience of nourishment: breastmilk taken from the mother's breast is simultaneously a nutritional, physical, thermic, microbial, emotional, genetic, and spiritual form of nourishment—the very definition of wholesome and whole-making, which taken to together, can only be called sacred.

Indeed, the word sacred literally means "to make holy," and the word holy shares an indivisible etymological root with the words "whole" and "heal" in proto-Indo European. This is, of course, before the sacred and the profane, the soul and the body, were considered irreconcilably opposed modes or states of being with the inception of dualistic thinking.

But the question still arises: how exactly does food makes us whole? That is, how does its arrangement of atoms possess any such power to put us into our presently miraculous form? It is the information within food that helps to explain this mystery. And quite literally, information means "to put form into."

THE CEREBRAL ASPECTS OF NUTRITION

The topic of food as information is a cerebral one, but so too is the act of eating, albeit in a slightly different way. The cephalic phase of nutrition, or the adaptive responses which prepare the body for the perception, digestion, and absorption of the food, literally means "in your head" (Greek from *kephalē* "head") (Zafra, Molina, & Puerto, 2006). This instrumental initiatory phase reflects how you are actually experiencing the food: Is it delicious? Are you feeling pleasure? These "subjective" aspects directly and profoundly affect the physiology of digestion and assimilation. Indeed, it has been estimated that the cephalic phase of digestion, or the "set of food intake-associated autonomic and endocrine responses to the stimulation of sensory systems mainly located in the oropharyngeal cavity," mediated largely by the efferent pathways of the vagus nerve, contributes greater than 50% to overall postprandial responses (Katschinski, 2000; Zafra, Molina, & Puerto, 2006, p. 1032).

Our experience of food, therefore, exists in a context that transcends merely physiochemical conditions and concerns. Just as the nocebo and placebo effects permeate the clinical setting of medicine and greatly affect patient outcomes, so too do psychogenic features apply to the realm of nutrition such that there exists intentionality and inseparability between observer-observed, or more aptly, the eater and what is eaten (Chavarria et al., 2017). And, therefore, it is difficult to ignore how this important layer of nutrition—the firsthand, experiential element—has been lost at the expense of fixation on the chemistry and reductionism of "objective" food science.

THE SOCIOCULTURAL MEANING OF FOOD

Food does not only equate to sustenance, but it is also inextricably intertwined with social, super-natural, and economic realms of life, carrying "with it a range of symbolic relationships between man and man, between man and his deities, and man and the natural environment" (Helman, 2007, p. 52). Although there exists intercultural variation when it comes to how food is cultivated, har-vested, marketed, prepared, served, and consumed, anthropologists such as Claude Levi-Strauss consider the perpetual transformation of raw food into cooked food to be one of the defining char-acteristics of human civilization, one that transcends arbitrary geopolitical demarcations and socio-cultural boundaries (Helman, 2007).

According to social anthropologist Cecil Helman (2007), the firsthand experience of food can be conceptualized in terms of the following six types of food classification systems, including, first and foremost, identification of edible versus nonedible. Cultural stamps of approval are required for consumption of foodstuffs, such that, "No group, even under conditions of extreme starvation, utilizes all available nutritional substances as food" (Peters & Niemeijer, 1987, p. 19). Food is fur-ther differentiated by the sacred versus the profane, whereby religious or spiritually encapsulated beliefs either encourage or deter consumption of specifically prescribed or prohibited foodstuffs, consistent with a broader moral framework of purity and abstentions (Helman, 2007). Third, food can be operationalized in terms of parallel food classifications, such that foods are organized into a binary classification system of "hot" and "cold." This dualistic system, which echoes early Greco-Islamic humoral theories of physiology and encompasses a system of beliefs and values spanning well beyond food, is epitomized by many cultural groups and traditional medical systems in Latin America, China, the Islamic world, and the Indian subcontinent (Helman, 2007).

With escalating concerns about food safety, food can further be delineated as poison, which is relevant in the context of modern concerns surrounding pasteurization, food irradiation, chemi-cal additives, xenoestrogens, antibiotics, dioxins, organophosphate pesticides, phthalates, bisphenol derivatives, artificial colors, acrylamide, genetically engineered food crops, microbial contamina-tion from factory farming operations, and other processes of industrial food production (Enticott, 2003). Next, foods are often imbued with social connotations, signifying an occasion for social intimacy, symbolizing social status or prestige, embodying the qualities of ritual symbols, and being used as instruments to engender and reinforce social relationships, solidarity, and cultural continu-ity (Helman, 2007). In this way, food serves as a form of social currency that is shared, exchanged, and ingested as a badge of group identity.

Finally, an ancient construct that is re-emerging in recent years is the revolutionary notion of food as medicine, a paradigm which incorporates ethnobotanical and scientific knowledge from lay, folk, and professional sectors of society. This final codification, which is being validated by contem-porary science, is also emblematic of the idea that food is information, which can dictate cellular bioenergetics via epigenetic change.

BACK TO THE "FOOD ITSELF"

We all eat when we are hungry. And we don't think that much about it after satisfying our craving. But without food, we soon become disabled and die. Consequently, nothing is more quintessential to the preservation of life. Therefore, nothing is more worthy of in-depth intellectual exploration than food. But to do so, perhaps we need to invoke the rallying cry of the early twentieth century school of thought known as phenomenology, whose founder, Edmund Husserl, named going "back to the things themselves" as the cardinal objective—implying a return to a careful exploration of the phenomenon itself, stripped of our overlain assumptions and projections (Husserl, 1900). And so, this requires we start at intellectual ground zero by asking the question anew: What is food?

Nutrition facts labels make it appear that not much is going on beyond caloric content and the pres-ence or absence of a relatively small set of essential nutrients such as carbohydrates, fats, proteins, vitamins, or minerals, defined by their molecular weight. Differences in quality, for instance, will never make it onto such a label.

Indeed, conventional nutritional principles are predicated upon an understanding of the nature of food that does not account for its informational properties. Food, within this outdated view, is either a source of energy (caloric content) or material building blocks (macro- and micronutrients). The fact that food contains signaling molecules that affect and actively regulate gene expression, and even contains gene-regulatory nucleic acids such as noncoding micro-RNAs, is not taken into account. When food is understood not just in terms of its material and energetic composition and value, but as a key factor in the regulation of the genome and epigenome, or as an instrument of biosemiosis, it begins to assume its original meaning: "that which puts form into" the human body.

THE OLD STORY OF FOOD AS A THING

Our concept of food is still generally constrained to the Newtonian view that all things are comprised of atoms, externally related to one another, and built up from there into molecules, organelles, cells, and increasingly complex structural and functional components which participate in the physiological symphony. When we eat things, digestion breaks them down into their constituent parts and our bodies then take these parts and build them back up. This strictly mechanical, simplistic view, while true in limited ways, no longer rings true in light of the new biology and science. Along with this view of food as matter is the concomitant perspective that food can be "burned" for energy and that like a furnace or a car, food provides "fuel" measured by calories to drive its engines along.

This reductionist view of food and its corollary principle, that envisions the body as a machine, is what I will call "the old story of food," and this narrative focuses on two primary dimensions.

FOOD AS MATTER

If we are examining the "material" aspects of food, we are looking at the physically quantifiable or measurable elements such as weight and size. You could not, for instance, objectively "measure" taste, as it differs qualitatively from person to person (so-called "subjective" experience). And so, nutritional science focuses on what is presumably "out there" objectively, namely, tangible quantities like the molecular weight of a given substance: for example, 50 mg of ascorbic acid, 10 grams of carbohydrate, or 200 mg of magnesium. In reality, these objective quantities are influenced by the type of measuring device we use—and so, there really are no ontologically pure (i.e., "really real") material aspects out there in and of themselves. But for the purposes of clarity, let us assume these material aspects are real, independent of the measuring device or person measuring. These material aspects, while providing information, are not considered to be "informational" in the sense of giving off distinct messages to the DNA in our body, altering their expression. They are considered part of the physical world, and therefore, while providing building blocks for our body, including its DNA, they are not understood to alter or control the expression of the DNA in a meaningful way. Food, therefore, is considered "dead," and not biologically meaningful, beyond its brick and mortar functions in constructing the body-machine.

The other primary dimension in this old view depicts food strictly as a source of caloric energy.

FOOD AS ENERGY

Energy is commonly defined as the power derived from the utilization of physical resources, especially to drive machines. In this view, food provides the fuel to power the body-machine. Food energy is conventionally defined in chemical terms. The basic concept is that animals, like humans, extract energy from their food and molecular oxygen through cellular respiration. That is, the body joins oxygen from the air with molecules of food through the vehicle of mitochondrial-based oxidative phosphorylation (aerobic respiration), or without oxygen, via cytosol-based glycolysis and fermentation, through reorganization of the molecules (Zeviar et al., 2014).

The system used to quantify the energy content of food is based on the "food calorie," "large calorie," or kilocalorie, equal to 4.184 kilojoules. One food calorie is the amount of heat required at a pressure of one atmosphere to raise the temperature of 1 g of water by 1°C. The alternate definition is the amount of food having an energy-producing value of one large calorie. The conventional way to ascertain the caloric content of a sample of food is using a calorimeter, which literally burns the food sample to a crisp, measuring the amount of heat given off (its caloric content). To account for the varying densities of material within a sample, such as fiber, fat, and water, a more complex algorithm is used today.

Again, in this view, while providing information in the form of caloric content, food is not an informational substance, but simply a source of energy which can fuel the life-sustaining activities of the body-machine.

THE NEW STORY: FOOD AS INFORMATION

The new view of food as replete with biologically important information is based on many relatively new discoveries in various fields of scientific research.

One of the first major indications that food possesses powerful "informational" properties came from Duhl's dietary methylation experiments with obese yellow mice, where feeding yellow-coated pregnant mice (with an unmethylated agouti gene) a methyl-rich diet caused their offspring to have a brown coat color (methylated agouti gene) (Duhl et al., 1994). Obviously if folate, vitamin B12, choline, and methionine—four food components—have the power to literally "shut off" the expression of genes, and profoundly alter the appearance of an animal's offspring, food can no longer be adequately comprehended via the energy/matter dichotomy. Nor can epigenetic inheritance systems such as methylation patterns be considered secondary in determining phenotype in offspring.

Since then, the field of nutrigenomics has expanded into a multidisciplinary exploration which not only investigates genomic (DNA and chromosomal damage/repair) and epigenomic alterations (DNA methylation and histone modification), but also RNA and micro-RNA expression (transcriptomics), protein expression (proteomics), and metabolite changes (metabolomics) (Fenech et al., 2011). In essence, the field acknowledges that food and/or food components have gene-regulatory properties whose significance is on par with the primary nucleotide sequences of protein coding genes. In other words, food can now be considered an instrument of biosemiosis, the process of communication among the components of living systems.

Nutrigenomics not only examines the effects of food constituents on the genome, but it also "has been defined by the influence of genetic variation on nutrition by correlating gene expression or single-nucleotide polymorphisms with a nutrient's absorption, metabolism, elimination, and/or biological effects" (Gonzalez et al., 2015, p. 2). In this way, the information conveyed by food is limited by what Dr. Roger Williams called a genetotrophic disease, where an individual's genetic predisposition necessitates higher levels of nutritional cofactors to overcome the reduced binding affinity of a polymorphic enzyme for its coenzyme (Williams, 2009).

It has been discovered that nutritional components can affect gene expression by changing concentrations of reactants or intermediates in metabolic pathways, by modifying signal transduction pathways, and by serving as ligands for transcription factor receptors (Gonzalez et al., 2015). According to Choi and Frisco, "It appears that nutrients and bioactive food components can influence epigenetic phenomena either by directly inhibiting enzymes that catalyze DNA methylation or histone modifications, or by altering the availability of substrates necessary for those enzymatic reactions" (Choi & Frisco, 2010, p. 8).

For example, butyrate, a short chain fatty acid from fermentable fiber, sulforaphane, an isothiocyanate in broccoli, and diallyl sulfide, an organosulfur compound contained in garlic, all inhibit histone acetyltransferase (HAT), whereas genistein from soy and green tea catechin affect DNA methyltransferases (DNMTs) (Choi & Frisco, 2010). Other molecular targets for epigenetic modifications by bioactive food components are histone deacetylases (HDACs), histone methyltransferases (HMTs), histone demethylases (HDMs), and microRNAs (miRNAs), which similarly affect chromatin remodeling and therefore influence accessibility of DNA for transcription (Choi & Frisco, 2010).

There is likewise a plethora of literature indicating that food agents can inhibit master transcription factors such as nuclear factor kappa beta (NFkB), the gatekeeper to expression of pro-inflammatory cytokines such as tumor necrosis factor (TNF) and cyclo-oxygenase (COX), the latter of which mediates expression of inflammatory prostaglandins and thromboxanes. For instance, nutrients such as quercetin, a bioflavonoid abundant in fruits and vegetables, kaempferol, a flavonol rich in broccoli, strawberries, beans, tea, and apples, and curcumin, found in the spice turmeric, down-regulate NF-kB, such that their use may be valuable in conditions where inflammatory cytokines play a pathophysiological role (García-Mediavilla et al., 2007; Şehirli et al., 2007; Henrotin et al., 2010; Somerset & Johannot, 2008). On the other hand, the nutritional components pterostilbene and resveratrol from red grapes enhance activity of peroxisome proliferator-activated receptors (PPARs), which favorably influence carbohydrate and fat metabolism as well as mitochondrial function, inducing improvements in metabolic parameters (Rimando et al., 2005; Floyd et al., 2008).

Nutrigenomics, the newfound discipline which epitomizes the informational nature of food, may usher in an era of personalized nutrition recommendations based on genotypes, following in the footsteps of previous schools of thought such as Dr. Roger Williams' biochemical individuality, Dr. Abram Hoffer's orthomolecular medicine, Dr. Jeffrey Bland's functional medicine, Dr. Bruce Ames' triage hypothesis, Dr. Michael Friedman and Dr. Denis Wilson's restorative medicine, and Dr. Michael Gonzalez's metabolic correction (Gonzalez et al., 2015).

Epigenetics, in particular, or the study of how nutritional elements induce somatically heritable changes in gene expression by altering chromatin structure without interfering with the nucleotide base pair sequence, is revolutionary in that it confirms that genes alone do not dictate physiological fate. Such a notion is validated by a recent study published in *Public Library of Science One* (PLoS One) entitled "Genetic Factors Are Not the Major Causes of Chronic Diseases," which identifies that the vast majority of non-communicable diseases are environmental, relating to epigenetic and exposome-related variables, whereas only a minority is attributable to genetics (Rappaport, 2016). In effect, the epigenetic effects of diet, via the many activators and suppressors of chromatin remodeling enzymes that food contains, can deprogram or reprogram vast quantities of genes regulating metabolic pathways, which in turn can influence the development of chronic, long-latency, and degenerative diseases.

Food's role as an epigenetic modulator of DNA expression is a powerful demonstration of its informational properties, but this is not the whole story.

Food, when not artificially sterilized, is comprised of other organisms; that is, all food has a microbiome. What's more, all organisms (except viruses) produce microvesicles, also known as exosomes, which function to deliver mitogenic lipids, signaling proteins, and RNAs for intercellular communication (Record, 2013). These exosomes contain non-coding RNAs, which can profoundly alter the expression of our DNA. In fact, there are estimated to be ~100,000 different sites in the human genome capable of producing noncoding RNAs, far eclipsing our 20–25,000 protein-coding genes (Iyer et al., 2015). It has been estimated that these RNAs orchestrate the expression of most of the genes in the body. They are, therefore, supervening forces largely responsible for maintaining our genetic and epigenetic integrity.

Food RNAs, particularly so-called micro-RNAs, can affect our RNA profiles, making them extremely impactful to our health. They are carried by virus-sized microvesicles called exosomes, secreted by all plant, animal, bacterial, and fungal cells found in all the food we eat, and are capable of surviving digestive processes to significantly alter our gene expression. In 2012, a groundbreaking study by Zhang and colleagues entitled "Exogenous Plant MIR168a Specifically Targets Mammalian LDLRAP1: Evidence of Cross-Kingdom Regulation by microRNA" found that exosomal miRNAs from rice altered LDL receptors in the livers of Chinese subjects (Zhang et al., 2012). The study, while controversial, appears to confirm that our gene expression can be profoundly affected by what we eat. It also appears to prove that cross-kingdom regulation by microRNA exists (Zhang et al., 2012). The ability of exosomes to mediate the transfer of miRNAs across kingdoms redefines our notion of the human species as genetically hermetically sealed off from others within the animal, plant, and fungi kingdoms. In this sense, foodborne exosomes are the mechanism through which all living things in the biosphere are interconnected, reminiscent of a key element of the Lovelock and Margulis Gaia hypothesis (Igaz & Igaz, 2015).

THE MICROBIOME OF FOOD

Acknowledging the microbiomes of food itself is a significant part of revising the conceptualization of food, from one circumscribed by constrained notions of energy/matter, to one inclusive of information. The genetic contribution of the bacteria, fungi, viruses, helminths, and archaea collectively represents a vast store of biologically meaningful information, which in the case of our human species eclipses the contribution of our genome alone by a factor of 99 or higher (Bordenstein & Theis, 2015). Everything we eat also contains a microbiome in its natural state, even if it is still largely unacknowledged by food and nutritional science.

One of the most powerful examples of how the food microbiome has profound implications for human health is the identification of a marine bacterial carbohydrate-active enzyme in the guts of Japanese people capable of digesting sulfated polysaccharides (Hehemann et al., 2010). This bacterial gene was identified as having been derived from bacteria living on edible seaweed (Porphyra spp. (nori)), and is believed to have "jumped" horizontally into a human gut bacterium sometime within the past few hundred years. The result is that its unique digestive enzyme capabilities were transferred to the microbiome of its Japanese hosts. In essence, the gene provided by these marine microbes vastly extended the genetic capability of our species. Suddenly, countless marine plants that were formerly indigestible became sources of food.

The human genome only contains about 17 carbohydrate-digesting enzyme templates, 9 of which have not yet been fully characterized, whereas the gut bacteria contains genetic information capable of helping to degrade thousands of different carbohydrates (Cantarel et al., 2012). In this sense, then, the microbiome is an information storehouse that radically transforms the definition of food from the matter/energy dichotomy to a living reservoir of vitally important genetic information.

This revelation has innumerable implications for human health. First and foremost, food technologies like cold pasteurization (gamma irradiated food) and chemical treatments that alter the microbiome dysbiotically will dramatically alter the qualitative/informational content of the food, even if this will never be visible or acknowledged via conventional metrics used to assess nutritional value.

FOOD TIMING AND QUALITY

Not only do the qualitative contents of food transfer information and microbes that activate or silence gene expression, as well as influence metabolic pathways, but food timing and quantity also deliver information capable of affecting bioenergetics and physiological functioning at a cellular level.

The ultimate manifestation of the effect of food quantity on human health is the longevity-promoting nature of caloric restriction (CR). Fasting, which has been an anchoring ritual in every major world religious doctrine, is rooted in evolutionary biology, as humans adapted to vacillating periods of feast and famine throughout evolutionary history. According to Mattson and colleagues (2016), "Because animals, including humans, evolved in environments where food was relatively scarce, they developed numerous adaptations that enabled them to function at a high level, both physically and cognitively, when in a food-deprived/fasted state" (Mattson, Longo, & Harvie, 2016, p. S1568).

Whereas caloric excess augments parameters of accelerated aging and chronic disease, CR represents the most empirically validated intervention for extending lifespan (Fontana, 2007; Genaro,

Sarkis, & Martini, 2009). Ad libitum eating predicts pathophysiological processes such as insulin resistance, visceral adiposity, and endothelial dysfunction, the precursors to contemporary chronic diseases, while CR has been scientifically proven to reduce morbidity and enhance longevity (Mattson et al., 2016). The disease-mitigating effects of CR are conserved from lower to higher life forms, since, according to Longo and Mattson (2014), the cytoprotective effects conferred by CR "have likely evolved billions of years earlier in prokaryotes attempting to survive in an environment largely or completely devoid of energy sources while avoiding age-dependent damage that could compromise fitness" (Longo & Mattson, 2014, p. 2).

For instance, the lifespan of *Escherichia coli* (*E. coli*) is quadrupled when it is switched from a nutrient-rich broth to a calorie-free medium (Gonidakis, Finkel, & Longo, 2010). In similar fashion, transitioning common brewer's yeast, *Saccharomyces cerevisiae* (*S. cerevisiae*) to water from a standard growth culture reliably multiplies its lifespan twofold and leads to dramatic increases in stress resilience (Longo et al., 1997, 2012). Moreover, deprivation or dilution of food consistently extends lifespan of both the common fruit fly, *Drosophila melanogaster* (*D. melanogaster*), and the nematode *Caenorhabditis elegans* (*C. elegans*) (Piper & Partridge, 2007; Lee et al., 2006; Kaeberlein et al., 2006).

At a biochemical level, the informatics conveyed by CR significantly inhibit inflammatory genes such as NFkB, AP1, COX-2, and iNOS (Choi & Frisco, 2010). Conversely, CR activates PPARs, and modulates intracellular sensors such as mechanistic target of rapamycin (mTORC) and adenosine monophosphate-activated protein kinase (AMPK), which integrate environmental input and assess nutrient accessibility to determine cell fate (Gonzalez et al., 2015; Laplante & Sabatini, 2012). That mTORC1 in particular is an essential positive determinant of the competency of regulatory T cell (Treg) populations, which establish peripheral immune tolerance, may be responsible for the benefits fasting confers in autoimmune diseases such as rheumatoid arthritis and multiple sclerosis (Sundqvist et al., 1982; Choi et al., 2016; Zeng et al., 2013).

CR activates gene expression patterns that improve biomarkers of cardiovascular health, cognition, executive function, and metabolic rate (Heilbronn & Ravussin, 2003). Periods of fasting likewise significantly reduce leptin, the pro-inflammatory adipokine implicated in type 1 diabetes, autoimmune hepatitis, psoriasis, rheumatoid arthritis, systemic lupus erythematosus, multiple sclerosis, Behcet's disease, and ulcerative colitis, which has the effect of up-regulating immunosuppressive Treg subsets (Hutcheson, 2015; Liu et al., 2012). Further, fasting improves other metabolic biomarkers such as lipids, glucose, and adiponectin, while favorably influencing insulin sensitivity, adipose tissue lipolysis, hepatic glycogenolysis, and anabolic activity in muscle, all of which cumulatively promote metabolic correction (Longo & Mattson, 2014; Mattson et al., 2016).

The absence of food also transmits information at the cellular level that facilitates DNA-based repair mechanisms, stem cell-derived regeneration, mitochondrial biogenesis, and autophagy-mediated clearance of dead cells, cellular debris, and misfolded proteins such as amyloid beta plaques and tau tangles which contribute to neurodegenerative disease (Mattson et al., 2016). Fasting similarly promotes neurological health via enhancements in neurogenesis, synaptic plasticity, neurotrophic factor synthesis, and attenuation of inflammation (Longo & Mattson, 2014; Mattson et al., 2016).

On a related note, consumption of food during restricted windows imparts information at a cellular level, such that, "It is hypothesized that some fasting regimens and time-restricted feeding impose a diurnal rhythm in food intake, resulting in improved oscillations in circadian clock gene expression that reprogram molecular mechanisms of energy metabolism and body weight regulation" (Patterson et al., 2015, p.7). Strategic food timing may moderate energy intake via changes in appetite-regulating hormones including xenin, ghrelin, and leptin, leading to lowered risk of obesity, cardiovascular disease, diabetes, and cancer, since abnormal meal timing may induce circadian desynchronization and interfere with restorative sleep (Patterson et al., 2015). Lastly, CR and time-restricted feeding may promote healthier composition of the colonic microbiota, leading to normalization of microbiota diurnal fluctuations, derangements in which are associated with obesity and glucose intolerance (Thaiss et al., 2014). A healthier microbiome may also result in less harvesting of energy from the diet by commensal flora, which in turn may influence energy storage and expenditure in a favorable direction (Patterson et al., 2015; Thaiss et al., 2014).

Hence, both the presence and absence of food, as well as meal timing, can serve as environmental cues to modulate both profiles of gene expression and levels of molecular signals, resulting in either benefits or detriments to human health. Therefore, the definition of food as information must be expanded to encompass the manner, frequency, and quantity in which food is ingested.

POWERFUL IMPLICATIONS FOR THE FUTURE OF FOOD

When food is perceived as a vital source of biologically important information which directly informs and affects the expression of our genome, it is much easier to understand how our ancestors considered its creation, production, harvest, cooking, and consumption to be sacred—that is, sustaining of life itself.

Understanding food as information makes it easier to comprehend that food is a highly targeted and powerful form of medicine, capable of altering the expression of thousands of genes in a manner not reproducible via synthetic medicines.

Also, once the exosomal non-coding RNAs in the plants, animals, fungi, and bacteria in the "outside" world we use as food are acknowledged to be essential for maintaining and regulating our species' own genetic and epigenetic template for well-being, no longer can we callously destroy or alter the biosphere without affecting ourselves, and the overall destiny of our species.

Today, with anthropogenic climate change, genetic engineering, and a wide range of industrial farming technologies changing the quality (and informational component) of our food, it is no longer sufficient to examine the material aspects of these changes alone. Food irradiation technology, genetic modification, pesticides, soil quality, processing, and a wide range of other factors may greatly alter the informational state and quality of a food without being reflected in overt changes in grosser qualities like caloric and materially defined dimensions.

BIOPHOTONS: THE HUMAN BODY EMITS, COMMUNICATES WITH, AND IS MADE FROM LIGHT

Increasingly, science agrees with the poetry of direct human experience: we are more than the atoms and molecules that make up our bodies, but beings of light as well. Decades ago, authors described "an envelope of radiation surrounding living organisms" (Van Wijk & Van Wijk, 2005). It was later discovered that biophotons are emitted by the human body, can be released through mental intention, and may modulate fundamental processes within cell-to-cell communication and DNA.

Nothing is more amazing than the highly improbable fact that we exist. We often ignore this fact, oblivious to the reality that instead of something, there could be nothing at all; that is, why is there a universe (poignantly aware of itself through us) and not some void completely unconscious of itself?

Consider that from light, air, water, basic minerals within the crust of the Earth, and the at least 3-billion-year-old information contained within the nucleus of one diploid zygote cell, the human body is formed, and within that body a soul capable of at least trying to comprehend its bodily and spiritual origins.

Given the sheer insanity of our existential condition, and bodily incarnation as a whole, and considering that our earthly existence is partially formed from sunlight and requires the continual consumption of condensed sunlight in the form of food, it may not sound so farfetched that our body emits light.

Indeed, the human body emits quanta of electromagnetic energy called biophotons, also known as biophoton emission (BPE) or ultraweak photon emissions (UPE), with a visibility 1,000 times lower than the sensitivity of our naked eye. While not visible to us, these particles of light (or waves, depending on how you are measuring them) are part of the visible electromagnetic spectrum (380–780 nanometers) and are detectable via sophisticated modern instrumentation (Schwabl et al., 2005). Although characterized by a very low emission intensity of hundreds of photons per second, this low-level chemiluminescence is theorized to be intrinsic to cellular energetics and physiology, and is correlated with energetically demanding processes such as cell metabolism, oxidative stress, phagocytosis, and neurological activity (Devaraj, Usa, & Inaba, 1997; Kataoka et al., 2001).

In fact, this photonic emission is hypothesized to be a heuristic and global indicator for health or debility, as BPE has been found to be associated with an array of pathological states, including cancer, multiple sclerosis, hyperlipidemia, and hemiparesis (Hossu & Rupert, 2006). Photon emission has been characterized from topical injuries, active wounds, and sites of skin disease (Cohen & Popp, 1997). In addition, subjects with hypothyroidism or surgically removed thyroid glands have less BPE than controls, which underscores the connection between biophoton release and metabolic rate (Van Wijk & Van Wijk, 2005). Further, left-right symmetry of UPE from hands is distorted in patients with hemiparesis compared to healthy controls, suggesting that asymmetry in photon emission may be a surrogate marker for pathology (Jung et al., 2003).

UPE may be modulated by mental intention, as some subjects are able to increase the magnitude of emission intensity via vibratory movements and deep breathing, such that a subject's efforts to increase their "energetic field" is proportional to the increase in the signal their body emanates (Van Wijk & Van Wijk, 2005). On the other hand, some data indicate that intentional attempts to decrease photonic emissions result in decreases in mean photon counts, or that the spectral characteristics of BPE can be altered by intentionality (Van Wijk & Van Wijk, 2005).

Further, the therapeutic efficacy of complementary and alternative medicine (CAM) interventions, including acupuncture, chiropractic, cranio-sacral therapy, reflex therapy, and Reiki may make sense in the context of BPE, which has been shown to be affected not only locally but distally by different bodywork techniques (Hossu & Rupert, 2006). However, the effects of another mind–body practice, Qigong, on BPE, has demonstrated mixed results (Nakamura et al., 2000). In essence, there seems to be wide inter- and intra-individual variation when it comes to manipulating BPE with mind–body approaches characteristic of traditional medical systems.

Although energy medicine has conventionally been relegated to the realm of placebo, researchers state, "The quantum behavior of the high energy processes of the human body that constitute the source of BPE are altered in some way by energy-based interventions" (Hossu & Rupert, 2006, p. 123). Not only does CAM influence the energetically intensive pathways in the body, but it also induces changes in the Q value, a measure of the coherence of the photonic field (Hossu & Rupert, 2006). That CAM therapies affect BPE both proximal and distal to the sites of intervention suggests, "direct energetic input to the local tissue and the body's reaction to that stimulation" may both be at play (Hossu & Rupert, 2006, p. 123).

Instead of eliciting its effect directly on physical structure, the efficacy of CAM interventions may lie in their interaction with BPE, and their effects on global regulatory processes (Curtis & Hurtak, 2004). In this way, the body of literature on biophotons challenges the prevailing lenses of the biomedical paradigm, reductionism and materialism, and constructs a foundation for CAM modalities that utilize bioinformation transfer carried by extremely minute energy signals, including spiritual healing, acupuncture, homeopathy, and electromedicine (Curtis & Hurtak, 2004). For instance, researchers postulate that the meridian grid system of Traditional Chinese Medicine may represent "a possible point of consonance and therefore a gateway of interaction" between the chemical-molecular body and the electromagnetic body that creates a standing wave surrounding the corporeal form (Curtis & Hurtak, 2004, p. 34).

Thus, recent developments are beginning to validate David Bohm's vision, articulated decades ago, that life is comprised of a perpetual "holomovement" or endless sea of light, whereby matter can be regarded as the crystallized manifestation of light energy (Curtis & Hurtak, 2004).

THE PHYSICAL AND "MENTAL" EYE EMITS LIGHT

The eye itself, which is continually exposed to ambient powerful photons that pass through various ocular tissues, emits spontaneous and visible light-induced ultraweak photon emissions

(Wang et al., 2011). It has even been hypothesized that visible light induces delayed bioluminescence within the exposed eye tissue, providing an explanation for the origin of the negative afterimage (Bókkon et al., 2011).

These light emissions have also been correlated with cerebral energy metabolism and oxidative stress within the mammalian brain (Kobayashi et al., 1999; Kataoka et al., 2001). And yet, biophoton emissions are not necessarily epiphenomenal.

Bókkon's hypothesis suggests that photons released from chemical processes within the brain produce biophysical pictures during visual imagery, and a recent study found that when subjects actively imagined light in a very dark environment, their intention produced significant increases in ultraweak photon emissions (Dotta et al., 2012). This is consistent with an emerging view that biophotons are not solely cellular metabolic byproducts, but rather, because biophoton intensity can be considerably higher inside cells than outside, it is possible for the mind to access this energy gradient to create intrinsic biophysical pictures during visual perception and imagery (Bókkon et al., 2010).

OUR CELLS AND DNA USE BIOPHOTONS TO STORE AND COMMUNICATE INFORMATION

It has been observed that biophotons are used by the cells of many living organisms, including bacteria, plants, and kidney cells and neutrophil granulocytes from animal cells, to communicate, which facilitates transfer of energy and information that is several orders of magnitude faster than chemical diffusion.

In a study by Sun and colleagues, for instance, researchers were able to demonstrate that "...different spectral light stimulation (infrared, red, yellow, blue, green, and white) at one end of the spinal sensory or motor nerve roots resulted in a significant increase in the biophotonic activity at the other end" (Sun, Wang, & Dai, 2010, p. 315). Researchers interpreted their findings to suggest that conduction of biophotons along nerve fibers, secondary to light stimulation, serves as a transduction mechanism for neural signals (Sun et al., 2010).

In addition, blood has been demonstrated to be a constant source of biophotons, one which stores energy in the form of the electron excitation that occurs as a byproduct of reactive oxygen species (ROS) production in normal metabolic pathways (Voeikov, 2000). Within this model, whereby neutrophil-generated ROS play an essential transformative role regarding the molecular oxygen transported by erythrocytes, the electron excited states (EES) within the blood exhibit exquisite sensitivity to infinitesimal fluctuations in the external photon field (Curtas & Hurtak, 2004). In addition, the propensity of blood to store energy as EES enables it to behave as a coordinated nonlinear and non-equilibrium system, whose contiguous units embody properties of holism, acting "with a conscious purpose as a whole system or organ rather than an aggregate of cells" (Curtas & Hurtak, 2004, p. 29).

Even when we go down to the molecular level of our genome, DNA can be identified as a source of biophoton emissions as well. One author proposes that DNA is so biophoton-dependent that it has excimer laser-like properties, enabling it to exist in a stable state far from thermal equilibrium at threshold (Popp et al., 1984).

Technically speaking, a biophoton is an elementary particle or quantum of light of non-thermal origin in the visible and ultraviolet spectrum emitted from a biological system. They are generally believed to be produced because of energy metabolism within our cells, or more formally, as a "byproduct of biochemical reactions in which excited molecules are produced from bioenergetic processes that involve active oxygen species" (Kobayashi, Kikuchi, & Okamura, 2009). Given the pivotal role that biophotons play in cell physiology, Einstein's enigmatic statement a century ago that he would prefer to spend the rest of his life contemplating the matter of light is particularly astute (Curtas & Hurtak, 2004).

THE BODY'S CIRCADIAN BIOPHOTON OUTPUT

Because the metabolism of the body changes in a circadian fashion, biophoton emissions also vary along the axis of diurnal time (Kobayashi et al., 2009). Research has likewise mapped out distinct anatomical locations within the body where biophoton emissions are stronger and weaker, depending on the time of the day.

Van Wijk and van Wijk (2005) articulate, "Generally, the fluctuation in photon counts over the body was lower in the morning than in the afternoon. The thorax-abdomen region emitted lowest and most constantly. The upper extremities and the head region emitted most and increasingly over the day" (van Wijk & van Wijk, 2005, p. 96). In addition, it was found that the major spontaneous emission from the palms, forehead, and superior ventral region of the right leg occurred at wavelengths of 470–570 nm, whereas the central palm emitted between 420 and 470 nm, congruent with the range of UPE emission from the hand in the autumn and winter (van Wijk & van Wijk, 2005).

Thus, in addition to temporal variations in photon emission throughout the day, BPE exhibits seasonal periodicity. In a different experiment, subjects produced lower bilateral photonic emission readings at all points of measurement in the winter compared to the summer (Bieske, Gall, & Fisch, 2000). Age may be another governing factor for BPE, since Sauermann and colleagues (1999) found that elderly subjects had elevated levels of spontaneous photon emission (SPE) from their hands, which the authors attribute to increased oxidative stress in the stratum corneum proteins of the integumentary system of aging skin.

MEDICAL APPLICATIONS OF BIOPHOTON EMISSIONS

Because biophoton emission may be reflective of the cumulative physiological or pathological state of living organisms, technology that evaluates SPE can be employed in disease prevention and monitoring of health outcomes (Zhao et al., 2017). For instance, based on their observations of the diurnal and seasonal periodicity of BPE, researchers concluded that spectral analysis of photonic emissions can illustrate *in vivo* trends in peroxidative and antioxidative processes (van Wijk & van Wijk, 2005). This has profound implications for routine evaluation of antioxidant capacity, peroxidative processes, and oxidative status of the skin, in particular, since current methodologies are invasive and labor-intensive (Van Wijk & Van Wijk, 2005).

Another potential application of technologies that measure SPE is cancer detection. Studies have indicated that SPE projected from lesion sites can differentiate human breast cancer-bearing mice from controls, and can predict tumor occurrence even in the absence of overt morphological disturbances (Zhao et al., 2017). Researchers state that as an optical methodology, SPE "may contribute to the preliminary screening of breast cancer, especially for early diagnosis, and it may play a critical role in curtailing the effects of breast cancer and improving the survival of patients in the future" (Zhao et al., 2017, p. 232).

In addition, spectral discrimination in photoinduced delayed luminescence (DL) has been observed between normal and leukemic serum samples (Chen et al., 2012). Delayed luminescence similarly allows tissues containing adenocarcinoma and squamous cell carcinoma lung cancer to be differentiated from adjacent normal tissue (Kim et al., 2005). A significant difference between the BPE intensity from tumorigenic mice harboring ovarian cancer cells and control mice has likewise been observed (Kim et al., 2006). Further evidence that BPE could be used in cancer imaging comes from mouse studies showing that biophoton intensity is correlated with tumor size after carcinoma cell transplantation (Takeda et al., 2004).

Another disease state in which biophoton release may represent an avenue for disease assessment is rheumatoid arthritis (RA), since mouse models of RA have demonstrated higher UPE after arthritis is instigated with repeated co-administration of type II collagen and lipopolysaccharide (van Wijk et al., 2013). UPE detection has also been shown to distinguish healthy subjects from those with the common cold via spectral peaks and spectral emission ratios, such that it could be used in the development of novel optical diagnostic tools (Yang et al., 2015).

Fundamentally, the paradigm-shifting reconception of human beings as bodies of light may pave the way for newfound modalities of detecting and treating myriad diseases, since, "ultra-weak photon emission is a common phenomenon and carries information about its generating processes, and is closely related to photosynthesis, lipid peroxidation, catabolism, free radical reactions, radiation effects, detoxification and carcinogenic effects, aging and death process" (Yang et al., 2015, p. 1331).

In addition, because UPE is an intrinsic attribute of all biological systems, resulting from the relaxation of electronically excited species stemming from metabolic processes, UPE evaluation has been considered an opportunity for assessment of food quality and medicinal properties of herbs (Hossu, Ma, & Chen, 2010; Pang et al., 2016).

MEDITATION AND HERBS AFFECT BIOPHOTON OUTPUT

Research has found an oxidative stress-mediated difference in biophoton emission among mediators versus non-meditators. Those who meditate regularly tend to have lower ultra-weak photon emission (UPE), which is believed to result from the lower level of free radical reactions occurring in their bodies (van Wijk et al., 2006). This is confirmed by studies documenting that the spectrum of UPE ranges from 450 to 630 nm, wavelengths which correspond to that exemplified by lipid peroxidation processes and production of oxygen-paired molecules in animal tissue (van Wijk et al., 2006). In one clinical study involving practitioners of transcendental meditation (TM), researchers found that experienced meditators exhibited the lowest UPE intensities (van Wijk et al., 2006).

Further, the authors conceptualize UPE as a partial representation of free radical reactions in living systems. They discuss, "It has been documented that various physiologic and biochemical shifts follow the long-term practice of meditation and it is inferred that meditation may impact free radical activity" (Van Wijk et al., 2006, p. 31). Thus, researchers hypothesize that the lower levels of photonic emission from transcendental meditators is correlated with lower stress levels, and that meditation may favorably alter the oxidative status of the body (Van Wijk et al., 2006).

Interestingly, an herb called rhodiola, well-known for its use in stress reduction (including inducing measurable declines in cortisol), and associated heightened oxidative stress, has been tested clinically in reducing the level of biophotons emitted by human subjects. In fact, a study published in 2009 in the journal *Phytotherapeutic Research* found that those who took the herb for one week had a significant decrease in photon emission in comparison with the placebo group, which was correlated with a significant decrease in fatigue (Schutgens et al., 2009).

THE ELECTROMAGNETIC BODY AND CONSCIOUSNESS

Biophotonic processes are further beginning to demystify such elusive phenomena as consciousness and the electromagnetic body, the latter of which is both disparate from the chemical body and described as a "light circulatory system operating on an energetic level," obeying fundamentally different laws and behaving in a fashion distinct from its bioplasmic counterparts" (Curtis & Hurtak, 2004, p. 27). In other words, although conventional biology has failed to incorporate quantum physics and has extracted bodies from the energy matrices in which they are embedded, biophysics is acknowledging light-based modes of energetic communication and information transmission in the body apart from the physical nervous, blood, and lymphatic systems (Curtis & Hurtak, 2004).

Researchers suggest that this circulatory system of biophotonic light, which is connected to a conduit of internal current running through the bodily meridians illuminated by Traditional Chinese Medicine, is the mechanism through which acupuncture works (Curtis & Hurtak, 2004). For instance, after acupuncture treatments, the left-right asymmetry in BPE is significantly reduced in subjects with hemiparesis (Choi et al., 2002). Emission intensity has also been observed to be higher from moxa and acupuncture points, and insertion of a needle or laser beam needle into acupuncture points leads to increases in BPE from non-stimulated acupuncture points (Yanagawa et al., 2000; Inaba, 1999a, 1999b, 2000).

Concepts of the electromagnetic body, which researchers speculate may be a medium through which consciousness is projected, incorporate knowledge on mitogenetic radiation (MGR), also known as UPE from living systems, and work from the Vernadsky–Gurwitsch–Bauer school of thought concerning the morphogenetic field (Curtis & Hurtak, 2004). According to the ground-breaking work of Gurwitsch (1944), MGR, which consists of energetic transfers that induce cell division via UPE, cannot occur without one photon of ultraviolet (UV) light (Voeikov, 2003). Not only do biophotons promote cell growth and differentiation, but they are also required for cell-to-cell communication (Popp, 1979; Chang et al., 2000).

Because the photon emissions are ultra-weak, the order of the radiation, and not its intensity, is what is integral to biophoton dynamics. It has likewise been established that biophotons embody the property of coherence, whereby biologic efficiency is inversely related to intensity, such that the coherence of biophotons exceeds even that of manufactured lasers (Voeikov, 2003). Within this model, the human body exhibits not only entropy, adhering to the second order of thermodynamics, but behaves in a dynamic consistent with centropy, the inverse of entropy whereby order increases, and matter is electrified (Curtis & Hurtak, 2004). In this sense, the body is understood to deviate from thermodynamic equilibrium and embody properties of chaos and dissipation (Curtis & Hurtak, 2004, p. 29).

This pioneering body of work also postulates that the body operates more as an energy biocomputer than as a mechanistic Descartes-style machine, and that biophotons, quantum coherence, and electron excitation comprise the essence of life (Curtas & Hurtak, 2004). In this view, because the body functions under nonequilibrium thermodynamics, it exhibits receptivity to bioenergetic fields and energetic forms of consciousness "that interpenetrate and commingle to form the totality that we call the human being" (Curtis & Hurtak, 2004, p. 28).

As such, a novel scientific jargon, elucidating many types of light, including superluminal, consciousness light, and photonic or particulate light, is emerging and redefining what it is to be human. This brave new world of research, which is recognizing the human body as both a biotransducer for energy fields and a quasi-light body, which transduces internal and extraneous signals locally and nonlocally, may pave the way for future biophoton therapeutic applications (Gariaev, Tertishny, & Leonova, 2000; Hurtak, 1996).

HUMAN SKIN MAY CAPTURE ENERGY AND INFORMATION FROM SUNLIGHT

Perhaps most extraordinary of all is the possibility that our bodily surface contains cells capable of efficiently trapping the energy and information from ultraviolet radiation. A study published in the *Journal of Photochemistry and Photobiology* in 1993, for example, discovered that when light from an artificial sunlight source was applied to fibroblasts from either normal subjects or individuals with the condition xeroderma pigmentosum, characterized by deficient DNA repair mechanisms, it induced far higher emissions of ultraweak photons (10–20 times higher) in the xeroderma pigmentosum group. The researchers concluded from this experiment, "These data suggest that xeroderma pigmentosum cells tend to lose the capacity of efficient storage of ultraweak photons, indicating the existence of an efficient intracellular photon trapping system within human cells" (Niggli et al., 1993, p. 281). More recent research has also identified measurable differences in biophoton emission between normal and melanoma cells (Niggli et al., 2005).

The concept that the body is capable of directly harvesting the energy of the sun has received increased interest over the past decade. For instance, in a seminal paper published in 2008 in the *Journal of Alternative and Complementary Medicine*, Goodman and Bercovich (2008) offer a thought-provoking reflection on the topic in their discussion of the animal pigment melanin, which possesses complex physico-chemical qualities and is unique in its absorption across the ultraviolet-visual spectrum (Goodman et al., 2008).

Melanin appears in the skin, eyes, hair, feathers, and scales, as well as internal, extracutaneous areas associated with pathology such as the mammalian cochlea and sites in the central nervous system such as the leptomeninges, cerebral hemisphere, and medulla oblongata (Goldgeier et al., 1984; Goodman & Bercovich, 2008). Although traditionally confined to roles in skin protection and signaling, it has been discovered that melanocytes contain enzymes that act as carrier proteins for lipophilic compounds such as thyroid hormone and bilirubin, and that melanin likely serves endocrine functions as well (Takeda, Takahashi, & Shibahara, 2007). The physiological roles of melanin are complex, as it can absorb heavy metal cations, scavenge free radicals, play a role in charge transfer, and exhibit properties of both conductors and semiconductors (Goodman et al., 2008).

Birds, which have unique anatomical characteristics to overcome gravity, contain an intra-ocular, melanised organ called the pecten, comprised of a fan-like pleated lamina which projects into the vitreous from the optic disc (Goodman & Bercovich, 2008). The pecten, enclosed by a peripectenial membrane, contains pigmented melanocytes which anastomose with networks of capillaries (Goodman & Bercovich, 2008). Not only does an oxygen gradient exist from pecten to retina, but the pecten also contains high concentrations of alkaline phosphatase and carbonic anhydrase, which signal metabolic activity (Pettigrew, Wallman, & Wildoset, 1990; Bawa & YashRoy, 1972; Amemiya & Yoshida, 1980). Pigment exposure is further maximized as the capillaries that intertwine with melanocytes support the latter (Goodman & Bercovich, 2008).

The pecten, which is enlarged in birds enduring hypoxia, thirst, and hunger during long-distance migrations, may serve as an adaptive coping mechanism to meet "energy and nutrient needs under extreme conditions, by a marginal but critical, melanin-initiated conversion of light to metabolic energy, coupled to local metabolite recycling" (Goodman & Bercovich, 2008, p. 190). This is substantiated by data showing that pheomelanin can be reduced to molecular oxygen (Ye et al., 2006). In addition, the lability and polymeric heterogeneity of melanin, stacked in a disordered nano-aggregate architecture, helps to explain its "thermodynamically cheap means for broadband light absorption" (Goodman & Bercovich, 2008, p. 197). In other words, micro-spatial changes in melanin conformation can produce instability in electron states, causing alterations in the direct biochemical milieu of melanin that instigate repletion of metabolic intermediates and up-regulate local anaplerosis (Goodman & Bercovich, 2008). Especially critical is that light can stimulate NADPH by way of melanin, and generate oxygen and water through catalase via the hydrogen peroxide flowing through the pecten (Goodman & Bercovich, 2008).

The pecten-mediated transformation of radiation into energy may not only support avian brain function during flight, but also help resolve what have remained mysteries in bird energetics, flight mechanics, and avian metabolism (Goodman & Bercovich, 2008). In addition, the authors discuss how the augmentation of melanin and reduction in body hair, which occurred in Central Africa during the course of human evolution, may have generated a process called photomelanometabolism (Goodman & Bercovich, 2008). Goodman and Bercovich (2008) speculate that this evolutionary event would not only have reduced energy expenditure required for hunting and gathering, but it would also have enabled the expansion of the energy-demanding cerebral cortex, leading to the development of higher cognition, which would pave the way for advancement of the human race (Goodman & Bercovich, 2008).

It is known that melanin can transform ultraviolet light energy into heat in a process known as "ultrafast internal conversion" (Meng et al., 2008). As a result, more than 99.9% of the absorbed UV radiation can be transformed from potentially genotoxic (DNA-damaging) ultraviolet light into harmless heat. Melanin, therefore, constitutes simultaneously both a "sun blocking" and energy conversion function.

Photomelanometabolism is thus so fundamental to our metabolism that is has been hypothesized that human hairlessness can be explained through it. Hairlessness was a mutational/adaptive event, occurring approximately 2 million years ago, which traded off the protective and endothermically ideal hair covering for the metabolic advantages of melanin-mediated sunlight harvesting. This would also explain why the encephalization event most characteristic of our species began $\sim$ 2 mya as well (Mathewson, 2015).

If melanin can convert light into heat, could it not also transform UV radiation into other biologically/metabolically useful forms of energy? This notion may not seem so farfetched when one considers that even gamma radiation, which is highly toxic to most forms of life, is a source of sustenance for certain types of heavily melanized fungi and bacteria (Dadachova & Casadevall, 2008).

In fact, ionizing radiation exposure has been shown to enhance growth of certain melanized fungal species that inhabit nuclear reactors, space stations, and the Antarctic mountains (Dadachova et al., 2007). Researchers note that the existence of melanized organisms in high radiation conditions "combined with phenomenon of 'radiotropism' raises the tantalizing possibility that melanins have functions analogous to other energy harvesting pigments such as chlorophylls" (Dadachova & Casadevall, 2008, p. 525).

Another indication that the body can harvest sunlight directly came in 2014, when a *Journal of Cell Science* study exemplified the role that chlorophyll pigments play in converting photonic energy into adenosine triphosphate (ATP) (Xu et al., 2014). It has been known that chlorophyll molecules, produced by the semi-autonomous mitochondrial analogs known as plant chloroplasts, can transform light energy into ATP. Likewise, studies have illuminated that chlorophyll metabolites, generated via plant consumption, retain capacity to absorb light in wavelengths of the visible spectrum that are able to penetrate animal tissues (Xu et al., 2014).

However, this study found that a metabolite of chlorophyll is taken up by mammalian mitochondria and is capable of capturing photons and, consequently, photo-energizing mitochondrial ATP production (Xu et al., 2014). When exposed to light, ATP concentrations produced in isolated mammalian tissue and mitochondria incubated with chlorophyll metabolites exceeded those of animal tissues not exposed to the metabolites (Xu et al., 2014). As a corollary, when this chlorophyll-derived metabolite was administered to the worm *Caenorhabditis elegans*, an increase in ATP production was generated upon light exposure with a concomitant increase in lifespan (Xu et al., 2014). Revolutionarily, Xu and colleagues (2014) likewise showed that a variety of mammals, including rats, mice, and pigs, can transform light into energy, as evidenced by the accumulation of chlorophyll metabolites in these mammals when a chlorophyll-rich diet is administered.

At a molecular level, dietary chlorophyll metabolites modulate reservoirs of mitochondrial ATP by catalyzing the reduction of coenzyme Q, the fat-soluble coenzyme of the electron transport chain that is instrumental to oxidative phosphorylation and is responsible for shuttling electrons to cytochrome C reductase of the respiratory chain (Xu et al., 2014). Importantly, the researchers speculate, "Photonic energy capture through dietary-derived metabolites may be an important means of energy regulation in animals" (Xu et al., 2014).

Moreover, despite the increased output, the expected increase in reactive oxygen species (ROS) that normally attends increased mitochondrial function was not observed; in fact, a slight decrease was observed (Xu et al., 2014). This is a highly significant finding because simply increasing mitochondrial activity and ATP output, while good from the perspective of energy, may accelerate aging and other ROS-induced, oxidative stress-related adverse cellular and physiological effects. Chlorophyll, therefore, appeared to make animal mitochondria function in a healthier way.

Researchers articulate that the transfer of photosensitized electrons originating "from excited chlorophyll-type molecules is widely hypothesized to be a primitive form of light-to-energy conversion that evolved into photosynthesis" (Xu et al., 2014, p. 394). This, in concert with the fact that sunlight-derived photons of red light have resided within nearly every mammalian tissue throughout evolution, lends credence to the notion that mammalian life harbors conserved molecular mechanisms designed to harness photonic energy (Xu et al., 2014). Fundamentally, this study reveals that animals are not just glucose-burning biomachines, but are light-harvesting hybrids. Technically, that knocks us out of the category of heterotrophs into photoheterotrophs.

THE BODY'S BIOPHOTON OUTPUTS ARE GOVERNED BY SOLAR AND LUNAR FORCES

It appears that modern science is only now coming to recognize the ability of the human body to receive and emit energy and information directly from the light given off from the sun (Slawinski et al., 2005).

There is also a growing realization that the sun and moon affect biophoton emissions through gravitational influences. Recently, biophoton emissions from wheat seedlings in Germany and

Brazil were found to be synchronized transcontinentally according to rhythms associated with the lunisolar tide (Gallep et al., 2013). In fact, the lunisolar tidal force, to which the sun contributes 30% and the moon 60% of the combined gravitational acceleration, has been found to regulate many features of plant growth upon Earth (Barlow et al., 2012).

WATER AS AN ALTERNATIVE CELLULAR FUEL SOURCE

Besides melanin, another conduit through which human beings exploit light energy may be water. Although the majority of our planet's surface and our body's interior is comprised of water, the orchestrated response of water molecules to light, and the coordinated organization of water molecules, has until recently remained a mystery.

In a dramatic departure from traditional schools of thought, which partitioned water into solid, liquid, and gaseous phases, a fourth phase of water has been unearthed by Dr. Gerald Pollack and colleagues (Pollack, 2013). This liquid-crystalline phase occurs proximate to hydrophilic, water-loving surfaces, which are surfaces typically capable of hydrogen bonding that thermodynamically favor interactions with other polar substances relative to hydrophobic, water-fearing solvents. This extensive fourth phase of water, which is ubiquitous in both nature and the human body, expands with absorption of electromagnetic energy in the form of light.

Radiant energy, ultimately emanating from the sun, transforms bulk water into fourth phase structured water, such that the magnitude of the fourth phase is directly related to the quantity of light absorbed (Pollack, 2015). Customary bulk water spontaneously absorbs ultraviolet, visible, and infrared wavelengths and is converted into this liquid crystalline water, also called "exclusion zone" or "EZ" water due to its exceptional omission of solutes (Pollack, 2015).

With a molecular formula H_3O_2, this "ordered" or "structured" fourth phase contains more molecular oxygen than H_2O, and hence is both denser and possesses a negative charge (Pollack, 2015). Although near infrared energy is most capable, the absorption of any spectrum of radiant energy splits water molecules into positive and negative moieties, with the former binding water molecules to create freely diffusing hydronium ions, and the latter constituting the elementary units that build the EZ (Pollack, 2015).

There is remarkable symmetry between this process, whereby additional assimilation of light energy engenders further charge separation, and the principal step of photosynthesis. In the process by which plants harness solar energy, hydrophilic chromophores, or light-absorbing molecules generally attached to a proteinaceous structure, catalyze the splitting of water molecules into oxygen and hydrogen (Fassioli et al., 2014). Light absorption by the chromophores transitions these antenna molecules from a ground state to a transient energetically excited state, and the excitation is transferred between chromophores until it ultimately arrives at a reaction center, where it induces a charge separation (Fassioli et al., 2014). A wide diversity of light-harvesting antenna structures exist in nature, such as chlorophyll, bilins, and carotenoids; however, each of these complexes retain the capacity to "convert the photo-generated excitations to charge separation with very high efficiency" (Fassioli et al., 2014, p. 2).

In the analogous process by which EZ water is generated, Pollack (2015) describes how any generic hydrophilic surface, from a dissolved molecule to a large polymer, can serve as the catalyst in the hydrolysis of water. In plants, segregation of charges delivers energy via a series of successive electron transfer reactions which enable photosynthetic energy transduction from a photo excited reaction center (Fassioli et al., 2014). This separation of charges, which generates energy via a battery-like configuration, operates not only in the plant kingdom, but also in EZ water.

The consequences of Pollack's revolutionary insights for human health are limitless, since 50%–75% of the body mass is water, and because two-thirds of the total body water resides in the intracellular compartment (Bianchetti, Simonetti, & Bettinelli, 2009). Further, 99% of molecules in the human body are water molecules, which were formerly regarded as secondary compared to nucleic acids and proteins, the latter of which were considered more important due to their contribution to the central dogma of biology (Pollack, 2015). In sharp divergence from the antiquated view that considers water to be the background carrier of these other molecules, structured water has been found to envelop every macromolecule, and to be quintessential to every cellular process (Pollack, 2001).

IMPLICATIONS OF EZ WATER FOR CIRCULATORY FLOW

For instance, the potential energy stored in water and amplified by additional incident light energy can power work in the form of flow. Experiments have elucidated that submerging hydrophilic tubes in water produces perpetual flow because of the radiant energy the water contains, with additional energy input eliciting faster flow (Pollack, 2013; Rohani & Pollack, 2013). Thus, Pollack (2015) demonstrates not only that EZ water can drive vascular flow in plants, but also rectifies the paradox of why pressure gradients across human capillary beds are negligible—radiant energy helps impel flow through capillaries, which would otherwise necessitate high driving pressure to overcome total peripheral resistance and to enable red blood cells to navigate capillaries with smaller diameters than the cells themselves. In a sense, then, both sauna therapy and sunlight exposure constitute previously unexplored sources of vascular force via their contribution to the construction of the body's structured water zones (Pollack, 2015).

IMPLICATIONS OF EZ WATER FOR SKELETAL MUSCLE STRUCTURE

In addition, Pollack (2015) explains that EZ water is the reason why joint sockets do not squeak because of frictional resistance during rotation under pressure, despite being situated at sites where bones abut one another. Hyaline cartilage, a semirigid avascular connective tissue consisting of a matrix of protein fibers in a gel-like ground substance, cocoons the ends of the bones to provide a sliding surface at joint articulations. Joints are in turn lined by fibrous areolar connective tissue enclosed by a layer of cuboidal or squamous epithelial cells devoid of a basement membrane called the synovial membrane, which consists of cells that secrete synovial fluid to decrease friction in the joint cavity. Because cartilage is a highly charged polymeric-like gel material, cartilage grows layers of EZ water in response to light (Pollack, 2015).

According to Pollack (2015), a concentrated population of hydronium ions are confined in the joint capsule, which repel one another maintaining distance between surfaces even in the presence of heavy loads, guaranteeing low frictional resistance. The double-layered joint capsule, comprised of a dense fibrous layer of connective tissue and an inner synovium, in turn ensures that the repelling hydronium ions do not disperse, which would jeopardize joint lubrication and cause asperities to make contact (Pollack, 2015).

With tissue injury and joint dislocation in particular, the full osmotic draw of EZ water is brought to bear. In theory, cells should generate an enormous osmotic water-attractant force since their cytoplasms are chock full of negatively charged proteins. However, the water-to-solids ratio of the cell normally remains at 2:1, versus 20:1 or higher for many gels, due to its complex cytoskeletal biopolymers such as actin filaments, microtubules, and intermediate filaments, which confer stiffness and establish cell architecture (Pollack, 2015; Fletcher & Mullins, 2010). The eukaryotic cell can resist deformation, adopt morphological changes during motility, transport intracellular cargo, and abstain from expansion to its full osmotic potential as a consequence of this cross-linking tubular network (Fletcher & Mullins, 2010).

However, when these cytoskeletal forces, which spatially organize the cell contents, are disrupted or contorted with injury, dramatic expansion occurs as an influx of EZ layers allows the tissue to massively hydrate (Pollack, 2015). Thus, healing, and reduction of swelling, will only take place with the successive reparation of these dynamic and adaptive cytoskeletal filaments and with the restoration of matrix mechanics.

Consequences of EZ Water for Human Health

Although hydration status and water homeostasis are recognized as critical determinants of health, researchers state, "Beyond these circumstances of dehydration, we do not truly understand how hydration affects health and well-being, even the impact of water intakes on chronic diseases" (Popkin, D'Anci, & Rosenberg, 2010). The pioneering paradigm of the fourth phase of water may fill in the gaps in this knowledge base. In essence, Pollack (2015) notes that the higher dipole moment of EZ water translates into better rehydration of cells, such that optimizing EZ water dynamics may be a future clinical priority.

He likewise states that EZ water may explicate the therapeutic properties of renowned healing bodies of waters such as the Lourdes and Ganges, which are fed by glacial melt or underground springs, many of which experience pressure from above that assembles ordered water from liquid water (Pollack, 2015). Further proof that these bodies of water build EZ water comes from studies that demonstrate that some glacial melt and spring waters exhibit a spectrometric peak at 270 nm, which is reflective of the ultraviolet wavelength at which EZ water absorbs light (So, Stahlberg, & Pollack, 2011).

Lastly, Pollack's groundbreaking work on structured water shines a spotlight on the role of antioxidants. Pollack (2015) speculates that humans bear net negative charge, since cells, which comprise 60% of the mass of the body, and components of the extracellular matrix, such as elastin and collagen, all possess negative polarity and adsorb EZ water. In contrast, those bodily compartments that bear positive charge, or have low pH, include expired air, perspiration, urine, and the gastrointestinal system, which function to eliminate positive charge in the form of excess protons from the body (Pollack, 2015). While plants can discharge positive charge via direct connection to the negatively charged earth, animals require antioxidants to counteract oxidation—the molecular process by which electrons are lost, robbing molecules of their net negative charge.

In this way, food can again be envisioned as imparting information, this time in the form of antioxidants which preserve health by reducing molecules via electron donation to help maintain proper bodily negativity. Accumulation of free radicals, which are highly reactive molecular species with an unpaired electron in an atomic orbital, in the absence of antioxidants to neutralize them, culminates in oxidative stress, which mediates disease pathology via damage to proteins, lipids, and nucleic acids (McCord, 2000). Whereas synthetic antioxidants have proven deleterious to human health, food-based antioxidants from spices, medicinal plants, and traditional Indian cuisine in particular "prevent free radical induced tissue damage by preventing the formation of radicals, scavenging them, or by promoting their decomposition" (Lobo et al., 2010).

Can Human Cells Exploit Photosynthesis?

Thus, it can be argued that human beings utilize a process akin to photosynthesis, in that we use light energy to create work through the vehicle of water. In this sense, water can be reconceptualized as an alternative to the traditional energy currency of the cell, ATP. Again, melanin may figure prominently in the conversion of light energy into chemical energy mediated by EZ water, in that this molecule absorbs the visible wavelengths and concentrates photons in such a way as to drive metabolic pathways (Herrera et al., 2015). Pollack (2015) further proposes that melanin could emit the absorbed energy in the infrared band, which in turn could power establishment of the EZ, division of charges, and generation of cellular energy.

Rather than merely engulfing and bathing the more integral molecular figures in the biochemical symphony, water constitutes a central player in the physiological orchestra and represents an informational powerhouse. Thus, investigating the clinical applications of structured water may yield future dividends for improving health.

INTENTION IS A LIVING FORCE OF PHYSIOLOGY

Even human intention itself, the so-called ghost in the machine, may have an empirical basis in biophotons. This notion was echoed by Max Planck, the German theoretical physicist who was awarded the Nobel Prize for his discovery of energy quanta, who conceived of matter as a derivative of consciousness (Curtis & Hurtak, 2004).

A recent commentary published in the journal *Investigación Clínica* addressed this connection. Bonilla (2008) discusses how biophoton emission is the vehicle through which intention, or a targeted train of thoughts meant to engender certain courses of action, elicits its effects. Rather than serving as mere epiphenomena, "Direct intention manifests itself as an electric and magnetic energy producing an ordered flux of photons" (Bonilla et al., 2008, p. 595). Thus, the directed emission of streams of photons, which are stored in the genetic material and may be altered in states of ill health, can send messages from one body part to another and to the extraneous environment.

As highlighted by Bonilla (2008), "Our intentions seem to operate as highly coherent frequencies capable of changing the molecular structure of matter" (Bonilla, 2008, p. 595). Therefore, abstract and esoteric phenomena such as hypnosis, extrasensory perception, stigmata, the placebo effect, the efficacy of prayer, and instances of spontaneous remission or remote healing may be conceptualized in terms of the power of beliefs and intention, mediated by photonic light particles. Moreover, because BPE is synchronized with macrocosmic-level gravitational, diurnal, and geomagnetic forces, its healing power could theoretically be harnessed by taking advantage of the lunar, solar, and seasonal cycles. This seems to fit the hypothesis advanced by Ji (2017) in his article, "Waves as the Symmetry Principle Underlying Cosmic, Cell, and Human Languages," that cellular, human, and cosmic languages are connected through waves: electromagnetic, mechanical, chemical concentration, and gravitational.

THE BIOELECTROMAGNETIC BODY

The notion of what it means to be human, and the nature of our body, is also being redefined by research exploring bioelectromagnetic interactions between individuals. Not only does the human body radiate light in the form of ultra-weak biophotonic emissions, but it also emits electromagnetic fields, since electromagnetic waves are generated when electrical charges move, according to Maxwell's equation. Our corporeal bodies, therefore, cannot only be perceived as entities of light, but also as beings of electricity.

That there is "an incredible amount of activity at levels of magnification or scale that span more than two-thirds of the 73 known octaves of the electromagnetic spectrum" in the human body elucidates how bodily systems are entrained to operate as a globally coherent system rather than displaying discordant and erratic behavior (Rosch, 2014). This integrated coherence, whereby body systems both function autonomously and collaborate interdependently with the whole, is responsible for defining qualities of living systems including exquisite sensitivity to signals, efficient energy transfer, and far-ranging coordination of activities (Ho, 2005). This coherence of the body, according to Rosch (2014), has implications for the energetic nature of social interactions, the contribution of bioelectromagnetism to physiological processes, the role of positive emotionality in health, and the interaction between people and the electromagnetic field in which the earth is enmeshed.

Positive emotions are associated with greater degrees of coherence, defined as more stable and harmonious interactions in the rhythmic activity of the oscillatory systems of the body (Rosch, 2014; Tiller, McCraty, & Atkinson, 1996). For instance, when an individual employs coherence-building techniques by exuding positive emotionality to produce feelings of gratitude, the synchronization between the alpha waves of their brains and their cardiac cycle significantly increases (McCraty, 2002). In addition to synchronization between the parasympathetic and sympathetic branches of the autonomic nervous system, which also occurs with physiological coherence, Rosch (2014) notes that entrainment can occur between cardiac, respiratory, digestive, neurological, and craniosacral rhythms, as well as other biological oscillators including fluctuations in blood pressure and the electrical conductance measured in the skin. This occurs because the subsystems of the body begin to vibrate at the resonant frequency of the holistic system (Rosch, 2014). These notions can be reconciled with the idea promulgated by Petoukhov, that organisms are systems of resonant oscillators, or operate in a way akin to musical instruments (Petoukhov & Petukhova, 2017).

A constellation of evidence is also evolving to demonstrate that group communication, social unity, and collective group intentions can be explained by an unseen bioenergetic field that connects and informs behavior of members in highly coherent groups (Rosch, 2014). Rosch's coherence construct is reinforced by a theory proposed by neuroscientist Karl Pribram and sociologist Raymond Bradley, who hypothesized that bioenergetic interconnectivity is the global thread that organizes group members into governing social hierarchies and a fabric of coherent social networks (Rosch, 2014).

This mechanism may function through the electromagnetic field radiated by a person's heart, which encodes frequency spectra that communicates information about an individual's emotional state into the social milieu (Rosch, 2014). Research in neurocardiology is confirming that the heart, which has metaphorically been conceived as the seat of emotional experience, behaves as a sensory organ, transmits afferent signaling to higher cognitive centers that are critical to integration and processing of emotional stimuli, and is capable of executive decisions independent of the cerebral cortex (Rosch, 2014; McCraty, 2002). The heart, which produces an electromagnetic field 5,000 times stronger than that of the brain, communicates with the brain via immune-mediated humoral pathways, neurological pathways, and bioelectromagnetic and biophysical (pulse wave) modes of signal transduction (Rosch, 2009, p. 304).

The heart in particular mediates inter-individual bioelectromagnetic communication, conveys emotional information, and can promote synchronicity in physiological rhythms between individuals, as evidenced by experiments showing that couples in stable and long-term relationships exhibit heart rhythm synchrony while they sleep (Rosch, 2014). Social rituals can likewise cement heart rhythm synchronicity, as illustrated by a Spanish fire-walking ritual where synchronized arousal developed between participants and related spectators (Konvalinka et al., 2011). Morris, in contrast, found that heart rhythm synchronization was dependent upon degree of bonding between subjects (Morris, 2010). Because the heart's signal can be transferred via radiation, even individuals sitting next to each other have a propensity to develop similar heart rhythms (Rosch, 2009).

Bioelectromagnetic communication between people and animals has also been confirmed by experiments showing that a child consciously radiating feelings of love for his dog led to synchronous shifts in the heart rhythms of both the boy and his pet, despite lack of physical contact or interaction (Rosch, 2014). Resonance between a mother's brain waves and her infant's heartbeats, in the absence of physical touch, has also been detected, when the mother actively expended mental energy focusing on the baby (Rosch, 2014). In addition to group dynamics, bioenergetic processes can therefore account for the repulsion or attraction between people, as well as related phenomena such as empathy and the enhanced efficacy of an empathetic physician or therapist during a therapeutic encounter (Rosch, 2014; Rakel et al., 2009).

BIOFIELDS AND ENERGETIC MEDICINE

Biofields may similarly account for the success of energetic medicine, which has long been acknowledged by Eastern traditions but dismissed by the conventional biomedical paradigm. For instance, skin punch biopsy incised full-thickness dermal wounds healed significantly faster in subjects treated by a hidden therapeutic touch of a practitioner compared to those who received sham treatments (Wirth, 1990). Compared to ill controls who did not receive "laying on of hands," subjects who received this intervention produced statistically significant changes in hemoglobin values (Krieger, 1974). Further, a 70% average reduction of pain was exhibited by individuals with tension headaches who were subjected to therapeutic touch, compared to half that level of improvement witnessed in those who received placebo touch (Keller, 1986). Therapeutic touch also decreased state anxiety in hospitalized inpatients in a cardiovascular unit compared to patients receiving casual touch or no touch (Heidt, 1981).

Another biofield-based therapy, reconnective healing, has been shown to amplify the autonomic arousal and energy of both healer and healee, produce improvements in pain and range of motion, and potentially entrain the biofields of individuals when performed in a group setting (Baldwin & Trent, 2017). Further, both a Cochrane review and a separate systematic review of randomized controlled trials and quasi-experimental studies concluded that biofield therapies are supported for reducing pain (Jain & Mills, 2010; VanderVaart et al., 2009). Evidence also exists that biofield-based modalities implemented as an adjunctive therapy in cancer improve persistent fatigue, depression, diurnal cortisol rhythms, natural killer activity, and other biomarkers of clinical significance (Jain et al., 2015).

Energetic healing modalities, which may invoke physiological coherence, are likewise promising for dementia, heart disease, and arthritis, and are so powerful at a molecular level that they can even elicit changes in structure of water and DNA conformation (Rosch, 2014; Jain et al., 2015). Rosch (2014) catalogues how increased coherence within and between the bioelectromagnetic systems of the body, which can also be invoked with feelings of appreciation, is associated with enhanced hormonal profiles, humoral immunity, cognitive performance, psychological health, and improvements in disease states such as asthma, diabetes, congestive heart failure, HIV/AIDS, and hypertension.

THE "LIFE ENERGY" AND HOLISTIC HEALTH

Due to our enmeshment within the greater macrocosm of the solar system, cosmic, gravitational, diurnal, and geomagnetic forces entrain human biological rhythms such that energetic variations emanating from these fields have profound implications for human health and global behaviors (Rosch, 2014). These forces influence human biofields hand in hand with their effects on biophoton emission. For example, magnetically intense storms are correlated with an increase in psychiatric hospital admissions, and low-frequency electromagnetic fields are capable of suppressing melatonin secretion (Rosch, 2009). Further, changes in daily cyclic light may influence pineal gland synthesis of psychoactive neuropeptides such as dopamine and serotonin (Rosch, 2009). Thus, solar, lunar, and gravitational forces can elicit physiological aberrations associated with pathological states. This underscores the deeply rooted belief, emphasized by many traditional medical systems, that harmony with cosmic, planetary, and environmental forces is essential for health.

In summary, the bioelectromagnetic body is a reincarnation of the ancient notion of a "life energy" which pervades many traditional cultures. As articulated by Paul Rosch, "Variously called *qi* (*chi*), *ki*, the 'four humors,' *prana*, 'archaeus,' 'cosmic aether,' 'universal fluid,' 'animal magnetism,' and 'odic force,' among other names, this purported biofield is beginning to yield its properties and interactions to the scientific method" (Rosch, 2009, p. 297). In the future, these concepts may not only provide a firm evidence base for many of the energetic healing arts, intangible psychic and social phenomena, and food-as-medicine therapeutic approaches, but they may also be harnessed to enhance human health in myriad other ways.

While this research is only preliminary, and calls into question basic assumptions about cellular bioenergetics and human physiology, the truth is that we have been immersed in hoary assumptions of a mechanistic and reductionistic bent that no longer accurately describe the thing itself: the human body and what sustains it.

REFERENCES

Amemiya, T., and H. Yoshida. "In vivo synthesis of glycogen by phosphorylase system." *Histochemistry* 66, 1980: 301–5.

Baldwin, A.L., and N.L. Trent. "An Integrative Review of Scientific Evidence for Reconnective Healing." *The Journal of Alternative and Complementary Medicine* 23, no. 8, 2017: 590–8. doi: 10.1089/acm.2015.0218.

Barlow, P.W., and J. Fisahn. "Lunisolar tidal force and the growth of plant roots, and some other of its effects on plant movements." *Annals of Botany* 110, no. 2, 2012: 301–18. doi: 10.1093/aob/mcs038.

Bawa, S.R., and R.C. YashRoy. "Effect of light and dark adaptation on the retina and pecten of chickens." *Experimental Eye Research* 3, 1972: 92–7.

Bianchetti, M.G., G.D. Simonetti, and A. Bettinelli. "Body fluids and salt metabolism—Part I." *Italian Journal of Pediatrics* 35, no. 1, 2009: 36. doi: 10.1186/1824-7288-35-36.

Bieske, K., D. Gall, and J. Fisch. "Measurement of low level emissions: Investigations on human hands, wrists, and lower arms." In *Biophotonics and Coherent Systems*, edited by L. Beloussov., F.A. Popp, V. Voeikov, & R. Van Wijk, 397–403. Moscow: Moscow University, 2000.

Bókkon, I., V. Salari, J.A. Tuszynski, and I. Antal. "Estimation of the number of biophotons involved in the visual perception of a single-object image: Biophoton intensity can be considerably higher inside cells than outside." *Journal of Photochemistry and Photobiology B: Biology* 100, no. 3, 2010: 160–66. doi: 10.1016/j.jphotobiol.2010.06.001.

Bókkon, I., R.L.P. Vimal, C. Wang, J. Dai, V. Salari, F. Grass, and I. Antal. "Visible light induced ocular delayed bioluminescence as a possible origin of negative afterimage." *Journal of Photochemistry and Photobiology B: Biology* 103, no. 2, 2011: 192–99. doi: 10.1016/j.jphotobiol.2011.03.011.

Bonilla, E. [Evidence about the power of intention] [Article in Spanish]. *Investigación Clínica* 49, no. 4, 2008: 595–615.

Bordenstein, S.R., and K.R. Theis. "Host biology in light of the microbiome: Ten principles of holobionts and hologenomes." *PLoS Biology* 8, 2015: e1002226. doi: 10.1371/journal.pbio.1002226.

Cantarel, B.L., V. Lombard, and B. Henrissat. "Complex carbohydrate utilization by the healthy human microbiome." *PLoS One* 7, no. 6, 2012: e28742. doi: 10.1371/journal.pone.0028742.

Chang, J.J., Y. Liu, Y. Wang, and F.A. Popp. "Biocommunication and Bioluminescence of *Lampyridae*." In *Biophotons and Coherent Systems, Proceedings of the 2nd Alexander Gurwitsch Conference*. Moscow: Moscow University Press, 2000.

Chavarria, V., J. Vian, C. Pereira, J. Data-Franco, B.S. Fernandes, M. Berk, and S. Dodd. "The Placebo and Nocebo Phenomena: Their Clinical Management and Impact on Treatment Outcomes." *Clinical Therapies* 39, no. 3, 2017: 477–86. doi: 10.1016/j.clinthera.2017.01.031.

Chen, P., L. Zhang, F. Zhang, J.-T. Liu, H. Bai, G.-Q. Tang, and L. Lin. "Spectral discrimination between normal and leukemic human sera using delayed luminescence." *Biomedical Optics Express* 3, no. 8, 2012: 1787–792. doi: 10.1364/boe.3.001787.

Choi, C., W.M. Woo, M.B. Lee, J.S. Yang, K.S. Soh, G. Yoon, M. Kim, and J.J. Chang. "Biophoton Emission from the Hands." *Journal of the Korean Physicians Society* 41, no. 2, 2002: 275–78.

Choi, I.Y., L. Piccio et al., "A diet mimicking fasting promotes regeneration and reduces autoimmunity and multiple sclerosis symptoms." *Cell Reports* 15, no. 10, 2016: 2136–146. doi: 10.1016/j.celrep.2016.05.009.

Choi, S.-W., and S. Friso. "Epigenetics: A new bridge between nutrition and health." *Advances in Nutrition: An International Review Journal* 1, no. 1, 2010: 8–16. doi: 10.3945/an.110.1004.

Cohen, S., and F.A. Popp. "Biophoton emission of the human body." *Journal of Photochemistry and Photobiology B: Biology* 20, no. 2, 1997: 187–89.

Curtis, B.D., and J.J. Hurtak. "Consciousness and quantum information processing: Uncovering the foundation for a medicine of light." *The Journal of Alternative and Complementary Medicine* 10, no. 1, 2004: 27–34.

Dadachova, E., R.A. Bryan, X. Huang, T. Moadel, A.D. Schweitzer, P. Aisen, J.D. Nosanchuk, and A. Casadevall. "Ionizing radiation changes the electronic properties of melanin and enhances the growth of melanized fungi." *PLoS One* 2, no. 5, 2007: e457. doi: 10.1371/journal.pone.0000457.

Dadachova, E., and A. Casadevall. "Ionizing radiation: how fungi cope, adapt, and exploit with the help of melanin." *Current Opinions in Microbiology* 11, no. 6, 2008: 525–31.

Devaraj, B., M. Usa, and H. Inaba. "Biophotons: Ultraweak light emission from living systems." *Current Opinions on Solid State Matter Science* 2, 1997: 188–93.

Dotta, B.T., K.S. Saroka, and M.A. Persinger. "Increased photon emission from the head while imagining light in the dark is correlated with changes in electroencephalographic power: support for Bókkon's biophoton hypothesis." *Neuroscience Letters* 513, no. 2, 2012: 151–54.

Duhl, D.M.J., H. Vrieling, K.A. Miller, G.L. Wolff, and G.S. Barsh. "Neomorphic agouti mutations in obese yellow mice." *Nature Genetics* 8, no. 1, 1994: 59–65. doi: 10.1038/ng0994-59.

Enticott, G. "Lay immunology, local foods and rural identity: defending unpasteurised milk in England." *Sociologia Ruralis* 43, no. 3, 2003: 257–70.

Fassioli, F., R. Dinshaw, P.C. Arpin, and G.D. Scholes. "Photosynthetic light harvesting: excitons and coherence." *Journal of the Royal Society Interface* 11, no. 92, 2014: 1–22. doi: 10.1098/rsif.2013.0901.

Fenech, M., A. El-Sohemy, L. Cahill et al., "Nutrigenetics and nutrigenomics: Viewpoints on the current status and applications in nutrition research and practice." *Journal of Nutrigenetics and Nutrigenomics* 4, no. 2, 2011: 69–89. doi: 10.1159/000327772.

Fletcher, D.A., and R.D. Mullins. "Cell mechanics and cytoskeleton." *Nature* 463, no. 7280, 2010: 485–92.

Floyd, Z.E., Z.Q. Wang, G. Kilroy, and W.T. Cefalu. "Modulation of peroxisome proliferator–activated receptor ɣ stability and transcriptional activity in adipocytes by resveratrol." *Metabolism* 57, no. 1, 2008: S32–8 doi: 10.1016/j.metabol.2008.04.006.

Fontana, L. "Nutrition, adiposity and health." *Epidemiology Prevention* 31, no. 5, 2007: 290–4.

Gallep, C.M., T.A. Moraes, S.R. Dos Santos, and P.W. Barlow. "Coincidence of biophoton emission by wheat seedlings during simultaneous, transcontinental germination tests." *Protoplasma* 250, no. 3, 2013: 293–96.

García-Mediavilla, V., I. Crespo, P.S. Collado, A. Esteller, S. Sánchez-Campos, M.J. Tuñón, and J. González-Gallego. "The anti-inflammatory flavones quercetin and kaempferol cause inhibition of inducible nitric oxide synthase, cyclooxygenase-2 and reactive C-protein, and down-regulation of the nuclear factor kappaB pathway in Chang Liver cells." *European Journal of Pharmacology* 557, no. 2-3, 2007: 221–29. doi: 10.1016/j.ejphar.2006.11.014.

Gariaev, P.P., G.G. Tertishny, and K.A. Leonova. "The wave, probabilistic and linguistic representations of cancer and HIV." *Journal of Nonlocality and Remote Mental Interactions* 1, no. 2, 2000.

Genaro, P.S., K.S. Sarkis, and L.A. Martini. "Effect of caloric restriction on longevity." *Arquivos Brasileiros de Endocrinologia & Metabologia* 5, 2009: 667–72.

Goldgeier, M.H., L.E. Klein, S. Klein-Angerer, G. Moellmann, and J.J. Nordlund. "The distribution of melanocytes in the leptomeninges of the human brain." *Journal of Investigative Dermatology* 82, no. 3, 1984: 235–38. doi: 10.1111/1523-1747.ep12260111.

Gonidakis, S., S.E. Finkel, and V.D. Longo. "Genome-wide screen identifies Escherichia coli TCA-cycle-related mutants with extended chronological lifespan dependent on acetate metabolism and the hypoxia-inducible transcription factor ArcA." *Aging Cell* 9, no. 5, 2010: 868–81. doi: 10.1111/j.1474-9726.2010.00618.x.

Gonzalez, M.J., J.R. Miranda-Massari, J. Duconge, J.R. Rodriguez, K. Cintron, M.J. Berdiel, and J.W. Rodriguez. "Nutrigenomics, metabolic correction and disease: the restoration of metabolism as a regenerative medicine perspective." *Journal of Restorative Medicine* 4, no. 1, 2015: 74–82. doi: 10.14200/jrm.2014.4.0109.

Goodman, G., and D. Bercovich. "Melanin directly converts light for vertebrate metabolic use: Heuristic thoughts on birds, Icarus and dark human skin." *Medical Hypotheses* 71, no. 2, 2008: 190–202.

Gurwitsch, A.G. *The Theory of the Biological Field [in Russian]*. Moscow: Sovetskaya Nauka Publishing House, 1944.

Hehemann, J.H., G. Correc, T. Barbeyron, W. Helbert, M. Czjzek, and G. Michel. "Transfer of carbohydrate-active enzymes from marine bacteria to Japanese gut microbiota." *Nature* 464, no. 7290, 2010: 908–12. doi: 10.1038/nature08937.

Heidt, P. "Effect of therapeutic touch on anxiety level of hospitalized patients." *Nursing Research* 30, no. 1, 1981: 32–7.

Heilbronn, L., and E. Ravussin. "Calorie restriction and aging: review of the literature and implications for studies in humans." *American Journal of Clinical Nutrition* 78, no. 3, 2003: 361–9.

Helman, C.G. "Diet and nutrition." In *Culture, Health, and Illness* (5th ed.), edited by Joanna Koster, Sarah Purdy, Clare Weber, and Jane Tod, 52–80. United Kingdom: Hodder Arnold, 2007.

Henrotin, Y., A.L. Clutterbuck, D. Allaway, E.M. Lodwig, P. Harris, M. Mathy-Hartert, M. Shakibaei, and A. Mobasheri. "Biological actions of curcumin on articular chondrocytes." *Osteoarthritis and Cartilage* 18, no. 2, 2010: 141–49. doi: 10.1016/j.joca.2009.10.002.

Herrera, A.S., M.D.C.A. Esparza, G.Md. Ashraf, A.A. Zamyatnin, and G. Aliev. "Beyond mitochondria, what would be the energy source of the cell?." *Central Nervous System Agents in Medicinal Chemistry* 15, 2015: 32–41. doi: 10.2174/1871524915666150203093656.

Ho, M-W. *The Rainbow and the Worm: The Physics of Organisms*. Singapore: World Scientific Publishing Co, 2005.

Hossu, M., L. Ma, and W. Chen. "Nonlinear enhancement of spontaneous biophoton emission of sweet potato by silver nanoparticles." *Journal of Photochemistry and Photobiology B: Biology* 99, no. 1, 2010: 44–8. doi: 10.1016/j.jphotobiol.2010.02.002.

Hossu, M., and R. Rupert. "Quantum events of biophoton emission associated with complementary and alternative medicine therapies: a descriptive pilot study." *The Journal of Alternative and Complementary Medicine* 12, no. 2, 2006: 119–24. doi: 10.1089/acm.2006.12.119.

Hurtak, J.J. "The human body—its energy and resonance matrix." *Future History* 2, no. 1, 1996: 7–10.

Husserl, E. *Logical Investigations*, Edited by D. Moran. 2nd ed. London: Routledge, 2001 [1900/1901].

Hutcheson, J. "Adipokines influence the inflammatory balance in autoimmunity." *Cytokine* 75, no. 2, 2015: 272–79. doi: 10.1016/j.cyto.2015.04.004.

Igaz, I., and P. Igaz. "Possible role for microRNAs as inter-species mediators of epigenetic information in disease pathogenesis: Is the non-coding dark matter of the genome responsible for epigenetic interindividual or inter-species communication?." *Medical Hypotheses* 84, no. 2, 2015: 150–54. doi: 10.1016/j.mehy.2014.11.021.

Inaba, H. "Human sensing based on ultimate technology of optical measurement." *Optical and Electro-optical Engineering Contact* 37, 1999a: 251–67.

Inaba, H. "Measurement of ultra-weak biophotonic information." *Proceedings of the Institute of Electrostatics Japan* 22, 1999b: 245–52.

Inaba, H. "Measurement of biophoton from human body." *Journal of the International Society of Life and Informational Science* 18, 2000: 448–52.

Iyer, M.K., Y.S. Niknafs, R. Malik, U. Singhal, A. Sahu, Y. Hosonu, T.R. Barrette et al. "The landscape of long noncoding RNAs in the human transcriptome." *Nature Genetics* 47, no. 3, 2015: 199–208. doi: 10.1038/ng.3192.

Jain, S., R. Hammerschlag, P. Mills, L. Cohen, R. Krieger, C. Vieten, and S. Lutgendorf. "Clinical Studies of Biofield Therapies: Summary, Methodological Challenges, and Recommendations." *Global Advances in Health and Medicine* 4, Suppl, 2015: 58–66. doi: 10.7453/gahmj.2015.034.suppl.

Jain, S., and P.J.P. Mills. "Biofield therapies: helpful or full of hype? A best evidence synthesis." *International Journal of Behavioral Medicine* 17, no. 1, 2010: 1–16.

Ji, S.L. "Waves as the Symmetry Principle Underlying Cosmic, Cell, and Human Languages." *Information* 8, no. 1, 2017: 1–25. doi: 10.3390/info8010024 PDF at http://www.mdpi.com/2078-2489/8/1/24

Jung, H.H., W.M., Woo, J.M., Yang, C. Choi, J. Lee, G. Yoon, J.S. Yang, S. Lee, and K.S. Soh. "Left-right asymmetry of biophoton emission from hemiparesis patients." *Indian Journal of Experimental Biology* 41, no. 5, 2003: 452–56.

Kaeberlein, T.L., E.D. Smith, M. Tsuchiya, K. Linnea Welton, J.H. Thomas, S. Fields, B.K. Kennedy, and M. Kaeberlein. "Lifespan extension in Caenorhabditis elegans by complete removal of food." *Aging Cell* 5, no. 6, 2006: 487–94. doi: 10.1111/j.1474-9726.2006.00238.x.

Katoka, Y., Y. Cui, A. Yamagata, M. Niigaki, T., Hirohata, N. Oishi, and Y. Watanabe. "Activity-dependent neural tissue oxidation emits intrinsic ultraweak photons." *Biochemistry and Biophysics Research Community* 285, 2001: 1007–11.

Katschinski, M. "Nutritional implications of cephalic phase gastrointestinal responses." *Appetite* 34, no. 2, 2000: 189–96. doi: 10.1006/appe.1999.0280.

Keller, E. "Effects of therapeutic touch on tension headache pain." *Nursing Research* 35, no. 2, 1986: 101–05.

Kim, H.-W., S.-B. Sim, C.-K. Kim, J. Kim, C. Choi, H. You, and K.-S. Soh. "Spontaneous photon emission and delayed luminescence of two types of human lung cancer tissues: Adenocarcinoma and Squamous cell carcinoma." *Cancer Letters* 229, no. 2, 2005: 283–89. doi: 10.1016/j.canlet.2005.04.038.

Kim, J., J. Lim, H. Kim, S. Ahn, S.B. Smi, and K.S. Soh. "Scanning spontaneous photon emission from transplanted ovarian tumor of mice using a photomultiplier tube." *Electromagnetic Biologic Medicine* 25, 2006: 97–102.

Kobayashi, M., D. Kikuchi, and H. Okamura. "Imaging of Ultraweak Spontaneous Photon Emission from Human Body Displaying Diurnal Rhythm." *Public Library of Science One* 4, no. 7, 2009: 1–4. doi: 10.1371/journal.pone.0006256.

Kobayashi, M., M. Takeda, T. Sato, Y. Yamazaki, K. Kaneko, K. Ito, H. Kato, and H. Inaba. "In vivo imaging of spontaneous ultraweak photon emission from a rat's brain correlated with cerebral energy metabolism and oxidative stress." *Neuroscience Research* 34, no. 2, 1999: 103–13.

Konvalinka, I., D. Xygalatas, J. Bulbulia, U. Schjødt, E.M. Jegindø, S. Wallot, G. Van Orden, and A. Roepstorff. "Synchronized arousal between performers and related spectators in a fire-walking ritual." *Proceedings of the National Academy of Sciences* 108, no. 2, 2011: 8514–15.

Krieger, D. "Healing by the laying on of hands as a facilitator of bioenergetic change: The response of in-vivo human hemoglobin." *Psychoenergetic Systems* 1, 1974: 121–29.

Laplante, M., and D.M. Sabatini. "MTOR Signaling in Growth Control and Disease." *Cell* 149, no. 2, 2012: 274–93. doi: 10.1016/j.cell.2012.03.017.

Lee, G.D., M.A. Wilson, M. Zhu, C.A. Wolkow, R. de Cabo, D.K. Ingram, and S. Zou. "Dietary deprivation extends lifespan in Caenorhabditis elegans." *Aging Cell* 5, 2006: 515–24.

Liu, Y., Y. Yu, G. Matarese, and A. La Cava. "Cutting edge: fasting-induced hypoleptinemia expands functional regulatory T cells in systemic lupus erythematosus." *Journal of Immunology* 188, no. 5, 2012: 2070–73.

Lobo, V., A. Patil, A. Phatak, and N. Chandra. "Free radicals, antioxidants and functional foods: Impact on human health." *Pharmacognosy Review* 4, no. 8, 2010: 118–26. doi: 10.4103/0973-7847.70902.

Longo, V.D., L.M. Ellerby, D.E. Bredesen, J.S. Valentine, and E.B. Gralla. "Human Bcl-2 Reverses Survival Defects in Yeast Lacking Superoxide Dismutase and Delays Death of Wild-Type Yeast." *The Journal of Cell Biology* 137, no. 7, 1997: 1581–588. doi: 10.1083/jcb.137.7.1581.

Longo, V.D., and M.P. Mattson. "Fasting: Molecular Mechanisms and Clinical Applications." *Cell Metabolism* 19, no. 2, 2014: 181–92. doi: 10.1016/j.cmet.2013.12.008.

Longo, V.D., G.S. Shadel, M. Kaeberlein, and B. Kennedy. "Replicative and Chronological Aging in Saccharomyces cerevisiae." *Cell Metabolism* 16, no. 1, 2012: 18–31. doi: 10.1016/j.cmet.2012.06.002.

Mathewson, I. "Did human hairlessness allow natural photobiomodulation 2 million years ago and enable photobiomodulation therapy today? This can explain the rapid expansion of our genus's brain." *Medical Hypotheses* 84, no. 5, 2015: 421–28. doi: 10.1016/j.mehy.2015.01.032.

Mattson, M.P., V.D. Longo, and M. Harvie. "Impact of intermittent fasting on health and disease processes." *Ageing Research Reviews* 16, 2016: S1568–1637. doi: 10.1016/j.arr.2016.10.005.

McCord, J.M. "The evolution of free radicals and oxidative stress." *American Journal of Medicine* 108, 2000: 652–9.

McCraty, R. "Influence of cardiac afferent input on heart-brain synchronization and cognitive performance." *International Journal of Psychophysiology* 45, no. 1–2, 2002: 72–3.

Meng, S., and E. Kaxiras. "Mechanisms for ultrafast nonradiative relaxation in electronically excited eumelanin constituents." *Biophysics Journal* 95, no. 9, 2008: 4396–402. doi: 10.1529/biophysj.108.135756.

Morris, S.M. "Facilitating collective coherence: Group effects on heart rate variability coherence and heart rhythm synchronization." *Alternative Therapies in Health and Medicine* 16, no. 4, 2010: 10–24.

Nakamura, H., H. Kokubo, D.V., Parkhomtchouk, W. Chen, M. Tanaka, and N. Fukuda. "Biophoton and temperature changes of human hand during Qigong." *Journal of the International Society of Life and Informational Science* 18, 2000: 418–22.

Niggli, H.J. "Artificial sunlight irradiation induces ultraweak photon emission in human skin fibroblasts." *Journal of Photochemistry and Photobiology* 18, no. 2–3, 1993: 281–85.

Niggli, H.J., S. Tudisco, G. Privitera, L.A. Applegate, A. Scordino, and F. Musumeci. "Laser-ultraviolet-A-induced ultraweak photon emission in mammalian cells." *Journal of Biomedical Optometry* 10, 2, 2005: 024006.

Owen. *Food Chemistry.* Edited by O. W. Fennema. (3rd ed). Vol. 76. Wisconsin: University of Wisconsin, 1996.

Pang, J., J. Fu, M. Yang, X. Zhao, E. Van Wijk, M. Wang, H. Fan, and J. Han. "Correlation between the different therapeutic properties of Chinese medicinal herbs and delayed luminescence." *Luminescence* 31, no. 2, 2016: 323–27. doi: 10.1002/bio.2961.

Patterson, R.E., G.A. Laughlin, D.D. Sears, A.Z. LaCroix, C. Marinac, L.C. Gallo, S.J. Hartman et al., "Intermittent fasting and human metabolic health." *Journal of the Academy of Nutrition And Dietetics* 115, no. 8, 2015: 1203–12. doi: 10.1016/j.jand.2015.02.018.

Peters, C., and R. Niemeijer. *Protein-Energy Malnutrition and the Home Environment: A Study among Children in Coast Province, Kenya.* Food and Nutrition Planning Unit, Ministry of Planning and National Development, Nairobi, Kenya, and African Studies Centre, Leiden, Netherlands, 1987.

Petoukhov, S.V., and E.S. Petukhova. "The concept of systemic-resonance bioinformatics. Resonances and the quest for transdisciplinarity." In *Information Studies and the Quest for Transdisciplinarity*, edited by M. Burgin and W. Hofkirchner, 467–87. Hoboken, NJ: World Scientific, 2017.

Pettigrew, J.D., J. Wallman, and C.F. Wildsoet. "Saccadic oscillations facilitate ocular perfusion from the avian pecten." *Nature* 343, 1990: 362–63.

Piper, M.D.W., and L. Partridge. "Dietary restriction in drosophila: delayed aging or experimental artefact?" *PLoS Genetics* 3, 4, 2007: e57. doi: 10.1371/journal.pgen.0030057.

Pollack, G.H. *Cells, Gels and the Engines of Life a New, Unifying Approach to Cell Function.* Seattle, WA: Ebner & Sons, 2001.

Pollack, G.H. *The Fourth Phase of Water: Beyond Solid, Liquid, and Vapor.* Seattle, WA: Ebner & Sons, 2013.

Pollack, G.H. "Can humans harvest the sun's energy directly like plants?" GreenMedInfo LLC, June 1, 2015, http://www.greenmedinfo.com/blog/can-humans-photosynthesize-1.

Popkin, B.M., K.E. D'Anci, and I.H. Rosenberg. "Water, hydration, and health." *Nutrition Reviews* 68, no. 6, 2010: 439–58.

Popp, F.A. "Coherent photon storage in biological systems." In *Electromagnetic Bio-Information*, edited by H.L. Konig and W. Peschka, 123–49. Munich-Baltimore: Urban & Schwarzenberg, 1979.

Popp, F.A., W. Nagl, K.H. Li, W. Scholz, O. Weingärtner, and R. Wolf. "Biophoton emission." *Cell Biophysics* 6, no. 1, 1984: 33–52. doi: 10.1007/bf02788579.

Rakel, D.P., T.J. Hoeft, B.P. Barrett, B.A. Chewning, B.M. Craig, and M. Niu. "Practitioner empathy and the duration of the common cold." *Family Medicine* 41, no. 7, 2009: 494–501.

Rappaport, S.M. "Genetic factors are not the major causes of chronic diseases." *PLoS One* 11, no. 4, 2016: e0154387.

Record, M. "Exosome-like nanoparticles from food: protective nanoshuttles for bioactive cargo." *Molecular Therapy* 21, no. 7, 2013: 1294–296. doi: 10.1038/mt.2013.130.

Rimando, A.M., R. Nagmani, D.R. Feller, and W. Yokoyama. "Pterostilbene, a new agonist for the peroxisome proliferator-activated receptor α-isoform, lowers plasma lipoproteins and cholesterol in hypercholesterolemic hamsters." *Journal of Agricultural and Food Chemistry* 53, no. 9, 2005: 3403–407. doi: 10.1021/jf0580364.

Rohani, M., and G.H. Pollack. "Flow through horizontal tubes submerged in water in the absence of a pressure gradient: mechanistic considerations." *Langmuir* 29, no. 22, 2013: 6556–561. doi: 10.1021/la4001945.

Rosch, P.J. "Bioelectromagnetic and subtle energy medicine." *Annals of the New York Academy of Sciences* 1172, no. 1, 2009: 297–311. doi: 10.1111/j.1749-6632.2009.04535.x.

Rosch, P.J. *Bioelectromagnetic and Subtle Energy Medicine.* Boca Raton: CRC Press, 2014.

Sauermann, G., W.P. Mei, U. Hoppe, and F. Stäb. "Ultraweak photon emission of human skin *in vivo*: Influence of topically applied antioxidants on human skin." *Methods in Enzymology* 300, 1999: 419–28. doi: 10.1016/s0076-6879(99)00147-0.

Schutgens, F.W.G., P. Neogi, E.P.A. Van Wijk, R. Van Wijk, G. Wikman, and F.A.C. Wiegant. "The influence of adaptogens on ultraweak biophoton emission: a pilot-experiment." *Phytotherapy Research* 23, no. 8, 2009: 1103–108. doi: 10.1002/ptr.2753.

Schwabl, H., and H. Klima. "Spontaneous ultraweak photon emission from biological systems and the endogenous light field." *Forschende Komplementärmedizin/Research in Complementary Medicine* 12, no. 2, 2005: 84–9. doi: 10.1159/000083960.

Şehirli, Ö., Y. Ozel, E. Dulundu, U. Topaloglu, F. Ercan, and G. Şener. "Grape seed extract treatment reduces hepatic ischemia-reperfusion injury in rats." *Phytotherapy Research* 22, no. 1, 2007: 43–8. doi: 10.1002/ptr.2256.

Slawinski, J. "Photon emission from perturbed and dying organisms: biomedical perspectives." *Forschende Komplementärmedizin/Research in Complementary Medicine* 12, no. 2, 2005: 90–5. doi: 10.1159/000083971.

So, E., R. Stahlberg, and G.H. Pollack. "Exclusion zone as intermediate between ice and water." *Water and Society* 153, 2011: 3–11. doi: 10.2495/wsl10011.

Somerset, S.M., and L. Johannot. "Dietary flavonoid sources in Australian adults." *Nutrition and Cancer* 60, no. 4, 2008: 442–49. doi: 10.1080/01635580802143836.

Sun, Y., C. Wang, and J. Dai. "Biophotons as neural communication signals demonstrated by *in situ* biophoton autography." *Photochemical & Photobiological Sciences* 9, no. 3, 2010: 315. doi: 10.1039/b9pp00125e.

Sundqvist, T., F. Lindström, K.-E. Magnusson, L. Sköldstam, I. Stjernström, and C. Tagesson. "Influence of fasting on intestinal permeability and disease activity in patients with rheumatoid arthritis." *Scandinavian Journal of Rheumatology* 11, no. 1, 1982: 33–8. doi: 10.3109/03009748209098111.

Takeda, K., N. Takahashi, and S. Shibahara. "Neuroendocrine functions of melanocytes: beyond the skin-deep melanin maker." *Tohoku Journal of Experimental Medicine* 211, 2007: 201–21.

Takeda, M., M. Kobayashi, M. Takayama, S. Suzuki, T. Ishida, K. Ohnuki, T. Moriya, and N. Ohuchi. "Biophoton detection as a novel technique for cancer imaging." *Cancer Science* 95, no. 8, 2004: 656–61. doi: 10.1111/j.1349-7006.2004.tb03325.x.

Thaiss, C.A., D. Zeevi, M. Levy, G. Zilberman-Schapira, J. Suez, A.C. Tengeler, L. Abramson et al. "Transkingdom Control of Microbiota Diurnal Oscillations Promotes Metabolic Homeostasis." *Cell* 159, no. 3, 2014: 514–29. doi: 10.1016/j.cell.2014.09.048.

Tiller, W.A., R. McCraty, and M. Atkinson. "Cardiac coherence: A new, noninvasive measure of autonomic nervous system order." *Alternative Therapies in Health and Medicine* 2, no. 1, 1996: 52–65.

Van Wijk, E., M. Kobayashi, R. van Wijk, and J. van der Greef. "Imaging of ultra-weak photon emission in a rheumatoid arthritis mouse model." *Public Library of Science One* 8, no. 12, 2013: 1–6.

Van Wijk, E.P.A., H. Koch, S. Bosman, and R. Van Wijk. "Anatomic characterization of human ultra-weak photon emission in practitioners of transcendental meditation (TM) and control subjects." *Journal of Alternative and Complementary Medicine* 12, no. 1, 2006: 31–8.

Van Wijk, E.P.A., and R. Van Wijk. "Multi-site recording and spectral analysis of spontaneous photon emission from human body." *Forschende Komplementärmedizin / Research in Complementary Medicine* 12, no. 2, 2005: 96–106. doi: 10.1159/000083935.

VanderVaart, S., V.M.G.J. Gijsen, S.N. de Wildt, and G. Koren. "A systematic review of the therapeutic effects of Reiki." *Journal of Alternative and Complementary Medicine* 15, no. 11, 2009: 1157–69.

Voeikov, V.L. "Processes involving reactive oxygen species are the major source of structured energy for organismal biophotonic field pumping." In *Biophotons and Coherent Systems: Proceedings of the 2nd Alexander Gurwitsch Conference*, edited by L. Beloussov., F.A. Popp, V. Voeikov, and R. Van Wijk. Moscow: Moscow University Press, 2000.

Voeikov, V.L. "Mitogenetic radiation, biophotons and non-linear oxidative processes in aqueous media." In *Integrative Biophysics*, edited by F.A. Popp and L. Beloussov, 331–59, Netherlands: Kluwer Academic Publishers, 2003.

Wang, C., I. Bókkon, J. Dai, and I. Antal. "Spontaneous and visible light-induced ultraweak photon emission from rat eyes." *Brain Research* 1369, 2011: 1–9.

Williams, R.J. "Concept of genetotrophic disease." *Nutrition Reviews* 8, no. 9, 2009: 257–60. doi: 10.1111/j.1753-4887.1950.tb02469.x.

Wirth, D.P. "The effect of non-contact therapeutic touch on the healing rate of full thickness dermal wounds." *Subtle Energies* 1, no. 1, 1990: 1–20.

Xu, C., J. Zhang, D.M. Mihai, and I. Washington. "Light-harvesting chlorophyll pigments enable mammalian mitochondria to capture photonic energy and produce ATP." *Journal of Cell Science* 127, Pt 2, 2014: 388–99. doi: 10.1242/jcs.134262.

Yanagawa, T., H. Sakaguichi, M. Ueno, and K. Nitta. "Sustaining faculty of living functions and its biophoton observation." *Journal of the International Society of Life and Informational Science* 18, 2000: 423–37.

Yang, M., J. Pang, J. Liu, Y. Liu, H. Fan, and J. Han. "Spectral discrimination between healthy people and cold patients using spontaneous photon emission." *Biomedical Optical Express* 6, 2015: 1331–9.

Ye, T., L. Hong, J. Garguilo, A. Pawlak, G.S. Edwards, R.J. Nemanich, T. Sarna, and J.D. Simon. "Photoionization thresholds of melanins obtained from free electron laser–photoelectron emission microscopy, femtosecond transient absorption spectroscopy and electron paramagnetic resonance measurements of oxygen photoconsumption." *Photochemistry and Photobiology* 82, no. 3, 2006: 733. doi: 10.1562/2006-01-02-ra-762.

Zafra, M., F. Molina, and A. Puerto. "The neural/cephalic phase reflexes in the physiology of nutrition." *Neuroscience & Biobehavioral Reviews* 30, no. 7, 2006: 1032–044. doi: 10.1016/j.neubiorev.2006.03.005.

Zeng, H., K. Yang, C. Cloer, G. Neale, P. Vogel, and H. Chi. "mTORC1 couples immune signals and metabolic programming to establish T(reg)-cell function." *Nature* 499, no. 7459, 2013: 485–90. doi: 10.1038/nature12297.

Zeviar, D.D., M.J. Gonzalez, J.R. Miranda Massari, J. Duconge, and N. Mikirova. "The role of mitochondria in cancer and other chronic diseases." *Journal of Orthomolecular Medicine* 29, no. 4, 2014: 157–66.

Zhang, L., D. Hou, X. Chen, D. Li, L. Zhu, Y. Zhang, J. Li et al. "Exogenous plant MIR168a specifically targets mammalian LDLRAP1: evidence of cross-kingdom regulation by micro-RNA." *Cell Research* 22, no. 1, 2012: 107–26. doi: 10.1038/cr.2011/158.

Zhao, X., J. Pang, J. Fu, Y. Wang, M. Yang, Y. Liu, H. Fan, L. Zhang, and J. Han. "Spontaneous photon emission: A promising non-invasive diagnostic tool for breast cancer." *Journal of Photochemistry and Photobiology B: Biology* 166, 2017: 232–38. doi: 10.1016/j.jphotobiol.2016.12.009.

11 The Scientific Basis of Ayurvedic and Chinese Medicine

Peter Eckman

CONTENTS

Why Eastern Medicine Fulfills the Foundational Criteria for Science 319
Music, Resonance, and Frequencies in Eastern Medicine 320
Eastern versus Western Modes of Scientific Thought 321
    Eastern Science Does Not Exclude the Non-Material 321
Pulse Diagnosis 322
A Return to Original Nature 323
The Impact of Intention 325
Notes 326

WHY EASTERN MEDICINE FULFILLS THE FOUNDATIONAL CRITERIA FOR SCIENCE

The prestige attached to the various branches of Western (Occidental) medicine is rightly attributed to its self-defined foundation in science and the scientific method. On the other hand, the traditional medicines which developed in Asia, and which may collectively be called Eastern (Oriental) medicine, have an ancient history dating back to before the word *science* was actually coined, this term having its immediate ancestry in Middle English and Old French. Can a modern term be accurately applied to a discipline that preceded it by more than a thousand years? This is no idle question, as those who would scoff at Oriental medicine need do nothing more than to call it unscientific as a way to invalidate its practice in the eyes of the public. To answer the question then, of whether Oriental medicine is scientific, we must first ask what does the term science actually mean? The American Heritage Dictionary of the English Language lists three definitions of science as follows:

1. The observation, identification, description, experimental investigation, and theoretical explanation of phenomena.
2. A systematic method or body of knowledge in a given area.
3. *Archaic*, Knowledge, especially that gained through experience.[1]

The intention of this chapter is twofold: to show that at least two branches of Oriental medicine, Chinese medicine and Indian medicine (Ayurveda), clearly fulfill these criteria, and in addition to present a précis of the scientific nature of the classical teachings of these two medical systems. Due to the constraints of being a small chapter in a large book, this presentation can only investigate a small piece of the field I choose to call Oriental medicine. One should note that science, as defined here, does not mean merely the collection of observations of nature, nor merely a set of theories that are the standards against which truth is measured. Rather, science is a process through which observations and theories are constantly checked against each other in order to develop an ever more accurate understanding of nature. This characteristic developmental process of science has been true for both Eastern and Western branches of science, including in the medical domain. What most characteristically differentiates these two branches of science is the type of distinctions the practicing scientist makes: quantitative versus qualitative, deductive versus inductive, and analytic versus synthetic. As a corollary of this presentation, we may conclude that science itself has more than one mode of achieving its ends, and that the Oriental and Occidental modes are opposite in nature but complementary in providing us with the kinds of knowledge we need in order to deliver the most comprehensive approach to medical care. I will begin by discussing Chinese medicine and afterward describe a bridge that allows for incorporating Ayurvedic medicine into the same scientific paradigm as Chinese medicine.

MUSIC, RESONANCE, AND FREQUENCIES IN EASTERN MEDICINE

Joseph Needham, in his renowned publication *Science and Civilization in China*, remarked, "The Taoist philosophers, with their emphasis on Nature, were bound in due course to pass from the purely observational to the experimental."[2] That is to say, they were clearly fulfilling each of the three definitions of science given above. Needham added, "Chinese coordinative thinking was not primitive thinking in the sense that it was an alogical or pre-logical chaos in which anything could be the cause of anything else...It was a picture of an extremely and precisely ordered universe in which things 'fitted' so exactly that you could not insert a hair between them."[3] This picture the ancient Chinese developed of nature has been called correlative thinking and systematic correspondence by different authors, but these terms, which are crucial to the medical practices the Chinese developed, miss the hidden axiomatic basis for these ideas, namely gǎn yìng 感應 or resonance, which is important to understand if one wishes to examine Chinese medical teachings through a scientific lens. Axioms exist at the limits of science, where we may observe their manifestation via the postulates they propose (which can be tested and verified), but are not themselves subject to further investigation as to their mechanism of action. The classical presentation of resonance can be found in the Han dynasty text *Huai Nan Zi*, Chapter 6.[4] This Chapter 6, in fact, presents a well-known example of the kind of resonance known to Western science, that is, the acoustical phenomenon of one vibrating string on a musical instrument causing an accompanying vibration to occur in a separate instrument whose string is tuned to the same note (frequency). In passing I might mention that the ancient Chinese characters for music (樂) and for medicine (藥) differ only in the addition of the plant radical (艹) on top, indicating that medicines were viewed as acting in a similar way as music: via the principles of resonance and harmony, and certainly leaving open the possibility that vibratory phenomena were involved. The two most widely known foundational theories of Chinese medicine, yīn yáng (陰陽) and the five elements (wǔ xíng 五行) were alluded to in other ancient Chinese texts in relation to acoustical phenomena in their descriptions of the five bells and the six pitch pipes, reflecting yang (odd numbered) and yin (even numbered) musical notes, respectively.[5] These two theories nicely demonstrate major aspects of resonance as this concept is used in Chinese medicine: All phenomena that resonate with each other belong to the same category (lèi 類), thus the Chinese built up lists of terms that resonated with either yin or yang, and also lists of terms that resonated with each of the five elements. *Huai Nan Zi* Chapter 6 states, "Each thing is affected inasmuch as it resembles or partakes of the shapes (xíng 形) and categories (lèi 類) of other things." This statement portrays an attempt to formulate a scientific principle governing the assignment of membership to one of the resonant categories. Some people may interpret this statement as nothing more than magical thinking, but in fact it is very similar to modern scientific notions of fractals and holograms. It is also the operative principle in the "doctrine of signatures" which plays a role in both Chinese medicine and pre-modern Western medicine. A second aspect of resonance that can be seen in both yin yang and five element theories is the idea that members of any resonating category have definable and demonstrable effects on members of other categories. This aspect is revealed in the "laws" or principles that relate yin and yang to each other, and also the "laws" or principles that relate each of the five elements to the other four (primarily by reinforcing or opposing them). In summary, resonance theory serves as the axiomatic basis for "laws" of nature that depend on observation and investigation to construct a rational explanation of the natural world; in other words, it is the basis for a scientific mode of thought.

Musical notes are expressions of acoustical waves that have specific frequencies. They have no material substance of their own, but rather impose structural changes on the medium through which they are transmitted, be it air, water, or something else. Middle C has no mass. One generalization we can draw from the above description is that Chinese medicine is primarily a therapy that uses non-material qualities to influence the functioning of material entities. Another way of saying this is that Chinese medicine is based on the transmission of information. Such a view is obviously different from that of Western medicine. These two systems can be distinguished from each other in the following generalized comparison alluded to earlier: Western medicine is quantitative, analytic, and deductive, with its emphasis on the structure of the human organism as its central focus. Chinese medicine is qualitative, synthetic, and inductive, with its emphasis on the functioning of the human organism. This distinction of the different modes of scientific thought between Western and Chinese medicine has been pointed out by other scholars.[6]

EASTERN VERSUS WESTERN MODES OF SCIENTIFIC THOUGHT

EASTERN SCIENCE DOES NOT EXCLUDE THE NON-MATERIAL

One of the major differences between the sciences developed in the West and the East concerns the scope of nature that is subject to investigation. Western science rejects as inadmissible terms such as "spirit" because they have no tangible or measurable manifestations. Eastern science, however, starts from the proposition that there is a non-material realm of nature underlying the material realm[7] and that spirit is just one of numerous concepts that can only be understood from the vantage point of non-material reality. Some authors have used this difference to claim that Chinese medicine is not scientific, but rather a form of religious belief.[8] The error in this conclusion is that it conflates idealism (as a philosophical position) with religion (which is not a characteristic of Chinese medicine). Materialism can go only so far in explaining the natural world. The ultimate conclusion of the materialist paradigm leads to the proposition that human beings are nothing more than very complex machines; machines that have no free will, spirit, or even mind—separate from their being merely epiphenomena of biochemical and biophysical activities. Therefore, to understand Chinese medicine as a science, one must start with its concepts of non-being (wú jí 無極) and being (tài Jí 太極), literally without a pole and great pole. Although these two expressions found their height of development in the Song dynasty (c. 1000 CE),[9] they had already been discussed by the early Daoist thinkers Lao Zi and Zhuang Zi[10] (roughly contemporaneous with the earliest strata of Chinese medicine). And if medicine is to fulfill its purpose in treating all the ills to which humans are subject, then it must recognize disturbances of mind and spirit as primary pathological states, rather than as epiphenomena of altered brain activity.

In Chinese, the word xīn 心 means both heart and mind, the distinction being made possible only by context, and even then the translational choice can be controversial. Almost all the terms in Chinese that relate to human consciousness have this heart character depicted in the way they are themselves written. Returning to the concept of resonance introduced earlier, both gǎn 感 and yìng 應 have this heart/mind radical as their basis, for example. Thus at its most fundamental, axiomatic level, Chinese medicine is based on a non-material aspect of reality, but it is one that allows Chinese medicine to deal with a broader terrain than Western medicine, as it does not exclude social factors, emotional factors, mental factors, or spiritual factors from the doctor's realm of knowledge and therapeutics.

If we start with the assumption that the term science does not automatically exclude non-material considerations, then it is possible to explain such things as the failure of anatomists to find reproducible evidence for concepts like the meridians (or channels) of acupuncture. While some phenomena accompanying acupuncture treatments, for example, may be explainable in Western scientific terms,[11] the attempt to reduce the clinical practice of acupuncture to such explanations is bound to be a failure, as it must eliminate acupuncture's conceptual basis in the non-material realm, that is in turn based on resonance. Although *Huai Nan Zi* proposed that the mechanism of resonance was not subject to any deeper explanation,[12] the example it cites, of vibrating musical strings, allows us to speculate on the medium through which this resonance occurs. The ancient Chinese also formed speculations, and the well-known answer they proposed was the concept of qì 氣, commonly translated as breath or energy, among other possible renditions. Qì is then the field through which the resonant waves propagate. Music consists of acoustical waves which can propagate through various physical media like air or water, but other types of waves, such as light and related electromagnetic phenomena, can propagate through a vacuum, so it is not surprising that the Chinese concept of qì does not yield to Western science's quantitative, analytical, and deductive research methods aimed at demonstrating its existence as a substance with mass, since like resonance, it emanates from the non-material realm. What the Chinese applied in their investigation of qì were qualitative, synthetic, and inductive methods of research.

Thus far, this presentation has been rather abstract, at least with regard to medical practice, but there is a link that allows us to make the transition from Chinese philosophy to Chinese medicine. I have already alluded to the similarity of the Chinese characters for music and medicine, and there have been various claims reporting the use of musical tones to treat problems of the 12 organ functions of Chinese medicine, which is certainly an area that could be explored by scientific experimentation. Although the weight of thousands of years of successful clinical practice based on careful observations reported by countless doctors constitutes evidence that Chinese medicine in its various modalities is a scientific form of therapy (by the dictionary definition of science at least), those trained in Western medicine have by and large remained skeptical about such a designation. Having devoted more than 40 years to the study and practice of acupuncture, I am of the opinion that the best way to establish the scientific nature of Chinese medicine is through research into the clinical practice of pulse diagnosis for the following reason. Pulse diagnosis, being one of the oldest and most characteristic methods employed in Chinese medicine, lends itself to explanations based on resonance theory. The arterial pulses consist of waveform fluctuations perceptible to a practitioner's palpating fingers, and the obvious analogy between pulse waves and acoustic waves makes the investigation of this procedure a logical place on which to base an investigation of Chinese medicine's scientific nature that might be more convincing to the aforementioned skeptics.

PULSE DIAGNOSIS

Pulse diagnosis was discussed in the cannon of Chinese medicine, the *Huangdi Neijing*, approximately 2000 years ago, and there are even earlier references to it in other works, so I think it is fair to conclude that it is one of the pillars on which this system of medicine is founded. Numerous books and commentaries have expounded on various aspects of pulse diagnosis in the ensuing years, two of the most important being the *Nanjing* (*Classic of Difficulties*) and the *Mai Jing* (*Classic of the Pulses*). The topic of pulse diagnosis is much too large to be dealt with in any great detail in this chapter, but I will present some basic teachings that can serve as a starting point for anyone interested in pursuing the subject in more depth. Some of what I'll present is standard knowledge in the field of Chinese medicine, but some additional insights will also be included that are the author's own discoveries. Like any scientific claim, these ideas about pulse diagnosis need to be replicated and validated by the experiences of other practitioners and researchers, but they have proven invaluable guides to a successful acupuncture practice in the author's long career. Classically, there are a number of different methods of pulse diagnosis used in Chinese medicine, but the most widely practiced method is the examination of a section of the radial artery proximal to the wrist, called the "qì mouth," where practitioners place index, middle, and ring fingers to gather information by palpating the pulse waves.[13] These three fingers used to examine a patient's left and right radial artery provide resonant information about the 12 organ systems of Chinese medicine, and their 12 connected meridians (or channels), along which acupuncture is performed in order to induce a (resonant) response in the patient's correlated organ systems. Each of the six fingers (three on the left radial artery and three on the right radial artery) provides data on these 12 organ functions, so each finger transmits information specifically about two of these organ functions. Each organ function, in turn, is associated with one of the five elements, and with either yin or yang. Thus, radial pulse diagnosis is directly connected to both of the major theories of Chinese medicine that are themselves based on the resonance paradigm. It is possible to use radial pulse diagnosis, by itself, to formulate efficacious acupuncture treatment strategies to deal with virtually any clinical problem, since the acupuncture needles act to transmit homeostatic information to the abnormally functioning organ systems with which they are in resonance. This simple (to describe in overview, if not so simple to perfect in practice) diagnostic procedure has been a mainstay of Chinese medicine for several millennia and is ideally suited for scientific investigation using qualitative, synthetic, and inductive standards of research.

Up to this point I have focused on Chinese medicine as one relatively well-known branch of Oriental medicine. Ayurvedic medicine is perhaps not as well-known in the Western world, but as I hope to demonstrate, it shares common core tenets with Chinese medicine and also has an ancient origin with a long history of clinical success based on observation, identification, description, experimental investigation, and theoretical explanation of phenomena, thereby satisfying the criteria for being "scientific."

At first glance, Ayurvedic medicine and Chinese medicine might appear to be unrelated approaches to healthcare. Ayurvedic medicine is characterized by a humoral system based on the three doshas, vata, pitta, and kapha, while Chinese medicine has no obvious humoral counterpart. However, if we look at the historical setting in which these two disciplines originated, we discover that there was commerce and exchange of ideas between the whole range of the Indo-European cultures, including parts of China and India, along the Silk Road at a time when their medical systems were in a developmental stage.[14] Thus, the feasibility for a shared philosophical and practical approach to healthcare existed, and it only remains to explicate the relationship of India's humoral system to China's non-humoral approach in order to establish a solid basis for hypothesizing that these two systems originated from a shared understanding of the nature of reality.

As a preliminary introduction to the relationship of Ayurvedic medical concepts to the Chinese ones I've discussed, the importance of sound cannot be stressed too highly. The Sanskrit word svanah, meaning sound or tone, generally refers to a type of synchronization, that is, resonance. This forms a basis for the following statements found on the website of the California College of Ayurveda: "In the Vedas, sound was understood to have a healing effect on its listener and, not surprisingly, various instruments were used to enable particular vibrations of sounds to prevent increases in particular doshas. For example, the instrumental sounds of the bamboo flute are thought to prevent the increase of vata. The bamboo flute emits soft notes and has a soothing effect on its listener. Pitta needs a strong quality to catch its attention and the sitar is believed to possess that with its nasal overtones and rich sound. The sarod is a classical Indian lute-like instrument and, with its deep and 'awakening' sound and clear tones, is said to help balance and enliven the kapha dosha."

A RETURN TO ORIGINAL NATURE

Like Chinese medicine, Ayurvedic medicine has a five-element theory, but these two theories, which share the same label, are not equivalent, and any attempt to correlate one with the other will only lead to erroneous results. Therefore, when mentioning five-element theory in this chapter, I am always referring to the Chinese version, in order to avoid confusion. On the other hand, a number of other theoretical premises of Ayurvedic medicine and Chinese medicine are similar enough to effectively be interchangeable. Some examples would include the concepts of Avyakta and Vyakta paralleling non-being and being, and Purusha and Prakriti paralleling the concepts of spirit and essence, respectively. These examples show that Ayurvedic medicine is also based on an idealistic rather than a materialistic understanding of nature, and in fact shed insight into the clinical implications of the Chinese terminology. Purusha is a term meaning pure consciousness that can be compared to the Chinese concept of spirit (shén 神), while Prakriti is a term meaning primordial nature that can be compared to the Chinese concept of essence (jīng 精). These terms are the key to understanding the nature of health and illness in both these systems of medicine. We inherit our unique physical constitution from our parents (via the fertilization of the gametes, which are classified as essences in Chinese medicine, coming from the material Earth realm), but we acquire our unique spirit from the non-material realm of pure consciousness, referred to as coming from Heaven in Chinese medicine. I have not seen any discussion in English concerning why a given individual's shén happens to unite with their particular jīng at the moment of conception, but the principle of resonance provides a reasonable explanation for the clinical reality that diagnoses based on bodily constitution and those based on a more intangible set of signs (such as five element acupuncture's focus on the spirit) generally reach similar conclusions (i.e., an individual's essence and spirit form a resonant pair). When there are differences, I believe they are due to the focus of some treatment styles (such as the Eight Diagnostic Categories of Traditional Chinese Medicine, or TCM) on the present pattern of signs and symptoms (called the Vikruti in Ayurvedic medicine), as opposed to the underlying constitution (called the Causative Factor or CF in five element acupuncture, and called the Prakriti in Ayurvedic medicine) in other treatment styles. These different approaches to treatment highlight the importance of having a clear understanding of the criteria of health and illness if any medical system is aiming to follow scientific principles. For this reason I propose the following definitions, which I believe are consistent with the teachings of both Ayurvedic and Chinese medicines. At conception, we are endowed with our original nature (both material and non-material), which dictates the relative strengths and weaknesses of our organ systems (that are in turn responsible for both our physical and mental/spiritual life functions). As long as we keep this arrangement of strengths and weaknesses corresponding to our original nature, we can be said to be healthy (we feel like ourselves). Illness occurs when, for whatever reason, we lose this arrangement of our original nature (we no longer feel like ourselves). Medical treatment for the purpose of recovery of health, in a holistic rather than symptomatic sense, is therefore best aimed at encouraging a restoration of original nature by any means possible (we feel like ourselves again). In Ayurvedic medicine this can imply returning our doshas to their original Prakriti states, while in Chinese medicine it can imply returning our hierarchy of elements and organ functions to their original states. One of the valuable aspects of Ayurvedic medicine is that its method of pulse diagnosis has several specific ways of determining one's Prakriti, or original nature,[15] while Chinese medicine has not had a similar method of diagnosing original nature via the pulses, at least not in the English literature to date, to the best of my knowledge. This lack of a pulse diagnostic method for identifying original nature in the practice of acupuncture has been addressed by Kuon Dowon, starting in the 1960s, when he developed an approach he called Korean Constitutional Acupuncture.[16] His research is still an ongoing endeavor, but one aspect that has never varied is his discovery that there are exactly eight different patterns in people's pulses, which are invariant during their lifetimes, not changing with age or health status. The eight pulse types therefore must reflect something at their constitutional level, since they stay the same from birth until death of the individual. These remarks on pulse diagnosis bring the discussion back to its prior focus on pulses as vibrational wave signals that can be viewed as conveying resonant information as part of a scientific paradigm. One unusual finding is that the eight unique pulse types discovered by Kuon are felt at the same location as are the Ayurvedic pulses, being approximately three finger breadths proximal to the place where the traditional Chinese pulses are felt at qì kǒu. The observation that these two locations for pulse diagnosis each use three fingers, and are separated by the same three fingerbreadth distance, suggests that we are indeed dealing with some kind of standing wave phenomenon, wholly in keeping with the prior exposition on music and resonance. In Ayurvedic medicine the pulses felt by the index, middle, and ring fingers, respectively, correspond to the vata, pitta, and kapha doshas, a simplified explanation that is necessary to present in order to understand the subsequent material in this chapter, but which in reality is a rather complex subject that requires extensive study and practical experience to master.

Most scholars and practitioners have considered Ayurvedic medicine and Chinese medicine to be entirely unrelated practices, primarily because the humoral system of doshas has no counterpart in Chinese medicine. In 2014, I published a concordance between the doshas of Ayurvedic medicine and the organ system imbalances of Chinese medicine that resulted from my studies with another Korean innovator, Yoo Tae Woo, originator of Korean Hand Acupuncture and its diagnostic approach known as three constitutions theory (sam il che jil).[17] This chapter is not the place to reprise the evidence for such a concordance, but interested readers can find a detailed explanation of how it was derived in my previous publication.[18] By means of this concordance, it has been possible to translate Chinese medical diagnoses into Ayurvedic medical diagnoses, and vice versa, at both the constitutional and conditional levels.

There is one further discovery I made of a concordance between Ayurvedic medicine and Chinese medicine. To present a somewhat more detailed picture of Ayurvedic diagnoses of the current condition (the Vikruti), as revealed by the pulse, one must look deeper than simply evaluating the balance of the three doshas. Each dosha is in fact subdivided into five separate subdoshas, which can be differentiated by the location of the place on the examiner's fingers where the pulse waves strike most clearly. Again, the teachings about subdosha pulses are part of various oral traditions, and the one I learned is slightly different from that communicated by Lad in the book cited previously. What I discovered is that the order of the subdoshas on each of the examining fingers is exactly correlated with the control cycle (xiāng kè 相剋) order of the Chinese five elements. This order from distal to proximal is metal, wood, earth, water, and when two subdoshas are simultaneously present on any finger, it corresponds to the element fire. The reason for including this second set of concordances between Ayurvedic and Chinese diagnoses is that such findings make no sense, to me at least, outside of the resonant wave explanation. Although my findings constitute anecdotal evidence at this point, they are uniquely suited to be studied by other practitioners who attempt to replicate them. Such an endeavor is a good example of how Oriental medical propositions can be validated or rejected on a scientific basis. Most studies of Oriental medical findings, whether based on Ayurvedic medicine, Chinese medicine, or other branches, have been statistical reports of the efficacy of one or another form of treatment for any number of medical conditions, but precious few studies have been carried out with the aim of investigating the underlying scientific postulates of these disciplines.

There is one caveat that applies to any research involving pulse diagnosis. There needs to be strict sets of agreed-upon protocols for determining finger positions and methods of palpation, so that uniformity of the findings can be maximized. This is certainly not the case yet, in any branch of Oriental medical pulse diagnosis that I have studied. With this requirement in mind, I published an article in the *Journal of Chinese Medicine* proposing one set of standards, but that is only the beginning of a discussion that needs to be addressed by the profession at large.[19] There are other methods of pulse diagnosis that have not been mentioned in this chapter, such as the comparison of the carotid and radial arterial pulses, which was the system that received the most detailed presentation in the *Huangdi Neijing*. It also needs a clearly defined set of standards for finger positions in palpating these pulses, but once having established agreed-upon standards, the exploration of the basic tenets (of Chinese medicine in this example) will be a possible topic of basic research in the field of Oriental medicine.

THE IMPACT OF INTENTION

This presentation would not be complete without some mention of the impact of intention on the part of the practitioner in determining the success or failure of any therapeutic encounter. There is no doubt that there is a certain degree of placebo effect in all forms of therapy, Eastern or Western. That situation does not prevent scientific investigations of Western therapies, and likewise should not be a barrier to investigations of Eastern therapies. However, the subject of intention (on the part of the practitioner) deserves special attention, since certain schools of acupuncture, for instance, teach that intention is the most important factor in the success or failure of treatment, and intention by its very nature is much less amenable to scientific study than is pulse palpation; for example, being in the non-material realm. A similar claim has often been made for the efficacy of emitted qì in what has been called "external qì gōng." This topic is by no means only a modern concern, but was implicitly discussed in Chapter 6 of *Huai Nan Zi*, under the name of "total resonance" by Le Blanc, who contrasted it with the type of resonance that has been discussed thus far, which Le Blanc called "relative resonance." The image presented in *Huai Nan Zi* of total resonance is the situation where by tuning one string in a special (unspecified) manner, its vibration can provoke a resonant vibration in all the other strings on the musical instrument, regardless of their tuning. I believe this reference is intimately connected with the idea of the power inherent in the non-material realm, epitomized by the ideal of emptiness, especially of the heart. Total resonance does not depend on shared shapes or categories (as does relative resonance), but rather on the original unity of all of creation in the primordial Dao from which everything is born, and to which it will eventually return. This original unity is never entirely absent, and I believe it is the explanation for how intention can evoke recognition of this connection to produce a resonant response, even in the absence of shared shapes or categories. Total resonance of this kind is possibly outside the bounds of scientific investigation, but it is important to mention because it probably plays a role in every patient-practitioner encounter. In Western medicine it is an aspect of "bedside manner," but Oriental medicine actually discusses ways that this therapeutic power can be maximized, and that is simply by emptying oneself of all preconceptions, prejudices, and expectations other than a desire to help our fellow sentient beings. I might call this the power of "intention by not trying," or wú wéi as the Daoists described it.

There is much more that could, and should, be written about the scientific basis of Ayurvedic and Chinese medicines, but a chapter in a text such as this is naturally limited in scope. For readers who wish to explore the material I have presented in greater depth, my publications might be a useful place to begin. For a history of Chinese medicine, see *In the Footsteps of the Yellow Emperor; Tracing the History of Traditional Acupuncture* (South San Francisco: Long River Press, second edition, 2007). For details of pulse diagnosis in Chinese medicine and Ayurvedic medicine, see *The Complete Acupuncturist; A Guide to Constitutional and Conditional Pulse Diagnosis* (London: Singing Dragon, 2014). And for an analysis of the classical texts on which Chinese medicine is based, including a more detailed examination of resonance as presented in *Huai Nan Zi*, see *Grasping the Donkey's Tail; Unraveling Mysteries from the Classics of Oriental Medicine* (London: Singing Dragon, 2017).

I would like to close this chapter with a quote attributed to Albert Einstein, which I think conveys the essence of what I have tried to communicate in a few pithy words: "If I were not a Physicist, I would probably be a Musician. I often think in music. I live my daydreams in music. I see my life in terms of music. I get most of my joy in life out of music."[20]

NOTES

1. American Heritage® Dictionary of the English Language, Fifth Edition. Copyright © 2016 by Houghton Mifflin Harcourt Publishing Company. Published by Houghton Mifflin Harcourt Publishing Company.
2. Needham, J., *Science and Civilization in China*. Vol. 2. p. 34. Cambridge, UK: Cambridge University Press, 1956.
3. Ibid. p. 286.
4. Le Blanc, C., *Huai-Nan Zi, Philosophical Synthesis in Early Han Thought: The Idea of Resonance (Kan Ying) With a Translation and Analysis of Chapter Six*. Hong Kong: Hong Kong University Press, 1985.
5. *Guan Zi* (3rd c. BCE), "In antiquity, Huang Di generated the 5 tones on the basis of the slow and fast (soundings), thereby ordering the 5 bells. Once he had regulated the 5 tones, he established the 5 Agents to order the Heavenly seasons, and then he set up the 5 official ranks to order the positions of Man." The

5 Agents is one of the multiple English terms that I have rendered as five elements. Most scholars have opted for either five movements or five phases as preferable translations of wǔ xíng, but most acupuncture practitioners who use this concept as their main guideline refer to it as five elements. See also Chapter 78 of the *Ling Shu*, titled "The nine needles" which asserts that the classical types of acupuncture needles were fashioned after the properties corresponding to the natural integers from one to nine, including this musical reference: "Five accords with the law of the (pentatonic) notes, six accords with the law of the tones of the (six) pitch pipes." It is of interest that the term 法 (fǎ meaning law) is used in this passage, connoting a belief in natural law, one of the hallmarks of a scientific viewpoint. The musical metaphor can be seen as a fundamental aspect of the two main therapeutic modalities of Chinese medicine: herbal prescription and acupuncture.

6. See Porkert, M., *Classical Acupuncture: The Standard Textbook*. Phainon, 1995.
7. "All things under heaven sprang from It (i.e., the Dao) as existing (and named); that existence sprang from It as non-existent (and not named)." From *Dao De Jing* Chapter 40.
8. Rosenberg, Z, *An Interview with Paul Unschuld*. United Kingdom: JCM, No. 103, pp.1–8, 2013.
9. See the Diagrams of the Supreme Ultimate by Zhou Dunyi (1017–1023) and Chen Tuan (c. 950) CE.
10. See *Lao Zi* Chapter 25 and *Zhuang Zi* (Outer Chapters) 3 "Letting Be, and Exercising Forbearance."
11. Examples include the higher electrical conductivity at acupuncture points and both the "gate control" hypothesis for how acupuncture reduces pain (via neurological mechanisms) and the "release of endorphins" hypothesis (by biochemical mechanisms).
12. "Knowledge (zhi) cannot explain it, nor discussion (bian) unravel it."
13. qì kǒu 氣口 (meaning qi mouth or opening) is also referred to as mài kǒu 脈口 (meaning vessel or pulse mouth or opening) and cùn kǒu 寸口 (meaning inch mouth or inch opening).
14. Although the Han Chinese do not have Indo-European ancestry, the Yueh-chih tribes (Kushans) coming from Western China occupied Benares (Varenisi) in northeast India. They are considered to have been instrumental in forming the Silk Road sometime prior to 500 BCE.
15. Vasant Lad, one of the contributors of a chapter in this text, explained the method he learned as an oral lineage, in *Secrets of the Pulse: The Ancient Art of Ayurvedic Pulse Diagnosis*. Albuquerque, NM: Ayurvedic Press, 1966. My own teacher, M. J. Cravatta, taught a different method, also transmitted from her Indian teacher J. R. Raju, via an oral lineage.
16. Kuon, D., "A study of constitution-acupuncture." *Journal of the International Congress of Acupuncture and Moxibustion*, 10, 1965, pp.149–167.
17. Yoo T. W., *Koryo Hand Acupuncture*. Vol. 1 (ed. P. Eckman). Seoul: Eum Yang Mek Jin, 1983.
18. Eckman, P., *The Compleat Acupuncturist; A Guide to Constitutional and Conditional Pulse Diagnosis*. London: Singing Dragon, 2014.
19. Eckman, P., "Precision in finger placement for pulse diagnosis," *The Journal of Chinese Medicine*, 109, 2015, pp. 49–55.
20. Posted by anna salem on 6/30/2014 on PonderAbout.com.

12 Ayurvedic Medicine
An Integrative Approach

Vasant Lad

CONTENTS

Part One: Ayurveda and Fundamental Principles...329
History of Ayurveda...329
Five Elements and Three Doshas...331
    Ether or Space 331
    Air 331
    Fire 332
    Water 332
    Earth 332
Ayurvedic Anatomy and Physiology..333
Marma Points...333
Constitutional Types 334
Individual Harmony and Self-Healing...335
Part Two: Understanding the Doshas...336
Doshic Characteristics 336
    Vāta Characteristics 336
    Pitta Characteristics...337
    Kapha Characteristics..338
Personality and Behavior According to Doshic Characteristics 338
Food Preferences..339
Effects of Stress on Different Body Types...340
The Seasons 340
Part Three: Balancing the Doshas..342
Doshic Imbalances...342
The Role of the Mind in Health 343
Ayurvedic Concept of Disease...344
    Origins of Āma in the Body...344
    Traits and Effects of Agni and Āma..344
    Removal of Āma from the Tissues...344
Overview and Conclusion..345
Note...346

PART ONE: AYURVEDA AND FUNDAMENTAL PRINCIPLES

HISTORY OF AYURVEDA

The principles and philosophy of Ayurveda are explained in three important textbooks called the "great three." Among them, the first is Charaka Samhitā. Charaka, by his name, was a wanderer. Internal medicine, etiology, pathology, symptomatology, management of diseases, and the use of herbs are beautifully explained in Charaka Samhitā. The second compilation was by Sushruta, a follower of the Dhanvantari school and a great surgeon. He discussed various types of surgery, preoperative and postoperative measures, and herbs. He was actually the founder of plastic surgery and developed an acupressure system called marma chikitsā, which uses about 170,000 different energy points for diagnostic as well as therapeutic purposes. Vāgbhata was the third of these "great three" who developed his own unique, poetic, and melodious style of talking about the essence of the earlier teachings.

Ayurveda, the science of life, comes from the Vedic tradition and is based on the six philosophies of life, which arise from the ancient scriptures and knowledge of the sages of India. These philosophies seek to discern the truth about life and ways to alleviate pain and suffering for humankind. Ayurveda incorporates all six philosophies. Sānkhya philosophy posits 24 principles in the manifestation of the universe, which provides Ayurveda with an understanding of physical existence (Figure 12.1). Here we will briefly touch upon some of those principles.

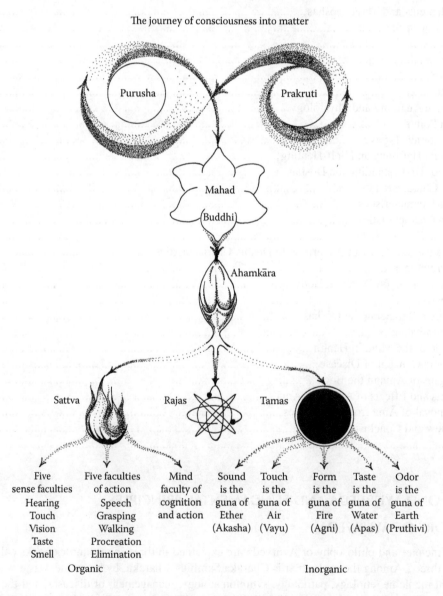

FIGURE 12.1   Illustrates the concepts of the journey of consciousness into matter.

FIVE ELEMENTS AND THREE DOSHAS

The structural aspects of the human body are derived from five basic elements: Ether, Air, Fire, Water, and Earth. These elements are the subtle elements that combine to form all material substances, including physical matter and also thoughts and emotions (Table 12.1).

ETHER OR SPACE

All spaces are related to the Ether element. Every cell contains space and in between two cells, there is intercellular space, through which one cell communicates with another. Without space, there is no communication and space gives freedom to move. Ether is nuclear energy, which comes from the spiritual energy of the soul. In other words, space is freedom, the extensive state of consciousness.

AIR

The next element is Air, the principle of movement. It can be compared to electrical energy. There is attraction between opposite, electrically charged atoms and there is repulsion between similar

TABLE 12.1
Doshas, Elements, and Gunas

Three Doshas	Five Elements	20 Gunas and Clinical Attributes
Vāta	*Ether*	Dry
	Nuclear Energy	Light
	Space	Cold
	Sattva	Mobile
	Air	Clear
	Electrical Energy	Subtle
	Rajas	Rough
		Attributes
		Dispersing
		Astringent (Taste)
Pitta	*Fire*	Hot
	Radiant Energy	Sharp, Penetrating
	Rajas	Light
	Sattva	Liquid
	Water	Oily
	Chemical Energy	Spreading
	Sattva	*Attributes*
	Tamas	Fleshy
		Sour, Pungent, Bitter (Tastes)
Kapha	*Water*	Heavy
	Chemical Energy	Slow
	Sattva	Cold
	Tamas	Oily
	Earth	Slimy, Smooth
	Physical Energy	Dense
	Earth	Soft
		Static, Stable
		Cloudy, Sticky
		Hard, Gross
		Attributes
		Sweet, Salty (Tastes)

atoms. On a subtle cellular level, movements are governed by positively and negatively charged ions that are vibrating, which is the principle of prāna or life energy. In our body, all sensory and motor movements are governed by the air element, and we breathe due to the air element.

FIRE

Where there is movement there is friction, which creates heat, so the next element is Fire. The Fire element regulates body temperature and gives color complexion to the skin, luster to the eyes, and warmth. Fire governs the digestion, absorption, assimilation, and transformation of food into energy, and matter into consciousness.

WATER

Next, the energy of consciousness liquefies, which is the Water element. Water is chemical energy because the liquid, cohesive, qualities make it a universal chemical solvent that governs all biochemical changes. Water element predominates in plasma, saliva, vitreous humor, cerebrospinal fluid, glandular secretions, urine, and sweat. It carries nutrients and maintains the hydration of cells.

EARTH

The final element is Earth, which is the ground of existence. It is the predominant element in most minerals, and in the muscles, bones, cartilage, bone marrow, tendons, hair, nails, and teeth.

The five elements govern the structural aspects of the human body, but the functional aspects are governed by the three energies or organizations called vāta, pitta, and kapha. Vāta is the biological combination of primarily ether and air elements; pitta is predominantly fire and water elements; kapha is mainly water and earth elements. These three doshas are present in every cell, tissue, organ, and system, and energetically they are present in every gene. According to Ayurveda, every biological substance has certain qualities and functions. Therefore, vāta, pitta, and kapha have definite qualities and, because of these attributes, they have particular functions.

Vāta is dry, light, cold, mobile, rough, subtle, and clear, and it has an astringent taste. We can see how these qualities manifest as certain functions at the cellular level. Due to its dry quality, vāta separates cells from one another. Light quality makes the cells and tissues light, so they can move. Cold quality helps to maintain optimal body temperature. Mobile quality governs all biological movement. Rough quality ensures that the muscle cells and bone cells do not stick together. Astringent helps mineral absorption and binds the stools.

Vāta is primarily present in the colon, pelvic cavity, bones, ears, and skin, and it governs the physiological functions of movement, ingestion, ejection, circulation, and respiration, as well as the sensory functions of touch, pain, and temperature.

Pitta is a biological combination of fire and water, so it is hot, sharp, light, oily, liquid, sour and slightly pungent, and it has a strong smell. The hot quality of pitta helps to maintain body temperature and creates appetite, thirst, hunger, and digestion, Because of its sharp quality, pitta penetrates into the subtle molecules of food and governs molecular digestion. Pitta is closely related to bile, which is oily, and this quality keeps the colon soft, lubricated, and allows regular bowel movements. Its liquid quality allows pitta to have a medium for digestive juices and enzymes. Hence, pitta people hardly ever have constipation whereas vāta types tend to become constipated easily. The sour attribute maintains the acid pH of the body and governs the digestive enzymes, most of which are acidic. Pitta is also pungent, so it aids digestion of fats and protein. Pitta has a strong smell and this makes the pitta person sensitive to strong smells.

Pitta is present particularly in the stomach, intestines, liver, spleen, sweat, sebaceous secretions, blood, eyes, and gray matter of the brain. Pitta governs digestion, metabolic activity, understanding, and comprehension. Pitta maintains luster, color complexion, vision and color perception, and normal body color and temperature.

Kapha is a biological combination of earth and water. It is heavy, dull, slow, cool, oily, liquid, slimy, dense, sticky, and has sweet and salty tastes. Its heavy quality creates growth. As it is dull and slow, kapha creates relaxation. The cool quality of kapha protects the stomach lining from burning, and the oily quality helps with lubrication of joints, muscles, bones, and tendons. Its liquid quality manifests in mucous and saliva. Because of its slimy quality, kapha makes the body flexible, while the dense attribute gives solidity and firmness. The sticky quality keeps things together in the body. The sweet attribute regulates blood sugar and gives energy, while the salty attribute bestows vigor and helps to maintain the water-electrolyte balance.

Kapha is present primarily in the stomach, chest, lungs, sinuses, blood plasma and lymphatic system, vitreous humor, white matter of the brain, and synovial fluid. Among other things kapha governs gastric mucus secretions, bronchial secretions, sinus secretions, and lubrication of the joints.

Vāta, pitta, and kapha have collective functional integrity. However, all bodily movements and catabolic functions are governed by vāta; all biochemical changes, thermodynamics, and metabolic functions are governed by pitta; and all building and anabolic functions, lubrication, and protection are governed by kapha.

AYURVEDIC ANATOMY AND PHYSIOLOGY

The human anatomy is comprised of seven bodily tissues, called dhātus. These are rasa, rakta, māmsa, meda, asthi, majjā, and either shukra or ārtava.

Rasa (plasma and lymph) governs nutrition of the body.
Rakta (blood cells) governs oxygenation, which is the function of bestowing life.
Māmsa (muscles, including skeletal, smooth, sphincter, cardiac, and hamstring muscles), covers and protects the vital organs, and governs bodily locomotion.
Meda (adipose or fatty tissue) has the function of lubrication of the skin, joints, and muscles, plus storage of energy and regulation of body temperature.
Asthi (bones, cartilage, and teeth) gives the body form and support.
Majjā (bone marrow and the nervous system) has two main functions. As bone marrow, it fills space (in the bones) and, as nerve tissue, it enables communication within the synaptic spaces.
Shukra (male reproductive tissue) and **ārtava** (female reproductive tissue) have the primary function of procreation.

These seven tissues also have functional integrity. For instance, physical and mechanical movements happen because of the integration between majjā, māmsa, and asthi. The nervous system carries a message to the muscles and they move the bones.

MARMA POINTS

A marma is a vital energy point located on the surface of the body. Like modern quantum physics, Ayurveda holds that a human being is not a solid, stable material structure but an ever-changing, dynamic collection of energy and intelligence in the larger field of energy and intelligence that is the universe. As the body is alive and pulsating with energy, there can be innumerable "energy points" within it and upon the surface, but Ayurveda texts have described 117 major marmas. These points are "vital" because they are infused with prāna, the life force, and imbued with consciousness. Consciousness expresses itself in lively, concentrated form at these points. Thus, marmas serve as a bridge or doorway between the body, mind, and soul and a source of balance and healing.[1]

Marma point therapy is of particular use in the first stages of management yet is helpful at almost any stage of illness. It is a diagnostic and therapeutic tool outlined by Sushruta in his ancient text,

Sushruta Samhita. The points on defined regions of the body relate to the subdoshas of vāta dosha and are used to treat disorders according to each subdoshas. Treatment can also be based on the individual's prakruti-vikruti paradigm using specified medicated oils according to doshic disorder. Marma therapy is a practical and noninvasive therapy that has been used for thousands of years in Ayurveda.

CONSTITUTIONAL TYPES

Prakruti or constitution is an individual's unique, psycho-physiological expression or nature. Right at the time of fertilization, each sperm carries specific qualities of the three doshas in a certain quantity from the father's body into the female genital organ. The ova also carry a unique quality and quantity of vāta, pitta, and kapha from the mother's body. When a single sperm mates with the ovum, these qualities and quantities of vāta, pitta, and kapha that are predominant in both parents combine to create a unique prakruti or individual constitution.

The way a person walks, the way they talk, the way they behave spontaneously and naturally, all depend on his or her constitution. In Ayurveda, the constitution is called prakruti, a unique expression of cosmic consciousness. Vāta, pitta, and kapha have a unique permutation and combination. If vāta is predominant, we can call that constitution vāta prakruti. The same is true for pitta and kapha.

There are seven body types:

- 3 monotypes: vāta, pitta, and kapha.
- 3 types of dual prakruti: vāta-pitta, pitta-kapha, and kapha-vāta.
- 1 sāma prakruti, or balanced prakruti.

With sāma prakruti, all three doshas are perfectly balanced, qualitatively and quantitatively, so we can say $vāta_3$, $pitta_3$, and $kapha_3$. Sāma prakruti is a very healthy prakruti. These people have perfect health; they live longer and can digest virtually any food without significant problems. This is because if one dosha goes out of balance due to dietary or environmental factors, the other two doshas are powerful enough to control it and immediately bring it back into balance.

Clinically, you do not see pure vāta, pitta, or kapha types. There are always minor percentages of the other doshas. Similarly, you cannot see pure dual types; there is always the third dosha, but there may be such a small percentage that it isn't very important.

On clinical grounds, we classify the constitution based on pulse analysis and individual characteristics. A simple system of annotation indicates the proportion of each dosha. For someone who has vāta predominant, pitta in a medium amount and less of kapha, we indicate that ratio as $vāta_3$, $pitta_2$, and $kapha_1$. Someone who has two doshas in equal proportions would be $vāta_1$, $pitta_3$, and $kapha_3$, and so on.

Prakruti indicates our disease proneness. It helps us to know possible future ailments and whether they will be easy, difficult, or impossible to cure. If we know our prakruti, we know how to live in harmony with nature. Vāta-predominant people are particularly prone to the vāta disorders and these are difficult to cure; pitta-predominant people are particularly prone to the pitta disorders, which are most problematic in a pitta person; and kapha-predominant people are particularly prone to kapha disorders, which are hardest to deal with in kapha prakruti.

That does not mean that every time a vāta person gets out of balance they will get a vāta disorder. Even a vāta person can get pitta or kapha diseases if the pitta or kapha provoking cause is frequent, intense, and repeated. However, such problems in a vāta person are easy to control. The same thing is true for pitta and kapha people with non-pitta and non-kapha disorders, respectively. These can be easily cured, because the doshas do not have an environment conducive to staying in the body.

The knowledge of prakruti not only shows us psychosomatic behavioral patterns, but it also helps us to understand how to achieve longevity and appropriate foods and medicines to use.

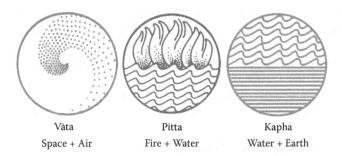

Vāta   Pitta   Kapha
Space + Air   Fire + Water   Water + Earth

FIGURE 12.2 Shows the combinations of elements in vata, pitta, kapha, and the elements.

Prakruti, determined at the time of fertilization, is a unique genetic code. However, due to the mother's diet, lifestyle, and emotional patterns during pregnancy, the doshas undergo changes. Suppose at the time of fertilization the person is vāta$_3$, pitta$_2$, and kapha$_1$, but because of these environmental, dietetic, and emotional changes vāta becomes 4. This altered state of the doshas that happens in intrauterine life or after birth is called vikruti.

Vikruti is the present state of the doshas, which may be responsible for congenital or otherwise acquired anomalies. Ideally, every individual should balance vikruti and prakruti. That is the basic Ayurvedic paradigm (Figure 12.2).

INDIVIDUAL HARMONY AND SELF-HEALING

Every individual has a unique qualitative and quantitative permutation and combination of the three doshas. They are the three organizations:

Vāta: principle of movement.
Pitta: principle of heat and transformation.
Kapha: building material of the body.

These three doshas are constantly exposed to environmental, seasonal, dietetic, and emotional. Due to all these changes, the outer ecological factors bombard the body, mind, and conscience. Instead of an external cause directly affecting the bodily tissues, organs, or systems, they hit a protective barrier, which are the doshas. So before an outer cause affects the nervous system, vāta becomes high. Before an outer cause affects the small intestines or liver, pitta becomes high. The same is true for an external cause directly affecting the lungs, which first disturbs kapha.

One meaning of the word dosha is fault and, in a way, the doshas are a fault in behavior, action, and past life karma. Your life is a beautiful expression of dynamic karmic force. There are cosmic karmas, maternal karmas, paternal karmas, individual karmas, and collective karmas. Karma means action. So looking is karma, listening is karma, breathing is karma, eating is karma, and any doing is karma. We carry the seeds of unresolved past life karma within our subtle or astral body, and these karmic forces or unresolved past life karmic seeds lie dormant in the astral body.

Even though a person's diet and lifestyle may be quite healthy, that person might become sick. People suffer from cancer even though there is no genetic history of cancer, no exposure to radiation or smoking. Why? Ayurveda says that disease happens through wrong diet, wrong lifestyle, wrong relationships, unhealthy emotional patterns, and unhealthy environment, as well as from the seeds of unresolved past life karma. These unresolved seeds lie dormant in the liver, kidney, heart, lungs, or other part of the body and one day they sprout. A person may suddenly get cancer of the lungs or liver.

Health is a process and disease is also a process. For self-healing, one has to keep a balance between these two processes. Even without doing anything, there are natural changes in the environment. Morning and evening are times of kapha, midday and midnight are pitta times, while dawn and dusk are times of vāta. Without you doing anything, the respective dosha becomes high at these times. The biological clock is governed by the doshas, and the Sun, Moon, and Earth govern the chronological clock.

Ayurveda speaks a great deal about dinācharya, which is the daily regime, as well as rutucharyā, the seasonal regime. These regimens maintain the harmony of our internal doshas. Self-healing occurs at every moment, by understanding the role of the doshas, their changes, and the flow of time. Accordingly, one has to amend one's own lifestyle and behavior to remain in harmony.

PART TWO: UNDERSTANDING THE DOSHAS

DOSHIC CHARACTERISTICS

Every individual has a unique body based on a combination of the three doshas. To detect one's body type, the guidelines below help.

VĀTA CHARACTERISTICS

Dry: Prone to dry skin, hair, nails, and lips; dry colon causes constipation; cracking and popping of the joints
Light: Light bones and muscles; underweight; prone to light-headedness
Cold: Cold hands and feet; poor circulation; love of warmth
Rough: Responsible for cracking of lips, heels, and elbows, as well as hemorrhoids, fissures, and fistula
Subtle: Goose bumps; nervous twitching of eyelids; muscle tremors; fear and anxiety
Mobile: Hyperactivity; muscle tremors, tics, and spasms; fast movement, talking, and eating
Clear: Clear, creative mind that easily forgets
Astringent: Choking sensation; often get hiccoughs while eating

Vāta people have prominent veins and minimal muscles and fat, so their bones are very visible. They have big joints that crack and pop, sunken cheeks, and often have a twisted nose and

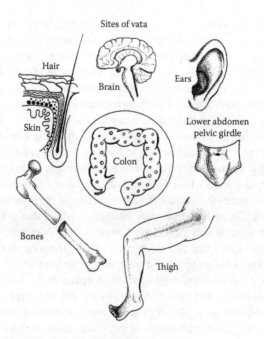

FIGURE 12.3   Illustrates the sites of vāta in the body.

protruding teeth. Vāta types are active and like to jog and hike, and love traveling, but they should limit these activities because they all aggravate vāta dosha. Vāta people should do yoga, walking, and gentle exercise that keeps them in harmony with nature. They need more rest than other body types (Figure 12.3).

PITTA CHARACTERISTICS

Hot: Strong appetite; excessive thirst; irritable; hair loss and premature graying

Sharp: Sharp eyes, nose, teeth, and nails; sharp memory and intellect

Light: Light to moderate weight; intolerance of bright light—lengthy exposure to both fluorescent lights and sunlight can cause headaches

Liquid: Loose stools; excessive urination and perspiration

Bitter: Nausea; food sensitivity

Spreading: Hives, rashes, urticaria, eczema, and acne; makes pitta people want to spread their name and fame, which makes them good public speakers, organizers, and leaders

Strong fleshy smell: Profuse sweating with a typical sulfuric smell; intolerance to strong smells, such as powerful perfumes and incense

Sour: Acidic saliva, urine, and sweat; prone to hyperacidity, acid indigestion, and inflammatory disorders such as gastritis, colitis, and dermatitis

Pungent: Strong appetite; quick digestion and absorption; heartburn; burning sensations

Pitta types are bright, brilliant, intellectual, delicate people who do not tolerate hard work. They can spend hours in front of a computer or reading and should take regular breaks and walk in the garden. Cooling, relaxing exercise is best, such as yoga, swimming, or walking in the morning or evening. However, many pitta people like to run in the middle of the day and play competitive sports, and this severely aggravates pitta (Figure 12.4).

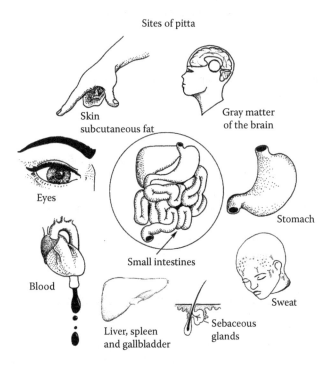

Sites of pitta

Skin subcutaneous fat

Gray matter of the brain

Eyes

Stomach

Small intestines

Blood

Liver, spleen and gallbladder

Sebaceous glands

Sweat

FIGURE 12.4 Illustrates the sites of pitta in the body.

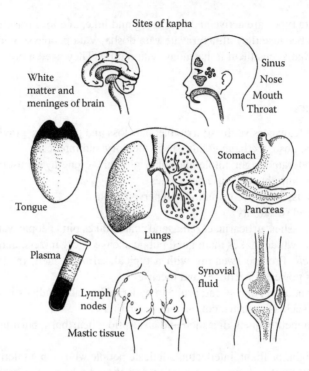

Sites of kapha

White matter and meninges of brain

Sinus
Nose
Mouth
Throat

Tongue

Stomach

Pancreas

Lungs

Plasma

Lymph nodes

Synovial fluid

Mastic tissue

FIGURE 12.5   Illustrates the sites of kapha in the body.

KAPHA CHARACTERISTICS

Heavy: Heavy bones, muscles, and body; easily put on weight

Slow: Slow digestion and metabolism; slow movements, slow speech, and slow mind

Soft: Soft skin; gentle nature

Oily: Oily skin

Slimy: Well-lubricated joints

Cold: Cool skin; hot inside and cool outside, which is why kapha types have a problem with emotional eating—they like cold drinks and iced water, but this lowers agni while not diminishing appetite

Dense: Thick skin; thick hair

Static: Enjoy eating or sitting and doing nothing

Cloudy: Foggy mind, especially in the morning and evening (kapha times)

Kapha types have thick, robust, muscular bodies, and muscles and fat blend to give padded heels, thighs, breasts, belly, and face. Kapha people are sedentary, loving to sit on the couch and watch TV. However, they should do brisk power-walking or other intense physical activity. Kapha types also need intellectual stimulus such as solving puzzles, but unlike pitta people, they don't like these activities and often fall asleep instead (Figure 12.5).

PERSONALITY AND BEHAVIOR ACCORDING TO DOSHIC CHARACTERISTICS

Personality and behavior can be studied by observing the expression of vāta, pitta, and kapha in an individual. We are not only a body, but also mind and consciousness. Every thought brings certain feelings and reactions, and these pass through the layers of vāta, pitta, and kapha. Emotions are the reactions of past memories to a current challenge. They are subjective mental feelings that drive most of our behavior, meeting any challenge as a doshic reaction.

Vāta individuals are highly creative, active, alert, attentive, flexible, and ready to change. They love traveling and enjoy jogging, jumping, and very active forms of exercise. They do not like to sit and do nothing; that is a punishment for a vāta person. They make money quickly and spend it quickly, usually on trivial items. A vāta person might typically go to a flea market and buy old furniture that is not really needed. Their rooms can be cluttered with antiques or junk and look chaotic, with shoes left lying in the kitchen and socks hanging on bookshelves. Vāta people are not disciplined and tidy, but in the disorder they find order. Vāta types also love staying inside, because they have fear and insecurity, and a highly active imagination about the future that can make them anxious.

Vāta people are hyperactive, quick thinking, and creative. They act quickly; they talk quickly and often answer without thinking, so they give a wrong answer with great conviction. Positive vāta mental qualities are creativity, happiness, flexibility, adaptability, and readiness to change. They love to change everything quickly because they get bored with the same thing. Under stress, vāta dosha can increase causing debilitating emotions such as fear, anxiety, nervousness, insecurity, loneliness, and ungroundedness.

Pitta individuals are typically bright, brilliant, intellectual, and disciplined people. You often see pitta types reading a book because they are typically bookworms. They read while traveling and even while walking. They love to take notes, solve problems, and do calculations. They usually have an analytical, calculating mind, which is why they are often research-oriented and make good researchers. They can have problems with judgment and criticism. If there is no one else appropriate for them to judge, they will judge themselves. They criticize themselves because, in the true sense, pitta individuals are perfectionists. They want to do everything meticulously and right on schedule. They want to control every situation. Pitta people keep everything in its right place, so their kitchen is usually as clean as an operating theatre.

Pitta people are generally bright, brilliant, intellectual types who think about matters deeply. They are well-organized, good speakers, and success-oriented. If they fail, they become severely depressed. Positive pitta mental qualities are dedication, commitment, and loyalty. Elevated pitta dosha can cause emotions such as judgment, criticism, comparison, competitiveness, aggression, and always wanting to be right, which leads to frustration, anger, hate, envy, and jealousy. Pitta people do not like to be told "no" and if you tell them, "You are wrong!" they will be upset.

Kapha individuals are generally loving, forgiving, and compassionate. They do not like physical activity and tend to walk, talk, and move slowly. They love eating, sitting doing nothing, watching TV, and sleeping. Kapha people have a sweet tooth and want to enjoy life. They are inclined to be honest people and if they adopt a schedule, they will follow it religiously. They have good strength and stamina with a strong sex drive and like to have the opposite gender around them. Forgiving people, they are likely to be quite spiritual with a deep profound faith. Everything for a kapha person is liable to be slow, sustained, and prolonged, including their emotions. They have a propensity to hold on to emotions.

Positive kapha mental qualities are trust, deep faith, compassion, forgiveness, sympathy, and acceptance. Even if you tell a kapha person, "You are wrong," he or she will accept it. However, increased kapha may cause negative emotions such as attachment, greed, possessiveness, and depression.

All people love, but a vāta person loves out of loneliness and insecurity; a pitta person loves out of desire for knowledge; and a kapha person has unconditional love but it may become attachment. We all have anger, attachment, and all the other emotions but are more prone to the ones common to our own doshic imbalance.

FOOD PREFERENCES

Biological needs and psychological or emotional cravings are two very different things. The constitutional doshas create biological cravings, but imbalanced doshas cause emotional, psychological, and perverted cravings.

- A healthy vāta person with balanced doshas prefers warm, oily food and loves to eat more sweet, sour, and salty foods to pacify vāta dosha.
- A healthy pitta person with balanced doshas loves cooling foods and eats more sweet, bitter, and astringent foods to calm pitta dosha.
- A healthy kapha person who has balanced doshas loves hot, spicy food and eats more bitter, pungent, and astringent foods to control kapha.

If a dosha is high, that dosha tries to stay in the body by creating imbalanced cravings for foods that actually increase the dosha. Additionally, increased doshas cause the following digestive problems:

- Imbalanced vāta makes people eat hurriedly and causes variable appetite and poor digestion.
- Imbalanced pitta causes cravings for stimulating, rajasic food. There is strong appetite but weak digestion.
- Imbalanced kapha creates a desire for sweets and dairy products. However, this is emotional hunger because there is low appetite and weak digestion.

The state of a person's agni is most important. When a vāta person craves sweet, sour, and salty things, we think it is good because these three tastes pacify vāta dosha. However, if vāta is high and there is low agni or vishama (irregular) agni, there will be poor digestion and formation of toxins. People with toxins crave sweet, sour, and salty things, which worsen the toxic load.

Before answering a craving, one should inquire whether there are toxins showing on the tongue, whether elimination is normal and there are good bowel movements, without bloating, constipation, diarrhea, or gas. Cravings created by toxins should never be satisfied.

EFFECTS OF STRESS ON DIFFERENT BODY TYPES

There is a physical stress, which is necessary for building the body, and psychological or emotional stress. Psychological stress is caused by repressed emotions. When we aren't able to deal with our emotions, we suppress them. The emotions are not completely resolved or understood, so they accumulate in the connective tissue and build stress.

Vāta and pitta people are delicate and do not respond so well to stress. Only kapha people can bear some stress.

Vāta people respond to stress with anxiety, insecurity, restlessness, insomnia, dark circles under the eyes, constipation, irritable bowel syndrome, ringing in the ear, sciatica, arthritis, tremors, spasms, muscle stiffness, and pain. They often feel tired and exhausted.

Pitta individuals tend to get hives, rashes, urticaria, eczema, psoriasis, conjunctivitis, hyperacidity, indigestion, peptic ulcers, ulcerative colitis, Crohn's disease, diarrhea, irritation, anger, and aggression. A pitta person becomes extremely hungry and, if there is no food, they can get hypoglycemia.

A kapha person under stress eats sweets, sleeps excessively, and often becomes obese. Stress creates false hunger, so kapha people are always snacking. Stress may be the cause of diabetes, high cholesterol, high triglycerides, high blood pressure, glaucoma, and many kapha disorders.

THE SEASONS

The seasons are governed by geographical location and the rotation of the Earth. In the Indian calendar, there are six seasons, translated as spring, summer, rainy, autumn, early winter, and late winter. We will focus on the four basic seasons used in much of the western world.

Summer: The season of the sun. It is hot, sharp, penetrating, and bright; hence, it is the season of pitta. People get sunburn, excess thirst, acid indigestion, diarrhea, ulcers, hives, rash, urticaria, itching, burning eyes, and other symptoms caused by high pitta. Summer tends to be an unhealthy season because the digestive fire is low, resulting in poor digestion.

Autumn: The trees drop their leaves and the weather is generally dry and windy. It is warm during daytime and cold at night and this abrupt drop in temperature disturbs vāta dosha, hence autumn is a season of vāta. Arthritis, sciatica, rheumatism, muscle aches, and pain all get worse and people experience more constipation, bloating, insomnia, anxiety, cracking and popping of the joints, and other vāta symptoms.

Winter: There is a lot of water in the form of either rain or snow, it is cold, and everything moves slowly. Hence, winter is a season of predominantly kapha dosha, but secondarily vāta. People get colds, congestion, cough, flu, and other kapha symptoms, as well as vāta problems such as arthritis, sciatica, constipation, anxiety, and muscle pain. Overall, winter is a healthy season because the digestive fire is pushed to the gastrointestinal (GI) tract, giving strong appetite and digestion.

Spring: In springtime, the trees and flowers begin to bloom as new life begins, so spring is a healthy season of rejuvenation, joy, and happiness. People are ready to change, they like to travel, and it is a more outgoing time. The early spring is kapha and late spring more pitta. Any snow starts melting in spring and similarly accumulated kapha starts melting, which can cause spring cold or allergies. It is a good time to cleanse but can also be a time of sinus congestion, hay fever, asthma, skin disorders, nausea, and poor digestion.

In the human body, there are biological times, which are the periods of vāta, pitta, and kapha. Chronological time is closely identified with biological time. Early morning and evening is kapha time, mid-day and midnight pitta, and early dawn and dusk is vāta period. This is the cyclical movement of the three doshas in one day (Figure 12.6). A bigger cycle is the seasons, governed by the movement of the Earth. Due to the tilt of the Earth's axis and the orbit of the Earth around the Sun, there are two solstices each year (winter and summer) when the Sun has no apparent northward or southward motion. This is an auspicious period, the starting point of the new season. Changes in the elements, attributes, colors, and directions are significant during each season. These changes influence bodily cells, organs, systems, and doshas. Even subtle emotional modifications can be experienced.

Ayurveda defines rutu sandhi as the transition between two seasons, the 15 days of the previous season and the 15 days of the future season. It is similar to when entering from outside to the inside. At the entrance, the outer space meets the inner one. This door is like the exit from one season and entry into another. During that period, you should remove your shoes, clothes, and attitudes of the old season. Then you are ready to enter into the next season. Ayurveda recommends that panchakarma should be undergone during rutu sandhi. The seasons are variable in the United States.

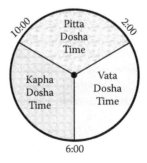

FIGURE 12.6   Shows the times of day of the dosha times.

Every region has a different timing. One must observe these specific changes. Depending on an individual's prakruti and vikruti, one can do the initial measures of panchakarma for 5 days, 7 days, or 15 days depending on the individual circumstances. Then you are ready for a specific cleansing operation.

Every state has a different season, every province has a different season, and every nation has a different season. We cannot go by the calendar that at a specific date the summer or winter will begin. Impossible! We have to see the nature and structure of the seasons. Some days there is so much fog and cold, it looks like winter. Then just behave like the winter season. Some days it becomes so hot, so bright, so like summer that you have to change your lifestyle on that day. During that very hot day, you can eat salad. That will cool down your system. You can eat yogurt. Nevertheless, on the foggy or cold days, don't eat salad. That will slow down your agni. Don't eat yogurt; that will create congestion. Once we know the general seasonal routine, then the same can be applied to every day. Within one day, you may get four seasons. Morning is springtime, the birds are singing, the sun is rising, and the flowers are blooming. Just like morning the whole season of spring is flowering. During midday, you might be having a hot summer day. The birds are exhausted and opening their beaks to drink water. Perhaps in the afternoon, fall may come with a sudden gust of wind with dry weather. At night when the sun sets, it could seem like winter.

So, dear friends, within one day, all four seasons can be experienced. We can understand daily cycles when we understand seasonal regimens as a whole. Although the seasons are changing, we know exactly what type of day it is and we can immediately change. This is the beauty of creating balance between external ecology and internal ecology. Just look at nature as it is. Once we study the standard nature of the seasons—winter, spring, summer, fall—then we can apply the principles according to the province, season, day, and time.

PART THREE: BALANCING THE DOSHAS

DOSHIC IMBALANCES

Prakruti is disease proneness, which means the inclination of the predominant doshas to go out of balance. If a person is vāta predominant, a vāta-provoking diet and lifestyle can easily cause vāta to go out of balance.

The colon is the primary site of vāta; the small intestines are the main site of pitta; and the upper part of the stomach and the lungs are the major kapha sites. Whenever a dosha goes out of balance, it will first accumulate in its site. Hence, vāta will accumulate in the colon, pitta in the intestine, and kapha in the stomach.

Vāta Symptoms: Irregular appetite, constipation, gases, bloating, distention, hemorrhoids, low backache; leads to cracking and popping of the joints, goose bumps, insomnia, anxiety, insecurity, ringing in the ears, sciatica, joint pain, muscle pain, backache, arthritis, osteoporosis, hyperactivity, excessive talking, and degenerative changes.

Causes: beans, raw vegetables, overly vigorous exercise, and overactivity.

Pitta Symptoms: Acid indigestion, hyperacidity, heartburn, gastritis, colitis, nausea, and vomiting; leads to chronic malabsorption, hives, rashes, urticaria, acne, eczema, psoriasis, fever, bleeding disorders, peptic ulcers, ulcerative colitis, yellowish discoloration of urine, feces, and sweat, and nearly all inflammatory disorders, such as oophoritis, vaginitis, orchitis, and conjunctivitis.

Causes: sour fruit, fermented food, chilies and other hot spices, alcohol, cigarettes, and working under the hot sun.

Kapha Symptoms: Cold, congestion, cough, low appetite, slow digestion, slow metabolism; leads to flu, pulmonary congestion, lymphatic obstruction, edema, swelling, asthma, diabetes, hypertension, high triglycerides, high cholesterol, and congestive diseases.

Causes: fatty or fried food, dairy products, watermelon, chilled drinks, excessive sleep, daytime naps, and sitting watching TV.

THE ROLE OF THE MIND IN HEALTH

The mind contains three gunas: sattva, rajas, and tamas.

- Sattva is the pure nature of the mind, which is clarity of perception resulting in direct knowledge.
- Rajas governs sensational movement and manipulates knowledge.
- Tamas attaches to knowledge, causing the ego to become fixed. Every experience is imprinted on the paper of the mind by the ink of tamas.

The three gunas are universal, nonlocalized energy fields whereas the doshas are individual, localized energy fields. An imbalance of the doshas creates physical ailments, but an imbalance of the psychological qualities (sattva, rajas, and tamas) creates mental disorders. Any dosha or guna that becomes overpowering can create mental imbalances such as illusion, delusion, hallucination, and depression (high tamas) or attention deficit disorder (high rajas). However, there is an intimate relationship between the doshas and gunas.

Pitta is partly sattvic and partly rajasic; vāta is also partly rajasic and partly sattvic; kapha is partly tamasic and partly sattvic. Tamas and kapha have similar qualities. They are both heavy, sluggish, and induce sleep. Pitta governs knowledge, understanding, and comprehension, which are all sattvic. However, pitta also brings judgment, criticism, and control, which are rajasic. Vāta is active, mobile, restless, ungrounded, and aggravated, and all these qualities are connected to rajas.

Psychosomatic disorders are nothing but the interchanging qualities of the doshas and the mind. That is why emotion is a reaction of the past to the present challenge. Every experience is recorded in memory. There is cellular memory in our body and every cell is a center of consciousness. Every cell has a mind, choice, intelligence, and memory. From that biochemical cellular memory, emotions enter the consciousness. Without the body and mind, there is no consciousness. Consciousness is like a vast ocean, but every vessel holds the ocean water according to its size and shape. Similarly, every person's body, mind, and doshas hold the oceanic consciousness as individual consciousness. Your consciousness identifies your cells with your body so you become somebody. Your consciousness identifies with your fear and you become fearful. Your consciousness identifies yourself with your anger and you become angry.

Consciousness is a pure, vast energy, in which there is a center, which is "I am." Around that center, the memory, thoughts, feelings, and emotions are moving. Whenever we respond to a challenge, we respond through the body and mind in the form of emotion. There is nothing wrong with emotions, but consciousness identifies through the ego and holds onto the emotions, storing them in the deeper layer of the subconscious. Therefore, we carry within our deep connective tissues many crystals of unresolved emotions. When emotion is not allowed to flow, it becomes stagnant and undergoes crystallization. These crystals accumulate in the deep connective tissue of organs like the heart, lungs, kidney, and brain creating khavaigunya, which are defective spaces. This is the start of the disease process.

The causes of disease are foods that are protagonistic to doshic aggravation and food that is antagonistic to tissue nutrition. Not eating according to one's constitution, in a timely manner, or having wrong habits, wrong diet, inappropriate emotional patterns, and physical and emotional trauma are the causes of disease. An imbalance of the doshas is the result, creating physical and emotional blockages. Emotional blockages become physical blockage. Nutrients do not flow and the tissues undergo congestion.

Our body is nothing but a journey of consciousness into matter. It is frozen consciousness, trapped light and crystallized energy. The physical body determines its genetic code at the time of fertilization, is structurally shaped by the tissues, and is governed functionally by doshas. There is no mind without body, and there is no body without mind. The mind is a subtler body, and the body a grosser mind. Does the mind live in the body or body live in the mind? Ayurveda says the body lives in the mind. There is a cosmic mind and cosmic consciousness, and an individual mind and individual consciousness.

Our physical body is created by the journey of consciousness through the five elements (Ether, Air, Fire, Water, and Earth). These five elements and the three gunas (sattva, rajas, and tamas) constitute the body. The body is made of the five elements. The mind is comprised of the qualities of the elements.

Pure universal consciousness has no attributes, but individual consciousness is colored by attributes. The five elements operate through consciousness, and consciousness operates through the five elements, in order to create structural and functional changes.

AYURVEDIC CONCEPT OF DISEASE

Disease occurs when aggravated doshas enter the tissues, affecting agni (digestive fire) and producing āma (toxins) that circulate throughout the body. Āma is undigested food that clogs the bodily channels and affects nutrition. It also enters into the mental faculty and clogs the flow of the mind. Āma is a good media for bacteria and virus growth. Disease is functional disintegration or disharmony between body, mind, and consciousness.

Origins of Āma in the Body

Proper nutrition is governed by healthy agni, the digestive fire. There are multiple types of agni, including jāthara (stomach) agni, bhūta (liver) agni, and dhātu (tissue) agni as well as cellular agni. As long as agni is healthy, proper, and robust, then there is wholesome nutrition and the person will have strength, health, and longevity. When agni becomes impaired, it creates undigested foodstuff that is not properly processed. Undigested, unprocessed food creates a toxic, morbid metabolic waste called āma. The word āma means raw, uncooked, unprocessed. Āma can build up in the body and is mainly created by low agni.

There are other sources of āma. The body has three malas (excreta)—urine, feces, and sweat. When they are not eliminated properly, the stagnated, accumulated mala can create āma. Āma can accumulate in the colon from chronic constipation, in the bladder from incomplete urination, and it can build up under the skin.

Āma can accumulate from bacterial, parasitic, or viral infection. When the dhātu agni of any of the seven dhātus is impaired, then the unprocessed, raw tissue is formed and that is called dhātu āma.

Āma can be caused by the buildup of impurities from imbalanced dosha, called āma dosha. Increased vāta dosha can create vishama (irregular) agni, causing an accumulation of āma in the colon and a blackish-brown coating on the tongue, gas, bloating, and foul-smelling flatus. Aggravated pitta dosha creates tīkshna (sharp, fast) agni, increasing āma in the small intestine, and creating a yellowish coating on the tongue as well as hives, rash, urticaria, eczema, and psoriasis. Imbalanced kapha dosha suppresses agni, producing manda (slow) agni and a thick, white coating on the tongue. This can lead to repeated colds, congestion, and lymphatic congestion.

Another type of āma comes from unresolved and unexpressed emotions such as anger, fear, hate, jealousy, and negative thinking. That is called mental āma.

Traits and Effects of Agni and Āma

Traits of Agni	Traits of Āma
Light, hot, dry, sharp	Heavy, cold, damp, dull, cloudy
Creates vigor, vitality, energy, fragrance, health	Creates fatigue, foul smell, debility

Removal of Āma from the Tissues

Āma is the root cause of all disease. It clogs the channels and becomes a media for bacteria and other infections to proliferate. Therefore, Ayurveda says we have to remove the āma from the bodily system. Ayurveda provides a multifaceted system for determining the state of the patient and the best methods to restore balance to that patient.

Depending on the strength, health, and age of the patient and the qualities of the disease as well as its stage of development, there are several measures of therapy. Palliative measures include dīpana, enkindling agni, and pāchana, and digesting āma directly.

Dīpana kindles the digestive fire before food is eaten. Using herbs to balance agni according to the person's current state, they kindle agni and prevent the formation of new toxins. This method particularly assists in cases of low agni.

Pāchana techniques will digest or burn the āma. The herbs are often the same as those used for dīpana but they are given in different amounts and after the meal to improve digestion and eliminate toxins (āma). Digestion overall will improve and help establish proper nutrition of the bodily tissues.

The cleansing measures known as shodhana are used when āma deposits into the deeper tissues of the body. The appropriate treatment plan is determined by a sophisticated, in-depth evaluation of the patient and the person's condition and strength to bear the treatments.

Preparatory methods, pūrvakarma, help to get the body ready. These techniques are designed to loosen āma from the tissues and encourage it to travel back to the digestive tract from where it can be eliminated by several methods. Typically, these are internal snehana (consumption of oil), external snehana (application of oil) via several methods including massage and other applications of medicated oils, and svedana (steam and other external heat therapies), as well as other measures such as dīpana and pāchana.

The goal of these methods is for the āma to return to the digestive tract where it will be eliminated by panchakarma or the five actions: vamana (emesis), virechana (purgation), basti (medicated enema), rakta moksha (bloodletting), and/or nasya (nasal administration of herb or medicated oils). Panchakarma, the five actions, is used for removal of accumulated toxins from the body.

Āma in the stomach is removed by vamana. Āma in the small intestine is removed by virechana, while that in the colon is eliminated by basti. If there is some lingering āma in the blood, then that can be removed by bloodletting, or the application of leeches. Vamana is for kapha dosha, virechana for pitta dosha, basti for vāta dosha, nasya for any residual dosha in the majjā dhātu, and rakta moksha removes āma from the hematopoietic system. Panchakarma is a part of a series of procedures called shodhana, detoxification. Shodhana makes the body free from āma.

The last step of detoxification is rasayana, rejuvenation. It is used to restore balance between the doshas, dhātus, and malas and body, mind and consciousness. After cleansing, rasayana stabilizes the gains and benefits from the detoxification process and special herbs and other therapies are used to bring about health, youthfulness, and vitality. Rasayana gives the patient a healthy body, mind, and tissues, and harmonious, functional integration between the organs.

OVERVIEW AND CONCLUSION

According to Ayurveda, every individual is a unique book; pages and pages have been written. Every Ayurvedic physician should learn the art of patient evaluation. Additionally, the patient's history is very important. Talk to the patient; ask him or her about their concerns and history. Collect the data based on signs and symptoms. These symptoms belong to a specific dosha. For example, constipation, gas, bloating, arthritis, and rheumatism are vāta symptoms. Pitta symptoms are hives, rashes, urticaria, and fever. Excess kapha can create cold, congestion, cough, edema, swelling, and some congestive changes such as water retention.

First, the Ayurvedic physician classifies these symptoms into vāta, pitta, or kapha type. Then he or she assesses the symptoms as they are related to the dhātus. Through this, you try to read that beautiful book, the patient. Then each person's prakruti (constitution) and vikruti (current state) should be understood. Now the physician knows which dosha is involved, the dhātu affected, and the organs involved. Based on that, the Ayurvedic physician can understand the samprāpti, the pathogenesis. Then he or she gives the proper diet, lifestyle, and herbal protocol, including shodhana and/or rejuvenation protocol, to heal the person.

Ayurveda hugs the human being completely. In that hugging, Ayurvedic medicine heals the body, mind, and consciousness. In one sense, Ayurvedic is the ancient art of longevity of life whose goal is for every individual to live more than 100 years.

NOTE

1. Vasant Lad and Anisha Durve, *Marma Points of Ayurveda: The Energy Pathways for Healing Body, Mind and Consciousness with a Comparison to Traditional Chinese Medicine* (Albuquerque, NM: The Ayurvedic Press, 2015), 17.

13 An Introduction to Ayurveda
Marma Therapy

Shekhar Annambhotla

CONTENTS

Marma Meditation 351
Classification of Marma Points on Doshas and Sub-Doshas 351
Technique of Marma Therapy 354
Clinical Application of Marma Therapy 354
Benefits of Marma Therapy 355

Marma points have been enumerated in the classical Ayurvedic treatise of 600 B.C., *Sushruta Samhita*, the textbook of surgical procedures and treatments. The term "*marma*" can be explained as the sensitive points of the body through which energy flows. These energy pathways facilitate the healing of the mind, body, and consciousness as the subtle energy, prana, flows through the marma points. There are 107 marma points described in Ayurveda, and they are all connected to the three major marma areas—Head (*Shira*), Heart (*Hrudaya*), and Bladder (*Basti*).

Marmas are junctions of various energy sources and are composed of one, two, or three of the following anatomical structures: muscles, veins, arteries, ligaments, bones, and joints. Further, the marma points are classified into five types according to their structure and composition of anatomical position.

1. Muscle-based marmas, which are fascia, sheaths, serous membranes, and muscles. Injury may lead to pain, tears, paralysis, atrophy, or swelling.
2. Vessel-based marmas, which supply energy through arteries, veins, and lymphatics. Injury may produce hemorrhage and/or blood loss, due to sharp penetration and surgical laceration.
3. Ligament-based marmas, which are related to tissues and structures and connect the bones and muscles. Injury produces damage of various organs, constant pain, and long-term deformity.
4. Bone-based marmas, which are related to bone tissue. Injury may lead to bone spurs, cracks, and breaks.
5. Joint-based marmas, which are related to various joints. Injury leads to immobility of joints, pain, and deformity of joints.

Injuries to marmas may be due to trauma, growths, or wounds. Signs and symptoms of injury are bleeding, pain, disorientation, loss of sensory damage, loss of coordination, and loss of consciousness, which can lead to short- to long-term disability and possibly death. When the marmas are afflicted, imbalances in vata, pitta, kapha, blood, prana, mind, and consciousness occur.

The marmas are again further classified based on their injury to a particular area. These are

1. Immediate-death causing marmas (*Sadhya Pranahara*): Death due to losing prana (life force). Significant injury to the head, heart, or bladder may lead to death. These are three heating energies (fire element) and significant injury may take away bodily warmth, circulation, or may lead to internal hemorrhage, irregular heartbeat, or rupture of bladder. Shock, pain, and death can happen in a short time.
2. Long-term death causing marmas (*Kalantara Pranahara*): Death happens over a period of time due to the marmas becoming filled with water and fire elements. Internal bleeding can occur in the vessels within the body.
3. Fatal-death-if-pierced marmas (*Vishalyaghna*): A foreign body (e.g., a bullet) lodged in the marma area can cause death to happen.
4. Disability-causing marmas (*Vaikalyakara*): The afflicted marmas lead to short-term to long-term disability.
5. Pain-causing marmas (*Rujakara*): Injury or trauma, either physical or psychological, leads to recurrent or constant pain.

Marmas can be afflicted by vata, pitta, and kapha doshas. When vata dosha afflicts a particular marma, it produces severe pain, sometimes all over the body. The person may experience fear, anxiety, insomnia, restlessness, tremors, constipation, nervous indigestion, and/or nervous agitation.

When pitta dosha affects the marma area, a feeling of heat, irritation, or redness manifests as generalized symptoms of fever, hyperacidity, skin problems, intolerance to light, and anger.

When kapha dosha afflicts the marma area, there will be swelling, edema, and congestion. Overall, there will be an increase in kapha symptoms, such as heaviness, lethargy, fatigue, and depression.

There are 22 yogic marmas corresponding to various locations (Figures 13.1 and 13.2):

1. *Adhipati Marma*—Crown on the head
2. *Sthapani Marma*—Middle of the eyebrows
3. *Apanga Marma*—Outer margin of the eyebrows
4. *Utkshepa Marma*—Above the ears
5. *Vidhura Marma*—Mastoid area
6. *Shankha Marma*—Temple area
7. *Phana Marma*—Root of the nose/both nostrils area
8. *Shringataka Marma*—Root of the tongue
9. *Nila Marma*—Base of the throat
10. *Hrudaya Marma*—Center of the heart
11. *Nabhi Marma*—Umbilicus
12. *Basti Marma*—Bladder area
13. *Vitapa Marma*—Perineum
14. *Nitamba Marma*—Middle of the buttocks
15. *Guda Marma*—Anus
16. *Urvi Marma*—Middle of the thigh
17. *Janu Marma*—Center of the knee joint
18. *Indra Basti Marma*—Middle of calf muscles
19. *Gulpha Marma*—Ankle joint
20. *Kurcha Shira Marma*—Calcaneus area
21. *Tala Hrudaya Marma*—Palmar area
22. *Kshipra Marma*—Web of the toes

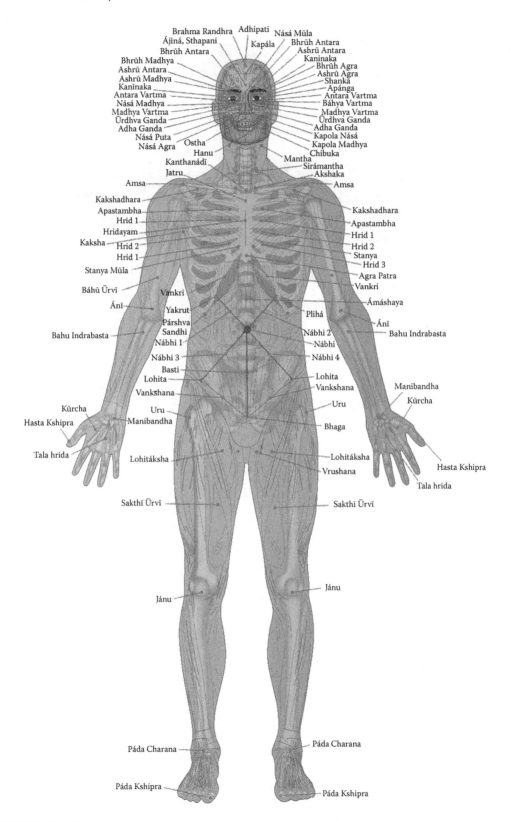

FIGURE 13.1 Marma points anterior view.

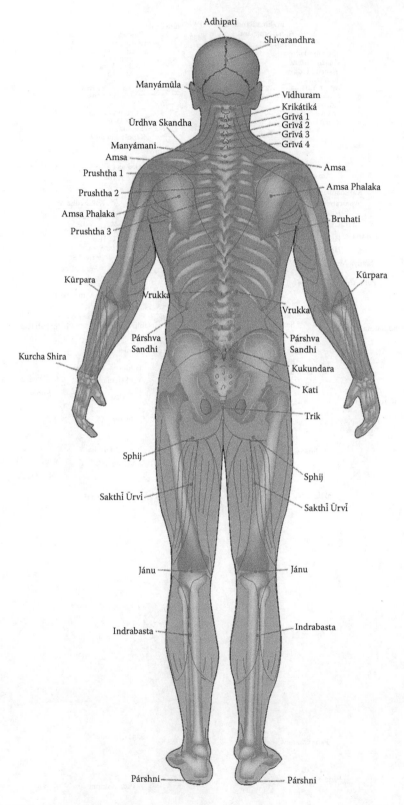

FIGURE 13.2   Marma points posterior view.

MARMA MEDITATION

Marma meditation is a unique technique to bring about awareness of pranic energy and consciousness to particular marma points and their surrounding areas. Spending 15–20 minutes meditation on various marma points brings calmness of mind, relaxation, and eases discomfort and pain.

CLASSIFICATION OF MARMA POINTS ON DOSHAS AND SUB-DOSHAS

Fifteen sub-doshas have been enumerated for the doshas. Vata Dosha's 5 sub-doshas are Prana, Udana, Samana, Apana, and Vyana (Figure 13.3).

Prana Vata is located above the clavicle and is responsible for bringing awareness, consciousness, creativity, and enthusiasm to the physiology. Particularly, Sthapani, Seemanta, and Adhipathi marmas are responsible for maintaining the balance of Prana Vata.

Udana Vata is located in the throat area and is responsible for bringing expressions, speaking, balancing the thyroid gland, and blood flow to the brain. Neela, Manya, and Sira Matrika marma points are responsible for bringing those benefits.

Samana Vata is situated in the stomach and intestines and is responsible for supporting the proper balance and support of the digestive process. The specific marma points, Nabhi and Apasthambha, are responsible for maintaining the balance.

Apana Vata is located in the pelvic area, lower extremities, and lower back. It is responsible for elimination, menstruation, delivery of fetus, and seminal flow or ejaculation. Nabhi, Basti, Vitapa, and Lohitaksha marma are essential for maintaining the balance.

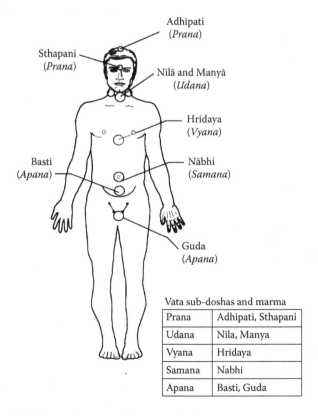

Vata sub-doshas and marma	
Prana	Adhipati, Sthapani
Udana	Nila, Manya
Vyana	Hridaya
Samana	Nabhi
Apana	Basti, Guda

FIGURE 13.3   Vata sub-doshas and marma points.

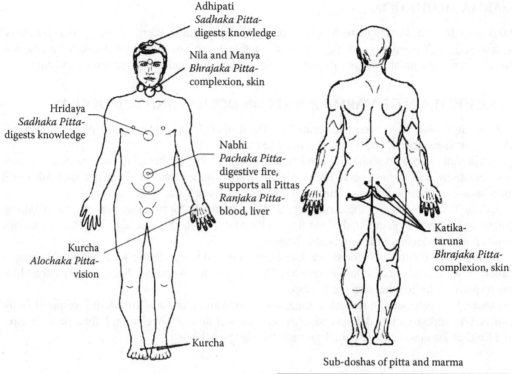

Adhipati
Sadhaka Pitta-
digests knowledge

Nila and Manya
Bhrajaka Pitta-
complexion, skin

Hridaya
Sadhaka Pitta-
digests knowledge

Nabhi
Pachaka Pitta-
digestive fire,
supports all Pittas
Ranjaka Pitta-
blood, liver

Kurcha
Alochaka Pitta-
vision

Kurcha

**Katika-
taruna**
Bhrajaka Pitta-
complexion, skin

Sub-doshas of pitta and marma

Sub pitta dosha	Marma	
Sadhaka	Hridaya, Adhipati	
Bhrajaka	Nila and Manya Katik tarun	
Pachaka	Nabhi	
Alochaka	Kurcha (Right great toe for spleen) Talahridaya	Kurchashira (Left great toe for liver)
Ranjaka	Nabhi	

FIGURE 13.4 Pitta sub-doshas and marma points.

Vyana Vata is located in the heart and all over the body, and its function is providing proper circulation to the entire body. The main points for Vyana Vata, Hrudaya, Lohitaksha, and Tala Hrudaya help provide proper circulation to the body.

There are 5 sub-doshas of Pitta—Pachaka, Ranjaka, Sadhaka, Alochaka, and Bhrajaka (Figure 13.4).

Pachaka Pitta is responsible for digestion and metabolism of food, and is located in the stomach. The marma points Nabhi and Apasthamba are responsible for maintaining proper functioning of Pachaka Pitta.

Ranjaka Pitta is located in the liver and spleen and is responsible for digestion of fats and maintaining hemoglobin levels. The marmas related to Ranjaka Pitta are Apasthamba and Nabhi.

Sadhaka Pitta is located in the heart and balances circulation and emotions. The responsible marma points are Hrudaya, Sthana Moola, and Sthana Rohita.

Alochaka Pitta is located in the eyes and is responsible for vision. The marma points Shanka, Apanga, Avartha, and Sthapani maintain and restore proper vision.

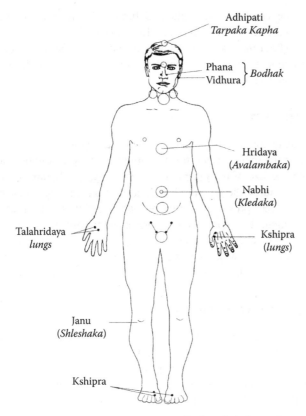

Kapha sub-doshas and marma points

Kapha sub-dosha	Marma	Comment
Tarpaka	Adhipati	Brain CNS
Avalambaka	Talahridaya/Hridaya	Heart—lungs
Kledaka	Nabhi/Apasthambha	Related to digestion
Bodhaka	Vidhura/Phana	Related to smell
Shleshaka	Janu	Many synovial bursae

FIGURE 13.5   Kapha sub-doshas and marma points.

Bhrajaka Pitta is located all over the skin and is responsible for proper nourishment and coloration of skin tissue. The marma points responsible for the skin are Hrudaya, Lohitaksha, Indra Basti, Apalapa, and Tala Hrudaya.

The 5 sub-doshas of Kapha are: Kledaka, Avalambaka, Bodhaka, Tarpaka, and Sleshaka (Figure 13.5).

Kledaka Kapha is located in the stomach and is responsible for initial digestion and metabolism of carbohydrates and moistening of food. The marma points responsible for assimilation of food are Nabhi and Apasthamba.

Avalambaka Kapha is located in the pericardium and protects the heart and balances the emotions. The marma points Hrudaya, Sthana Moola, Sthana Rohita, and Apalapa are responsible for proper nourishment of the heart and surrounding tissues.

Bodhaka Kapha is located in the mouth and is responsible for salivary secretions and supports the taste. The marma point responsible for these functions is Shringataka.

Tarpaka Kapha is located in the cerebrospinal fluid and brain. The related marma points Adhipathi, Seemantha, and Shamka are responsible for nourishment of brain tissues.

Sleshaka Kapha is located throughout the body, particularly in the joints, and is responsible for proper lubrication of joints and ligaments. The main marma points are Manibhanda, Koorpara, Lohitaksha, Kakshadhara, Gulpha, and Janu.

TECHNIQUE OF MARMA THERAPY

Ayurvedic practitioners use various techniques to balance the marma points. It is very important to keep a subtle and gentle touch on the marma point for maximum efficacy. In my practice, I use one or more fingers, depending on the size of the marma point. Initially, the therapy starts with a light touch, and gradually over 2–3 minutes, the pressure is increased to a firm touch of each marma point. Some marma points require direct pressure, and some marma points need circular movements. In general, a clockwise movement stimulates and invigorates the marma point, while a counterclockwise movement breaks up the blocked or congested energy within the marma point. After performing both clockwise and counterclockwise movements on the marma point, we must stabilize the energy by placing either one or two fingers on the marma point for a minimum of 1 minute.

CLINICAL APPLICATION OF MARMA THERAPY

Marma therapy is a unique therapy performed by Ayurvedic physicians from time immemorial, which offers tremendous healing benefits for modern chronic health problems. For example, for sinusitis condition, the specific marma points of Phana, Sthapani, Shanka, Apanga, and Avartha are stimulated to alleviate the symptoms of sinus problems and sinus allergies. A deep understanding of anatomy and physiology is required to correctly perform and administer marma therapy. Marma therapy can be learned hands-on under the guidance of a qualified ayurvedic physician who is well trained in marma therapy (Figure 13.6).

In my Ayurvedic practice, I see various chronic illnesses, including bronchial asthma, chronic sinusitis, varied neurological conditions, insomnia, and menstrual to menopausal conditions. After

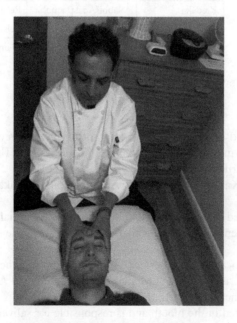

FIGURE 13.6   The author performing marma therapy in his practice.

performing marma therapy for a particular ailment, I administer herbal modalities—application of turmeric, boswellia, ginger, and cinnamon paste on particular marma points to relieve pressure and alleviate pain and tenderness. I also provide clients with certain herbal decoction teas according to their individual imbalances of doshas. The Ayurvedic herbs and herbal formulations are classified according to doshas. These herbs and herbal compound preparations alleviate symptoms and help to rectify the deep-seated imbalances in the tissues.

BENEFITS OF MARMA THERAPY

- Clears the channels of circulation—*srotas*
- Connects to consciousness
- Creates equilibrium of doshas
- Enhances alertness
- Enhances digestion and metabolism
- Enhances energy levels
- Enhances sexual energy
- Enhances tactile sensation
- Facilitates balanced release of waste products (*malas*)
- Improves attention span
- Improves breathing and heart rates
- Improves immune system
- Improves lymphatic circulation
- Improves meditation practice
- Improves memory
- Improves rejuvenation
- Increases emotional balance
- Increases pain tolerance
- Induces natural state of sleep
- Induces the easy flow of energy through the channels of circulation
- Maintains balance of mind–body–spirit
- Maintains homeostasis
- Nourishes and nurtures the body
- Produces deep relaxation
- Reduces blood pressure
- Regenerates tissue metabolism
- Relieves physical and mental blockages of energy
- Removes ama (endotoxins)
- Slows the aging process
- Strengthens the organ systems
- Supports proper development of tissues (*dhatus*)

Marma therapy as an ancient science offers immeasurable value to integrative medicine physicians and allied health practitioners today as a non-invasive modality for wellness and disease prevention. The incorporation of various Ayurvedic protocols, specifically marma therapy, improves individuals' overall health and consciousness of maintaining wellness, thereby contributing to the strength of communities and societies at a fundamental level.

14 Chinese Medicine and Acupuncture

Yemeng Chen

CONTENTS

Introduction 357
Philosophy of Chinese Medicine 357
Modalities of Chinese Medicine 358
    Chinese Herbology 358
    Tui Na (Chinese Manipulative Therapy) 359
    Chinese Dietary Therapy 359
    Energetic Exercises 360
Acupuncture 360
Chinese Medicine in an Integrative Way 361
References 361

INTRODUCTION

Chinese medicine is the science of healing based on the ancient philosophy of Taoism, Yin-Yang, and Five Phases. It provides a unique method of understanding human health, dysfunction, and disease through holistic approaches. Chinese medicine emphasizes maintaining a dynamic balance among body, mind, and spirit. This discipline acts to prevent and treat illnesses and diseases through its own integrated system of human physiology, pathology, and diagnosis. As an important aspect of Chinese culture, Chinese medicine evolved into a specialized system of medical theory through thousands of years of clinical practice under the influence and direction of ancient philosophy.

Traditional Chinese medicine (TCM) is another term that is commonly used when relating to Chinese medicine. In the United States, TCM sometimes refers to a style of practice characterized by modern approaches used by practitioners who studied Chinese medicine in Chinese medical colleges after 1956. In 2002, the White House Commission on Complementary and Alternative Medicine Policy designated TCM as an alternative healthcare system.[1] TCM is now listed as a complementary health approach by the National Center of Complementary and Integrative Health (NCCIH), under the National Institutes of Health (NIH).[2]

PHILOSOPHY OF CHINESE MEDICINE

Chinese medicine is grounded in the ancient philosophical concepts of Taoism, Yin-Yang, and Five Phases. It believes that the universe is in a constant dynamic balance and harmony between Yin and Yang, two opposing forces or energetic fields, and that the human body is a miniature version of this larger universe. The balance of Yin-Yang is the basis of health.

As translated by Paul U. Unschuld and Hermann Tessenow, *Yellow Emperor's Inner Classic*, the first completed work on Chinese medicine, states:

> *As for yin and yang, they are the Way of heaven and earth, the fundamental principles [governing] the myriad beings, father and mother to all changes and transformations, the basis and beginning of generating life and killing, the palace of spirit brilliance. To treat diseases, one must search for the basis.*[3]

Chinese medicine also utilizes the Five Phases theory, which describes the interactions between the basic elements of life: water, wood, fire, earth, and metal. These elements also symbolize all phenomena in the body such as organs, tissues, body fluids, functional activities, emotions, pathogenic factors, symptoms, and exterior presentations.

The key to Chinese medicine is its holistic view. Unity exists between the human body and the natural universe. The human body's close connection with nature is manifested by the fact that humans live in nature which provides conditions that are indispensable to humans' survival. Natural changes may influence the human body directly or indirectly, thereby causing a corresponding response. Holism also embraces the unity within the human body itself. The body is an integral whole composed of a variety of tissues and organs. Although each tissue and organ performs a specific function, they are inseparable and are conditioned by one another in physiology and interact with each other in pathology.

In the practice of Chinese medicine, diagnosis and therapeutic strategies are based on an overall analysis of syndromes (*zheng*). *Zheng*, which means comprehensive pattern differentiation, is not a mere combination of symptoms but a pathological generalization of diseases and disorders that takes into consideration their stage, location, etiology, nature, and the relationship between the body's resistance and pathological agents.

TCM differs from Western medicine in its fundamental principle of determining therapeutic protocols based on comprehensive pattern differentiation, also known as differential diagnosis, when recognizing and treating diseases and disorders. Principles such as "treating the same disease with different methods" or "treating different diseases with the same method" were established based on this pattern differentiation. For example, two asthma patients could have different patterns depending on their constitutions and symptoms. Therefore, their treatment approaches would be different. On the other hand, Western medicine may consider two symptoms as unrelated, whereas they may have the same pattern according to Chinese medicine. For example, a 50-year-old woman complains of dry eyes and blurred vision, easily-broken fingernails, and irregular menstrual cycles. Based on Chinese medicine, these four symptoms all fit the pattern differentiation of "liver blood deficiency." A treatment plan derived from the root pattern will aid in the alleviation of all the above-mentioned symptoms.

MODALITIES OF CHINESE MEDICINE

Chinese medicine modalities include Chinese herbology, acupuncture, *tuina* (Chinese manipulative therapy), dietary therapy, and energetic exercises such as *tai chi* and *qi gong*. Acupuncture will be introduced in a separate section due to its more prevalent use in the United States.

CHINESE HERBOLOGY

Chinese herbology is based on Chinese medicine's fundamental philosophies and theories and also utilizes its own unique principles. Chinese herbs are derived from natural resources such as botanicals (most common), minerals, and animal products for medicinal use. Historically, Chinese herbal medicine has been the main healthcare system in China for thousands of years. Over the course of several millennia, different specialties of practice developed with rich literature describing Chinese herbology's therapeutic effects in areas such as internal medicine, external medicine, gynecology, pediatrics, traumatology, ENT (ear, nose, and throat), optometry, oral disorders, and so on.

Compared to any other system of herbal practice, Chinese herbology has the most extensively studied, organized, and defined material medica beyond just empirical cases. The herbs are individually characterized by their properties (cold, hot, cool, and warm), tastes (sour, bitter, sweet, pungent, and salty), and the meridians that they enter. The characteristics are a summary of an herb's functions and multiple therapeutic actions. According to Yin-Yang and Five Phases theory, herbs rebalance the body by utilizing the above-mentioned characteristics to treat pathogenic factors.

Herbal formula composition is another key aspect of Chinese medicine. Herbal prescriptions are created by combining different herbs to act as the chief, deputy, assistant, or envoy ingredient. This design enhances therapeutic effects, promotes herbal interactions, moderates herbal properties, and/or regulates toxicities.

Although an herbal decoction's taste is often unpleasant, there are less side effects due to the herbs' harmonious and cooperative actions. In addition to decoction, many other forms of herbal products exist such as pills, tablets, powders, syrups, plasters, tinctures, and so on. Currently, concentrated powders are the most convenient and widely used form.

Contemporary herbal pharmaceutical research is advanced. Chemical components with therapeutic effects are extracted from raw herbs to create new drugs. In 2015, Dr. Youyou Tu won the Nobel Prize in Physiology or Medicine because of her extraordinary research on artemisinin, an extract from the Chinese herb *Qing Hao* (*Artemisia carvifolia*), which inhibits the malaria parasite. This extract became a novel therapy against malaria and aided in saving and improving the health of millions of people.[4]

In the United States, Chinese herbs are listed as dietary supplements under the Dietary Supplement Health & Education Act (DSHEA) of 1994. Thus far, 22 states have included Chinese herbology into the scope of practice of acupuncturists. Despite this, Chinese herbology faces many challenges including overdose and inappropriate use (e.g., ephedra and Chinese herbal products containing aristolochic acid). In addition to ensuring herbal quality and safety, the protection of both botanical and animal endangered species is important to today's society.

Tui Na (Chinese Manipulative Therapy)

Tui Na is a special therapeutic method for external treatment based on the principles of Chinese medicine as well as acupoints and meridian theory. Although the name means pushing and pulling, Tui Na mainly manipulates and stimulates acupoints, meridian pathways, and other surface areas on the body by practitioners without the application of any herbs or medications. Tui Na is typically performed after acupuncture treatment to enhance both modalities' therapeutic effects, especially for musculoskeletal disorders.

Tui Na is not only limited to treating musculoskeletal disorders but is also effective for both chronic or acute internal organ disorders and gynecological problems. Infant Tui Na is a unique form of therapy which utilizes special points and manipulations to treat different conditions found in babies and toddlers. Expecting mothers can learn infant Tui Na techniques to perform by themselves in times of need. The most common indications for infant Tui Na treatment include indigestion, diarrhea, torticollis, and so on.

Tui Na is often mistaken as a form of massage even though its concept, techniques, and stimulating areas are drastically different. Although other forms of manipulative therapy, such as Shiatsu and Amma, are similar, they are not identical to Tui Na. Tui Na's numerous techniques and methods include acupressure, a commonly used form of treatment. Although, Tui Na is not individually licensed in the United States, licensed acupuncturists can legally practice most forms of Tui Na.

Chinese Dietary Therapy

Chinese dietary therapy is a healthy way of eating based on an understanding of the different effects of food on the human body. Having the same concept as Chinese herbology, all foods are classified into different categories based on their properties such as warm, cool, hot, and cold. Different foods are recommended according to an individual's constitution and state of health to help rebalance and restore the body's energy and functions.

Despite herbs and food deriving from the same natural resources, dietary therapy's effects are mild and cannot fully replace herbs for therapeutic purposes. However, dietary therapy is very important for everyday health and well-being. Due to different cultural practices and preferences, dietary therapy is most applicable for Chinese or East-Asian communities.

ENERGETIC EXERCISES

Qi Gong is a way of energy cultivation through the coordination of body posture and movement, breathing, and meditation. Although there are many diversified forms of Qi Gong, all forms emphasize promoting harmony and balance among the body, mind, and spirit. According to research, Qi Gong provides health benefits for cancer survivors and patients with chronic pain, stress, anxiety, and hypertension.[5–8]

Tai Chi, another form of energetic exercise, is popular in the United States. Data from the 2012 National Health Interview Survey (n = 34,525) showed that the lifetime and 12-month prevalence of Tai Chi/Qi Gong practice were 3.1% and 1.2%, respectively.[9] Recent studies demonstrate that Tai Chi exercises help Parkinson's Disease patients with balance and fall prevention, postmenopausal women with bone health, and fibromyalgia patients in dealing with musculoskeletal pain, depression, and attaining a better quality of life.[10–13]

ACUPUNCTURE

Acupuncture is a healing art that employs Chinese medicine theory, especially Meridian Theory, to insert needles into acupoints, specific points on the body, accompanied with manipulation and/or stimulation with pressure, heat, light, or electricity. In recent years, new acupuncture treatment principles have developed based on anatomical structure, such as dry needling. Despite its similarity to *Ashi Point Puncture*, which has been used for thousands of years, dry needling is a standalone method and also belongs under acupuncture's scope of practice. The original modality was called "acupuncture and moxibustion." Moxibustion, also known as moxa, is the application of burning mugwort toward acupuncture points on the body, either individually or in addition to acupuncture needles. Since the burning herb creates smoke, it is restricted in office buildings with central air conditioning and fire alarm systems.

Since the 1970s, acupuncture has been legally regulated by and practiced in 47 states and the District of Columbia. In 1997, the National Institutes of Health sponsored a landmark Consensus Development Conference, during which the panel concluded: "Acupuncture may be effective as an adjunct therapy, an acceptable alternative, or as part of a comprehensive treatment program…The data in supporting acupuncture is as strong as those for many accepted western medical therapies. One of the advantages of acupuncture is that the incidence of adverse effects is substantially lower than that of many drugs or other accepted medical procedures used for the same conditions." The conference also posted research-backed indications, where acupuncture was found to have therapeutic effects on such indications as addiction, stroke rehabilitation, headache, menstrual cramps, tennis elbow, fibromyalgia (general muscle pain), low back pain, carpal tunnel syndrome, and asthma.[14]

It is clear that the efficacy of acupuncture is more far reaching than the above-mentioned conditions. In 2003, the World Health Organization published a report on acupuncture clinical trials in which more than 100 indications were discussed and divided into four groups according to the strength of existing evidence.[15] Acupuncture is well known for its therapeutic effect of pain management. One systemic review was conducted to identify randomized controlled trials (RCTs) of acupuncture for chronic pain in which allocation concealment was determined unambiguously to be adequate. Individual patient data meta-analyses were conducted using data from 29 of 31 eligible RCTs, totaling 17,922 patient cases. This review indicated the significant differences between true and sham acupuncture and concluded that acupuncture is effective for the treatment of chronic pain. Therefore, acupuncture is not just a placebo effect but a reasonable referral option for pain management.[16]

Acupuncture is recommended for both acute and chronic low back pain (LBP) as one of the first lines of therapy recommended by the Clinical Practice Guidelines from the American College of Physicians (ACP). Treatment for acute LBP, pain that lasts less than 3 months, includes heat, massage, acupuncture, or spinal manipulation. For chronic LBP, pain that lasts more than 3 months, treatments are exercise, rehabilitation, acupuncture, mindfulness stress reduction, tai chi, yoga, and so on.[17]

In 2014, a paper published in *The Journal of the American Medical Association* that was criticized for its rationale, stated that the authors' research findings do not support laser or needle acupuncture for moderate or severe chronic knee pain.[18,19] A recent landmark study concluded that acupuncture provides pain relief and improves the functional abilities of people with osteoarthritis of the knee and serves as an effective complement to standard care. This study, the largest Phase III clinical trial of acupuncture for knee osteoarthritis, was funded by the National Center for Complementary and Integrative Health (NCCIH) and the National Institute of Arthritis and Musculoskeletal and Skin Diseases, both components of the National Institutes of Health.[20]

Besides pain management, acupuncture has been applied to treat mental-emotional disorders, women's health, and cancer survivors supporting care. According to the Memorial Sloan-Kettering Cancer Center's Integrative Medicine Service, symptoms commonly experienced by cancer patients that may be treated with acupuncture include dyspnea, post-chemotherapy chronic fatigue, chemotherapy-related nausea and vomiting, xerostomia, lymphedema, hot flashes, postoperative ileus in colon cancer patients, pain, dysfunction, and so on.[21,22]

In 2005, the American Medical Association issued four current procedural terminology (CPT) codes for acupuncture and electro-acupuncture, which make it possible for third-party reimbursement of acupuncture.[23] On May 10, 2017, the Food and Drug Administration (FDA) released proposed changes to its blueprint on educating healthcare providers about treating pain. The guideline recommends that doctors be knowledgeable about and, when appropriate, refer patients to acupuncture and chiropractic care as complementary therapies that might help avoid long-term opioid prescriptions in pain management.[24] It is foreseeable that acupuncture has the potential and will continue to advance into other clinical fields as endorsed by the FDA.

CHINESE MEDICINE IN AN INTEGRATIVE WAY

Although Chinese medicine has over 3000 years of practice and heritage, it has become integrated into the contemporary healthcare system since its philosophy and therapeutic values have become more accepted and recognized by Western society. Integrative medicine is an increasing trend in healthcare, encouraged by the Institute of Medicine, a branch of the Academy of Science, and pioneered in several world-renowned medical centers. Integrative medicine provides care that is patient-centered, healing oriented, emphasizes therapeutic relationships, and uses therapeutic approaches originating from conventional medicine and alternative medicine.[25] Both conventional medicine and Chinese medicine practitioners should understand each other's modalities and use one another's strengths to find the best treatment plan for patient care. For example, acupuncture has become more involved with in-vitro fertilization procedures after a German study showed that concurrent acupuncture treatments increased the success rate of IVF from 26.3% to 42.5%.[26] Special protocols have now been established for acupuncture treatments along different phases of the IVF process.

Chinese medicine is trying to establish a common language to better communicate with fellow healthcare providers in a multidisciplinary setting. This will also enable Chinese medicine to engage in more evidence-based research to ensure its accuracy and efficacy and to meet contemporary needs while keeping its philosophical essence and foundation.

REFERENCES

1. White House Commission on Complementary and Alternative Medicine Policy. *Final Report*, March 2002, P. 9. https://ods.od.nih.gov/Health_Information/White_House_CAM_Commission.aspx.
2. https://nccih.nih.gov/health/whatiscam/chinesemed.htm.
3. Unschuld PU and Tessenow H. 2011. *Huang Di Nei Jing Su Wen: An Annotated Translation on Huang Di's Inner Classic—Basic Questions*. Berkeley, CA, and London: University of California Press.
4. https://www.nobelprize.org/nobel_prizes/medicine/laureates/2015/tu-facts.html.

5. Fong SS, Choi AW, Luk WS et al. 2016. Bone mineral density, balance performance, balance self-efficacy, and falls in breast cancer survivors with and without qigong training. *Integr Cancer Ther* Dec 1:1534735416686687.

6. Holmberg C, Farahani Z, and CWitt CM. 2016. How do patients with chronic neck pain experience the effects of qigong and exercise therapy? A qualitative interview study. *Evid Based Complement Alternat Med* 2016: Article ID 8010891.

7. Wang CW, Chan CH, Ho RT et al. 2014. Managing stress and anxiety through qigong exercise in healthy adults: A systematic review and meta-analysis of randomized controlled trials. *BMC Complement Altern Med* Jan 9;14:8.

8. Xiong X, Wang P, Li X et al. 2015. Qigong for hypertension: A systematic review. *Medicine* 94(1):1–14.

9. Lauche R, Wayne PM, Dobos G et al. 2016. Prevalence, patterns, and predictors of T'ai Chi and Qigong use in the United States: Results of a nationally representative survey. *J Altern Complement Med* 22(4):336–42.

10. Li F, Harmer P, and Fitzgerald K. 2012. Tai Chi and Postural stability in patients with Parkinson's disease. *N Engl J Med* 366:511–519.

11. Shen C-L, Chyu M-C, Pence BC et al. 2010. Green tea polyphenols supplementation and tai chi exercise for postmenopausal osteopenic women: Safety and quality of life report. *BMC Complement Altern Med* 10(1):76.

12. Wang C, Schmid CH, Rones R et al. 2010. A randomized trial of tai chi for fibromyalgia. *N Engl J Med* 363(8):743–754.

13. Yeh GY, Kaptchuk TJ, and Shmerling RH. 2010. Prescribing tai chi for fibromyalgia—are we there yet? *N Engl J Med* 363(8):783–784.

14. NIH Consensus Development Panel on Acupuncture. 1998. Acupuncture. *JAMA* 280(17):1518–24.

15. http://apps.who.int/medicinedocs/pdf/s4926e/s4926e.pdf.

16. Vickers AJ, Cromin AM, Maschino AC et al. 2012. Acupuncture for chronic pain: Individual patients data meta-analysis. *Arch Intern Med* 172(19):1444–53.

17. Berman BM, Lao L, Langenberg P et al. 2004. Effectiveness of acupuncture as adjunctive therapy in osteoarthritis of the knee: A randomized, controlled trial. *Ann Intern Med* 141(12):901910.

18. Hinman RS, McCrory P, Marie Pirotta M et al. 2014. Acupuncture for chronic knee pain a randomized clinical trial. *JAMA* 312(13):1313–22.

19. Fan Y, Zhou K, Gu S et al. 2016. Acupuncture is effective for chronic knee pain: A reanalysis of the Australian acupuncture trial. *Altern Ther Health Med* 22(3):32–36.

20. Qaseem A, Wilt TJ, McLean RM et al. 2017. Noninvasive treatments for acute, subacute, and chronic low back pain: A clinical practice guideline from the American college of physicians. *Ann Intern Med* 166(7):514–530.

21. Javdan B and Cassileth B. 2015. Acupuncture research at Memorial Sloan Kettering Cancer Center. *J Acupunct Meridian Stud* 8(3):115–121.

22. Deng GE, Cassileth BR, Cohen L et al. 2007. Integrative oncology practice guidelines. *J Soc Integr Oncol* 5(2):65–84.

23. Wells D. 2005. New CPT codes for acupuncture are here! *Acupuncture Today* 6(2):16–17, 19.

24. https://www.fda.gov/downloads/Drugs/NewsEvents/UCM557071.pdfone.

25. Maizes V, Rakel D, and Niemiec C. 2009. Integrative medicine and patient-centered care. *Explore* 5(5):277–89.

26. Paulus WE, Zhang M, Strehler E et al. 2002. Influence of acupuncture on the pregnancy rate in patients who undergo assisted reproduction therapy. *Ferti Steril* 77(4):721–4.

15 Yoga and Healing
Yogic Asanas, Breath, Mudras, and Their Relation to Human Anatomy and Subtle Anatomy

Virender Sodhi

CONTENTS

Definition of Yoga 364
Philosophy of Yoga 364
Yoga in the United States 365
My Fascination with Yoga...366
Yoga and Heart..366
Yoga Reverses Arterial Stiffness 368
Yoga and Gastroesophageal Reflux Disease 368
Yoga and Irritable Bowel Syndrome (IBS) 369
Yoga and Diabetes...371
Yoga and Depression and Anxiety 373
Yoga and Sickle Cell Anemia 374
Yoga and Eating Disorders..374
Yoga and Arthritis 375
Yoga and Asthma 376
Yoga and Cystic Fibrosis 378
Yoga and PMS...379
Yoga and Homocysteine..379
Yoga and Endometriosis 380
Yoga and Menopause 380
Yoga and Hormones..381
Yoga and PCOS...382
Yoga and Cancer 382
Yoga during Chemotherapy 383
Yoga and Osteoporosis..384
Yoga and Obesity 385
Yoga and Hypothyroidism 385
Yoga and Post-Traumatic Stress Syndrome 386
Yoga and Insomnia..386
Yoga and Autism...387
Left and Right Nostril Variations 387
References 388

Yoga means union. It is derived from the Sanskrit word, *Yuj*, which means "to join"; join the body with the mind or in other words "create harmony between the body and the mind." The aim of yoga is to create a union between the individual and his or her true self. Yogic practices are very ancient, and the first written book of the world, *Rig Veda*, mentioned the yogic practices. Yoga is a science. It is based on timeless scientific principles that are beyond the understanding of current scientific thought. It is science that needs to catch up with yoga. Yoga does not need to catch up with science as it is understood today. Still, the goal of this chapter is to present an understanding of yoga using the current scientific paradigm, to set a framework for future research into yoga and to give clinicians an outline of how yoga can be used to help heal many chronic diseases of the body and mind for which western medicine has no effective cure.

DEFINITION OF YOGA

Yoga is defined in the *Yoga Sutras* by Patanjali as the quieting of the mind by restraint of the agitation of thoughts. Continuous thinking keeps us stuck in an endless loop. Yoga helps create space for the mind to step outside of the endless loop of thoughts, which in turn brings harmony to the body and the life of the person practicing yoga in its true form.

PHILOSOPHY OF YOGA

Around the third century BC, Patanjali systematized the yoga practices, and rooted the philosophy of yoga based on the Samkhya School of Philosophy. He narrated the yoga sutras. Sound mind in a sound body is what yoga stands for. Patanjali first mentioned *Ashtanga* yoga or eight limbs of yoga, namely: (1) Yama; (2) Niyama; (3) Asana; (4) Pranayama; (5) Pratyahara; (6) Dharana; (7) Dhyana; and (8) Samadhi.

1. *Yama*: The first limb of yoga symbolizes ethical morals of yoga. The five yamas include the following: *ahimsa* or nonviolence; *satya* or truthfulness; *asteya* or non-stealing; *brahmacharya* or abstinence; and *aparigraha* or non-greedy or non-covetousness.
2. *Niyama*: The second limb of yoga is associated with self-discipline and spiritual rituals. For example, following a routinely meditation practice is a *niyama*. The five *niyamas* are: *saucha* or purity; *samtosa* or happiness or contented; *tapas* or asceticism or spiritual rigor; *svadhyaya* or study of the holy scriptures and your own inner self; and *isvara pranidhana* or surrendering yourself to divinity.
3. *Asana*: The third limb of yoga represents the physical postures of yoga practice. Via asana practice, we acquire order and proficiency of concentration, which is necessary for the preparation of meditation.
4. *Pranayama*: The fourth limb of yoga unites the breath of life with mind and sensations. The word pranayama means extension of prana or life force. Pranayama invigorates the body and promotes longevity.
5. *Pratyahara*: The fifth limb of yoga means withdrawal from external stimulus. We practice transcendence of the senses by exercising detachment. We practice withdrawal from those factors of life which are injurious to our health and well-being.
6. *Dharana*: The sixth limb of yoga refers to concentration or intention. Dharana comes before meditation. This custom entails slowing down thoughts by concentrating on one object perceptually such as a photo of a God or Goddess. Other examples of dharana include silent recital of a mantra or giving awareness to an energetic chakra in the body.
7. *Dhyana*: The seventh limb of yoga is meditation or reflection. It is a natural flow of concentration. Whereas dharana practices one-pointed awareness, dhyana is a state of awareness apart from concentration. Your mind is silent, as no thoughts exist in the mind during meditation or dhyana.

8. *Samadhi*: The eighth limb of yoga is bliss or ecstasy. Here, the practice allows a human to unite and transcend the self with the universe.

According to Samkhya philosophy, the mind rides on five horses of five senses. It is very difficult to bring control over all five senses if you are not in balance. The yoga practices override these five sensual experiences, and peek through a different sense and establish a connection with the whole universe. That is the gist of yoga.

Patanjali collected all the Vedic and the Upanishadic literature around 300 BC, and turned them into yoga sutras or the threads of yoga. Sutra means thread. Neither the yoga techniques nor the philosophy were his original contributions. He just collected and published the yoga sutras. Patanjali mainly used Samkhya philosophy, and he adapted it to yoga and meditation. That's why the yoga and Samkhya philosophies are so similar. Samkhya philosophy gives us the goal and yoga philosophy helps us to attain that goal.

YOGA IN THE UNITED STATES

Yoga was brought to the West by Swami Vivekananda in 1893, when he came to deliver a lecture at the World Parliament of Religions in Chicago. His famous speech where he addressed the "sisters and brothers of America" attracted a huge population. The audience were so impressed that they all gave him a standing ovation. This started the love affair of West with the East. There was a steady flow of Eastern influence on the West thereafter.

In 1920, Paramahansa Yogananda came in to address a conference of Religious Liberals in Boston. He was sent by his guru, the ageless Babaji, to spread the message of Kriya Yoga to the West. In 1924, the United States government imposed an immigration ban, and there was a quota of Indian immigrants coming into the United States. At that time, the westerners travelled to India to seek the teachings. One of the earliest was Theos Burnett, who returned from India in 1947, and published the *Hatha Yoga*, a report of his personal experience. It was a major source of yoga in the 1950s and is still read.

In the early 1950s, Indra Devi opened a yoga studio in Hollywood. She was a follower of Shri Krishnamacharya, who was the first to bring his lineage to the West, and whose students included B.K.S. Iyengar and T.K.V. Desikachar. An early American to introduce yoga to the United States was Richard Hittleman, who in 1950 returned from India, and taught yoga in New York. He sold millions of copies of his books, and he also pioneered yoga on the television in 1961. He became a trendsetter for yoga in the United States. He was a student of sage Ramana Maharshi.

Yoga was established in the West Coast in the mid-1950s with Walt and Magana Baptiste's San Francisco studio. Walt's father had been influenced by Vivekananda, and Walt and Magana were students of Yogananda.

In 1958, Indian-born Swami Vishnudevananda, who was a disciple of Swami Sivananda Saraswati, was sponsored by artist Peter Max. His book, *The Complete Illustrated Book of Yoga*, was published in 1960, and became an essential guidebook for many practitioners in the West. He founded Sivananda Yoga Vedanta Center, which is one of the largest networks of yoga schools in the world.

In the early 1960s, Maharishi Mahesh Yogi began teaching Transcendental Meditation (TM), and he trained almost 40,000 teachers in TM. He has reached out to more than 4 million practitioners in over 100 countries. He founded more than 1,000 TM centers worldwide.

In 1966, B.K.S. Iyengar published the book, *Light on Yoga*, in the United States. Iyengar publicized yoga in India and all around the world. He was the founder of Iyengar yoga, a style of hatha yoga.

In 1965, the U.S. law was modified, and the Indian immigration opened. In 1966, Yogi Amrit Desai founded the Yoga Society of Pennsylvania, and later, Kripalu Yoga Ashram. Also, Swami Rama established his foundation in the 1970s. In 1966, Swami Satchidananda, another Swami

Sivananda disciple, arrived in New York, and ended up staying permanently. His Internal Yoga Institute had more than 40 branches worldwide. Satchidananda opened the Woodstock Festival in 1969 echoing Vivekananda's greeting of "my beloved sisters and brothers" 75 years later, looking like an aging hippie himself with flowing hair and a beard. He provided a living example of life dedicated to spirit.

By the 1970s, the yoga and spiritual teachings were taught almost all over the United States. Baba Hari Dass founded Mount Madonna Center in California, to provide a residential yoga program in the 1970s. In 1975, the first issue of *Yoga Journal* was published. This is a brief history of yoga in the United States.

MY FASCINATION WITH YOGA

My interest in yoga started as a young child. I was encouraged by my parents to explore yoga. My mom used to do yoga herself, and she would teach us simple yoga postures at home. My father was very keen about pranayama. He used to talk to us about pranayama, and how the pranayama has amazing powers to heal almost every disease.

When I went to medical school, I certainly got deeper into yoga, and started learning from our teacher. Since then I have continued my practice of yoga on a daily basis. I have found it to have a profound effect on my personal health. I used to have asthma myself, and after practicing yoga for almost four to five months, my asthma completely went away. And this is around 30 years ago. I have had amazing success in my allergies. The practice of yoga helped me to get my allergies under control. When I was a student at medical college, I was a part of a power lifting team and weight lifting team, and injured my back. Later, I discovered that I have spondylolisthesis, but my yogic practices kept me moving. Yet, even today, I can do all my postures, and I am very active. I garden. I go walking. I go hiking. I do weight training to keep my muscle mass fit. I contribute my fitness to my yogic practices.

In my medical practice for 36 years, one of my key elements of healing has been assigning my patients yogic practices of pranayama (breathing exercises), and simple yogic postures. I found that by doing simple yogic practices, patients have amazing success from diabetes to rheumatoid arthritis to insomnia, even cancer.

I began considering research that has been published regarding yoga, breathing exercises, and meditation. I was surprised to find there was a lot of literature available on yogic practices and their amazing effects on health and well-being.

In the next sections, we will talk about the research on yoga regarding different health conditions.

YOGA AND HEART

Dr. Dean Ornish was the first to publish data on heart disease and lifestyle changes in showing the reversal of coronary artery disease. The Lifestyle Heart Trial was the first randomized clinical trial to investigate whether ambulatory patients could be motivated to make and sustain comprehensive lifestyle changes (yoga and stress reduction) and whether the progression of coronary atherosclerosis can be stopped or reversed without using lipid-lowering drugs, as measured by coronary arteriography. After one year, the experimental group was able to make and maintain an intensive lifestyle change. They had 37.2% reduction in the LDL cholesterol and 91% reduction in the frequency of anginal episodes. Average person time stenosis regressed from 40% at baseline to 37.8% after one year. In contrast, in the usual-care control group, the LDL level went up by 6%, and had 165% increase in the frequency of angina. Also, the stenosis increased from 42.7% to 46.1%. The study was extended for four more years, and the feasibility of patients maintaining intensive changes in diet and lifestyle for longer times was measured along with the effects of these changes on risk factors such as coronary atherosclerosis and other cardiac events (Ornish et al., 1998).

Data on the cardiac events were obtained from 48 patients. Cardiac events included myocardial infarction, coronary angioplasty, coronary artery bypass, surgical cardiac-related hospitalization, and cardiac-related death. At five years, there were more cardiac events in the control group, 45 for 20 patients or 2.0 per patient. In the experimental group, the number was 25 for 28 patients, almost 1.0 per patient. Control group patients were more likely to have undergone coronary angiography and bypass, and they were more likely to have been hospitalized for cardiac events than the experimental group (Ornish et al., 1998).

What was more notable in the study was that even after 5 years, there was less stenosis in the experimental group in contrast to the control group. There were twice as many cardiac events in the control rather than the experimental group. The LDL cholesterol level dropped by 40% the first year. By 5 years, there was a 20% reduction. And these results are very comparable to cholesterol lowering drugs. The frequency of angina reduced after 1 year, and it continued to sustain even after 5 years. After 5 years, there was a slight decrease in the diameter of the blood vessel whereas in the control group, it increased (Ornish et al., 1998).

In summary, after 5 years, with the diet and lifestyle changes, there was more regression of the coronary artery atherosclerosis, whereas in the control group, there was a progression of the coronary artery disease. There were twice as many cardiac events in the control group rather than in the experimental group. It demonstrated extraordinary results with the yoga and lifestyle changes. These experimental group patients were put on 10% vegetarian fat diet, moderate aerobic exercise, stress and management training like yoga, smoking cessation, and group psychological support. The control group was asked to follow the advice of their personal physician regarding their lifestyle changes (Ornish et al., 1998).

In a randomized control study, 40 patients (30% of them were females with heart failure) were randomized to have an intervention for 12 weeks, either doing yoga or hydrotherapy twice a week for 45–60 minutes. Evaluation was done at baseline and after 12 weeks with a self-reported health-related quality of life, a 6-minute walk test, a sit-to-stand test, and symptoms of anxiety and depression. Yoga therapy and hydrotherapy had an equal impact on the quality of life, exercise capacity, clinical outcome, and symptoms of anxiety and depression improved (Hagglund et al., 2017).

Patients in yoga groups significantly improved their health, as reported by the self-reported, health-related quality of life assessment. The symptoms of depression were decreased in the yoga therapy group. It was concluded that yoga might be an alternative or complementary choice to established styles of exercise training including hydrotherapy for improvement in health-related quality of life and may decrease depressive symptoms in heart failure patients. The findings confirmed previous studies demonstrating that yoga has the potential to balance both the physical and mental dimensions as well as be an alternative therapeutic exercise strategy in patients with heart failure (Hagglund et al., 2017).

In another study, effectiveness of personalized lifestyle interventions was determined for cardiovascular disease risk reduction. Using published literature on risk factor reduction via diverse lifestyle interventions—group therapy for "stopping smoking," Mediterranean diet, aerobic exercise (walking), and yoga—the risk reduction was calculated. Yoga was very effective with a large 10-year cardiovascular disease risk reduction. There was an absolute risk reduction of 16.7% in the highest risk individuals with yoga. Walking was ranked second with 11.4% risk reduction, followed by a Mediterranean diet (9.2%) and group therapy for "stopping smoking" (1.6%). You can see yoga was found to be one of the most effective forms of cardiovascular disease prevention. If you combine all the four factors such as yoga, walking, Mediterranean style diet, and "stopping smoking" strategies, the effects can be compounding (Chu et al., 2016).

In a randomized control study, 80 stable coronary artery disease patients below 65 years of age of both sexes were selected and randomized into two groups of 40 each. Group one was given a yoga regimen for 3 months, which consisted of yoga postures, pranayama breathing, exercise, and dietary modifications, along with their conventional medications. Group two only got conventional medicine. Lung function including diffusion capacity was recorded three times in both groups—the first day at the baseline, on the 22nd day, and the 90th day—with computerized cardio-respiratory instruments. The yoga regimen was found to enhance lung functions and diffusion capacity in coronary artery disease patients apart from improving cardiovascular functions. It was concluded that yoga can be used as a complementary therapy along with conventional medicine for treatment and rehabilitation (Yadav et al., 2015).

In another meta-analysis, 3,168 participants were included and the effects of yoga on modifiable biological cardiovascular disease risk factors was assessed. Yoga improved systolic blood pressure by 5.8 mm Hg and diastolic blood pressure by 4.12 mm Hg. Heart rate improved by 6.59 beats per minute. Respiratory rate was enhanced, and waist circumference was improved. The waist to hip ratio improved. The total cholesterol dropped. There was a drop of an average of 13.09 mg/dl of the total cholesterol. The HDL was increased. The LDL dropped. The triglycerides dropped by 20.97 mg/dl. There was an improvement in the glycated hemoglobin, and insulin resistance was reduced. The meta-analysis indicated evidence for clinically important effects of yoga on cardiovascular disease (Cramer et al., 2014).

YOGA REVERSES ARTERIAL STIFFNESS

Arterial stiffness is increasingly recognized as an important prognostic index and potential therapeutic target in patients with hypertension. It is closely linked to raised blood pressure, and its physiopathology is still not fully understood. Aortic stiffness and arterial pulse wave reflections are key determinants of elevated central systolic pressure and are associated with adverse cardiovascular outcomes, independent of blood pressure.

Forty-three (23 normal body mass index or BMI; 20 overweight/obese) apparently healthy participants completed an 8-week yoga intervention. Body composition was estimated via dual energy x-ray absorptiometry and arterial stiffness was measured via brachial ankle pulse wave velocity, and health-related quality of life was assessed via RAND 36-Item Short Form survey at baseline and at the end of the 8-week intervention. Eight weeks of yoga decreased brachial-ankle pulse wave velocity and weight ($P < 0.05$) in overweight/obese participants. Only no changes were observed in people with normal BMI. Essentially, the quality of life and emotional well-being improved ($P < 0.05$) in both groups (Hunter et al., 2016).

YOGA AND GASTROESOPHAGEAL REFLUX DISEASE

Gastroesophageal reflux disease (GERD), also known as acid reflux disease, is one of the most common gastric problems confronted. Proton pump inhibitors (PPIs) can be effective in treating symptoms of GERD, but in serious cases of GERD, conventional medications fail to treat the disease. PPIs combined with yoga can improve symptoms of severe GERD as well as assist in delaying or avoiding the need of invasive procedures (Shah et al., 2013).

There was a 62-year-old male with a history of heartburn. In the beginning, the patient was put on high doses of PPIs. However, the symptoms did not improve. The patient was asked to continue treatment with high doses of PPIs. When in combination with PPIs, the patient began doing yoga daily, the symptoms of GERD alleviated. A routinely yoga practice of Kapalbhati Pranayama and Agnisar Kriya was advised to the patient. After 6 months, a follow-up visit demonstrated that esophagitis grade improved to Grade A from preliminary Grade D esophagitis according to Los Angeles classification of esophagitis (Shah et al., 2013).

To confirm these findings, the Bravo study was conducted. The Bravo study showed a noticeable progress in DeMeester scores; the day one score improved from 81.1 to 12 and the day two score improved from 35.1 to 17. These findings indicate that the patient had considerable symptomatic recovery after 6 months of combined regimen of yoga and PPI, which were noncompliant to high doses of PPIs alone. The patient's heartburn and dysphagia symptoms got better in terms of severity as well as rate of recurrence (Shah et al., 2013).

It was concluded that this patient has shown the effect of regular practice of a Kapalbhati Pranayama and Agnisar Kriya on severe GERD. Kapalbhati is a type of Pranayama (breathing control technique) in which inspiration is passive and expiration is active through abdominal muscles. This act clears the respiratory passage and strengthens the diaphragm. Agnisar Kriya is a method of contracting or "flapping" abdominal muscles inside and outside, and hence, it enhances digestion and gastrointestinal motility, thereby decreasing the reflux episodes experienced in GERD. After adding regular yoga exercises to the ongoing treatment of high doses of PPIs, the patient in this case study demonstrated tremendous clinical improvement proven by both the reduction of Bravo scores and improvement in esophagitis grading (Shah et al., 2013).

Even with PPI therapy, a large percentage of patients do not achieve full symptomatic relief and can worsen to esophagitis, esophageal ulcers, strictures, laryngeal disease, chronic cough, Barrett's esophagus, and adenocarcinoma. Recently, the positive impact of yoga has been seen in studies on functional dyspepsia, irritable bowel syndrome, and inflammatory bowel disease (Shah et al., 2013).

Yoga practices increase diaphragmatic tone, thus decreasing reflux from the stomach to esophagus. Furthermore, an increase in stress has demonstrated an increase in gastric-acid secretion, which is linked to developing peptic ulcer. Yoga lowers the stress response of the digestive tract, and is a potential treatment for GERD and peptic ulcers (Shah et al., 2013).

YOGA AND IRRITABLE BOWEL SYNDROME (IBS)

Irritable bowel syndrome (IBS) is a set of symptoms established as a functional gastrointestinal (GI) disorder in which patients experience abdominal pain, discomfort, and bloating that is normally eased with passing a stool. IBS is usually connected with a host of secondary chronic conditions including anxiety, depression, headaches, and fatigue. In a review, the basic concept of Pancha Kosha, which refers to "five sheaths of human existence," was investigated. Pancha Kosha comes from an Indian scripture, Taittiriya Upanishad. Also, the pathophysiology of a disease from the yoga approach, Yoga Vasistha's Adhi as "originated from mind" and Vyadhi or "ailment/disease concept" was explored. A parallel was drawn between the ancient idea of Adhi-Vyadhi and modern scientific stress-induced dysregulation of the brain-gut axis, as it impacts IBS. Based on these aspects, it was concluded that a possible yoga element ought to be considered as a remedial therapy to better manage the primary and secondary symptoms of IBS (Kavuri et al., 2015).

A systematic review was conducted to study the effects of yoga on symptoms of IBS, pain, quality of life, mood, stress, and safety in patients with IBS. Randomized controlled trials were conducted for patients with IBS. The primary outcomes were gastrointestinal symptoms, quality of life, and pain. Anxiety, mood, and safety were identified as secondary outcomes (Schumann et al., 2016).

A qualitative analysis was performed based on six randomized controlled trials with a total of 273 patients. There was evidence for a favorable effect of a yogic intervention in contrast to conventional treatment in IBS, with decreased levels of bowel symptoms, IBS severity, and anxiety. There were noticeable enhancements in quality of life, global improvement, and physical functioning after yoga in contrast to no treatment. The findings of this systematic review indicate that yoga might be a feasible and safe integrative treatment for patients with IBS (Schumann et al., 2016).

Another study was performed to evaluate the impact of a 6-week, twice per week Iyengar yoga (IY) program on IBS symptoms in adolescents and young adults (YA) with IBS in contrast to a usual-care control group. Evaluations of symptoms, global improvement, pain, health-related quality of life, psychological distress, functional disability, fatigue, and sleep were gathered before and after treatment. Every week ratings of pain, IBS symptoms, and global improvement were also documented up to a 2-month follow-up mark. A total of 51 people participated in the study, 29 in the yoga group and 22 in the usual-care control group (Evans et al., 2014).

The baseline attrition rate in the IY program based study was 24%. The yoga group attended an average of 75% of classes. Comparative to controls, the adolescents ages 14–17 years who were allocated to yoga accounted for a substantial improvement in physical functioning, while the YA ages 18–26 years designated to yoga showed significant improvement in IBS symptoms, global improvement, disability, psychological distress, sleep quality, and fatigue. Even though the level of abdominal pain was statistically the same, 44% of adolescents and 46% of YA reported a negligibly clinically significant reduction in pain following yoga, and one-third of YA reported clinically significant levels of global symptom improvement. The results indicate that a brief IY intervention is a practical and harmless complementary treatment for young people with IBS, beneficial in many IBS-specific and general working areas for YA (Evans et al., 2014).

A novel pilot study of yoga treatment in children with functional abdominal pain (FAP) and IBS was conducted. The purpose of this pilot study was to assess the effect of yoga exercises on the rate of recurrence of pain as well as intensity and on quality of life in children with FAP. Patients of IBS or FAP were included in the study. There were 20 children patients, aged 8–18 years, who received 10 yoga lessons. Pain intensity and pain frequency were measured, and quality of life was assessed with the Kidscreen quality of life (KQoL) questionnaire (Brands et al., 2011).

It was found that group pain frequency dropped in the 8- to 11-year-old group and the 11- to 18-year-old group by the end of therapy as compared to baseline. After 3 months there was a substantial decline in pain frequency in the younger patient group and a marginally substantial decline in pain frequency in the total group. The parents of participating children informed a substantially higher KQoL-score after yoga treatment. Based on this pilot study, it was concluded that yoga exercises are helpful for children ages 8–18 years with FAP, with the outcome of a substantial reduction of pain intensity and frequency, particularly in 8- to 11-years-old children (Brands et al., 2011).

In a further interesting study, evidence for clinical applications of yoga among the pediatric population was evaluated. An electronic literature search was operated. Randomized controlled trials (RCTs) and nonrandomized controlled trials (NRCTs) were chosen and involved yoga or yoga-based interventions for persons ages 0 to 21 years. Data was obtained and articles were analytically reviewed (Birdee et al., 2009).

Thirty-four controlled studies published between 1979 and 2008 were classified, with 19 RCTS and 15 NRCTs. The clinical subjects for which yoga was examined include IBS, physical fitness, cardiorespiratory effects, motor skills/strength, behavior and development, mental health and psychological disorders, as well as birth outcomes following prenatal yoga. There was a presence of limited information on the clinical applications of yoga among the pediatric population. Most of the published controlled trials indicated beneficial results, but they are based on low quantity and quality of trials. An additional investigation of yoga for children by using a greater criterion of methodology and reporting will assure results (Birdee et al., 2009).

Adolescents suffering from IBS often feel a hindrance with their daily activities. Mind–body tactics including yoga have been suggested as therapy for patients with IBS. Even though results of yoga therapy in adults with IBS have been favorable, there have been limited inquiries studying the effectiveness of yoga in young pediatric subjects (Kuttner et al., 2006).

A randomized trial of yoga for adolescents with IBS was organized. The core mission of this study was to perform a preliminary randomized study of yoga as treatment for adolescents with IBS. Twenty-five adolescent patients with IBS, aged 11–18 years, were randomly allocated to either a yoga or wait list control group. Prior to the intervention, the two groups filled out questionnaires evaluating gastrointestinal symptoms, pain, functional disability, coping, anxiety, and depression. The yoga group participated in a 1-hour training session, demonstration and practice, along with 4 weeks of daily home practice as channeled by a video. At the completion of 4 weeks, adolescents once again filled out the baseline questionnaires. At this point, the wait list control group obtained the yoga intervention and after 4 weeks completed a supplementary set of questionnaires (Kuttner et al., 2006).

The results were encouraging. The adolescents who participated in the yoga group informed declined levels of functional disability, a lower practice of emotion-focused avoidance, and less anxiety following the yoga therapy as compared to the adolescents in the control group. Upon analyzing the pre- and post-intervention data for the two groups, adolescents had considerably lower scores for gastrointestinal symptoms and emotion-focused avoidance after participating in the yoga therapy. Yoga was beneficial to these adolescents, and they revealed that they would continue the practice to cope with their IBS. It was concluded that yoga is a promising instrument for adolescents with IBS (Kuttner et al., 2006).

An alternative study was performed to evaluate the fundamental effect of yogic and conventional treatment in diarrhea-predominant IBS in a randomized control plan. There were 22 participating males, ages 20–50 years, with a confirmed diagnosis of diarrhea-predominant IBS. The conventional group received symptomatic treatment with loperamide 2–6 mg/day for two months. In contrast, the yogic intervention group performed a set of 12 asanas or yogic poses (including Vajrasana, Shashankasana, Ushtrasana, Marjariasana, Padhastasana, Dhanurasana, Trikonasana in two variations, Pawanmuktasana, and Paschimottanasana) along with Surya Nadi pranayama (right-nostril breathing) two times a day for 2 months. All participants were tested at three proportional intervals, at the beginning of the study—0 month, 1 month, and 2 months of receiving the intervention. The subjects were examined for bowel symptoms, autonomic symptoms, autonomic reactivity, surface electrogastrography, and anxiety profile by Spielberger's Self Evaluation Questionnaire, which assessed trait and state anxiety (Taneja et al., 2004).

After 2 months of both conventional and yogic intervention, there was a noticeable decline in bowel symptoms and state anxiety. This result was supplemented by an increase in electrophysiologically recorded gastric activity in the conventional group and an enhanced parasympathetic reactivity, as computed by heart rate parameters, in the yogic intervention group. The research demonstrated a positive outcome of yogic intervention over conventional treatment in diarrhea-predominant IBS (Taneja et al., 2004).

A pilot study was conducted to understand the therapeutic effects of yoga and walking for patients with IBS. It was hypothesized that the medications are not very efficient for symptom relief of IBS, so non-medication treatments might play a significant role to treat IBS. The goal of this study was to evaluate the efficiency of two self-regulation techniques for alleviation of symptoms and mood controlling in IBS patients. Thirty-five adult patients of IBS were registered for the study. Of the 35 participants, 27 (77%) finished treatment and before and after-treatment visits (89% women, 11% men), and 20 of the 27 (74%) finished a 6-month follow-up. The participants were randomly allocated to 16 biweekly group sessions of Iyengar yoga or a walking schedule. There was no substantial group by time effect on IBS severity (Shahabi et al., 2016).

Investigative analyses of secondary outcomes assessed change separately for each treatment condition. From before- to after-treatment, yoga demonstrated a noteworthy decline in IBS severity measures, visceral sensitivity, and severity of somatic symptoms. Walking demonstrated a significant decrease in overall GI symptoms, negative effect, and state anxiety. After 6 months, follow-up occurred, and general GI symptoms for walking persistently decreased. For yoga, GI symptoms rebounded toward baseline levels. In conclusion, yoga and walking (which involve movement) are self-regulatory behavioral treatments that can have various impacts and are both valuable for IBS patients. Although, maintenance of a self-regulated walking schedule may be more feasible and, hence, more effectual in the long run (Shahabi et al., 2016).

YOGA AND DIABETES

Type 2 diabetes is a multifaceted and challenging chronic disease. Even though the male to female ratio among patients with diabetes is approximately equal in India, women are distinctively and more rigorously affected. Coping with type 2 diabetes requires extensive skill for the patient in the management of drugs, diet, and exercise. In a low, middle-income country like India, it is important to analyze low-cost interventions that can empower the patient and construct on accessible resources to assist in the management of diabetes. A feasibility study was performed as a randomized controlled trial of the effect of yoga and peer support on glycemic outcomes in women with type 2 diabetes mellitus in India (Sreedevi et al., 2017).

As a methodology, an open label parallel three-armed randomized control trial was led with 124 recruited women with diabetes for 3 months. Block randomization with a block length of six was executed with each group containing at least 41 women. In the yoga limb, an instructor coordinated sessions comprising a group of postures along with breathing for an hour, two days a week. In the peer support limb, each peer mentor visited women with diabetes weekly after training, followed by a phone call. The meeting entailed incorporating disease management or prevention plans into everyday life (Sreedevi et al., 2017).

There was a pattern in decreasing of fasting plasma glucose in the peer and yoga group and of glycosylated hemoglobin (HbA1c) in the yoga group only. A significant reduction was noted in diastolic blood pressure and hip circumference in the yoga group. The procedure specified that almost 80% of the women in the yoga group attended classes regularly and 90% of the women in the peer group reported that peer mentoring was beneficial. In conclusion, the influence of yoga and peer support on glycemic results was cumulative (Sreedevi et al., 2017).

Another study examined the adherence to yoga and its resultant effects on blood glucose in type 2 diabetes in a community-based follow-up study. The purpose of this study was to determine the adherence to yoga and its effects on blood glucose parameters in patients with type 2 diabetes mellitus. A single group longitudinal study was operated at VASK yoga center in Bangalore, India over a period of 6 months. Fasting blood sugar (FBS), postprandial blood sugar levels, glycosylated hemoglobin, and a qualitative in-depth interview of the participants and therapist were directed at baseline, end of the 3rd month, and end of 6 months. Intermediate observations were led at the end of every month. Patients who participated in the yoga program had significantly lower HbA1c (end of the 3rd month). At the end of 6 months, yoga adherence was substantially negatively correlated with FBS and stress (Angadi et al., 2017).

Moreover, there was a trend toward those who dropped out having higher FBS, in relationship to their medication intake, higher stress levels, and dietary inclinations. Qualitative data disclosed that most of the participants joined and finished the yoga program to cure their diabetes. Some participants left the yoga program early for subjective reasons such as travel, ill-health, and increased personal work-load. In conclusion, a devout practice of yoga has an effect on the blood glucose parameters in diabetes. Therefore, tactics to inspire participants to undergo lifestyle modification practices, such as an increased dedication to yoga practice, ought to be the emphasis to experience any healing effects of yoga (Angadi et al., 2017).

In the research study, "Impact of a 10 minute Seated Yoga Practice in the Management of Diabetes," the investigators prospectively assessed the impact of a 10-minute seated yoga program in addition to ordinary complete diabetes care on glucose control and heart health in the critically ill, medically complex diabetic patients. A group of 10 patients with type 2 diabetes, ages 49–77, with length of diabetes >10 years and hemoglobin A1C >9% (75 mmol/mol) was studied. Patients who were randomly selected for the yoga group were educated on a 10-minute seated yoga practice, granted an instructive DVD and a fold-out pocket guide to encourage practice at home, and were directed to integrate the yoga practice as much as plausible. The participants in the control limb were offered information on the existing yoga classes on campus only (Mullur et al., 2016).

At a 3-month clinical follow up, the average reduction in fasting capillary blood glucose (CBG) was 45% among yoga participants. Heart rate (HR) declined by 18% and diastolic blood pressure (BP) fell by 29% in the yoga intervention limb. There were no substantial statistically significant changes in the hemoglobin A1C, systolic blood pressure, weight, or body mass index in either group. This minute pilot study reinforces the current medical evidence supporting the practice of yoga alongside standard care, to improve health results in diabetes patients (Mullur et al., 2016).

The next study is a prospective cohort study from India which evaluates the correlation between adjunctive naturopathy and improved glycemic control along with a reduction in the need for medications among type 2 diabetes patients. There are approximately 65 million diabetes mellitus (DM) patients in India, ranking as second worldwide in conditions of DM burden. The stress of current medical practice in the treatment of DM has been on pharmacotherapy. However, even with the best combination therapies, achieving glycemic control (reduction of blood sugar to desirable levels) is a challenge. The "Integrated Naturopathy and Yoga" (INY) is an alternative system of medicine that outlines the role of diet and physical exercise in achieving healthy outcomes. In this paper, the short-term effects of INY as an adjunct to pharmacotherapy on glycemic control among type 2 DM patients were evaluated (Bairy et al., 2016).

In this prospective cohort study with a 3-month follow-up, DM patients were successively admitted to a hospital in India from May–October 2014 for either 15 or 30 days. They were given INY therapy with a vegetarian diet (with no added oil, sugar, or salt), a yoga-based exercise program, patient counselling, and rest. A "favorable outcome" was identified as glycemic control (glycosylated hemoglobin [HbA1c] <7% or absolute reduction by 1%) along with at least 50% reduction in anti-diabetes medications at 3 months comparative to baseline. Obedience to dietary regimen was recorded by self-report (Bairy et al., 2016).

Out of 101 patients with 3-month follow-up data, 65 achieved a favorable outcome—with 19 stopping medication while maintaining glycemic control. Factors associated with favorable outcome were baseline HbA1c and obedience to diet, which showed a substantial linear relationship with mean HbA1c reductions of 0.4%, 1.1%, and 1.7% in relation to poor, moderate, and excellent dietary obedience, respectively. In conclusion, INY, as an integrative approach to pharmacotherapy, was linked with a significant beneficial effect on glycemic control and decreased the overall need for anti-diabetes medications. These results are encouraging (Bairy et al., 2016).

YOGA AND DEPRESSION AND ANXIETY

A systematic review of yoga for major depressive disorder was performed. The goal of this review was to examine the effectiveness and safety of yoga interventions in treating patients with major depressive disorder. MEDLINE, Scopus, and the Cochrane Library were sifted through December 2016. Randomized controlled trials (RCTs) comparing yoga to inactive or active parallels in patients with major depressive disorder were considered suitable. Primary results entailed remission rates and severity of depression. Anxiety and adverse events composed secondary outcomes (Cramer et al., 2017a,b).

Seven RCTs with 240 participants comprised the study. Risk of bias was uncertain for most RCTs. In comparison to aerobic exercise, there were no short- or medium-term group differences in depression severity. Higher short-term depression severity was discovered for yoga compared to electro-convulsive therapy; remission rates were not different between groups. No short-term group dissimilarities struck when yoga was contrasted to antidepressant medications. Inconsistent evidence was found when yoga was compared to attention-control interventions, or when yoga as an add-on to antidepressant medications was compared to medication alone. Only two RCTs measured adverse events and testified that no treatment-related adverse events occurred. This review discovered some support for positive effects of yoga beyond placebo and comparable effects as compared to evidence-based interventions. Nevertheless, organizational problems and the ambiguous risk-benefit ratio prevent definitive advice for or against yoga as an adjunct treatment for major depressive disorder (Cramer et al., 2017a,b).

Up to approximately 50% of patients with major depressive disorder who take antidepressant medications do not receive complete healing. A recent study has further substantiated that yoga is helpful in lowering symptoms of depression in patients with major depressive disorder. The core purpose of the study was to evaluate the benefits of an Iyengar postural yoga intervention and coherent breathing at about five breaths per minute in patients with major depressive disorder. The participants between ages 18–64 years were randomized into two groups and scored for 12 weeks: a high-dose group (HDG) consisting of 15 patients or a low-dose group (LDG) consisting of 15 patients as well. The HDG attended three, 90-minute yoga classes per week along with a home practice composed of four, 30-minute yoga sessions per week. The LDG attended two, 90-minute yoga classes per week alongside a home practice composed of three, 30-minute yoga sessions per week (Streeter et al., 2017).

In both groups, there was a remarkable reduction in depressive symptoms. There were no significant variations between the two groups based on response or remission after the 12-week intervention. It was noted that the group with higher dosage of yoga demonstrated lower depressive symptoms and an enhanced mood improvement. In comparison to mood changing medications, the yoga intervention is valuable in relieving symptoms of depression as well as precluding added side effects of drugs such as antidepressants. It was concluded that patients of depression must do yoga and coherent breathing at least two times a week to diminish symptoms of depression (Streeter et al., 2017).

YOGA AND SICKLE CELL ANEMIA

Sickle cell disease (SCD) vaso-occlusive crisis (VOC) is a significant reason for acute pain in pediatrics, and it is a normal SCD complication. Most suggestions for pain management in SCD involve nonpharmacological interventions. One nonpharmacological intervention which has helped in pain reduction in some groups of patients is yoga. Conversely, there is proof missing for the effectiveness of yoga in children with VOC (Moody et al., 2017).

A randomized trial was conducted to compare the validity of yoga versus an attention control on pain in children with VOC. The goal was to compare the outcome of yoga with an attention control on anxiety, length of stay (LOS), and opioid use in this population. Eligible patients had a diagnosis of SCD, were between ages 5 and 21 years old, were hospitalized for uncomplicated VOC, and had an admission pain score >7. Participants were divided based on disease severity and randomized to the yoga or control group (Moody et al., 2017).

In comparison to the control group, children in the yoga group has a significantly greater reduction in mean pain score after the first yoga session. However, there were no substantial differences in anxiety, LOS, or opioid use between the two groups. The researchers concluded that yoga is a suitable, viable, and accommodating intervention for hospitalized children with VOC. Further research is necessary to study yoga for children with SCD pain in inpatient and outpatient settings (Moody et al., 2017).

YOGA AND EATING DISORDERS

A pilot study was organized to study the utilization of yoga in outpatient eating disorder treatment. Patients who suffer from eating disorders along with co-morbid psychiatric disorders try to control symptoms via vigorous exercises that increase caloric outflow. For such patients, yoga is a safe method of participating in physical activity that offers an outlet for disease-associated symptoms (Hall et al., 2016).

The primary objective of this pilot study was to assess the function of yoga practice in an outpatient setting and its effect on anxiety, depression, and body image disturbance in adolescents with eating disorders. Participants included a group of 20 adolescent girls who were enrolled from an urban eating disorders clinic. The girls practiced weekly yoga classes at a local studio, and additionally applied themselves to standard multidisciplinary care. Yoga instructors were given training regarding this group of patients. As a prerequisite to the initial yoga class as well as after finishing 6 and 12 classes, participants filled out questionnaires focused on anxiety, depression, and body image disturbance (Hall et al., 2016).

In participants who completed the study, a statistically significant decrease in anxiety, depression, and body image disturbance was seen. Spielberger State anxiety mean scores decreased after the completion of 7–12 yoga classes as did the anorexia nervosa scale scores, Beck depression scale scores, and weight and shape concern scores. No substantial differences in body mass index were seen throughout the trial. Yoga therapy along with outpatient eating disorder treatment demonstrated a decline in anxiety, depression, and body image disturbance without negatively impacting weight. The results from this pilot study recommend yoga to be a promising adjunct treatment tactic, alongside standard multidisciplinary care (Hall et al., 2016).

YOGA AND ARTHRITIS

A pilot randomized controlled trial was organized to study the management of knee osteoarthritis (OA) with yoga or aerobic/strengthening exercise programs in older adults. Even though exercise is often suggested for patients with OA, limited evidence-based exercise options are available for older adults with OA. This investigation studied the effects of Hatha yoga (HY) and aerobic/strengthening exercises (ASE) on knee OA. A randomized controlled trial with three groups was used: HY, ASE, and education control. The HY and ASE groups comprised 8, weekly, 45-minute group sessions with 2–4 days/week home practice sessions. The control group received OA education brochures and weekly phone calls from researchers. OA symptoms, physical function, mood, spiritual health, fear of falling, and quality of life were measured at baseline, 4 weeks, and 8 weeks (Cheung et al., 2017).

Eighty-three adults with symptomatic knee OA completed the study. Approximately 84% were females. The mean age was 71.6 ± 8.0 years. Retention rate was 82%. Compared to the ASE group at 8 weeks, subjects in the HY group had a significant improvement from baseline with regard to OA symptoms, anxiety, and fear of falling. There were no differences in class/home practice groups between HY and ASE. Three minor negative events were reported from the ASE group. The HY seemed helpful for older adults with knee OA (Cheung et al., 2017).

Another study was conducted in Ottawa on the management of knee OA with mind–body exercise programs. The aim of the study was to identify effective mind–body exercise programs and offer doctors and patients with updated, high-quality suggestions regarding nontraditional exercises for knee OA. Four high-quality investigations showed that various mind–body exercise programs are capable of aiding in helping knee OA. Hatha yoga showed substantial improvement for pain relief and physical function. The study concluded that mind–body exercises are optimistic ways to reduce pain, as well as to improve physical function and quality of life for knee OA patients (Brosseau et al., 2017).

OA is a widespread and incapacitating chronic condition. Physical activity is crucial in OA management. There was a focused review study on the effects of yoga on symptoms, physical function, and psychosocial outcomes in adults with OA. Yoga is a trendy mind–body exercise that enhances flexibility, strength, endurance, and balance. The goal of this focused review was to scrutinize the effects of yoga on OA symptoms as well as physical and psychosocial outcomes. A complete search was organized using seven electronic databases. Exactly 589 patients with OA-related symptoms participated in the study. Hatha and Iyengar yoga were the ordinary styles of yoga practiced. Yoga was practiced from once a week to six days a week. The sessions were 45–90 minutes long per session for 6–12 weeks. The results included a decrease in pain, stiffness, and swelling. (Cheung et al., 2016).

A qualitative study was conducted to explore community yoga practice in adults with rheumatoid arthritis (RA). It was hypothesized that yoga may enhance physical function and lower disease symptoms in adults with RA. Participants completed a semistructured telephone interview. Thematic analysis was used to analyze interview transcripts. A convenience sample of 17 adult patients with RA who had practiced yoga within the past year were asked about the decision to start, continue, and stop yoga. They were further interviewed about their perception on the benefits of yoga as well as general thoughts about yoga as it relates to RA. The patients with RA explained how yoga practice helped improve physical and psychosocial symptoms related to their ailment. It was concluded that yoga practice can be helpful for adults with RA even though yoga may not be helpful for every adult with RA (Greysen et al., 2017).

Another study analyzed the effect of Iyengar yoga on quality of life in young women with RA. The goal of this study was to assess the impact of a 6-week, twice a week Iyengar yoga program on health-related quality of life (HRQoL) of young adults with RA compared with a usual-care waitlist control group. Evaluations were collected pretreatment, posttreatment, and at 2 months after treatment. Weekly ratings of anxiety, depression, pain, and sleep were also recorded (Evans et al., 2013).

Twenty-six participants completed the intervention (yoga = 11; usual-care waitlist = 15). All participants were female with an average age of 28. Overall attrition was low at 15%. No adverse events were reported. In contrast to the usual-care waitlist, women assigned to the yoga program showed significantly greater improvement on measures of HRQoL, pain disability, general health, mood, fatigue, and acceptance of chronic pain. The research suggested that a brief Iyengar yoga intervention is a feasible and safe integrative treatment for young people with RA (Evans et al., 2013).

YOGA AND ASTHMA

Asthma entails chronic inflammation of the airways which causes occurrences of wheezing, breathlessness, chest tightness, and coughing. Many studies have testified positive effects of yoga on bronchial asthma, specifically pulmonary functions, quality of life, and reduction in medication use. A randomized controlled study was conducted to understand the effect of yoga on biochemical profile of asthmatics (Kant et al., 2014).

Exactly 276 patients of mild to moderate asthma, between ages 12 and 60 years, were recruited. The participants were randomly assigned to two groups. The first group was the yoga group, where patients received general medical treatment and yogic intervention. The second group was the control group where patients received general medical treatment without yogic intervention. After 6 months, 35 participants dropped out. Out of 276 subjects, only 241 subjects completed the entire study. A total of 121 subjects were from the yoga group, and 120 subjects were from the control group. A biochemical evaluation was carried out at baseline and after 6 months (Kant et al., 2014).

The yoga group demonstrated a substantial improvement in the proportion of hemoglobin and antioxidant superoxide dismutase in contrast to the control group. There was also a significant reduction in the total leukocyte count (TLC) and differential leukocytes count in contrast to the control group. The yoga group demonstrated a significant improvement in biochemical variables in comparison to the control group. It was concluded that yoga can be practiced as an adjunctive therapy along with normal inhalation therapy to help ease the symptoms of asthma (Kant et al., 2014).

Many asthma patients perform breathing exercises even though they are slightly challenging to perform in their health condition. A study was conducted to evaluate the effectiveness of a modified breathing exercise program for asthma patients. The participants in the study were between ages 18 and 65 and had a diagnosis of asthma. Three unique breathing exercises were taught to participants: yoga pranayama techniques, diaphragmatic breathing, and pursed lip breathing. Patients were scheduled to complete their breathing exercise in less than 10 minutes per day (Karam et al., 2017).

The patients participated in the Asthma Control Test (ACT) and a mini-Asthma Quality of Life Questionnaire (AQLQ) at baseline and after 1 month of being enrolled in the study. Additionally, the patients participated in a survey that asked them to grade the efficacy and complexity of the breathing exercises, as well as whether they would suggest them to others in the future. Exactly 74 participants were registered in this investigation. The intervention enhanced breathing for 52.9% of the participants, whereas 67.6% felt that their daily activity was enhanced, and 66.1% pointed out that the breathing exercises permitted a reduced use of a rescue inhaler. Around 80.9% of the participants suggested breathing exercises as a supplemental therapy for asthma and 79.4% of the participants claimed that the exercises took not more than 10 minutes of their time per day. In general, the ACT scores improved noticeably post-exercise with a statistically nonsignificant improvement in AQLQ scores (Karam et al., 2017).

An alternative investigation analyzed the effectiveness of naturopathy and yoga in bronchial asthma. The purpose of the investigation was to test the effectiveness of a 1-month in-patient naturopathy and yoga program for asthma patients. A data analysis of 159 bronchial asthma patients, participating in the naturopathy and yoga program, was carried out. The measures in the analysis included Forced Vital Capacity, Forced Expiratory Volume at the end of 1 second, and Maximum Voluntary Ventilation and Peak Expiratory Flow Rate during baseline, 11th day, on discharge, and once in three months for 3 years (Rao et al., 2014).

There was a significant rise in the Forced Vital Capacity and Forced Expiratory Volume from baseline up to the 6th month. Maximum Voluntary Ventilation escalated substantially between baseline and the date of discharge. The Peak Expiratory Flow Rate ascended substantially from baseline until the 36th month of follow-up. These results reinforced and confirmed the advantageous outcome of combining naturopathy and yoga in managing bronchial asthma (Rao et al., 2014).

Numerous investigations have demonstrated invaluable advantages of yoga for patients with bronchial hyperreactivity in correlation with a decrease in the usage of medications, a rise in exercise capacity, and an improved lung function. In an investigation, an assessment was carried out to understand the advantages of yoga in children with exercise-induced bronchoconstriction (EIB). The nature of the investigation was prospective, and there was no control group. Subjects were randomly selected (Tahan et al., 2014).

The study took place in the Pediatric Allergy Unit, in Kayseri, Turkey. There were two sets of children with asthma, ages 6–17 years, registered. The first group consisted of 10 children with positive responses to an exercise challenge, and the second group was comprised of 10 children with negative responses. Both groups joined for 1-hour sessions of yoga training twice a week for 3 months. Spirometric measurements were directed to all children pre- and immediately post-participation in an exercise task. The measurements were recorded at baseline as well as at the end of the investigation (Tahan et al., 2014).

In the group of children with positive responses to an exercise challenge, the researchers detected a noteworthy improvement. It was interesting that all exercise response-positive asthmatic patients became exercise response-negative asthmatic patients after the yoga training. The researchers concluded that yoga posed positive outcomes in children with EIB. Hence, based on this research, yoga training can complement drug therapy in treatment of asthmatic children (Tahan et al., 2014).

Yoga is quite trendy worldwide as an integrative approach to treating bronchial asthma with medicine. In a randomized trial, an evaluation was carried out to understand the consequences of yoga on the quality of life of patients with bronchial asthma. A total of 120 non-smoking patients of asthma between ages 17 and 50 years were randomized into two groups: yoga group and control group. Both groups of patients consumed their prescribed medications. Only the yoga group patients participated in yoga breathing exercises for 8 weeks (Sodhi et al., 2014).

The following factors were measured via the Asthma Quality of Life Questionnaire (AQLQ) and a diary record: quality of life, number and severity of asthmatic attacks, and the dosage of the medication necessary at baseline and after 8 weeks. The yoga group demonstrated a statistically significant progress symptomatically as well as in the activities and environmental areas of AQLQ after 8 weeks of yoga practice. There was a substantial decline in the everyday number and severity of attacks as well as the dose of medication necessary at 4 and 8 weeks in contrast to the baseline. The research team inferred that the yoga breathing exercises when integrated with the ordinary medical treatment for bronchial asthma substantially enhanced the quality of life in these patients (Sodhi et al., 2014).

Even though physical exercise is advised in patients with asthma, proof for the clinical benefits of exercise in the lives of these subjects is still lacking. A systematic review and meta-analysis research found the impact of exercise training (EXT) on quality of life (QoL), bronchial hyperresponsiveness (BHR), exercise-induced bronchoconstriction (EIB), lung function, and exercise capacity, in addition to the elements impacting changes in QoL and exercise capacity in patients with asthma after some EXT. A computerized search was conducted in MEDLINE, EMBASE, and CINAHL databases and a review was performed (Eichenberger et al., 2013).

EXT was defined as training for ≥ 7 days, ≥ 2 times per week, ≥ 5 training sessions in total and a minimum of one of the following factors were measured: QoL, airway hyperreactivity, forced expiratory volume in one second (FEV_1), peak expiratory flow (PEF), inflammatory parameters, exercise capacity, or exercise endurance. Out of 500 potentially relevant articles, 13.4% or 67 studies encompassing 2059 subjects were eligible for additional analyses (Eichenberger et al., 2013).

A meta-analysis of all the eligible RCTs was performed. Moreover, relative pre/post-changes were examined. Also, multiple linear regression models were applied to measure the influence of relative changes in airway hyperreactivity (BHR or EIB), lung function (FEV$_1$ or PEF), and training hours on QoL and exercise performance (Eichenberger et al., 2013).

In 17 studies encompassing 599 participants, meta-analyses demonstrated a significant improvement in days without asthma symptoms, FEV$_1$ and exercise capacity while BHR only tended to improve. There was a 17% improvement in QoL, 53% in BHR, 9% in EIB, and 3% in FEV$_1$ in contrast to the control group. EXT demonstrated an improvement in asthma symptoms, QoL, exercise capacity, BHR, EIB, and FEV$_1$ in asthma patients. Therefore, physical activity including yoga ought to be advised as an integrative approach to treating asthma in conjunction with medication (Eichenberger et al., 2013).

Prana is the cosmic life-force energy, and when this self-energizing life force in the body is combined with the extension, expansion, and control of breathing techniques, it is called pranayama. In theory, pranayama may impact the environment in the bronchioles and alveoli in lungs, especially at the alveolo-capillary membrane during facilitated diffusion as well as gas transportation. Pranayama also assists in enhancing the oxygenation at the tissue level. In a research study, the impact of yoga on pulmonary function tests including transfer factor of lung for carbon monoxide (TLCO) in asthma patients was explored. The core objective of the study was to compare pulmonary functions and diffusion capacity in patients with bronchial asthma prior to yogic intervention and following yogic intervention of 2 months. A total of 60 stable asthmatic-patients were randomly selected and distributed into two groups of 30 subjects each: yoga training group and control group (Singh et al., 2012).

Lung functions were documented in all patients at baseline and then after 2 months. Patients in the yoga training group demonstrated a statistically significant improvement in TLCO, forced vital capacity (FVC), forced expiratory volume in the 1st sec (FEV$_1$), peak expiratory flow rate (PEFR), maximum voluntary ventilation (MVV), and slow vital capacity (SVC) after yoga practice. Also, the quality of life of patients enhanced notably. The research unit concluded that pranayama and yoga postures play an important role in increasing respiratory stamina, relaxing the chest muscles, expanding the lungs, elevating energy levels, and calming the body (Singh et al., 2012).

In a randomized trial, the impact of an integrative medicine approach was measured in managing asthma in adults on disease-related quality of life and pulmonary function. The aim of this study was to examine the efficacy of integrative medicine in controlling asthma symptoms in contrast to orthodox clinical care on quality of life (QoL) and clinical outcomes. Subjects were asthma patients between ages 18 and 80 years. The intervention was comprised of six group sessions and involved nutritional manipulation, yoga techniques, and journaling. Subjects also took nutritional supplements such as fish oil, vitamin C, and a standardized hops extract. The control group obtained standard medical care. The following outcomes were measured: Asthma Quality of Life Questionnaire (AQLQ), The Medical Outcomes Study Short Form-12 (SF-12), and standard pulmonary function tests (PFTs) (Kligler et al., 2011).

A total of 154 patients were randomized into two groups: 77 in the treatment group and 77 in the control group. Subjects in the treatment group demonstrated a higher level of improvement than controls at 6 months for the AQLQ total score as well as for three subscales of Activity, Symptoms, and Emotion. The treatment group also exhibited a higher level of improvement than controls on all three of the SF-12 subscales including physical functioning, role limitations, and social functioning. The cumulative scores in the physical and mental health outcomes were also greater for the treatment group. The PFTs indicated no change in either group. It was concluded that a low-cost, group-oriented integrative medicine intervention can improve the quality of life in patients with asthma (Kligler et al., 2011).

YOGA AND CYSTIC FIBROSIS

Evidently, yoga has demonstrated significant improvement in the health of asthmatics. What about cystic fibrosis (CF) patients? A prospective pilot study was conducted to study yoga as a therapy for adolescents and young adults with CF. Subjects were between ages 12 and 25 years and participated in a 50-minute yoga session twice a week for 8 weeks. The primary outcome measures were safety and tolerability. The secondary outcome measures were respiratory symptoms, the Cystic Fibrosis Quality of Life instrument (CFQ-R), lung function, Ease of Breathing Score (a measure of exercise tolerance), and weight. Exactly 10 subjects finished the study. The 8-week yoga program was safe and well tolerated among the participating CF patients with mild to moderate lung disease. Further controlled trials would be required to verify greater benefits (Ruddy et al., 2015).

YOGA AND PMS

Many women with premenstrual syndrome attend yoga classes. An interesting study was performed in Taiwan to understand the impact of yoga on premenstrual symptoms among a group of female employees. Researchers scrutinized the impact of a 12-week yoga intervention on premenstrual symptoms in menstruating females in Taiwan. A total of 64 females participated in the study. The participants filled out a structured self-report questionnaire on their demographics, personal lifestyle, menstrual status, menstrual pain scores, premenstrual symptoms, and health-related quality of life, before and after the yoga intervention (Tsai, 2016).

Out of 64 participants, 90.6% reported feeling menstrual pain during their menses. At the completion of the yoga intervention, participants informed of a reduced utilization of analgesics during menses as well as reduced moderate or severe impact of menstrual pain at work. The yoga practice was linked to an improvement in physical function and bodily pain, substantially reduced abdominal swelling, breast tenderness, abdominal cramps, as well as cold sweats. Overall, there was a tremendous improvement in physical function, bodily pain, general health acuity, vitality/energy, and social function, as well as mental health. The research team concluded that yoga might significantly lower premenstrual distress and improve women's health (Tsai, 2016).

A single-blind, randomized controlled trial was organized as an effort to study the impact of yoga practice on menstrual cramps and menstrual distress in undergraduate students suffering from dysmenorrhea. Exactly 40 undergraduate nursing students were randomly selected and 20 were assigned to an exercise group, while the remaining 20 were placed in a control group. The subjects in the exercise group participated in a yoga program for 1 hour, once a week, for 12 weeks. The intervention was comprised of physical exercise in combination with relaxation and meditation (Yang et al., 2016).

Menstrual cramps and menstrual distress levels were measured. Data were analyzed statistically. Menstrual pain intensity and menstrual distress levels declined significantly in the experimental group in comparison to the control group. The findings denoted that yoga interventions may decrease menstrual cramps and menstrual distress in female undergraduate students suffering with dysmenorrhea (Yang et al., 2016).

YOGA AND HOMOCYSTEINE

In a cohort of adolescent women with primary dysmenorrhea and normal healthy controls, yoga was investigated to understand its impact on the serum levels of homocysteine and nitric oxide (NO) levels. Participants in this community-based study, a prospective controlled trial, included 35 women with primary dysmenorrhea in the experimental group and 35 healthy controls. Menstrual Distress Questionnaires (MDQs) were directed to measure the menstrual symptoms (Chien et al., 2013).

All subjects were given a yoga intervention, two times a week for 30 minutes/session, successively for 8 weeks. Blood samples were collected from each woman on the third day of their menses. Evaluations of MDQs and blood samples to reveal the levels of homocysteine and NO concentrations were executed at baseline and within the first 3 days of their next menses upon completing the yoga intervention. A total of 30 women from the dysmenorrheal group and 30 women from the control group finished the study (Chien et al., 2013).

The levels of homocysteine were more elevated in those with dysmenorrhea in parallel to healthy controls before yoga intervention. No statistically significant differences were found between the two groups after 8 weeks of yoga training. After 8 weeks of yoga intervention, the homocysteine strengths in the dysmenorrheal group declined by 51.37% and in the control group by 46.46%. There were no statistically significant gaps in NO levels between the two groups at baseline and post-yoga therapy. Yoga intervention was linked with a decrease in dysmenorrhea severity. The researchers concluded that yoga might be helpful in lowering serum homocysteine levels. Also, yoga therapy might be effective in restoring endothelial function in women (Chien et al., 2013).

YOGA AND ENDOMETRIOSIS

In a research study, the effect of the practice of Hatha yoga on the treatment of pain associated with endometriosis was explored. The primary objective of this randomized controlled trial was to understand chronic pelvic pain, menstrual patterns, and quality of life (QoL) in women with endometriosis. One group completed the 8-week yoga intervention and the second group did not participate in the 8-week yoga intervention (Goncalves et al., 2017).

The study took place in Brazil. There was a total of 40 women, out of which 28 participated in the yoga intervention and 12 did not practice yoga. The participants attended 90-minute scheduled yoga sessions two times per week for 8 weeks. An Endometriosis Health Profile (EHP)-30 questionnaire was also requested from the subjects to assess the women's QoL at baseline and 8 weeks later, at the end of the yoga program. Additionally, menstrual and daily pain patterns were measured. The amount of daily pain was considerably less in the women who practiced yoga in contrast to the control group (Goncalves et al., 2017).

With regard to the EHP-30 domains, pain, impotence, well-being, and image from the central questionnaire, and work and treatment from the modular questionnaire were quite dissimilar between the study groups over time. With respect to the diary of menstrual patterns, there was no significant gap between the two groups. However, yoga practice was related to a decline in chronic pelvic pain and an improvement in QoL in women with endometriosis (Goncalves et al., 2017).

YOGA AND MENOPAUSE

During menopause, females often sense discomfort and show an array of symptoms. Yoga therapy is a powerful tool in stress reduction, health improvement, and fitness enhancement, as well as in the controlling of symptoms of a wide spectrum of disorders. A comparative assessment was led to understand the effects of Hatha yoga and physical exercise on biochemical functions in perimenopausal women. The study entailed understanding the impact of Hatha yoga therapy and regular physical exercise on the fasting blood sugar (FBS), glycated hemoglobin (GHB), thyroid stimulating hormone (TSH), serum cortisol, and total plasma thiol levels in perimenopausal women (Chaturvedi et al., 2016).

The participants included 216 women with perimenopausal symptoms, 111 in the test group (Hatha yoga) and 105 in the control group (physical exercise). The intervention occurred for 45 minutes daily for 12 weeks. Blood samples were taken before and after the intervention. FBS and GHB demonstrated a major reduction in post-yoga therapy. In the control group, cortisol levels increased considerably during the post-intervention period. In the Hatha yoga therapy group, the cortisol levels remained about the same between the two time periods. The total plasma thiols level, on the other hand, demonstrated an increase in the post-intervention period: there was a significant increase in the control group but not a significant increase in the experimental group. The TSH levels did not change in either group. The examiners concluded that exercise is beneficial in maintaining the sugar levels, but the calming effects of yoga are essential for stress relief as well as the improvement of overall health in perimenopausal women (Chaturvedi et al., 2016).

Another study was conducted to confirm the effects of yoga and aerobic exercise on actigraphic sleep parameters in midlife menopausal women with hot flashes. The influence of yoga and aerobic exercise was compared with normal activity on objective assessments of sleep in midlife women. In this randomized controlled trial, secondary analyses were carried out through the Menopause Strategies: Finding Lasting Answers for Symptoms and Health (MsFLASH) network (Buchanan et al., 2017).

Exactly 186 late transition and postmenopausal women between the ages of 40 and 62 years with hot flashes were randomized to either a 12 weeks of yoga group, an aerobic exercise group, or a normal activity control group. The mean and coefficient of variation (CV) of change in actigraphic sleep measures from each of the experimental groups were compared to the normal activity group. Variations in the actigraphic sleep outcomes from beginning to weeks 11–12 were small, and did not fluctuate much between groups. There was a plausibly better sleep stability with yoga in menopausal women who self-identified themselves initially with poor sleep quality (Buchanan et al., 2017).

Yoga practice precisely involves a set of psychophysical methods. Many former studies have demonstrated the positive effects of yoga for health and rehabilitation as well as advances in quality of life. A randomized controlled trial studied the impact of Hatha yoga practice on menopause symptoms and quality of life. The objective of this study was to explore the psychophysiological effects of Hatha yoga routinely practiced in post-menopausal women (Jorge et al., 2016).

A total of 88 post-menopausal women participated in this 12-week study. The subjects were randomly allocated into (1) control group (no intervention), (2) exercise group, or (3) yoga group. Questionnaires were completed by the subjects to assess climacteric syndrome, stress, quality of life, depression, and anxiety. Physiological changes were also measured via hormone levels including cortisol, follicle stimulating hormone (FSH), LH, progesterone, and estradiol (Jorge et al., 2016).

At 12 weeks, yoga participants indicated statistically significant scores for less menopausal symptoms, lower stress levels, and decreased depression symptoms, alongside significantly higher scores in quality of life in contrast to control and exercise groups. The control group was the only cluster showing a significant increase in cortisol levels. The yoga and exercise groups demonstrated reduced levels of FSH and LH in contrast to the control group. These findings implied that yoga promotes positive psychophysiological changes in postmenopausal women and can be utilized as a complementary therapy in this group (Jorge et al., 2016).

YOGA AND HORMONES

In a case report, it was found that yoga increased serum estrogen levels in postmenopausal women. The purpose of this study was to assess 4 months of yoga practice on the quality of life (QoL) and estradiol levels of two postmenopausal women. The two subjects had FSH levels more than or equal to 30 mIU/mL and a body mass index of less than 30 kg/m. The subjects observed yoga for 4 months, twice a week, in increments of 60-minute sessions. The subjects had an unusual increase in estrogen levels after 4 months of yoga practice and demonstrated QoL improvements. It was concluded that in some cases, the ritual of yoga can have an impact on the female neuroendocrine system, elevating estrogen, and hence, improving QoL (Afonso et al., 2016).

A double-blind, randomized, placebo-controlled trial examined the effects of dehydroepiandrosterone (DHEA) in unity with exercise on bone mass, muscle strength, and physical function in frail, older women. The subjects included 99 women with low sulfated DHEA (DHEAS) levels, low bone mass, and frailty. Partakers were given DHEA or a placebo for 6 months, while all the subjects got calcium and cholecalciferol. The women joined in 90-minute exercise routines, twice a week (Kenny et al., 2010).

Hormone levels, bone mineral density (BMD), bone turnover markers, body composition, upper and lower extremity strength, and physical performance were measured. Out of 99 women, 87 finished the program for 6 months. There were no extensive changes in BMD or bone turnover markers. DHEA supplementation led to improvements in lower extremity strength. There were noteworthy changes in all hormone levels, including DHEAS, estradiol, estrone, and testosterone. There was a decrease in sex hormone-binding globulin levels in women taking DHEA. Overall,

DHEA supplementation enhanced lower extremity strength and function in older, frail women who participated in a gentle exercise program of chair aerobics or yoga (Kenny et al., 2010).

Another double-blind, randomized, placebo-controlled study evaluated the effects of DHEA on cardiovascular risk factors in older women with frailty characteristics. A total of 99 women with low DHEA-S level and frailty participated in this study. Subjects were given 50 mg/day DHEA or placebo for 6 months, while all of them received calcium and cholecalciferol. The women followed exercise routines for 90 minutes twice per week, performing either chair aerobics or yoga (Boxer et al., 2010).

An evaluation of outcome factors consisted of hormone levels (DHEA-S, oestradiol, oestrone, testosterone, and sex hormone-binding globulin [SHBG]), lipid profiles (total cholesterol, HDL cholesterol, LDL cholesterol, and triglycerides), body composition, glucose levels and blood pressure (BP). Exactly 87 women finished 6 months of study. There were major changes in all hormone levels (including DHEA-S, oestradiol, oestrone, and testosterone) and a decrease in SHBG levels in those taking DHEA supplements (Boxer et al., 2010).

Even though the hormone levels transformed, there were no notable modifications in cardiovascular risk factors such as lipid profiles, body or abdominal fat, fasting glucose, or BP. The researchers concluded that even though recent research has not demonstrated steady effects of DHEA on cardiovascular risk, this investigation complements existing information that short-term therapy with DHEA along with an exercise routine such as yoga is safe for older women relative to cardiovascular risk factors (Boxer et al., 2010).

An inquiry on shifts in cardiovascular risk factors and hormones took place for three months in a comprehensive residential kriya yoga training program. Moreover, a routine of a low-fat lacto-vegetarian diet was followed. A significant risk factor reduction was found. Body mass index, total serum and LDL cholesterol, fibrinogen, and blood pressure declined considerably, particularly in those with elevated levels. Urinary excretion of adrenaline, noradrenaline, dopamine, and aldosterone, as well as serum testosterone and luteinizing hormone levels declined, while cortisol excretion was substantially higher in subjects (Schmidt et al., 1997).

YOGA AND PCOS

A prospective, randomized, active controlled trial was conducted to understand the impact of a holistic yoga program on endocrine health factors in adolescents with polycystic ovarian syndrome (PCOS). The primary purpose of this trial was to compare the impact of a holistic yoga program with a traditional exercise program in adolescent PCOS patients. A total of 90 adolescent females between the ages of 15 and 18 who met the prerequisites of the study were selected from a residential college in India. The subjects were randomized into two groups: yoga group and control group. The yoga group followed a holistic yoga routine, whereas the control group participated in physical exercises for 60 minutes/day, for 12 weeks (Nidhi et al., 2013).

Anti-mullerian hormone (AMH-primary outcome), LH, FSH, testosterone, prolactin, body-mass index (BMI), hirsutism, and menstrual frequency were measured at baseline and after 12 weeks. The testosterone levels were relatively different among the two groups. The shifts in FSH and prolactin post-intervention were not so different amid the two groups. Body weight and BMI did not demonstrate any significant changes between the two groups, whereas changes in menstrual frequency were substantially different among the two groups. The investigation also concluded that a holistic yoga program for 12 weeks is far nobler than physical exercise in reducing AMH, LH, and testosterone, mFG score for hirsutism, and enhancing menstrual frequency alongside promoting insignificant fluctuations in body weight, FSH, and prolactin in adolescents with PCOS (Nidhi et al., 2013).

YOGA AND CANCER

A program was designed for high-grade glioma patients and their caregivers. In a single-arm pilot trial, patients participated in a 12-session yoga program across the course of their radiation. The intervention focused on breathing exercises, gentle movements, and guided meditations. Progress was tracked for cancer-related symptoms (MD Anderson Symptom Inventory), depressive symptoms (Centers for Epidemiological Studies-Depression scale), fatigue (Brief Fatigue Inventory), sleep disturbances (Pittsburgh Sleep Quality Index [PSQI]), and overall mental and physical quality of life (36-item Short-Form Survey [SF-36]) at baseline and post-dyadic yoga program, which was at the end of radiotherapy (Milbury et al., 2017).

All patients received benefit from the program. Paired t tests revealed a marginally significant, yet a clinically meaningful, decrease in patients' cancer symptoms ($t = 2.32$, $P = 0.08$; MDASI mean; pre $= 1.75$, post $= 1.04$). There were clinically significant reductions in patient sleep disturbances (PSQI mean: pre $= 10.75$, post $= 8.00$) and improvements in patient and caregiver mental quality of life (MCS of SF-36 mean: pre $= 42.35$, post $= 52.34$, and pre $= 45.14$, post $= 51.43$, respectively). This novel supportive care program can be used for both patients and caregivers, and it is safe, feasible, acceptable, and subjectively useful for high grade glioma patients and their caregivers (Milbury et al., 2017).

A search of peer reviewed journal articles published between January 2009 and July 2014 was conducted. The goal of this systematic review was to determine the effect of yoga therapy in the treatment of breast cancer. Patients' physical and psychosocial quality of life measures were determined. Yoga therapy showed benefits in anxiety, emotional and social functioning, stress, depression, and quality of life. Yoga decreased salivary cortisol, and improved sleep quality and lymphocyte apoptosis. Benefits in these areas were linked strongly with the yoga interventions, in addition to significant improvement in overall quality of life (Galliford et al., 2017).

A review of nonrandomized and randomized controlled trials of yoga interventions for children and adults undergoing treatment for cancer was administered. Findings most consistently supported improvement in depression, distress, and anxiety. Studies also found that yoga enhanced quality of life, and improved sleep and fatigue. However, in pediatric oncology, evidence was not as strong (Danhauer et al., 2017).

Another meta-analysis found moderate-quality evidence confirming the recommendation of yoga as a supportive intervention for breast cancer victims in improving health-related quality of life as well as reducing fatigue and sleep disturbances when compared with no therapy. There was also a reduction in depression, anxiety, and fatigue in breast cancer patients. Yoga might be as effective as other exercise interventions and might be utilized as an alternate to other exercise programs (Cramer et al., 2017a,b).

An alternative study demonstrated that participation in yoga provides benefits for posture and strength in women with breast cancer related lymphedema. The improvements were attributed to the concentration of yoga on overall postural and functional movement patterns (Loudon et al., 2016).

YOGA DURING CHEMOTHERAPY

Fatigue is the most common side effect of chemotherapy. Yoga has shown to enrich quality of life of patients undergoing chemotherapy. A study demonstrated that yoga practice improved fatigue in colorectal cancer patients receiving chemotherapy. Yoga Skills Training (YST), consisting of four, 30-minute in-person sessions, was executed during chemotherapy. YST was implemented while in the chair during chemotherapy infusions for colorectal cancer patients with suggested daily home practice for 8 weeks (Sohl et al., 2016a,b).

Therapeutic goals of the YST included lowering fatigue, circadian disruption, and psychological distress. Elements of the YST were awareness meditation, gentle seated movement, breathing practice, and relaxation meditation. Attention, comfort, and ease were also emphasized. This account of a protocol for incorporating yoga with conventional cancer treatment notified future study designs and clinical practice. The design of the YST was innovative, because it applied yoga individually during clinical care (Sohl et al., 2016a,b).

A study that was a randomized, partially blinded, controlled trial compared a standardized yoga intervention to standard care. It was conducted at three medical centers in Montreal, Canada. Participants were given yoga practices consisting of 23 gentle yoga poses, 2 breathing exercises (pranayama), corpse poses (shavasanas), and psycho-educational themes. Participants attended 8 weekly sessions lasting 90 minutes each and received a DVD for home practice with 20- and 40-minute sessions. Yoga intervention showed beneficial effects in reducing and preventing the worsening of depression symptoms during chemotherapy treatment (Dupuis et al., 2016).

Fatigue and other treatment-related symptoms such as sleep disturbance are serious targets for enhancing quality of life in patients enduring chemotherapy. Yoga may help alleviate such symptoms. In a randomized controlled pilot study, a short yoga intervention for colorectal cancer was examined during chemotherapy. The researchers randomized adults with colorectal cancer to a short YST group or an attention control (AC) group (Sohl et al., 2016a,b).

The interventions and assessments were employed one-on-one in the clinic while patients obtained chemotherapy. Both interventions were comprised of three sessions as well as suggested home practice. The primary outcome was feasibility (accrual, retention, adherence, data collection). Self-reported outcomes (i.e., fatigue, sleep disturbance, quality of life) and inflammatory biomarkers were also explained. This inquiry showed the viability of performing a larger randomized controlled trial to assess YST among patients receiving chemotherapy for colorectal cancer (Sohl et al., 2016a,b).

An investigation was performed studying self-directed yoga practice at home in women with breast cancer during chemotherapy. The study showed improvement in cognitive functions of patients receiving chemotherapy due to breast cancer. Cognitive loss with chemotherapy is serious and is often known as chemo-brain. Yoga can be a non-pharmacological approach to improving chemo-brain (Komatsu et al., 2016).

In a randomized control trial, the effects of a yoga program were compared with supportive therapy on self-reported symptoms of depression in breast cancer patients undergoing conventional treatment. A total of 98 breast cancer patients with stage II and III disease from a cancer center were randomly assigned to receive yoga (n = 45) and supportive therapy (n = 53) over a 24-week period during which they underwent surgery followed by adjuvant radiation or chemotherapy or both. Yoga and supportive therapy both decreased depression. There was a significant decrease in depression scores in the yoga group as compared to controls following surgery, radiation, and chemotherapy (P < 0.01). There was a positive correlation (P < 0.001) between depression scores with symptom severity and distress during surgery, radiation, and chemotherapy. Yoga practices showed antidepressant effects in breast cancer patients undergoing conventional radiation and chemotherapy (Rao et al., 2015).

YOGA AND OSTEOPOROSIS

A 12-minute daily yoga regimen reversed osteoporotic bone loss in a 10-year study. A total of 741 Internet-recruited volunteers participated in the study. The pre-yoga bone mineral density changes were compared with the post-yoga bone mineral density changes. DEXA scans, radiographs of hips and spine as well as a bone quality study were conducted. Bone mineral density improved in the spine, hips, and femur of the 227 moderately and fully compliant patients (Lu et al., 2016).

In another research study, 30 females in the age group of 45–62 years suffering from postmenopausal osteoporosis with a DEXA score of ≤-2.5 underwent 6 months of a fully supervised yoga session. There was an improvement in T-score of DEXA scans of -2.55 ± 0.25 at post-training versus a pretraining score of -2.69 ± 0.17. Yoga practices included weight bearing and nonweight bearing postures, breathing exercises (pranayama), and sun salutation (suryanamaskar), all of which assisted in improving bone mineral density in postmenopausal osteoporotic females (Bedekar et al., 2016).

YOGA AND OBESITY

Women ages 34–39 years from the Australian Longitudinal Study on Women's Health were surveyed regarding body satisfaction, weight control behaviors, and yoga and meditation practice. The objective of the study was to analyze whether yoga or meditation use is associated with body (dis) satisfaction and weight control methods in Australian women. Associations of body satisfaction and weight control methods with yoga/meditation practice were analyzed using chi-squared testing and multiple logistic regression modelling (Lauche et al., 2017).

Of the 8,009 women, 49% were overweight or obese. The 65% percent of women with normal body mass index (BMI) and approximately 95% of the overweight women with obesity wanted to lose weight. At least one in four women with normal BMI was dissatisfied with body weight and shape, as were more than two in three women with overweight/obesity. The most common weight control methods included exercising (82.7%), cutting down meal sizes (76.8%), and cutting down sugars or fats (71.9%). Yoga/meditation was practiced frequently by 688 women (8.6%) and occasionally by 1176 women (14.7%) (Lauche et al., 2017).

Yoga/meditation users with normal BMI were less likely to be dissatisfied with body weight and shape. All yoga/meditation users more likely exercised and followed a low glycemic diet or diet books. Women with obesity occasionally used yoga/meditation and more likely utilized fasting or smoking to lose weight. Yoga/meditation users with normal BMI appeared to be more satisfied with their body weight and shape than non-yoga/meditation users. It was concluded that while women with normal BMI or overweight tend to rely on healthy weight control methods, women with obesity occasionally using yoga/meditation may more likely utilize unhealthy weight control methods (Lauche et al., 2017).

Obesity has become a serious problem all over the world. Obesity leads to diabetes, heart disease, hypertension, hormonal imbalances, and even cancer. Yoga practice reduces the stress which may improve the eating habits and help in weight reduction. In a randomized control trial for 14 weeks of yoga training, obese adult males were studied. Improvements were noticed in anthropometric and psychological parameters such as weight, percentage body fat, and stress (Rshikesan et al., 2016a,b).

A similar study was done on women and the focus was abdominal obesity, as it is a major risk factor for morbidity and mortality. After a 12-week yoga intervention, abdominal circumference was significantly reduced, and there were improvements in waist/hip ratio, body weight, body mass index, body fat percentage, body muscle mass percentage, mental and physical well-being, self-esteem, subjective stress, body awareness, and trust in bodily sensations. There were no serious adverse events. The highlight of this research investigation is that none of the subjects embarked on a low-calorie diet while participating in the study (Cramer et al., 2016).

YOGA AND HYPOTHYROIDISM

The thyroid gland is under attack due to pollution, lack of iodine, and the presence of halogens such as chlorine and bromine as well as radiation from x-rays, cell phones, PDAs, and computers. Hypothyroidism is characterized by elevated lipid profiles and thyroid stimulation hormone (TSH). It is also a comorbid factor for coronary artery disease, obesity, depression, osteoporosis, sleep apnea, and many more. A 6-month yoga training was devised for 22 household women suffering from hypothyroidism between the ages of 30 and 40 (mean $\pm$ SD; 36.7 $\pm$ 3.2) years, with an average of 4 $\pm$ 1.12-year history of hypothyroidism (Nilakanthan et al., 2016).

Patients with known cardiac issues, hypertension history, recent surgery, and degenerative disc disease were excluded from the study. All the women were on thyroxine (mean 65.78 $\pm$ 22.74 mcg). All the women did yoga for 1 hour for 4 days/week for 6 months. Lipid profile, thyroxine dosage, and serum TSH levels were assessed before and after intervention. There was a significant reduction in total cholesterol (p = 0.006; −8.99%), LDL (p = 0.002; −9.81%) and triglycerides (p = 0.013; −7.6%), and improvement in HDL (p = 0.02; +9.65%) along with a reduction in TSH levels (p = 0.452; −9.72%). There was a 15.30% decline in the doses of thyroxine (Nilakanthan et al., 2016).

In my clinical practice of 36 years, I have seen several thousand patients with hypothyroidism. Many patients have been able to bring their thyroid function back to normal and come completely off the medications. They were at least able to reduce the usage of medications up to 50% with yoga and herbal supplements.

YOGA AND POST-TRAUMATIC STRESS SYNDROME

Yoga has been found to be an effective post-traumatic stress disorder (PTSD) treatment for a variety of trauma survivors, including females with chronic conditions. A 20-week trauma-sensitive yoga treatment in women with chronic treatment-resistant PTSD (N = 9) showed a reduction in dissociation symptoms over several assessment periods, suggesting that more intensive trauma-sensitive yoga treatment for longer duration and home practice may be more advantageous for individuals with severe and chronic PTSD. The implications of the findings are enormous, as so many veterans suffer with PTSD, and the pharmaceutical approach has not helped at all (Price et al., 2017).

A randomized controlled study was carried out on 60 women with chronic, treatment-resistant PTSD and associated mental health problems stemming from prolonged or multiple trauma exposures. After 10 sessions of yoga, participants exhibited statistically significant decreases in PTSD symptoms severity and a greater likelihood of loss of PTSD diagnosis, significant decreases in engagement in negative tension reduction activities (e.g., self-injury), and greater reductions in dissociative and depressive symptoms when compared with the control (Metcalf et al., 2016).

Participants from a randomized controlled trial were invited to participate in long-term follow-up assessments approximately 1.5 years after study completion to assess whether the initial intervention and/or yoga practice after treatment was associated with additional changes. A group of 49 women completed the long-term follow-up interviews. Continuing yoga practice significantly predicted greater decreases in the severity of PTSD symptoms and depression symptoms as well. There was also a greater likelihood of a loss of PTSD diagnosis with a routine yoga practice (Rhodes et al., 2016).

In a pilot randomized control study, 80 individuals with current PTSD symptoms participated in Kundalini yoga practices. Two groups were compared: Kundalini yoga (KY) group and a waitlist control group. Both groups demonstrated changes in PTSD symptomology. However, yoga participants showed greater changes in measures of sleep, positive affect, perceived stress, anxiety, stress, and resilience (Jindani et al., 2015). Furthermore, a meta-analysis of 19 studies showed a moderate level of evidence for efficacy of yoga in PTSD (Metcalf et al., 2016).

YOGA AND INSOMNIA

Sleep deprivation is reported to affect two-thirds of American adults and is considered an important public health concern. Sleep experts recommend adults to receive 7–9 hours of sleep a night for good health and optimum performance. Yet, most adults get considerably less sleep (Kennedy, 2014). Sleeping pills are not helpful either. Sleeping pills swallowed by millions every night could be linked to up to 500,000 deaths a year. Approximately 35,000 people were tracked for 2.5 years. Here is what was learned: If you take 132 sleeping pills a year, you are 5.3 times as likely to die as non-users. The heaviest uses of Zolpidem (also known as Ambien) boosts the risk of death up to 5.7 times and Temazepam (also known as Restoril) raises the risk of death to 6.6 times. Heavy sleeping pill users also have a 35% greater chance of cancer (Kripke et al., 2012).

Daily yoga treatment was evaluated in a chronic insomnia population consisting of sleep-onset and/or sleep-maintenance insomnia and primary or secondary insomnia. Participants maintained sleep-wake diaries during a pretreatment 2-week baseline and a subsequent 8-week intervention, in which they practiced the treatment on their own, following a single in-person training session with subsequent brief in-person and telephone follow-ups. Sleep efficiency, total sleep time, total wake time, sleep onset latency, wake time after sleep onset, number of awakenings, and sleep quality measures were derived from sleep-wake diary entries and were averaged in 2-week intervals. For 20 participants completing the protocol, statistically significant improvements were observed in sleep efficiency, total sleep time, total wake time, sleep onset latency, wake time after sleep onset, number of awakenings, and sleep quality at end-treatment as compared with pretreatment values (Khalsa, 2004).

YOGA AND AUTISM

Autism spectrum disorder (ASD) is a complex neurodevelopmental disorder with deficiencies in many developmental milestones during the infantile childhood. Early behavior intervention is a must for ASD children that primarily affects the psychological level. A research studied the contributions of yoga to alleviate such problems. It was concluded that yoga is a noninvasive and alternative therapy that brings change in both physiological and psychological levels of a child affected by ASD (Narasingharao et al., 2016).

A classroom yoga program among children with ASD was devised. The intervention group received the yoga program daily for 16 weeks, and the control group engaged in their standard morning routine. Challenging behaviors and behavior coding were measured before and after intervention. Students in the yoga program showed significant decreases ($p < 0.05$) in teacher ratings of maladaptive behavior, as measured with the Aberrant Behavior Checklist, compared with the control participants (Koenig et al., 2012).

Moreover, a case focused on a 7-year-old boy with Apert and Asperger's syndrome who attended 8, 45-minute multisensory yoga sessions, twice a week, during a 4-week camp. Results from the pre- and post-tests on Treatment and Research Institute for Autism Social Skills Assessment showed improvements in the total score changes from 19 to 7 for disruptive behaviors. Sparks Target Behavior Checklist scores changed from 8 to 1 showing progression in ability to stay on task. He revealed a positive development in expressive emotions, social engagement, and decline in looking around. Outside class, parents and school behavioral specialists reported the improved ability of this child to self-regulate stress using lion's breath and super brain yoga. He showed improvements in behaviors that influenced the physical performance, emotional expression, and social interaction after yoga training (Scroggins et al., 2016).

LEFT AND RIGHT NOSTRIL VARIATIONS

An investigation researched the effects of uninostril and alternate nostril pranayamas on cardiovascular constraints and reaction time. Many previous studies have denoted that the differential physiological and psychological effects of yogic uninostril breathing (UNB) and alternate nostril breathing (ANB) techniques are phenomenal. The purpose of this study was to determine differential effects of these techniques on reaction time (RT), heart rate (HR), and blood pressure (BP) (Bhavanani et al., 2014).

Twenty yoga-trained persons were called to a lab setting on six distinctive days. Their RT, HR, and BP were documented randomly pre- and post-nine rounds of right UNB (surya nadi [SN]), left UNB (chandra nadi [CN]), right initiated ANB (surya bhedana [SB]), left initiated ANB (chandra bhedana [CB]), nadi shuddhi (NS), and normal breathing (NB) (Bhavanani et al., 2014).

A general comparison of percent changes demonstrated statistically significant differences between groups for all constraints. There was a total decline in HR- and BP-based parameters following CB, CN, and NS with a simultaneous rise following SB and SN. The consequences of right nostril initiated (SB and SN) and left nostril initiated (CB, CN, and NS) UNB and ANB techniques were recorded. Variations following NB were insignificant in all aspects. The overall evaluation of percent changes for RT exhibited statistically significant differences between groups that were significantly lowered following both SB and SN. This study offered proof of sympathomimetic effects of right nostril initiated pranayamas with sympatholytic/parasympathomimetic effect following left nostril initiated pranayamas (Bhavanani et al., 2014).

The authors proposed that the main effect of UNB and ANB techniques is regulated by the nostril utilized for inspiration instead of the one utilized for expiration. It was concluded that right and left yogic UNB and ANB techniques have important physiological effects which are in sync with the traditional swara yoga notion that air flow through the right nostril (SN and pingala swara) is activatory in nature, whereas the flow through the left nostril (CN and ida swara) is calming (Bhavanani et al., 2014).

My fascination for yoga from early childhood, later as personal and clinical experience of 36 years with my patients has given me the firm belief that yoga is an integral part of healing. Simple yogic techniques like asana, pranayama, and meditation provide great healing regardless of what healing modality you use for your patients.

REFERENCES

Afonso, R. F., E. H. Kozasa, D. Rodrigues, H. Hachul, J. Roberto Leite, and S. Tufik. "Yoga Increased Serum Estrogen Levels in Postmenopausal Women—A Case Report." *Menopause* 23.5, 2016: 584–86. Web.

Angadi, P., A. Jagannathan, A. Thulasi, V. Kumar, K. Umamaheshwar, and N. Raghuram. "Adherence to Yoga and Its Resultant Effects on Blood Glucose in Type 2 Diabetes: A Community-based Follow-up Study." *International Journal of Yoga* 10.1, 2017: 29. Web.

Bairy, S., A. M. V. Kumar, M. Raju, S. Achanta, B. Naik, J. P. Tripathy, and R. Zachariah. "Is Adjunctive Naturopathy Associated with Improved Glycaemic Control and a Reduction in Need for Medications among Type 2 Diabetes Patients? A Prospective Cohort Study from India." *BMC Complementary and Alternative Medicine* 16.1, 2016: 290. Web.

Bedekar, N., Z. Motorwala, S. Kolke, P. Panchal, P. Sancheti, and A. Shyam. "Effects of Yogasanas on Osteoporosis in Postmenopausal Women." *International Journal of Yoga* 9.1, 2016: 44–8. Web.

Bhavanani, A., D. Pushpa, M. Ramanathan, and R. Balaji. "Differential Effects of Uninostril and Alternate Nostril Pranayamas on Cardiovascular Parameters and Reaction Time." *International Journal of Yoga* 7.1, 2014: 60. Web.

Birdee, G. S., G. Y. Yeh, P. M. Wayne, R. S. Phillips, R. B. Davis, and P. Gardiner. "Clinical Applications of Yoga for the Pediatric Population: A Systematic Review." *Academic Pediatrics* 9.4, 2009: 212–220. Web.

Boxer, R. S., A. Kleppinger, J. Brindisi, R. Feinn, J. A. Burleson, and A. M. Kenny. "Effects of Dehydroepiandrosterone, DHEA) on Cardiovascular Risk Factors in Older Women with Frailty Characteristics." *Age and Ageing* 39.4, 2010: 451–58. Web.

Brands, M. M. M. G., H. Purperhart, and J. M. Deckers-Kocken. "A Pilot Study of Yoga Treatment in Children with Functional Abdominal Pain and Irritable Bowel Syndrome." *Complementary Therapies in Medicine* 19.3, 2011: 109–14. Web.

Brosseau, L., J. Taki, B. Desjardins, O. Thevenot, M. Fransen, et al. "The Ottawa Panel Clinical Practice Guidelines for the Management of Knee Osteoarthritis. Part One: Introduction, and Mind-body Exercise Programs." *Clinical Rehabilitation* 31.5, 2017: 582–595. Web.

Buchanan, D. T., C. A. Landis, C. Hohensee, K. A. Guthrie, J. L. Otte, et al. "Effects of Yoga and Aerobic Exercise on Actigraphic Sleep Parameters in Menopausal Women with Hot Flashes." *Journal of Clinical Sleep Medicine* 13.01, 2017: 11–8. Web.

Chaturvedi, A., G. Nayak, A.G. Nayak, and A. Rao. "Comparative Assessment of the Effects of Hatha Yoga and Physical Exercise on Biochemical Functions in Perimenopausal Women." *Journal of Clinical and Diagnostic Research* 10.8, 2016: KC01–C04. Web.

Cheung, C., J. Park, and J. F. Wyman. "Effects of Yoga on Symptoms, Physical Function, and Psychosocial Outcomes in Adults with Osteoarthritis: A Focused Review." *American Journal of Physical Medicine & Rehabilitation* 95.2, 2016: 139–51. Web.

Cheung, C., J. F. Wyman, U. Bronas, T. Mccarthy, K. Rudser, and M. A. Mathiason. "Managing Knee Osteoarthritis with Yoga or Aerobic/strengthening Exercise Programs in Older Adults: A Pilot Randomized Controlled Trial." *Rheumatology International* 37.3, 2017: 389–98. Web.

Chien, L.-W., H.-C. Chang, and C.-F. Liu. "Effect of Yoga on Serum Homocysteine and Nitric Oxide Levels in Adolescent Women With and Without Dysmenorrhea." *The Journal of Alternative and Complementary Medicine* 19.1, 2013: 20–3. Web.

Chu, P., A. Pandya, J. A. Salomon, S. J. Goldie, and M. G. Myriam Hunink. "Comparative Effectiveness of Personalized Lifestyle Management Strategies for Cardiovascular Disease Risk Reduction." *Journal of the American Heart Association* 5.3, 2016: 16. Web.

Cramer, H., D. Anheyer, R. Lauche, and G. Dobos. "A Systematic Review of Yoga for Major Depressive Disorder." *Journal of Affective Disorders* 213, 2017a: 70–77. Web.

Cramer, H., R. Lauche, H. Haller, N. Steckhan, A. Michalsen, and G. Dobos. "Effects of Yoga on Cardiovascular Disease Risk Factors: A Systematic Review and Meta-analysis." *International Journal of Cardiology* 173.2, 2014: 170–83. Web.

Cramer, H., R. Lauche, P. Klose, S. Lange, J. Langhorst, and G. J. Dobos. "Yoga for Improving Health-related Quality of Life, Mental Health and Cancer-related Symptoms in Women Diagnosed with Breast Cancer." *Cochrane Database of Systematic Reviews* 1, 2017b: CD010802. Web.

Cramer, H., M. S. Thomas, D. Anheyer, R. Lauche, and G. Dobos. "Yoga in Women With Abdominal Obesity— A Randomized Controlled Trial." *Deutsches Arzteblatt International* 113.39, 2016: 645–52. Print.

Danhauer, S. C., E. L. Addington, S. J. Sohl, A. Chaoul, and L. Cohen. "Review of Yoga Therapy during Cancer Treatment." *Supportive Care in Cancer* 25.4, 2017: 1357–1372. Web.

Dupuis, G., R. Marcaurell, M. Bali, D. Lanctot, and A. S. Anestin. "The Effects of the Bali Yoga Program, BYP-bc) on Reducing Psychological Symptoms in Breast Cancer Patients Receiving Chemotherapy: Results of a Randomized, Partially Blinded, Controlled Trial." *Journal of Complementary and Integrative Medicine* 13.4, 2016: 405–12. Web.

Eichenberger, P. A., S. N. Diener, R. Kofmehl, and C. M. Spengler. "Effects of Exercise Training on Airway Hyperreactivity in Asthma: A Systematic Review and Meta-Analysis." *Sports Medicine* 43.11, 2013: 1157–170. Web.

Evans, S., K. C. Lung, L. C. Seidman, B. Sternlieb, L. K. Zeltzer, and J. C. I. Tsao. "Iyengar Yoga for Adolescents and Young Adults With Irritable Bowel Syndrome." *Journal of Pediatric Gastroenterology and Nutrition* 59.2, 2014: 244–53. Web.

Evans, S., M. Moieni, K. Lung, J. Tsao, B. Sternlieb, M. Taylor, and L. Zeltzer. "Impact of Iyengar Yoga on Quality of Life in Young Women With Rheumatoid Arthritis." *The Clinical Journal of Pain* 29.11, 2013: 988–97. Web.

Galliford, M., S. Robinson, P. Bridge, and M. Carmichael. "Salute to the Sun: A New Dawn in Yoga Therapy for Breast Cancer." *Journal of Medical Radiation Sciences* 64.3, 2017: 232–238. Web.

Goncalves, A. V., N. F. Barros, and L. Bahamondes. "The Practice of Hatha Yoga for the Treatment of Pain Associated with Endometriosis." *The Journal of Alternative and Complementary Medicine* 23.1, 2017: 45–52. Web.

Greysen, H. M., S. Ryan Greysen, K. A. Lee, O. S. Hong, P. Katz, and H. Leutwyler. "A Qualitative Study Exploring Community Yoga Practice in Adults with Rheumatoid Arthritis." *The Journal of Alternative and Complementary Medicine* 23.6, 2017: 487–493. Web.

Hall, A., N. A. Ofei-Tenkorang, J. T. Machan, and C. M. Gordon. "Use of Yoga in Outpatient Eating Disorder Treatment: A Pilot Study." *Journal of Eating Disorders* 4.1, 2016: 38–46. Web.

Hagglund, E., I. Hagerman, K. Dencker, and A. Stromberg. "Effects of Yoga versus Hydrotherapy Training on Health-related Quality of Life and Exercise Capacity in Patients with Heart Failure: A Randomized Controlled Study." *European Journal of Cardiovascular Nursing* 16.5, 2017: 381–389. Web.

Hunter, S. D., M. S. Dhindsa, E. Cunningham, T. Tarumi, M. Alkatan, N. Nualnim, and H. Tanaka. "Impact of Hot Yoga on Arterial Stiffness and Quality of Life in Normal and Overweight/Obese Adults." *Journal of Physical Activity and Health* 13.12, 2016: 1360–363. Web.

Jindani, F., N. Turner, and S. B. S. Khalsa. "A Yoga Intervention for Posttraumatic Stress: A Preliminary Randomized Control Trial." *Evidence-Based Complementary and Alternative Medicine* 2015, 2015: 1–8. Web.

Jorge, M. P., D. F. Santaella, I. M. O. Pontes, V. K. M. Shiramizu, E. B. Nascimento et al. "Hatha Yoga Practice Decreases Menopause Symptoms and Improves Quality of Life: A Randomized Controlled Trial." *Complementary Therapies in Medicine* 26, 2016: 128–35. Web.

Kant, S., S. Kumar, R. Mishra, S. Mishra, and S. Agnihotri. "Impact of Yoga on Biochemical Profile of Asthmatics: A Randomized Controlled Study." *International Journal of Yoga* 7.1, 2014: 17. Web.

Karam, M., B. P. Kaur, and A. P. Baptist. "A Modified Breathing Exercise Program for Asthma Is Easy to Perform and Effective." *Journal of Asthma* 54.2, 2017: 217–222. Web.

Kavuri, V., N. Raghuram, A. Malamud, and S. R. Selvan. "Irritable Bowel Syndrome: Yoga as Remedial Therapy." *Evidence-Based Complementary and Alternative Medicine* 2015, 2015: 1–10. Web.

Kennedy, S. L. "Yoga as the "next Wave" of Therapeutic Modalities for Treatment of Insomnia." *International Journal of Yoga Therapy* 24, 2014: 125–29. Print.

Kenny, A. M., R. S. Boxer, A. Kleppinger, J. Brindisi, R. Feinn, and J. A. Burleson. "Dehydroepiandrosterone Combined with Exercise Improves Muscle Strength and Physical Function in Frail Older Women." *Journal of the American Geriatrics Society* 58.9, 2010: 1707–714. Web.

Khalsa, S. B. S. "Treatment of Chronic Insomnia with Yoga: A Preliminary Study with Sleep-Wake Diaries." *Applied Psychophysiology and Biofeedback* 29.4, 2004: 269–78. Web.

Kligler, B., P. Homel, A. E. Blank, J. Kenney, H. Levenson, and W. Merrell. "Randomized Trial of the Effect of an Integrative Medicine Approach to the Management of Asthma in Adults on Disease-related Quality of Life and Pulmonary Function." *Alternative Therapies In Health and Medicine* 17.1, 2011: 10–15. Print.

Koenig, K. P., A. Buckley-Reen, and S. Garg. "Efficacy of the Get Ready to Learn Yoga Program Among Children With Autism Spectrum Disorders: A Pretest-Posttest Control Group Design." *American Journal of Occupational Therapy* 66.5, 2012: 538–46. Web.

Komatsu, H., K. Yagasaki, H. Yamauchi, T. Yamauchi, and T. Takebayashi. "A Self-directed Home Yoga Programme for Women with Breast Cancer during Chemotherapy: A Feasibility Study." *International Journal of Nursing Practice* 22.3, 2016: 258–66. Web.

Kripke, D. F., R. D. Langer, and L. E. Kline. "Hypnotics' Association with Mortality or Cancer: A Matched Cohort Study." *BMJ Open* 2.1, 2012: 2: e000850. Web.

Kuttner, L., C. T. Chambers, J. Hardial, D. M. Israel, K. Jacobson, and K. Evans. "A Randomized Trial of Yoga for Adolescents with Irritable Bowel Syndrome." *Pain Research and Management* 11.4, 2006: 217–24. Web.

Lauche, R., D. Sibbritt, T. Ostermann, N. R. Fuller, J. Adams, and H. Cramer. "Associations between Yoga/meditation Use, Body Satisfaction, and Weight Management Methods: Results of a National Cross-sectional Survey of 8009 Australian Women." *Nutrition* 34, 2017: 58–64. Web.

Loudon, A., T. Barnett, N. Piller, M. A. Immink, D. Visentin, and A. D. Williams. "The Effects of Yoga on Shoulder and Spinal Actions for Women with Breast Cancer-related Lymphoedema of the Arm: A Randomised Controlled Pilot Study." *BMC Complementary and Alternative Medicine* 16.1, 2016: 343. Web.

Lu, Y-H., B. Rosner, G. Chang, and L. M. Fishman. "Twelve-Minute Daily Yoga Regimen Reverses Osteoporotic Bone Loss." *Topics in Geriatric Rehabilitation* 32.2, 2016: 81–87. Web.

Metcalf, O., T. Varker, D. Forbes, A. Phelps, L. Dell, A. Dibattista, N. Ralph, and M. O'donnell. "Efficacy of Fifteen Emerging Interventions for the Treatment of Posttraumatic Stress Disorder: A Systematic Review." *Journal of Traumatic Stress* 29.1, 2016: 88–92. Web.

Milbury, K., S. Mallaiah, A. Mahajan, T. Armstrong, S-P. Weathers, K. E. Moss, N. Goktepe, A. Spelman, and L. Cohen. "Yoga Program for High-Grade Glioma Patients Undergoing Radiotherapy and Their Family Caregivers." *Integrative Cancer Therapies* January 2017: 1534735417689882. Web.

Moody, K., B. Abrahams, R. Baker, R. Santizo, D. Manwani, V. Carullo, D. Eugenio, and A. Carroll. "A Randomized Trial of Yoga for Children Hospitalized with Sickle Cell Vaso-Occlusive Crisis." *Journal of Pain and Symptom Management* 53.6, 2017: 1026–1034. Web.

Mullur, R. S., and D. Ames. "Impact of a 10 Minute Seated Yoga Practice in the Management of Diabetes." *Journal of Yoga & Physical Therapy* 06.01, 2016: 1000224. Web.

Narasingharao, K., B. Pradhan, and J. Navaneetham. "Sleep Disorder, Gastrointestinal Problems and Behaviour Problems Seen in Autism Spectrum Disorder Children and Yoga as Therapy: A Descriptive Review." *Journal of Clinical and Diagnostic Research* 10.11, 2016: VE01–E03. Web.

Nidhi, R., V. Padmalatha, R. Nagarathna, and R. Amritanshu. "Effects of a Holistic Yoga Program on Endocrine Parameters in Adolescents with Polycystic Ovarian Syndrome: A Randomized Controlled Trial." *The Journal of Alternative and Complementary Medicine* 19.2, 2013: 153–60. Web.

Nilakanthan, S., K. Metri, N. Raghuram, and N. Hongasandra. "Effect of 6 Months Intense Yoga Practice on Lipid Profile, Thyroxine Medication and Serum TSH Level in Women Suffering from Hypothyroidism: A Pilot Study." *Journal of Complementary and Integrative Medicine* 13.2, 2016: 189–193. Web.

Ornish, D. "Intensive Lifestyle Changes for Reversal of Coronary Heart Disease." *JAMA* 280.23, 1998: 2001. Web.

Price, M., J. Spinazzola, R. Musicaro, J. Turner, M. Suvak, D. Emerson, and B. Van Der Kolk. "Effectiveness of an Extended Yoga Treatment for Women with Chronic Posttraumatic Stress Disorder." *The Journal of Alternative and Complementary Medicine* 23.4, 2017: 300–309. Web.

Rao, R., N. Raghuram, H. R Nagendra, M. R. Usharani, K. S. Gopinath, R. Diwakar, S. Patil, N. Rao, and R. Bilimagga. "Effects of an Integrated Yoga Program on Self-reported Depression Scores in Breast Cancer Patients Undergoing Conventional Treatment: A Randomized Controlled Trial." *Indian Journal of Palliative Care* 21.2, 2015: 174–81. Web.

Rao, Y. C., A. Kadam, A. Jagannathan, N. Babina, R. Rao, and H. R. Nagendra. "Efficacy of Naturopathy and Yoga in Bronchial Asthma." *Indian Journal of Physiology and Pharmacology* 58.3, 2014: 233–39. Print.

Rhodes, A., J. Spinazzola, and B. Van Der Kolk. "Yoga for Adult Women with Chronic PTSD: A Long-Term Follow-Up Study." *The Journal of Alternative and Complementary Medicine* 22.3, 2016: 189–96. Web.

Rshikesan, P. B., and P. Subramanya. "Effect of Integrated Approach of Yoga Therapy on Male Obesity and Psychological Parameters–A Randomised Controlled Trial." *Journal of Clinical and Diagnostic Research* 10.10, 2016a: KC01–C06. Web.

Rshikesan, P. B., P. Subramanya, and R. Nidhi. "Yoga Practice for Reducing the Male Obesity and Weight Related Psychological Difficulties–A Randomized Controlled Trial." *Journal of Clinical and Diagnostic Research* 10.11, 2016b: OC22–C28. Web.

Ruddy, J., J. Emerson, S. Mcnamara, A. Genatossio, C. Breuner, T. Weber, and M. Rosenfeld. "Yoga as a Therapy for Adolescents and Young Adults with Cystic Fibrosis: A Pilot Study." *Global Advances in Health and Medicine* 4.6, 2015: 32–36. Web.

Schmidt, T., A. Wijga, A. Von Zur Muhlen, G. Brabant, and T. O. Wagner. "Changes in Cardiovascular Risk Factors and Hormones during a Comprehensive Residential Three Month Kriya Yoga Training and Vegetarian Nutrition." *Acta Physiologica Scandinavica. Supplementum* 640, 1997: 158–62. Print.

Schumann, D., D. Anheyer, R. Lauche, G. Dobos, J. Langhorst, and H. Cramer. "Effect of Yoga in the Therapy of Irritable Bowel Syndrome: A Systematic Review." *Clinical Gastroenterology and Hepatology* 14.12, 2016: 1720–731. Web.

Scroggins, M., L. Litchke, and T. Liu. "Effects of Multisensory Yoga on Behavior in a Male Child with Apert and Asperger Syndrome." *International Journal of Yoga* 9.1, 2016: 81. Web.

Shah, S., A. Mishra, H. Patel, N. Patel, P. Sangwan, A. Chodos, Z. Brelvi, and D. Kaswala. "Can Yoga Be Used to Treat Gastroesophageal Reflux Disease?" *International Journal of Yoga* 6.2, 2013: 131. Web.

Shahabi, L., B. D. Naliboff, and D. Shapiro. "Self-regulation Evaluation of Therapeutic Yoga and Walking for Patients with Irritable Bowel Syndrome: A Pilot Study." *Psychology, Health & Medicine* 21.2, 2016: 176–88. Web.

Singh, S., R. Soni, K. P. Singh, and O. P. Tandon. "Effect of Yoga Practices on Pulmonary Function Tests including Transfer Factor of Lung for Carbon Monoxide, TLCO) in Asthma Patients." *Indian Journal of Physiology and Pharmacology* 56.1, 2012: 63–68. Print.

Sodhi, C., S. Singh, and A. Bery. "Assessment of the Quality of Life in Patients with Bronchial Asthma, before and after Yoga: A Randomised Trial." *Iranian Journal of Allergy, Asthma and Immunology* 13.1, 2014: 55–60. Print.

Sohl, S. J., G. S. Birdee, S. H. Ridner, A. Wheeler, S. Gilbert, D. Tarantola, J. Berlin, and R. L. Rothman. "Intervention Protocol for Investigating Yoga Implemented During Chemotherapy." *International Journal of Yoga Therapy* 26.1, 2016a: 103–11. Web.

Sohl, S. J., S. C. Danhauer, G. S. Birdee, B. J. Nicklas, G. Yacoub, M. Aklilu, and N. E. Avis. "A Brief Yoga Intervention Implemented during Chemotherapy: A Randomized Controlled Pilot Study." *Complementary Therapies in Medicine* 25, 2016b: 139–42. Web.

Sreedevi, A., U. A. Gopalakrishnan, S. K. Ramaiyer, and L. Kamalamma. "A Randomized Controlled Trial of the Effect of Yoga and Peer Support on Glycaemic Outcomes in Women with Type 2 Diabetes Mellitus: A Feasibility Study." *BMC Complementary and Alternative Medicine* 17.1, 2017: 100–108. Web.

Streeter, C. C., P. L. Gerbarg, T. H. Whitfield, L. Owen, J. Johnston et al. "Treatment of Major Depressive Disorder with Iyengar Yoga and Coherent Breathing: A Randomized Controlled Dosing Study." *The Journal of Alternative and Complementary Medicine* 23.6, 2017: 236–243. Web.

Tahan, F., E. H. Gungor, and E. Bicici. "Is Yoga Training Beneficial for Exercise-induced Bronchoconstriction?" *Alternative Therapies in Health and Medicine* 20.2, 2014: 18–23. Print.

Taneja, I., K. K. Deepak, G. Poojary, I. N. Acharya, R. M. Pandey, and M. P. Sharma. "Yogic Versus Conventional Treatment in Diarrhea-Predominant Irritable Bowel Syndrome: A Randomized Control Study." *Applied Psychophysiology and Biofeedback* 29.1, 2004: 19–33. Web.

Tsai, S-Y. "Effect of Yoga Exercise on Premenstrual Symptoms among Female Employees in Taiwan." *International Journal of Environmental Research and Public Health* 13.7, 2016: 721. Web.

Yadav, A., S. Singh, K. P. Singh, and P. Pai. "Effect of Yoga Regimen on Lung Functions including Diffusion Capacity in Coronary Artery Disease Patients: A Randomized Controlled Study." *International Journal of Yoga* 8.1, 2015: 62. Web.

Yang, N-Y., and S-D. Kim. "Effects of a Yoga Program on Menstrual Cramps and Menstrual Distress in Undergraduate Students with Primary Dysmenorrhea: A Single-Blind, Randomized Controlled Trial." *The Journal of Alternative and Complementary Medicine* 22.9, 2016: 732–38. Web.

16 Mind–Body Medicine

Jacqueline Proszynski and Darshan H. Mehta

CONTENTS

Introduction 393
Historical Perspectives and Development 394
Epidemiology 395
    Age Variations 395
    Sociodemographic and Ethnic Variations 396
Advances in Research 397
    Psychosocial MBT Research 398
    Physiological MBT Research 400
    Neuroimaging MBT Studies 401
    Genomic Research 403
    Composite Markers 404
Health Outcomes 406
    Pain, Neurological, and Autoimmune Disorders 406
    Cancer 406
    Mental Health 406
    Gastrointestinal (GI) Health 408
    Cardiovascular Health 409
    Metabolic and Endocrine Health 410
    Side Effects and Risks of MBT 410
Economic Considerations 411
Barriers and Facilitators of MBT Use 412
Summary 413
References 413

INTRODUCTION

Mind–body medicine, a relatively young discipline within the field of clinical research and care, focuses on the interactions between the brain, mind, body, and behavior, to promote physical health and well-being through the power of emotional, mental, social, spiritual, and behavioral factors. It integrates principles of traditional medicine into modern medical practice and encompasses a wide range of treatments, known as mind body therapies (MBTs) designed to facilitate the mind's capacity to affect health. MBTs are used across the world for the purposes of disease treatment and prevention, and health promotion. Techniques such as yoga, mindful meditation, guided imagery, tai chi, qigong, hypnosis, prayer, and deep breathing exercises work to down-regulate the body's natural stress response via mental and biological mechanisms.

Although MBTs have a common goal of increasing mental focus while deterring external sources of distraction and stress, the wide range of MBTs provides many options to tailor treatment plans based on patient interests, needs, and preferences. MBTs are found in a variety of health care settings and can be used in conjunction with conventional modern therapeutics, including procedure-based, technology-based, and pharmacologically based therapies. For example, they may ease symptoms worsened by stress or brought on by side effects of medications (Rosen, Gardiner, and Lee 2013). However, researchers are just beginning to understand the mechanistic pathways through

TABLE 16.1

Common Mind–Body Therapies

	Direction	Focus	Action	Body	Practice
Transcendental Meditation	Self-directed; initially trained	Focused	Indirect	Little emphasis	Daily 2x for 20 min
Mindfulness Meditation	Externally directed, eventually self-directed	Focused, later wider focus	Indirect	Little emphasis	Supervised programs with daily practice
Hypnosis	Externally directed	Focused	Indirect	Little emphasis	Supervised programs as needed
Guided Imagery	Externally directed or self-directed with recording	Focused	Indirect	Little emphasis	Daily for 20/30 min
Biofeedback	Self-directed with assistance of an expert	Focused	Direct	Emphasis	Supervised programs as needed
Relaxation Therapy	Externally directed	Focused	Direct	Emphasis	Supervised programs for 15/20 min
Combination Therapies	Self-directed or externally directed	Focused	Direct or indirect	Emphasis or little emphasis	As needed
Yoga (all types)	Externally directed, later self-directed	Focused	Direct	Emphasis	Supervised session with daily practice
Tai Chi or Qigong	Externally directed, later self-directed	Focused	Direct	Emphasis	Taught lesson with daily practice

which MBTs catalyze positive psychological and physiological change. Table 16.1 categorizes the most common forms of MBTs based on their universal components: (1) self-directed versus instructor-directed, (2) narrow focus versus wide focus of attention, (3) direct action versus indirect action and intervention, (4) body-oriented versus mind-oriented, and (5) recommended amount of practice (adapted from Barrows and Jacobs 2002).

HISTORICAL PERSPECTIVES AND DEVELOPMENT

Traditions from the present-day countries of China and India have attested to the powerful interplay between the mind and body for thousands of years. Scientific advances during the Renaissance and Enlightenment, however, ignited fundamental changes in the way societies approached medicine and the treatment of disease. Rene Descartes and other great philosophers of the time began to distinguish the mind from the body, which subsequently influenced the ideologies of various medical fields. The onset of this Cartesian Dualism recalibrated patient care to fit a disease-based model, void of the spiritual and psychological aspects of healing.

Philosophers and practitioners alike maintained this dualistic perspective for centuries until novel insights on pain control and stress occurred in the early twentieth century. Walter Cannon's work brought attention to the existence of a self-regulatory system within the body and its connection to the autonomic nervous system during stressful situations, known as the *fight or flight response* (Cannon 1915, 1929), or the *stress response*. The stress response consists of generalized increases in sympathetic nervous system activity and catecholamine production along with rises in blood pressure, heart and respiratory rates, and musculoskeletal blood flow (Abrahams, Hilton, and Zbrozyna 1960; Cannon 1914). In essence, Cannon's work reinstated the idea of the mind–body connection, rather than a distinction, by showing that physiological activation and emotion have a joint response to a stimulating event.

Over the proceeding decades, physicians, clinicians, and academics began to reconsider the mind's role in physiological and biological functions. Dr. Herbert Benson, one of the first physicians to bring spirituality and healing into modern medical practice, viewed this vastly underdeveloped field as a path vastly deserving of scientific exploration. Benson identified common patterns across a host of mind–body techniques: they all appeared to evoke an altered state of consciousness and a physiologically relaxed state of the body, what he later coined the *Relaxation Response (RR)* (Wallace and Benson 1972). The RR is associated with decreases in oxygen consumption, respiratory rate, and blood pressure, along with an increased sense of well-being (Wallace, Benson, and Wilson 1971). A closer look into the mechanisms governing this reaction showed decreases in sympathetic nervous system (SNS) activation and an integrated hypothalamic response (Benson 1982).

Benson's work exploring the physiological effects of transcendental meditation illustrated that the RR can be voluntarily elicited and, as such, it may be highly beneficial to integrate relaxation techniques into clinical care settings. Thus, he and his colleagues demonstrated that behavioral processes not only cause physiological changes in reaction to stimulating events, but they can also lead to the alleviation and reversal of some of the predisposing features of illness (Benson 1982).

At roughly the same time, Jon Kabat-Zinn founded mindfulness-based stress reduction (MBSR) in 1979, which involves intensive training in mindfulness meditation and its integration into the challenges and adventures of everyday life. MBSR aims to teach individuals how to use innate resources and abilities to respond more effectively to pressure, pain, and illness. In his preliminary work, Kabat-Zinn demonstrated considerable improvement in chronic pain over the course of a 10-week MBSR training program (Kabat-Zinn 1982), with multiple decades worth of support since.

Within the past 30 years, the medical world has come to embrace the value of mind–body medicine and MBTs in both clinical research and practice. Mind–body clinics, institutes, departments, and centers have steadily begun to appear in hospitals and academic institutions across the world, accompanied by tremendous leaps in our understanding of MBTs. MBT practices are now more widely available, making them more accessible to clinical populations as well as increasing their popularity with the general public.

EPIDEMIOLOGY

Approximately 33% of the U.S. adult population reported complementary and integrative medicine (CAM) practice in 2012 (Clarke et al. 2015). MBTs are among the top 10 CAM therapies used by adults and children, with yoga and meditation being some of the most popular mind–body methods (Cramer et al. 2016). Results from the 2012 National Health Interview Survey (NHIS) show adults most frequently reported using mind–body techniques such as deep breathing (10.9%), yoga, tai chi, or qigong (10.1%), and meditation (8.0%) (Clarke et al. 2015) as displayed in Figure 16.1.

Over the past 13 years, there has been a steady increase in the practice of yoga as seen in Figure 16.2. In 2012, 9.5% of Americans practiced yoga, up from 5.1% in 2002 and from 6.1% in 2007. Prevalence of yoga hovered around 13.2% for lifetime use and 8.9% for 12-month use (Cramer et al. 2016). The reported lifetime and 12-month prevalence rates for tai chi were 3.1% and 1.2%, respectively, based on the 2012 NHIS data (Lauche, Wayne, and Dobos 2016). Reported rates of guided imagery, acupuncture, and massage use remained steady over the same period, while progressive muscle relaxation techniques have become less popular over the past 12 years (Barnes, Bloom, and Nahin 2004, 2008; Peregoy et al. 2014; Clarke et al. 2015; Ni, Simile, and Hardy 2002).

AGE VARIATIONS

Mind–body use was most popular among individuals aged 50–59 years old (44.1%), followed by 60–69 years (41%) and 40–49 years (40.1%) (Barnes, Bloom, and Nahin 2008). MBTs are used by several million children in the United States each year. The current research suggests that early mind–body training is as a useful tool that can help prevent or manage certain health problems (Ndetan, Evans, and Williams 2014). According to the 2012 NHIS, 3.7% of children ages 4–17 years in the United States used mind–body approaches, which were most popular among youth between

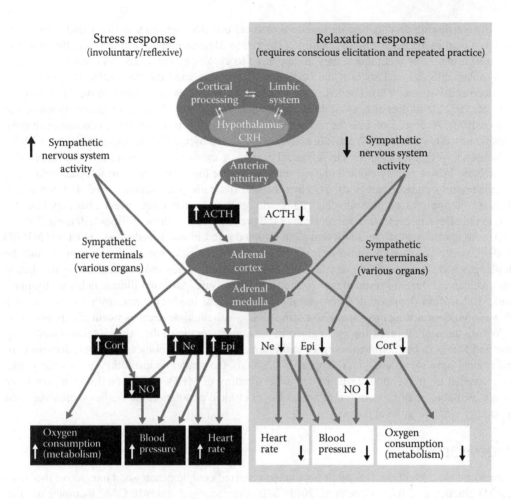

FIGURE 16.1   Dusek and Benson's (2009) stress physiology conceptual model.

the ages of 13–17 years (Black et al. 2015). If children experiencing pain-related conditions or emotional, behavioral, or mental conditions received mental health care, they were more likely to use MBTs. The most common reasons for the use of mind–body approaches were to improve overall health and feel better physically, to reduce stress level or relax, for general wellness or disease prevention, and to feel better emotionally (McClafferty et al. 2016).

SOCIODEMOGRAPHIC AND ETHNIC VARIATIONS

Some of the strongest predictors of MBT use include sociodemographic variables. Estimates from the 2012 NHIS Alternative Medicine Supplement examining sociodemographic predictors of engagement in meditation, yoga, tai chi, and qigong found higher education, higher socioeconomic status (SES), younger age, better health status, being female, and living on the West Coast were associated with increased mindfulness practices (Olano et al. 2015; Lauche, Wayne, and Dobos 2016). As with many forms of medical care, women were twice as likely to engage in an MBT (5.7% vs. 1.7%) (Olano et al. 2015; Cramer et al. 2016) regardless of age (McClafferty et al. 2016). Sadly, vulnerable populations with worse health outcomes were less likely to use MBTs even though these groups could benefit the most. Minority status was also predictive of decreased MBT use among non-Hispanic blacks and Hispanics (Olano et al. 2015).

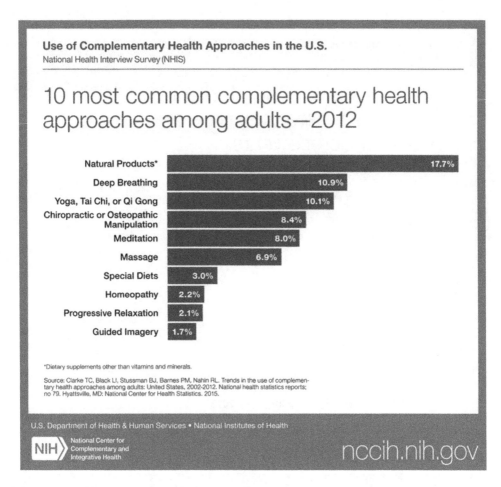

FIGURE 16.2   Ten most common CAM approaches in 2012.

However, sociodemographic factors may influence which MBT method an individual prefers. Tai chi, for instance, was found to have proportionally higher 12-month prevalence rates for individuals of Asian, African American, or other ethnic descent and for individuals 30 years or older. Tai chi or qigong has seen a great increase over the past decade in the number of participants from minority backgrounds, relative to those from non-minority backgrounds (Lauche, Wayne, and Dobos 2016). Yoga use in minority and all age groups has increased as well (Barner et al. 2010; Cramer et al. 2016). Given that minorities tend to be at higher risk for health complications, the increase in MBT use among these groups may bring on positive changes in health outcomes.

ADVANCES IN RESEARCH

Technology continues to expand the scope of analytic possibilities. Psychosocial, physiological, neurological, and genomic methods name a few of the various ways to objectively measure the impacts of MBTs. Given these advances, further research still must refine how best to measure constructs of the mind as they relate to health outcomes. A handful of multi-factorial models have been developed to help tease apart this complex relationship. Dr. Peter Wayne et al.'s (2013) model, for example, describes the components contributing to the effect of a tai chi practitioner's work (Wayne et al. 2013), shown in Figure 16.3.

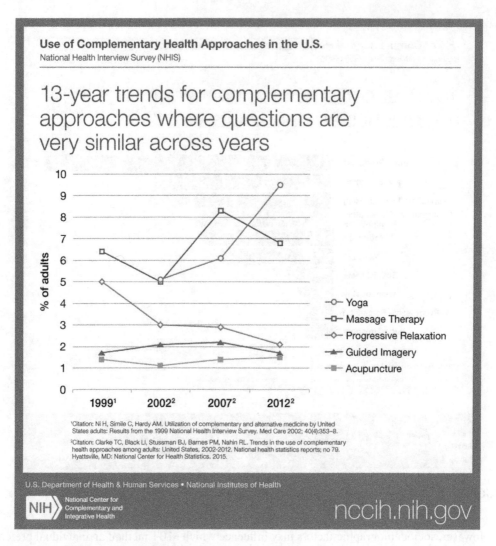

FIGURE 16.3   Thirteen-year trends in CAM use.

PSYCHOSOCIAL MBT RESEARCH

Because of definitional ambiguities, there has been great debate in the literature on how best to measure the effects of MBTs. Thus far, MBT research has established its ability to reduce perceived stress and burnout, elevate mindfulness, and ease symptoms of depression and anxiety, all of which are mediators to health outcomes across multiple disciplines and domains. Table 16.2 summarizes the most commonly studied psychosocial markers of MBT research. All MBTs incorporate these active ingredients, however, to varying degrees.

Perceived stress. One of the most common psychometric outcome measures used in MBT clinical trials is perceived stress, which is defined as the feelings or thoughts that an individual has about their own stress during a designated period of time (Cohen, Kamarck, and Mermelstein 1983). The most widely used measure of perceived stress is the Perceived Stress Scale (PSS) (Cohen, Kamarck, and Mermelstein 1983), which aims to capture the extent to which life is generally appraised as stressful, overloaded, unpredictable, and uncontrollable over the previous month, and one's ability to handle such stress. Reductions in perceived stress are often

TABLE 16.2
Common Psychosocial Markers Used in MBT Research

Marker	Common Scale	Association with Clinical Conditions	Recent Studies
Perceived Stress	Perceived Stress Scale (PSS) Perceived Stress Questionnaire (PSQ)	Community sample	White Jiang, Hall, Katz, Zimmerman, Sliwinski, and Lipton (2014). Higher Perceived Stress Scale scores are associated with higher pain intensity and pain interference levels in older adults.
Mindfulness	Five-Facet Mindfulness Questionnaire (FFMQ) Cognitive and Affective Mindfulness Scale–Revised (CAMS-R) Mindful Attention and Awareness Scale (MAAS)	Clinical and healthy samples	Zimmaro et al. (2016). Association of dispositional mindfulness with stress, cortisol, and well-being among university undergraduate students.
Burnout	Maslach Burnout Inventory (MBI)	Medical student residents	Rosenbluth, Freymiller, Hemphill, Paull, Stuber, and Friedlander (2017). Resident well-being and patient safety: Recognizing the signs and symptoms of burnout.
Depression	Beck Depression Inventory (BDI)	Major Depressive Disorder (MDD)	Streeter et al. (2017). Treatment of major depressive disorder with Iyengar yoga and coherent breathing: A randomized controlled dosing study.
Anxiety	Beck Anxiety Inventory (BAI)	Anxiety disorders	Kocovski et al. (2015). Mindfulness and acceptance-based group therapy and traditional cognitive behavioral group therapy for social anxiety disorder: Mechanisms of change.

accompanied by improvements in symptom severity, sense of well-being, and overall quality of life. Conversely, higher perceived stress scores have been associated with elevated symptom severity, poorer health outcomes, and decreased quality of life (White et al. 2014). In all, perceived stress may be an indicator of the quality and effectiveness of an intervention in research as well as in practice.

Mindfulness. Mindfulness has generally been defined as "the awareness that emerges through paying attention on purpose, in the present moment, and non-judgmentally to things as they are" (Williams et al. 2007, p. 47). It is a state of heightened consciousness or awareness that may mediate the effects of MBT training on mental health outcomes (Deckro et al. 2002; Baer, Carmody, and Hunsinger 2012). Increases in mindfulness scores on these scales tend to describe improvements in openness, internal state awareness, positive and pleasant affect, and well-being, and decreases in neuroticism, anxiety, stress, and rumination (T. Park, Reilly-Spong, and Gross 2013). In a study of overly stressed adults with chronic pain, improvements in mindfulness skills preceded improvement in perceived stress, suggesting that mindfulness may be a mechanism of change in psychosocial MBT research (Baer, Carmody, and Hunsinger 2012). Thus, like perceived stress, mindfulness scales are often used as a gauge of MBT treatment efficacy. Common mindfulness measures include the Five-Facet Mindfulness Questionnaire (FFMQ; Baer et al. 2006), the Cognitive and Affective Mindfulness Scale–Revised (CAMS-R; Feldman et al. 2007), and the Mindful Attention and Awareness Scale (MAAS; Brown and Ryan 2003).

Burnout. Burnout is associated with a host of negative psychosocial and physical health consequences related to persistent, relentless work-related stress. It is characterized by emotional exhaustion, depersonalization, cynicism, cognitive numbness and/or boredom, disengagement, memory impairment, reduced feelings of accomplishment, and most drastically, suicide (Freudenberger 1974; Renzo Bianchi, Schonfeld, and Laurent 2014). Over time, symptoms may lead physical health consequences such as increased risk of coronary heart disease, extreme fatigue, type 2 diabetes, and more (Williams et al. 2015; Toker et al. 2012). The rapid rise in prevalence of burnout makes it especially important to thoroughly investigate treatment methods. Professions that tend to experience burnout at the highest rate include those in healthcare, law, and finance.

One major obstacle in assessing burnout is its close resemblance to depression. Work by Bianchi, Schonfeld, and Laurent (2014) suggests that burnout could be classified as a depressive syndrome after finding that 90% of workers displaying classic signs of burnout also met DSM-5 criteria for a depressive disorder (Williams et al. 2015; Bianchi and Laurent 2015). There are many instruments used to measure burnout in research, the most well-known being the Maslach Burnout Inventory (MBI; Maslach and Jackson 1981). The MBI has strong reliability and validity, interpreting burnout as a progressive syndrome that begins with emotional exhaustion and advances to depersonalization (Maslach, Leiter, and Schaufeli 2008). More research is needed to further increase the efficacy and understanding of MBTs in relation to burnout prevention and intervention.

Physiological MBT Research

As with psychosocial outcomes, MBTs bring on physiologic changes in the body through relaxation. Understanding the stress–inflammation relationship is important for improving MBTs by treating the complex system of physiological mechanisms underlying disease rather than viewing each as an isolated illness (Yan 2016). In non-stressed states, individuals typically experience decreases in oxygen consumption, carbon dioxide elimination, respiratory rate, heart rate, and blood pressure, and increases in nitric oxide production and low frequency heart rate oscillations (Wallace et al. 1971; Dusek et al. 2008). Figure 16.4 shows Dusek and Benson's (2009) conceptual model that integrates differing physiological patterns of change when an individual is in stressed and relaxed states (Dusek and Benson 2009). This comparative view illustrates the complex interplay between physiological, endocrinological, and molecular parameters.

Heart rate variability (HRV) and skin conductance. Studies on the physiological effects of MBTs consistently report a reduction in autonomic sympathetic activation as measured by skin conductance, heart rate, and heart rate variability (Krygier et al. 2013; Van der Zwan et al. 2015). Both HVR and skin conductance are frequently used physiological markers in MBT trials as an assessment of autonomic balance and regulation (Tyagi and Cohen 2016). Higher HVR and lower skin conductance indicate better functioning. Yogic breathing techniques and meditation, for example, have been shown to significantly improve autonomic function by increasing HVR (Tyagi and Cohen 2016) and decreasing skin conductance (Delgado-Pastor et al. 2015).

Cortisol. Cortisol is a steroid hormone produced by the adrenal glands and regulated by the hypothalamic–pituitary–adrenal axis (HPA) and a frequently used biomarker of stress in MBT research. It is the most widely used biomarker of stress, stress reduction, and HPA activity within MBT research as meditation, yoga, tai chi, and many other MBT practices are associated with reductions in cortisol levels (Paul-Labrador et al. 2006; Sanada et al. 2016), decreases blood pressure (Nyklicek et al. 2013) and induces immune responses (Iseri et al. 2005; Biyikli et al. 2006). Studies on the physiological effects of MBTs consistently report improvements in hormone levels and metabolism, measured by cortisol levels in plasma, saliva, urine, and hair samples. However,

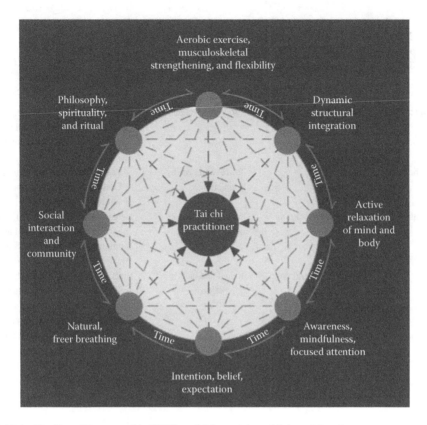

FIGURE 16.4 Dr. Peter Wayne et al.'s (2013) multi-factorial model describing the components contributing to the effect of a tai chi practitioner's work.

clinicians and researchers should keep in mind that cortisol level is sensitive to time of collection, typically peaking in the morning and steadily declining over the course of the day.

Proinflammatory cytokines. Several lines of evidence suggest that individuals experiencing psychosocial stress have increased markers of inflammation. Experiencing a stressful life event, economic hardship, or academic stress, for instance, elevates the circulating pro-inflammatory cytokines like C-Reactive Protein (CRP), IL-6, and soluble tumor necrosis factor-alpha (TNF-alpha) receptor I (Shearer et al. 2001; Haack, Sanchez, and Mullington 2007) suggesting chronic inflammation (Maes et al. 1998; Song et al. 1999; Brydon et al. 2004; Gemes, Ahnve, and Janszky 2008). MBTs have demonstrated their ability to counteract inflammatory responses and strengthen immunity in a host of samples and studies (Black and Slavich 2016; Walsh, Eisenlohr-Moul, and Baer 2016). Still, many of the aforementioned studies differ in the methods of measurement, the time of day the studies took place, and the extent of participant experience with MBTs thus creating a need for further research. Table 16.3 details common physiological biomarkers in MBT research explored thus far.

NEUROIMAGING MBT STUDIES

Neuroimaging studies have begun to explore the neural mechanisms underlying MBTs, especially meditation. Gray matter density, hippocampal volume, and amygdala activation have received the most attention.

Gray matter density. Anatomical MRI studies show that experienced meditators exhibit a denser gray matter structure in multiple brain regions when compared to non-meditating individuals (Lazar et al. 2005; Holzel et al. 2008; Grant et al. 2010; Luders et al. 2013; Fox et al. 2014;

TABLE 16.3
Common Physiological Biomarkers in MBT Research

Marker	MBT Studied	Association with Clinical Conditions	Recent Studies
Blood pressure	MBSR	Highly stressed adults	Nyklíček et al. (2013). Mindfulness-based stress reduction and physiological activity during acute stress: A randomized controlled trial.
Heart rate variability	Yoga	Clinical and healthy populations	Mantovani et al. (2016). Immediate effect of basic body awareness therapy on heart rate variability.
Skin conductance	Mindfulness training	Chronically stressed adults	Delgado-Pastor et al. (2015). Dissociation between the cognitive and interoceptive components of mindfulness in the treatment of chronic worry.
Cortisol	Mindfulness training	Clinical and healthy populations	Black et al. (2017). Mindfulness practice reduces cortisol blunting during chemotherapy: A randomized controlled study of colorectal cancer patients.
Proinflammatory cytokines	Mindfulness training	Depression	Walsh, Eisenlohr-Moul, and Baer (2016). Brief mindfulness training reduces salivary IL-6 and TNF-α in young women with depressive symptomatology.

Marchand 2014). MBSR practice has also been linked to similar changes in neural structure and function as are associated with meditation training. Compared to waitlist controls, the MBSR group reported positive changes in stress that have been correlated with changes in gray matter density in several brain regions, including the amygdala (Holzel, Carmody, and Evans 2010; Gotink et al. 2016).

Hippocampal volume. The hippocampus plays a significant role in both long-term and working memory processes, yet it is highly sensitive to stress (Lazarov and Hollands 2016). Maintained or increased hippocampal volume may be a major benefit of meditation-induced stress reduction, in addition to better autonomic regulation and immune system functioning (Luders et al. 2013). Larger hippocampal volume in frequent meditators may be partially responsible for the cognitive skills and mental capacities associated with the practice of meditation. These findings extend to clinical samples as well. In an RCT of meditation for mild cognitive impairment, the meditation group showed increases in functional connectivity and a halt in hippocampal volume atrophy. Thus, meditation may benefit the regions of the brain most tied to dementia and Alzheimer's disease (Wells et al. 2013; Larouche, Hudon, and Goulet 2015).

Amygdala activation. The amygdala is well-known to mediate stress and anxiety (LeDoux 2000), and has been implicated in both the detection of stressful and threatening stimuli along with the initiation of adaptive coping responses (LeDoux 2000; Hasler et al. 2007). MBTs may help to dampen amygdala activity during situations perceived as threatening, negative, and stressful. A recent RCT found that individuals in an awareness-based compassion meditation group showed significant improvements in anxiety and lower amygdala activity during and after negative emotional processing (Leung et al. 2017). MBT-induced changes in amygdala activity were maintained outside of the intervention setting as well, which has important implications for stress tolerance and management (Gotink et al. 2016; Leung et al. 2017). Table 16.4 summarizes commonly studied brain regions used in neuroimaging-based MBT research.

TABLE 16.4
Common Biomarkers Used in MBT Neuroimaging Research

Marker	MBT Studied	Association with Clinical Condition	Recent Studies
Gray matter density	Meditation MBSR	Clinical and healthy populations Parkinson's	Kumar et al. (2014). Effect of SOHAM meditation on human brain: A voxel-based morphometry study.
Hippocampal volume	Meditation	Clinical and healthy populations	Luders et al. (2013). Global and regional alterations of hippocampal anatomy in long-term meditation practitioners.
Amygdala	Meditation	Clinical and healthy populations	Leung et al. (2017). Meditation-induced neuroplastic changes in amygdala activity during negative affective processing.

GENOMIC RESEARCH

Genomics-based investigations of MBTs have revolutionized the understanding of their mechanistic pathways and effects on human physiology. The developing field of functional genomics unites genomics, epigenomics, transcriptomics, proteomics, and metabolomics to uncover molecular pathways and determinants involved in the changes brought about, in this context, by MBTs. The vast majority of functional genomic studies use methods in transcriptomics, such as assessing gene expression by partially or fully sequencing the transcriptome of peripheral white and red blood cells. Other commonly used genomic analyses involve microarray technologies that measure the expression levels of many genes simultaneously or to genotype multiple regions of a genome. Table 16.5 describes frequently used genomic biomarkers in MBT studies.

Nuclear factor-kappa B (NF-kB). In general, the effects of MBTs on functional genomics revealed intriguing connections to the immune system through the nuclear factor-kappa B (NF-kB)

TABLE 16.5
Common Biomarkers in MBT Genomic Research

Marker	MBT Studied	Association with Clinical Conditions	Recent Studies
NF-kB	Meditation Yoga	Dementia Alzheimer's healthy population	Black et al. (2013). Yogic meditation reverses NF-κB and IRF-related transcriptome dynamics in leukocytes of family dementia caregivers in a randomized controlled trial.
Peripheral blood	Mindful mediation	Diseased and healthy population	Kaliman et al. (2014). Rapid changes in histone deacetylases and inflammatory gene expression in expert meditators.
Telomere length	Meditation	Depression PTSD	Rao et al. (2015). Antiaging effects of an intensive mind and body therapeutic program through enhancement of telomerase activity and adult stem cell counts.
DNA methylation	Yoga	Chronic stress	Harkess, Ryan, Delfabbro, and Cohen-Woods (2016). Preliminary indications of the effect of a brief yoga intervention on markers of inflammation and DNA methylation in chronically stressed women.

cascade, to telomere maintenance, and to apoptotic regulation (Niles et al. 2014). Study results link MBTs to changes in cellular processes of inflammation, apoptosis, ubiquitin-dependent protein catabolism, telomere regulation, and epigenetic change. Downregulation of the NF-kB pathway as a result of MBT has been documented in multi-week interventions (Antoni et al. 2012; Black et al. 2013; Bower et al. 2014; Bhasin et al. 2017) and in rapid-response gene transcription following MBT (Kaliman et al. 2014; Bhasin et al. 2017).

Telomere length. Telomere length is a measure of cellular aging at the chromosomal level (Epel et al. 2009; Zhang et al. 2014). A recent review summarized evidence that magnitude and duration of traumatic stress, depression, and post-traumatic stress disorder (PTSD) are associated with higher oxidative stress, lower telomerase activity, and shorter peripheral blood mononuclear cell (PBMC) telomere length. Supporting this result, a longitudinal randomized controlled study (n = 34) with distressed breast cancer survivors recently reported that an 8-week MBT consisting of mindfulness meditation combined with Hatha yoga and group therapy improved telomere length and maintenance (Carlson et al. 2014). The anti-anxiety effects of oxytocin, the peptide involved with trust formation and pro-approach behaviors, has anti-stress effects as well suggesting it may contribute to the beneficial health effects of MBTs. Reviews of the literature indicate that mindfulness meditation and yogic breathing have been associated with decreased stress arousal, shown to reduce the rate of telomere shortening and upregulation of hormonal factors that may promote telomere maintenance (Epel et al. 2009; Jacobs et al. 2011; Lavretsky et al. 2013).

DNA methylation. More and more, MBT RCTs involve epigenomic analyses, using histone modification analysis and DNA methylation sequencing technologies. DNA methylation is an epigenetic mechanism though which cells control and down-regulate the expression of genes. Increasing our understanding of epigenetic change resulting from MBT interventions paints a fuller picture of how DNA methylation correlates with other psychological and biological markers and creates lasting effects in those who practice (Niles et al. 2014). In fact, one study found links between psychological variables and methylation of IL-6 and C-reactive proteins in a sample of 111 chronically stressed women after an 8-week yoga group (Harkness et al. 2016). However, these findings are limited to a small number of trials and relatively small sample sizes. More rigorous randomized controlled trials of healthy subjects and specific disease states are warranted.

COMPOSITE MARKERS

Resilience. Recently, there has been focus on assessing the role of resilience in health outcomes. Resilience is the ability of a dynamic, adaptable system to withstand threats to its stability, viability, or development (Charney 2004; Krasner et al. 2009; Pipe et al. 2012; Mehta et al. 2016). Regarding mind–body medicine, resilience is the ability of an individual to adapt and bounce back from psychological or physiological stressors and return to a state of homeostasis and well-being (Baer 2011). MBTs with an emphasis on communication, stress management, and resilience may provide individuals with beneficial insights on relaxation and stress reduction (Ruotsalainen et al. 2014; Williams et al. 2015). Studies of resilience-enhancing group interventions for health care providers (Mealer et al. 2014; Mehta et al. 2016) and psychiatric populations (Southwick and Charney 2012; Sveinbjarnardottir, Kolbrun Svavarsdottir, and Wright 2013; Miller et al. 2015; Waugh and Koster 2015) have found growth in numerous aspects of well-being. Such programs include the Relaxation Response Resiliency Program (3RP; Park et al. 2013), and Resilient Warrior (Sylvia et al. 2015), a stress management group to improve psychological health in service members.

The complexity of defining resilience as a scientific construct has been widely recognized and creates considerable difficulties when developing an operational model (Luthar, Cicchetti, and Becker 2000; Masten 2007). However, Southwick and Charney's (2012) model is widely known and accepted. It incorporates the cognitive/behavioral, emotional, social, physical, and neurobiological components of resilience, and how therapeutic interventions foster the protective factors of resilience. Although it was initially developed for patients with depression, this model is generalizable to

Health component	Health risk factor	MBT	Resilience protective factor
Cognitive/behavioral	Poor executive functioning and coping skills; negative appraisal of events rigid cognitive style	MBSR MBCT	Strong executive functioning and coping abilities; positive appraisal of events, optimism
Emotional	Poor affect regulation, such as high stress reactivity and anhedonia	Meditation Yoga MBSR	Strong affect regulation, such as delayed gratification and rapid stress recovery
Social	Lack of social skill, social network, and/or positive role model	Yoga Tai Chi Qigong	Presence of a strong social support network, positive role model, and social skills
Physical	Low physical fitness and activity level; poor nutrition and sleep hygiene habits; obesity;	Yoga Tai Chi Qigong Meditation	Good physical fitness; good nutrition and sleep habits;
Neurobiological	Dysregulated SNS and HPA axis; decreased grey matter density; hyperactive limbic system	Mediation MBSR	Proper regulation of the SNS and HPA axis in response to stress; strong prefrontal cortex executive functioning; regulated limbic system

FIGURE 16.5 Components of resilience in MBTs. (Adapted from Southwick et al. 2012. *Science* 338 (6103): 79–82.)

nearly all conditions. Figure 16.5 shows the components of resilience in relation to MBTs, adapted from Southwick and Charney (2012). Multiple scales have been created to measure resilience as a process, such as the Connor–Davidson Resilience Scale (CD-RISC; Connor and Davidson 2003), the Resilience Scale (RS; Wagnild and Young 1993), the Brief Resilience Scale (BRS; Smith et al. 2008), and the Positive and Negative Affect Schedule (PANAS; Watson, Clark, and Tellegan 1988). Though currently there is no gold-standard for a resiliency measure, the CD-RISC, the RS, and the BRS received the best psychometric ratings (Windle, Bennett, and Noyes 2011).

Allostatic load. Allostatic load describes the increased susceptibility to disease because of the cumulative stress-induced deterioration of the body (McEwen and Stellar 1993). This leads to elevated stress hormones and subsequent strain on many biological systems that is measurable using an index of biomarkers. The Allostatic Load Index consists of a set of neuroendocrine, metabolic, cardiovascular, and immune system biomarkers that reflect dysregulation across many physiological systems and provide an informed estimate of the effects of chronic stress on the body (Seeman et al. 1997). While individuals can adapt mentally and physically to small levels of stress, relentless environmental demands activate the HPA axis, dysregulate proper homeostatic balance, and can result in chronic alterations in these systems.

Importantly, previous research has determined that the Allostatic Load Index is associated with all-cause mortality in several populations, regardless of race or ethnicity (Borrell, Dallo, and Nguyen 2010). The use of multiple markers has the benefit of decreasing overall error due to a single incorrect measurement. A composite measure can provide a better assessment of risk than individual measures; for example, cardiologists use a composite measure of lab results and clinical findings to assess risk and make recommendations for treatment (Adult Treatment Panel III, 2001). Moreover, using an index helps to eliminate confounds like time of day, recent cigarette use, activity level, medication use, recent food intake, and collection technique that may obscure test results.

HEALTH OUTCOMES

MBTs are beneficial for patients from many walks of life with various treatment goals. Thus far, MBTs have been used to manage diseases and pain of neurological and autoimmune; psychiatric; gastrointestinal; cardiovascular; and metabolic origin. Systematic reviews have shown that MBTs may ease symptom severity for many mental and physical disorders that are caused or exacerbated by stress. These therapies work by improving coping skills, reducing tension and pain, and lessening the need for medication. Experience with MBTs will provide physicians with nonpharmacologic treatment options for use as an adjunct to other therapies or as a primary treatment method. Only a small fraction of this body of work is described below.

PAIN, NEUROLOGICAL, AND AUTOIMMUNE DISORDERS

Reviews of MBTs find positive effects on symptoms in the treatment of pain, neurological, and autoimmune disorders. Evidence suggests that migraine and post-traumatic headache populations greatly benefit from biofeedback-based MBTs, especially thermal and EMG biofeedback methods (Fraser et al. 2017), as well as yoga and meditation (Millstine, Chen, and Bauer 2017). Patients often report significant reductions in monthly headache frequency, headache intensity, and improved daily functioning. Yoga has also been shown to reduce fatigue associated with multiple sclerosis and help to better-manage epileptic seizures, largely due to the relaxing effects of the practice (Panebianco, Sridharan, and Ramaratnam 2015; Bauer et al. 2016; Abbott et al. 2017). Individuals with fibromyalgia, rheumatoid arthritis, and osteoarthritis may find solace in practicing tai chi and MBSR as they have been shown to ease symptom severity, disease-specific pain, and to elevate overall quality of life (Chen et al. 2015; Theadom et al. 2015; Del Rosso and Maddali-Bongi 2016; Lauche, Wayne, and Dobos 2016), with reports of benefits maintained at 3-year follow-up (Grossman et al. 2007). Table 16.6 describes common diseases and disorders studied in MBT research.

CANCER

Introducing an MBT practice, such as yoga, to patients with cancer can help to build coping skills to help manage physical and psychological side effects of treatment. MBT techniques can be easily incorporated into oncological care and demonstrated the ability to increase the quality of life for both patients and providers (Sisk and Fonteyn 2016). The Society for Integrative Oncology outlines clinical practice guidelines (Deng et al. 2013) on the use of integrative therapies for specific clinical indications during and after cancer treatment, strongly recommending MBT use as part of a multidisciplinary approach to cancer care. Music therapy, meditation, stress management, yoga, and the likes are suggested for anxiety, stress, and depressive symptom control and for their ability to ease cancer pain, nausea, and vomiting related to chemotherapy (Greenlee et al. 2017). Table 16.7 describes common types of cancers studied in MBT research.

MENTAL HEALTH

MBTs have a powerful effect on mental health and well-being. Even compared to other complementary and alternative medicine (CAM) techniques, individuals using MBTs are more likely to demonstrate improved cognitive functioning (Wayne, Walsh et al. 2014), emotional functioning, and levels of perceived stress (Luberto et al. 2014; Quaglia, Goodman, and Brown 2015). There is consistent,

TABLE 16.6
Conditions Treated with MBTs: Pain, Neurological, and Autoimmune Disorders

Health Condition	MBT Studied	Intervention Effects	Recent Studies
Migraine/headache	Yoga meditation biofeedback	Significan reductions in monthly headache frequency, headache intensity and improved daily functioning.	Millstine et al. (2017). Complementary and integrative medicine in the management of headache.
Lower back pain	Yoga MBSR Tai Chi	Practice moderately associated with alleviation of pain.	Morone et al. (2016). A mind–body program for older adults with chronic low back pain: a randomized clinical trial.
Multiple sclerosis	Tai Chi Yoga mindful meditation	Helps to improve balance, coordination, fatigue and to lessen depressive symptoms.	Burschka et al. (2014). Mindfulness-based interventions in multiple sclerosis: Beneficial effects of Tai Chi on balance, coordination, fatigue and depression.
Fibromyalgia	MBSR Tai Chi	Increased quality of life and decreased reports of pain, anxiety, depression, and somatic complaints.	Del Rosso and Maddali-Bongi (2016). Mind body therapies in rehabilitation of patients with rheumatic diseases.
Osteoarthritis	Mindfulness training MBSR Tai Chi	Improved disease-specific symptoms of pain, stiffness, pain coping, and knee extensor strength.	Lee, Harvey, Price, Morgan, Morgan and Wang (2017). Mindfulness is associated with psychological health and moderates pain in knee osteoarthritis.

TABLE 16.7
Conditions Treated with MBTs: Cancers

Health Condition	MBT Studied	Intervention Effects	Recent Studies
Breast cancer	Yoga meditation	Moderate-quality evidence supports the recommendation of yoga and meditation as supportive interventions for improving health-related quality of life and reducing fatigue and sleep disturbances when compared with no therapy, as well as for reducing depression, anxiety and fatigue.	Cramer et al. (2017). Yoga for improving health-related quality of life, mental health, and cancer-related symptoms in women diagnosed with breast cancer.
Lung cancer	Yoga MBSR	Reduced anxiety, mood disturbance, sleep disturbance, fatigue, chronic or acute pain, chemotherapy-induced nausea and vomiting in lung cancer patients experiencing the symptoms and improve quality of life.	Deng et al. (2013). Complementary therapies and integrative medicine in lung cancer: diagnosis and management of lung cancer: American College of Chest Physicians evidence-based clinical practice guidelines.

good-quality patient-oriented evidence confirming the efficacy of MBTs in the treatment of anxiety, depression, insomnia, substance use, and more as outlined in Table 16.8. Mindfulness-based cognitive therapy (MBCT) is a frequently used and effective MBT in clinical settings for individuals experiencing symptoms of anxiety and mood disorders, substance use disorder, insomnia, and eating disorders (Katterman et al. 2014; Schoenberg and David 2014; Shallcross and Visvanathan 2016; Sarkar and Varshney 2017). Other MBTs such as meditation are useful therapeutic modalities as well, especially for those unresponsive to cognitive-based psychotherapies. Yoga has demonstrated its ability to aid in the detoxification process of substance use disorder treatment, and likewise decreases drug use relapse rates (Sarkar and Varshney 2017). It is important to note that an MBT may need to be adapted to cater to the needs and sensitivities of the clinical concern at hand, especially those related to trauma. Where other forms of therapy may cause distress, for instance, trauma sensitive yoga for women with post-traumatic stress disorder (Nolan 2016), as well as depression-specific yoga for treatment resistant depression (Pradhan et al. 2015) appear to have merit.

GASTROINTESTINAL (GI) HEALTH

It is useful to discuss MBTs with patients being treated for indigestion, irritable bowel syndrome (IBS), inflammatory bowel disease (IBD), ulcerative colitis, gastroesophageal reflux disease (GERD), Crohn's disease, and heartburn. GI symptoms are often exacerbated by psychological burdens such as stress and anxiety, thus the stress-reducing components of MBTs may be particularly useful for GI symptom management (Mallorquí-Bagué et al. 2016). IBS and IBD are the most

TABLE 16.8
Conditions Treated with MBTs: Mental Health

Health Condition	MBT Studied	Intervention Effects	Recent Studies
Anxiety disorders	MBSR Yoga biofeedback	Improvements in symptom severity, stress reactivity, and coping.	Hoge et al. (2013). Randomized controlled trial of mindfulness meditation for generalized anxiety disorder: effects on anxiety and stress reactivity.
Depression	Yoga MBCT	Short-term improvements in symptom severity with yoga practice.	Streeter et al. (2017). Treatment of major depressive disorder with Iyengar yoga and coherent breathing: A randomized controlled dosing study.
Post-traumatic stress disorder	Biofeedback MBSR Yoga	Reductions in anxiety, depression, and anger, and increases in pain tolerance, self-esteem, energy levels, ability to relax, and ability to cope with stressful situations.	Colgan et al. (2016). The body scan and mindful breathing among veterans with PTSD: Type of intervention moderates the relationship between changes in mindfulness and post-treatment depression.
Insomnia	MBCT meditation	Improvements in patient-reported sleep quality, sleep disturbance, and mood.	Shallcross and Visvanathan (2016). Mindfulness-Based Cognitive Therapy for Insomnia.
Substance use disorders	Yoga	May aid in short-term detoxification and long-term management of substance use via stress reductions, increased coping skills, and additional pro-social support networks.	Nakamura et al. (2015). Investigating impacts of incorporating an adjuvant mind–body intervention method into treatment as usual at a community-based substance abuse treatment facility: A pilot randomized controlled study.
Eating disorders	Mindful meditation	Effectively decreases binge eating and emotional eating in populations engaging in this behavior.	Pacanowski et al. (2017). Yoga in the treatment of eating disorders within a residential program: A randomized controlled trial.

TABLE 16.9

Conditions Treated with MBTs: Gastrointestinal Disorders

Health Condition	MBT Studied	Intervention Effects	Recent Studies
Irritable bowel syndrome	Yoga	Decreased bowel symptoms, IBS severity, and anxiety. Significant improvements in quality of life, global improvement, and physical functioning.	Sharma, Saito, and Amit (2014). Mind–body medicine and irritable bowel syndrome: A randomized control trial using stress reduction and resiliency training.
Inflammatory bowel disease	9-week relaxation response mind–body group intervention	Decreased pain catastrophizing, symptom severity, trait anxiety, and improved quality of life.	Kuo et al. (2015). Genomic and clinical effects associated with a relaxation response mind–body intervention in patients with irritable bowel syndrome and inflammatory bowel disease.

frequently studied GI conditions in MBT trials, described in Table 16.9. A review of studies focusing on psychological therapies for IBS patients indicates that somatization affects the perception of their illness and the outcome and the efficacy of treatment more than actual symptom severity (Reed-Knight et al. 2016). Relative to controls, these patients also tended to score higher on symptom catastrophizing measures, and this significantly predicted reports of gastrointestinal symptoms related to pain. CBT, gut-directed hypnotherapy, guided imagery, yoga, and meditation have shown beneficial short-term effects in improving gastrointestinal symptoms of patients acting through these psychosomatic mechanisms (Kuo et al. 2015; Reed-Knight et al. 2016; Schumann et al. 2016).

CARDIOVASCULAR HEALTH

There are well-known links between stress and cardiovascular diseases: chronic stress predicts the occurrence of coronary heart disease, hypertension, high cholesterol, atherosclerosis, stress cardiomyopathy, and can worsen atrial fibrillation symptoms (Steptoe and Kivimäki 2012; Lakkireddy et al. 2013). Acute psychological stress may induce transient myocardial ischemia among patients with coronary heart disease, and more importantly, long-term stress can elevate the risk of death. The stress-reducing capabilities of MBTs aid in the relaxation of the physiological mechanisms responsible for cardiovascular health. Table 16.10 outlines conditions frequently studied in MBT research.

TABLE 16.10

Conditions Treated with MBTs: Cardiovascular-Related Conditions

Health Condition	MBT Studied	Intervention Effects	Recent Studies
Cardiovascular disease	Meditation Tai Chi Qigong	Decreases in blood triglycerides, blood pressure, and increases in quality of life and physical functioning.	Khobragade et al. (2016). Meditation as primary intervention strategy in prevention of cardiovascular diseases.
Hypertension	Yoga meditation	Reductions in systolic and diastolic blood pressure.	Cramer (2016). The efficacy and safety of yoga in managing hypertension.
Atrial fibrillation	Yoga meditation	Improvements in arrhythmia burden, heart rate, blood pressure, anxiety and depression scores, and several domains of quality of life.	Lakkireddy et al. (2013). Effect of yoga on arrhythmia burden, anxiety, depression, and quality of life in paroxysmal atrial fibrillation: the YOGA My Heart Study.

The impacts of MBTs as complementary interventions for hypertension have been observed. Yoga specifically reduced systolic blood pressure by 10 mm/Hg and diastolic blood pressure by roughly 8 mm/Hg (Cramer 2016) and decreased arrhythmia burden and symptom severity in patents with atrial fibrillation (Lakkireddy et al. 2013). The breathing and meditative components of the practice, rather than physical movement, seem to be the active part of yoga interventions for patients. This suggests that meditation could also be highly beneficial. These findings are limited to yoga as an adjunctive treatment, and further research will be needed to investigate this in larger samples. All forms of meditation, tai chi, and qigong demonstrate capabilities for decreasing blood triglycerides, and systolic and diastolic blood pressure, while boosting quality of life and physical functioning in patients with cardiovascular disease (Wang et al. 2016).

METABOLIC AND ENDOCRINE HEALTH

Chronic stress can dysregulate the neuroendocrine system, potentially leading to metabolic and hormonal abnormalities (Corey et al. 2014). MBTs have demonstrated their psychological benefits in patients with diabetes and thyroid complications by reducing depression, anxiety, and distress symptoms, thus at the very least may be considered as add-on interventions for symptoms management (Rosen, Gardiner, and Lee 2013; Kumar et al. 2016). Recent systematic reviews of randomized controlled trials (RCTs) investigating the effect of yoga on glycemic control in diabetic patients, for instance, found moderate support for its ability to improve fasting glucose, lipid profile, fasting blood sugar (FBS), postprandial blood sugar (PPBS), and glycosylated hemoglobin (HBA1C) compared to standard care alone (Vizcaino and Stover 2016; Kumar et al. 2016).

Although there is little support for direct improvements of thyroid functioning, it may be of benefit to discuss MBTs with patients with hypothyroidism as they can help to ease side effects, such as weight gain, constipation, and fatigue (Rosen, Gardiner, and Lee 2013). Still, the literature provides mixed evidence for the clinical effectiveness of MBTs in treating such health concerns (Noordali, Cumming, and Thompson 2015). More long-term follow-up studies with consistent, standardized outcome measures are needed to develop an accurate understanding of any lasting physiological changes to better inform practitioners about their use in clinical practice. Table 16.11 lists metabolic and endocrine conditions that may benefit from MBTs based on the literature.

SIDE EFFECTS AND RISKS OF MBT

MBTs are generally considered safe and low-impact treatments. Overall, yoga, tai chi, qigong, and guided imagery are safe when practiced appropriately under the supervision of a certified instructor. There have been little side effects and low risk of serious injury using MBTs, yet certain conditions

TABLE 16.11

Conditions Treated with MBTs: Metabolic and Neuroendocrine Conditions

Health Condition	MBT Studied	Intervention Effects	Recent Studies
Diabetes	Yoga	Improved fasting glucose, blood sugar lipid profile, postprandial blood sugar and glycosylated hemoglobin.	Gainey et al. (2016). Effects of Buddhist walking meditation on glycemic control and vascular function in patients with type 2 diabetes.
Thyroid disease	Various MBTs	As adjunctive therapies, eased side effects, such as weight gain, constipation, and fatigue.	Rosen, Gardiner, and Lee (2013). Effectiveness of mindfulness-based interventions on physiological and psychological complications in adults with diabetes: A systematic review.

may limit the extent of use (Cramer 2016). Physical injuries or the presence of cardiopulmonary disease may present a barrier to participation in trauma survivors (Carlson and Nitz 1991). In a yoga practice, types of stroke as well as pain from nerve damage are among the rare possible side effects. It is advised that women who are pregnant, and people with certain medical conditions, such as high blood pressure, glaucoma, and sciatica, should modify or avoid certain postures especially when starting a yoga practice.

There have been rare reports that meditation could cause or worsen certain anxiety and depression-related symptoms (i.e., intrusive thoughts, flashbacks; Kim, Kravitz, and Scheneider 2012). Tai chi and qigong appear to be safe practices, yet clinicians should advise against self-taught tai chi or qigong given that the movements are done correctly or safely, especially for beginners. These MBTs may be associated with minor musculoskeletal aches and pains, though unlikely to cause any injury when performed correctly (Wayne et al. 2014). As with all health care practice, it is important to speak with patients about any complementary or integrative health approaches they may use to ensure coordinated and safe care.

ECONOMIC CONSIDERATIONS

The dramatic impact of MBTs has become the forefront of healthcare research, with much focus on the economic benefits associated with stress reduction. The negative consequences of stress on health and well-being drive a great deal of healthcare utilization, especially when accompanied by a lack of physical and psychological resilience in response to stress. With more frequent primary care visits, recurrent hospitalizations, and increases in the numbers of prescribed medications comes a hefty financial burden on the recipients and providers of these healthcare services. A 2015 report estimated that the cost of depression alone in the United States rose by 21.5% between 2005 and 2010 from $173.2 to $210.5 billion a year (Greenberg et al. 2015). Over 90% of people suffering severe and mild mental disorders such as mood disturbances, depression, or dysthymia more regularly seek treatment from their family physician and are frequent utilizers of non-psychiatric care (Greenberg et al. 2015). Sixty percent of all medical visits were by the "worried well" with no diagnosable disorder, which make up roughly 70% of physicians' caseloads and significantly raise costs for insurance companies, employers, and most importantly patients (Stahl et al. 2015).

Physical symptoms resulting from psychological distress, such as headaches, insomnia, gastroesophageal reflux disease, irritable bowel syndrome, and chest discomfort are some of the most common reasons people seek medical care. In patients with anxiety, meditation significantly reduced mental health visits and missed work days, with more practice time related to greater benefit (Hoge et al. 2017). A study using a whole group analysis at 1 year post-MBT intervention found significant decreases in utilization (−43%), clinical encounters (−41.9%), imaging (−50.3%), lab encounters (−43.5%), and procedures (−21.4%). Emergency department (ED) visits decreased from 3.6/year to 1.7/year while hospital and urgent care visits became indistinguishable from controls (Stahl et al. 2015). A Kaiser Permanente study showed that patients who participated in psychotherapeutic interventions decreased their in-hospital length of stay by 77.9%, decreased their hospitalization rate by 66.7%, decreased office visits by 47.1%, decreased ER visits by 45.3%, and decreased prescriptions written by 4% (Sobel 2000). Some estimates find that every dollar spent on mental health care saves $6 in healthcare utilization, with weekly claims dropping by 64%, surgical costs decreasing by 48.9%, and overall medical costs shrinking by 18%–44% (Greenberg et al. 2015).

MBTs typically cost only a few hundred dollars to the patient or insurer, not a substantial amount in comparison to the resources consumed during a visit to the emergency department, a high-resolution imaging study, or repeated office visits. In fact, it is possible to recoup the extra cost of the psychotherapy sessions or group interventions within 6 months (Guthrie et al. 1999), and see overall cost savings over a 5-year period (Klatt et al. 2016). As such, it seems appropriate to reevaluate the role that mind–body interventions play in healthcare. If MBTs make clinical symptoms more manageable, reduce anxiety and stress, and increase patients' resilience to new stressors, they should in turn help prevent individual healthcare problems from evolving into critical ones, improve quality of life, and reduce healthcare utilization.

BARRIERS AND FACILITATORS OF MBT USE

As with nearly all therapeutic modalities used in clinical practice, MBTs come with their own set of perks and challenges. Though successful, clinically tested MBT treatments exist, barriers to MBT use persist much like those associated with other treatment options. Stigma is one of many factors that prevent individuals from seeking the care they need, especially mental health services (Corrigan, Druss, and Perlick 2014). In a review of 144 studies, with 90,189 participants, internalized and treatment stigma were most highly correlated with reduced help-seeking and treatment use. Moreover, those most impacted by stigma-related treatment deterrence include men, youth, minorities, those in the military, and, ironically, healthcare professionals (Clement et al. 2015). Being aware of stigma and actively trying to combat it may be vital in clinicians' attempts to increase help-seeking and treatment engagement (Corrigan, Druss, and Perlick 2014; Clement et al. 2015). Discussing MBTs with patients may help to decrease the stigma associated with care seeking; however, effectiveness is highly dependent on the care provider's knowledge, time, and training.

Instructor training is yet another impediment on the use of MBTs and with a lack of adequately trained health care providers comes a lack in patient access to MBT services. Regardless of specialty, clinicians report that a lack of training, inadequate expertise, and insufficient clinic time significantly impact their ability to incorporate mind–body techniques into their practice. These concerns are often higher among family physicians than among psychiatrists, most likely due to the training emphasis and nature of their respective field. However, family physicians are likely the first care provider people turn to when seeking treatment (Sierpina et al. 2007). Practitioners may lack the time needed to receive training on and properly integrate MBTs into appointments considering the already dense caseloads and schedules (Burhenn et al. 2016; McGuire, Gabison, and Kligler 2016). Likewise, they may also fear that recommending them to patients might lead them to feel that their symptoms were being discounted. Yet taking a few moments to discuss the empirical evidence backing these treatment modalities can help to legitimize mind–body practices for the patient, promote self-care practices, and ultimately reduce the frequency of non-routine health care visits. Clinician gender did play an influential role in the use of MBTs in practice, with female physicians being significantly more likely to use MBTs, in practice and in personal life, and reporting stronger trust in the benefits of MBTs for various health concerns (Sierpina et al. 2007).

There appears to be frequent miscommunication between patients and their providers about MBTs since they are not typically treated in the same manner as other treatment interventions. Because most MBTs are publicly accessible, patients may not think to ask a physician for information, and those who have already established a mind–body practice may neglect to discuss it with their clinician. At the same time, providers may not emphasize mind–body practices during appointments, and if they are mentioned it may only mean having the individual fill out paperwork without any follow up discussion (Rosen, Gardiner, and Lee 2013). It is important for health care professionals to inquire about any patient MBT use to gain a comprehensive understanding of their patient's health practices and inform treatment recommendations. This includes both patient-based and practitioner-based therapies.

Regardless of these barriers, there has been exponential growth in the public interest in MBT use, particularly yoga. Several factors jointly sparked this cultural shift toward recognizing the importance of self-care, well-being, and use of use of relaxation techniques for recreation or treatment.

Social media, mobile applications, and websites, along with the advent of fitness watches and physiology trackers have made MBTs more accessible than ever, especially for the younger tech-savvy generations. While there may be concerns about the media's slight commercialization of MBTs, these platforms may help to increase patients' familiarity with the various types of mind–body based treatment options and facilitate clinical research. Researchers in the field have begun testing the efficacy of MBTs delivered through mobile apps and video conferencing for a variety of mental health conditions including stress, anxiety, and depression (Mani 2017), as well as physical symptoms like chronic lower back and neck pain (Blodt et al. 2014). A small-scale systematic review of 8 MBT clinical trials found substantial support for the efficacy of MBTs in reducing perceived stress via online platforms and other virtual modalities, methods of increasing demand and popularity as technology continues to advance (Jayewardene et al. 2016).

Mobile applications can help to deliver MBTs on a more consistent, regular basis when patients are not in the presence of their PCP or care provider. This may help to address some of the challenges of effectively delivering mindfulness training to highly vulnerable or busy individuals and likewise assist the patient in developing MBT-based self-care practices.

The U.S. government has been responsive to the demand for MBTs and other complementary and integrative medicine techniques over the past two decades (Brower 2006). In 1992, the Office of Alternative Medicine (OAM) was created to facilitate empirical research on complementary and alternative medical practices in hopes of extending this knowledge to the public, MBTs included. Just six years later, Congress elevated the status of OAM to that of an official NIH center, establishing the National Center for Complementary and Alternative Medicine (NCCAM). NCCAM has since been renamed the National Center for Complementary and Integrative Health (NCCIH), which better represents the ideology of an integrative approach to health and wellness within health care settings in the United States.

With the increase in federal attention, and possible grant funding opportunities, there has been a growing collection of medical schools, graduate programs, and centers equipped with departments devoted to MBT research. Universities such as Harvard, Columbia, UCLA, and the University of Pittsburgh are a few among the many. Likewise, many training programs for residents, physicians, and other hospital employees are now incorporating MBT techniques into their curriculum, for both clinical training purposes as well as a means to help manage the stress brought on by these programs and careers (Brower 2006). This way, healthcare professionals become better acquainted with these treatment modalities on a clinical and personal level and are thus able to extend this knowledge to their patients.

SUMMARY

Though its ideological influences have a rich history spanning thousands of years, researchers have only just begun investigating the benefits of mind–body medicine and MBTs. Innovative studies are more consistently demonstrating the efficacy of MBTs in their ability to improve health and well-being. However, extensive research is still warranted to establish a more comprehensive understanding of the mechanisms through which MBTs work. Openly discussing MBTs such as yoga, meditation, tai chi, and qigong with patients and catering these therapies to their condition, preferences, and existing health care routine is an important step to minimize barriers of MBT use.

REFERENCES

Abbott, R.A., A.E. Martin, T.V. Newlove-Delgado, A. Bethel, J. Thompson-Coon, R. Whear, and S. Logan. 2017. Psychosocial Interventions for Recurrent Abdominal Pain in Childhood. *The Cochrane Library.* 3: CD010972

Abrahams, V.C., S.M. Hilton, and A. Zbrozyna. 1960. Active Muscle Vasodilatation Produced by Stimulation of the Brain Stem: Its Significance in the Defence Reaction. *The Journal of Physiology* 154 (3): 491.

Antoni, M.H., S.K. Lutgendorf, B. Blomberg, C.S. Carver, S. Lechner, A. Diaz, J. Stagl, J.M.G. Arevalo, and S.W. Cole. 2012. Cognitive-Behavioral Stress Management Reverses Anxiety-Related Leukocyte Transcriptional Dynamics. *Biological Psychiatry* 71 (4): 366–372.

Baer, R.A. 2011. Measuring Mindfulness. *Contemporary Buddhism: An Interdisciplinary Journal* 12 (1): 241–61.

Baer, R.A., J. Carmody, and M. Hunsinger. 2012. Weekly Change in Mindfulness and Perceived Stress in a Mindfulness-Based Stress Reduction Program. *Journal of Clinical Psychology* 68 (7): 755–65.

Baer, R.A., G.T. Smith, J. Hopkins, J. Krietemeyer, and L. Toney. 2006. Using Self-Report Assessment Methods to Explore Facets of Mindfulness. *Assessment* 13 (1): 27–45.

Barner, J.C., T.M. Bohman, C.M. Brown, and K.M. Richards. 2010. Use of Complementary and Alternative Medicine for Treatment among African-Americans: A Multivariate Analysis. *Research in Social and Administrative Pharmacy* 6 (3): 196–208.

Barnes, P.M., B. Bloom, and R.L. Nahin. 2004. Complementary and Alternative Medicine Use among Adults: United States, 2002. *Seminars in Integrative Medicine* 2 (2): 54–71.

Barnes, P.M., B. Bloom, and R.L. Nahin. 2008. Complementary and Alternative Medicine Use among Adults and Children: United States, 2007. *National Health Statistics Reports* 12:12–24.

Barrows, K.A. and B.P. Jacobs. 2002. Mind-Body Medicine: An Introduction and Review of the Literature. *Medical Clinics of North America* 86 (1): 11–31.

Bauer, B.A., J.C. Tilburt, A. Sood, G. Li, and S. Wang. 2016. Complementary and Alternative Medicine Therapies for Chronic Pain. *Chinese Journal of Integrative Medicine* 22 (6): 403–11.

Benson, H. 1982. The Relaxation Response: History, Physiological Basis and Clinical Usefulness. *Medica Scandinavica* 211 (S660): 231–37.

Bhasin, M.K., J.A. Dusek, B-H. Chang, M.G. Joseph, J.W. Denninger, G.L. Fricchione, H. Benson, and T.A. Libermann. 2017. Correction: Relaxation Response Induces Temporal Transcriptome Changes in Energy Metabolism, Insulin Secretion and Inflammatory Pathways. *PloS One* 12 (2): e0172873.

Bianchi, R. and E. Laurent. 2015. Emotional Information Processing in Depression and Burnout: An Eye-Tracking Study. *European Archives of Psychiatry and Clinical Neuroscience* 265: 27–34.

Bianchi, R., I.S. Schonfeld, and E. Laurent. 2014. Is Burnout a Depressive Disorder? A Reexamination with Special Focus on Atypical Depression. *International Journal of Stress Management* 21 (4): 307–24.

Biyikli, N.K. et al. 2006. Effect of Alzheimer Caregiving Stress and Age on Frailty Markers Interleukin-6, C-Reactive Protein, and D-Dimer. *Peptides* 27 (9): 2249–57.

Black, D.S., S.W. Cole, M.R. Irwin, E. Breen, N.M. St. Cyr, N. Nazarian, D.S. Khalsa, and H. Lavretsky. 2013. Yogic Meditation Reverses NF-KB and IRF-Related Transcriptome Dynamics in Leukocytes of Family Dementia Caregivers in a Randomized Controlled Trial. *Psychoneuroendocrinology* 38 (3): 348–355. doi:10.1016/j.psyneuen.2012.06.011.

Black, D.S., C. Peng, A.G. Sleight, N. Nguyen, H-J Lenz, and J.C. Figueiredo. 2017. Mindfulness Practice Reduces Cortisol Blunting during Chemotherapy: A Randomized Controlled Study of Colorectal Cancer Patients. *Cancer* 123(16): 3088–3096. doi:10.1002/cncr.30698/full.

Black, D.S. and G.M. Slavich. 2016. Mindfulness Meditation and the Immune System: A Systematic Review of Randomized Controlled Trials. *Annals of the New York Academy of Sciences* 1373 (1): 13–24.

Black, L.I., T.C. Clarke, P.M. Barnes, B.J. Stussman, and R.L. Nahin. 2015. Use of Complementary Health Approaches among Children Aged 4–17 Years in the United States: National Health Interview Survey, 2007–2012. *National Health Statistics Reports*, 78: 1.

Blodt, S., D. Pach, S. Roll, and C.M. Witt. 2014. Effectiveness of App-Based Relaxation for Patients with Chronic Low Back Pain (Relaxback) and Chronic Neck Pain (Relaxneck): Study Protocol for Two Randomized Pragmatic Trials. *Trials* 15 (1): 490.

Borrell, L.N., F.J. Dallo, and N. Nguyen. 2010. Racial/Ethnic Disparities in All-Cause Mortality in U.S. Adults: The Effect of Allostatic Load. *Public Health Rep* 125 (6): 810–816.

Bower, J.E., G. Greendale, A.D. Crosswell, D. Garet, B. Sternlieb, P.A. Ganz, M.R. Irwin, R. Olmstead, J. Arevalo, and S.W. Cole. 2014. Yoga Reduces Inflammatory Signaling in Fatigued Breast Cancer Survivors: A Randomized Controlled Trial. *Psychoneuroendocrinology* 43: 20–29.

Brower, V. 2006. Mind–body Research Moves towards the Mainstream. *EMBO Reports* 7 (4): 358–361.

Brown, K.W. and R.M. Ryan. 2003. The Benefits of Being Present: Mindfulness and Its Role in Psychological Well-Being. *Journal of Personality and Social Psychology* 84 (4): 822.

Brydon, L., S. Edwards, V. Mohamed-Ali, and A. Steptoe. 2004. Socioeconomic Status and Stress-Induced Increases in Interleukin-6. *Brain, Behavior, and Immunity* 18 (3): 281–90.

Burhenn, P.S., B. Ferrell, S. Johnson, and A. Hurria. 2016. Improving Nurses' Knowledge About Older Adults With Cancer. In *Oncology Nursing Forum*. Vol. 43. http://search.ebscohost.com/login.aspx?direct=tru e&profile=ehost&scope=site&authtype=crawler&jrnl=0190535X&AN=116230058&h=2wkycoWIB sm3ElGzRm9%2BKNEuJJbSD6BmPxppaW56WZ60Py5pZsQ9vEXdWpkNEoWzF35iJ311xB2QTRE VIZrxqQ%3D%3D&crl=c.

Burschka, J.M., P.M. Keune, U.H. Oy, P. Oschmann, and P. Kuhn 2014. Mindfulness-Based Interventions in Multiple Sclerosis: Beneficial Effects of Tai Chi on Balance, Coordination, Fatigue and Depression. *BMC Neurology* 14 (1): 165.

Cannon, W.B. 1915. *Bodily Changes in Pain, Hunger, Fear, and Rage: An Account of Recent Researches into the Function of Emotional Excitement.* D. Appleton and Company, New York.

Cannon, W.B. 1914. The Emergency Function of the Adrenal Medulla in Pain and the Major Emotions. *American Journal of Physiology-Legacy Content* 33 (2): 356–72.

Cannon, W.B. 1929. Bodily Changes in Pain, Hunger, Fear and Rage. *Southern Medical Journal* 22 (9): 870.

Carlson, C.R. and A.J. Nitz. 1991. Negative Side Effects of Self-Regulation Training: Relaxation and the Role of the Professional in Service Delivery. *PubMed, Biofeedback Self Regul* 16 (2): 191–97.

Carlson, L.E., T.L. Beattie, J. Giese-Davis, P. Faris, R. Tamagawa, L.J. Fick, E.S. Degelman, and M. Speca. 2014. Mindfulness-Based Cancer Recovery and Supportive-Expressive Therapy Maintain Telomere Length Relative to Controls in Distressed Breast Cancer Survivors. *Cancer* 121 (3): 476–84.

Charney, D.S. 2004. Psychobiological Mechanisms of Resilience and Vulnerability. *American Journal of Psychiatry* 161 (2): 195–216.

Chen, Y-W., M.A. Hunt, K.L. Campbell, K. Peill, and W. Darlene Reid. 2015. The Effect of Tai Chi on Four Chronic Conditions—cancer, Osteoarthritis, Heart Failure and Chronic Obstructive Pulmonary Disease: A Systematic Review and Meta-Analyses. *British Journal of Sports Medicine* 50:397–407. doi:10.1136/bjsports-2014–094388.

Clarke, T.C., L.I. Black, B.J. Stussman, P.M. Barnes, and R.L. Nahin. 2015. Trends in the Use of Complementary Health Approaches among Adults: United States, 2002–2012. *National Health Statistics Report* 79: 1.

Clement, S., O. Schauman, T. Graham, F. Maggioni, S. Evans-Lacko, N. Bezborodovs, C. Morgan, N. Rüsch, J.S. Brown, and G. Thornicroft. 2015. What is the Impact of Mental Health-Related Stigma on Help-Seeking? A Systematic Review of Quantitative and Qualitative Studies. *Psychological Medicine* 45 (1): 11–27.

Cohen, S., T. Kamarck, and R. Mermelstein. 1983. A Global Measure of Perceived Stress. *Journal of Health and Social Behavior*, 24 (4): 385–396.

Colgan, D.D., M. Christopher, P. Michael, and H. Wahbeh. 2016. The Body Scan and Mindful Breathing among Veterans with PTSD: Type of Intervention Moderates the Relationship between Changes in Mindfulness and Post-Treatment Depression. *Mindfulness* 7 (2): 372–383.

Connor, K.M. and J.R.T. Davidson. 2003. Development of a New Resilience Scale: The Connor-Davidson Resilience Scale (CD-RISC). *Depression and Anxiety* 18 (2): 76–82.

Corey, S.M., E. Epel, M. Schembri, S.B. Pawlowsky, R.J. Cole, M.R.G. Araneta, E. Barrett-Connor, and A.M. Kanaya. 2014. Effect of Restorative Yoga vs. Stretching on Diurnal Cortisol Dynamics and Psychosocial Outcomes in Individuals with the Metabolic Syndrome: The PRYSMS Randomized Controlled Trial. *Psychoneuroendocrinology* 49: 260–71.

Corrigan, P.W., B.G. Druss, and D.A. Perlick. 2014. The Impact of Mental Illness Stigma on Seeking and Participating in Mental Health Care. *Psychological Science in the Public Interest* 15 (2): 37–70.

Cramer, H. 2016. The Efficacy and Safety of Yoga in Managing Hypertension. *Experimental and Clinical Endocrinology & Diabetes* 124 (02): 65–70.

Cramer, H., R. Lauche, P. Klose, S. Lange, J. Langhorst, and G. Dobos. 2017. Yoga for Improving Health-related Quality of Life, Mental Health and Cancer-related Symptoms in Women Diagnosed with Breast Cancer. *The Cochrane Library* 1, CD010802–CD010802.

Cramer, H., L. Ward, A. Steel, R. Lauche, G. Dobos, and Y. Zhang. 2016. Prevalence, Patterns, and Predictors of Yoga Use; Results of a U.S. Nationally Representative Survey. *American Journal of Preventative Medicine* 50 (2): 230–35. doi:10.1016/j.amepre.2015.07.037.

Deckro, G.R., K.M. Ballinger, M. Hoyt, M. Wilcher, J. Dusek, P. Myers, B. Greenberg, D.S. Rosenthal, and H. Benson. 2002. The Evaluation of a Mind/Body Intervention to Reduce Psychological Distress and Preceived Stress in College Students. *Journal of American College Health* 50 (6): 281–87.

Del Rosso, A. and S. Maddali-Bongi. 2016. Mind Body Therapies in Rehabilitation of Patients with Rheumatic Diseases. *Complementary Therapies in Clinical Practice* 22: 80–86.

Delgado-Pastor, L.C., L.F. Ciria, B. Blanca, J.L. Mata, M.N. Vera, and J. Vila. 2015. Dissociation between the Cognitive and Interoceptive Components of Mindfulness in the Treatment of Chronic Worry. *Journal of Behavior Therapy and Experimental Psychiatry*, 48 (2015):192–199.

Deng, G.E., S.M. Rausch, L.W. Jones, A. Gulati, N.B. Kumar, H. Greenlee, C. Pietanza, and B.R. Cassileth. 2013. Complementary Therapies and Integrative Medicine in Lung Cancer: Diagnosis and Management of Lung Cancer: American College of Chest Physicians Evidence-Based Clinical Practice Guidelines. *Chest* 143 (5): e420S–e436S.

Dusek, J. and H. Benson. 2009. Mind-Body Medicine: A Model of the Comparative Clinical Impact of the Acute Stress and Relaxation Responses. *Minnesota Medicine* 92 (5): 47–50.

Dusek, J.A., P.L. Hibberd, B. Buczynski, B.-H. Chang, K.C. Dusek, J.M. Johnston, A.L. Wohlhueter, H. Benson, and R.M. Zusman. 2008. Stress Management versus Lifestyle Modification on Systolic Hypertension and Medication Elimination: A Randomized Trial. *The Journal of Alternative and Complementary Medicine* 14 (2): 129–138.

Epel, E., J. Daubenmier, J.T. Moskowitz, S. Folkman, and E. Blackburn. 2009. Can Meditation Slow Rate of Cellular Aging? Cognitive Stress, Minfulness, and Telomeres. *Annals of the New York Academy of Sciences* 1172 (1): 34–53.

Feldman, G., A. hayes, S. Kumar, J. Greeson, and J. Laurenceau. 2007. Mindfulness and Emotion Regulation: The Development and Initial Validation of the Cognitive and Affective Mindfulness Scale-Revised (CAMS-R). *Journal of Psychopathy and Behavioral Assessment* 29 (3): 177–90.

Fox, K.C., S. Nijeboer, M.L. Dixon, J.L. Floman, M. Ellamil, S.P. Rumak, P. Sedlmeier, and K. Christoff. 2014. Is Meditation Associated with Altered Brain Structure? A Systematic Review and Meta-Analysis of Morphometric Neuroimaging in Meditation Practitioners. *Neuroscience and Biobehavioral Reviews* 43: 48–73.

Fraser, F., Y. Matsuzawa, Y.S. Christine Lee, and M. Minen. 2017. Behavioral Treatments for Post-Traumatic Headache. *Current Pain and Headache Reports* 21 (5): 22.

Freudenberger, H.J. 1974. Staff Burn-Out. *Journal of Social Issues* 30 (1): 159–65.

Gainey, A., T. Himathongkam, H. Tanaka, and D. Suksom. 2016. Effects of Buddhist Walking Meditation on Glycemic Control and Vascular Function in Patients with Type 2 Diabetes. *Complementary Therapies in Medicine* 26: 92–97.

Gemes, K., S. Ahnve, and I. Janszky. 2008. Inflammation a Possible Link between Economical Stress and Coronary Heart Disease. *European Journal of Epidemiology* 23 (2): 95–103.

Gotink, R.A., R. Meijboom, M.W. Vernooij, M. Smits, and M.G. Myriam Hunink. 2016. 8-Week Mindfulness Based Stress Reduction Induces Brain Changes Similar to Traditional Long-Term Meditation Practice–a Systematic Review. *Brain and Cognition* 108: 32–41.

Grant, J.A., J. Courtemanche, E.G. Duerden, G.H. Duncan, and P. Rainville. 2010. Cortical Thickness and Pain Sensitivity in Zen Meditators. *Emotion* 10 (1): 43–53.

Greenberg, P.E., A-A Fournier, T. Sisitsky, C.T. Pike, and R.C. Kessler. 2015. The Economic Burden of Adults with Major Depressive Disorder in the United States (2005 and 2010). *The Journal of Clinical Psychiatry* 76 (2): 155–162.

Greenlee, H., M.J. DuPont-Reyes, L.G. Balneaves, L.E. Carlson, M.R. Cohen, G.E. Deng, J.A. Johnson et al. 2017. Clinical Practice Guidelines on the Evidence-based Use of Integrative Therapies during and after Breast Cancer Treatment. *CA: A Cancer Journal for Clinicians* 67: 194–232.

Grossman, P., U. Tiefenthaler-Gilmer, A. Raysz, and U. Kesper. 2007. Mindfulness Training as an Intervention for Fibromyalgia: Evidence of Postintervention and 3-Year Follow-up Benefits in Well-Being. *Psychotherapy and Psychosomatics* 76: 226–33.

Guthrie, E., J. Moorey, F. Margison, H. Barker, S. Palmer, G. McGrath, B. Tomenson, and F. Creed. 1999. Cost-Effectiveness of Brief Psychodynamic-Interpersonal Therapy in High Utilizers of Psychiatric Services. *Archives of General Psychiatry* 56 (6): 519–526.

Haack, M., E. Sanchez, and J.M. Mullington. 2007. Elevated Inflammatory Markers in Response to Prolonged Sleep Restriction Are Associated with Increased Pain Experience in Healthy Volunteers. *Sleep* 30 (9): 1145–52.

Harkness, K.N., J. Ryan, P.H. Delfabbro, and S. Cohen-Woods. 2016. Preliminary Indications of the Effect of a Brief Yoga Intervention on Markers of Inflammation and DNA Methylation in Chronically Stressed Women. *Translational Psychiatry* 6 (11): e965. doi:10.1038/tp.2016.234.

Hasler, G., S. Fromm, R.P. Alvarez, D.A. Luckenbaugh, W.C. Drevets, and C. Grillon. 2007. Cerebral Blood Flow in Immediate and Sustained Anxiety. *Journal of Neuroscience* 27 (23): 6313–19.

Hoge, E.A., E. Bui, L. Marques, C.A. Metcalf, L.K. Morris, D.J. Robinaugh, J.J. Worthington, M.H. Pollack, and N.M. Simon. 2013. Randomized Controlled Trial of Mindfulness Meditation for Generalized Anxiety Disorder: Effects on Anxiety and Stress Reactivity. *The Journal of Clinical Psychiatry* 74 (8): 786.

Hoge, E.A., B.M. Guidos, M. Mete, E. Bui, M.H. Pollack, N.M. Simon, and M.A. Dutton. 2017. Effects of Mindfulness Meditation on Occupational Functioning and Health Care Utilization in Individuals with Anxiety. *Journal of Psychosomatic Research* 95: 7–11.

Holzel, B.K., J. Carmody, and K.C. Evans. 2010. Stress Reduction Correlated with Structural Changes in the Amygdala. *Social Cognitive and Affective Neuroscience* 5 (1): 11–17.

Holzel, B.K., U. Ott, T. Gard, H. Hempel, M. Weygandt, K. Morgen, and D. Vaitl. 2008. Investigation of Mindfulness Meditation Practitioners with Voxel-Based Morphometry. *Social Cognitive and Affective Neuroscience* 3 (1): 55–61.

Iseri, S.O. et al. 2005. Oxytocin Protects against Sepsis-Induced Multiple Organ Damage: Role of Neutrophils. *Journal of Surgical Research* 126 (1): 73–81.

Jacobs, T.L., E. Epel, J. Lin, E. Blackburn, O.M. Wolkowitz, D.A. Bridwell, A.P. Zanesco et al. 2011. Intensive Meditation Training, Immune Cell Telomerase Activity, and Psychological Mediators. *Psychoneuroendocrinology* 36 (5): 664–81.

Jayewardene, W.P., D.K. Lohrmann, R.G. Erbe, and M.R. Torabi. 2016. Effects of Preventative Online Mindfulness Intervetnions on Stress and Mindfulness: A Meta-Analysis of Randomized Controlled Trials. *Preventative Medicine Reports.*

Kabat-Zinn, J. 1982. An Outpatient Program in Behavioral Medicine for Chronic Pain Patients Based on the Practice of Mindfulness Meditation: Theoretical Considerations and Preliminary Results. *General Hospital Psychiatry* 4 (1): 33–47.

Kaliman, P., M.J. Álvarez-López, M. Cosín-Tomás, M.A. Rosenkranz, A. Lutz, and R.J. Davidson. 2014. Rapid Changes in Histone Deacetylases and Inflammatory Gene Expression in Expert Meditators. *Psychoneuroendocrinology* 40 (February): 96–107. doi:10.1016/j.psyneuen.2013.11.004.

Katterman, S.N., B.M. Kleinman, M.M. Hood, L.M. Nackers, and J.A. Corsica. 2014. Mindfulness Meditation as an Intervention for Binge Eating, Emotional Eating, and Weight Loss: A Systematic Review. *Eating Behaviors* 15 (2): 197–204.

Khobragade, Y., A.B. Lutfi Abas, B. Ankur, and others. 2016. Meditation as Primary Intervention Strategy in Prevention of Cardiovascular Diseases. *International Journal of Research in Medical Sciences* 4 (1): 12–21.

Kim, S.H., L. Kravitz, and S.M. Scheneider. 2012. PTSD & Exercise: What Every Exercise Professional Should Know. *IDEA Fitness Journal* 9: 20–23.

Klatt, M.D., C. Sieck, G. Gascon, W. Malarkey, and T. Huerta. 2016. A Healthcare Utilization Cost Comparison between Employees Receiving a Worksite Mindfulness or a Diet/Exercise Lifestyle Intervention to Matched Controls 5 Years Post Intervention. *Complementary Therapies in Medicine* 27: 139–44.

Kocovski, N.L., J.E. Fleming, L.L. Hawley, M-H. Ringo Ho, and M.M. Antony. 2015. Mindfulness and Acceptance-Based Group Therapy and Traditional Cognitive Behavioral Group Therapy for Social Anxiety Disorder: Mechanisms of Change. *Behaviour Research and Therapy* 70: 11–22.

Krasner, M.S., R.M. Epstein, H. Beckman, A.L. Suchman, B. Chapman, C.J. Mooney, and T.E. Quill. 2009. Association of an Educational Program in Mindful Communication with Burnout, Empathy, and Attitudes among Primary Care Physicians. *JAMA* 302 (12): 1284–93.

Krygier, J.R., J.A.J. Heathers, S. Shahrestani, M. Abbott, J.J. Gross, and A.H. Kemp. 2013. Mindfulness Meditation, Well-Being, and Heart Rate Variability: A Preliminary Investigation into the Impact of Intensive Vipassana Meditation. *International Journal of Psychophysiology* 89 (3): 305–13.

Kumar, U., A. Guleria, S.S. Kunal Kishan, and C. L. Khetrapal. 2014. Effect of SOHAM Meditation on Human Brain: A Voxel-Based Morphometry Study. *Journal of Neuroimaging* 24 (2): 187–190.

Kumar, V., A. Jagannathan, M. Philip, A. Thulasi, P. Angadi, and N. Raghuram. 2016. Role of Yoga for Patients with Type II Diabetes Mellitus: A Systematic Review and Meta-Analysis. *Complementary Therapies in Medicine* 25: 104–12.

Kuo, B., M. Bhasin, J. Jacquart, M.A. Scult, L. Slipp, E.I. Kagan Riklin, and V. Lepoutre. 2015. Genomic and Clinical Effects Associated with a Relaxation Response Mind-Body Intervention in Patients with Irritable Bowel Syndrome and Inflammatory Bowel Disease. *PloS One* 10 (4): e0123861.

Lakkireddy, D., D. Atkins, J. Pillarisetti, K. Ryschon, S. Bommana, J. Drisko, S. Vanga, and B. Dawn. 2013. Effect of Yoga on Arrhythmia Burden, Anxiety, Depression, and Quality of Life in Paroxysmal Atrial Fibrillation: The YOGA My Heart Study. *Journal of the American College of Cardiology* 61 (11): 1177–82.

Larouche, E., C. Hudon, and S. Goulet. 2015. Potential Benefits of Mindfulness-Based Interventions in Mild Cognitive Impairment and Alzheimer's Disease: An Interdisciplinary Perspective. *Behavioural Brain Research* 276: 199–212.

Lauche, R., P.M. Wayne, and G. Dobos. 2016. Prevalence, Patterns, and Predictors of t'ai Chi and Qigong Use in the United States: Results of a Nationally Representative Survey. *US National Library of Medicine National Institutes of Health Search Database, Journal of Alternative and Complementary Medicine* 22 (4): 336–342.

Lavretsky, H., E. Epel, P. Siddarth, N. Nazarian, N.S. Cyr, D.S. Khalsa, J. Lin, E. Blackburn, and M.R. Irwin. 2013. A Pilot Study of Yogic Meditation for Family Dementia Caregivers with Depressive Symptoms: Effects on Mental Health, Cognition, and Telomerase Activity. *International Journal of Geriatric Psychiatry* 28 (1): 57–65.

Lazar, S.W., C.E. Kerr, R.H. Wasserman, J.R. Gray, D.N. Greve, M.T. Treadway, M. McGarvey et al. 2005. Meditation Experience is Associated with Increased Cortical Thickness. *Neuroreport* 16 (17): 1893–97.

Lazarov, O. and C. Hollands. 2016. Hippocampal Neurogenesis: Learning to Remember. *Progress in Neurobiology* 138: 1–18.

LeDoux, J.E. 2000. Emotion Circuits in the Brain. *Annual Review of Neuroscience* 23: 155–84.

Lee, A.C., W.F. Harvey, L.L. Price, L.P.K. Morgan, N.L. Morgan, and C. Wang. 2017. Mindfulness Is Associated with Psychological Health and Moderates Pain in Knee Osteoarthritis. *Osteoarthritis and Cartilage* 25 (6): 824–831.

Leung, M-K., W.K.W. Lau, C.C.H. Chan, S.S.Y. Wong, A.L.C. Fung, and T.M.C. Lee. 2017. Meditation-Induced Neuroplastic Changes in Amygdala Activity during Negative Affective Processing. *Social Neuroscience* 2017:1–12.

Luberto, C.M., S. Cotton, A.C. McLeish, C.J. Mingione, and E.M. O'Bryan. 2014. Mindfulness Skills and Emotion Regulation: The Mediating Role of Coping Self-Efficacy. *Mindfulness* 5 (4): 373–380.

Luders, E., P.M. Thompson, F. Kurth, Jui-Y. Hong, O.R. Phillips, Y. Wang, B.A. Gutman, Y-Y. Chou, K.L. Narr, and A.W. Toga. 2013. Global and Regional Alterations of Hippocampal Anatomy in Long-term Meditation Practitioners. *Human Brain Mapping* 34 (12): 3369–75.

Luthar, S.S., D. Cicchetti, and B. Becker. 2000. The Construct of Resilience: A Critical Evaluation and Guidelines for Future Work. *Child Development* 71 (3): 543–62.

Maes, M., C. Song, A. Lin, R. De Jongh, A. Van Gastel, G. Kenis, E. Bosmans et al. 1998. The Effects of Psychological Stress on Humans: Increased Production of pro-Inflammatory Cytokines and a Th1-like Response in Stress-Induced Anxiety. *Cytokine* 10 (4): 313–18.

Mallorquí-Bagué, N., A. Bulbena, G. Pailhez, S.N. Garfinkel, and H.D. Critchley. 2016. Mind-Body Interactions in Anxiety and Somatic Symptoms. *Harvard Review of Psychiatry* 24 (1): 53–60.

Mani, M. 2017. *E-Mindful Health: Evaluation of Mobile Apps for Mindfulness.* Queensland University of Technology. Brisbane, Australia. https://eprints.qut.edu.au/102651/.

Mantovani, A.M., C.E.P. Teles Fregonesi, R. Modolo R. Lorençoni, N.U. Savian, M. Romanholi Palma, A. Shiguemi I. Salgado, L.V. Franco de Oliveira, and R.B. Parreira. 2016. Immediate Effect of Basic Body Awareness Therapy on Heart Rate Variability. *Complementary Therapies in Clinical Practice* 22: 8–11.

Marchand, W.R. 2014. Neural Mechanisms of Mindfulness and Meditation: Evidence from Neuroimaging Studies. *World Journal of Radiology* 6 (7): 471–79.

Maslach, C. and S.E. Jackson. 1981. The Measurement of Experienced Burnout. *Journal of Organizational Behavior* 2 (2): 99–113.

Maslach, C., M.P. Leiter, and W. Schaufeli. 2008. Measuring Burnout. http://www.oxfordhandbooks.com/view/10.1093/oxfordhb/9780199211913.001.0001/oxfordhb-9780199211913-e-005.

Masten, A.S. 2007. Resilience in Developing Systems: Progress and Promise as the Fourth Wave Rises. *Development and Psychopathology* 19 (03): 921–30.

McClafferty, H., E. Siblanga, M. Bailey, T. Culbert, J. Weydert, and M. Brown. 2016. Mind-Body Therapies in Children and Youth. *Pediatrics* 138(3): e1–e15.

McEwen, B.S. and E. Stellar. 1993. Stress and the Individual. Mechanisms Leading to Disease. *Archives of Internal Medicine* 153 (18): 2093–2101.

McGuire, C., J. Gabison, and B. Kligler. 2016. Facilitators and Barriers to the Integration of Mind-Body Medicine into Primary Care. *The Journal of Alternative and Complementary Medicine* 22 (6): 437–42.

Mealer, M., D. Conrad, J. Evans, K. Jooste, J. Solyntjes, B. Rothbaum, and M. Moss. 2014. Feasability and Acceptability of a Resilience Training Program for Intensive Care Unit Nurses. *American Journal of Critical Care* 23 (6): e97–105.

Mehta, D.H., G.K. Perez, L. Traeger, E.R. Park, R.E. Goldman, V. Haime, E.H. Chittenden, J.W. Denninger, and V.A. Jackson. 2016. Building Resiliency in a Palliative Care Team: A Pilot Study. *Journal of Pain and Symptom Management* 51 (3): 604–608.

Miller, K.M., E. Chad-Friedman, V. Haime, D.H. Mehta, V. Lepoutre, D. Gilburd, D. Peltier-Saxe et al. 2015. The Effectiveness of a Brief Mind-Body Intervention for Treating Depression in Community Health Center Patients. *Global Advances in Health and Medicine* 4 (2): 30–35.

Millstine, D., C.Y. Chen, and B. Bauer. 2017. Complementary and Integrative Medicine in the Management of Headache. *BMJ* 357: j1805. doi:10.1136/bmj.j1805.

Morone, N.E., C.M. Greco, C.G. Moore, B.L. Rollman, B. Lane, L.A. Morrow, N.W. Glynn, and D.K. Weiner. 2016. A Mind-Body Program for Older Adults with Chronic Low Back Pain: A Randomized Clinical Trial. *JAMA Internal Medicine* 176 (3): 329–337.

Nakamura, Y., D.L. Lipschitz, E. Kanarowski, T. McCormick, D. Sutherland, and M. Melow-Murchie. 2015. Investigating Impacts of Incorporating an Adjuvant Mind–Body Intervention Method Into Treatment as Usual at a Community-Based Substance Abuse Treatment Facility: A Pilot Randomized Controlled Study. *SAGE Open* 5 (1): 2158244015572489.

Ndetan, H., M.W. Jr. Evans, and R.D. Williams. 2014. Use of Movement Therapies and Relaxation Techniques and Management of Health Conditions among Children. *US National Library of Medicine National Institutes of Health, Alternative Therapies in Health and Medicine* 20 (4): 44–50.

Ni, H., C. Simile, and A.M. Hardy. 2002. Utilization of Complementary and Alternative Medicine by United States Adults: Results from the 1999 National Health Interview Survey. *Medical Care* 40 (4): 353–358.

Niles, H., D.H. Mehta, A.A. Corrigan, M.K. Bhasin, and J.W. Denninger. 2014. Functional Genomics in the Study of Mind-Body Therapies. *The Ochsner Journal* 14 (4): 681–695.

Nolan, C.R. 2016. Bending without Breaking: A Narrative Review of Trauma-Sensitive Yoga for Women with PTSD. *Complementary Therapies in Clinical Practice* 24: 32–40.

Noordali, F., J. Cumming, and J.L. Thompson. 2015. Effectiveness of Mindfulness-Based Interventions on Physiological and Psychological Complications in Adults with Diabetes: A Systematic Review. *Journal of Health Psychology* 22 (8): 965.

Nyklicek, I., P. Mommersteeg, S. Van Beugen, C. Ramakers, and G.J. Van Boxtel. 2013. Mindfulness-Based Stress Reduction and Physiological Activity during Acute Stress: A Randomized Controlled Trial. *Health Psychology* 32 (10): 1110.

Olano, H.A., D. Kachan, S.L. Tannenbaum, A. Mehta, D. Annane, and D.J. Lee. 2015. Engagement in Mindfulness Practices by US Adults: Sociodemographic Barriers. *The Journal of Alternative and Complementary Medicine* 21 (2): 100–102.

Pacanowski, C.R., L. Diers, R.D. Crosby, and D. Neumark-Sztainer. 2017. Yoga in the Treatment of Eating Disorders within a Residential Program: A Randomized Controlled Trial. *Eating Disorders* 25 (1): 37–51.

Panebianco, M., K. Sridharan, and S. Ramaratnam. 2015. Yoga for Epilepsy. *Cochrane Database of Systematic Reviews* 25 (1): 37–51 doi:10.1002/14651858.CD001524.pub2.

Park, E.R., L. Traeger, A-M. Vranceanu, M. Scult, J.A. Lerner, H. Benson, J. Denninger, and G.L. Fricchione. 2013. The Development of a Patient-Centered Program Based on the Relaxation Response: The Relaxation Response Resiliency Program (3RP). *Psychosomatics* 54 (2): 165–174.

Park, T., M. Reilly-Spong, and C.R. Gross. 2013. Mindfulness: A Systematic Review of Instruments to Measure an Emergent Patient-Reported Outcome (PRO). *Quality of Life Research* 22 (10): 2639–59.

Paul-Labrador, M., D. Polk, J.H. Dwyer, I. Velasquez, S. Nidich, M. Rainforth, R. Schneider, and C.N. Merz. 2006. Effects of a Randomized Controlled Trial of Transcendental Meditation on Components of the Metabolic Syndrome in Subjects with Coronary Heart Disease. *Archives of Internal Medicine* 166 (11): 1218–24.

Peregoy, J.A., T.C. Clarke, L.I. Jones, B.J. Stussman, and R.L. Nahin. 2014. Regional Variation in Use of Complementary Health Approaches by US Adults. *NCHS Data Brief* 146: 1.

Pipe, T.B., V.L. Buchda, S. Launder, B. Hudak, L. Hulvey, K.E. Karns, and D. Pendergast. 2012. Building Personal and Professional Resources of Resilience and Agility in the Healthcare Workplace. *Stress and Health* 28 (1): 11–22.

Pradhan, B., T. Parikh, R. Makani, M. Sahoo, and M. Sahoo. 2015. Ketamine, Transcranial Magnetic Stimulation, and Depression Specific Yoga and Mindfulness Based Cognitive Therapy in Management of Treatment Resistant Depression: Review and Some Data on Efficacy. *Depression Research and Treatment.* Article ID 842817

Quaglia, J.T., R.J. Goodman, and K.W. Brown. 2015. From Mindful Attention to Social Connection: The Key Role of Emotion Regulation. *Cognition and Emotion* 29 (8): 1466–1474.

Rao, K.S., S.K. Chakrabarti, V.S. Dongare, K. Chetana, C.M. Ramirez, P.S. Koka, and K.D. Deb. 2015. Antiaging Effects of an Intensive Mind and Body Therapeutic Program through Enhancement of Telomerase Activity and Adult Stem Cell Counts. *Journal of Stem Cells* 10 (2): 107.

Reed-Knight, B., R.L. Claar, J.V. Schurman, and M.A.L. vanTilburg. 2016. Implementing Psychological Therapies for Functional GI Disorders in Children and Adults, *Expert Review of Gastroenterology & Hepatology* 10 (9): 981–984.

Rosen, J.E., P. Gardiner, and S.L. Lee. 2013. Complementary and Integrative Treatments: Thyroid Disease. *Otolaryngologic Clinics of North America* 46 (3): 423–35.

Rosenbluth, S.C., E.G. Freymiller, R. Hemphill, D.E. Paull, M. Stuber, and A.H. Friedlander. 2017. Resident Well-Being and Patient Safety: Recognizing the Signs and Symptoms of Burnout. *Journal of Oral and Maxillofacial Surgery* 75 (4): 657–59.

Ruotsalainen, J.H., J.H. Verbeek, A. Marine, and C. Serra. 2014. Preventing Occupational Stress in Healthcare Workers. *Cochrane Database Systematic Reviews*: CD002892–CD002892.

Sanada, K., J. Montero-Marin, M.A. Diez, M. Salas-Valero, M.C. Perez-Yus, H. Morillo, M.M.P. Demarzo, M. Garcia-Toro, and J. Garcia-Campayo. 2016. Effects of Mindfulness-Based Interventions on Cortisol in Healthy Adults: A Meta-Analytical Review. *Frontiers in Physiology* 7: 471.

Sarkar, S. and M. Varshney. 2017. Yoga and Substance Use Disorders: A Narrative Review. *Asian Journal of Psychiatry* 25: 191–96.

Schoenberg, P.L.A. and A.S. David. 2014. Biofeedback for Psychiatric Disorders: A Systematic Review. *Applied Psychophysiology and Biofeedback* 39 (2): 109–135.

Schumann, D., D. Anheyer, R. Lauche, G. Dobos, J. Langhorst, and H. Cramer. 2016. Effect of Yoga in the Therapy of Irritable Bowel Syndrome: A Systematic Review. *Clinical Gastroenterology and Hepatology* 14 (12): 1720–30.

Seeman, T.E., B.H. Singer, J.W. Rowe, R.I. Horwitz, and B.S. McEwen. 1997. Price of Adaptation—Allostatic Load and Its Health Consequences. MacArthur Studies of Successful Aging. *Archives of Internal Medicine* 157 (19): 2259–68.

Shallcross, A.J. and P. Visvanathan. 2016. *Mindfulness-Based Cognitive Therapy for Insomnia. Mindfulness-Based Cognitive Therapy*, Springer International Publishing, Cham, Switzerland. 19–29.

Sharma, V., Y. Saito, and S. Amit. 2014. Mind-Body Medicine and Irritable Bowel Syndrome: A Randomized Control Trial Using Stress Reduction and Resiliency Training. *The Journal of Alternative and Complementary Medicine* 20 (5): A94–A94.

Shearer, W.T., J.M. Reuben, J.M. Mullington, N.J. Price, B.N. Lee, E.O. Smith, M.P. Szuba, H.P. Van Dongen, and Dinges D.F. 2001. Soluble TNF-Alpha Receptor 1 and IL-Plasma Levels in Humans Subjected to the Sleep Deprivation of Spaceflight. *The Journal of Allergy and Clinical Immunology* 107 (1): 165–70.

Sierpina, V., R. Levine, J. Astin, and A. Tan. 2007. Use of Mind-Body Therapies in Psychiatry and Family Medicine Faculty and Residents: Attitudes, Barriers, and Gender Differences. *EXPLORE: The Journal of Science and Healing* 3 (2): 129–35.

Sisk, A. and M. Fonteyn. 2016. Evidence-Based Yoga Interventions for Patients with Cancer. *Clinical Journal of Oncology Nursing* 20 (2): 181–86.

Smith, B., J. Dalen, K. Wiggins, E. Tooley, P. Christopher, and J. Bernard. 2008. The Brief Resilience Scale: Assessing the Ability to Bounce Back. *International Journal of Behavioral Medicine* 15 (3): 194–200.

Sobel, D.S. 2000. The Cost-Effectiveness of Mind-Body Medicine Interventions. *Progress in Brain Research* 122: 393–412.

Song, C., G. Kenis, A. van Gastel, E. Bosmans, A. Lin, R. de Jong, H. Neels et al. 1999. Influence of Psychological Stress on Immune-Inflammatory Variables in Normal Humans. Part II. Altered Serum Concentrations of Natural Anti-Inflammatory Agents and Soluble Membrane Antigens of Monocytes and T Lymphocytes. *Psychiatric Research* 85 (3): 293–303.

Southwick, S.M. and D.S. Charney. 2012. The Science of Resilience: Implications for the Prevention and Treatment of Depression. *Science* 338 (6103): 79–82.

Stahl, J.E., M.L. Dossett, A. Scott LaJoie, J.W. Denninger, D.E. Mehta, R. Goldman, G.L. Fricchione, and H. Benson. 2015. Relaxation Response and Resiliency Training and Its Effect on Healthcare Resource Utilization. *PLos ONE* 10 (10): e0140212.

Steptoe, A. and M. Kivimäki. 2012. Stress and Cardiovascular Disease. *Nature Reviews Cardiology* 9 (6): 360.

Streeter, C.C., P.L. Gerbarg, T.H. Whitfield, L. Owen, J. Johnston, M.M. Silveri, M. Gensler et al. 2017. Treatment of Major Depressive Disorder with Iyengar Yoga and Coherent Breathing: A Randomized Controlled Dosing Study. *The Journal of Alternative and Complementary Medicine* 23 (3): 201–207.

Sveinbjarnardottir, E.K., E.K. Svavarsdottir, and L.M. Wright. 2013. What Are the Benefits of a Short Therapeutic Conversation Intervention with Acute Psychiatric Patients and Their Families? A Controlled before and after Study. *International Journal of Nursing Studies* 50 (5): 593–602.

Sylvia, L.G., E. Bui, A.L. Baier, D.H. Mehta, J.W. Denninger, G.L. Fricchione, A. Casey, L. Kagan, E.R. Park, and N.M. Simon. 2015. Resilient Warrior: A Stress Management Group to Improve Psychological Health in Service Members. *Global Advances in Health and Medicine* 4 (6): 38–42.

Theadom, A., M. Cropley, H.E. Smith, V.L. Feigin, and K. McPherson. 2015. Mind and Body Therapy for Fibromyalgia. *Cochrane Database of Systematic Reviews.* (4): CD001980–CD001980. doi:10.1002/14651858.CD001980.pub3.

Toker, S., S. Melamed, S. Berliner, D. Zeltser, and I. Shapira. 2012. Burnout and Risk of Coronary Heart Disease: A Prospective Study of 8838 Employees. *Psychosomatic Medicine* 74: 840–47. doi:10.1097/PSY.0b013e31826c3174.

Tyagi, A. and M. Cohen. 2016. Yoga and Heart Rate Variability: A Comprehensive Review of the Literature. *International Journal of Yoga* 9 (2): 97.

Van der Zwan, J.E., W. de Vente, A.C. Huizink, S.M. Bogels, and E.I. de Bruin. 2015. Physical Activity, Mindfulness Meditation, or Heart Rate Variability Biofeedback for Stress Reduction: A Randomized Controlled Trial. *Applied Psychophysiology and Biofeedback* 40 (4): 257–68.

Vizcaino, M. and E. Stover. 2016. The Effect of Yoga Practice on Glycemic Control and Other Health Parameters in Type 2 Diabetes Mellitus Patients: A Systematic Review and Meta-Analysis. *Complementary Therapies in Medicine* 28: 57–66.

Wagnild, G. and H. Young. 1993. Development and Psychometric. *Journal of Nursing Measurement* 1 (2): 165–78.

Wallace, R.K. and H. Benson. 1972. The Physiology of Meditation. *Scientific American* 226(2): 84–90. http://psycnet.apa.org/psycinfo/1972-22284-001.

Wallace, R.K., H. Benson, and A.F. Wilson. 1971. A Wakeful Hypometabolic Physiologic State. *The American Journal of Physiology* 221 (3): 795–99.

Walsh, E., T. Eisenlohr-Moul, and R.A. Baer. 2016. Brief Mindfulness Training Reduces Salivary IL-6 and TNF-α in Young Women with Depressive Symptomatology. *Journal of Consulting and Clinical Psychology* 84 (10): 887–97.

Wang, X-Q., Y-L. Pi, P-J. Chen, Y. Liu, R. Wang, X. Li, B-L Chen, Y. Zhu, Y-J. Yang, and Z-B. Niu. 2016. Traditional Chinese Exercise for Cardiovascular Diseases: Systematic Review and Meta-Analysis of Randomized Controlled Trials. *Journal of the American Heart Association* 5 (3): e002562.

Watson, D., L.A. Clark, and A. Tellegan. 1988. Development and Validation of Brief Measures of Positive and Negative Affect: The PANAS Scales. *Journal of Personality and Social Psychology* 54 (6): 1063–70.

Waugh, C.E. and E.H.W. Koster. 2015. A Resilience Framework for Promoting Stable Remission from Depression. *Clinical Psychology Review* 41: 49–60.

Wayne, P.M., D. Berkowitz, D.E. Litrownik, J.E. Buring, and G.Y. Yeh. 2014. What Do We Really Know about the Safety of Tai Chi?: A Systematic Review of Adverse Event Reports in Randomized Trials. *Archives of Physical Medicine and Rehabilitation* 95 (12): 2470–83.

Wayne, P.M., B. Manor, V. Novak, M.D. Costa, J.M. Hausdorff, A.L. Goldberger, A.C. Ahn et al. 2013. A Systems Biology Approach to Studying Tai Chi, Physiological Complexity and Healthy Aging: Design and Rationale of a Pragmatic Randomized Controlled Trial. *Contemporary Clinical Trials* 34 (1): 21–34.

Wayne, P.M., J.N. Walsh, R.E. Taylor-Piliae, R.E. Wells, K.V. Papp, N.J. Donovan, and G.Y. Yeh. 2014. Effect of Tai Chi on Cognitive Performance in Older Adults: Systematic Review and Meta-Analysis. *Journal of American Geriatrics Society* 62 (1): 25–39.

Wells, R.E., G.Y. Yeh, C.E. Kerr, J. Wolkin, R.B. Davis, Y. Tan, R. Spaeth et al. 2013. Meditation's Impact on Default Mode Network and Hippocampus in Mild Cognitive Impairment: A Pilot Study. *Neuroscience Letters* 556: 15–19.

White, R.S., J. Jiang, C.B. Hall, M.J. Katz, M.E. Zimmerman, M. Sliweinski, and R.B. Lipton. 2014. Higher Perceived Stress Scale Scores Are Associated with Higher Pain Intensity and Pain Interference Levels in Older Adults. *Journal of the American Geriatrics Society* 62 (12): 2350–56.

Williams, D., G. Tricomi, J. Gupta, and A. Janise. 2015. Efficacy of Burnout Interventions in the Medical Education Pipeline. *Academic Psychiatry* 39 (1): 47–54.

Williams, M., J.D. Teasdale, Z.V. Segal, and J. Kabat-Zinn. 2007. *The Mindful Way through Depression: Freeing Yourself from Chronic Unhappiness.* Guilford Press, New York.

Windle, G., K.M. Bennett, and J. Noyes. 2011. A Methodological Review of Resilience Measurement Scales. *Health and Quality of Life Outcomes* 9 (1): 8.

Yan, Qing. 2016. *Psychoneuroimmunology: Systems Biology Approaches to Mind-Body Medicine.* Springer, Cham, Switzerland.

Zhang, L., X.Z. Hu, X. Li, H. Li, S. Smerin, D. Russell, and R.J. Ursano. 2014. Telomere Length—a Cellular Aging Marker for Depression and Post-Traumatic Stress Disorder. *Medical Hypotheses* 83 (2): 182–85.

Zimmaro, L.A., P. Salmon, H. Naidu, J. Rowe, K. Phillips, W.N. Rebholz, J. Giese-Davis et al. 2016. Association of Dispositional Mindfulness with Stress, Cortisol, and Well-Being among University Undergraduate Students. *Mindfulness* 7 (4): 874–885.

17 Meditation, Neurobiological Changes, Genes, and Health
A New Paradigm for the Healthcare System

Marjorie H. Woollacott

CONTENTS

Introduction 423
Definition 424
Historical Context 425
Physiological Effects of Meditation in Health and Disease 427
    Cardiovascular Effects (Cardiovascular Disease/Hypertension) 427
    Neurobiological Effects of Meditation in Health and Disease 429
    Modulation of Pain Pathways by Meditation 432
    Immune System Improvements and Genetic Changes in Health and Disease 432
        Gene Expression 433
Summary 434
References 435

INTRODUCTION

Meditation and its related forms of mind–body therapy, such as yoga, tai chi, and chi-gong, has become increasingly studied by researchers during the last 30 years as a complementary medicine used to reduce stress and to treat a variety of disorders. These include mental/emotional problems, such as ADHD, depression, anxiety, and obsessive-compulsive disorder (OCD), cardiovascular disease, and immune function issues (including psoriasis and other autoimmune diseases), among others (Grossman et al. 2004; Hofmann et al. 2010; Goyal et al. 2014; O'Reilly et al. 2014; Bai et al. 2015). As you will see throughout this chapter, research on meditation has consistently demonstrated a positive effect on a number of physiological variables resulting in the amelioration of many diseases. However, despite this research, meditation as a therapeutic tool is still not widely recommended by medical doctors (Hammerman et al. 2016).

In this chapter we explore the evidence for meditation as an important complementary medical practice. In the medical profession, "evidence-based" practice is an important guiding principle. David Sackett defines evidence-based practice as integrating the best available research evidence with clinical expertise and patient preference (Sackett et al. 2000). Thus, when we talk about evidence-based clinical practice, we mean using research (and one's own clinical experience) to inform, transform, and guide clinical decisions regarding assessment and treatment in an individual patient.

However, there are a number of barriers to implementing evidence-based practice within clinicians themselves and within the profession. One such barrier is discussed by Sheldon and his colleagues. They say, "The degree to which clinicians see even good quality research as able to be implemented will depend on the extent to which the results conflict with their own professional experience and belief" (Sheldon et al. 1998, 142). For example, a clinician may hear of a new research study providing evidence that mindfulness meditation reduces symptoms of attentional deficit hyperactivity disorder (ADHD) in children. But in medical school he or she was taught that pharmaceuticals are the optimal approach to managing ADHD symptoms, and so, based on this, the clinician may simply write a prescription, rather than investigating research related to mindfulness training as a complementary tool for ADHD, or, in some cases, as an alternative to a pharmaceutical approach. This chapter explores the evidence to support the use of meditation and other mind–body therapies to aid healing for a variety of disorders.

A second barrier to translating research into practice is a lack of an appropriate framework for understanding the implications of the research for benefiting practice. For example, most physicians are trained to treat patients according to a theoretical framework that makes the assumption that the field of medicine is materially based. A materially based model assumes that the neurons in the brain are the sole producers of our consciousness or mental activity. It is what could be defined as a bottom-up model, as activity goes one way, from the neurons toward awareness. Thus to treat ADHD, a pharmaceutical which would affect neurotransmitters would be the treatment of choice. But in complementary medicine a second model is considered: a mind–brain continuum model, where there is a two-way interaction between the mind and the brain, so that our thoughts or mental training can also affect our brain function. If a clinician accepts this model, then he or she would be interested in using a treatment involving mental training, as the model includes a two-way interaction between mind and brain. I will talk about these alternative models later in the chapter.

In the following pages of this chapter we will first explore what we mean by meditation and mind–body therapies and explain the historical context from which they were developed, as well as how they have come to be used as healing aids in the medical field.

We will then discuss the physiological benefits of meditation, including improvements to cardiovascular, neurophysiological, and immunological function, examine the effects of meditation on gene expression, and discuss specific research on its healing capacity with respect to different diseases.

DEFINITION

The medical dictionary defines meditation as "a practice of concentrated focus upon a sound, object, visualization, the breath, movement, or attention itself in order to increase awareness of the present moment, reduce stress, promote relaxation, and enhance personal and spiritual growth" (medical-dictionary.thefreedictionary.com/meditation).

One of the goals of meditation is to become anchored in one's own *awareness* of what is happening inside oneself, and more specifically, letting go of identifying with one's feelings and thoughts, and with the various outer situations or dramas of life. The meditator learns to simply watch or witness them. When we realize that we are not our thoughts, feelings, or sensations, but are the one watching our thoughts, we become much more capable of finding a state of equipoise, and of effectively and compassionately addressing what needs to be done in the moment.

Many meditation traditions distinguish between what they call "concentrative" forms of meditation, in which one focuses on an object, like the breath, and what they call "open-awareness" meditation, in which there is not an attempt to focus, but to simply be aware of the contents of consciousness, that is, to simply observe the contents of the mind, as discussed above. In fact, most meditation traditions have students begin their practice with an object of focus, for example, the breath, and then eventually move to open-awareness, as the person becomes more skilled in their practice or as they continue within the meditation period.

In addition to sitting forms of meditation, various movement-oriented practices also have meditative aspects. For example tai chi, considered a moving form of meditation, is a Chinese exercise system that uses slow, smooth body movements to achieve a state of relaxation of both body and mind. Chi gong combines movement, meditation, and breath regulation to balance the flow of chi (considered the life energy of the body). And yoga typically involves both postures (asanas), used to strengthen and align the body and bring blood flow to all the organs, and breathing exercises, in addition to sitting meditation, to quiet and discipline the mind (medical-dictionary: thefree-dictionary.com).

HISTORICAL CONTEXT

Meditation is a practice that has been part of many cultures for thousands of years. Archeologists have found art from the Indus Valley civilization dating from about 5000–3000 BCE, depicting people sitting in meditation postures. There are also texts of Vedanta from India dating back about 3500 years, giving descriptions of meditation techniques. Texts from China show that meditation also developed there between 600 and 500 BCE, in the form of Taoism and Buddhism. One of the most well-known early texts on meditation is the *Yoga Sutras* of Patanjali, which outlines eight limbs of the yogic practice of meditation, designed to quiet the mind. These include, among others, posture, control of the breath, withdrawal of the senses from focusing on external objects, concentration, meditation, and deep meditative absorption. One of the first sutras, or verses in the text states that yoga (the word used for meditation) is the stilling of the thought-waves of the mind (Feuerstein 1989).

The practice of meditation spread to Europe in the third century, with the teachings of Plotinus (Gerson 1996); many spiritual traditions have incorporated its concepts, including Sufism, Judaism, and Christianity, in the form of the practice of centering prayer. Today there are many different variations on meditative practice, but the central goal is typically stilling the thoughts of the mind, so that one can experience the clear and peaceful state of simple awareness in the present moment. It is only in recent years that researchers have investigated the effect of this practice on physiological parameters in the body.

In fact, many research studies have shown the physiological benefits of meditation; as a result, a number of scientists and clinicians have developed secular forms of meditation practice, in order to adapt it for use in the medical setting. Jon Kabat-Zinn, of the University of Massachusetts Medical Center, was one of the first persons to develop a clinically based form of meditation practice, which is called Mindfulness-Based Stress Reduction (MBSR) (Kabat-Zinn 1990). It is designed to address a number of chronic health problems and diseases. Other clinicians have also adapted these meditation tools in creating such programs as Mindfulness-Based Cognitive Therapy (MBCT) (a combination of MBSR and cognitive behavior therapy) to treat depression (Kabat-Zinn 1990), Clinically Standardized Meditation (CSM) (Ospina et al. 2007), developed by Patricia Carrington, and Respiratory ONE, by Herbert Benson (Benson, 1976). See the text boxes for summaries of these clinical applications of meditation.

Though these clinical training methods in meditation vary as to what aspects of the meditation process are emphasized, there are still many aspects that are similar to those practiced in classical meditation methods. These include (1) assuming a steady and comfortable upright sitting posture with arms comfortably on the lap, often with one palm resting upright on the other (though a walking meditation is a variation on sitting meditation), (2) breathing evenly and naturally, and (3) choosing an approach to absorbing the mind within, such as focus on the breath, on a set of syllables or mantra, or simply letting go of thoughts. The most important quality to hold in one's awareness is a gentle intention to go within to a space of quiet awareness, and to let go of thoughts. Learning to quiet the mind takes practice, as does any skill, and patience is key.

**BOX 17.1   MINDFULNESS-BASED STRESS REDUCTION
(JON KABAT-ZINN, U. OF MASS. MEDICAL SCHOOL)**

This is taught in the form of a course which meets 2 1/2 hours once per week for 8 weeks, in addition to an all-day weekend class between weeks 6 and 7 of the course. There is also a homework assignment of 45–60 minutes each day, which includes listening to 4 home-practice CDs and working with a home-practice workbook. The classes include:

- Guided instruction in mindfulness meditation practices
- Gentle stretching and mindful yoga
- Group dialogue and discussions aimed at enhancing awareness in everyday life
- Individually tailored instruction

Adapted from U. Massachusetts Medical School website: umassmed.edu

**BOX 17.2   RESPIRATORY ONE METHOD OF MEDITATION
(HERBERT BENSON, HARVARD MEDICAL SCHOOL)**

This is taught as a set of steps to elicit what is called the Relaxation Response (RR). They are

1. Sit quietly in a comfortable position.
2. Close your eyes.
3. Deeply relax all your muscles, beginning at your feet and progressing up to your face. Keep them relaxed. [Relax your tongue—and thoughts will cease.]
4. Breathe through your nose. Become aware of your breathing. As you breathe out, say the word "one"* silently to yourself. For example, breathe in, and then out, and say "one,"* in and out, and repeat "one."* Breathe easily and naturally.
5. Continue for 10–20 minutes. You may open your eyes to check the time, but do not use an alarm. When you finish, sit quietly for several minutes, at first with your eyes closed and later with your eyes opened. Do not stand up for a few minutes.
6. Do not worry about whether you are successful in achieving a deep level of relaxation. Maintain a passive attitude and permit relaxation to occur at its own pace. When distracting thoughts occur, try to ignore them by not dwelling on them and return to repeating "one."*
7. With practice, the response should come with little effort. Practice the technique once or twice daily, but not within two hours after any meal, since the digestive processes seem to interfere with the elicitation of the Relaxation Response.*

From Benson's book, The Relaxation Response, 1976, 162–163

---

* Choose any soothing, mellifluous sounding word, preferably with no meaning or association, in order to avoid stimulation of unnecessary thoughts.

> **BOX 17.3   CLINICALLY STANDARDIZED MEDITATION (PATRICIA CARRINGTON, YALE UNIVERSITY)**
>
> Clinically Standardized Meditation uses the mental repetition of a sound selected from a list of sounds (or self-created), which is allowed to move at its own pace. That is, it is not systematically liked with the breath. It is considered to be an adaptation of the practices of Transcendental Meditation (TM) for the clinic.

In the next sections we will discuss the research on meditation and the physiological benefits of meditation, including improvements to cardiovascular, neurophysiological, and immunological function, and associated medical disorders.

PHYSIOLOGICAL EFFECTS OF MEDITATION IN HEALTH AND DISEASE

Meditation has been shown to be effective in improving the function of a variety of systems, including the attentional systems of the brain (improving attentional abilities in normal young adults, and ameliorating symptoms of Attentional Deficit Hyperactivity Disorder [ADHD] and Mild Cognitive Impairment [MCI]), the cardiovascular system (reducing blood pressure and cardiovascular disease), and the immune system (reducing cortisol levels and ameliorating the symptoms of autoimmune diseases) and in reducing symptoms of chronic pain.

CARDIOVASCULAR EFFECTS (CARDIOVASCULAR DISEASE/HYPERTENSION)

Cardiovascular disease is a major problem in the United States. It is ranked number one in causes of mortality (Lozano et al. 2012; World Health Organization 2010). Statistics indicate that persons with symptoms of acute coronary syndrome and myocardial infarction make up about 10% of hospital emergency room visits and about 25% of hospital admissions The costs for treating patients with cardiovascular disease is about $286 billion each year, which is about 17% of total healthcare expenditures (Ray et al. 2014). Many research studies have shown that there are a number of psychological risk factors contributing to cardiovascular disease, including anxiety, depression, and hostility. Increases in psychological stress directly contribute to pathophysiological processes leading to cardiovascular disease. These include increases in sympathetic nervous system activation, evaluated by increased norepinephrine in the blood, impairment in platelet function, increased cortisol levels, and the exacerbation of atherosclerosis (Rozanski et al. 1999; Schwartz et al. 2012).

Can meditation and other mind/body therapies, which reduce stress factors, such as anxiety, depression, and hostility, reduce cardiovascular disease? Many carefully designed studies have shown that meditation does reduce both the psychological and physiological risk factors related to heart disease (Zeidan et al. 2010; Ray et al. 2014). For example, a randomized controlled clinical trial (RCT) on patients with cardiovascular disease and depression by Delui et al. (2013) compared three groups: a meditation training group, a relaxation training group, and a control (no intervention) group. Training consisted of 10 sessions of progressive muscle relaxation (PMR) or of meditation. Meditation training resulted in significant reductions in depression scores on the Beck depression scale, as well as reduced systolic blood pressure in the patients with cardiovascular disease, compared to the control group, while relaxation training was not effective.

In addition to reductions in blood pressure, meditation also modulates sympathetic nervous system activity, reducing norepinephrine levels in the blood. This is significant as norepinephrine is known to be a factor indicative of cardiovascular disease progression, cardiovascular mortality, hospitalization for congestive heart failure, ischemic events, and myocardial infarction (Curiati et al. 2005).

Studies on prehypertensive patients have shown similar results. For example, a randomized controlled trial compared 8 weeks (2.5 hrs/week) of training in MBSR to PMR in 56 patients with unmedicated hypertension. As you see in Figure 17.1, the meditation training resulted in a significantly greater (4.8 mmHg) reduction in systolic blood pressure (BP) compared to the relaxation group (0.7 mmHg). The authors note that it has been shown that BP changes of this size are relevant for public health and, if they can be sustained over a period of time, may result in reduced incidence of myocardial infarction, stroke, and death (Hughes et al. 2013).

These two studies are of importance in that they suggest that simple relaxation as practiced in PMR training is not enough to improve the measures of the physiological variables associated with heart disease. Thus, meditation is not acting through simple relaxation, but a mechanism that is more profound.

Similar results have been found in studies using Transcendental Meditation (TM) training (Rainforth et al. 2007). In fact, a systematic review and meta-analysis of various approaches to stress reduction in patients with elevated blood pressure concluded that TM showed BP reductions of -5 to -2.8 mmHg, across a series of well-designed studies. These reductions were similar to or greater than other lifestyle modifications such as aerobic exercise, weight-reduction, and so on. The authors of this meta-analysis also note that another meta-analysis (Schneider et al. 2005) of randomized controlled trials of subjects with elevated BP and an average follow-up of eight years showed a 23% decrease in all-cause mortality and a 30% decrease in CVD mortality in the TM group compared to controls. They note that this is significant because no other stress reduction or lifestyle modification that has been recommended for hypertension has been shown to reduce mortality rates in RCTs (Chobanian et al. 2003; Rainforth et al. 2007).

A second systematic review and meta-analysis of the effectiveness of mind–body practices on ameliorating diagnosed heart disease (Younge et al. 2015a) evaluated 13 randomized controlled clinical trials, including 793 patients, carried out in six different countries. The mind–body practices they evaluated were MBSR, TM, other forms of meditation, and PMR; interventions were from 4 to 26 weeks in duration. For systolic blood pressure, they found an average medium statistically significant effect of $d = 0.48$, while for diastolic blood pressure it was lower (0.36) but still significant. This was accompanied by average medium effect sizes for psychological variables such as depression, anxiety, and quality of life ($d = 0.61$, 0.52 and 0.45, respectively).

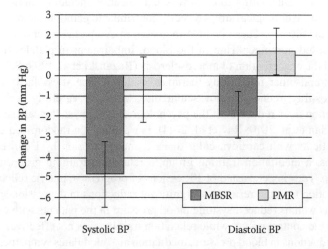

FIGURE 17.1 Mean change in clinic systolic and diastolic blood pressure from pretreatment to post-treatment. Error bars represent the standard error of the mean. PMR = progressive muscle relaxation. MBSR = mindfulness-based stress reduction. (Adapted from Hughes et al. 2013. *Psychosom Med* 75:721–728, Figure 3.)

The authors of this meta-analysis conclude that "even though the American Heart Association (AHA) has recognized the importance of psychosocial interventions as a core component in cardiac rehabilitation programmes, these interventions have only been integrated in a limited number of settings. Furthermore, only 25%–31% of eligible patients participate in these comprehensive programmes" (Younge et al. 2015a, 1396).

Is tai chi also effective in reducing both psychological and physiological risk factors for heart disease? A number of studies suggest that it is. A meta-analysis (Yeh et al. 2009) reported that four randomized controlled clinical trials, with typically a 12-week tai chi intervention, resulted in a significant reduction in blood pressure in patients with hypertension (Young et al. 1999; Sheng and Su 2000; Tsai et al. 2003; Thomas et al. 2005). One RCT involving 8 weeks of tai chi training (Robins et al. 2015) measured biological variables associated with heart disease. At 2 months post intervention they found that tai chi helped significantly down-regulate proinflammatory cytokines associated with underlying cardiovascular disease (CVD) risk.

As the data reported above suggest that meditation and tai chi, a moving form of meditation, are helpful in ameliorating both psychological and physiological variables associated with heart disease, one might ask if there is a specific point at which intervention or prevention is recommended. In fact, research suggests that stress is related to heart disease along the continuum of disease progression, from the development of arteriosclerosis to acute cardiac events, which occur as part of the chronic disease state (Steptoe and Kivimaki 2012; Thurston et al. 2013).

A study from Rotterdam examined the association between mind–body practices (meditation, yoga, etc.) and cardiometabolic risk factors in a healthy population of 2579 participants, free from cardiovascular disease (Younge et al. 2015b). They found that those participants (15%) who were involved in a form of mind–body practice had a significantly lower body-mass index, lower log-transformed triglyceride levels, and fasting glucose levels. They were also less likely to have metabolic syndrome. The authors thus concluded that persons who practiced mind–body interventions had a significantly better cardio-metabolic risk profile compared with those who did not. This suggests that meditation and other mind–body practices should be practiced throughout life as a preventative measure for reducing the risk of cardiovascular disease.

NEUROBIOLOGICAL EFFECTS OF MEDITATION IN HEALTH AND DISEASE

Studies on both behavioral and neurobiological changes associated with meditation practice show benefits across the lifespan, from children to older adults. In healthy persons these include improved ability to focus attention (involving executive attention networks), increased emotional regulation, and for persons with attentional, memory, or emotional disorders, meditation leads to significant improvements in these areas (Lutz et al. 2008; Tang et al. 2015). Studies have also investigated the specific neural changes associated with these improvements in attention, memory, and emotional regulation.

Executive attention is a key aspect of cognitive ability. It involves the ability to deal with conflicting impulses and choose that which is beneficial in the long term rather than what is only pleasurable in the moment. Areas of the brain involved in the executive attention network include the prefrontal cortex and the anterior cingulate cortex (ACC). It has been shown that AAC size is highly correlated with success in the world. It is the best predictor of how well children resolve conflict (Fjell et al. 2012). And conflict resolution or effortful control at four years of age is highly correlated with success later in life (health, income, social relationships, criminality). Most importantly, the size of the ACC is modifiable through meditation (Grant et al. 2010).

For example, one study (Grant et al. 2010) asked whether meditation increased cortical thickness in attentional regions of the brain. They hypothesized that, because meditation is a form of mental training, it would cause significant changes in the cortical structure in the attentional regions engaged in this mental exercise. Using magnetic resonance imaging (MRI), they compared 19 Zen meditators to 20 control subjects and found that the meditators had higher cortical thickness in several areas, including the ACC. In a second study (Grant et al. 2013) they found that cortical thickness is actually correlated with years of meditation practice, including areas of the parietal cortex, prefrontal cortex, and the ACC. A study by Lazar and colleagues (Lazar et al. 2005) found similar results and, interestingly, differences between groups in prefrontal cortex were greatest in the older participants. This suggests that meditation may reduce age-related thinning of the cortex.

Our own lab has also shown that both meditation and tai chi, a moving form of meditation, have greater ability to improve executive attention and the underlying neural networks, than aerobic activity, when compared to a sedentary control group (Hawkes et al. 2014). EEG activity was measured while participants performed a complex computer game (a spatial switch task, in which rules changed every two trials). The long term meditation and tai chi groups not only had better performance on the task than the other groups, but also showed significantly larger P3b event related potentials (ERPs), as you see in Figure 17.2. P3b ERPs are attentionally associated EEG activity occurring 300 ms after the onset of the stimulus on the computer screen, which triggered a given switch trial. Larger ERPs are associated with greater attention given to the task, so this demonstrates the greater attentional network activity in the tai chi and meditation groups (Hawkes et al. 2014). What areas of the brain are associated with this improvement in executive attentional networks? We determined this using independent component analysis, which separates the ERP into its sources from different regions of the cortex. The ACC showed one of the greatest contributions to the differences in ERP size between groups.

In addition to executive attention functions, meditation has been shown to improve emotional regulation (Tang et al. 2007; Lutz et al. 2016). For example, in an RCT, Tang et al. (2007) showed that, compared to a control group (given relaxation training), students trained in meditation showed significant improvements in the Profile of Mood states (POMS) scales of anger-hostility, depression-dejection, fatigue-inertia, tension-anxiety, and vigor-activity post-training. Lutz et al. (2016) have shown that meditation training is associated with increased activation in the dorsomedial prefrontal cortex in response to presentation of blocks of positive or negative self-selected

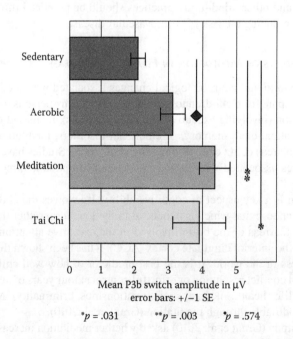

FIGURE 17.2 Mean P3b event-related potential (ERP) switch trial amplitude for the tai chi, meditation, aerobic, and sedentary adult groups, while performing an attentional spatial switch task. Note that only tai chi and meditation groups show significantly higher EEG ERP amplitudes than controls. (From Hawkes et al. 2014.)

adjectives, suggesting increased awareness, and mindful self-regulation of self-criticism and self-praise in long-term meditators.

If meditation can increase attentional abilities and cortical thickness in healthy individuals, can it also improve these same abilities in persons with cognitive impairment? Research is just beginning in this area, but results of initial studies are promising. Initial research in this area shows that, first, there is cortical thinning in attentional areas of persons who have Attentional Deficit Hyperactivity Disorder (ADHD). A study by Shaw and colleagues (2006) showed that when comparing cortical thickness in different regions associated with attention (e.g., the ACC), there was an inverse correlation for cortical thickness in meditators and persons with ADHD, with meditators showing increased, and persons with ADHD decreased, cortical thickness in the ACC (Grant et al. 2013).

Since mindfulness training improves ACC thickness and attentional function in normal subjects, it suggests that it may be possible to improve ACC function and structure in persons with ADHD as well. To test this hypothesis, Hepark et al. (2015) performed an RCT with 103 persons with ADHD randomized to a treatment or waitlist control group. They were given 12 weeks of Mindfulness-based Cognitive Therapy (MBCT) three times per week, and their ADHD symptoms were measured before versus after the training. Using the Conners Adults ADHD Rating Scale (CAARS-INV), and the Behaviour Rating Inventory of Executive Function scale (BRIEF-ASR), they showed significant improvements for those who participated in the MBCT Treatment versus the waitlist control group, as you see in Table 17.1.

Researchers are also beginning to ask whether meditation training can improve other disorders, such as mild cognitive impairment (MCI), which is a precursor to dementia and Alzheimer's Disease (AD) and in fact progresses to dementia in 50% of cases. Currently there are no known therapies to prevent the progression of MCI toward dementia. It is also of interest that high baseline stress levels may increase the probability of persons developing MCI and AD. A pilot RCT by Wells et al. (2013) aimed to determine if MBSR training would improve MCI and the connectivity in attention and memory areas of the brain as compared to usual care. Results indicated that after the training, MBSR participants showed increased functional connectivity between the posterior cingulate cortex and medial prefrontal cortex and hippocampus compared to control subjects. The authors also noted that MBSR participants had trends toward less hippocampal atrophy than the control group. This thus gives support for the use of meditation to help in slowing the decline of cognitive abilities with aging.

Major depressive disorder (MDD) is considered the leading cause of disease burden according to the World Health Organization. And statistics show that depression is a recurring problem: the risk of recurrence after one depressive episode is approximately 50%, and this increases to 70%–80%

TABLE 17.1

Differences in Scores for Persons with Attentional Deficit Hyperactivity Disorder (ADHD) on Tests of Executive Function: Effect of Mindfulness-Based Cognitive Therapy (MBCT) Treatment versus Control

	MBCT Treatment	Waitlist Control	Difference in Improvement between Groups
CAARS-INV-Baseline	29.3	29.0	
CAARS-INV Post-treatment	21.5	28.0	$p < 0.01$
Executive Fn. (Brief-ASR) Baseline	150.3	156.7	
Executive Fn. (Brief-ASR) Post-treatment	132.2	153.8	$p < 0.01$

Source: Data from Hepark et al. 2015.

after two or three depressive episodes (Godfrin et al. 2010). Many studies have been conducted to determine the effect of mindfulness practices on anxiety and depression.

A recent meta-analysis (Khoury et al. 2013) examining 209 studies with a total of 12,145 participants, states that Mindfulness Based Therapies (MBT) showed large and clinically significant effects in treating anxiety and depression, and the gains were maintained at follow-up. For example, in an RCT by Godfrin et al. (2010), MBCT was added to treatment as usual to determine its efficacy in preventing relapse or recurrence in depression in patients who had at least 3 prior depression episodes. The results show that participation in the MBCT program decreased the percentage of patients who relapsed at least once within 14 months by more than half, from 68.1% to 30%. In addition, the risk of relapse was decreased by 77%. In addition, the patients who were in the treatment as usual group had a smaller time to relapse/recurrence, while MBCT increased the period to the first relapse by about 15 weeks. Finally, the authors note that adding MBCT to treatment as usual decreased the severity of the remaining symptoms of depression and improved the participants' quality of life and mood states (Godfrin et al. 2010).

MODULATION OF PAIN PATHWAYS BY MEDITATION

Does meditation also modulate pain pathways and thus help control pain in chronic disease states? A substantial amount of research has been performed in this area (Bohlmeijer et al. 2010; Reiner et al. 2013). In fact, MBSR was originally created by Jon Kabat-Zinn to improve the self-management of chronic pain in patients (Kabat-Zinn 1982). Research shows significant correlations between higher levels of mindfulness and lower pain intensity ratings in patients with chronic pain (McCracken and Thompson 2009). A recent review of eight controlled studies evaluated the evidence of the effect of mind–body interventions on pain intensity ratings in clinical trials (Reiner et al. 2013). The clinical trials that were included involved patients with fibromyalgia, chronic back pain, rheumatoid arthritis, and other patients with chronic pain. Of the eight controlled studies, six concluded that pain intensity showed greater reductions in the mind–body intervention group compared to the control group. One of the studies showed comparable pain reduction for the mind–body (MB) intervention and cognitive behavioral therapy, while one showed no difference in the MB intervention and usual care. Interestingly, follow-up assessments, performed in three of the studies, showed that the effect was lasting, with pain intensity reductions maintained over 3 months to 3-year follow-up periods. Finally, the authors note that MB interventions resulted in medium effect sizes for reduction in pain intensity (Reiner et al. 2013). Thus, this research provides strong evidence to support the effectiveness of mind–body therapies such as meditation in controlling the intensity of chronic pain in a variety of patient populations, with good long-term benefit.

IMMUNE SYSTEM IMPROVEMENTS AND GENETIC CHANGES IN HEALTH AND DISEASE

One of the first studies on the effects of meditation on immune function was performed by Richard Davidson and his colleagues at the University of Wisconsin Madison in 2003 (Davidson et al. 2003). It was a cleverly designed study in which the authors vaccinated all the subjects in both the meditation (MBSR) group and the wait-list control group at the end of an eight-week meditation training. They hypothesized that, if meditation improves immune function, the meditation group would show increased antibody titers in response to the vaccine when compared with the control group. In fact, this is precisely what they found. Figure 17.3 shows a graph of the Log Transformed Antibody Rise from 3 to 5 weeks to 8 to 9 weeks post-vaccination. Note that the meditation group has a significantly greater rise than the control group. A further RCT by the lab (Rosenkranz et al. 2013) compared an MBSR training group to an active control group, which was given a Health Enhancement Program (HEP) training; they examined the response of individuals to an inflammation-inducing topical application of capsaicin cream to the arm, after a stress-inducing test, the Trier Social Stress

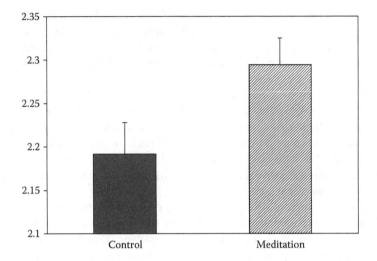

FIGURE 17.3 Log transformed antibody rise from 3–5 weeks to 8–9 weeks post-vaccination for flu virus in meditation versus control group. (Adapted from Davidson et al. 2003. *Psychosom Med* 65:564–570, Figure 5.)

Test. The MBSR training resulted in a significantly smaller post-stress inflammatory response compared to HEP training. They conclude that interventions, like meditation, which reduce emotional reactivity, may be helpful in controlling chronic inflammatory conditions.

A recent meta-analysis of studies on the effects of meditation on immune function reviewed 20 RCTs totaling 1602 participants (Black and Slavich 2016). From examining the results of the 20 studies, the authors concluded that mindfulness meditation appears to be associated with decreases in proinflammatory processes, increases in cell-mediated defense parameters, and increases in the telomerase enzyme activity that guards against cell aging.

Does meditation help oppose the negative effects of cancer and auto-immune diseases? A study examining the effects of MBSR on quality of life and immune system parameters in breast and prostate cancer patients found significant improvements in quality of life and symptoms of stress, as well as an increase in T cell production of IL-4, and a decrease in IFN-gamma, as well as a reduction in the production of IL-10 by natural killer (NK) cells, used by the body in counteracting disease (Carlson et al. 2003). Interestingly, the immune system profile also shifted from one associated with depression to one that was more normal. The authors conclude that this was the first paper to show changes in cancer-related cytokine production associated with MBSR.

In addition, a review of studies on the effect of mind–body medicine on the auto-immune disease of multiple sclerosis (MS) found high quality trials (yoga, mindfulness, relaxation, and biofeedback) which were helpful for a variety of MS symptoms, including quality of life, fatigue, depression and anxiety. Some of the studies also found improvements in both balance and in pain intensity (Senders et al. 2012). Finally, a study on the effect of meditation and yoga (8 wk intervention) on inflammatory bowel disease, including Crohn's disease, also found improvements in arthralgia and intestinal colic pain, as well as state and trait anxiety (Sharma et al. 2015).

Gene Expression

The exploration of changes in gene expression through mindfulness-based therapies is just in its infancy. However, recent reviews of the literature have noted that training in MBSR was associated with reduced oxidative stress, DNA damage, and cytokine secretion, and increased natural killer cell activity (Carlson et al. 2003; Kaliman et al. 2014). Studies have also shown that the expression of genes related to cellular metabolism and oxidative stress pathways in blood cells is positively affected by mind–body therapies (Dusek et al. 2008; Bhasin et al. 2013).

In one of these studies, Dusek and colleagues (2008) asked whether differences in gene expression may be an underlying factor in the physiological and psychological changes associated with meditation training. They examined both long-term meditators as well as control subjects. They found that there were significant differences in the gene expression profiles among individuals with a long-term meditation practice compared to controls. They also noted that when the control group was given 8 weeks of meditation practice, there were significant changes within the gene expression profiles of these individuals over the 8-week period. Using gene ontology and gene set enrichment analyses, the authors found significant alterations in cellular metabolism, oxidative phosphorylation, generation of reactive oxygen species, and response to oxidative stress in both the long-term meditators and the group of individuals given an 8-week meditation training. This suggests that these modifications may counteract cellular damage related to chronic psychological stress.

In a further study, the authors (Bhasin et al. 2013) explored whether there were acute changes in gene expression of short- or long-term meditators within one session of meditation practice. A control group of nonmeditators was used as a comparison. Blood samples were collected at three different time points, as participants listened to a meditation CD (or a health-related CD in controls). Results showed that within a single meditation session both short- and long-term meditators showed significant gene expression changes, with greater changes being seen for long-term meditators. A single meditation session increased expression of genes related to telomere maintenance, energy metabolism, mitochondrial function, and insulin secretion and decreased expression of genes related to stress-related pathways and the inflammatory response. All of these changes are associated with increased well-being and health.

A similar study by Kaliman et al. (2014) found that experienced meditators show a rapid reduction in the expression of pro-inflammatory genes at the end of an intensive day of meditation practice. Lower levels of these genes also predicted a better recovery from a social stress test, which was given before and after the meditation session. In comparison to a control group (engaged in leisure activities during the day), the meditators showed greater reductions in the inflammatory gene expression and better cortisol recovery. This suggests that meditation promotes anti-inflammatory processes that contribute to healthy resilience in response to the stresses and challenges of life. These studies provide strong preliminary evidence to suggest that meditation has a profound influence on gene expression; while effects are apparent after even a single session, long-term meditation practice gives more profound and enduring effects.

SUMMARY

In summary, the research evidence regarding the effects of meditation on cardiovascular, neurophysiological, and immune function, and the control of chronic diseases associated with these systems is positive. Studies show improvements in symptoms associated with many disorders, including cardiovascular disease, ADHD, depression, and auto-immune diseases, with many studies showing medium effect-sizes, comparable to more conventional management, such as pharmaceutical therapies. New data suggest that meditation improves immune function through altering expression of genes related to stress pathways, inflammatory responses, mitochondrial function, and energy metabolism.

How do mind–body therapies promote these positive changes in health? Evidence suggests that the mental training associated with meditation affects, in a top-down manner, the neural and endocrine pathways related to stress reduction, and positive emotional and attentional regulation. The number of carefully designed studies and positive results give substantial evidence supporting the use of these mind–body therapies in the healthcare setting. As mind–body therapies are low in cost and can often be implemented in the home environment after an initial training period they are both a useful and cost-effective set of therapies than can be used to complement other medical treatments. The question remains, given the strong supporting evidence, "Why aren't mind–body therapies more frequently recommended by healthcare professionals?" An important research priority is the exploration of the barriers to the implementation of complementary medical practices.

REFERENCES

Bai, Z., J. Chang, C. Chen, P. Li, K. Yang, and I. Chi. 2015. Investigating the effect of transcendental meditation on blood pressure: A systematic review and meta-analysis. *J Hum Hypertens* 29:653–662.

Benson, H. 1976. *The Relaxation Response*. New York: Avon Books.

Bhasin, M.K., J.A. Dusek, B.H. Chang et al. 2013. Relaxation response induces temporal transcriptome changes in energy metabolism, insulin secretion and inflammatory pathways. *PLoS One* 8:e62817.

Black, D.S. and G. M. Slavich. 2016. Mindfulness meditation and the immune system: A systematic review of randomized controlled trials. *Ann N Y Acad Sci* 1373:13–24.

Bohlmeijer, E., R. Prenger, E. Taal, and P. Cuijpers. 2010. The effects of mindfulness-based stress reduction therapy on mental health of adults with a chronic medical disease; a meta-analysis. *J Psychosom Res* 68:539–544.

Carlson, L.E., M. Speca, K.D. Patel, and E. Goodey 2003. Mindfulness-based stress reduction in relation to quality of life, mood, symptoms of stress, and immune parameters in breast and prostate cancer outpatients. *Psychosom Med* 65:571–581.

Chobanian, A.V., G.L. Bakris, H.R. Black et al. 2003. The seventh report of the joint national committee on prevention, detection, evaluation, and treatment of high blood pressure: The JNC VII report. *JAMA* 289:2560–2572.

Curiati, J.A., E. Bocchi, J.O. Freire et al. 2005. Meditation reduces sympathetic activation and improves the quality of life in elderly patients with optimally treated heart failure: A prospective randomized study. *J Altern Complement Med* 11:465–472.

Davidson, R.J., J. Kabat-Zinn, J. Schumacher et al. 2003. Alterations in brain and immune function produced by mindfulness meditation. *Psychosom Med* 65:564–570.

Delui, M.H., M. Yari, G. Khouyinezhad, M. Amini, and J. H. Bayazi. 2013. Comparison of cardiac rehabilitation programs combines with relaxation and meditation techniques on reduction of depression and anxiety of cardiovascular patients. *Open Cardiovasc Med J* 7:99–103.

Dusek, J.A., H. H. Otu, A.L. Wohlhueter et al. 2008. Genomic counter-stress changes induced by the relaxation response. *PLoS One* 3:e2576.

Feuerstein, G. 1989. *The Yoga-Sutra of Patanjali*. Rochester, VT: Inner Traditions, International.

Fjell, A.M., K.B. Walhovd, T.T. Brown et al. 2012. Multimodal imaging of the self-regulating developing brain. *Proc Natl Acad Sci U S A* 109:19620–19625.

Gerson, L.P. 1996. *The Cambridge Companion to Plotinus*. Cambridge: Cambridge University Press.

Godfrin, K.A. and C. van Heeringen 2010. The effects of mindfulness-based cognitive therapy on recurrence of depressive episodes, mental health and quality of life: A randomized controlled study. *Behav Res Ther* 48:738–746.

Goyal, M., S. Singh, E.M. Sibinga et al. 2014. Meditation programs for psychological stress and well-being: A systematic review and meta-analysis. *JAMA Intern Med* 174:357–368.

Grant, J.A., J. Courtemanche, E.G. Duerden, G. H. Duncan, and P. Rainville. 2010. Cortical thickness and pain sensitivity in Zen meditators. *Emotion* 10:43–53.

Grant, J.A., E.G. Duerden, J. Courtemanche, M. Cherkasova, G.H. Duncan, and P. Rainville. 2013. Cortical thickness, mental absorption and meditative practice: Possible implications for disorders of attention. *Biol Psychol* 92:275–281.

Grossman, P., L. Niemann, S. Schmidt and H. Walach. 2004. Mindfulness-based stress reduction and health benefits. A meta-analysis. *J Psychosom Res* 57:35–43.

Hammerman, O., D. Mostofsky, Y. Louria, G. Ifergane, and Y. Ezra. 2016. "Tested, but not tried"—why is behavioral medicine rarely implemented in clinical practice? [Article in Hebrew]. *Harefuah* 155:119–123, 130.

Hawkes, T.D., W. Manselle, M.H. Woollacott. 2014. Tai Chi and meditation-plus-exercise benefit neural substrates of executive function: A cross-sectional, controlled study. *J Complement Integr Med* 11:279–288.

Hepark, S., L. Janssen, A. de Vries et al. 2015. The efficacy of adapted MBCT on core symptoms and executive functioning in adults With ADHD: A preliminary randomized controlled trial. *J Atten Disord* pii: 1087054715613587. [Epub ahead of print].

Hofmann, S.G., A.T. Sawyer, A.A. Witt and D. Oh. 2010. The effect of mindfulness-based therapy on anxiety and depression: A meta-analytic review. *J Consult Clin Psychol* 78:169–183.

Hughes, J.W., D.M. Fresco, R. Myerscough, M.H. van Dulmen, L.E. Carlson, and R. Josephson. 2013. Randomized controlled trial of mindfulness-based stress reduction for prehypertension. *Psychosom Med* 75:721–728.

Kabat-Zinn J. 1982. An outpatient program in behavioral medicine for chronic pain patients based on the practice of mindfulness meditation; Theoretical considerations and preliminary results. *Gen Hosp Psychiatry* 4:33–47.

Kabat-Zinn J. 1990. *Full Catastrophe Living: Using the Wisdom of Your body and Mind to Face Stress, Pain, and Illness.* New York, NY: Random House.

Kaliman, P., M.J. Alvarez-López, M. Cosín-Tomás, M.A. Rosenkranz, A. Lutz, and R.J. Davidson. 2014. Rapid changes in histone deacetylases and inflammatory gene expression in expert meditators. *Psychoneuroendocrinology* 40:96–107.

Khoury, B., T. Lecomte, G. Fortin et al. 2013. Mindfulness-based therapy: A comprehensive meta-analysis. *Clin Psychol Rev* 33:763–771.

Lazar, S.W., C.E. Kerr, R.H. Wasserman et al. 2005. Meditation experience is associated with increased cortical thickness. *Neuroreport* 16:1893–1897.

Lozano, R., M. Naghavi, K. Foreman et al. 2012. Global and regional mortality from 235 causes of death for 20 age groups in 1990 and 2010: A systematic analysis for the Global Burden of Disease Study 2010. *Lancet* 380:2095–2128.

Lutz, A., H.A. Slagter, J.D. Dunne, and R.J. Davidson. 2008. Attention regulation and monitoring in meditation. *Trends Cogn Sci* 12:163–169.

Lutz, J., A.B. Brühl, N. Doerig et al. 2016. Altered processing of self-related emotional stimuli in mindfulness meditators. *Neuroimage* 124:958–967.

McCracken L.M. and M. Thompson. 2009. Components of mindfullness in patients with chronic pain. *J Psychopathoi Behav Assess* 31:75–82.

Medical-dictionary.thefreedictionary.com/meditation (accessed August 10, 2016).

O'Reilly, G.A., L. Cook, D. Spruijt-Metz, and D.S. Black. 2014. Mindfulness-based interventions for obesity-related eating behaviours: A literature review. *Obes Rev* 15:453–461.

Ospina, M.B., K. Bond, M. Karkhaneh et al. 2007. Meditation practices for health: State of the research. *Evid Rep Technol Assess (Full Rep)* June (155):1–263.

Rainforth, M.V., R.H. Schneider, S.I. Nidich, C. Gaylord-King, J.W. Salerno, and J.W. Anderson. 2007. Stress reduction programs in patients with elevated blood pressure: A systematic review and meta-analysis. *Curr Hypertens Rep* 9:520–528.

Ray, I.B., A.R. Menezes, P. Malur, A.E. Hiltbold, J.P. Reilly, and C.J. Lavie. 2014. Meditation and coronary heart disease: A review of the current clinical evidence. *The Ochsner Journal* 14:696–703.

Reiner, K., L. Tibi, and J.D. Lipsitz. 2013. Do mindfulness-based interventions reduce pain intensity? A critical review of the literature. *Pain Med* 14:230–242.

Robins, J.L., R.K. Elswick Jr, J. Sturgill, and N.L. McCain. 2015. The effects of Tai Chi on cardiovascular risk in women. *Am J Health Promot* 30:613–622.

Rosenkranz, M.A., R.J. Davidson, D.G. Maccoon, J.F. Sheridan, N.H. Kalin, and A. Lutz. 2013. A comparison of mindfulness-based stress reduction and an active control in modulation of neurogenic inflammation. *Brain Behav Immun* 27:174–184.

Rozanski, A., J.A. Blumenthal, and J. Kaplan. 1999. Impact of psychological factors on the pathogenesis of cardiovascular disease and implications for therapy. *Circulation* 99:2192–2217.

Sackett D., S.E. Straus, W. Richardson et al. 2000. *Evidence-Based Practice: How to Practice and Teach EBM.* 2nd Ed. Thousand Oaks, CA: Sage Publications.

Schneider, R.H., C.N. Alexander, F. Staggers et al. 2005. Long-term effects of stress reduction on mortality in persons >55 years of age with systemic hypertension. *Am J Cardiol* 295:1060–1064.

Schwartz, B.G., W.J. French, G.S. Mayeda et al. 2012. Emotional stressors trigger cardiovascular events. *Int J Clin Pract* 66:631–639.

Senders, A., H. Wahbeh, R. Spain, and L. Shinto. Mind-body medicine for multiple sclerosis: A systematic review. *Autoimmune Dis* 2012:567324.

Sharma, P., G. Poojary, D.M. Vélez, S.N. Dwivedi, and K.K. Deepak. 2015. Effect of Yoga-Based Intervention in Patients with Inflammatory Bowel Disease. *Int J Yoga Therap* 225:101–112.

Shaw, P., J. Lerch, D. Greenstein et al. 2006. Longitudinal mapping of cortical thickness and clinical outcome in children and adolescents with attention-deficit/hyperactivity disorder. *Archives of General Psychiatry* 63:540–549.

Sheldon, T.A., G.H. Guyatt, and A. Haines. 1998. When to act on the evidence. *British Med J* 317(7151):139–142.

Sheng, Z.S. and X.H. Su. 2000. The effect of Tai Chi Qigong form 18 on hypertension. *Modern Rehabil* 4:33–34.

Steptoe, A. and M. Kivimaki. 2012. Stress and cardiovascular disease. *Nat Rev Cardiol* 9:360–370.

Tang, Y.Y., B.K. Hölzel, and M.I. Posner. 2015. The neuroscience of mindfulness meditation. *Nat Rev Neurosci* 16:213–225.

Tang, Y.Y., Y. Ma, J. Wang et al. 2007. Short-term meditation training improves attention and self-regulation. *Proc Natl Acad Sci U S A* 104:17152–17156.

Thomas, G.N., A.W.L. Hong, B. Tomlinson et al. 2005. Effects of tai chi and resistance training on cardiovascular risk factors in elderly Chinese subjects: A 12-month longitudinal, randomized, controlled, intervention study. *Clin Endocrinol* 63:663–669.

Thurston, R.C., M. Rewak, and L.D. Kubzansky. 2013. An anxious heart: Anxiety and the onset of cardiovascular diseases. *Prog Cardiovasc Dis* 55:524–537.

Tsai, J.C., W.H. Wang, P. Chan et al. 2003. The beneficial effects of Tai Chi Chuan on blood pressure and lipid profile and anxiety status in a randomized controlled trial. *J Altern Complement Med* 9:747–754.

Wells, R.E., G.Y. Yeh, C.E. Kerr et al. 2013. Meditation's impact on default mode network and hippocampus in mild cognitive impairment: A pilot study. *Neurosci Lett* 556:15–19.

World Health Organization. 2010. *Global status report on non-communicable diseases 2010*, http://whqlibdoc.who.int/ publications/2011/9789240686458_eng.pdf (2011, accessed July 31, 2013).

Yeh, G.Y., C. Wang, P.M. Wayne, and R. Phillips. 2009. Tai chi exercise for patients with cardiovascular conditions and risk factors: A systematic review. *J Cardiopulm Rehabil Prev* 29:152–160.

Young, D.R., L.J. Appel, and S.H. Lee. 1999. The effects of aerobic exercise and T'ai Chi on blood pressure in older people: Results of a randomized trial. *J Am Geriatr Soc* 47:277–284.

Younge, J.O., R.A. Gotink, C.P. Baena, J.W. Roos-Hesselink, and M.G. Hunink. 2015a. Mind-body practices for patients with cardiac disease: A systematic review and meta-analysis. *Eur J Prev Cardiol* 22:1385–1398.

Younge, J.O., M.J. Leening, H. Tiemeier et al. 2015b. Association Between mind-body practice and cardiometabolic risk factors: The Rotterdam Study. *Psychosom Med* 77:775–783.

Zeidan, F., S.K. Johnson, N.S. Godon, and P. Goolkasian. 2010. Effects of brief and sham mindfulness meditation on mood and cardiovascular variables. *J Altern Complement Med* 16:867–873.

18 The Fourth Phase of Water
Implications for Energy, Life, and Health

Gerald H. Pollack

CONTENTS

Does Water Transduce Energy? 440
Applications in Natural Science...441
Practical Applications 442
Applications in Medical Science 443
Water and Healing...444
Negative Charge and Antioxidants...445
Information in Water? 445
The Future...446
References..447

Can drinking water supply energy? Is water merely another kind of food? How does water relate to health?

Answering these and related questions requires an understanding of the nature of water. Many presume that water must be completely understood, given its simplicity and pervasiveness through nature, but in fact precious little has been known about how water molecules organize themselves and interact with one another—until recently.

Students learn that water has three phases: solid, liquid, and vapor. But there is something more: in our laboratory at the University of Washington we have uncovered a *fourth* phase. This phase occurs next to water-loving (hydrophilic) surfaces. It is surprisingly extensive, projecting out from surfaces by up to millions of molecular layers. And it exists almost everywhere throughout nature, including your body. In fact, it fills your cells.

This newly identified phase of water has been described in *The Fourth Phase of Water: Beyond Solid, Liquid, and Vapor* (Pollack 2013). The book documents the basic findings and presents many applications beyond the ones mentioned above. It also deals with water's well-recognized anomalies, turning those anomalies into easily explained features.

The existence of a fourth phase may seem unexpected. However, it should not be entirely so: a century ago, the physical chemist Sir William Hardy argued for the existence of a fourth phase, and many authors over the years have found evidence for some kind of "ordered" or "structured" phase of water. Fresh experimental evidence not only confirms the existence of such an ordered, liquid-crystalline phase, but also details its properties. It is more viscous, dense, and alkaline than H_2O and has relatively more oxygen since its formula is H_3O_2. As a result, it has a negative charge and, like a battery, can hold energy as well as deliver that energy when needed. These properties explain everyday observations and answer questions ranging from why gelatin desserts hold their water to why teapots whistle.

The presence of the fourth phase carries many implications. Here, I will outline some basic features of this phase, and then deal with several of those implications including energetic aspects. We obtain energy from food; however, we can also get energy from water. I will touch briefly on atmospheric science implications because everyone has interest in the weather, and then focus on some biological and health applications.

DOES WATER TRANSDUCE ENERGY?

The energy for building water structure comes from the sun. Radiant energy converts ordinary bulk water into ordered water, building this ordered zone. We found that all wavelengths ranging from ultraviolet, through visible, to infrared can build this ordered water. Near-infrared energy is the most capable. Water absorbs infrared energy freely from the environment; it uses that energy to convert bulk water into liquid-crystalline water (fourth phase water)—which we also call "exclusion zone" or "EZ" water because it profoundly excludes solutes. Hence, buildup of EZ water occurs naturally and spontaneously from environmental energy. Additional energy input creates additional EZ buildup.

Of particular significance is the fourth phase's charge: commonly negative (Figure 18.1). Absorbed radiant energy splits water molecules; the negative moiety constitutes the building block of the EZ, while the positive moiety binds with water molecules to form free hydronium ions, which spread diffusely throughout the water. Adding additional light (radiant energy) stimulates more charge separation.

This process resembles the first step of photosynthesis. In that step, energy from the sun splits water molecules. Hydrophilic chromophores catalyze that splitting. The process considered here is similar but more generic: any hydrophilic surface may catalyze the splitting of water. Some surfaces work more effectively than others.

The separated charges resemble a battery. That battery can deliver energy in a manner similar to the way the separated charges in plants deliver energy. Plants, of course, comprise mostly water, and it is therefore no surprise that similar energy conversion takes place in water itself.

The stored electrical energy in water can drive various kinds of work, including flow. An example is the axial flow through tubes. We found that immersing tubes made of hydrophilic materials into water produces flow through those tubes, similar to blood flow through blood vessels (Figure 18.2).

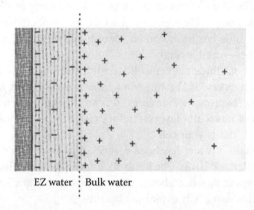

EZ water ⋮ Bulk water

FIGURE 18.1 Diagrammatic representation of EZ water, negatively charged, and the positively charged bulk water beyond. Hydrophilic surface at left.

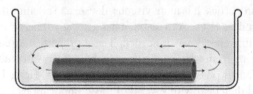

FIGURE 18.2 Practically incessant flow occurs through hydrophilic tubes immersed in water.

The driving energy comes from the radiant energy absorbed and stored in the water. Nothing more. Flow may persist undiminished for many hours, even days. Additional incident light brings faster flow. This is not a perpetual motion machine: incident radiant energy drives the flow—in much the same way that it drives vascular flow in plants and powers water from the roots to nourish trees taller than the length of a football field.

APPLICATIONS IN NATURAL SCIENCE

The water-based energy conversion framework is rich with implication for many systems involving water. These systems may range from biology and chemistry all the way to atmospheric science and engineering. The fourth phase appears nearly everywhere: all that's needed is water, radiant energy, and a hydrophilic surface. The latter can be as large as a slab of polymer or as small as a dissolved molecule. The liquid-crystalline phase inevitably builds—and its presence plays some integral role in the system's behavior.

Let me provide a few representative examples.

One example is...you. By volume, two thirds of your cells' content is water. However, the water molecule is so small that making up that two-thirds volume requires 99% of all your molecules. Modern cell biology considers that 99% molecular fraction as mere background carriers of the "important" molecules of life such as proteins and nucleic acids. Conventional wisdom asserts that 99% of your molecules don't do very much.

However, EZ water envelops every macromolecule in the cell. Those macromolecules are so tightly packed that the EZ water largely fills your cells. In other words, most of your cell water is EZ water. This water plays a central role in everything the cell does—as elaborated in my earlier book, *Cells, Gels and the Engines of Life* (Pollack 2001).

What's new is the role of radiant energy: incident radiant energy powers many of those cellular functions. An example is the blood flowing through your capillaries. That blood eventually encounters high resistance: capillaries are often narrower than the red blood cells that must pass through them; in order to make their way through, those red cells need to contort. Resistance is high. You'd anticipate the need for lots of driving pressure, yet the pressure gradient across the capillary bed is negligible. The paradox resolves if radiant energy helps propel flow through capillaries in the same way that it propels flow through hydrophilic tubes. Radiant energy may constitute an unsuspected source of vascular drive, supplementing cardiac pressure.

Why you feel good after a sauna now seems understandable. If radiant energy drives capillary flow and ample capillary flow is important for optimal functioning, then sitting in the sauna will inevitably be a feel-good experience. The infrared energy associated with heat should help drive that flow. The same if you walk out into sunlight: we presume that the feel-good experience derives purely from the psychological realm, but the evidence above implies that sunlight may build your body's EZs. Fully built EZs around each protein seem necessary for optimal cellular functioning.

A second example of the EZ's central role is weather. Common understanding of weather derives from two principal variables: temperature and pressure. Those two variables are said to explain virtually everything we experience in terms of weather. However, the atmosphere also contains water—micrometer-scale droplets commonly known as aerosol droplets or aerosol particles. Those droplets make up atmospheric humidity. When the atmosphere is humid, the many droplets scatter considerable light, conferring haze; you can't see clearly through that haze. When the atmosphere contains only a few droplets, you may see clearly, over long distances.

The Fourth Phase book presents evidence for the structure of those droplets. It shows that EZ water envelops each droplet, while hydronium ions occupy the droplets' interiors. Repelling one another, those hydronium ions create pressure, which pushes against the robust shell of EZ water. That pressure explains why droplets tend toward roundness.

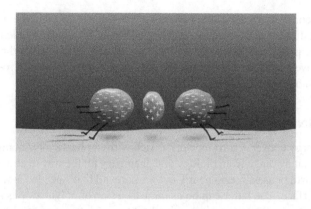

FIGURE 18.3   Like-charged entities attract because of an intermediate of opposite charge.

How do those aerosol droplets condense to form clouds? The droplets' EZ shells bear negative charge. Negatively charged droplets should repel one another, precluding any condensation into clouds. Those like-charged aerosol droplets should remain widely dispersed throughout the atmosphere. However, droplets *do* condense into clouds, and the question is how that can happen.

The reason they condense is because of the unlike charges that lie in between the droplets. Richard Feynman, the legendary Nobel Prize physicist of the late twentieth century, understood the principle, opining: "like-likes-like because of an intermediate of unlikes." The like-charged droplets "like" one another, so they come together; the unlike charges lying in between those droplets constitute the attractors (Figure 18.3).

The like-likes-like principle has been widely appreciated, but also widely ignored: after all, how could like charges conceivably *attract*? A reason why this powerfully simple concept has been ignored is that the source of the unlike charges has been difficult to identify. We now know that the unlike charges can come from the splitting of water—the negative components building EZ shells, while the corresponding positive components provide the unlike attractors. With enough of those attractors, the negatively charged aerosol droplets may condense into clouds.

These two phenomena, radiant energy-induced biological function and like-likes-like cloud formation, provide examples of how water's energy can account for phenomena not otherwise explained. The fourth phase is the key building block that allows for construction of an edifice of understanding.

PRACTICAL APPLICATIONS

Beyond scientific, the discovery of the fourth phase has practical applications. They include flow production (already mentioned), electrical energy harvesting, and even filtration. I briefly mention the latter two applications.

Filtration occurs naturally because the liquid-crystalline phase massively excludes solutes and particles in much the same way as does ice. Accordingly, fourth phase water is essentially solute free. Collecting it provides solute-free and bacteria-free water. A patented working prototype has confirmed this expectation. Purification by this method requires no physical filter: the fourth phase itself does the separation, and the energy comes from the sun.

Energy harvesting seems straightforward: light drives the separation of charge, and those separated charges constitute a battery. Harvesting electrical energy should be realizable with proper electrodes. This (patented) technology development has the potential to replace standard photovoltaic systems with simpler ones based on water. More detail on these practical applications can be found on the Pollack laboratory homepage: http://faculty.washington.edu/ghp/.

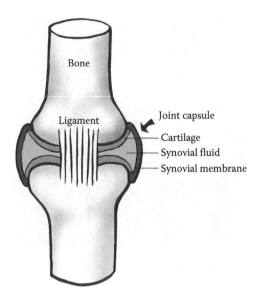

FIGURE 18.4 Enveloping the joint, the capsule ensures that the fluid's hydronium ions don't disperse. The concentrated hydronium ions repel, keeping surfaces apart and ensuring low friction.

APPLICATIONS IN MEDICAL SCIENCE

Practical applications also exist within our bodies, and I present two of them: why your joints don't squeak and why dislocated or sprained joints will swell *within seconds*.

Joints are sites at which bones press upon one another (Figure 18.4). The bones may also rotate, as during deep-knee bends and push-ups. You'd think that rotation under pressure might elicit squeaky frictional resistance, but joint friction remains remarkably modest. Why so?

The ends of bones are lined with cartilage. Those cartilaginous materials do the actual pressing. Hence, the issue of joint friction reduces to the issue of the cartilaginous surfaces and the synovial fluid lying in between. How does this system behave under pressure?

Cartilage is made of classic gel materials: highly charged polymers and water; therefore, cartilage is a gel. Gel surfaces bear EZs, so cartilage surfaces should likewise bear EZs. The splitting of water associated with EZ buildup creates many hydronium ions in the synovial fluid in between. Additional hydronium ions come from the molecules within that fluid, creating their own EZs and protons. Thus, many hydronium ions will lie in the area where two cartilaginous surfaces lie across from one another. The repulsive force coming from those hydronium ions should keep the cartilage surfaces apart—some investigators maintain that the cartilage surfaces never touch, even under heavy loads. That separation means that any rough spots, or asperities, will never come into contact with one another as the respective surfaces shear past one another, and that in turn means low friction.

For such a mechanism to actually work, some kind of built-in restraint should be present to keep the repelling hydronium ions in place. Otherwise, those hydronium ions may be forced out of the local region, thereby compromising lubrication. Nature provides that safety net: a structure known as the joint capsule envelops the joint. By constraining the dispersal of hydronium ions, that encapsulation ensures low friction. That's why your joints don't ordinarily squeak.

Regarding swelling, the second issue under consideration here, osmosis evidently plays a role. Since the cell is packed with negatively charged proteins, the cytoplasm should generate an osmotic draw similar to the osmotic draw generated by diapers or gels. Physiologists know that it does.

A peculiar feature of cells, however, is their relatively modest water content. Compared to 20:1 or higher for many common gels, the cell's water-to-solids ratio is only about 2:1. The many negatively charged macromolecules of the cell should generate a strong osmotic draw; yet the water content in

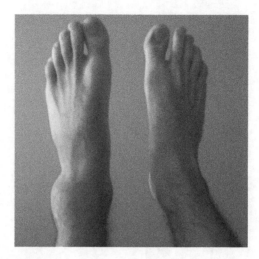

FIGURE 18.5 Example of post-injury swelling.

the cell remains surprisingly low. That limited water content may come because of the macromolecular network's stiffness: cellular networks typically comprise tubular or multi-stranded biopolymers tightly cross-linked to one another. The resultant stiffness prevents the network from expanding to its full osmotic potential.

If those cross-links were to disrupt, however, then the full power of osmotic draw would take effect; the tissue could then build many EZ layers and therefore hydrate massively, bringing huge expansion (Figure 18.5). That's what happens when body tissues are injured, especially with dislocations. The injury disrupts fibrous macromolecules and cross-links, eliminating the restraining forces that keep osmosis at bay; EZ buildup can then proceed virtually unimpeded.

The reason why swelling can be so impressive is that the cross-link disruption occurs progressively. Breaking one cross-link results in higher stress on neighboring cross-links, so disruption progresses in a zipper-like fashion. When that happens, the osmotic rush of water into the tissue can continue practically without restraint, resulting in the enormous immediate swelling that is often seen. The tissue will return to normal only when cross-links repair and the matrix returns to its normally restraining configuration.

WATER AND HEALING

During childhood illness, grandmothers and doctors will often advise: "drink more water." In his now-classical book, titled *Your Body's Many Cries for Water: You Are Not Sick, You Are Thirsty* (Batmanghelidj 1997), the Iranian physician Fereydoon Batmanghelidj confirms the wisdom of this quaint advice. The author documents years of clinical practice showing reversal of diverse pathologies simply by drinking more water. Hydration is critical.

Batmanghelidj's experience meshes with evidence of healing from special waters such as those from the Ganges and Lourdes. Those waters most often come from deep underground springs or from glacial melt. Spring waters experience pressure from above; pressure converts liquid water into EZ water because of EZ water's higher density. EZ water differs from bulk water in that it absorbs light in the UV region of 270 nanometers on spectrometry. The more light in this sector that is absorbed, the higher the concentration of EZ water in the sample. Specimens from the above and certain spring waters show a peak in this 270-nanometer zone, suggesting that relatively high EZ concentrations could contribute to their therapeutic benefits.

The same for mountain water: it too should have high EZ content. Our studies have shown that ice formation requires an EZ intermediate. That is, bulk water does not convert directly to ice; it converts to EZ, which then converts to ice. Similarly for melting, melting ice forms EZ, which subsequently converts to bulk water. Fresh ice melt contains abundant EZ water.

For spring water and fresh ice melt, then, the high EZ content may explain the recognized health benefits. EZ water should rehydrate tissues better than ordinary water because of its higher dipole moment. To appreciate this argument, picture a bean with positive charge localized at one end, negative at the other. The positive end of that dipole orients toward the negatively charged cell, which then strongly draws in that dipole. The larger the dipole, the stronger will be the draw. Since EZs contain masses of separated charges, or large dipoles, EZ water should hydrate cells better than ordinary water. That's why EZ water may particularly promote good health.

NEGATIVE CHARGE AND ANTIOXIDANTS

Humans are considered neutral, but I suggest that we bear net negative charge.

Physical chemists reasonably presume that all systems tend toward neutrality because positive charge attracts negative charge. The human body being one of those "systems," we assume that the body must be neutral.

Not all systems are neutral, however. The earth bears net negative charge, while the atmosphere bears net positive charge. Water itself can bear charge: Anyone watching MIT professor Walter Lewin's stunning demonstration of the Kelvin water dropper, http://www.youtube.com/watch?v=oYleyLEo8_A&feature=related, where separated bodies of water eventually discharge onto one another, will immediately see that bodies of water *can* bear net charge. If any doubt remains, then the experience of getting an electric shock from touching certain kinds of drinking water (which my colleagues and I have personally experienced) should eliminate that doubt.

Charges can remain separated if input energy keeps them separated—something like recharging your cell phone battery and creating separated negative and positive terminals. Since we constantly absorb external energy from the environment, the theoretical possibility exists that we may bear net charge.

Consider the arithmetic. Cells make up some 60% of your body's mass, and they are negatively charged. Extracellular tissues such as collagen and elastin are next in line, and those proteins bear negative charge and adsorb negatively charged EZ water. Only some of the smaller compartments are positively charged with protons (low pH), and they commonly *expel*: urine, gastrointestinal system, sweat, and expired air (containing hydrated CO_2 or carbonic acid). They help *rid* the body of positive charge.

So, the arithmetic shows not only that our body bears net negative charge, but also that the body makes every effort to maintain that negativity by ridding itself of protons. It is as though maintaining negativity is a "goal" of life. Plants do it easily: they connect directly to the negatively charged earth; animals need to struggle a bit more to maintain their body's charge, in exchange for greater mobility.

How does our body's negative charge relate to the benefits of antioxidants?

Answering this question returns us to basic chemistry. Recall that "reduction" is the *gain* of electrons, while "oxidation" means electron *loss*. Oxidation strips molecules of their negative charge, working against the body's attempt to maintain high negativity. To guard against that loss we employ *anti*oxidants. Antioxidants may keep us healthy simply by maintaining proper negativity.

INFORMATION IN WATER?

The question of the "memory of water" first became widely known from the studies of the late Jacques Benveniste, once a world-class French immunologist. In mid-career, Benveniste inadvertently turned from orthodoxy to controversy. He had been studying basophils, a type of white blood cell that secretes histamine when exposed to a particular antibody. Someone in his lab found an odd result: even when that antibody suspension had been diluted so extensively that not even a single antibody molecule could theoretically remain, exposure of that extremely diluted suspension produced the same response as did the original. Pouring what amounted to pure water elicited the same response as pouring the antibody.

Benveniste made the tragic mistake of labeling the phenomenon "water memory." The essentially pure water appeared to have retained "memory" of the molecules with which it had previously had contact; otherwise, how could the water have elicited so specific a response? However, water molecules are known to jitter randomly many times each nanosecond; how possibly could actively dancing molecules retain information? Clearly, they cannot.

Before I recount the Galileo-like saga that befell Benveniste, I should mention that his results have been confirmed in multiple laboratories (Belon et al. 1999). Furthermore, a possible physical-chemical basis for understanding how water could hold information is now evident: it may lie in water's liquid-crystalline fourth phase. The idea of water memory is no longer a scientific joke but, among some groups, a phenomenon ripe for exploration and one that is now being actively pursued.

In 1989, however, water memory was heresy. Benveniste's attempts to publish his lab's findings in the respected journal *Nature* were thwarted multiple times by the editor, Sir John Maddox. Finally, under pressure to publish a collective submission by several groups reporting the same result, Maddox relented. He'd publish the submission under one condition: he'd send a committee of peers to look over the shoulders of those French scientists to see what they were really about. The committee of peers would then report their findings to the readers of *Nature*. Seeing vindication on the horizon, Benveniste accepted Maddox's offer.

Several weeks later the committee arrived in Paris. Not exactly a committee of "peers," the visitors consisted of a threesome: Maddox himself, a journalist with limited experience in biology; Walter Stewart, a professional fraud sleuth from the National Institutes of Health; and "The Amazing Randi," a world-class magician. Randi's fame came partly from his own genius at magic and partly from his ability to uncover the basis of other magicians' tricks.

The committee's makeup sent signals of Maddox's intent. Since "water memory" seemed nigh unto impossible, clearly the French were engaging in some kind of duplicity, and what better committee than the one assembled could uncover the nature of their trick?

Although the "trick" was never specifically identified, the committee managed to find what it was looking for and the subsequent report to *Nature*'s readers dubbed water memory a "delusion." The impact was practically instantaneous. Water memory became a scientific joke, and Benveniste became the community's laughing stock—having trouble remembering? Why not drink some of Benveniste's memory water?

Benveniste never recovered. While pressing on with experiments showing that the stored information could be transmitted even over the Internet, he found himself unable to secure funds to support his work. His laboratory soon collapsed. He became demoralized, and finally succumbed following a routine surgical procedure.

Nevertheless, Benveniste opened the field of information storage in water, including the therapeutic use thereof, as championed by Nobelist Luc Montagnier (Montagnier et al. 2009). A possible key to understanding may lie in the fourth phase water, which is liquid crystalline. Crystals are stable. Molecules don't bounce around in the same way as ordinary liquid molecules. Indeed, the ordered array of oxygen molecules resembles the ordered array of molecules in digital memories. In the latter case, molecules may take on either of two states, denoting zero or one. The oxygen molecules of water can do even better—theoretically assuming any of the five possible oxidation states, from negative two all the way to positive two. Hence the capacity of the water memory mechanism may be superior to that of the standard digital memory.

It remains to be seen whether the water memory phenomenon will assume a dominant role in medical therapy and diagnosis, or will be rejected by a community that has already decided that the phenomenon cannot be true and is therefore unworthy of exploration.

THE FUTURE

Water's centrality for health is nothing new, but it has been progressively forgotten. With the various sciences laying emphasis on molecular, atomic, and even sub-atomic approaches, we have lost sight of what happens when the pieces come together to form the larger entity. The whole may indeed exceed the sum of its parts. About 99% of those parts are water molecules. To think that 99% of our molecules merely bathe the "more important" molecules of life ignores centuries of evidence to the contrary. Water plays a central role in all features of life.

Until recently, the understanding of water's properties has been constrained by the common misconception that water has three phases. We now know it has four. Considering this fourth phase allows many of water's "anomalies" to vanish: those anomalies turn into predictable features. Water becomes more understandable, and so do entities made largely of water, such as oceans, clouds, and, indeed, human beings.

Various hour-long talks describe these fresh understandings. One of them is a University of Washington public award lecture, http://www.youtube.com/watch?v=XVBEwn6iWOo. Another was delivered more recently, http://www.youtube.com/watch?v=JnGCMQ8TJ_g&list=PLwOA YhBuU3Ufr53AnJv9RLousgVN4G_uX&index=8. A third is a recent TEDx talk, http://youtu.be/i-T7tCMUDXU.

A much fuller, well-referenced understanding of these phenomena and more appears in the previously-mentioned book, *The Fourth Phase of Water: Beyond Solid, Liquid, and Vapor* (Pollack 2013), www.ebnerandsons.com.

REFERENCES

Batmanghelidj F. *Your Body's Many Cries for Water: You Are Not Sick, You Are Thirsty. Don't Treat Thirst with Medications.* Falls Church: Global Health Solutions, 1997.

Belon P, Cumps J, Ennis M, Mannaioni, PF. Inhibition of human basophil degranulation by successive histamine dilutions: Results of a European multi-centre trial. *Inflammation Research* 48:S17, 1999.

Montagnier L, Aissa J, Montagnier J-L, Lavallee C. Electromagnetic signals are produced by aqueous nanostructures derived from bacterial DNA sequences. *Interdisciplinary Sciences: Computational Life Sciences* 1:81–90, 2009.

Pollack G. *Cells, Gels and the Engines of Life: A New Unifying Approach to Cell Function.* Seattle, WA: Ebner and Sons, 2001.

Pollack G. *The Fourth Phase of Water: Beyond Solid, Liquid, and Vapor.* Seattle, WA: Ebner and Sons, 2013.

19 Sound Healing, Theory, and Practice

John Beaulieu and David Perez-Martinez

CONTENTS

Introduction 449
Theory 451
Vibration 451
Consciousness 455
Mindful Listening 456
Mantras: Ancient Sound Healing for Modern Times 457
Sound Healing Practice 458
Sound Healing Tools and Instruments 460
    Part I: Psychoacoustics 461
        Music 461
        Voice 461
        Singing Bowls and Gongs 461
        Drums, Rattles, Percussive Instruments 462
        Tuning Forks 462
    Part II: Vibroacoustic Sound Healing 465
Summary 466
Notes 468
Sound Healing Training Programs 468
References 469
Bibliography 470

INTRODUCTION

Sound healing is the practice of using sound and listening in a mindful manner to transform and expand consciousness to enhance the body's natural drive to regenerate and heal itself. The basic premise and theoretical foundation of sound healing is that *all existence is vibratory in nature and, therefore, it is the underlying vibratory field that sustains and imbues everything that exists with structure and form.* The goal of a sound healing practice is to promote high-level wellness through the restoration of balance at all levels of existence. Sound is a perfect tool for healing practices and personal growth because it *mimics the vibratory nature of existence* and affects individuals at all levels: anatomical, physiological, emotional, psychological, and spiritual. It can be integrated into almost any wellness or medical therapy. Used in conjunction with visualization, mindful listening, mantra, and other meditation practices, sound can create spaces for individuals to experience themselves in meditative and hyperconscious states that are conducive to healing.

Sound has been used continuously throughout time and in all cultures as a therapeutic agent in medical and healing practices. Healing with sound and music is recognized in all the traditional natural healing systems, including Oriental, Ayurvedic, Tibetan, and Hermetic medicine. The ancient Rishis of India created mantras as a means of expanding consciousness and obtaining a high-level wellness that they called enlightenment. Based on Pythagorean mathematics, the ancient

Greeks used sonic intervals to positively affect consciousness to stimulate dreams and heal traumas. Shamans of all indigenous traditions have used vocal sounds, whistles, rattles, drums, didgeridoos, flutes, and other kinds of sound-making instruments to enter into altered states of consciousness or spiritual realms in their quest for healing individuals and entire communities. These traditions have in common a universal view of consciousness and healing based on an understanding of sound and vibration.

Modern medical training has unfortunately divorced itself from both sound and healing practices despite its history and value. Modern doctors have become highly specialized and compartmentalized, limited to their particular area of attention and expertise at the expense of the whole. It is our intention to demonstrate how we have brought healing back to the practice of medicine using sound. Healing means to be whole, balanced, and complete—of *sound* mind and body. Healing is not something that happens to us or that is done to us, but rather a manifestation of our nature as living beings. Life seeks to maintain and sustain itself. All living organisms have a way of repairing themselves in their quest for survival and higher states of being. Healing occurs within organisms, vibrationally interacting with their environments. Sound healing practices seek to strengthen the natural drive of living organisms toward wholeness and balance. The ultimate goal is to help both practitioners and clients see themselves as powerful and active agents who are continuously projecting their consciousnesses as co-creators of the reality they experience.

We use the term sound healing in two different yet related ways. As practitioners, we use sound as a therapeutic agent that can be easily integrated into all healing practices. As educators and theorists, we use the vibrational dynamics of sound to illustrate healing principles that are universal to all healing and healing arts practices. It is not by accident that the term healing means "to be of sound mind and body." Because the use of sound or its vibrational dynamics is not ordinarily discussed in medical education, it is necessary to define a few terms to better understand this chapter, as well as to give you the confidence as a healing arts practitioner to be inspired to integrate sound into your practice.

Sound is a perception created in the central nervous system by the effect of pressure waves (vibration) on the auditory system and on the body as a whole. The auditory nerve has a vestibular branch that processes vibration and movement directly from inside and outside the body and a cochlear branch that converts pressure waves in the tympanic membrane into electrical impulses in the brain. These are then experienced as sounds, words, music, and associated emotional and psychological states. This division of the auditory nerve produces what sound healers have referred to as the vibroacoustic (vestibular, vibrational) versus psychoacoustic (cochlear, emotional, psychological) effects of sound.

Music is the appreciation of *organized* sound. Organization and appreciation point to the existence of an underlying consciousness. Music is thus a creation of human consciousness and, therefore, all sounds have the potential to become "music to our ears." It is important to differentiate sound from structured music. Everyone can make and use sound in all aspects of their lives and practices. In contrast, structured music requires years of specialized training and a specific type of listening.

Listening is the act of paying attention to sounds. It is the active, mindful experience of focused awareness of sound that has the potential to transform the act of listening into a harmonious experience with profound biological and psychological effects.

Harmony is the experience of merging with sound and of perceiving a greater relationship with the whole through sound. The Greek root *harmos* refers to the process of joining together objects, people, concepts, and so on, that previously had separate existences. Harmony in this sense is the continual journey to wholeness through a constant joining with the whole.

Healing is the intrinsic drive of all living organisms to repair themselves by reestablishing a natural state of homeostasis, or balance, between constituent parts. "To be healed" means to be balanced, of sound mind and body.

THEORY

The mechanisms of action underlying the usefulness of sound as a healing/therapeutic agent are derived from the nature and manifestations of vibration and consciousness and the effect of that interaction on energy, matter, and living organisms. Vibration has organizational and design properties observed at every level of existence that are manifestations of its ability to alter the physical and chemical properties of atoms (Beaulieu 2018). Human consciousness manifesting as intention alters the behavior of sub-atomic particles with every thought or physical action. Intention is the prime mover in sound healing. It is the state of consciousness that empathetically drives one individual toward compassion, the desire to help and serve others, and another toward the formation of a therapeutic alliance with the former with the intent of being helped. Mindful listening, mantra repetition, and other meditative techniques facilitate the ability to quiet or silence the mind. Silencing the mind allows an expansion of consciousness into hyperconscious states that have been shown in clinical research to produce behavioral, physical, emotional, psychological, and morphological changes in the brain (Chiesa and Serretti 2010).

VIBRATION

Everything in the universe is constantly moving, vibrating, creating vibrations and vibrations within vibrations. Since its creation, matter has been organized and designed into a myriad of forms by underlying *vibrational blueprints* (Lincoln 2013). These blueprints direct matter to configure into specific structural forms by altering the physical and chemical properties of its constitutional elements and hence its *vibratory signature*. Swiss physician Dr. Hans Jenny developed a procedure called *cymatics* to help us intuitively understand vibrational blueprints and how vibration creates structural forms (Jenny 1974). Dr. Jenny performed cymatic experiments by putting substances such as sand, fluid, and powder onto a metal plate attached to an oscillator which had its vibratory rate controlled by a frequency generator. During these experiments, Dr. Jenny could hear and simultaneously see the sound as it created a cymatic form on the vibrating plate. By changing the frequency of the underlying vibratory field in the plate, he was able to observe in real time and to effectively demonstrate the organizing and designing nature of vibration in the creation of the plethora of structural forms observed in nature from the micro to the macrocosm.

Specific vibratory frequencies and amplitudes of sound waves create unique structures that can be precisely recreated each time, as seen in Dr. Jenny's high-speed cymatic photographs.

Each of the following images began as a small pile of sand on a metal plate Figures 19.1 and 19.2.

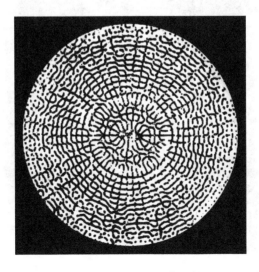

FIGURE 19.1 Hans Jenny's high-speed photograph of sand vibrating on a metal plate.

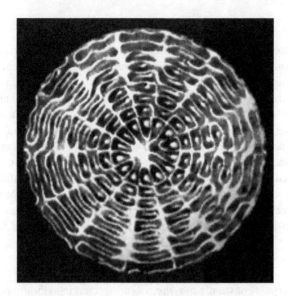

FIGURE 19.2   Hans Jenny's high-speed photograph of sand vibrating on a metal plate.

Each of the following images began as a drop of water on a metal plate Figures 19.3 and 19.4.

When the plate is vibrated to an audible frequency, the sand or water will consistently move into the same geometric pattern based on the frequency. Although the photos appear to have been drawn, the geometric patterns are all created by vibration. If one were to attempt to change or rearrange the geometric pattern without changing the vibrational frequency of the field, the original geometric pattern would always return.

The organizational properties of vibration are exemplified by the fact that cymatically created structures are at times indistinguishable from structures observed in nature at both micro and macro levels of organization (Lauterwasser 2002). For example, there is a numeric sequence called the *Fibonacci number series/frequencies* that is observed in nature as an organizing principle at all levels of organization from the structures of DNA and brain microtubules, the shape of our galaxy and

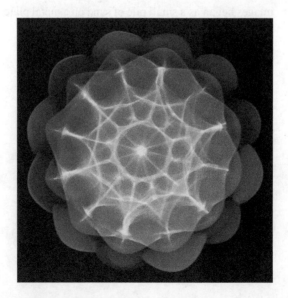

FIGURE 19.3   Hans Jenny's high-speed photograph of water vibrating on a metal plate.

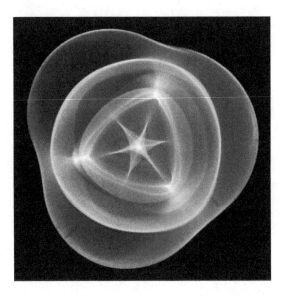

FIGURE 19.4 Hans Jenny's high-speed photograph of water vibrating on a metal plate.

hurricane clouds, breeding patterns of rabbits and bees, to the structure of certain chemical compounds, stock market patterns, and the spacing of leaves in plants and teeth in our mouths. When we look at patterns in nature, human-made architectural designs, and specifically, the geometric design patterns of our body, we tend to disassociate the visual pattern from its vibrational and wave components. It is these very patterns that substantiate the premise that it is the underlying vibratory field which sustains matter and gives it form and structure.

The pictures below are of a church window (Figure 19.5), a top-down view of DNA (Figure 19.6), and a cymatics photograph of water (Figure 19.7).

These three photographs compare similarities between the geometric patterns of a church window (Figure 19.5), a DNA molecule (Figure 19.6), and the high-speed photograph of water vibrating on a metal plate (Figure 19.7).

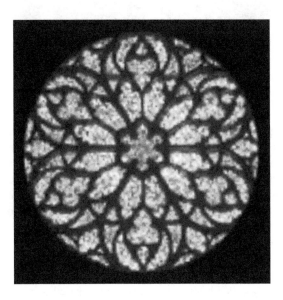

FIGURE 19.5 Stained glass church window.

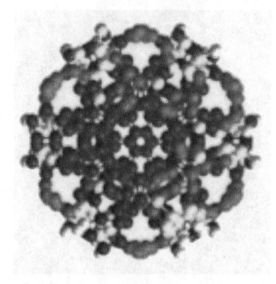

FIGURE 19.6   Top down view of DNA.

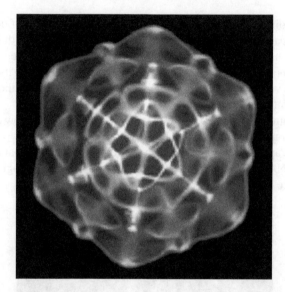

FIGURE 19.7   Cymatics frequency in water.

Another important aspect of vibration that is central to the work of sound healers was discovered by Dutch physicist Christian Huygens in 1665. He observed that autonomously vibrating entities with complementary (resonant) frequencies in close proximity to each other have the tendency to conserve energy by synchronizing their vibratory rates. In his now classic experiment, he observed that clock pendulums in close proximity to each other, initially moving at different rates, always ended up aligning and moving in synchronicity. This inherent tendency observed at all levels of existence in physical and biological systems in close proximity to synchronize their vibratory patterns is called *entrainment,* which is a variant of resonance.

All life is subject to rhythmic cycles and entrainment is, therefore, found everywhere in nature. Every biological activity with periodicity is subject to entrainment. In the brain, the specific vibratory frequencies collectively called brain waves that are measured using an electroencephalogram (EEG), as well as the rhythmic firing of muscle cells in the heart as measured in electrocardiograms

(EKG), are subject to entrainment. In the sound healing process, the ability of vibrations and sound to alter physiological processes, as well as emotional and psychological states in individuals, is called *sonic entrainment*. This is an important part of the mechanism of action underlying the practice of sound healing.

In general, it has been demonstrated that sound and music affect cardiac variability and blood pressure, respiratory rate, pain, and multiple physiological markers that are considered to reflect immunologic functions, and the organism's ability to manage and recuperate from stress, anxiety, and other pathological emotional and physical states. The powerful effect of sound on emotions suggests significant influence over the neural circuitry and chemistry underlying its manifestations. Sound promotes neuroplastic changes in the brain through the formation of new neurons, glial cells, neurological connections, and alterations of existing neural pathways via the process of synapse formation, elimination, dendritic remodeling, and axonal pruning and sprouting (Munte et al. 2002; Kays et al. 2012).

Clinical research has demonstrated that sound and music, which has been more researched, can either increase or decrease blood pressure and heart rate variability, depending also on the state of consciousness of the individual (Iakovides et al. 2004). It can cause peripheral vasodilation, perhaps by stimulating the release of nitric oxide (NO) which is an integral part of the defense against stress and a contributor to psychiatric illness when not properly regulated (Reif et al. 2009; Wass et al. 2009). In 2003, Dr. Beaulieu and collaborators published a peer-reviewed article suggesting that NO provides the physiological pathways through which sound and music operate to create a relaxation response (Beaulieu et al. 2003).[1] Sound also plays a role in the management of stress and anxiety by its ability to increase or decrease both cortisol and norepinephrine (Kreutz 2006; Levitin and Chanda 2013) and by its related ability to decrease arousal due to stress (Pelletier 2004). It affects the immune system by stimulating the production of IgA and NK cells (Kreutz 2006).

CONSCIOUSNESS

The statement that sound mimics the vibratory nature of existence is illustrated by the relationship between cymatics and quantum theory. The universe that can be perceived by our senses and their manufactured extensions is only a minute part of the totality of existence. The basic structure of the known universe consists of unknown vibrating, subatomic particle/waves that are collectively referred to as the *quantum field*. It is a ubiquitous, continuous, interconnected vibrating whole that does not behave according to the laws of classical physics or according to what the mind perceives as normal reality. The quantum universe behaves in ways that defy our perceptions of reality. In the quantum field, particles are also waves. This is called wave-particle duality. A cymatic pattern mimics wave-particle duality. Cymatic images are distinct structures corresponding to specific vibratory parameters of tone and frequency and are simultaneously part of a bigger pattern of structural forms (vibrational blueprints) that are constantly changing. The cymatic image is, like a particle, confined to a small region of space, but sound waves spread out in every direction creating a myriad of fluid structural forms. In the quantum reality, interactions between particles are not subject to or limited by distance, time, or space. This is called the *principle of non-locality* or *quantum entanglement*. Cymatic patterns mimic quantum entanglement in that the sound wave has the potential to recreate the same pattern at another distant location or locations. If the frequency of the wave were to change, then the patterns in distant locations would simultaneously change.

The last aspect of quantum behavior to mention is that the nature of existence is configured by the interaction between the consciousness of the observer and the observed. Physicists call this the *uncertainty principle*. According to quantum theory, human beings are connected to the basic structure of the universe through consciousness. Mind and matter are intrinsically and causally connected. Quantum theory was originally conceived to address the fact that there is no law or explanation in the deterministic view of classical physics that explains the existence of consciousness and the fact that every human thought or action initiated either automatically, unconsciously, or volitionally, creates changes at the quantum level. Thoughts and physical changes create quantum fluctuations in fundamental particles that precede all observed changes from the molecular to the anatomical level.

Consciousness, though not yet well understood, is therefore a fundamental manifestation of the universe and the driving force behind sound healing. Consciousness carries information and uses sound as a vehicle to manifest itself. In humans, it connects the body to the mind, creating a sense of self and an awareness of self and of one's sense of reality and definition of existence. It gives one the ability to alter one's internal physiochemical environment from the subatomic to the physical level. This fact is most evident in our own bodies, where thoughts and emotions have been observed to create very specific changes in brain chemistry and morphology. Sound mimics the vibratory nature of reality on the one hand, and the role and nature of consciousness on the other.

This does not mean that consciousness can be reduced to physiological processes in the brain or to anything else for that matter. Modern medicine as a healing art is conceptually stuck in the mechanistic, deterministic view of Newtonian and classical physics that conceptualizes the human organism as a passive sophisticated machine comprised of several independent though connected component systems. It has not updated itself either to the current or ancient understanding of humans as vibrating, sonic entities with consciousness: We are active agents able to exercise will and choose a particular course of action that influences outcomes in observed events at all levels of existence.

MINDFUL LISTENING

Mindful listening is the most fundamental skill required of sound healers and patients. Mindful listening is the ability to be aware of and to consciously enter into sounds by focusing one's awareness on the present moment while calmly accepting thoughts, feelings, and body sensations without judgment. If you are mindfully listening to a sound, you are practicing sound healing in its simplest form since *all sounds have the potential to be healing*. In this sense, the principles of sound healing are universal and can be practiced by anyone simply by learning to listen mindfully. When our conscious awareness is mindfully focused on a sound, we simultaneously entrain with that sound. As our inner experience of reality comes into entrainment with the sound, our consciousness and inner awareness expands, and our rational-objective mind becomes an aware yet passive observer. This opens the possibility for healing via a change in consciousness that creates an inner sense of balance, harmony, and well-being.

The following mindful listening experience was shared by a client who was struggling with an issue and couldn't make a decision. This story illustrates the point.

> I was in the middle of an empty football field on a warm day. A wind came up and the ropes on the flag-poles began to clang against the metal poles. The flag poles were all around the stadium and, depending on how the wind came through the stadium, the sounds would be different. Something came over me and I laid on the ground, closed my eyes, and listened. I let go into the sounds. I was simultaneously all sound even though they were coming from different directions. The sense of unity, beauty, and connectedness was almost overwhelming. When I opened my eyes, I knew what decision I needed to make.

The next story was shared by a client who was feeling alone and isolated and looking for a sense of connection in her life.

> I was sitting near a waterfall talking with my friends. Suddenly, something within the sound of the waterfall caught my ears. I tried to ignore it because I wanted to talk with my friends. The sound kept coming back. Finally, I excused myself and sat on a rock very near the waterfall. The rock felt like "my rock" and sitting on it gave me an immense sense of security. I just let go and dissolved into the sounds of the flowing water. I kept discovering new sounds, and all of the sounds were somehow related to each other in the most intimate ways. I became a sound flowing with the other sounds. I realized that there were trillions upon trillions of sounds and that we were all flowing and communicating as one.

These experiences are transformative, self-transcendent events that allow individuals to experience themselves as the consciousness that they are. When engaged in mindful listening, the mind becomes silent, physiological activity slows, awareness increases, and consciousness changes to create a new perspective and relationship to life events. This case illustrates the possibilities.

> Maria is a 54-year-old uneducated immigrant Mormon from Ecuador who worked as a house cleaner and faced many severe psychosocial stressors. After approximately two years of charity psychiatric care for depression and anxiety with limited success, she inquired one day about all of those singing bowls and tuning forks in my office. It was explained that these are healing instruments. She then became visibly upset and asked, "Why haven't you tried that on me? I like sound." We proceeded to have a session using Himalayan singing bowls and BioSonic tuning forks with the intention of inducing a mindful state of relaxation and well-being that changes consciousness and creates a sense of balance in mind and body. As she sat with her eyes closed during the session, she was instructed to adopt an attitude of mindful listening—a non-judgmental, detached observation of her body and mind. No explanations were given to her other than the initial statement that sound and vibration are used as healing tools. When the session ended she stated that it had been years since she had last felt so relaxed.
>
> When she was seen again a month later she walked in asking, "Doctor, what did you do to me? Since I left your office a month ago my life has changed completely. I don't know why, but since I left your office I no longer feel depressed or anxious. About two weeks ago, I stopped taking the antidepressant and pain medication and all my body pains are gone. I'm sleeping through the night without pills. I generally feel calm and happy. Now I'm walking around singing all the time and my family is worried. They're asking me what's wrong because they think I'm not acting like my usual self."

A sound healing treatment had never been considered for Maria because it was assumed that it would be something too weird and strange, too much outside of her expectations and worldview. It was also assumed that her Mormon faith would lead her to suspect or reject these "Eastern"-sounding practices as being in opposition to her religion. As we saw, however, with no knowledge or idea about sound healing, Maria was able to surrender and go deep into the sound. She was able to change her consciousness and experience of herself from that of a sad, worried, depressed person with little hope, to a joyous and calm person, still walking around facing a lot of serious problems but with a different outlook (change in consciousness). Three months after the session, she terminated treatment herself stating, "Although I love coming here for these sessions, I feel that I don't need them anymore and at this point I feel like I'd be abusing your generosity if I kept coming."

Never underestimate the capacity of any individual to change their consciousness. Changes in consciousness affect emotions, neural circuitry, and physiology. Knowledge and educational status are not predictive of success in a person's ability to use sound and to change consciousness in a way conducive to healing. It's possible, in fact, that knowledge and education can even be a potential hindrance for certain individuals. Highly educated intellectuals may find it difficult to let go, to silence the "rational mind," to favor intuition and the experiential expansion of consciousness that Einstein and many others have identified as the true source of new knowledge.

MANTRAS: ANCIENT SOUND HEALING FOR MODERN TIMES

Mantras are sounds that were discovered in deep meditation by the great saints of India thousands of years ago. Mantras form the basis of an ancient sound healing system that combines meditation, chanting, and mindfully listening to the sound of a mantra. Mantra meditation has been used for centuries to attain deep relaxation and hyperconscious states of awareness, to improve both mental and physical health, and to enhance overall functioning and a sense of well-being. Millions of people around the world now practice mantra meditation and its healing and other beneficial effects have been extensively researched (NCCIH 2012). The research literature on mantra meditation suggests that it may be useful in treating attention deficit disorder and in improving the ability to regulate emotions and to increase self-awareness (Benson et al. 1974). Research has also demonstrated that repeating a mantra changes the electrical activity of the brain (entrainment) and enhances immune function (Davidson et al. 2003). These research findings are important because they establish the universal nature of the practice of mantra. Although the practice comes from an Indian religious tradition, its effects are part of a universal/transcultural sound healing system that is best explained by the interaction between consciousness and vibration in a living organism. In other words, the efficacy and legitimacy of mantra practices are not dependent on a *specific* spiritual tradition or belief. The only requirements are sound (a mantra that can be inwardly repeated or chanted), the ability to enter a state of mindfulness by sitting calmly while observing the contents of the mind in a detached manner, and the belief that doing these things is beneficial. This belief can take many forms. It can be based on the trust that a client has in a practitioner with whom there is a strong therapeutic alliance, trust in the scientific research on mantra, or belief in a higher power, which can also be conceived in many ways. The ancient sound healing systems were always conceived as being part of a larger understanding of energy or of a higher interconnected power grid in the universe that is similar in concept to modern quantum theory (Capra 1999). For this reason, mantras are often associated with spiritual traditions because the cultures in which the mantra sound healing system developed did not separate universal energy principles from mind and body as we tend to do in modern times.

The physical and psychological effects of different mantras and sounds are well documented. Mantras and sounds are used in the natural healing systems of India, China, Japan, and Tibet, as well as used by shamanistic practitioners from indigenous cultures throughout the world. It is common for a traditional physician or shaman in these healing traditions to give a mantra or sound to cure different physical and mental conditions. Because the mantra or sound is always given as part of an integrative sound healing system that includes mindfulness and belief, it is inaccurate to do research just on the sound. However, researchers who have used meaningless sounds or words, such as the number one, to focus the mind have found that they were not as effective as a sound that the person identifies with in a positive way (Benson and Proctor 2003). We hypothesize that as technology advances we will be able to better understand the structural patterns of sound and their psychological, biological, and quantum effects. We also believe that taking a sound out of the context of mindfulness and belief will limit the therapeutic effect of the sound even though it may be shown to have therapeutic value.

SOUND HEALING PRACTICE

The practice of sound healing begins with establishing environmental and personal safety. When individuals are ill and imbalanced, they are usually vulnerable, fearful, and apprehensive. It is therefore of the utmost importance that they each feel safe and comfortable with the therapist and the therapeutic space, as well as to the sound healing treatment itself and to the instruments being offered. Every client will be different, just as every individual who flies in an airplane will have a different level of comfort and ability to trust and to let go during the flight.

The key to the creation of this sense of safety is the therapeutic alliance, which is usually congruent with and reflective of the therapist's intentions and compassion when approaching the client. Safety in the treatment being offered is a major concern in sound healing practices because sounds have powerful physical and psychological effects on humans. Most individuals have a neutral listening range, outside of which they can feel uncomfortable and unable to mindfully listen to sounds. A neutral sound, in the broadest sense, is any sound the listener can listen to without mental or physical tension. Research is currently being conducted to define which frequency and dynamic range of sound might signal vagal arousal leading to a flight or fight response (Porges 2011). The general clinical practice rule is to try a sound and then observe the body's response to the sound. If there is any tension, this is not the right sound. No matter how much you may like a sound or think that it's good, if there is tension, it's not right for that person. Once a neutral range is determined, it can be used to fine-tune other sounds within the neutral range, either for a specific outcome or as a baseline for the expansion of the neutral range.

Sound healing requires that practitioners be empathically bonded with their clients while simultaneously being able to play sounds that are best for them. Driven by compassion, the sound healer's objective is to embed sounds with healing intentions that are congruent or resonant with their client's needs. The most fundamental attitude required of sound healers and indeed of all healers is the ability to exercise compassion to facilitate the intuitive empathic contact that leads to the possibility of healing. In the practice of sound healing, success is determined by the consciousness of subject and practitioner as manifested in the intention underlying their actions and interactions together. The practitioner's intention must be driven by compassion and the subject must be able to form a therapeutic alliance. The following case study illustrates how sound healing can be integrated into a psychiatric practice within a safe environment in which the therapeutic alliance has been professionally established.

CASE HISTORY

Joe is a 34-year-old Hispanic fashion retailer from New York City with a history of sporadic treatment for depression and anxiety since adolescence when he began experiencing panic attacks. He was sexually molested from the ages of 7–12 by an older, distant cousin who lived in his home part of that time. He remembers feeling terrified of the cousin yet drawn to him and guilty through the years over the fact that part of him enjoyed the attention and the excitement of the encounters. He developed a feeling of shame and walked around feeling overly self-conscious, often imagining that people, including strangers, were talking about him. His biggest fear throughout adolescence was that people would discover his past, judge, and then reject him.

His first panic attack occurred when he was 16 years old in response to a bullying incident. He convinced himself that everyone knew about him and then panicked just before going home to face his family.

He presented initially with complaints of depression, insomnia, nausea, restlessness, dizziness, weakness, general malaise, pains all over the body, severe anxiety, and, according to him, daily panic attacks in response to a situation at work. He was informed by another employee that his current boss, who was a former personal friend, was spreading false rumors about him to the staff. She was allegedly stating that the patient was into black magic and was performing witchcraft on people at work.

He requested initially to be put on medical disability, expressing an inability to deal with the situation, and admitted later that he had come to the visit primarily for that reason. He believed that his problem was totally created by the fact that he had to be in this toxic place every day and if he could just avoid that he would be fine. He usually was, after all, fine when not at work or thinking about it.

In the first session, the patient's anxiety was so severe that it was decided to start him on an antidepressant/antianxiety drug and an anxiolytic to be used as needed to abort panic attacks. He was also given a sound healing session with deep breathing and mindfulness meditation exercises. Because of the intensely physical manifestations of the anxiety, the patient was instructed to lay down with his eyes covered. He was then exposed to a sound drone as he received instructions for mindfulness and breathing. After 15 minutes the patient was then treated vibroacoustically with the Otto 128 and a large Himalayan singing bowl. The Otto 128 was used to activate the parasympathetic nervous system and to impart the frequency of a perfect fifth throughout the skeletal system. The singing bowl targeted the muscles as well as his abdominal cavity. The session ended with a protocol (C-G-F-A) for anxiety, designed by John Beaulieu, using the regular (psychoacoustic) tuning forks close to the ears and then with a final period of quiet relaxation (water fountain in background). After this first session, the patient stated that he had never felt this relaxed in his life and had only come close to it previously when he took alprazolam. He was also "shocked" that after the session all of his physical symptoms had disappeared.

In the next few sessions, however, it was noticed that the patient always came in in an extremely anxious state and was basically unable to engage in therapy. At times he would go into some kind of dissociative state, his mind going blank and exhibiting thought blocking. We decided, therefore, to start all visits with a relaxing sound healing session for the first half hour and then talk therapy and medication management for the rest of the hour. This made it possible to engage in cognitive restructuring interventions that allowed him to see that his fears were essentially self-created and were unfounded distortions of the trauma he experienced in childhood.

He was able to see clearly that, even though this situation had been going on for almost two years, no harm had ever come to him. The underlying thought driving his behavior and emotions over the past two years was that he was unable to manage the situation at work, was unable to be at peace, and was assuming that people were thinking badly of him. The turning point of his condition and in the treatment came when he finally realized and saw clearly that the position that he was currently in was exactly the same one he had been in since he could remember. He had been feeling fearful, judged, misunderstood, powerless, and victimized by powerful individuals and yet angry and guilty that somehow all this was a measure of how worthless he was. Once he made that shift in his consciousness, all his symptoms began to disappear, and he basically stopped taking sleeping and antianxiety medications. About five months into treatment, the patient left the job for a lower paying one where he nevertheless felt calmer and happier.

This case illustrates perfectly how sound healing practices can be integrated with cognitive behavioral therapy, mindful listening, and psychopharmacological interventions. The sound healing intervention changed certain physiological parameters that set the stage for the changes in consciousness required for the other interventions to work. Experiencing himself in a relaxed state initiated the process of changing his state of mind from "Nothing can change my situation, there's nothing I can do" to "I can relax myself. I see how my own fears and insecurities led to the negative thoughts that I used to keep myself in the nervous condition that I was in."

The sound facilitated his ability to enter a meditative state and to adopt the mindful listening attitude of *detached observance* of mental and physical phenomena. This detached observance, which indicates a change in consciousness, in turn, helped and complemented the cognitive behavioral techniques. Medication also played an important role in this case. The initial level of suffering, the intensity of the symptoms and the looming sense of crisis called for psychopharmacological intervention. Besides its biochemical effect, the medication influenced the patient's consciousness by giving him a sense of security that also facilitated the sound work and cognitive behavioral therapy (CBT).

SOUND HEALING TOOLS AND INSTRUMENTS

An important part of sound healing practice is to develop basic sound making skills by learning to use different musical instruments and/or sound making materials. For sound healers, *anything that makes sound is potentially a sound healing instrument.* A sound healer must know how to play his or her instrument, must develop a feel for tonal dynamics, have a sense of space and tone, and develop the ability to mindfully listen. Knowledge of music, music theory, and reading music is not necessary and can even be an obstacle. For this reason, sound healers often use instruments that are easy to learn and control, such as tuning forks, crystal and Himalayan singing bowls, gongs, whistles, didgeridoos, flutes, frame drums, rain sticks, the voice, and so on. The general rule is: Be like a child and have fun making and mindfully listening to sounds.

PART I: PSYCHOACOUSTICS

Music

Sound healers view and use music as a tool for healing; they approach it as if it's just another sound healing instrument. Although it's a fact that different cultures and individuals have predilections for specific musical styles, all music has the potential to be useful as a sound healing tool. Composers and musicians arrange and play sounds to create specific musical styles that listeners can identify with and build preferences for. Sound healers, on the other hand, listen to the sound dynamics of a style or a particular piece of music and observe how it affects the listener. The sound healer must work with musical styles that resonate with the client and recommend listening depending on the desired effect. Everyone does this intuitively on their own. We are always choosing different music depending on our moods, state of mind, or the nature and level of the activity we engage in. For example, if we want to wake up and get motivated or exercise, we listen to fast, syncopated music. But if what we want is to calm down and relax or go to sleep, we listen to soft, slow, flowing music.

Voice

The voice is arguably the most powerful sound healing instrument of all. The use of the voice in healing sessions can be passive—that is, clients just listen and absorb—or active by engaging clients in humming, toning, chanting, singing, and multiple other vocal exercises. *Mindfully listening to the sound of one's own voice expands consciousness and opens the door to self-awareness and the possibility of healing.* The voice is also a great assessment tool for practitioners to evaluate their client's mental and emotional state and certain personality traits such as self-confidence, self-esteem, and so on (Beaulieu 1987).

Singing Bowls and Gongs

Singing bowls and gongs are some of the most popular and widely used sound healing instruments today. A major mode of sound healing therapy that is quickly proliferating is the so-called "sound bath" where individuals or groups typically lay or sit and mindfully listen for an extended period of time. Singing bowls are either Himalayan (metallic) or made of quartz crystal. The quartz crystal bowls are psychoacoustic (Figure 19.8). The Himalayan bowls are both psychoacoustic and vibro-acoustic. The bowls and gongs are excellent tools for toning, humming, chanting, and as aids to facilitate meditation. Many individuals spontaneously report increased ability to quiet the mind and relax and to engage in mindful listening with the sounds of the bowls.

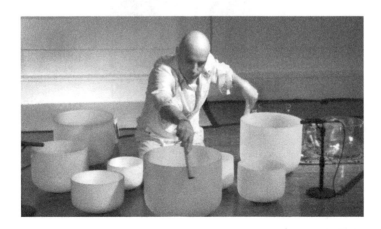

FIGURE 19.8   Sound Healer Philippe Garnier playing crystal bowls during a sound healing concert.

Drums, Rattles, Percussive Instruments

Everything that exists has a characteristic rhythm, frequency, or vibratory pattern. Drums and percussion instruments are useful sound healing tools that, in groups, can increase social connectedness and cohesiveness and, in individuals, can change physiological parameters such as electrical conduction in the brain (EEG) and heart rate. These are examples of entrainment. Drums can have both psychoacoustic or vibroacoustic effects, as we will see ahead.

Tuning Forks

Tuning forks are versatile and neutral sound healing instruments. They are neutral because they are used by musicians all over the world to tune their instruments and are not associated with any specific culture or style of music. They are versatile because they are always in tune, are lightweight, can be easily carried in your pocket, and are easy to learn and use. They lend themselves to research and consistent results with clients because of their tuning accuracy. In general, when tuning forks are tapped with healing intentions, their effects are quick and can be integrated with and enhance every therapy. Hospitals are stressful places and doctors, nurses, therapists, and support staff have a lot to do. Tapping a tuning fork, even just for a moment, is a way of shifting gears with a patient and then moving on to the next patient, knowing that the sound will serve to enhance whatever therapies the patient is receiving.

The two primary tuning fork systems used in the world today by sound healers are the Acutonic and the BioSonic tuning forks. Acutonic tuning forks were developed by acupuncturist Donna Carey and are designed to be used vibroacoustically over acupuncture and trigger points as well as foci of pain in the body. BioSonic tuning forks were developed by Dr. John Beaulieu and include both vibroacoustic (Otto) and psychoacoustic forks. Their use is discussed in depth in his book *Human Tuning: Sound Healing with Tuning Forks* (Beaulieu 2010). The primary BioSonic tuning forks are C256 cps, G384 cps, and Otto 128 cps. As part of the Fibonacci series, the C and G create an interval of a perfect fifth (a perfect 2/3 ratio) when sounded (Figure 19.9). The Otto 128 cps (the difference tone obtained by subtracting C256 from G384) spreads the vibration of the

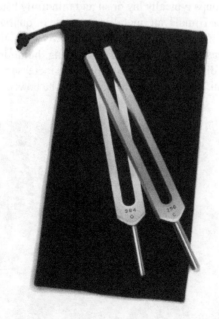

FIGURE 19.9   G and C tuning forks.

perfect fifth vibroacoustically through the body when placed directly on any tissue, but especially bone (Figure 19.10). The goal of treatment is to create a state of balance by entraining the person's nervous system to the vibratory rate of a perfect fifth (Figures 19.11 and 19.12). The sound (psychoacoustic) and vibratory (vibroacoustic) effects of this entrainment operate by triggering a relaxation response that, as stated earlier, is hypothesized to be related to the nitric oxide stimulation observed with the use of the tuning forks (Beaulieu 2002; *Otto128 Tuning Fork and Nitic Oxide Response.* Unpublished raw data set).

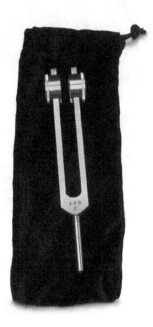

FIGURE 19.10   Otto 128 tuning fork.

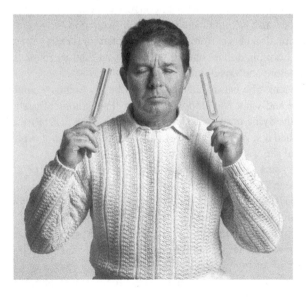

FIGURE 19.11   Dr. John Beaulieu listening to C and G tuning forks.

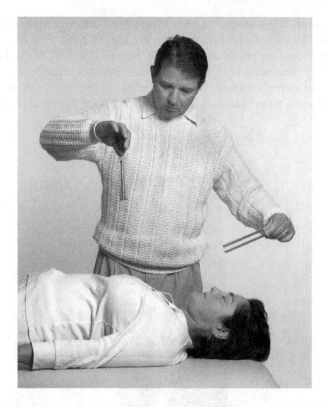

FIGURE 19.12 Dr. Beaulieu sounding C and G tuning forks, which are tapped together during an integrative sound healing session.

CASE HISTORY

Betty is a hospice patient in the last stages of congestive heart failure. She is agitated, suffering from panic attacks, and is angry. She is taking lorazepam (Ativan) to control her anxiety and to sleep. If the situation gets extreme or nears a behavioral emergency, she is given a dose of liquid morphine. Looking at her chart, it was apparent that her panic attacks came later in the evening or just before she was going to sleep.

I met Betty at 10 a.m. She was awake, calm, and happy to have someone sit with her. We talked about her life and what was important to her. Psychologically, she was clearly in the bargaining stage of the dying process as defined by Kübler-Ross (1969) and not ready to let go. That evening Betty had a severe panic attack and was given liquid morphine. I saw her again the next morning and she was still agitated.

I said, "Betty, are you aware of what happens to you when you start getting tired and thinking about going to sleep?" She said in an angry voice, "I do not want to go to sleep. I know the nurses want me to go to sleep so that I'll die and not be a problem anymore."

Betty was frail and worn down by the progression of her congestive heart failure. I was amazed at the level of anger and resolve she was able to express. It was clear that Betty was a fighter and that she was using what had to be the last of her inner strength to hold on rather than to face her fear of letting go. Psychologically, she was caught in a loop of bargaining, anger, and fear. She knew she was dying and was not ready to accept it, and she was afraid she would lose control at night and die in her sleep.

I asked Betty if I could visit her in the evening. She smiled and said, "That would be wonderful." Then she whispered in a quiet, secretive voice, "You can help me with those nurses."

When I visited Betty in the evening I brought a set of four tuning forks, C, F, G, and A, that can be played much like a harp. I showed them to Betty and asked if I could play them for her. She smiled and said, "Oh, I would love that." I held the C in my left hand and the F, G, and A in my right hand. Using the C to tap, I tuned into Betty and created a mini-healing sound event. When I finished Betty was asleep. I left very quietly and the nurse, who had been listening, said, "Is she really asleep?"

I said, "I think so."

Betty slept through the night without drugs. I saw her briefly the next morning and she said, "What did you do to me?" I said, "Do you remember the sounds?"

She said, "Yes, I remember listening and then a sense of safety came over me."

I said, "And you woke up this morning just fine."

She said, "Yes."

I said, "I'll play for you again tonight." She replied with a smile, "I'd like that."

That evening before I played, Betty said, "I want to go further with the sounds tonight. They are my friends. What will happen?"

I held her hand and said, "You'll be taking a chance. The sounds may take you to a place where you'll just keep going and will not have any interest in coming back."

She said, "I thought so. It's ok. I'm ready."

I played for her again and she went to sleep. That night she passed away peacefully without drugs.

Today there are many harp therapy programs in which musicians learn to play harps at the bedsides of sick and dying patients with amazing results (Briggs 2002). The advantage of a sound healing approach in contrast to a music approach is that normal musical training and tuning instruments are not necessary. After Betty passed away, the hospice nurses requested an in-service training on how to use the tuning forks with dying patients. They were able to learn the basics in a day and immediately began to integrate sound healing with their nursing skills. To be clear, each approach works and brings healing and comfort to patients, as well as staff. One requires years of musical training and the other requires mindful listening and basic sound making skills. Both require the ability to understand the patient's needs and to establish a therapeutic alliance.[2]

PART II: VIBROACOUSTIC SOUND HEALING

Vibroacoustic sound healing techniques consist of the direct transmission of vibration from a vibrating sound healing instrument to the body to stimulate "skin hearing." Vibroacoustic sound healing practices are thousands of years old and are found in every culture. For example, it is common for indigenous shamans to use drums as vibroacoustic instruments, combined with singing, chanting, or blowing onto specific areas of the skin to affect healing (Cohan 2010). Although these practices may appear strange and the language used to describe them is far from technical, they nevertheless create brain responses via a skin/ear pathway that we are only now beginning to understand.[3] Today, a growing body of research is creating a new understanding that we hear with our skin as well, or perhaps even better, than we hear with our ears (Derrick et al. 2009; Frenzel et al. 2012).

Vibroacoustic sound healing practices are a combination of music and sound (psychoacoustic) with sinusoidal sound waves that transmit vibrations directly to the body. The majority of the vibroacoustic equipment and techniques available today combine the direct transmission of vibration to the body simultaneously with music and/or sounds (Figure 19.13). Vibroacoustic therapy began to be formulated by pioneers such as Olav Skille sometime in the late 1960s and started to be used

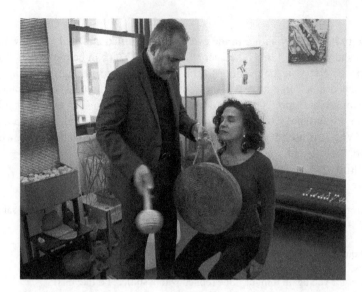

FIGURE 19.13 Dr. Perez-Martinez using a gong as a vibroacoustic sound healing instrument.

clinically by 1980. Although much of the evidence for the efficacy of vibroacoustics is anecdotal or based on observed response, there is a growing body of clinical research that suggests beneficial results on a wide range of conditions from pain management, muscular tension and spasms, anxiety and emotional regulation, to cardiovascular conditions and osteoporosis (Wellmes 2016).

A recent vibroacoustic study conducted in Japan using a mattress embedded with auditory and vibrational devices studied the effectiveness of using vibroacoustic sound healing working with nursing home patients with symptoms of depression (Yoshihisa et al. 2012). The study concluded that vibroacoustic therapy provided relaxation effects of elderly nursing home residents and improved depressive symptoms. Another study using a vibroacoustic chair to treat autism spectrum disorder (ASD) was conducted in a hospital in Sweden. The study concluded that sitting in the vibroacoustic chair for 10 minutes significantly reduced challenging behaviors related to ASD and developmental disabilities (Lundqvist et al. 2009). A pilot study conducted at the University of Toronto used a vibroacoustic chair to treat Alzheimer's patients. The patients sat in a vibroacoustic chair twice a week. They were given a 40 Hz frequency based on gamma brain waves found in healthy brains. The study concluded that the short-term effects of vibroacoustic stimulation had a positive effect on Alzheimer's patients and suggested that the vibroacoustic chair was a viable treatment to support other therapies (Clements-Cortes et al. 2016).

Another instrument of vibroacoustic sound healing is the BioSonic Otto 128 cps tuning fork (Figure 19.14). Many medical students are taught how to use the Otto tuning forks as part of a neurological and auditory exam. The same tuning fork can be repurposed for different forms of vibroacoustic healing. It can be used directly on the body to stimulate nerves, relieve tension, and trigger a sense of deep relaxation in the targeted area. It is especially effective when placed on bones and has the ability to relieve muscle tension, spasms, and pain, and to improve circulation by relaxing constricting muscle tissue and causing increased blood flow. The Otto 128 cps is a very efficient way to stimulate acupuncture, trigger and reflex points, and can be easily integrated with those therapies.

SUMMARY

Vibration, sound, and consciousness are fundamental manifestations of the universe that largely define the nature of existence and the structure and organization of everything that exists. The

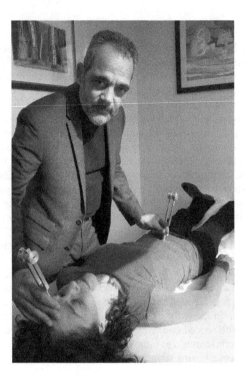

FIGURE 19.14 Dr. Perez-Martinez demonstrating vibroacoustic application of BioSonic 128 cps tuning forks.

human organism is a sonorous instrument that operates in a musical manner, like much of nature, and is designed to transport and process information about movement (vibration) and sounds into consciousness. The auditory nerve has a vestibular (vibroacoustic) branch that processes movement and balance and a cochlear (psychoacoustic) branch that processes sound. The hearing apparatus, however, is now understood to encompass the entire body and not just the ear and auditory nerve. The musical nature of our organism is manifested, for example, in the way behavior-specific neural networks in the human brain are organized into harmonic patterns that are observed everywhere in nature (Atasoy et al. 2016). And, recently, using a procedure called *sonification*, scientists have been able to improve their ability to analyze biochemical processes by converting data about proteins into musical melodies or sounds (Bywater and Middleton 2016).

The practice of sound healing is based on the fact that all biological processes have characteristic *vibrational signatures* that collectively define the nature of specific organisms and the vibratory parameters and dynamics that define it when in a state of balance. Hearing, listening, and making sounds and music are integral parts of healthy living, functioning, and development. Sound is an integral part of the mechanisms necessary for down-regulating stress and restoring the body to balance, as well as the system involved in arousal and alertness to potential or actual danger. Sound healing, especially when integrated with mindfulness and breathing practices, is in our experience, *the quickest and most effective way to achieve relaxation*. There are virtually no medical conditions, states of imbalance, or individuals that cannot benefit from relaxation. Likewise, there is no one who can manage stress, pain, or tension without sound. When in pain, we scream or moan to restore balance. When sad, we cry. When happy, we laugh. Imagine touching a hot iron and not making a sound. Without the release of sound, the body would tighten and go further out of balance. Sound is necessary in restoring the body to a balanced state and that is why today we are rediscovering the sound healing procedures of past cultures, subjecting them to evidence-based research, and integrating sound healing into mainstream medical and wellness practices to fulfill the objective of bringing healing back into the practice of medicine.

NOTES

1. Relaxation during sound healing is hypothesized by Dr. Beaulieu and collaborators to be the result of a very specific response related to neural processes and their coupling to constitutive nitric oxide. Dr. Beaulieu and collaborators published a peer-reviewed article suggesting that NO provides the physiological pathways through which sound and music operate by hypothesizing that sound stimulates the release of anandamide, an endogenous endocannabinoid that in turn stimulates the release of cNO in immune cells, neural tissues, and human vascular endothelial cells (Beaulieu et al. 2003). In technical terms, nitric oxide is a "gaseous diffusible modulator" that moves through the entire body and central nervous system in waves or puffs of gas. The release of nitric oxide counteracts the negative effects of adrenergic overstimulation. Adrenergic stimulation in the presence of norepinephrine/adrenaline results in a racing heart, high blood pressure, anxiety, and greater vulnerability to pain. This in turn triggers a relaxation response to sound by the effects of a wave of nitric oxide gas that signals a reduction in blood pressure, lowers heart rate, increases pain tolerance, and an overall lowering of metabolism. This positive reaction also appears to affect the immune system by stimulating the production of IgA and NK cells.
2. Although more research needs to be done, it appears that sound, when used in the right environment and therapeutic alliance, can act in a similar manner as psychotropic drugs by triggering endogenous molecules that create similar effects. In the 1970s, Dr. Stanislav Grof conducted research about the use of psychotropic substances such as LSD and mescaline to treat terminal cancer, alcoholism, and other serious diseases in a controlled setting. When research with psychotropic drugs was stopped by the federal government in the early 1970s, the research team turned to sound and music to induce similar states as those experienced on the psychotropic substances. Helen L. Bonney, a music therapist and a member of the research team, developed GIM, Guided Imagery and Music, to facilitate healing states of consciousness using sound and music and to help cancer patients in the dying process (Burns 2001).
3. Dr. Alfred Tomatis, a French audiologist and a pioneer in sound healing, proposed that our skin is a piece of differentiated ear that translates the potential of vibrational stimuli that come from the skin, to the brain. He hypothesized that the special sensory cells of the organ of Corti produce nerve impulses in response to sound vibrations that are similar to mechanoreceptor cells found in our skin (Tomatis 1989).

SOUND HEALING TRAINING PROGRAMS

Certificate in Sound, Voice, and Music in the Healing Arts
California Institute of Integral Studies
San Francisco, CA 94103
www.ciis.edu

Integrative Sound and Music Institute
Integrative Sound and Music Practitioner Training
NY Open Center
New York, NY
www.opencenter.org

Certificate in Integrative Sound Healing
Polarity Zentrum
Zürich, Switzerland
www.polarity.ch

BioSonic Enterprises, Ltd.
Integrative Sound Healing Classes
Stone Ridge, NY
www.biosonics.com

REFERENCES

Atasoy, S., I. Donnelly, and J. Pearson. 2016. Human brain networks function in connectome-specific harmonic waves. *Nature Communications*. http://www.nature.com/articles/ncomms10340.

Beaulieu, J. 1987. *Music and Sound in the Healing Arts*. New York: Station Hill Press.

Beaulieu, J. 2010. *Human Tuning*. Stone Ridge, NY: Biosonic Enterprises, Ltd.

Beaulieu, J. 2018. The nature of healing sound and its design. *Psychology's New Design Science and The Reflective Practitioner*. Editors: Susan Imholz and Judy Sachter. River Bend, NC: LibraLab Press.

Beaulieu, J., G.B. Stefano, E. Salamon, and M. Kim. 2003. Sound therapy induced relaxation: Down regulating stress processes and pathologies. *Medical Science Monitor* 9, 116–121.

Benson, H., J.F. Beary, and M.P. Carol. 1974. The relaxation response. *Psychiatry* 37, 37–46.

Benson, H. and W. Proctor. 2003. *The Break-Out Principle*. New York: Scribner. 221–224.

Briggs, T. 2002. *Grace Notes: Reflections on the Harp and Healing*. Minnesota: Medical Reflections Press.

Burns, D.S. 2001. The effect of the Bonny Method of guided imagery and music on the mood and life quality of cancer patients. *Journal of Music Therapy*, 38, 51–65.

Bywater, R.P. and J.N. Middleton. 2016. Melody discrimination and protein fold classification. *Bioinformatics* https://www.ncbi.nlm.nih.gov/pmc/articles/PMC5079661/.

Capra, F. 1999. An exploration of the parallels between modern physics and Eastern mysticism. *Tao of Physics*. Massachusetts: Shambhala Publications.

Chiesa, A. and S. Serretti. 2010. A systematic review of neurobiological and clinical features of mindfulness meditations. *Psychol. Med.* Aug 40(8), 1239–1252. doi: 10.1017/S0033291709991747. Epub: Nov 27 2009.

Clements-Cortes, A., H. Ahonen, M. Evans, M. Freedman, and L. Bartel. 2016. Short-term effects of rhythmic sensory stimulaton in Alzheimer's disease: An exploratory pilot study. *Journal of Alzheimer's Disease* 52, 651–660.

Cohan, J.A. 2010. *The Primitive Mind and Modern Man*. Potomac, MD: Bentham Books. 104.

Davidson, R.J., J. Kabat-Zinn, J. Schumacher et al. 2003. Alterations in brain and immune function produced by mindfulness meditation. *Psychosomatic Medicine* July–Aug, 564–570.

Derrick, D., P. Anderson, and S. Green. 2009. Characteristics of air puffs produced in english 'pa': Experiments and simulations. *Journal of the Acoustical Society of America* 125(4), 2272–2281.

Frenzel, H., J. Bohlender, K. Pinsker et al. 2012. A genetic basis for mechanosensory traits in humans. *Journal of PLOS Biology* DOI: 10.137 May 1 http://journals.plos.org/plosbiology/article?id=10.1371/journal.pbio.1001318.

Iakovides, S.A., V. Th Iliadou, V. Th Bizeli, S.G. Kaprinis, K.N. Fountoulakis, and G.S. Kaprinis. 2004. Psychophysiology and psychoacoustics of music: Perception of complex sound in normal subjects and psychiatric patients. *Annals of General Hospital Psychiatry* 3(6) Web: https://annals-general-psychiatry.biomedcentral.com/track/pdf/10.1186/1475-2832-3-6?site=annals-general-psychiatry.biomedcentral.com.

Jenny, H. 1974. *Cymatics: The Structure and Dynamics of Wave Phenomena and Vibrations*. Two-volume compilation re-issued 2001. Eliot, ME: MACROmedia Publishing. www.cymaticsource.com.

Kays, J.L., R.A. Hurley, and K.H. Taber. 2012. The dynamic brain: Neuroplasticity and mental health. *The Journal of Neuropsychiatry and Clinical Neuroscience*, 24(2), 118–124.

Kreutz, P. 2006. Effects of choir singing and listening on secretory immunoglobulin a, cortisol, and emotional state. *Journal of Behavioral Medicine* 23, 171–179.

Kübler-Ross, E. 1969. *On Death and Dying: What the Dying Have to Teach Doctors, Nurses, Clergy and Their Own Families*. New York: Scribner.

Lauterwasser, A. 2002. *Water Sound Images: The Creative Music of the Universe*. English edition published 2006. Eliot, ME: MACROmedia Publishing. www.cymaticsource.com.

Levitin, D.J. and M.L. Chanda. 2013. The neurochemistry of music. *Trends in Cognitive Sciences* 17.4 (2013), 179–93. Web.

Lincoln, Don. 2013. The good vibrations of quantum field theories. *The Nature of Reality*. www.pbs.org/wgbh/nova/blogs/physics/2013/08/the-good-vibrations-of-quantum-field-theories.

Lundqvist, L-O., G. Andersson, and J. Viding. 2009. Effects of vibroacoustic music on challenging behaviors in individuals with autism and developmental disabilities. *Research in Autism Spectrum Disorders* 3(2), 390–400.

Munte, T.F., E. Altenmuller, and L. Jancke. 2002. *The Musician's Brain as a Model of Neuroplasticity*. Nature Publishing Group. nature.com.

NCCIH (National Center for Complementary and Integrative Health), National Health Interview Survey. 2012. https://nccih.nih.gov/research/statistics/NHIS/2012/mind-body/meditation.

Pelletier, C.L. 2004. The effect of music on decreasing arousal due to stress: A meta-analysis. *Journal of Music Therapy* 41(3), 192–214.

Porges, S.W. 2011. Neurophysiological foundations of emotions, attachment, communication, and self-regulation. *The Polyvagal Theory*, Editors: Allan N. Schore and Daniel J. Siegel New York: W.W. Norton Co. 133–202.

Reif, A., C.P. Jacob, D. Rujescu et al. 2009. Influence of functional variant of neuronal nitric oxide synthase on impulsive behaviors in humans. *Archives of General Psychiatry* 41.

Tomatis, A. A. 1989. *About the Tomatis Method*. Editors: Timothy M. Gilmore et al. Canada: Listening Centre Press. 214–216.

Wass, C., D. Klamer, K. Fejgin et al. 2009. The importance of nitric oxide in social dysfunction. *Behavioral Brain Research*, 113–116.

Wellmes, D. 2016. 7 *Health Benefits of Vibroacoustic (Sound & Vibration) Therapy, Wake Up World*. http://wakeup-world.com/2016/03/18/7-health-benefits-of-vibroacoustic-sound-vibration-therapy.

Yoshihisa, K., H. Mitsuyo, T. Yukie, S. Kazuhiko, N. Reiko, and K. Yoshio. 2012. Effects of vibroacoustic therapy on elderly nursing home residents with depression. *Journal of Physical Therapy Science* 24(3), 291–294 4p. CINAHL Complete, EBSCOhost (accessed December 6, 2015).

BIBLIOGRAPHY

Beck, F. 2008. Synaptic quantum tunneling in brain activity. *NeuroQuantology* 6(2) 140–251.

Bhoria, R. and S. Gupta. 2012. A study of the effect of sound on EEG. *International Journal of Electronics and Computer Science Engineering*. Vol 2. 120–124

Gold, C., M. Voracek, and T. Wigram. 2004. Effects of music therapy for children and adolescents with psychopathology: A meta-analysis. *J Child Psychol & Psychiat Journal of Child Psychology*, Vol. 58, 586–594. Web.

Hermanns, W. 1983. *Einstein and the Poet: In Search of the Cosmic Man*. Wellesley MA: Branden Books.

Holten, S. 2004. Music therapy for people with Parkinson's. *Parkinson's Disease*. Web.

King, L.K., Q.J. Almeida, and H. Ahonen. 2009. Short-term effects of vibration therapy on motor impairments in Parkinson's disease. *NeuroRehabilitaion*, 297–306.

Kotchoubey, B., Y.G. Pavlov, and B. Kleber. *Music in Research and Rehabilitation of Disorders of Consciousness: Psychological and Neurophysiological Foundations*. Institute for Medical Psychology and Behavioural Neurobiology, University of Tübingen, Tübingen, Germany.

Kyoiku, O., M. Yamakawa, N. Tanaka, H. Murakami, and S. Hori. 2010. Influence of sound and light on heart rate variability. *Journal of Human Ergology* 34, 25–34.

Levitin, D.J. 2006. *This Is Your Brain on Music. The Science of a Human Obsession*. New York, New York: Dutton.

Loewy, J. 2004. Integrating music, language and the voice in music therapy. *Voices: A World Forum for Music Therapy* 4(1).

Maratos, A., M.J. Crawford, and S. Procter. 2011. Music therapy for depression: It seems to work, but how? *The British Journal of Psychiatry*, 92–93. Web.

Nieizen, S., O. Olsson, and R. Öhman. 1993. On perception of complex sound in schizophrenia and mania. *Psychopathology* 26(1), 112–23.

Riganello, F., A. Candelieri, M. Quintieri, and G. Dolce. 2010. Heart rate variability, emotions, and music. *Journal of Psychophysiology*, 112–119.

Rudhyar, D. 1982. *The Magic of Tone and the Art of Music*. Boulder CO: Shambhala.

Rüütel, E. 2002. The psychophysiological effects of music and vibroacoustic stimulation. *Nordic Journal of Music Therapy*, 16–26.

Sahu, S., S. Ghosh, D. Fujita, and A. Bandyopadhyay. 2014. Live visualizations of single isolated tubulin protein self-assembly via tunneling current: Effect of electromagnetic pumping during spontaneous growth of microtubule. *Scientific Reports* 4(7303).

Silverman, M.J. 2007. Evaluating current trends in psychiatric music therapy: A descriptive analysis. *Journal of Music Therapy*, 388–414.

Stapp, H.P. 2007. Quantum approaches to consciousness. *The Cambridge Handbook of Consciousness*. New York, NY: Cambridge University Press.

Stefano, G.B., G.L. Fricchione, B.T. Slingsby, and H. Benson. 2001. The placebo effect and the relaxation response: Neural processes and their coupling to constitutive nitric oxide. *Brain Research Reviews* 35.

Tufail, Y., A. Yoshihiro, S. Pati, M.M. Li, and W.J. Tyler. 2011. Ultrasonic neuromodulation by brain stimulation with transcranial ultrasound. *Nature Protocols* 6, 1453–1470.

Wass, C. and A. Andreazza. 2013. The redox brain and nitric oxide: Implications for psychiatric illness. *Journal of Pharmacology and Clinical Toxicology* 1(1), 1008.

Yanagihashi, R., M. Ohira, T. Kimura, and T. Fujiwara. 1997. Physiological and psychological assessment of sound. *International Journal of Biometeorology* 40(3), 151–161.

Yau, J.M., A. Weber, F.J. Dammann, and S.J. Bensamia. 2011. Pitch and loudness interactions between audition and touch. *The Journal of the Acoustical Society of America* 1(5).

20 Healing with Light

Anadi Martel, Wesley Burwell, and Magda Havas

CONTENTS

Introduction 474
Living Organisms are Electromagnetic Beings of Light 474
Phototherapy Backgrounder 475
    What is Light Therapy? 475
    Light Application 475
    Light Placement 476
    Color 476
    Dosage 477
    Exposure Parameters 478
    Modulation 478
    Light Source for Photobiomodulation 479
    Medical Devices and Government Acceptance 481
Mechanisms of Photobiomodulation 481
    Nitric Oxide (NO) 482
    Adenosine Triphosphate (ATP) 482
Potential Applications of Photobiomodulation 483
    Circulation and Pain 483
    Inflammation 484
    Wound Healing 484
    Attention Deficit Hyperactivity Disorder (ADHD) 485
    Traumatic Brain Injury (TBI) 485
    Post-Traumatic Stress Disorder (PTSD) 485
    Athletic Performance and Recovery 486
    Wrinkles and Anti-Aging 486
Chronobiological Applications of Light 486
Chromotherapy and the Importance of Color 488
Principles of Chromotherapy 491
Tools and Methods of Chromotherapy 492
    A Sample of Chromotherapy Methods 492
    Spectro-Chrome Method 493
    Syntonic Phototherapy 493
    Colorpuncture 494
    Chromatothérapie 494
    Emotional Transformation Therapy 495
    Lateral Light Therapy 495
    Sensora 495
    Van Obberghen Color Therapy 495
    Monocrom Method 496
Conclusions 496
Notes 496
References 497

INTRODUCTION

Our relationship with light and especially with light from the sun has gone through several cultural transformations. Early civilizations worshipped the sun. Around the time of Hippocrates, sunlight was used for healing (heliotherapy) and was prescribed along with thermal baths and rest. In the middle ages, since peasants worked the fields and aristocrats stayed indoors, or were otherwise sheltered from the sun, fair skin was viewed as a sign of wealth and privilege leading to the peaches–and–cream complexion so valued among British maidens. During the industrial revolution, a growing population worked in factories and received little sun exposure while the rich could afford vacations in southern climates. So, a tan was associated with wealth and leisure. Today, most people associate the sun with skin cancer, which bodes well for the sunscreen industry that encourages us to cover up and get as little direct sun exposure as possible.

Similarly, our relationship with artificial light has gone through several revolutions with the first, and perhaps most profound, being the use of fire, which morphed from wood to animal fat to kerosene to candles as the source of fuel. The second revolution came a century ago with Edison's incandescent light bulb. Concern about fossil fuel reserves and climate change prompted a move toward energy efficiency, and several countries banned incandescent light bulbs in favor of energy efficient fluorescent lights and light emitting diodes (LED).

We are currently witnessing the third revolution of light as a source of information that can be used and deciphered by living cells. Light has been used as a tool for healing and promoting optimal health for millennia. Recent advances in lasers, LEDs and other forms of light emissions, combined with research on the mechanisms involved with light therapy at the cellular and tissue level, have catapulted us into a new era of medical treatments within the field of energy medicine. This chapter is about the use of light therapy to heal and to promote optimal health. It includes light treatments that act primarily through the body and light that passes through the retina.

Emphasis is placed on non-invasive light therapy and does not require the use of chemical reagents. Consequently, invasive use of laser therapy (intravenous, interstitial, intra-articular), extracorporeal light treatment of fluids that are transfused back into the body, and photodynamic therapy (PDT) that relies on the interaction of light with photosensitive chemical reagents are not discussed. Nor are other important biological effects associated with neonatal jaundice, vitamin D production, pulsed electromagnetic field (PEMF) therapy that uses frequencies well below the visible spectrum, the role of coherent *biophotons* (photons emitted by biological organisms), photoperiod effects, and Meares–Irlen Syndrome. The harmful effects of artificial light are discussed in Chapter 22 of this book.

LIVING ORGANISMS ARE ELECTROMAGNETIC BEINGS OF LIGHT

Health care practitioners who learn and practice western medicine take classes in morphology, physiology, biochemistry, chemistry, pathology, and so on. They learn how various systems of the body function or malfunction and are taught with an emphasis on chemical pathways and transformations. Few medical schools pay sufficient attention to the electromagnetic activities of the body even though these are involved in all metabolic functions and are an indicator of life itself (pulse, brain wave activity).

In essence, living organisms are "beings of light."[1] Yet this concept is viewed as "new age" thinking and not taken seriously by many health care practitioners well versed in western medicine primarily because it is not taught in medical schools. Advances in quantum physics, the concept of the morphogenetic field, and the role of coherent biophotons provide interesting new insights into how the body functions from an electromagnetic perspective.

A physician once said that he looks for three things when he is treating patients. Do they have all the essential chemicals/nutrients their body requires? Do they have toxins that need to be removed? Are there chemical blockages to communication that need to be resolved?

The same can be said about electromagnetic energy. Does the body have the essential frequencies? Is the body exposed to toxic frequencies? Are there blockages to electromagnetic communication within the body?

Communication is essential for any system to function smoothly. The late Ross Adey (2004) said that cells are whispering to each other electromagnetically. Whatever interferes with this communication results in illness and whatever facilitates this communication promotes healing.

PHOTOTHERAPY BACKGROUNDER

WHAT IS LIGHT THERAPY?

Light therapy refers to treatments that involve using the sun (heliotherapy) or artificial forms of light (phototherapy) consisting of one (monochromatic) or more (polychromatic) colors (chromotherapy) at specific wavelengths (measured as nm) of the visible spectrum (red to blue) and extending to near infrared (NIR) and near ultraviolet (NUV) radiation. There are three main modalities for light therapy: low-level light therapy (LLLT), bright light therapy, and chromotherapy.

While various terms exist for LLLT, the one recommended following a nomenclature consensus meeting of the North American Association for Light Therapy and the World Association for Laser Therapy is *photobiomodulation*—defined as:

> A form of light therapy that utilizes non-ionizing forms of light sources, including lasers, LEDs, and broadband light, in the visible and infrared spectrum. It is a nonthermal process involving endogenous chromophores eliciting photophysical (i.e., linear and nonlinear) and photochemical events at various biological scales. This process results in beneficial therapeutic outcomes including but not limited to the alleviation of pain or inflammation, immunomodulation, and promotion of wound healing and tissue regeneration (Anders et al. 2015).

Photobiomodulation therapy is now an accepted term in the Medical Subject Headings (MeSH) of the National Library of Medicine and, while it is the preferred term for LLLT, in this chapter we employ various terms that are used in the literature.

LIGHT APPLICATION

Phototherapy is applied via two main pathways: directly on the body and skin for an action on cellular metabolism, and through the eyes for an action on the visual system. Both pathways are the subject of intensive ongoing medical research.

Major mechanisms for the first pathway (light on skin) have been elucidated since the 1990s through the work of pioneering researchers such as Prof. Tiina Karu in Russia (Karu 2007). *Photobiomodulation*, which denotes the ability of light to modulate biological functions and accelerate cellular metabolism, is mainly activated by red and near-infrared colors. Other light-on-skin modalities make use of the photooxidative properties of light to sterilize and destroy infectious pathogens, mainly with blue, violet, and ultraviolet colors.

The profound influence of the second pathway (light through the eyes) has been medically recognized only since the early 2000s, following the discovery of what is now known as the *non-visual, or non-image-forming (NIF)* optic pathway. This previously unknown pathway reveals a direct link between the eye's retina and the hypothalamus, at the core of the brain. Through it, light controls our circadian rhythm and our hormonal balance. These powerful chronobiological effects are mostly driven by the blue part of the spectrum.

Both pathways can also be used to apply colored light or *chromotherapy*. In this modality, the influence exerted by light is not so much related to the purely biochemical effects mentioned above, but rather to the interaction of specific colors with biofields (when shone on the body) as well as with cognition (through the visual system).

LIGHT PLACEMENT

For light received primarily through the eyes, this can be done with exposure to direct light or to reflected light. With applications through the skin, another consideration is the placement of light. One obvious limitation is the size of the light beam. Lasers provide an intense narrow beam ideal for acupuncture points, whereas the area covered by LEDs depends on the number of LEDs within the array used. A few systems exist that expose the entire body (back and front) to light simultaneously in large chambers.

Generally, lights are placed directly at the area that requires treatment. In other cases, acupuncture points are used on the body, ear, hand, and foot generally with low intensity lasers. The light can be placed near specific organs or glands (liver, kidney, thyroid, lymph nodes, etc.) as well as in the mouth (for dentistry). Treatment of the head can be done transcranially or through the nose (intranasal). Light can penetrate the skull at longer wavelengths provided it has sufficient intensity. Intranasal exposure is beneficial because this part of the body is highly vascularized and a portion of that blood enters the brain. Certain chemicals that would otherwise be delayed or possibly be destroyed going through the digestive system can be introduced to the body through nasal sprays.

A 20- to 30-minute intranasal light treatment exposes the blood in the entire body several times to light. Nasal light therapy was originally used for rhinitis and sinusitis and later to treat the cardiovascular, central nervous, and immune systems. This type of exposure may benefit patients who have neurological brain disorders like depression, anxiety, multiple sclerosis, Parkinson's disease, attention deficit disorder (ADD/ADHD), or who have experienced traumatic brain injury or post-traumatic stress disorder (PTSD) (Naeser et al. 2014).

COLOR

Color[2] is a function of wavelength and frequency as shown in Table 20.1. Higher frequencies and shorter wavelengths have more energy and beyond the near UV this "light" has enough energy to break chemical bonds. In other words, blue light has a higher frequency, a shorter wavelength, and

TABLE 20.1
Wavelength, Frequency, and Photon Energy from Infrared, Visible and Ultraviolet Light

Color	Wavelength nm	Frequency THz	Energy eV
Mid to far infrared	>2500	<120	<0.5
Near infrared	2500–700	120–430	0.5–1.8
Red	700–620	430–480	1.8–2.0
Orange	620–590	480–510	2.0–2.1
Yellow	590–570	510–530	2.1–2.2
Green	570–495	530–610	2.2–2.5
Blue	495–450	610–670	2.5–2.8
Violet	450–400	670–750	2.8–3.1
Near ultraviolet	400–320	750–950	3.1–4.0

Note: Values are approximate.

The visible spectrum wavelength in nm

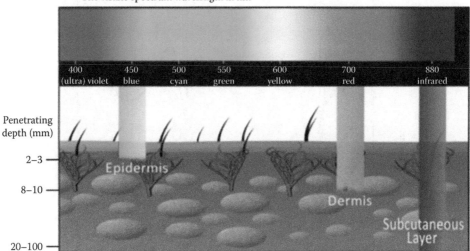

FIGURE 20.1 Depth of visible light penetration at different wavelengths. The longer the wavelength (red and infrared), the deeper the penetration. Blue light tends to be used for surface skin tissues and red/infrared for improved circulation and pain reduction.

more energy than red light. Most light therapies use light at either end of the visible spectrum (red/infrared and blue/violet), although with LEDs and filters more color options are available and green and yellow lasers are also now available.

Depth of penetration is a function of color (wavelength) and skin pigmentation. Longer waves (infrared/red) penetrate more deeply into the body than shorter (blue/violet) wavelengths (Figure 20.1), and intermediate wavelengths (yellow/green) have intermediate depths of penetration. Consequently, blue/violet lights are used for skin problems and red/infrared lights are used to promote deep tissue circulation and to stimulate mitochondrial adenosine triphosphate (ATP) production.

Different molecules in the body preferentially absorb different wavelengths and it is this absorbed energy that has biological effects. Knowing the absorption spectrum is necessary to determine the effect of the various colors. Optimal absorption of water, for example, is blue light (405 nm) and of hemoglobin and melanin is green and yellow light (~532 nm) (Figure 20.2).

According to Weber (2015), red light stimulates the immune system, increases ATP production, and has photosensitizing effects on hematoporphyrins and chlorines. Yellow light has a detoxifying and antidepressive effect and boosts serotonin and vitamin D metabolism and photosensitizing effect on hypericin. Green light increases oxygen supply and mitochondrial ATP production. Blue light increases nitric oxide (NO) production, stimulates microcirculation, and has an antibacterial effect.

DOSAGE

While depth of penetration is color dependent, the amount of light that reaches the tissue or cell is a function of intensity and duration of exposure. High intensity lasers (also referred to as "hard" class IV lasers) provide photon energies that may be damaging to the skin and tissue and are used, for example, in medical surgical settings by licensed practitioners. Low intensity (soft) lasers providing between 1 and 500 mW of power are class III lasers and are classified as low-level laser therapy (LLLT).

The longer the exposure time the more energy that reaches the cells. However, more is not necessarily better when it comes to intensity and/or exposure time as with dosage of certain types of medication. In most cases, exposures consist of a 5- to 20-minute treatment several times a week for

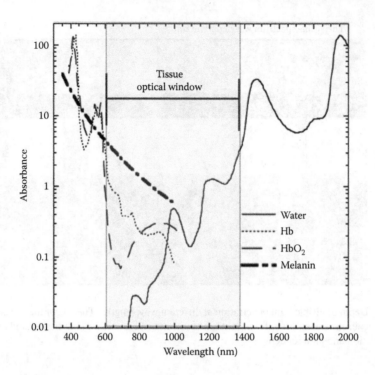

FIGURE 20.2 Absorption spectra of the main chromophores in living tissue on a log scale showing the optical window where visible and near infrared (NIR) light can penetrate deepest into tissue. (From Huang Y-Y. et al. 2009. *Dose Response* 7(4): 358–383.)

as many weeks as are necessary for the desired benefits. In some cases, a single 20-minute treatment may be enough to reduce swelling and improve circulation (Plate 20.1, Table 20.2).

EXPOSURE PARAMETERS

Exposure parameters that need to be considered are time of day since the body has its own circadian rhythm. Blue light at night reduces melatonin production and can impair sleep. However, exposure to white light with a high blue to red spectral ratio in the morning or during the day provides cognitive stimulation and enhances wakefulness.

MODULATION

Light can be modulated or pulsed and some believe this makes the light therapy even more effective. Indeed, therapeutic devices that use pulse electromagnetic field (PEMF) without light provide similar therapeutic benefits as those discussed in this chapter for light. Lights can be modulated at different frequencies and with different waveforms or wave shapes (sinusoidal, square wave, saw toothed wave, etc.) that have additional biological effects. Parameters that can be manipulated with the pulse structure are peak power (mW), pulse frequency (Hz), pulse width (ns), and duty cycle (% of time the pulse is on vs. off). A duty cycle of 100% implies that there is no pulse modulation of the light and the light is constantly "on."

Pulsation patterns are built in with certain devices and may include:

1. The earth's Schumann resonance frequencies (~8 Hz and harmonics 16, 32, 64, etc.);
2. Brain wave frequencies that correspond to deep, dreamless sleep (delta 1–3 Hz); drowsy, light sleep (theta 4–8 Hz); relaxed, meditative state (alpha 9–14 Hz); awake, alert, actively engaged (beta 15–30 Hz); and hyperactive (gamma >30 Hz) brain waves;

3. Nogier frequencies that resonant with different parts of the body (292 Hz for cellular vitality resonates with ectoderm; 584 Hz for nutritional metabolism resonates with endoderm; 1168 Hz for movement resonates with mesoderm; 2336 Hz for balancing both sides of the brain; 4672 Hz for nerves, spinal and skin disorders and pain control; harmonics of 73 Hz for emotional reactions resonates with subcortical or lower regions of the brain; and harmonics of 146 Hz for intellectual organization, resonates with cerebral cortex.)

LIGHT SOURCE FOR PHOTOBIOMODULATION

The light source can be coherent (lasers) or incoherent (solar, halogen, fluorescent, or LED lights) and may be linearly or circularly polarized. At low power (less than 500 mW) it is referred to as LLLT. Light sources differ in irradiance as measured by power density (mW/cm²).

While there is considerable controversy as to whether lasers or other light sources—like LEDs—provide the best therapy, what is safe to say is that they all work provided they are applied at the appropriate wavelength (color), intensity, and dose for the condition treated to either stimulate or inhibit a particular reaction.

Disadvantages of lasers is that they can damage eyes and are much more expensive with fewer color choices than LEDs or halogen lights (Starwynn 2004). A disadvantage of some LEDs is that they may not have enough photon energy to elicit a response.

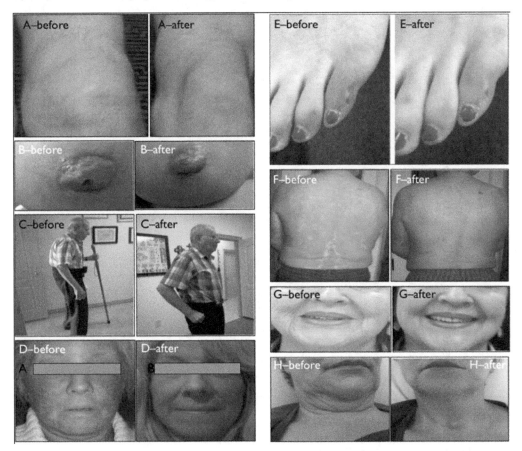

PLATE 20.1 Before and after light therapy for (A) swelling; (B) infection and scar tissue MRSA; (C) back problems; (D) scleroderma; (E) bruising; (G) wrinkles; and (H) sagging skin. Light treatments ranged from one 20-minute session (E) to several months of weekly treatments (C). For treatment parameters refer to Table 20.2.

TABLE 20.2

Treatments Applied to Patients in Plate 20.1 Using LED Lights

		Placement of LED Lights	Exposure per Treatment (minutes)	Number of Treatments	Comments
A	Swollen knee	Wrapped pad around knee	20	1 session	
B	Breast with MRSA infection	Initially with red/infrared & then with blue/infrared	20	3 per week for 3.5 weeks	One week after the last photo was taken, the infection had completely healed.
C	Posture issues	Pads placed on the whole spine	15	4 sessions over a period of 3.5 weeks	86-year-old diabetic male; able to stand straighter with no lower back brace and no cane; able to reduce insulin injections by 50%.
D	Scleroderma	Applied to face (normally multiple areas of application on various body parts for a total of 60 minutes with 20 minutes per area of application)	60	Daily for 8.5 months	Patient was prescribed prednisone, methyltrexate, and zithromax and symptoms cleared but started showing liver and kidney damage. She was weaned off medication over a period of 8.5 months and is now using only light therapy to control her symptoms.
E	Bruise on toe	Applied to toes	20	1 session	31-year-old diabetic.
F	Psoriasis	Applied to area affected and to liver	60	14 sessions	Major complaint was pain especially when lying down; all medications had failed; after 7 sessions pain resolved; after 14 sessions area had cleared; no additional treatment given and psoriasis has not recurred.
G	Facial wrinkles	Applied to face	20	2 per week for 5 weeks	
H	Sagging skin	Applied to neck	20	2 per week for 5 weeks; before bed (should be daily before bed for 5 weeks)	

Response to light energy is biphasic, which means that stimulation occurs above a certain low-level energy threshold and increases to a maximum. Further increases in irradiance decrease beneficial effects and, above an upper energy threshold, may damage cells.

MEDICAL DEVICES AND GOVERNMENT ACCEPTANCE

The Food and Drug Administration (FDA) in the United States defines a medical device that requires a 510(k) as, "an instrument, implement, machine, contrivance, implant, *in vitro* reagent or other similar or related article, including a component part, or accessory which is intended to affect the structure or ANY function of the body of man ...." Phototherapeutic devices fall within this category.

A device that has low risk (colored eye glasses, colored film for reading) are *medically exempt*. A device that the FDA has determined to be substantially equivalent to another legally marketed device may receive *FDA clearance*, and a device that requires *approval* is generally reserved for high-risk medical devices that involve more rigorous premarket review than the 510(k) pathway.

Classification of a medical device is based on its intended use and the risk it places on a patient or user. Class I devices have the lowest risk and Class III devices the greatest risk. Various light therapeutic devices have FDA 510(k) clearance as a Class II medical device for reducing pain and increasing circulation.

In Canada approval comes from the Medical Devices Bureau within the Therapeutic Products Directorate of Health Canada. Health Canada "is the federal authority that regulates pharmaceutical drugs and medical devices for human use. Prior to being given market authorization, a manufacturer must present substantive scientific evidence of a product's safety, efficacy and quality as required by the *Food and Drugs Act and Regulations*" (Health Canada 2014). Private citizens can purchase devices that don't have medical clearance if these devices are restricted to personal use.

In Europe, phototherapeutic devices require a CE-Certification. The European Union Medical Devices Directive is currently undergoing revisions.

Health care practitioners need to select devices that have federal approval if they want to treat patients. A growing number of health care practitioners use light therapy including medical doctors, acupuncturists, chiropractors (pain), dentists (disinfection with lasers; temporomandibular joint dysfunction or TMJD), estheticians (wrinkles), naturopaths (wellness), physiotherapists (pain, inflammation), psychologists (depression or anxiety) as well as veterinarians (pain and wound healing). Indeed, veterinarians have used light therapy, particularly on racehorses, since the 1980s and provided much of our early understanding of the physiologic influence of light on living tissue. These devices are also used by people with chronic pain and limited mobility as well as by top-level athletes who want to recover quickly following strenuous physical exercise.

MECHANISMS OF PHOTOBIOMODULATION

The fundamental principle of LLLT is that for the treatment to have an effect on a living system, the photon has to be absorbed by a photoacceptor or chromophore (Sutherland 2002). *Chromophore* refers to a group of atoms or molecules whose presence is responsible for the color of the compound. Chromophores work in one of two ways. Either they absorb photons of light (NIR to UV) that cause electrons to move from their ground state to an excited state (electronic transition) or they absorb photons that cause them to resonantly vibrate or twist in response to infrared radiation.

Common biologically important compounds that have an electronic transition include chlorophyll in plants, oxy- and deoxy-hemoglobin, melanin, vitamin B12, cytochrome-c-oxydase, NADH-dehydrogenase, and so on; while water is an example of a vibrational transition. The specific wavelengths that are absorbed by different chromophores are referred to as the action spectrum.

Knowledge of the action spectrum for each chromophore helps determine which mechanisms are stimulated by various colors. For example, the respiratory chain in the mitochondria begins with NADH-dehydrogenase that absorbs blue light, and ends with cytochrome-c-oxydase that absorbs red/infrared light (Weber 2015). So, a combination of red and blue lights may have a greater effect on mitochondrial respiration than either red or blue lights alone.

Light therapy works at the subcellular level by increasing production of NO and ATP. Both NO and ATP are critical for virtually all metabolic activities in cells and tissues and thus they affect many physiological and biochemical functions within the body. An excellent discussion paper (Amat et al. 2006) hypothesizes that the electric field induced by light explains cellular responses to electromagnetic energy. Examples are provided regarding the mechanisms involved that include not only the production of ATP and NO but other reactive oxygen species (ROS) as well as effects on the Na^+/K^+ ATPase pump, intracellular Ca^{2+} concentrations, and on enzymatic activity that occurs in the presence or absence of chromophores like cytochrome c.

Nitric Oxide (NO)

Nitric oxide (NO) is a free radical that exists as a gas with a half-life of less than 1 second. It is one of the most important signaling molecules in the body of mammals, including humans. Robert F. Furchgott, Louis J. Ignarro, and Ferid Murad won the Nobel Prize for Physiology or Medicine in 1998 for their discoveries concerning nitric oxide as a major signaling molecule in the cardiovascular system. Indeed, NO plays many critical roles in the human body:

1. Cardiovascular system: vasodilatation (improved circulation and increases blood supply to cells), blood cell regulation, myocardial contractility, microvascular permeability;
2. Peripheral nervous system: nerve-mediated relaxation;
3. Central nervous system: learning and memory, pain sensitization, neurodegeneration, blood pressure control;
4. Reproduction: penile erection, pre-term labor;
5. Respiratory system: asthma, bronchodilation;
6. Immunology: unspecific immunity, increases phagocytosis, increases in monocyctes and lymphocytes, inhibition of viral replication, transplant rejection;
7. Cell proliferation: apoptosis, angiogenesis, increases RNA–DNA synthesis;
8. Cell regeneration: mobilization and targeted differentiation of stem cells, enhanced wound healing;
9. Skeletal system: increases bone mineralization (reduces osteoporosis);
10. Lymphatic system: increases lymphatic activity (decreases swelling in extremities).

Levels of NO generated by nitric oxide synthase (NOS) decrease with age. An insufficient amount of NO can result in atherosclerosis, Alzheimer's disease, chronic inflammation, erectile dysfunction, immune dysfunction, hypertension, peripheral artery disease, thrombosis, and uncontrolled cell proliferation (cancer) (Bryan 2015).

With evidence that light promotes NO production, the potential benefits of light therapy go well beyond just circulation and pain.

Adenosine Triphosphate (ATP)

Cells require energy to do work and this energy is generated within the mitochondria and stored as ATP. ATP is required for cellular metabolism, nerve conduction, muscle contraction, and cellular replication, and is the energy currency of the cell. ATP production is reduced when circulation is poor. In the absence of enough ATP, nerve cells express pain and hyper-excitability, wound healing is slowed, and cell death occurs more rapidly (aging). "Mitochondrial dysfunction" is a good indicator of chronic fatigue syndrome (Myhill et al. 2009) and may be linked to cardiovascular disease, diabetes, aging, Alzheimer's disease and Parkinson's disease (Greenamyre et al. 1999, Onyango et al. 2016). Since light therapy promotes mitochondrial activity it may also benefit these illnesses. Clearly more research is needed in this area.

Near infrared to red light activates the electron transport chain in mitochondrial membranes and stimulates ATP production by up to 150% (Hode and Tunér 2014). Increases in ATP result in enhanced cellular activity, improved muscle contraction, increased body energy levels, and improved nerve conduction. Low power lasers using monochromatic visible light stimulate DNA production, promote normal cell growth and many basic functions of living organisms (Karu 1989).

Combined with the beneficial effects of NO production and increased circulation, oxygenation of the cells, pain reduction and accelerated wound healing, light can be a powerful agent in promoting health by stimulating biochemical changes within the body rather than masking symptoms more common with certain drugs.

POTENTIAL APPLICATIONS OF PHOTOBIOMODULATION

The FDA has cleared some phototherapeutic devices for improved circulation and pain reduction, but improved circulation can have multiple benefits other than pain relief. Some of those potential applications are provided here. See Plate 20.1 for images related to some of the applications below.

A short guide that outlines therapeutic protocols for light (Cartier 2013) lists the following applications in the table of contents. Note that protocols vary with different devices.

1. Periarticular disorder: bursitis, TMJ, chronic inflammatory conditions, tendonitis, plantar fasciitis, epicondylitis, skin splints, neuritis, synovitis;
2. Neuralgia: Bell's palsy, post hepatic herpes zoraster;
3. Other: Tinea corporis, cellulitis, osteomyelitis;
4. Range of motion deficits: frozen shoulder, contractures;
5. Orthopedic: non-union joint fractures, degenerative disc disease, low back pain, intervertebral disc herniation;
6. Post-surgical: total knee arthroplasty, total hip arthroplasty, rotator cuff repair, knee surgery–bursitis and injury, foot surgery;
7. Trauma: bruise, strain, sprain;
8. Wounds: venous stasis, pressure ulcers (arterial), diabetic ulcers, venous insufficiency;
9. Circulation conditions (Plate 20.1);
10. Fibromyalgia: pain management;
11. Nerve entrapments;
12. Carpal tunnel syndrome;
13. Scleroderma (Plate 20.1);
14. Hypothyroid;
15. Acne (Plate 20.1).

CIRCULATION AND PAIN

Photobiomodulation devices are known to improve circulation and to reduce pain. Impaired circulation, chronic or acute, deprives cells of oxygen and other vital nutrients, allows the buildup of waste products, and is often signaled as pain. Light can be used to manage pain or, in some cases, to eliminate it entirely. Light can be used to treat neuropathy, trigeminal neuralgia, somatic pain, headaches, muscle spasms, radioculopathy, and lumbago (Harkless et al. 2006).

INFLAMMATION

Inflammatory disorders (-itis) can benefit from light therapy including cardiovascular disease that is considered to have an inflammatory basis, peripheral vascular disease, arthritis, tendonitis, cellulitis, plantar fasciitis, rheumatoid arthritis, psoriasis, and eczema.

According to Avci et al. (2013), inflammatory diseases such as psoriasis and acne can be managed with light therapy that is noninvasive with almost complete absence of side effects.

"The mechanism for relieving joint pain in RA [rheumatoid arthritis] by low-level light therapy (LLLT) may involve reducing the level of pro-inflammatory cytokines/chemokines produced by synovialcytes. This mechanism may be more general and underlie the beneficial effects of LLLT on other inflammatory conditions" (Yumara et al. 2009).

Interestingly, cytokines and chemokines have been linked to depression, which may explain at the biochemical level why people with chronic pain are depressed. One of the co-authors (WB) observed improved mood among people treated for chronic pain with light therapy. This mood enhancement may be due to pain relief and/or to the reduction in the inflammatory markers that contribute to depression. So, a "side effect" of light therapy may be a more cheerful mood.

WOUND HEALING

The three stages of post-trauma wound healing include inflammation, proliferation, and remodeling. Inflammation involves mast cells, leukocytes, and macrophages and may take up to 3 or 4 days if there is no infection. Proliferation involves fibroblasts and endotheliocytes and may take between 3 and 21 days. Remodeling during which time fibroblasts are transformed into myofibroblasts may take between 10 days and 6 months depending on the extent and severity of the injury. Light therapy accelerates the first two stages of wound healing but may have little impact on remodeling (Wunsch 2016a,b).

By enhancing circulation, light therapy is known to promote wound healing and that includes diabetic wounds especially in the feet and legs, surgical incisions, bruises, acne, scar tissue, pressure ulcers, stretch marks, and burns (Plate 20.1).

Significant improvements have been observed in second-degree burns treated right away for a few minutes with blue light. Pain is immediately reduced and blistering and other signs of physical damage are less noticeable 24 hours post-injury.

Polarized-light therapy (400–2000 nm, 40 mW/cm^2, 2.4 J/cm^2) has been successfully used to treat deep dermal burns that would otherwise require surgery (Monstrey et al. 2002). "Polarized-light irradiation resulted in a significantly shorter healing time, with almost no hypertrophic scarring, and optimal aesthetic and functional results at long-term follow-up." Wound closure was achieved within 12–21 days depending on the age of the patient, with older patients taking longer to recover.

Diabetic wounds are often called "non-healing wounds" because circulation is poor and mitochondrial function of the cell tissue surrounding the non-healing wound is sluggish. The application of lights for a period of 6–8 weeks has been shown to accelerate the healing of such diabetic wounds or ulcers to the point that surgical amputations of digits and limbs has been averted (Havas 2016). Poor circulation in diabetics can result in peripheral neuropathy and infections like gangrene, both of which can be treated with light therapy (Kochman et al. 2002; Schindl et al. 1998).

With *surgical incisions*, application of lights can help promote healing and reduce scar formation (Agrawal et al. 2014).

Bruises are the result of trauma to the tissue that breaks the underlying blood vessels. Lights increase blood flow to the damaged tissue and stimulate the growth of new blood vessels reducing bruising. In one study, laser treatment resulted in a 63% mean improvement in bruising within 48–72 hours following facial cosmetic surgery (DeFatta et al. 2009).

Scar tissue is the result of inadequate circulation and interrupted cellular replication and can interfere with the flow of molecules and energy within the body. Light can significantly reduce scar formation that is often noticeable after just one treatment (Barolet and Boucher 2010).

Acne can be due to excessive production of testosterone, bacterial infection, and reactions to various foods or chemicals in the environment. When the primary cause is bacterial, application of blue light creates a cytotoxic environment and supports the antibacterial, immune response (Momen and Al-Niaimi 2015).

Pressure ulcers are wounds caused by unrelieved pressure on boney prominences of the body and typically occur in facilities and situations where people are bed bound and unable to move without help. The unrelieved pressure stops the circulation to the tissue and results in cell/tissue death. Light that promotes circulation and angiogenesis promotes healing and reduces pain.

Hematomas are similar to bruises and are the result of trauma to the tissue breaking blood vessels under the skin resulting in blood pooling and coagulation. Lights increase circulation of the nutrients and chemicals necessary to dissolve and repair the damage (Calderhead et al. 2015).

Non-union *bone fractures* have been treated for decades with pulsed electromagnetic fields (Bassett et al. 1981). Red and infrared lights penetrate more deeply into the tissue than light at shorter wavelengths (blue) and release nitric oxide that stimulate bone remineralization and facilitate bone fracture healing (Trelles and Mayayo 1987; Shakouri et al. 2010).

ATTENTION DEFICIT HYPERACTIVITY DISORDER (ADHD)

Evidence strongly suggests a reduction in blood flow in the prefrontal cortex for ADHD individuals, which is what happens in a highly stressed normal adult. This region can be likened to a "braking" region in the brain, in which inhibitory judgment and control of behaviors is thought to occur. Therefore, under activity in this critical brain region, either via deficiency in blood flow or chemical signaling agents and processes is thought to reduce the ability of the individual to inhibit unwanted responses and behaviors. As a result, impulsive behavior, which is a hallmark characteristic of ADHD, is more likely to occur if this brain region is underactive. Light treatment results are rapid, generally within a few minutes, but need to be repeated for lasting benefits.

TRAUMATIC BRAIN INJURY (TBI)

Traumatic brain injury is the result of a significant physical trauma to the head. According to Defense Advance Research Project Agency (DARPA), light therapy applied just after the injury, during the "golden window," may prevent TBI physiologic and behavioral effects. In one study with 5 veterans who had multiple TBI, the vascular pathways in the brain were mapped, and after 12 weeks of light therapy administered 3 times a week changes were significant. Areas that were hyperactive were calmed down and other areas showed revascularization. Significant improvements were also noted in behavior of the veterans. Most of these veterans also had PTSD and there were vast improvements in these symptoms as well. Authors concluded, "These results show statistically significant, preclinical outcomes that support the use of NIR treatment after TBI [traumatic brain injury] in effecting changes at the behavioral, cellular, and chemical levels," (Quirk et al. 2012).

POST-TRAUMATIC STRESS DISORDER (PTSD)

Historically, PTSD was thought to be a mental disorder. Current research shows PTSD to be a physical malady that has both psychological and physical manifestations. PTSD pathology functions as a physiologic disturbance of the autonomic nervous system. In one study (Kim et al. 2007), PTSD patients showed a decreased cerebral blood flow in the right thalamus. Light therapy can increase blood flow and when applied to the skull will pass transcranially (through the skull and to the brain) and may provide some relief from those suffering from PTSD and could be used in conjunction with other therapeutic modalities.

ATHLETIC PERFORMANCE AND RECOVERY

Athletes are using light therapy to enhance their performance and recovery after strenuous physical activity. Light therapy applied before resistance exercise can enhance contraction function, reduce the fatigue response, and prevent exercise-induced cell damage. Optimal time is 3 hours before exercising. Phototherapy administered before resistance exercise has been found to have both ergogenic benefits by enhancing physical performance, stamina, and/or recovery and prophylactic benefits to skeletal muscle. In one study (Vanin et al. 2016), pre-exercise LLLT, with 50 J dose, significantly increased performance and improved biochemical markers related to skeletal muscle damage and inflammation.

Light therapy applied after resistance exercise can delay the onset of fatigue and improve post-exercise recovery of strength and function. Sore muscles and stiffness the day following strenuous exercise can be virtually eliminated with post-exercise light therapy. In one study, Ferraresi et al. (2016), used red, NIR, and red/NIR and reported that photobiomodulation increased muscle mass gained after training, and decreased inflammation and oxidative stress in muscle.

WRINKLES AND ANTI-AGING

"The treated subjects experienced significantly improved skin complexion and skin feeling, profilometrically [PBM] assessed skin roughness, and ultrasonographically measured collagen density. PBM has demonstrated efficacy and safety for skin rejuvenation and intradermal collagen increase when compared with controls" (Wunsch and Matuschka 2014). Results are noticeable with ultrasound scans after 15 light treatments (Wunsch 2016a,b).

> LED, which is a novel light source for non-thermal, non-ablative skin rejuvenation, has been shown to be effective for improving wrinkles and skin laxity (Plate 20.1).

In summary, light therapy increases ATP and nitric oxide production, which in turn improves circulation and wound healing; reduces inflammation, pain, muscle spasms and muscular tension; and improves post-exercise recovery. Light therapy is an effective, non-invasive tool that can be used to promote wellness and to treat both chronic and acute injury.

CHRONOBIOLOGICAL APPLICATIONS OF LIGHT

Chronobiology is the science of biological rhythms controlled by the cycles of nature, the primary one being that of the day—the *circadian* rhythm, driven by the light of the sun. Its effect is so fundamental that nearly half of all the activity of our genes is under its influence (Zhang et al. 2014).

Since early in the twentieth century biologists suspected that light's circadian influence extended beyond our sense of vision (Hollwich 1948), but it was only from 2000 that its mechanisms were finally elucidated. A new pathway within the optic nerve was discovered, distinct from the main visual pathway linking the retina to the visual cortex at the back of the brain. This non-visual pathway directly connects the retina to a central region of the brain, the *suprachiasmatic nucleus* (SCN), the area of the hypothalamus that governs our internal clock (Hattar et al. 2002; Figure 20.3a).

The non-visual pathway originates from specialized photoreceptors within the retina, distinct from the rods and cones photoreceptors used for the sense of vision. These non-visual receptors, named *intrinsically photoreceptive retinal ganglion cells* (ipRGC), are mostly sensitive to the blue part of the spectrum in the range of 460–490 nm (Brainard et al. 2001). Sunlight has an abundant proportion of this blue color only during midday, providing a clear signal to entrain and synchronize

(a)

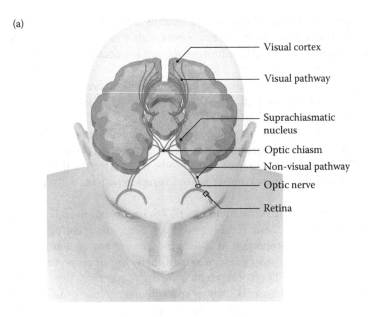

(b)

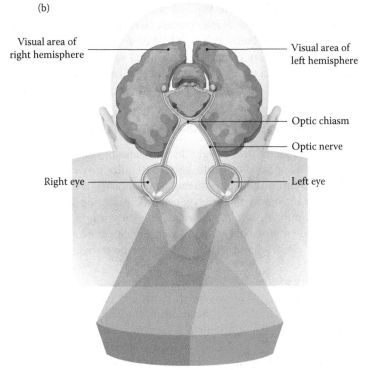

FIGURE 20.3 (a) The two pathways of the optic nerve: visual (in red) and non-visual (in blue); (b) the laterality of the visual system.

our inner clock with the circadian rhythm. The SCN, in turn, controls our master glands and regulates the secretion cycles of key hormones, such as melatonin (the "darkness hormone") from the pineal, and ACTH from the pituitary (which ultimately controls cortisone, the "stress hormone").

This intimate relation between our hormonal balance and light has led to one of the most famous types of light therapy, known as *bright light therapy (BLT)*, which simply consists of looking at a source of intense light. Practiced since the pioneering work of Dr. Norman Rosenthal in the 1980s (Rosenthal et al. 1984), bright light therapy is now widely recognized as an effective treatment for *seasonal affective disorder* (SAD), a form of depression occurring during winter and caused by a chronic lack of light (Golden et al. 2005). Typically, this is done with a 10,000 lux light box for periods of 30–90 minutes; studies have also demonstrated good results with light intensities reduced to as low as 2500 lux (Alotaibi et al. 2016). As a comparison, indoor light is approximately 50–200 lux, while sunlight can be as bright as 100,000 lux.

BLT is being applied in the treatment of many disorders besides SAD, including sleep disorders (Van Maanen et al. 2016), jet-lag, bipolar disorders, eating disorders, and Parkinson's disease (Willis et al. 2012). BLT has also been shown to be more effective than one of the most common pharmacological anti-depressants (fluoxetine or Prozac) in patients suffering from major depressive disorders (Lam et al. 2016).

To properly entrain our circadian rhythm, a BLT source needs to emit a sufficient amount of blue light to stimulate the retina's ipRGC photoreceptors. Since the spectrum of classical incandescent bulbs only contains a low proportion of blue light, they are not very effective for this application. Fluorescent and LED emitters can generate a significantly higher proportion of blue and are therefore preferred for BLT. Some LED models producing pure blue or cyan light require less intensity than white sources for equal effectiveness, as their spectrum more closely matches that of the ipRGCs.

Conversely, the blue-enriched light emitted by fluorescent and LED sources is considered problematic in some ambient-lighting applications because of its increased potential to interfere with the viewers' circadian rhythm. This is, for example, the case with indoor lighting in the evening or at night, where LED or fluorescent light bulbs with high blue content (corresponding to correlated color temperatures above 3000 K) can delay or prevent the natural secretion of melatonin linked to the onset of sleep (Chang et al. 2015). In the long term, such circadian disruption can have an influence on numerous pathologies including obesity, diabetes, heart problems, and cancer (Zubidat et al. 2015).

CHROMOTHERAPY AND THE IMPORTANCE OF COLOR

One of the most important characteristics of light that regulates physiological response is its color. Ever since the sense of vision appeared on Earth, about 540 million years ago, color has played an essential role in biology. Within a short time span, in evolutionary terms, life developed a great number of *chromophores*, or biological molecules capable of interacting with light and colors. Many creatures, both vegetal and animal, became adorned with the most brilliant colors to stand out sharply from the background environment and attract or threaten more effectively. In parallel with this, animal eyes and their related brain structures became better adapted at perceiving all the subtleties of color.

This heightened sensitivity to color is wired in our own brains as well: the most brilliant colors inescapably captivate our attention. Who among us is not entranced by the lustrous hues of the rainbow? In many ancient cultures, this fascination naturally led to an association of color with quasi-supernatural properties. The Cro-Magnons, for example, carefully placed vividly colored beads in their tombs among the precious objects needed in the afterlife. The painters of Lascaux had already mastered the art of preparing colored pigments for their masterpieces 17,000 years ago. The Egyptians had a highly refined science of color, and the monochromatic iridescence of the scarab gave it divine status as a representation of Khepri, a solar aspect of the great god Ra (Egyptian sun god).

The therapeutic use of sunlight, known as *heliotherapy*, was common in antiquity, whether in Egypt, Greece, or Rome. Separately from this use of the sun's white full-spectrum light, there gradually emerged sophisticated systems of healing with colors, or *chromotherapy*. Some of the earliest records can be found in India's Ayurvedic medicine: the Atharvan Veda, dating from 1500 bce,[3] which describes the healing powers of colored light and is considered as important as food and medicinal remedies. China's traditional medicine associates each organ with a specific color.

Closer to us, the great Arabian physician Avicenna ascribed much importance to the role of color for both diagnostic and treatment purposes, as attested to in his *Canon of Medicine* from 1025 CE.[4] Avicenna had devised a special treatment alcove where he would expose his patients to the sun's rays filtered by tinted glass panels—a new technological advance recently perfected by famed Arabian glass workers which produced light of unprecedented chromatic purity. Their techniques soon migrated to Europe and led to the wondrous stained-glass windows of the great cathedrals, the colored rays of which were considered to be a source of healing.

The advent of the scientific age brought new attempts to understand the nature of light and color. Early pioneers, such as Newton and Goethe, were among the first to analyze the properties of colors and to organize them along circular diagrams known as chromatic wheels or color circles (Figure 20.4). In Goethe's version both ends of the rainbow spectrum, the deep red and the violet, merge into magenta, a new synthetic color nowhere to be found in the rainbow itself.

Many nineteenth century researchers explored the effects of colored light on plants, animals, and humans, notably the Americans Augustus Pleasanton and Seth Pancoast in the 1870s. Perhaps the most influential of these early researchers was Dr. Edwin Babbitt, whose 1878 treatise *Principles of Light and Color* inspired the following generation of chromotherapy pioneers in the early twentieth century. This period was a true golden age for light therapy, as light was being applied to numerous medical treatments by physicians such as Dr. Auguste Rollier, Dr. John Harvey Kellogg, and most famously by Dr. Niels Ryberg Finsen, who was awarded the 1903 Nobel Prize in medicine for his work on healing *Lupus vulgaris* (skin condition), which is caused by tuberculosis bacteria, using primarily ultraviolet light.

During this time, new, more sophisticated chromotherapy systems also appeared. One of the most significant was the *Spectro-Chrome* system developed from the 1920s by Dinshah Ghadiali, who defined a set of 12 standardized colors covering the visible spectrum and assigned specific therapeutic properties to them (Figure 20.5). Dinshah devised treatments (which he called *tonations*) for a wide variety of conditions, involving the projection of colored light on various parts of the body during sessions lasting up to an hour.

The optometrist Harry Riley Spitler, a contemporary of Dinshah, was one of the first to systematically explore the therapeutic applications of colored light via the eyes. His *Syntonic phototherapy* method was based on the use of color to re-establish the equilibrium of the autonomous nervous system (ANS), a key factor in many chronic illnesses (Figure 20.6). Spitler observed that

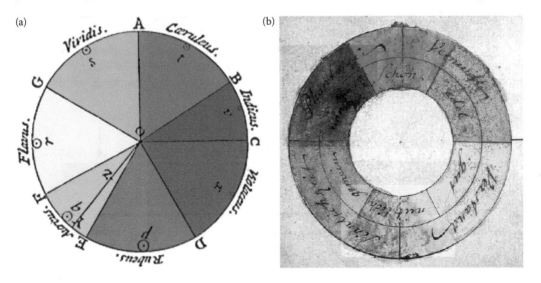

FIGURE 20.4 (a) Newton's chromatic wheel with seven colors (1660s) and (b) Goethe's chromatic wheel with six colors (1809).

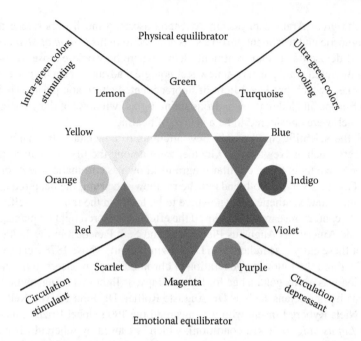

FIGURE 20.5 Dinshah's Spectro-Chrome chromatic wheel.

the long-wavelength end of the spectrum (red, orange, yellow) appeared to stimulate the sympathetic branch of the ANS, while the short-wavelength end (blue, indigo, violet) stimulated the parasympathetic branch.

This era of chromotherapeutic creativity was to be short-lived. Following the discovery of new powerful biochemical drugs (such as antibiotics in 1937 that could act more rapidly and reliably than the subtler light-based modalities) and the subsequent rise of the pharmaceutical industry, light therapy was gradually eclipsed along with most other "alternative" methods like naturopathy or homeopathy. In the United States, the FDA sued light therapists such as Spitler and Dinshah and outlawed their equipment (Dinshah was actually sentenced to three years of jail in 1947 and all his documents ordered destroyed). By the 1950s most traces of light-based treatments were erased from the medical system, and light therapy was considered as quackery for much of the remainder of the twentieth century.

Only recently has this situation changed, due to major discoveries—notably those of photobiomodulation and of the non-visual optic pathway mentioned previously—which have restored the fundamental importance of light for health. The early twenty-first century is witnessing an

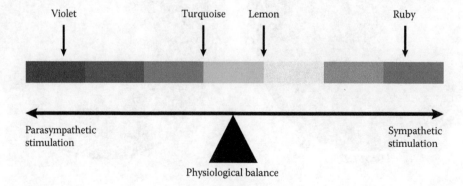

FIGURE 20.6 Spitler's Syntonic physiological balance of the ANS.

unprecedented expansion in research on the biological effects of light and the establishment of a new light medicine. Despite this, the therapeutic role of colors remains somewhat of an enigma for modern medicine. The main reason for this is that the perception of color is not purely a physiological occurrence but also a cognitive one and consequently affects the mind as well as the body, rendering its study particularly challenging.

PRINCIPLES OF CHROMOTHERAPY

Color is an especially complex phenomenon because it acts simultaneously in multiple dimensions: biophysical, energetic, and cognitive.

The *biophysical influence* of color is connected to the action of specific wavelengths of light on the biochemistry of the living cell, the optic pathways, and our hormonal balance. This aspect is readily amenable to the reductionist study of light medicine.

The *energetic influence* of color is connected to the action of light on the systems of "subtle energy" within living organisms. Most models of this biofield recognize that it is closely related to electromagnetic phenomena and therefore readily susceptible to interaction with light photons. This can be conceived, for example, as interplay between light and the acupuncture meridians of traditional Chinese medicine (TCM) which is at the basis of many modern chromotherapy methods.

The *cognitive influence* of color is of the psychological and symbolic order. It is mediated primarily by our sense of vision and derives from different factors, such as ancient evolutionary color associations, cultural color biases, and also our own individual history leading to personal color preferences and aversions. It is also likely exerted through other non-visual optic pathways conveying color information from the retina to various brain areas: the *retinohypothalamic pathway* (the NIF optic pathway introduced earlier in this chapter, reaching the hypothalamus where it can affect mood and alertness) (LeGates et al. 2014), the *retinotectal pathway* (linked to brain structures involved in unconsciously perceived emotional stimuli such as the superior colliculus and the amygdala) (Tamietto and Gelder 2010), and the *accessory optic tract* (connected to the brainstem which regulates physiological functions such as sleep, heart rate, and breathing) (Hill and Marg 1963). Color therefore reaches into every level of our cerebral processes, both conscious and unconscious.

Given this complexity, it is to be expected that the influence of color defies simple definitions and quantification. And, indeed, most biologists and psychologists who studied the subject agree on its intricacy, not least because it depends on so many variables that are difficult to control in a clinical setting, including wavelength, intensity, and the context in which colors are presented (Meier et al. 2012). Studies on the effects of colors on the ANS, cognitive performance (Mehta and Zhu 2009), or cardiorespiratory synchronization (Edelhäuser et al. 2013), for example, often reach opposite conclusions. Therefore, chromotherapy, in its current state, mostly rests on the empirical evidence accumulated by generations of practitioners.

The multidimensionality of the effects of colors also explains why various chromotherapy systems may assign different properties to each color, depending on the level at which they operate. Despite this variety, however, there exists a consensus shared by essentially all modern chromotherapy methods regarding some general principles.

One basic principle is the existence of two main categories of colors: those said to be *warm*, considered to be stimulating, tonic, activating, and those said to be *cool*, considered to be calming, sedative, analgesic. In most systems warm colors range from red to orange and yellow, while cool colors range from green (or turquoise) to blue and indigo. Many systems share Spitler's contention that warm colors stimulate the sympathetic ANS, while the cool ones stimulate the parasympathetic. Mapping these colors on a chromatic wheel reveals two intermediate color ranges: one centered on lime and green, and one around magenta (Figure 20.7). These transition colors are generally considered to have a balancing effect.

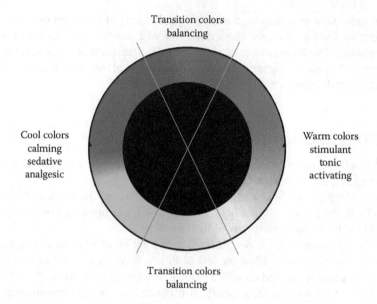

FIGURE 20.7   The warm colors, the cool colors, and the transition colors of chromotherapy.

Another significant principle of chromotherapy is that of *complementary colors*. When a color is found to exert an influence on a specific aspect of health, there usually is an opposite, or complementary, color exerting this influence in the opposite direction. The pair can therefore be used to either amplify or reduce the quality under influence. The exact pairing of complementary colors is usually obtained through the chromatic wheel, either from diagonal opposites or through mirroring, and may vary depending on the chromotherapy method.

TOOLS AND METHODS OF CHROMOTHERAPY

Most chromotherapy methods are based on the application of colored light and require instruments capable of generating and delivering light with precision. These instruments are as varied as are the modalities of chromotherapy. Some are designed to shine light in the eye (as in Syntonic phototherapy), on specific body areas (as in Spectro-Chrome), on specific acupuncture points, on the whole body and biofield, or indirectly through a projection screen.

Two main techniques are available to produce specific colors. The first one relies on a wide-spectrum white light source (such as an incandescent, halogen, or xenon light bulbs) coupled with colored filters. The second uses narrow-band sources such as LEDs (or lasers) which in themselves produce pure colors.

The first technique affords more flexibility in the spectra and bandwidths of end colors, depending on the type and sharpness of the color filter used. While the second technique has a more restricted choice of colors (since commercially available LEDs are manufactured in a limited range of wavelengths), it has the advantage of delivering semi-monochromatic colors.

A SAMPLE OF CHROMOTHERAPY METHODS

There are today a vast number of forms of light therapy based on the influence of colors. We can only list here a few of the major ones having clinical relevance, which are representative of the wide range of modern chromotherapy methods. Some are derivatives of energy medicine modalities, such as acupuncture, and similarly address a general range of pathologies. Some have more specialized applications, for example, treatments targeting the visual system. Some address psychotherapy while others are applied for overall wellness.

Most of these methods fall within two main categories: those that use *light on the skin*, making use of the biophysical and energetic influences of color, and those that use *light through the eyes*, making use of the powerful roles of our optic pathways. And a few combine both modalities to use the global influence of light.

SPECTRO-CHROME METHOD

The Spectro-Chrome method was developed by Dinshah Ghadiali between 1920 and 1940 and enjoyed a substantial following during that period, when it was practiced by many physicians. It was thoroughly discredited after Dinshah's indictment by the FDA in the 1940s and remains today much misunderstood. In the eyes of many light therapists this is unfortunate, and the basic principles of the effects of colors established by Dinshah remain at the core of most contemporary chromotherapy methods.

Dinshah applied colored light on various parts of the body according to protocols he had developed for over 300 pathologies. While few today ascribe such wide-ranging powers to colors, many modern therapists have optimized some of his methods and original instruments and apply them with a significant degree of success in certain applications, such as treating burns and skin problems. The 12 main colors of Spectro-Chrome (www.spektrochrom.de) are now available as standardized filter gels manufactured by Roscolene. Dinshah Ghadiali's son, Darius Dinshah, founded the Dinshah Health Society (www.dinshahhealth.org), which continues to provide educational material (Dinshah 2012) on the Spectro-Chrome method.

SYNTONIC PHOTOTHERAPY

Syntonic phototherapy is another one of the oldest methods of light medicine. Its instigator, Dr. Spitler, founded the *College of Syntonic Optometry* in 1933 (www.collegeofsyntonicoptometry.com), and it has been active ever since. He proposed that applying certain frequencies of light through the eyes could restore balance within the body's regulatory centers, thereby correcting visual dysfunctions at their source. Syntonic phototherapy is mostly employed in the alleviation of ophthalmological and visual problems, but it can also be helpful in a wider range of applications such as improving memory and learning, alleviating ADHD and migraines, as well as accelerating the recovery from head injuries and strokes. An estimated 1300 optometrists from all over the world practice this therapy today.

The instrument Spitler originally designed to shine colored light into the eyes of his patients, the "Syntonizer," has inspired many generations of light therapists who created improved versions as technology progressed. Notable among those were Dr. Jacob Liberman's "Spectral Receptivity Trainer" and Dr. John Downing's "Lumatron" in the 1980s (Plate 20.2). The most advanced versions available today include instruments such as the "PhotonWave" (www.photonwave.be) and the "Photon Stimulator" (www.photonstimulator.com).

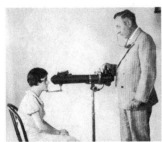 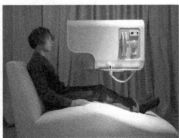 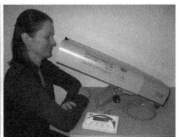

PLATE 20.2 Eye stimulation instruments—Spitler's Syntonizer (1933, left), Downing's Lumatron (1986, center), PhotonWave (2005, right).

COLORPUNCTURE

Colorpuncture™ is a method unifying light and acupuncture (Plate 20.3). It was developed in the 1980s by the German naturopath Peter Mandel (1986) and has since evolved into a sophisticated healing modality called Esogetics™. It involves applying colored light with great precision to acupuncture points, enabling either stimulation or sedation of these points with complementary colors. Its assumption is that deeper layers of the organism can be reached through the transmission of *information* by light. Mandel has established protocols that are appropriate for numerous treatments, both on the physical and energetic levels. Colorpuncture is taught throughout the world (www.esogetics.com, www.colorpunctureusa.org) and numbers about 2500 practitioners. The *Mandel International Institute* is now directed by Mandel's son, Markus Wunderlich.

CHROMATOTHÉRAPIE

Chromatothérapie™ is a sophisticated system combining light with concepts derived from traditional Chinese medicine, developed by the French neuropsychiatrist Christian Agrapart. It has different modalities applying light either through the eyes, on affected body zones, or, in its most advanced form, on acupuncture points. As a basis for his system, Dr. Agrapart associated colors to TCM's four *climatic factors*: red with *heat*, orange with *cold*, green with *dryness*, and blue with *humidity*. Chromatothérapie is presented as a complete medical system (Agrapart 2016), not

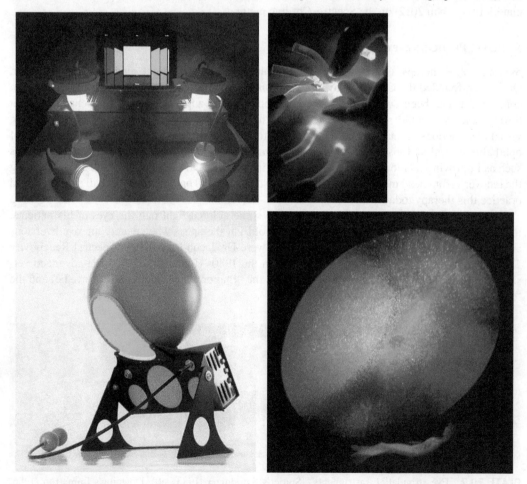

PLATE 20.3   Various devices using color therapy.

in conflict with traditional medicine but rather in complementarity. Its practitioners undergo several years of training (www.chromatotherapie.com) and achieve remarkable results with numerous pathologies, including severe burns, joint inflammation, and brain trauma.

EMOTIONAL TRANSFORMATION THERAPY

Developed by Dr. Steven Vazquez in the United States, Emotional Transformation Therapy (or ETT®) (Vazquez 2014) is a form of psychotherapy based on brain stimulation through the visual pathway. The technique uses pulsing colored light under therapist supervision to access and resolve core emotional memories. ETT involves the application of precise visual stimulation at the exact time emotional distress is active, enabling specific brain mechanisms responsible for a symptom, such as sadness, to be directly targeted resulting in rapid change. Dr. Vazquez's school (www.ett-center.com) has trained over 1000 therapists now practicing the method around the world. ETT is used to treat acute stress, PTSD, addiction, depression, bipolar disorder, anxiety conditions, ADHT, schizophrenia and other psychotic states, insomnia, and chronic pain.

LATERAL LIGHT THERAPY

This powerful light therapy modality was developed in the 1990s by Ukrainian psychiatrist A.P. Chuprikov. It is based on the fact that each side of our visual field is linked to the visual cortex of the opposite brain hemisphere (due to the crossing of optic nerve fibers in the *optic chiasm*), thereby enabling the differential stimulation of each hemisphere through appropriate light patterns (Figure 20.3b). Dr. Chuprikov observed that numerous pathologies can be linked to an imbalance or lack of communication between the two brain hemispheres, and devised methods of rebalancing them with lateral light patterns featuring a stimulating color on one side and a sedative one on the other.

Lateral light therapy found validation in multiple clinical studies (Palienko 2001a) conducted in Ukraine on applications in psychiatry (Chuprikov 1994) as well as for the treatment of chronic illnesses as diverse as hypertension (Palienko 2000), arrhythmia (Palienko 2001b), and rheumatoid arthritis. It is unfortunately little known in the West, probably because most articles were published in Russian only. A few modern chromotherapy systems (such as *Sensora*) are starting to apply lateral light.

SENSORA

Sensora™ is a multisensorial system of integrative therapy. Developed by Canadian physicist Anadi Martel (a co-author of this chapter) and therapist Ma Premo, it combines visual, audio, and kinesthetic stimulation. Its chromotherapy aspect is generated by a *light modulation* process (Ross et al. 2013) in which low-frequency pulsations (in the range of 1/100–50 Hz) are embedded within light projections, enabling the entrainment of biorhythms such as brainwaves and the heartbeat. In addition, it uses light projectors with multiple channels capable of creating complex light patterns suitable for lateral light therapy applications (Plate 20.3).

The Sensora (www.sensora.com) is used as a complementary tool in psychotherapy, hypnotherapy, massage, post-operative convalescence, and palliative care. It can provide effective support in the treatment of depression, burnout, PTSD, insomnia, chronic pain, and fibromyalgia.

VAN OBBERGHEN COLOR THERAPY

The color therapy method of Belgian Pierre Van Obberghen (www.color-institute.com) provides a complete psychological and symbolic interpretation of colors (Van Obberghen 2007) synthesizing the chromotherapeutic knowledge of multiple traditions including Western, Chinese, and Indian.

Van Obberghen has developed a variety of instruments and techniques for the application of colored light through the eyes, on the whole body or on reflex points, with the purpose of inducing physiological reactions that are favorable to the maintenance or the reestablishment of health (Plate 20.3).

Van Obberghen has also devised a *Color Test* method using attraction and aversion to colors to evaluate a person's state. The test provides insight in the emotional relationship that we have with colored objects and is a tool for analyzing personality.

MONOCROM METHOD

The Monocrom method relies on the aesthetic and psychological properties of *monochromatic light*, the light offering colors so highly saturated that their spectra are reduced to a very narrow bandwidth. It was developed by Swedish psychologist Karl Ryberg, who observed, what he calls, that this "super light" induces intense subjective experiences as higher brain functions readily respond to its stimulation. He devised many instruments (www.monocrom.se) capable of delivering monochromatic light (with bandwidth of the order of 10 nm) across the whole visual spectrum, based on wide-band light sources filtered through holographic gratings (Plate 20.3).

In Ryberg's method the user chooses the treatment colors on his or her own, rather than relying on the therapist to do so. Because of the concentrated sensory stimulus exerted by monochromatic light, Monocrom treatments are kept short (5–10 minutes). They are used for alleviating depression or stress and to induce general wellness.

CONCLUSIONS

Light therapy, in the form of heliotherapy and chromotherapy, has been used for thousands of years. Recent advances in lighting technology (LASERs and LEDs) and research on the biological effects of light have stimulated the production and testing of different phototherapeutic devices to treat illness. The FDA recognizes the effectiveness of phototherapy to promote circulation and reduce pain and it has cleared a number of these devices for use in the United States enabling doctors to treat their patients.

Unlike drugs that often mask symptoms, light therapy promotes well-being and healing at the cellular level by stimulating cellular energy production and the release of nitric oxide that creates a cascade of beneficial effects. In its bright light therapy modality, it contributes to restore the natural rhythms of our hormonal balance. Also unlike drugs, low-level light therapy is non-invasive and has virtually no adverse side effects.

While much is known about the effects of light on living tissue, more research is needed to optimize the beneficial effects of phototherapy since intensity, modulation, wavelength, waveform, time, and duration of exposure all influence the healing process. More research on the effects of color is also needed to bring many chromotherapy methods, which are still considered alternative, into the clinical field.

Because light affects us at all levels—cellular, hormonal, and cognitive—its application is remarkably suited to integrative medicine. This is particularly apparent in the case of intractable disorders like depression, with roots in both body and mind, that can be successfully tackled with multiple modalities of phototherapy (photobiomodulation, bright light therapy, and chromotherapy) each acting through a different channel.

As the percentage of people with chronic illness continues to increase and as a growing number of children are born who have physiological and developmental problems, we will need treatments that are effective, safe, and affordable. Phototherapy is one of those treatments.

NOTES

1. With "light" used here as representing the electromagnetic spectrum.
2. Wave length (m) × frequency (Hz) = the speed of light ($\sim 300 \times 10^6$ m/s).

3. BCE, before the Common Era, now replaces BC or before Christ.
4. CE, Common Era, now replaces AD or after death or *Anno Domini*.

REFERENCES

Adey WR. 2004. Potential therapeutic applications of nonthermal electromagnetic fields: Ensemble organization of cells in tissue as a factor in biological field sensing. In *Bioelectromagnetic Medicine*. ed. Rosch PJ and MS Markov. Boca Raton, FL: CRC Press/Taylor & Francis.

Agrapart C. 2016. *Se Soigner Par Les Couleurs*. Sully.

Agrawal T, GK Gupta, V Rai, JD Carroll, and MR Hamblin. 2014. Pre-conditioning with low-level laser (light) therapy: Light before the storm. *Dose Response*. 12(4):619–649.

Alotaibi M, M Halaki, and CM Chow. 2016. A systematic review of light therapy on mood scores in major depressive disorder: Light specification, dose, timing and delivery. *International Journal of Basic and Applied Sciences*, 5(1):30–37.

Amat A, J Rigau, RW Waynant, IK Ilev, and JJ Anders. 2006. The electric field induced by light can explain cellular responses to electromagnetic energy: A hypothesis of mechanism. *Journal of Photochemistry and Photobiology B: Biology* 82:152–160.

Anders JJ, RJ Lanzafame, and PR Arany. 2015. Low-level light/laser therapy versus photobiomodulation therapy. *Photomed Laser Surg*. 33(4):183–184.

Avci P, A Gupta, M Sadasivam et al. 2013. Low-level laser (light) therapy in skin: Stimulating, healing, restoring. *Semin Cutan Med Surg*. 32:41–52.

Barolet D and A Boucher. 2010. Prophylactic low-level light therapy for the treatment of hypertrophic scars and keloids: A case series. *Lasers Surg Med*. 42(6):597–601.

Bassett, CA, SN Mitchell and SR Gaston. 1981. Treatment of ununited tibial diaphyseal fractures with pulsing electromagnetic fields. *J Bone Joint Surg Am*. 63(4):511–523.

Brainard GC, JP Hanifin, JM Greeson et al. 2001. Action spectrum for melatonin regulation in humans: Evidence for a novel circadian photoreceptor. *The Journal of Neuroscience* 21(16):6405–6412.

Bryan NS. 2015. *Clinical Use of Nitric Oxide Therapy, American Academy of Ozonotherapy*. Dallas, TX, Feb 19–21, 2015.

Calderhead RG, WS Kim, T Ohshiro et al. 2015. Adjunctive 830 nm light-emitting diode therapy can improve the results following aesthetic procedures. *Laser Ther*. 24(4):277–289.

Cartier G. 2013. Simple protocols for light therapy. *Recommended Application Protocols and Suggested Treatment Parameters for Common Complaints for Clinicians & Practitioners*, 49 pp. http://vigishair.com/blog/wp-content/uploads/2017/02/Protocols-5142013.pdf

Chang AM, D Aeschbacha, JF Duffya, and CA Czeislera. 2015. Evening use of light-emitting eReaders negatively affects sleep, circadian timing, and next-morning alertness. *Proc Natl Acad Sci* 112(4):1232–1237.

Chuprikov AP, AN Linev, IA Marcenkovskij et al. 1994. *Lateral Therapy—Guide for therapists*. Kiev: Zdorovja.

DeFatta RJ, S Krishna and EF Williams 3rd. 2009. Pulsed-dye laser for treating ecchymoses after facial cosmetic procedures. *Arch Facial Plast Surg*. 11(2):99–103.

Dinshah D. 2012. *Let There Be Light*. Dinshah Health Society. 11th reprint, Malaga, New Jersey.

Edelhäuser F, F Hak, U Kleinrath et al. 2013. Impact colored light on cardiorespiratory coordination. *Evidence-Based Complementary and Alternative Medicine*, 2013, doi:10.1155/2013/810876, Article ID 810876.

Ferraresi C, YY Huang and MR Hamblin. 2016. Photobiomodulation in human muscle tissue: An advantage in sports performance? *J Biophotonics* 9(11–12):1273–1299.

Golden RN, BN Gaynes, RD Ekstrom et al. 2005. The efficacy of light therapy in the treatment of mood disorders: A review and meta-analysis of the evidence. *Am J Psychiatry* 162:656–662.

Greenamyre JT, G MacKenzie, T-I Peng, and SE Stephans. 1999. Mitochondrial dysfunction in Parkinson's disease. *Biochemical Society Symposia*, 66 85–97.

Harkless LB, S DeLellis, DH Carnegie, and TJ Burke. 2006. Improved foot sensitivity and pain reduction in patients with peripheral neuropathy after treatment with monochromatic infrared photo energy–MIRE. *J Diabetes Complications* 20(2):81–87.

Hattar S, HW Liao, M Takao et al. 2002. Melanopsin-containing retinal ganglion cells: Architecture, projections, and intrinsic photosensitivity. *Science* 295(5557):1065–1070.

Havas M. 2016. The role of electro smog and electrotherapy in diagnosing and treating diabetics with electrical hypersensitivity. *BAOJ Diabet* 2(22):014.

Health Canada. 2014. Therapeutic Products Directorate, http://www.hc-sc.gc.ca/ahc-asc/branch-dirgen/hpfb-dgpsa/tpd-dpt/index-eng.php, last updated 2014-02-27.

Hill RM and E Marg. 1963. Single-cell responses of the nucleus of the transpeduncular tract in rabbit to monochromatic light on the retina. *Journal of Neurophysiology* 26(2):249–257.

Hode L. and J. Tunér 2014. *Laser Phototherapy, Clinical Practice and Scientific Background.* Coeymans Hollow, New York: Prima Books.

Hollwich F. 1948. Untersuchungen über die Beeinflussung funktioneller Abläufe, insbesondere des Wasserhaushaltes durch energetische Anteile der Sehbahn. *Ber Dtsch Ophthal Ges Heidelberg* 54, 326.

Huang Y-Y, ACH Chen, JD Carroll, and MR Hamblin. 2009. Biphasic dose response in low level light therapy. *Dose Response* 7(4):358–383.

Karu TI. 1989. Photobiology of Low-power Laser Effects. Monochromatic visible light stimulated DNA production, growth of normal cells, and many other basic functions of living organisms. *Health Physics* 56:691–704.

Karu TI. 2007. *Ten Lectures on Basic Science of Laser Phototherapy.* Coeymans Hollow, New York: Prima Books.

Kim SJ, IK Lyoo, YS Lee et al. 2007. Decreased cerebral blood flow of thalamus in PTSD patients as a strategy to reduce re-experience symptoms. *Acta Psychiatr Scand.* 116(2):145–153.

Kochman AB, DH Carnegie, and TJ Burke. 2002. Symptomatic reversal of peripheral neuropathy in patients with diabetes. *J Am Podiatr Med Assoc.* 92:125–130.

Lam RW, AJ Levitt, RD Levitan et al. 2016. Efficacy of bright light treatment, fluoxetine, and the combination in patients with nonseasonal major depressive disorder: A randomized clinical trial. *JAMA Psychiatry* 73(1):56–63.

LeGates T, D Fernandez, and S Hattar. 2014. Light as a central modulator of circadian rhythms, sleep and affect. *Nature Reviews Neuroscience* 15 (7):443–454.

Mandel P. 1986. *Practical Compendium of Colorpuncture.* Germany: Medicina Biologica.

Mehta R and RJ Zhu. 2009. Blue or red? Exploring the effect of color on cognitive task performances. *Science* 323(5918):1226–1229.

Meier BP, RP D'Agostino, AJ Elliot et al. 2012. Color in context: Psychological context moderates the influence of red on approach– and avoidance-motivated behavior. *PLOS One* 7(7). https://doi.org/10.1371/journal.pone.00 40333

Momen S and F Al-Niaimi. 2015. Acne vulgaris and light-based therapies. *J Cosmet Laser Ther.* 17(3):122–128.

Monstrey S, H Hoeksema, H Saelens et al. 2002. A conservative approach for deep dermal burn wounds using polarised-light therapy. *British Journal of Plastic Surgery* 55:420–426.

Myhill S, NE Booth, and J McLaren–Howard. 2009. Chronic fatigue syndrome and mitochondrial dysfunction. *Int J Clin Exp Med.* 2(1):1–16.

Naeser MA, R Zafonte, MH Krengel et al. 2014. Significant improvements in cognitive performance post-transcranial, red/near-infrared light-emitting diode treatments in chronic, mild traumatic brain injury: Open-protocol study. *Journal of Neurotrauma* 31(11):1008.

Onyango IG, J Dennis, and SM Khan. 2016. Mitochondrial dysfunction in Alzheimer's disease and the rationale for bioenergetics based therapies. *Aging Dis.* 7(2):201–214.

Palienko IA. 2000. Hemodynamic effects of lateralized colored-light stimulation of the brain hemispheres in patients with essential hypertension (in Russian). *Ukr Kardiol Zh Nos.* 5/6 (Issue II), 46–48.

Palienko IA. 2001a. Modifications of the EEG activity upon lateralized stimulation of the visual inputs to the right and to the left brain hemispheres by light with different wavelengths. *Neurophysiology* 33(3):169–174.

Palienko IA. 2001b. Spectral analysis of heart rate responses to light and color stimulation of the cerebral hemispheres (in Russian). *Fiziol Zh (Ukraine)* 47(2):70–73.

Quirk BJ, M Torbey, E Buchmann et al. 2012. Near-infrared photobiomodulation in an animal model of traumatic brain injury: Improvements at the behavioral and biochemical levels. *Photomed Laser Surg.* 30(9):523–529.

Rosenthal NE, DA Sack, JC Gillin et al. 1984. Seasonal affective disorder, a description of the syndrome and preliminary findings with light therapy. *Arch Gen Psychiatry* 41:72–80.

Ross MJ, P Guthrie, and JC Dumont. 2013. The impact of modulated color light on the autonomic nervous system. *Advances in Mind-Body Medicine* 27(4):7–16.

Schindl A, M Schindl, H Schön et al. 1998. Low-intensity laser irradiation improves skin circulation in patients with diabetic microangiopathy. *Diabetes Care* 21:580–584.

Shakouri SK, J Soleimanpour, Y Salekzamani, and MR Oskuie. 2010. Effect of low-level laser therapy on the fracture healing process. *Lasers Med Sci.* 25(1):73–77.

Starwynn D. 2004. Laser and LED treatments: Which is better? *Acupuncture Today* 5(6):5 pp.

Sutherland JC. 2002. Biological effects of polychromatic light. *Photochem Photobiol.* 76(2):164–170.

Tamietto M and B de Gelder. 2010. Neural bases of the non-conscious perception of emotional signals. *Nature Reviews Neuroscience* 11:697–709.

Trelles MA and E Mayayo. 1987. Bone fracture consolidates faster with low-power laser. *Lasers in Surgery & Med.* 7:36–45.

van Maanen A, AM Meijer, KB van der Heijden and FJ Oort. 2016. The effects of light therapy on sleep problems: A systematic review and meta-analysis. *Sleep Medicine Reviews* 29:52–62.

Van Obberghen P. 2007. *Traité de Couleur Thérapie Pratique.* Paris, France: Guy Trédaniel Éditeur.

Vanin A, T De Marchi, S Silva Tomazoni et al. 2016. Pre-exercise infrared low-level laser therapy (810 nm) in skeletal muscle performance and postexercise recovery in humans, what is the optimal dose? A randomized, double-blind, placebo-controlled clinical trial. *Photomed Laser Surg.* 34(10):473–482.

Vazquez S. 2014. *Emotional Transformation Therapy.* Lanham, Maryland: Rowman & Littlefield Publishers.

Weber MH. 2015. Clinical Applications of Low-Intensity Lasertherapy, *Presentation*, Toronto April 2015. Weber Institute for Research and Laser Therapy, Lauenförde & Göttingen, Germany.

Willis GL, C Moore, and SM Armstrong. 2012. A historical justification for and retrospective analysis of the systematic application of light therapy in Parkinson's disease. *Rev Neurosci.* 23(2):199–226.

Wunsch A. 2016a. Skin, Light and Beauty, Light as a tool for wellness, anti-aging and tissue regeneration. *LSW 2016*, October 12–14, 2016, Wismar, Germany.

Wunsch A. 2016b. Photoendocrinology: How natural & artificial light is impacting human's endocrine system & hormones. *LSW 2016*, October 12–14, 2016, Wismar, Germany.

Wunsch A and K Matuschka. 2014. A controlled trial to determine the efficacy of red and near-infrared light treatment in patient satisfaction, reduction of fine lines, wrinkles, skin roughness, and intradermal collagen density increase. *Photomed Laser Surg.* 32(2):93–100.

Yumara M, M Yao, I Yanoslavsky et al. 2009. Low level light effects on inflammatory cytokine Production by Rheumatoid Arthritis Synoviocytes. *Lasers in Surgery and Medicine* 41:282–290.

Zhang R, NF Lahens, HI Balance et al. 2014. A circadian gene expression atlas in mammals: Implications for biology and medicine. *Proc Natl Acad Sci.* 111(45):16219–16224.

Zubidat AE, B Fares, F Fares, and A Haim. 2015. Melatonin functioning through DNA methylation to constricts breast cancer growth accelerated by blue LED light-at-night in 4T1 tumor-bearing mice. *Gratis Journal of Cancer Biology and Therapeutics* 1(2):57–73.

21 The Role of Light and Electromagnetic Fields in Maintaining Vascular Health

Stephanie Seneff

CONTENTS

Introduction 501
Sulfate Transport 504
eNOS: A Moonlighting Enzyme 505
Collagen and Heparan Sulfate 506
Ion Channels and Pumps 507
Iron, Sulfate, and Lysosomes 508
Streaming Potential 510
Glycocalyx Recycling as Glucose Buffering 512
Chlorophyll, Tryptophan, and Jumping Genes 512
Glyphosate's Disruption of Electrical Systems 513
    Sulfate Homeostasis 513
    Depletion of Aromatic Sulfate Transporters 514
    Cholesterol Sulfate, PPARγ, and the Liver 515
    Disruption of eNOS 516
    Sodium/Potassium ATPase and the Heart 516
Broader Consequences 517
References 518

INTRODUCTION

The human body is 99% water, by molecule count. Water not only is essential for life but also is a magical molecule that can form multiple crystalline configurations out of communities of water molecules to encode information and capture energy [1]. Water in the solid form, familiar to us as "ice," has a hexameric crystalline structure. Water vapor, the gas form, consists of individual water molecules chaotically moving about randomly in the air. But water in the liquid form has many possibilities for the formation and reformation of configurations containing four, five, or six water molecules loosely bound together. Most remarkable is the structured form of water that forms the "fourth phase" of water, as popularized by Prof. Gerald Pollack of Washington University, made of a regular crystalline lattice of hexamers, analogous to the lattice in ice crystals, producing a gel that is not quite liquid and not quite solid [2]. The energy to produce the structure can be supplied by sunlight, and this stored energy can later be released to perform useful work in a cell. Essentially, water can be used as a battery to store the energy in sunlight, and the human body exploits this remarkable biophysical feature of water to meet many of its energy needs [3,4].

Most of the water in our bodies is in this highly structured, largely immobile, gelled hexameric crystalline form. However, there is one huge exception, and this is the flowing blood. The body faces a remarkable challenge to be able to maintain highly structured, largely immobile, water everywhere except in the myriad blood vessels, including the tiny capillaries that supply nutrients to and remove waste from all the cells in the body. Human blood is a colloidal suspension in a water-based plasma, and its viscosity needs to be carefully controlled so as to be neither too thin nor too thick. The elderly population in particular face a tough challenge to try to avoid the opposing extremes of hemorrhage and thrombosis. The plasma consists of up to 95% water by volume, and it also contains dissolved proteins, clotting factors, glucose, electrolytes, hormones, and so on. The platelets in suspension are charged with the awesome responsibility to plug any leaks that develop in the artery walls, and to clot the blood that escapes the vasculature in an open wound to protect from excessive blood loss through hemorrhage. Yet a blood clot produced, for example, in the leg might travel to the lungs and lodge in a vein, producing a pulmonary embolism that could be fatal. The tasks of repeatedly producing and then dissolving blood clots without causing collateral damage become more arduous when there are multiple leaks in the artery walls due to a defective barrier.

The red blood cells (RBCs) deliver oxygen to the tissues and dispose of the carbon dioxide waste product of oxidative phosphorylation in the mitochondria, which produces fuel in the form of adenosine triphosphate (ATP) by oxidizing nutrients such as glucose and fats. The RBCs face a tough challenge to traverse the tiny capillaries that are often a tight squeeze for these cells. It is truly astonishing that RBCs are able to freely migrate through all the tiny capillaries of the body, seemingly sliding effortlessly from the arterioles to the venules. How is this feat accomplished?

Electromagnetic fields play an essential role in managing blood flow through capillaries. It is highly significant that nearly all the charged "particles" that are suspended in the blood are *negatively* charged. The RBCs, the platelets, the white blood cells, the low-density lipoprotein (LDL) and high-density lipoprotein (HDL) particles, and the major blood protein, serum albumin, are all maintained with a negatively charged surface field. Zeta potential (ZP) is a scientific term to capture the electrokinetic potential in colloidal dispersions such as the blood. The ZP of the blood is a useful measure of its potential to resist coagulation or flocculation. A high ZP reflects more negative charge on the suspended particles, and leads to a more stable and well-maintained colloidal suspension, because the particles' mutual negative charge will be a repulsive force that keeps them well separated. If ZP falls too low, there is imminent danger of disseminated intravascular coagulation, a catastrophic cascade leading to a no-flow situation and multiple-organ failure.

The pH of the blood drops when going from arteries to veins. Generally, the arteries have the highest pH, and the terminal watershed regions in the kidneys and the brain have the lowest pH. This means that there is a charge drop across the capillary such that the venous side is positively charged, relative to the arterial side. This charge differential acts like a battery terminal to attract the negatively charged suspended particles, such as the platelets and the RBCs. The walls of the capillary, on the other hand, are negatively charged, so they repel the negatively charged RBCs, helping to keep it from getting stuck to the side of the tube. The most acidic terminal watershed regions attract flow toward them like a magnet, allowing the water in the blood to leave the body as saliva in the head or urine in the groin.

The endothelial cells lining the walls of the capillaries rely on an extracellular matrix composed of complex proteoglycans to maintain a layer of structured water encircling the inner wall of the capillary and providing a slick, frictionless surface to allow the RBCs safe passage. The entire complex structure formed by these extracellular matrices in the vasculature is referred to collectively as the "glycocalyx," and the health of the vasculature as a whole critically depends on the health of the glycocalyx [5]. In turn, the health of the glycocalyx depends critically on its supply of negative charge, and on its ability to maintain the gelled water, both of which are achieved through the generous addition of *sulfate ions* to the matrix glycoproteins, in an irregular but non-random distribution pattern.

The membranes of the endothelial cells, and of most cells in the body, have proteins embedded in them which are able to form proteoglycans by attaching externally to glycosaminoglycans (GAGs) consisting of long unbranched polysaccharides that protrude into the space surrounding the cell. These GAGs are highly heterogeneous and information-bearing. Familiar variants include heparan sulfate, keratan sulfate, chondroitin sulfate, dermatan sulfate, and hyaluronic acid. Hyaluronic acid is the only one that is not sulfated. Figure 21.1 shows the general structure of heparan sulfate chains, which are typically attached to serine residues in a core protein that is inserted into the cell's plasma membrane. Each position, X, Y, and Z, in the individual units of the chain can be modified by addition of either a sulfate or an acetyl group. A low ratio of sulfate to acetyl groups is an indicator of sulfate deficiency.

With a highly sulfated glycocalyx, the capillary wall is shielded by a thick "exclusion zone" made up of multiple layers of water hexamers forming a structured water gel. The gel encasement conceals all the molecules dangling off the endothelial cells, and presents a smooth slick surface to the RBCs, sliding through the capillary, propelled by the positive charge field on the venous side and repelled by the negatively charged sulfates embedded in the gel. An RBC traversing a capillary is depicted in cross-section in Figure 21.2. The nearly frictionless surface of the gel layer greatly reduces the load on the heart to pump blood through the capillaries. And the exclusion zone also consists of almost pure water—excluding all the solutes in the blood and preventing them from accidentally leaking out into the interstitial spaces. The water in the gel is immobile, and therefore is separated from the flowing blood almost as if it is a separate substance from the unstructured water that forms the bulk of the flowing plasma. In fact, protons collect at the surface of the interface between the structured water in the glycocalyx and the unstructured water in the flowing blood. This is in part because each of the water hexamers in the EZ is short one proton—these extra protons that are released when the water molecules form a hexamer will be forced out and naturally gather at the edge of the exclusion zone, creating charge separation which can be turned into energy to fuel the cell.

Research by a team led by Prof. Gerald Pollack of Washington University has shown that exclusion zones grow by as much as fourfold in the presence of infrared light [6]. Incident radiant energy appears to be stored in the water as entropy loss and charge separation. This will directly increase the strength of the battery, thus capturing the energy in the light and making it available for useful work. Studies have shown that structured clustered water can retain low frequency information, such as that contained in infrared light, and this may also provide a platform to support meridian signaling that is invoked to explain the beneficial effects of acupuncture [7].

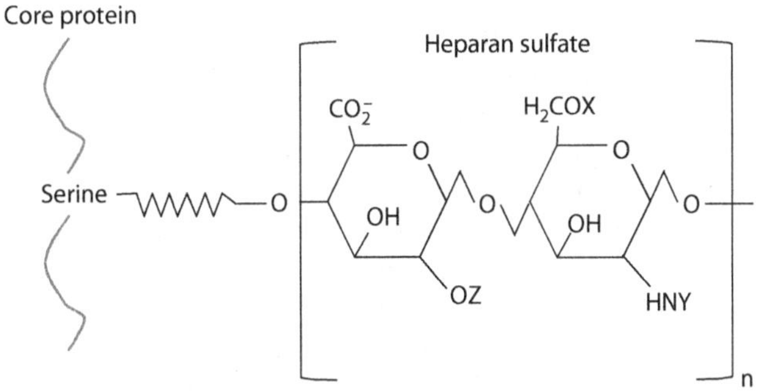

X:	H	H	SO_3^-	H	SO_3^-	H	SO_3^-
Y:	Ac	SO_3^-	Ac	Ac	SO_3^-	SO_3^-	SO_3^-
Z:	H	H	H	SO_3^-	H	SO_3^-	SO_3^-

FIGURE 21.1 Schematic of a capillary cross-section with an RBC traversing the capillary. The exclusion zone is made up of heavily sulfated glycosaminoglycans anchored to the endothelial plasma membranes. Excluded protons are attracted to the negative charge within the exclusion zone, and this achieves charge separation and battery formation. The red blood cell is negatively charged, due in part to the cholesterol sulfate that is embedded in its membrane. Only a small fraction of the water in the capillary actually flows due to the fact that the structured water in the exclusion zone behaves more like a solid than a liquid.

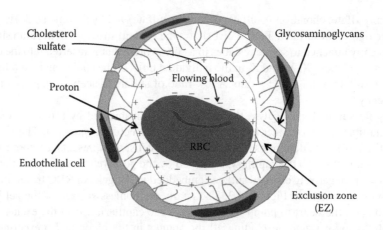

FIGURE 21.2 Schematic of a capillary cross section with an RBC traversing the capillary. The exclusion zone is made up of heavily sulfated glycosaminoglycans anchored to the endothelial plasma membranes. Excluded protons are attracted to the negative charge within the exclusion zone, and this achieves charge separation and battery formation. The red blood cell is negatively charged, due in part to the cholesterol sulfate that is embedded in its membrane. Only a small fraction of the water in the capillary actually flows due to the fact that the structured water in the exclusion zone behaves more like a solid than a liquid.

SULFATE TRANSPORT

Possibly the most overlooked factor in the issue of maintaining human health is the need for an adequate supply of sulfate to all the tissues, particularly the vasculature—both the cells lining the vessel walls and the cells travelling through the blood vessels. The major puzzle that presents itself to biological systems is that sulfate gels water: this is a feature once the sulfate anion is securely anchored in the membrane of some cell, but, during transit, gelling the free-flowing blood in the blood vessels will result in a no-flow crisis. The body has come up with ingenious solutions to this problem, but, unfortunately, as we will see later, toxic chemicals in the environment are derailing the body's clever solutions, and causing systemic diseases as a consequence. The levels of *free sulfate* in the blood are tightly regulated within a narrow concentration range centered around 1 millimolar. The so-called Jones–Ray effect shows that 1 millimolar concentration results in a minimum in surface tension [8]. Any more or any less is problematic, and any excess free sulfate will have to be flushed out through the kidneys even if there is a severe sulfate deficiency problem.

The clever solution that the body has devised is to produce a large variety of sulfate *transporters*: special molecules that can form a chemical bond with a sulfate anion, disperse the negative charge over a ring or two within the molecular structure of the carrier, and thereby prevent the sulfate anion from gelling the blood. Three major classes of sulfate transporters are the aromatic amino acids, polyphenols, and sterols. The aromatics are three essential amino acids that contain a benzene ring: tryptophan, tyrosine, and phenylalanine. Aromatic amino acids are able to absorb light due to their conjugated double bonds, and this is an important consideration in the capitalization of sunlight as a source of energy that we will revisit later.

The monoamine neurotransmitters are derived from the aromatic amino acids, and they also transport sulfate. It is well known that all of the monoamine neurotransmitters—serotonin, dopamine, noradrenalin, and adrenalin—as well as the metabolic derivative of serotonin that regulates the wake-sleep cycle, the hormone melatonin, are usually *sulfated* during transit. The related thyroid hormone is also sulfated. Other important sulfate transporters are the polyphenols found in fruits, vegetables, green tea, black tea, red wine, coffee, chocolate, olives, extra virgin olive oil, herbs, spices, and nuts, which are touted as being an important part of a healthy diet. These go by specific names such as flavonoids, isoflavones, and quercetin, which may be more familiar, and all of them contain multiple carbon rings. Curcumin, the spice that is a crucial active ingredient in turmeric used in curry dishes, is a polyphenolic compound with remarkable health benefits. Vitamin C, found in high concentration in certain tropical fruits, while not a polyphenol, is also a sulfate transporter. In fact, vitamin C may be able to facilitate sulfate transfer from one sulfated molecule to another, something that becomes very important for repopulating sulfate anions in the capillary glycocalyx.

But perhaps the most important sulfate transporter in the body is the sterol, cholesterol, essential for mammalian life. Cholesterol is not found in plants, and it can in fact be likened to chlorophyll in importance: cholesterol is what gives animals mobility and a nervous system. Cholesterol sulfate is known to be present in the blood in relatively high concentrations, but there seems to be remarkably little interest in understanding its role there. Cholesterol sulfate is synthesized in the skin in response to sunlight, along with vitamin D sulfate. It forms an important part of the skin barrier which keeps microbes out. The skin is also believed to be the most important supplier of cholesterol sulfate to the blood [9].

Cholesterol sulfate is an especially interesting molecule because the sulfate ligand provides the cholesterol molecule with water solubility, an extremely important point because this means that the cholesterol can travel freely in the blood rather than being hidden inside a lipid particle such as low-density lipoprotein (LDL) or high-density lipoprotein (HDL). Furthermore, sulfation is what allows cholesterol to leave lipid stores inside cells and get exported across the water-based cytoplasm into the blood. More importantly, the cholesterol half of cholesterol sulfate readily inserts itself into the membranes of red blood cells and platelets, helping them to build a layer of structured water around them that will protect their delicate membrane lipids from oxidative and glycation damage. At the same time, the sulfate half of these membrane-bound cholesterol sulfate molecules sticks out from the cell membrane and supplies the cell with negative charge, giving it the mobility it needs to easily navigate the capillaries in the electric field created by the voltage drop across the capillary, and also protecting it from agglomerating with other red blood cells or platelets.

There are many important sterols that are derived from cholesterol that also transport sulfate. Many of these are synthesized by the adrenal glands. But the gonads also produce estrogen, testosterone, and progesterone, all of which are sulfated in transit. Dehydroepiandrosterone (DHEA) sulfate, produced in large amounts by the adrenal glands, is generally present in high amounts in the blood, and it probably provides a good back-up system for cholesterol sulfate. Vitamin D is also derived from cholesterol, and its molecular structure is minimally different from that of cholesterol. It too is often sulfated in transit.

All of these bioactive molecules are *inactive* when sulfated, and this point has often been invoked to dismiss the utility of the sulfated versions to the body. However, I believe that one of their most important roles is to *deliver* sulfate to the tissues. When they arrive at their destination, a sulfatase detaches their sulfate and a sulfotransferase reattaches it to one of the sulfated GAGs in the extracellular matrix of the target cell, beefing up their sulfate supplies.

eNOS: A MOONLIGHTING ENZYME

The vasculature does not solely depend on sulfate *transport* to maintain adequate sulfate supplies because it can also synthesize sulfate *in place*. Together with collaborators, I have published two papers that explain how red blood cells, platelets, and endothelial cells can utilize the energy in sunlight as a catalyst to directly synthesize sulfate, and then incorporate it either into cholesterol sulfate or into sulfated GAGs in the extracellular matrix [4,10]. The enzyme we identified as being responsible for sulfate synthesis is endothelial nitric oxide synthase (eNOS), a fascinating protein with complex regulatory control.

eNOS is well known for its role in producing nitric oxide, a signaling gas which promotes vascular flow by relaxing the smooth muscle cells in the artery wall. It is also well established that eNOS, in an uncoupled state, produces superoxide instead of nitric oxide. eNOS is an orphan member of the important class of cytochrome P450 enzymes, and as such it contains a heme complex with bound iron. Tetrahydrobiopterin (BH4) is critical for inducing electron flow from eNOS-bound heme to L-arginine, the precursor to nitric oxide. When BH4 levels are insufficient, eNOS produces superoxide instead of nitric oxide, and this is generally viewed as a pathological condition [11]. However, under proper circumstances, the superoxide can be channeled into a cavity formed between the two eNOS molecules of an eNOS dimer, where it can be used to oxidize sulfane sulfur bound to conserved cysteines in eNOS, probably first producing sulfur dioxide and finally producing sulfate. Details can be found in [4,10]. It is likely, in fact, that hydrogen sulfide gas, either pulled directly from the air or produced through the breakdown of free cysteine molecules, is first oxidized to thiosulfate in the mitochondria. Subsequently, the thiosulfate supplies sulfur to form thiocystine (CSSH) in a cysteine residue of eNOS, leaving behind a sulfite molecule that is oxidized to sulfate via sulfite oxidase. Ultimately, the extra "S" in CSSH is also oxidized to sulfate through the oxidation process orchestrated by the eNOS dimer. Thus, two molecules of hydrogen sulfide gas are transformed into two molecules of sulfate, with thiosulfate serving as an intermediary.

Strong support for the idea that eNOS can produce sulfate as well as nitric oxide comes from the observation that red blood cells contain substantial amounts of eNOS [11–14]. This has presented a puzzle to researchers because any nitric oxide produced by RBC eNOS would nitrosylate hemoglobin, impairing its ability to transport oxygen. The eNOS in RBCs is found only in a membrane-bound configuration, and membrane-bound eNOS is inactive in nitric oxide production. Instead, I highly suspect that eNOS, when attached to the membrane, is able to attract superoxide ions that are mobilized *within* the structured water (exclusion zone) of the glycocalyx. The electrons are mobilized in response to sunlight, absorbing the energy in sunlight and converting it to kinetic energy as they become energized within the exclusion zone.

The growth of new blood vessels following myocardial infarction is an important part of the healing process. Neovascularization through angiogenesis restores healthy circulation. It was originally believed that angiogenesis induced by ischemia could be achieved by the endothelial cells already residing in the artery wall. However, through studies on mice that are deficient in eNOS, it has now been established that angiogenesis depends on recruitment of progenitor cells from the bone marrow [14]. Furthermore, eNOS plays an essential role both in the bone marrow to mobilize the stem cells and in the developing artery wall to promote vessel growth. Nitric oxide released by eNOS nitrosylates matrix metalloproteinases, thereby activating them. This promotes vascular remodeling through the breakdown of existing extracellular matrices. But eNOS is also essential for reconstructing the extracellular matrix around cells that have newly established residence in the budding vessel wall. This is because membrane-bound eNOS can produce sulfate to repopulate the matrix and promote the development of a healthy glycocalyx, in a continuing cycle of disassembly and renewal.

COLLAGEN AND HEPARAN SULFATE

Collagen is the most abundant protein in the body, representing approximately 25% of the total protein mass. Collagen forms a scaffold to provide strength, structure, and flexibility to the bones, muscles, skin, and tendons. An important member of the collagen family is collagen XVIII, which is almost always found as a proteoglycan with numerous heparan sulfate attachments [15]. The core protein has a molecular mass of 180 kDa, but an additional mass of 120 kDa is completely attributed to attached heparan sulfate chains. Collagen XVIII is found predominantly in the extracellular matrix of the basal laminae, in the lungs, the skin, the skeletal muscles, kidney tubules and glomeruli, cardiac muscle, blood vessels, and the pia mater, the innermost layer of the membranes surrounding the brain and spinal cord. Endostatin, an anti-angiogenic tumor-suppressing peptide, is identically the C-terminal part of collagen XVIII.

The basement membrane is the thin delicate membrane made up of protein fibers and glycosaminoglycans separating the epithelium from the underlying tissues. The dense layer closer to the connective tissue is called the lamina densa. It contains multiple collagen IV fibers coated with the heparan-sulfate rich proteoglycan, perlecan [16]. Perlecan also serves as a barrier between the circulating blood and the surrounding tissue [17]. It maintains the integrity of microvessels [18], and white blood cells must cross a perlecan barrier in order to extravasate into the surrounding tissues.

A close examination of the activities in cells directed toward maintenance of heparan sulfate suggests that cholesterol sulfate plays an essential role in providing sulfate to the glycans in the glycocalyx, and that this process is mediated by apolipoproteins. Apolipoproteins are proteins that populate the membrane of HDL and LDL particles, and their main function is to transport lipids. There are several different variants including Apolipoprotein (Apo) A1, B, C2, and E, that appear in different proportions in different lipid particles. Vascular ApoE, present in HDL particles, has anti-angiogenic properties. It also promotes the synthesis of heparan sulfate by endothelial cells [19]. Reduced levels of heparan sulfate in the glycocalyx are found in atherosclerotic arteries. Vessels with 50% less heparan sulfate have 4- to 5-fold more stored cholesterol. ApoE escorts cholesterol sulfate from the Golgi apparatus to the plasma membrane, and ultimately delivers it to HDL-A1 [19]. ApoE thus provides a direct link between cholesterol sulfate and heparan sulfate. It is highly likely that cholesterol sulfate supplies sulfate to the endothelial cell at the membrane, needed to produce the heparan sulfate that will reinforce the supply in the glycocalyx. It follows that a deficiency in cholesterol sulfate will lead to atherosclerosis.

The NaS1 sulfate transporter is an important regulator of sulfate levels in the body, as it actively transports sulfate across the gut border and returns sulfate back into circulation in the renal tubules. There is a high incidence of genetic variants in NaS1 among autistic children, associated with renal sulfate wasting [20]. Mice engineered to be NaS1$^{-/-}$ exhibited a 12-fold increased rate of tumor growth along with more than double the density of a tumor vascular supply compared to NaS1$^{+/+}$ mice [21]. Their tumors were also severely impoverished in collagen.

Collagen V produced by Schwann cells binds with high affinity to heparan sulfate at its N-terminal domain [22]. The Schwann cell surface contains attached glypican-1, a proteoglycan which is populated with heparan sulfate chains that bind securely to the collagen molecule. Tube-like extracellular matrix structures that surround axon-Schwann cell units during myelination contain collagen V. Suppression of either glypican-1 or collagen V expression significantly inhibits myelination during peripheral nerve terminal differentiation.

ION CHANNELS AND PUMPS

Much of the energy exploited by biological systems to do useful work is generated via voltage gradients and/or ion gradients across lipophilic membranes. Each cell has a large number of internal organelles, for example, mitochondria and lysosomes, and there are ion gradients and voltage gradients across all the membranes of these organelles. The internal space of the mitochondria is maintained at a high pH (7.8 or more). The internal space of lysosomes is highly acidic, as is the intermembrane space of the mitochondria. Thus, induction of a large voltage drop across the boundary between the interior and the intermembrane space of mitochondria drives the synthesis of ATP. There is also a voltage change across the plasma membrane of the cell. Resting cells typically have a voltage drop of about −70 millivolts, although this varies among cell types and is especially high for skeletal muscle cells at −95 millivolts.

Cells also make sure that strong ion gradients are maintained across their plasma membrane, especially for potassium which is highly concentrated internally and sodium which is kept at very low internal concentrations. When a cell is stimulated by acetylcholine, the receptors open up ion channels that essentially produce tunnels through the relatively impervious plasma membrane so that sodium and potassium can freely flow toward equilibrating the internal and external concentrations. This flow does not need to be fueled because the ion gradients naturally promote flow in one direction only—toward the region of lesser concentration. But these channels must be gated to make sure flow only happens under signaling control. The flowing ions create an electric current that can be exploited to perform useful work. There are several ion channels specializing in various metal cations, with sodium, potassium, and calcium channels probably being the most important ones. There are also several channels that co-transport metal ions along with organic nutrients. For example, many amino acids are imported into the cell along with sodium ions which help to facilitate the uptake of the amino acid.

Following stimulation by acetylcholine or another agonist of the acetylcholine receptor, the sodium ions and potassium ions must be restored to their original side of the boundary in order to maintain the ion gradients that support renewed rapid passive flow. This is a much slower process because it is working against the concentration gradient, and it also burns up ATP at the same time. Pumps require gates on both sides of the channel, and only one gate can be open at a time, whereas a channel only needs a single gate to block flow [23]. This is because a pump will be overwhelmed with back flow that will immediately defeat all its efforts if there is free passage in the reverse direction along the strong concentration gradient. The ions being moved are momentarily trapped inside the membrane, and, when the second gate opens, they can leave only in the direction that is against the gradient.

A hugely important protein, especially in the very active skeletal muscle cells and neurons, is the sodium-potassium ATPase pump (Na-K pump). This pump achieves multiple goals: (1) making sure there is a high ratio of potassium ions internally compared to the extracellular milieu, (2) making sure that the corresponding ratio for sodium is low, (3) making sure the cell is sufficiently polarized (maintaining the -70 millivolt drop across the membrane), and (4) making sure that the number of total buffering agents in solution in the interior is comparable to that in the exterior milieu. Item (4) is important because an imbalance will trigger the movement of water across the boundary to adjust for osmotic differences. If the cell pushes out too many ions compared to how many are drawn in, the ionic buffering in the cytoplasm will be too dilute, and this will cause water to leave the cell to reequilibrate the total concentration of solutes on both sides of the membrane.

The Na-K pump is estimated to consume 40%–50% of the ATP synthesized by the cell under normal conditions. It pulls two potassium ions inside for every three sodium ions that exit. Thus, it leads to a net decrease in internal positive charge, and can therefore restore the resting potential following depolarization. It also leads to a decrease in internal buffering capacity (with a net loss of one ion with each exchange), and this will cause water to also leave the cell. It's very interesting that the acetylcholine receptor induces the exact opposite effect of the Na-K pump, and therefore the pump can restore equilibrium after the receptor fires. The Na-K pump is very tightly regulated, because an overshoot—if it fires too much and/or too long—will be costly in terms of both loss of ATP and a hyperpolarized membrane. An overactive pump in the heart could lead to arrhythmias, cardiac arrest, and sudden death. We will revisit this topic later in this chapter.

IRON, SULFATE, AND LYSOSOMES

One of the many essential activities for the sulfate ions that are bound to the extracellular matrix glycoproteins is to support the role of iron in metabolizing and recycling cellular debris. Iron, because it has multiple redox states and is so abundant in nature, has been exploited for many uses in biological systems. However, it must be managed very carefully because it will react with hydrogen peroxide to produce superoxide via the Fenton reaction if the pH of the medium is too high. Superoxide can cause considerable damage to neighboring tissues if it is not able to be contained in a sequestered space. At a sufficiently low pH, water is produced instead of superoxide, and therefore the surrounding tissues are protected from collateral damage. Lysosomes are important organelles in cells with the responsibility to clean up cellular debris such as oxidized and glycated proteins. Iron sulfate is exploited in the lysosomes to provide adequate reaction strength to break down the bonds in the debris, and lysosomes use the sulfate to help maintain a very low pH to assure that the reaction product is water instead of superoxide. Sulfuric acid (hydrogen sulfate) is extremely acidic (low pH).

Lysosomes begin their life as caveolae ("little caves"). Caveolae are cavities (indentations) that appear in the membranes of multiple cell types, particularly muscle cells, which need considerable energy to maintain their ability to promote movement. The cytoskeleton is a network of protein fibers that give the cell physical strength but also likely double as electrical wires for transporting protons into organelles that are attached to the cytoskeleton, including lysosomes and mitochondria. The microtubules that form the cytoskeleton organize as hollow cylinders filled with structured water. The water is essential to maintain conductivity; without water, the tubule becomes an insulator. An imaginative paper by Sahu et al. has uncovered resonance phenomena in these tubules maintained through "electromagnetic resonant oscillation" that can encode information analogous to human-engineered wireless communication channels [24].

Research on the properties of the actin filaments that make up the cytoskeleton has revealed that they have a high concentration of negatively charged amino acids that imbue them with a unique property, relative to other proteins that were studied [25]. They showed experimentally that actin induces an unusual surrounding double-layer of water molecules with distinctly different properties, wherein the inner layer is immobile structured water, and the outer layer is highly mobile fluid water. It seems plausible that hydronium ions (carrying protons) concentrated on the edge of the glycocalyx would be attracted to the negatively charged actin filaments and easily traverse this fluid layer surrounding the tube to reach the organelles that are attached to the cytoskeleton and supply them with protons.

Prof. Pollack has shown that protons gather at the phase boundary between structured and unstructured water: they are attracted to the negatively charged water matrix of the structured gel, but the tight crystalline structure leaves them with no physical path to penetrate the barrier. So they slide along the edge and can be channeled into the caveolae to be trapped there as the cave is fully enclosed and then pinched off to become a free organelle within the cell's cytoplasm. The charge separation (excess protons at the boundary and excess electrons within the crystalline matrix) is essentially a battery and it can perform useful work, supplying electricity to the cell.

Thus, protons, originally concentrated in the extracellular matrix, are drawn into the caveolae, and then become trapped there, along with whatever debris has also been swept up, once the caveolae are pinched off to become intracellular organelles, or endosomes. Contained in the debris are also fragments of heparan sulfate that were extracted from the extracellular matrix with the help of nitric oxide. Oxidized LDL binds to heparan sulfate and stimulates endothelial secretion of heparanase, which thus further enables the heparan sulfate chains and the lipids to be swept up together into caveolae for internalization, clearance, and recycling [26].

Lysosomes and the intermembrane space of mitochondria operate at a much lower pH than the surrounding cytoplasm. These organelles are typically attached to the cytoskeleton, which, in turn is attached to the cell's plasma membrane. As schematized in Figure 21.3, the endosomes are guided along the cytoskeletal tracks, and gradually become more acidified as they mature into lysosomes. It is plausible that protons, originally concentrated along the boundary between the structured and unstructured water (EZ) in the extracellular matrix, can be channeled into the fluid outer water layer of cytoskeletal tubules in the form of hydronium ions and directed ultimately into these two classes of attached organelles to induce and maintain their low pH.

To the extent that mitochondria can obtain protons from this external source (the cytoskeleton), they will have to work less hard to pump protons out of their interior region. Thus, the process by which protons are flowing into the cell along the cytoskeletal pathways is entirely analogous to an electrical circuit supplying electricity to a house. All of this works because of the structured water that is maintained by the sulfates in the extracellular matrix and by the negatively charged amino acids in the actin cytoskeleton.

Remarkable support for this idea comes from a paper on tumor cells, which showed that the mitochondria in tumor cells are abnormally enriched in cholesterol [27]. Normally, mitochondrial membranes contain very little cholesterol. Cholesterol enrichment causes them to be much less permeable to protons. The mitochondrial membranes of cholesterol-enriched mitochondria in tumor

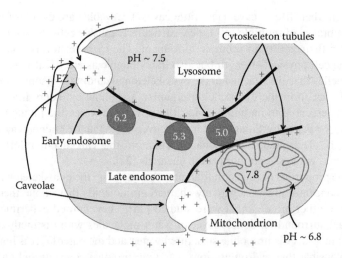

FIGURE 21.3 Cartoon schematic of a cell showing how protons gathering at the edge of the exclusion zone (EZ) outside the cell can be ushered into the caveolae, and then concentrated within endosomes that bud and get internalized and then later converted to lysosomes through further acidification. The tubules in the cytoskeleton are also immersed in EZ water with heavily acidified fluid water traveling along the outer channels. This concentrates protons that can then be more easily pumped into the lysosomes and the mitochondrial intermembrane space to maintain their acidic pH. The mobile protons essentially provide current to the cell.

cells were shown to have a significantly lower proton leak current, most especially in the outer mitochondrial membrane. Proton leaks should work against the proton pump that forces protons from the interior of the mitochondria across the inner membrane. But proton leaks in the outer membrane will be very effective if protons are pouring into the mitochondrial intermembrane space across this membrane in high concentration, supplied through "electrical wires" tracing the cytoskeletal tubules. This makes it much easier to maintain the voltage gradient across the inner membrane. Indeed, tumor cells have an impaired ability to produce ATP through the mitochondrial citric acid cycle, and instead derive most of their energy through aerobic glycolysis. I propose that tumors arise directly due to impaired supply of sulfate to the extracellular matrix, which shuts down the supply of electricity to the cell, disabling both mitochondrial ATP synthesis and lysosomal clearance of cellular debris.

If the sulfates are deficient, both the mitochondria and the lysosomes suffer. The mitochondria produce less ATP, and the lysosomes become unable to digest debris without causing collateral damage through the release of superoxide. With dysfunctional lysosomes, a cell is forced to accumulate debris that can eventually reach overwhelming levels. Lipofuscin is the term used to describe the clutter of damaged proteins that can eventually reach untenable levels. A cell in this situation is forced to choose one of two strategies: either clone itself to produce two cells, each with half the debris, or commit suicide through apoptosis, calling in macrophages to clear the cumulated debris.

STREAMING POTENTIAL

"Streaming potential" is the technical term used to describe the electromagnetic field that is generated by flowing charged particles, traveling through a channel with charged walls. Clearly, the moving suspended particles in the blood create a streaming potential, referred to more specifically as the "electrokinetic vascular streaming potential," which is a force that can be exploited to do useful work [28]. With every beat of the heart, the suspended, negatively charged particles in the blood are pushed forward. During the off cycle, when the force is removed, they slow down. Because these particles are charged, this constant acceleration and deceleration generates an electromagnetic field at a frequency that is equal to the heart rate. Remarkably, the endothelial cells lining the artery wall respond to the signal in this field by releasing nitric oxide. When the heart beats faster, the frequency goes up, and more nitric oxide is released. The nitric oxide, through gaseous signaling mechanisms, conveniently relaxes the vessel wall and opens up the flow. It also quickly oxidizes to nitrite, which can detach snippets of heparan sulfate from the glycocalyx (induce shedding) [29,30]. Further enzymatic oxidation by nitrite oxidase produces nitrate, which is a chaotrope, disordering water structure and reducing the viscosity of the flowing blood. This is in direct contrast to sulfate, which is a kosmotrope: a water-structuring molecule. The nitrate's chaotropic effects reach into the glycocalyx freeing up additional water to join the flowing blood and providing room for RBCs to pass through capillaries.

A paper by Van Teeffelen et al. is among the best in the literature for helping the reader to visualize the glycocalyx in action in capillaries and its modifications under varying conditions [31]. These authors estimate that the healthy living capillary glycocalyx in the absence of red blood cells traversing the capillary has a true thickness of up to 1.5 micrometers. When the red blood cells squeeze through the capillary, they naturally compress the glycocalyx, perhaps down to 0.9 micrometers when the flow rate is 10 RBCs per second. Drugs that release nitric oxide or stimulate nitric oxide synthesis in the endothelial wall cause a remarkable and rapid growth of the area within the capillaries that is accessible to solutes. This implies that nitric oxide induces the conversion of structured water along the edges of the capillary into unstructured water, that then participates in vascular flow. But its oxidation products could also actually degrade matrix glycoproteins, snipping off heparan sulfate proteoglycan fragments that can be taken up by the cells and utilized both to clear cellular debris and as a source of glucose (fuel) and of sulfate for the surrounding tissues. Endogenously produced nitric oxide would achieve both of these effects—destructuring the water and freeing up matrix glycoproteins—through its oxidation to nitrite and finally to nitrate, as discussed previously.

Thus, in the absence of nitric oxide, the flow rate of red blood cells—and of plasma—through the capillaries is greatly reduced. Nitric oxide and its oxidation products induce perfusion not just through the ability to relax smooth muscle cells lining the artery wall, but also through destructuring effects on the water and erosion of the matrix glycoproteins in the capillaries. By freeing matrix glycoproteins, it opens up access to the cells to deliver nutrients, and it makes room for new deposition of a fresh batch of heparan sulfate and other sulfated polysaccharides in the matrix, in a continual cycle of renewal and consumption of the buffered glycoproteins.

The heparan sulfate molecules in the matrix are constantly assembled and destroyed. They serve multiple functions for the cell lucky enough to take them up into its lysosomes. As we've seen, the sulfate provides the acidic environment that allows iron to safely break down molecular debris, generating water as a by-product rather than superoxide or the hydroxyl radical. It isn't until the very end of the digestive process in the lysosome that the sulfates are finally detached from the sugar molecules in the heparan sulfate. Now, the reducing action of the sugar can reduce the sulfate to sulfide, which likely reacts with common molecules like pyruvate to form mercaptopyruvate, and with cysteine to form cysteine persulfide (CSSH). These molecules are essentially carriers of hydrogen sulfide gas, just as molecules such as S-nitrosoglutathione (GSNO) are carriers of nitric oxide that can later be released.

Mathematically, the strength of the streaming potential electromagnetic signal is proportional to the heart rate and blood pressure, and inversely proportional to the viscosity of the blood. It is conceivable that the reason why blood pressure and heart rate tend to become elevated as we age is because a higher pressure will induce a stronger signal, releasing more nitric oxide and promoting blood flow and heparan sulfate recycling. This may compensate for an increase in blood viscosity with age due to the accumulation of oxidized and glycated proteins. Insufficient negative charge on the suspended particles is another factor, in turn related to deficiencies in cholesterol sulfate due to exposure to environmental toxicants.

GLYCOCALYX RECYCLING AS GLUCOSE BUFFERING

The gaseous signaling molecules, hydrogen sulfide and nitric oxide, are tightly coupled in human physiology. Cystathionine γ lyase (CSE) is a major source of hydrogen sulfide gas through cysteine metabolism. Mice engineered to be deficient in CSE (CSE knockout mice) have reduced levels of sulfide in the blood along with significant increases in oxidative stress [32]. Perhaps surprisingly, they also have reduced bioavailability of nitric oxide associated with impaired eNOS functioning. CSE knockout mice showed a reduction in nitrite levels, attributed to impaired phosphorylation of eNOS, leading to susceptibility to myocardial injury. Thus, hydrogen sulfide gas plays an essential role in promoting the release of nitric oxide, which, as we've seen, will lead to a stripping of the extracellular matrix glycoproteins.

Hydrogen sulfide can be oxidized to thiosulfate in the mitochondria [33], and then to sulfate via membrane-bound eNOS [4], ultimately resupplying the glycocalyx with a renewal of the heparan sulfate that was depleted due to the catalytic effects of nitrite. Thus, hydrogen sulfide and nitric oxide work in concert to constantly build up and break down the glycocalyx, which serves as a temporary storage bin for sulfated sugars. When the turnover rate of heparan sulfate chains is lowered, for example, due to impaired supply of hydrogen sulfide or to impaired mitochondrial function, the cell is less able to buffer sugars and therefore is more dependent on glucose supplied directly by the blood. This impaired buffering of sulfated sugars may be an indirect cause of elevated blood sugar because the cells cannot process sugar as efficiently when they can't store half of what they take in externally in the extracellular matrix. The temporary buffering of glucose within heparan sulfate chains allows the cell to survive the fasting period between meals.

CHLOROPHYLL, TRYPTOPHAN, AND JUMPING GENES

Most people are well aware that an abundance of dietary fresh green vegetables is beneficial to human health. Remarkably, a recent paper by Zhang et al. reveals a very novel direct benefit of the chlorophyll found in fresh green vegetables. These authors found that a metabolite of chlorophyll, specifically, pyropheophorbide-a (P-a), was able to enhance the ability of mitochondria to produce ATP in the presence of light, while at the same time maintaining or even reducing the amount of reactive oxygen species produced by the mitochondria [34]. This beneficial effect was achieved through catalysis of the reduction of coenzyme Q through the capture of photonic energy in the red frequency range of light. They demonstrated the effect in isolated mouse mitochondria, homogenates of mouse brain, heart and lens, and, most remarkably, in the live *Caenorhabditis elegans* worm species. Furthermore, they showed that worms exposed to light had a 17% increase in life span if they were also administered P-a.

Although the subject of "jumping genes" is tangential to the rest of this chapter, a chapter on sunlight's role in human physiology would not be complete without mentioning the unique role of tryptophan, mediated by sunlight, in evolution. An emerging and not yet fully understood story involves jumping genes, which likely are a key driver behind environmentally induced genetic evolutionary processes in response to stressors. Remarkably, these jumping genes make up 17% of our genome. Most of the copies are inert, although up to 100 of them are capable of jumping to a new location within the genome and then becoming actively expressed as novel genomic material. The essential aromatic amino acid, trytophan, plays a key role in activating these jumping genes, and this activation is mediated by sunlight [35]. Tryptophan is "fluorescent," meaning that it is capable of absorbing light and using it to excite an electron that induces a chemical reaction.

In response to both visible light and UV light, tryptophan is converted to 6-formylindolo[3,2-b] carbazole (FICZ). FICZ is the most likely endogenous activator of the aryl hydrocarbon receptor. This receptor induces the expression of multiple cytochrome P450 (CYP) enzymes in the liver that are essential for degrading xenobiotics [36]. Intriguingly, the aryl hydrocarbon receptor has been considered to be promiscuous in its response to multiple xenobiotics, including clinical drugs, food additives, industrial compounds, pesticides, and metals. However, it is likely that these all act indirectly by inhibiting the metabolism of FICZ through CYP hydroxylation and subsequent sulfation [37]. The receptor responds to FICZ at extremely low concentrations, and, if FICZ cannot be metabolized, the receptor will continue to induce CYP enzyme expression until successful clearance of the offending xenobiotic.

However, perhaps the most important role of FICZ is in priming these jumping genes for actually jumping within the genome to create new genetic expression. It is intriguing that cocaine and methamphetamine, two drugs that are widely abused, also activate jumping genes in neuronal cells in a manner that is identical to the process by which tryptophan activates them [38]. It is possible that a deficiency in tryptophan leads to a dependency on these mood-altering drugs. Indeed, the deficits in decision-making and cognition of chronic amphetamine abusers is inducible in normal subjects through a tryptophan-restricted diet [39].

GLYPHOSATE'S DISRUPTION OF ELECTRICAL SYSTEMS

Glyphosate is the active ingredient in the pervasive herbicide, Roundup®. Much recent research has shown that glyphosate is far more toxic to humans than we have been led to believe. The arguments for its benign effects on humans is based on the fact that a key mechanism of its toxicity to plants involves a biological pathway that human cells do not possess—the shikimate pathway. However, our gut microbes do have this pathway and they utilize it to supply us with essential amino acids that human cells are unable to synthesize for themselves. These are the aromatic amino acids, tryptophan, tyrosine, and phenylalanine, and their many biologically important derivatives can be expected to be deficient as well in the presence of chronic glyphosate poisoning. A tryptophan deficiency will impair aryl hydrocarbon receptor signaling, and this may explain the observed suppression of CYP enzyme expression by glyphosate in rat liver [40].

A seminal paper by Swanson et al. shows remarkably strong and highly significant correlations between the rise in glyphosate usage on core crops in the United States and the concurrent rise in the incidence of a large number of chronic, debilitating diseases and conditions, including diabetes, obesity, Alzheimer's disease, liver disease, kidney failure, inflammatory bowel disease, autism, pancreatic cancer, and thyroid cancer [41]. A paper recently published by Anthony Samsel and myself has shown how glyphosate's likely ability to substitute for glycine by mistake during protein synthesis can explain how glyphosate could cause all of these diseases [42]. A precedent for this concept has been set by at least four naturally produced toxins that work by acting as analogues for four distinct coding amino acids to cause diseases like amyotrophic lateral sclerosis (ALS) and multiple sclerosis. Glyphosate, however, is never found in nature, but only available through its synthesis in the chemistry lab.

In this section, I will describe several different ways in which glyphosate's pathological effects on human physiology can induce sulfate insufficiency, and also disrupt critical ion pumps and ion channels, impairing the cells' ability to regulate their internal ion concentrations and their membrane voltage gradients. This results in a significant impairment of the electrical system, systemically, leading to multiple disease states.

SULFATE HOMEOSTASIS

It is notable that several enzymes involved in sulfate metabolism in *Escherichia coli* are downregulated by glyphosate, as shown in Table 21.1. These include enzymes involved with sulfate transport, sulfate reduction, sulfation, and sulfate binding [43].

A glycine-to-aspartate mutation at residue 473 in sulfite oxidase impairs dimerization [44] and results in severe reduction in the enzyme's catalytic activity. This effect was believed to be due to the negative charge and the large size of aspartate. Since glyphosate has similar properties, it can be predicted that glyphosate substituting for this key glycine residue would have a similar catastrophic

TABLE 21.1

Genes Expressed by *E. coli*, Involved in Sulfate Homeostasis, Whose Activity is Suppressed by Glyphosate

Suppressed Protein	Fold Change
cysH 3-phosphoadenosine 5-phosphosulfate reductase	−3.75
cysM; ATP:sulfurylase (ATP:sulfate adenylyltransferase), subunit 2	−2.65
pdxJ; adenosine 5-phosphosulfate kinase	−2.55
yibN; predicted rhodanese-related sulfur transferase	−2.27
Sbp; sulfate transporter unit	−2.55
potG; periplasmic sulfate-binding protein	−3.39

Source: For details, see Lu W et al. *Mol. BioSyst.* 2013; 9: 522–530. Supplementary Table S2. Functional description of genes downregulated in response to glyphosate shock.

effect. Sulfotransferases contain a highly conserved GxxGxxK motif that is required for binding to the activated sulfate donor [45]. Clearly, substitution of glyphosate for either of the two glycines in this motif would disrupt its ability to transfer sulfate ligands.

Collagen, which forms a crucial component of the basement membrane and which is often gly-cosylated, contains a huge amount of glycine in its peptide sequence. A triple GXX motif is a multiple repeat unit in long stretches of collagen, and overall about 25% of collagen consists of glycine residues. Substitution of glyphosate for these residues will cause impaired double-helix formation of the collagen matrix, impairing its elastic and tensile strength properties and likely also disrupting its role in maintaining structured water.

DEPLETION OF AROMATIC SULFATE TRANSPORTERS

The monoamine neurotransmitters include serotonin, melatonin, dopamine, and epinephrine, and they are crucial for proper brain function. They regulate emotion and arousal, and are involved in memory retention, and implicated in multiple psychiatric disorders, such as depression, schizophrenia, and anxiety. All of the monoamine neurotransmitters are derived from the aromatic amino acids, phenylalanine, tyrosine, and tryptophan. These essential amino acids are all products of the shikimate pathway, which glyphosate inhibits [46]. Since we depend on our gut microbes to provide these essential nutrients, chronic exposure to glyphosate will lead to a deficiency in their supply.

The gut-brain axis is a bidirectional communication channel between the microbiome and the brain, and it plays a significant role in health and disease. There is an epidemic in the United States today in multiple gut disorders, including inflammatory bowel diseases, irritable bowel syndrome, Celiac disease (gluten intolerance), and gastroesophageal reflux disease (GERD). Glyphosate likely is a significant contributor to gut disorders, due to its ability to alter the distribution of microbes in the gut toward an overgrowth of pathogens, as well as its ability to chelate minerals making them unavailable to both the gut microbes and the human cells. Crucial to glyphosate's negative effects is the disruption of the shikimate pathway and therefore of the bioavailability of the aromatic amino acids and their derivatives, the monoamine neurotransmitters.

A central role in the communication channel between the gut and the brain is played by tryptophan and its derivatives. Serotonin is synthesized predominantly in the gut from tryptophan by intestinal enterochromaffin cells, and it is crucial for maintaining intestinal secretory, sensory, and motor function. Serotonin is also transported to the brain as serotonin sulfate, and thus it can serve as an important supplier of sulfate to the brain. In the brain, serotonin is converted to melatonin in the pineal gland in the evening, and the melatonin is also sulfated before being shipped out via the cerebrospinal fluid to the neurons of the brain. This supply of sulfate may be very important for enhancing the brain's ability to clear cellular debris at night during sleep [47]. Melatonin is also synthesized in the gut, and in fact the gut provides most of the melatonin supply to the body.

CHOLESTEROL SULFATE, PPAR-γ, AND THE LIVER

Oxysterol sulfates are derivatives of cholesterol that have been oxidized by CYP enzymes and then sulfated by sulfotransferases (SULTs). They are produced in the liver, and it has recently become apparent that they are regulatory signaling molecules with dramatic responses when present at low concentrations [48]. In the liver, they have remarkably beneficial effects in suppressing the release of nuclear factor kappa-light-chain-enhancer of activated B cells (NF-κB) and pro-inflammatory cytokines following exposure to lipopolysaccharides (LPS) and tumor necrosis factor α (TNFα). They reduce the build-up of lipid stores in the liver (fatty liver disease), protect from apoptosis, and promote proliferation of liver cells. They also promote bile flow, which is essential for the digestion of dietary fats, among many other roles. In many cases, the same oxysterols, when unsulfated, have the opposite effect.

Peroxisome proliferator activated receptors (PPARs) are nuclear receptors that sense cellular cholesterol and lipid levels and elicit changes in gene expression to maintain lipid homeostasis and protect from lipid overload [49]. Remarkably, a novel highly sulfated oxysterol, with *three* liganded sulfates, has recently been identified and found to have potent regulatory properties, involving control of lipid metabolism, inflammation, and cell proliferation [49]. This unique sulfated oxysterol substantially increased expression of PPAR-γ in the liver, decreasing hepatic triglyceride and cholesterol levels. In vitro experiments on glyphosate exposure to fibroblasts revealed that glyphosate formulations at environmentally realistic levels suppressed expression of PPAR-γ [50]. This can be predicted to lead directly to elevated serum LDL. As shown in Figure 21.4, serum LDL levels have risen steadily in the U.S. population in the last two decades, in step with the rise in glyphosate usage

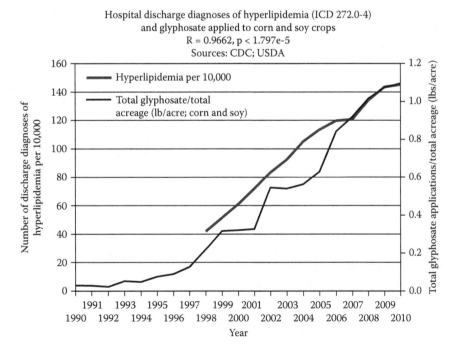

FIGURE 21.4 Temporal trends in hyperlipidemia according to the U.S. CDC's hospital discharge data plotted together with upward trends in glyphosate usage on corn and soy crops.

on core crops. Whether this effect of glyphosate is a direct consequence of its impairment of sulfation pathways is not clear.

Disruption of eNOS

It was previously described how eNOS produces sulfate in response to sunlight exposure when it is bound to the plasma membrane at cavaeolae. eNOS binding is orchestrated through a highly conserved terminal glycine residue via a process termed myristoylation [51].

If this residue is replaced with alanine (a single extra methyl group), myristoylation is thwarted and the molecule is unable to attach to the membrane at all. Furthermore, another highly conserved glycine residue is essential for NOS dimer formation [52]. Dimerization is required for sulfate synthesis [4]. Therefore, if glyphosate substitutes for either of these essential glycines by mistake during protein synthesis, eNOS will be derailed in its ability to synthesize sulfate. eNOS is also an orphan member of the CYP family, and as such it can be expected to be inhibited by glyphosate [40,53]. The pathological state of eNOS that produces superoxide instead of NO [54,55] is likely induced by glyphosate exposure.

Sodium/Potassium ATPase and the Heart

There is an epidemic today in attempted suicide among agricultural workers by drinking glyphosate-based formulations, and they often succeed [56]. These formulations contain, in addition to glyphosate, surfactants such as polyethoxylated tallow amine (POEA) which act as adjuvants to increase glyphosate uptake into cells. The surfactants have a direct effect on cells that increases the permeability of the membrane to ions—in particular, exposure to surfactant will induce sodium leaks into the cell which will activate the Na-K pump. A recent study by Prof. Seralini's team in France showed that over-expression of this pump leads to arrhythmias and cardiac arrest following exposure of perfused rat hearts in vitro to glyphosate-based herbicide [57]. The crucial role that the Na-K pump plays in cellular physiology was previously described.

If glyphosate can substitute for glycine during protein synthesis, as proposed in [42], it can be predicted that regulation of the Na-K pump will be highly disturbed. In particular, the pump will work harder and longer than it should. There are at least three other proteins involved in regulating the pump, all of which contain highly conserved glycines that play essential roles. One of these, phospholemman, is normally attached to the pump in the membrane, and it suppresses its activity level by about a factor of two. Disruption of its two highly conserved glycines [58] by glyphosate will prevent it from anchoring in the membrane, essentially disabling its function altogether. The second protein is a kinase which phosphorylates and inactivates phospholemman. Glyphosate's substitution for glycine in the active site of the kinase can be predicted to *increase* its activity [42], thus disabling phospholemman's suppression of the pump even when the phospholemman is not itself contaminated with glyphosate.

Finally, a third protein, the glycine-rich ZNRF2, controls the degradation of the Na-K pump. Disruption of its conserved glycines will cause the pump to linger longer than it should, thus exhausting ATP supplies and causing the cell to reach a hyperpolarized state, with too much internal potassium and too little internal sodium. ZNRF2 interacts with the Na-K pump to induce ubiquitylation and subsequent degradation of the molecule [59]. It has a highly conserved glycine at its N-terminal end which is essential for myristoylation. Myristoylation, in turn, is essential for it to be able to secure itself to the membrane, just as is the case for eNOS. A substitution of alanine for glycine (one extra methyl group) leads to impaired function, and, as a consequence, Na/K ATPase accumulates. The same thing can be predicted to occur if glyphosate substitutes for glycine at the same location.

The net result of all of this disruption by glyphosate is that exposed cells become hyperpolarized and depleted in electrolytes and ATP. Osmosis will drive water out of the cell to rebalance the electrolyte buffering. This will cause epithelial cells in the gut lining exposed to glyphosate to shrink, opening up the tight junctions and allowing penetration of the glyphosate and the surfactant (along with undigested proteins and other allergenic molecules) into the vasculature and the lymph system.

Once in the vasculature, the surfactants and glyphosate, working in concert, will cause a similar effect in the vascular wall. This will open up vascular leaks allowing the poisons to infiltrate the pleural cavity, along with blood plasma and small proteins. This will cause pleural effusion and allow access of the poisons to the heart and lungs via the interstitial fluids. The danger becomes acute when cardiac cells over-express the Na-K pump, because this leads to long QT syndrome, arrhythmias such as tachycardia and bradycardia (slow heart rate), and cardiac arrest. These are well-known consequences of acute poisoning by glyphosate-based herbicides [56].

A precipitous drop in blood pressure is also a common observation following acute glyphosate exposure, due to both the loss of blood volume through vascular leaks and impaired cardiac capacity due to the arrhythmias and depleted ATP supplies. Furthermore, the hyperpolarization of endothelial cells in the cardiac arteries leads to acidification of the artery, and therefore a reduction in the battery strength attributed to the pH drop across capillaries. Due to all these disruptions, a no-flow situation with disseminated intravascular coagulation and multiple organ failure are possible outcomes.

While acute glyphosate poisoning is a rare occurrence, chronic low-dose glyphosate exposure is almost universal in the United States. Glyphosate usage has grown exponentially over the past two decades, in step with the widespread adoption of glyphosate-resistant crops. Over time, one can anticipate that glyphosate will insidiously accumulate in the tissues, and will be continuously recycled into new proteins with unpredictable consequences.

The skeletal muscle cells are a major storage site for potassium, and, due to their enhanced need for ionic currents to induce contraction, they are abundantly supplied with Na-K pumps [60]. Under conditions of intense exercise and/or adrenalin stimulation, Na-K pumps are activated in the muscle cells to restore internal potassium levels. With chronic glyphosate poisoning, there is a serious risk of these pumps going into overdrive and severely depleting potassium levels in the blood. This effect can take place in a matter of seconds, and there is a serious threat of cardiac arrest and sudden death as a consequence. This may explain the epidemic we're seeing in sudden infant death syndrome (SIDS) [3] and in sudden cardiac death of a young athlete following an adrenalin rush, such as has happened in intense athletic events [61]. Race horses dying at the finish line is likely the same phenomenon [62].

Worldwide, 3 million people suffer from sudden cardiac death each year, and 1/6 of them are under 50 years old [60]. In one study, hypokalemia was associated with a 10-fold higher risk of death among hospitalized patients. Low serum potassium increases the risk to ventricular fibrillation by 5-fold. Low potassium is associated with long QT syndrome and with increased heart rate. Beta adrenergic agonists used to treat asthma patients carry a serious risk to sudden death due to hypokalemia. Non-potassium sparing diuretics and insulin therapy are also associated with a risk of arrhythmia and sudden cardiac death.

As many as 20% of hospitalized patients and 40% of patients on diuretics suffer from hypokalemia. Certainly a diet enriched in foods that are high in potassium is protective, but a more important preventive measure is to consume a certified organic diet in order to reduce glyphosate exposure.

BROADER CONSEQUENCES

We suffer from many painful and debilitating autoimmune diseases today, including type-1 diabetes, rheumatoid arthritis, lupus, multiple sclerosis, chronic fatigue syndrome, irritable bowel disease, and many others. I propose that all of these diseases are characterized by an autoimmune attack on a specific organ or organ system with the goal of retrieving sulfate in order to maintain a working circulatory system. Inflammation, thrombohemorrhagic phenomena, colloidal instability, and cardiac arrhythmias, with high mortality risk, can arise from low serum zeta potential and streaming potential due to impaired supply of sulfated glycoproteins and sterols [3]. Without sulfate, the immune cells cannot adequately clear infectious microbes, and the red blood cells cannot easily traverse the capillaries. Blood stagnates and coalesces, producing thrombosis events that can lead to a fatal pulmonary embolism. The heart must work much harder to force the suspended particles through capillaries when the blood is too viscous and there is not enough negative charge on the suspended particles, and a thinner glycocalyx leads to equally damaging threats of hemorrhage. Cells are unable to clear debris that then accumulates as lipofuscin or amyloid beta, leading to neurological diseases such as Alzheimer's that are very costly to society, both emotionally and financially.

There is hope for the future, however, and it is especially gratifying that the path toward good health involves natural solutions that are relatively easy to implement. It should be a global policy to work toward finding new efficient ways to grow food organically and sustainably, removing our dependence on toxic herbicides, particularly glyphosate, and perhaps facing up to the fact that we need to put more manual labor back into agriculture. With the increased sophistication of robotics, it may be possible to develop a robotic solution to killing weeds without the use of toxic chemicals, and this is where research is desperately needed. A dietary change from heavily processed, chemically laden foods to organic whole foods that are rich in cholesterol, sulfur, ascorbate, and polyphenols will promote healing and hasten a return to good health.

A crucial component of a healthy lifestyle is adequate sun exposure, as sunlight energy can be utilized to synthesize sulfate, capturing energy, oxygen, and sulfur in a form that is vital to the homeostasis of water and the production of electricity in the body. The battery that is created in the structured water and charged up in the presence of sunlight ultimately provides energy that fuels the Na-K pump, by promoting the flow of protons into the intermembrane space of the mitochondria. The mitochondria use this energy to synthesize ATP, and the Na-K pump depletes the ATP as it moves ions across the plasma membrane against their concentration gradient. The moonlighting enzyme, eNOS, plays the dual role of providing sulfate and nitrate to promote the continual recycling of heparan sulfate proteoglycans. The essential extracellular matrix glycoproteins with attached heparan sulfate chains facilitate the entry of nutrients into the cell and the clearance of infectious microbes and of cellular debris via the lysosomes.

REFERENCES

1. Davidson RM, Lauritzen A, Seneff S. Biological water dynamics and entropy: A biophysical origin of cancer and other diseases. *Entropy* 2013; 15(9): 3822–3876.
2. Pollack GH. *The Fourth Phase of Water: Beyond Solid, Liquid, and Vapor.* Ebner and Sons Publishers, Seattle, WA, 2013.
3. Davidson RM, Seneff S. The initial common pathway of inflammation, disease, and sudden death. *Entropy* 2012; 14: 1399–1442.
4. Seneff S, Lauritzen A, Davidson R, Lentz-Marino L. Is endothelial nitric oxide synthase a moonlighting protein whose day job is cholesterol sulfate synthesis? Implications for cholesterol transport, diabetes and cardiovascular disease. *Entropy* 2012; 14: 2492–2530.
5. Reitsma S, Slaaf DW, Vink H, van Zandvoort MAMJ, oude Egbrink MGA. The endothelial glycocalyx: Composition, functions, and visualization. *Pflugers Arch - Eur J Physiol* 2007; 454: 345–359.
6. Chai B, Yoo H, Pollack GH. Effect of radiant energy on near-surface water. *J Phys Chem B* 2009; 113(42): 13953–13958.
7. Pan J, Zhu K-N, Zhou M, Wang ZY. Low resonant frequency storage and transfer in structured water cluster. *IEEE International Conference on Systems, Man and Cybernetics 2003.* (Volume 5) 5–8 Oct. 2003, Washington DC, USA.
8. Petersen PB, Johnson JC, Knutsen KP, Saykally RJ. Direct experimental validation of the Jones-Ray effect. *Chem Phys Lett* 2004; 397(1): 46–50.
9. Strott CA, Higashi Y. Cholesterol sulfate in human physiology: What's it all about? *J Lipid Res* 2003; 44(7): 1268–1278.
10. Seneff S, Davidson RM, Lauritzen A, Samsel A, Wainwright G. A novel hypothesis for atherosclerosis as a cholesterol sulfate deficiency syndrome. *Theor Biol Med Model* 2015; 12: 9.
11. Kuzkaya N, Weissmann N, Harrison DG, Dikalov S. Interactions of peroxynitrite, tetrahydrobiopterin, ascorbic acid, and thiols: Implications for uncoupling endothelial nitric-oxide synthase. *J Biol Chem* 2003; 278(25): 22546–22554.

12. Kleinbongard P, Schulz R, Rassaf T et al. Red blood cells express a functional endothelial nitric oxide synthase. *Blood* 2006; 107: 2943–2951.
13. Kang ES, Ford K, Grokulsky G, Wang YB, Chiang TM, Acchiardo SR. Normal circulating adult human red blood cells contain inactive NOS proteins. *J Lab Clin Med* 2000; 135: 444–451.
14. Aicher A, Heeschen C, Mildner-Rihm C, Urbich C, Ihling C, Technau-Ihling K, Zeiher AM, Dimmeler S. Essential role of endothelial nitric oxide synthase for mobilization of stem and progenitor cells. *Nat Med* 2003; 9(11): 1370–1376.
15. Halfter W, Dong S, Schurer B, Cole GJ. Collagen XVIII Is a Basement Membrane Heparan Sulfate Proteoglycan. *JBC* 1993; 273(39): 25404–25412.
16. Noonan DM, Fulle A, Valente P, Cai S, Horigan E, Sasaki M, Yamada Y, Hassell JR. Sequence of perlecan, a basement membrane heparan sulfate proteoglycan, reveals extensive similarity with laminin A chain, low density lipoprotein-receptor, and the neural cell adhesion moleculgcale. *J Biol Chem* 1991; 266(34): 2293947.
17. Farach-Carson MC, Warren CR, Harrington DA, Carson DD. Border patrol: Insights into the unique role of perlecan/heparan sulfate proteoglycan2 at cell and tissue borders. *Matrix Biol* 2014; 34: 64–79.
18. Gustafsson E, Almonte-Becerril M, Bloch W, Costell M. Perlecan maintains microvessel integrity in vivo and modulates their formation in vitro. *PloS One* 2013; 8:53715.
19. Paka L, Kako Y, Obunike JC, Pillarisetti S. Apolipoprotein E Containing High Density Lipoprotein Stimulates Endothelial Production of Heparan Sulfate Rich in Biologically Active Heparin-like Domains. A potential mechanism for the anti-atherogenic actions of vascular apolipoprotein E. *JBC* 1999; 274(8): 4816–4823.
20. Bowling FG, Heussler HS, McWhinney A, Dawson PA. Plasma and urinary sulfate determination in a cohort with autism. *Biochem Genet* 2013; 51(1–2): 147–153.
21. Dawson PA, Choyce A, Chuang C, Whitelock J, Markovich D, Leggatt GR. Enhanced tumor growth in the NaS1 sulfate transporter null mouse. *Cancer Sci* 2010; 101(2): 369–373.
22. Chernousov MA, Rothblum K, Stahl RC, Evans A, Prentiss L, Carey DJ. Glypican-1 and alpha4(V) collagen are required for schwann cell myelination. *J Neurosci* 2006; 26(2): 508–517.
23. Gadsby DC. Ion channels versus ion pumps: The principal difference, in principle. *Nat Rev Mol Cell Biol* 2009; 10(5): 344–352.
24. Sahu S, Ghosh S, Ghosh B, Aswani K, Hirata K, Fujita D, Bandyopadhyay A. Atomic water channel controlling remarkable properties of a single brain microtubule: Correlating single protein to its supramolecular assembly. *Biosens Bioelectron* 2013; 47: 141–148.
25. Kabir SR, Yokoyama K, Mihashi K, Kodama T, Suzuki M. Hyper-mobile water is induced around actin filaments. *Biophys J* 2003; 85: 3154–3161.
26. Pillarisetti S. Lipoprotein modulation of subendothelial heparan sulfate proteoglycans (perlecan) and atherogenicity. *Trends Cardiovasc Med* 2000; 10(2): 60–65.
27. Baggetto LG, Clottes E, Vial C. Low mitochondrial proton leak due to high membrane cholesterol content and cytosolic creatine kinase as two features of the deviant bioenergetics of Ehrlich and AS30-D tumor cells. *Cancer Res* 1992; 52(18): 4935–4941.
28. Trivedi DP, Hallock KJ, Bergethon PR. Electric fields caused by blood flow modulate vascular endothelial electrophysiology and nitric oxide production. *Bioelectromagnetics* 2013; 34(1): 22–30.
29. Mani K, Jönsson M, Edgren G, Belting M, Fransson LA. A novel role for nitric oxide in the endogenous degradation of heparan sulfate during recycling of glypican-1 in vascular endothelial cells. *Glycobiology* 2000; 10(6): 577–586.
30. Vilar RE, Ghael D, Li M, Bhagat DD, Arrigo LM, Cowman MK, Dweck HS, Rosenfeld L. Nitric oxide degradation of heparin and heparan sulphate. *Biochem J* 1997; 324: 473–479.
31. Van Teeffelen JWGE, Constantinescu AA, Brands J, Spaan JAE, Vink H. Bradykinin- and sodium nitroprusside-induced increases in capillary tube haematocrit in mouse cremaster muscle are associated with impaired glycocalyx barrier properties. *J Physiol* 2008; 586(13): 3207–3218.
32. King AL, Polhemus DJ, Bhushan S et al. Hydrogen sulfide cytoprotective signaling is endothelial nitric oxide synthase-nitric oxide dependent. *PNAS* 2014; 111(8): 3182–3187.
33. Hildebrandt TM, Grieshaber MK. Three enzymatic activities catalyze the oxidation of sulfide to thiosulfate in mammalian and invertebrate mitochondria. *FEBS J* 2008; 275: 3352–3361.
34. Xu C, Zhang J, Mihai DM, Washington I. Light-harvesting chlorophyll pigments enable mammalian mitochondria to capture photonic energy and produce ATP. *J Cell Sci* 2014; 127: 388–399.
35. Okudaira N, Iijima K, Koyama T, Minemoto Y, Kano S, Mimori A, Ishizaka Y. Induction of long interspersed nucleotide element-1 (L1) retrotransposition by 6-formylindolo[3,2-b] carbazole (FICZ), a tryptophan photoproduct. *PNAS* 2010; 107(43): 18487–18492.

36. Diani-Moore S, Labitzke E, Brown R, Garvin A, Wong L, Rifkind AB. Sunlight generates multiple tryptophan photoproducts eliciting high efficacy CYP1A induction in chick hepatocytes and in vivo. *Toxicol. Sci.* 2006; 90(1): 96–110.

37. Wincent E, Bengtsson J, Bardboria AM, Alsberg T, Luecke S, Rannug U, Rannug A. Inhibition of cytochrome P450l-dependent clearance of the endogenous agonist FICZ as a mechanism for activation of the aryl hydrocarbon receptor. *Proc Natl Acad Sci U S A* 2012; 109(12): 4479–4484.

38. Okudaira N, Ishizaka Y, Nishio H. *Retrotransposition of long interspersed element 1 induced by methamphetamine or cocaine.* JBC Papers in Press, July 22, 2014, DOI 10.1074/jbc.M114.559419

39. Rogers RD, Everitt BJ, Baldacchino A et al. Dissociable deficits in the decision-making cognition of chronic amphetamine abusers, opiate abusers, patients with focal damage to prefrontal cortex, and tryptophan-depeleted normal volunteers: Evidence for monoaminergic mechanisms. *Neuropsychopharmacology* 1999; 20: 322339.

40. Hietanen E, Linnainmaa K, Vainio H. Effects of phenoxyherbicides and glyphosate on the hepatic and intestinal biotransformation activities in the rat. *Acta Pharmacol Toxicol (Copenh)* 1983; 53(2): 103–112.

41. Swanson NL, Leu A, Abrahamson J, Wallet B. Genetically engineered crops, glyphosate and the deterioration of health in the United States of America. *J Org Syst* 2014; 9(2): 6–37.

42. Samsel A, Seneff S. Glyphosate, pathways to modern diseases V: Amino acid analogue of glycine in diverse proteins. *J Biol Phys Chem* 2016; 16: 9–46.

43. Lu W, Li L, Chen M, Zhou Z, Zhang W, Ping S, Yan Y, Wang J, Lin M. Genome-wide transcriptional responses of Escherichia coli to glyphosate, a potent inhibitor of the shikimate pathway enzyme 5-enolpyruvylshikimate-3-phosphate synthase. *Mol. BioSyst.* 2013; 9: 522–530. Supplementary Table S2. Functional description of genes downregulated in response to glyphosate shock.

44. Wilson HL, Wilkinson SR, Rajagopalan KV. The G473D mutation impairs dimerization and catalysis in human sulfite oxidase. *Biochemistry* 2006;45(7): 2149–2160.

45. Komatsu K, Driscoll WJ, Koh YC, Strott CA. A P-loop related motif (GxxGxxK) highly conserved in sulfotransferases is required for binding the activated sulfate donor. *Biochem Biophys Res Commun* 1994; 204(3): 1178–1185.

46. de Maria N, Becerril JM, Garca-Plazaola JI, Hernández A, De Felipe MR, Fernandez-Pascual M. New insights on glyphosate mode of action in nodular metabolism: Role of shikimate accumulation. *J Agric Food Chem* 2006; 54(7): 2621–2628.

47. Seneff S, Swanson N, Li C. Aluminum and glyphosate can synergistically induce pineal gland pathology: Connection to gut dysbiosis and neurological disease. *Agricultural Sciences*, 2015; 6: 42–70.

48. Ren S, Ning Y. Sulfation of 25-hydroxycholesterol regulates lipid metabolism, inflammatory responses, and cell proliferation. *Am J Physiol Endocrinol Metab* 2014; 306: E123–E130.

49. Ren S, Kim JK, Kakiyama G, Rodriguez-Agudo D, Pandak WM, Min H-K, Ning Y. Identification of novel regulatory cholesterol metabolite, 5-cholesten, 3b,25-diol, disulfate. *PLOS ONE* 2014; 9(7): e103621.

50. Martini CN, Gabrielli M, Brandani JN, del C Vila M. Glyphosate inhibits PPAR gamma induction and differentiation of preadipocytes and is able to induce oxidative stress. *J Biocem Molecular Toxicol* 2016 [Epub ahead of print].

51. Kamps MP, Buss JE, Sefton BM. Mutation of NH2-terminal glycine of p60src prevents both myristoylation and morphological transformation. *Proc Natl Acad Sci U S A*. 1985; 82(14): 4625–4628.

52. Cho HJ, Martin E, Xie Q, Sassa S, Nathan C. Inducible nitric oxide synthase: Identification of amino acid residues essential for dimerization and binding of tetrahydrobiopterin. *Proc Natl Acad Sci USA* 1995; 92(25): 11514–11518.

53. Samsel A, Seneff S. Glyphosate's suppression of cytochrome P450 enzymes and amino acid biosynthesis by the gut microbiome: Pathways to modern diseases. *Entropy* 2013; 15: 1416–1463.

54. Hijmering EM, van Zandvoort M, Wever R, Rabelink TJ, van Faassen EE. Origin of superoxide production by endothelial nitric oxide synthase. *FEBS Lett* 1998; 438(3): 161–164.

55. Vásquez-Vivar J, Kalyanaraman B, Martásek P, Hogg N, Siler Masters BS, Karoui H, Tordo P, Pritchard KA Jr. Superoxide generation by endothelial nitric oxide synthase: The influence of cofactors. *Proc Natl Acad Sci USA* 1998; 95: 9220–9225.

56. Lee HL, Chen KW, Chi CH, Huang JJ, Tsai LM. Clinical presentations and prognostic factors of a glyphosate-surfactant herbicide intoxication: A review of 131 cases. *Acad Emerg Med* 2000; 7(8): 906–910.

57. Gress S, Lemoine S, Puddu P-E, Séralini G-E, Rouet R. Cardiotoxic electrophysiological effects of the herbicide roundup in rat and rabbit ventricular myocardium in vitro. *Cardiovasc Toxicol* 2015; 15: 324–335.

58. Mahmmoud YA, Cramb G, Maunsbach AB, Cutler CP, Meischke L, Cornelius F. Regulation of Na,K-ATPase by PLMS, the phospholemman-like protein from shark: Molecular cloning, sequence, expression, cellular distribution, and functional effects of PLMS. *JBC* 2003; 278(39): 37427–37438.

59. Hoxhaj G, Najafov A, Toth R, Campbell DG, Prescott AR, MacKintosh C. ZNRF2 is released from membranes by growth factors and, together with ZNRF1, regulates the Na+/K+ATPase. *J Cell Sci* 2012; 125(19): 4662–4675.

60. Kjeldsen K. Hypokalemia and sudden cardiac death. *Exp Clin Cardiol* 2010; 15(4): e96–e99.

61. Koester MC. A review of sudden cardiac death in young athletes and strategies for preparticipation cardiovascular screening. *J Athl Train* 2001; 36(2): 197–204.

62. Physick-Sheard PW, McGurrin MKJ. Ventricular arrhythmias during race recovery in standard bred racehorses and associations with autonomic activity. *J Vet Intern Med* 2010; 24: 1158–1166.

22 Electromagnetic Hygiene

Magda Havas

CONTENTS

Introduction..524
An Historical Overview 525
What is Electromagnetic Pollution?...530
    Basic Properties of Electromagnetic Energy...530
What Are the Different Types of Non-Ionizing Radiation (NIR) That Are of Concern?.............530
Biological Effects of Electrosmog 532
    Cancer 532
    Reproduction 534
        ELF Electromagnetic Fields...534
        Dirty Electricity and Intermediate Frequencies..535
        RF/MW..535
        Effects on Sperm 535
        Adverse Pregnancy Outcomes..536
        Effects on Offspring 536
        Antennas and Reproduction 537
    Electrohypersensitivity (EHS)...537
        Provocation Testing 538
        Mitigation Testing 539
What Do Authorities Say about Electrosmog? 540
What Can We Do to Protect Ourselves from Electrosmog? 541
    Electromagnetic Hygiene: Specific Recommendations 541
        ELF Magnetic Field 541
        Dirty Electricity..542
        Radio Frequency and Microwave Radiation 542
    Here Are a Few Things You Need to Know about a Few Commonly Used Devices.................543
        Cell Phones...543
        Cordless Phones 543
        Internet Access: Computer, Wi-Fi Router, Tablets 544
        Wireless Baby Monitors 544
        Smart Meter...544
        Smart Appliances..545
        Gaming Systems..545
        Energy Efficient Light Bulbs..545
        Bluetooth 545
        Clock Radio 547
        Electric Equipment...547
        Electrical Panel and Utility Room..547
        Electric Blanket and Waterbed 547
        Turn Bedroom Power Off..547
        Monitoring Your Exposure 547
Acknowledgments..547
References 547

INTRODUCTION

Ever since Ignaz Semmelweis discovered that physicians who washed their hands with a disinfectant prior to helping with deliveries had greater success of a healthy outcome for both mother and child, we have recognized the importance of hand hygiene. Clean hands, clean water, clean air, and clean food that is not genetically modified or contaminated with microbes or toxic chemicals provide the backbone to and is the basis for healthy living. However, there is one form of pollution that virtually goes unnoticed—electromagnetic pollution.

Electromagnetic pollution, commonly referred to as electrosmog, is an invisible silent killer that has been studied for decades but which the western medical establishment has not yet accepted. And just as it took time for the medical establishment to accept Semmelweis's warning—that microorganisms, tiny creatures that we can't see, can make us sick—the same is true regarding electrosmog.

Semmelweis's concepts in 1847 combined with the use of the microscope and Alexander Fleming's discovery of penicillin in 1927 led to the field of microbiology, a respected field of research taught in medical schools. It also laid the foundations for the pharmaceutical industry resulting in the survival of many who would have otherwise died from bacterial infections.

The health effects of electrosmog, tiny waves that can make us ill, is hotly denied by anyone who has even a vague understanding of physics. Yet the research in this area is becoming increasingly more convincing to anyone who has an open mind and is not set on protecting the status quo. This is what Thomas Kuhn (1962) refers to as the scientific revolution and is the primary way that science advances.

As with any environmental pollutant—where health, money, legal issues, and politics come into play—we often have controversy, some of which is scientifically justified due to inadequate information and some of which is based on financial benefits to those who produce the pollutant. To differentiate between scientific controversy and financial controversy is not always obvious and can often be done only by those intimately familiar with the field of study. Most doctors don't have the time for this research; most journalists don't have the scientific credentials for this type of investigative reporting; and most scientists can't be bothered getting involved in the controversy. Policy makers often use disagreements among scientists to delay updating policy, which delays incorporation of scientific information into useful medical procedures and medical education.

The early warning scientists and physicians, who notice a problem and bring attention to it, are often criticized and attempts are made to discredit them. This has happened with asbestos (Irving Selikoff—who pressured the Occupational Health and Safety Association [OHSA] to limit worker asbestos exposures); DDT (Rachel Carson—whose popular book *Silent Spring* brought the dangers of DDT to public attention), and lead (Sam Epstein—who gave expert testimony to the U.S. Senate among others about lead toxicity in children). Decades later—with continued research—society benefits as the scientific information is eventually accepted.

According to Arthur Schopenhauer …

All truth passes through three stages.
First, it is ridiculed.
Second, it is violently opposed.
Third, it is accepted as being self-evident.

This will continue to happen, so it is critical for those in the health care profession to make up their own minds and become familiar with the literature. This is easier said than done due to time constraints. The purpose of this chapter is to summarize the research that documents the harmful effects of electrosmog and to provide useful tips on how to minimize exposure and thus delay or prevent injury, and how to help those who are already adversely affected by exposure to electromagnetic pollution.

AN HISTORICAL OVERVIEW

Our exposure to electromagnetic energy generated by anthropogenic sources has been increasing since the beginning of the twentieth century. Edison's invention of the incandescent electric light bulb (1879) combined with Tesla's invention of alternating current (1888) brought electric light and electricity to the world. By 1895, Niagara Falls was able to distribute electricity to Buffalo, NY and—with the construction of transmission lines and distribution lines—electricity is now available virtually in every urban and rural center. In addition to the electric light bulb, we now have many devices that rely on electricity from stoves to refrigerators and freezers, washers and dryers, to simple motors that run a power tool or a hair dryer. Our consumption of electricity has increased greatly. No matter how the electricity is generated, by hydroelectric power or by fossil fuels or by renewable energy, anything that is plugged into an electric outlet generates an electric field and anything that is turned on and consuming power generates a magnetic field. Consequently, our exposure to power frequency electric and magnetic fields started with the electric light bulb and has been increasing ever since. This type of energy is classified as extremely low frequency (ELF) and referred to as *power frequency* because of its reliance on electric power.

Our exposure to radio frequency radiation began with the discovery of radio waves and the invention of the radio. Marconi made the first long distance trans-Atlantic wireless transmission by radio in 1891 from St. John's Newfoundland to Cornwall in the U.K. Radio broadcasting of the human voice and music started around the 1920s when there were only a few radio stations operating for only a few hours each day. Today, there are literally hundreds of thousands of radio stations operating at any one time around the world.

The next major step in broadcasting was television that involved sending picture as well as sound wirelessly. The British Broadcast Corporation (BBC) began transmitting the world's first regular public high-definition service from the Victorian Alexandra Palace in north London on November 2, 1936 and is known as the birthplace of TV broadcasting.

Both radio and television broadcasting rely on radio frequency radiation to send a message to a receiver that is an antenna or now, more commonly, a satellite dish on top of a building or tower. With the increase in the number of stations and expansion of parts of the electromagnetic spectrum used for transmission, our exposure to radio frequency radiation continues to increase.

In 1888 Heinrich Hertz discovered that radio waves could be bounced off objects. This led to the third major invention, radar, used for the first time during World War II. The U.S. Navy coined the term RADAR in 1940 as an acronym for RAdio Detection And Ranging. Radar is part of the radio frequency spectrum but at higher frequencies than radio and television broadcasting. It uses microwave frequencies between 300 MHz and 300 GHz except for over-the-horizon (OTH) coastal radar (3–30 MHz) at high frequency (HF) and long range, ground-penetrating radar (30–300 MHz) at very high frequency (VHF).

Originally radar was used exclusively by the military and then for aviation and naval detection of airplanes and sea vessels. Exposure was occupational. A "by chance" observation that radar could melt a chocolate bar eventually led to the radar range, or the modern microwave oven in 1971. This was the first use of microwaves in residential settings. These ovens were designed not to leak, but leak they did, exposing families to microwave radiation when they were turned on.

New telecommunication technologies such as Wi-Fi, cell phones, and smart meters are exposing the population to higher levels of microwave radiation. Figure 22.1 shows Wi-Fi networks in 2006 and again in 2016. Combine this with cell phone towers and other telecommunication antennas and it is clear to see that the world in 2018 is quite different than just even 10 years earlier.

As the generation of radio frequency and microwave radiation began to increase, safety guidelines were needed. Since this radiation is non-ionizing, it was assumed to be safe if the intensity (power density) was low enough not to heat the body. This calculation of the thermal guideline was based on an average military man in top physical condition exposed for a few hours each day. It

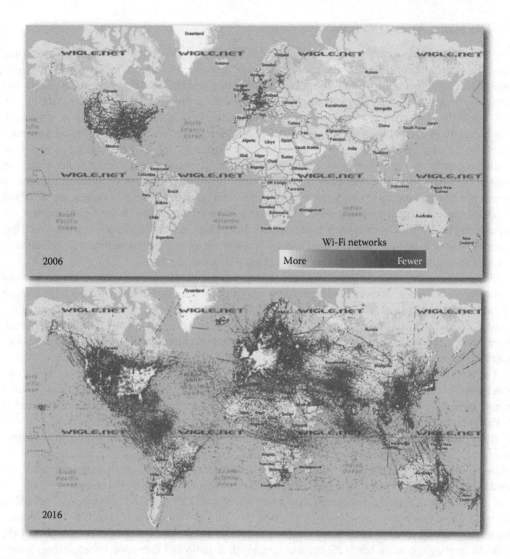

FIGURE 22.1   Global distribution of Wi-Fi Networks in 2006 and 2016. (From www.wigle.net.)

was not designed to protect the heating of an infant or a pregnant woman exposed potentially for 24 hours daily. The thermal guideline is expressed as the specific absorption rate (SAR) or dose and as power density (μW/cm^2) or exposure. The guidelines recommended by International Commission on Non-Ionizing Radiation Protection (ICNIRP, 1998) and various other authorities are provided in Table 22.1. These guidelines vary by orders of magnitude because some include non-thermal biological effects.

One of the key concerns about electromagnetic pollution is that our exposure is increasing rapidly, and more devices are being invented each year that rely on this energy. Light bulb manufacturers are designing light bulbs that can be turned on and off with a cell phone. These light bulbs emit unnecessary microwave radiation even when they are not communicating with a cell phone.

Home appliances that emit microwave radiation are being manufactured without concern about how much radiation a human body can tolerate. Smart appliances (air conditioners, furnaces, refrigerators, freezers, stoves, washers, driers) have special chips that allow them to communicate wirelessly with the electric smart meter, now required on most homes and buildings. These smart meters have replaced the analog hour-watt meters that recorded the amount of electricity used. They send the information wirelessly to the electric utility. Some communities also have smart water meters

TABLE 22.1
National and International Radio Frequency Exposure Guidelines, Exposures, and Biological Effects

Power Density μW/cm²	Frequency MHz	Exposure Guidelines, Typical Exposures, and Effects
		National and International Guidelines
10,000	300–300,000	**U.S. Standard** C95.1-1966 (occupational exposure); first standard limiting exposure to microwaves in Western world
		ICNIRP International Guidelines (1998); new revision expected in 2018 http://www.icnirp.org/cms/upload/ publications/ICNIRPemfgdl.pdf
1,000	1,500–15,000	These guidelines are based on biological effects of short-term, high-level
450	900	exposures only, also referred to as thermal effects: e.g. Germany (1996), USA (1997), Japan (1997), Switzerland (2000), Australia (2002), Finland (2002), Sweden (2002), UK (2004), Austria (2006)
		Canada, Safety Code 6 (2015); https://www.canada.ca/en/health-canada/ services/environmental-workplace-health/reports-publications/radiation/ safety-code-6-health-canada-radiofrequency-exposure-guidelines-environmental-workplace-health-health-canada.html
535	2,400	new limit about 50% lower than previous one from 2009
274	900	new limit about 60% lower than the previous one from 2009
~10	range	**Toronto Board of Health**, Canada (1999); Prudent Avoidance Policy for Siting of Cell Phone Base Stations, voluntary in 2013; http://app.toronto.ca/tmmis/ viewAgendaItemHistory.do?item=2013.HL25.5
		Russia, Ministry of Health Standard (2003), exposure limit for general public; http://www.tesla.ru/english/protection/standards.html
		Italy, Council of Ministries (2003), decree precautionary attention level not to be exceeded in sensitive areas; http://www.who.int/peh-emf/publications/ reports/en/italy.pdf
		Switzerland, Ordinance on Protection against non-ionizing radiation (1999), precautionary cell tower exposure limit for sensitive areas; https://www.admin. ch/opc/de/classified-compilation/19996141/index.html
		ECOLOG Institute, Germany (2000); https://www.ecolog-institut.de/ startseite/arbeitsbereiche/technik-umwelt/
~1	range	Precautionary recommendation based on review of scientific literature
0.3	range	Emissions from single RF sources (e.g. cell tower) at max. 30% of precautionary limit
0.17	range	**Seletun Consensus Statement** (2010), Precautionary recommendations; http:// www.iemfa.org/seletun-statement/
0.1	range	**Salzburg Resolution** on mobile telecommunication base stations (2000) precautionary recommendation; https://www.salzburg.gv.at/gesundheit_/ Documents/proceedings_(32)_salzburg_resolution.pdf
0.001	GSM sum total	**Salzburg,** precautionary for outdoor environments (Salzburg, Austria 2002); https://www.salzburg.gv.at/das_salzburger_modell_langfassung-2.doc
		Parliamentary Assembly of Council of Europe, Resolution 1815 (2011), Precautionary for indoor environments; http://assembly.coe.int/nw/xml/XRef/ Xref-XML2HTML-en.asp?fileid=17994
		Austrian Antenna System Siting Guidelines (2012, updated 2015), precautionary target threshold level inside and outside buildings; https://www. wko.at/branchen/gewerbe-handwerk/elektro-gebaeude-alarm-kommunikation/ Leitfaden_Senderbau.html
0.0001	GSM sum total	**Salzburg,** precautionary for indoor environments (Salzburg, Austria, 2002)

(Continued)

TABLE 22.1 (*Continued*)
National and International Radio Frequency Exposure Guidelines, Exposures, and Biological Effects

Power Density μW/cm²	Frequency MHz	Exposure Guidelines, Typical Exposures, and Effects
		Typical Exposures
≤1000	cell phone	RF radiation exposure from cell phone handset held next to head
100	cell phone	RF radiation exposure from cell phone handset at 1 foot (~30 cm)
10–40	DECT phone	DECT cordless phone at 1 foot (~30 cm)
10–20	Wi-Fi	Wi-Fi access points/client at 8 inches (~20 cm)
0.1–10	cell tower	within 400 m radius of cell tower
0.000,000,001 –0.000,000,1	cell phone	Minimum power level required for cell phone communication
~0.000,000,001	30–30,000	Stormy sun
~0.000,000,000,1		Natural background
		Effects—Increased Risk
0.2–8	range	increased risk of leukemia in children; Hocking 1996; https://www.ncbi.nlm.nih.gov/pubmed/8985435
3	2,400	Havas et al. (2010); heart palpitations in controlled experiments; https://scholar.google.ca/citations?user=Q56SGDQAAAAJ&hl=en
0.5–0.1	range	Kundi (2009), Health effects observed in populations near cell towers, cardiac effects, headaches, sleep problems
<0.01288	1	Increased incidence of fatigue, depression, sleeping disorders, concentration difficulties, cardiovascular problems near cell towers (Oberfeld 2004); http://www.vws.org/documents/Cell-Project-Documents/OberfeldSpanishstudy.pdf
0.003–0.02	range	Children and adolescents (8–17 years) short-term exposure associated with headache, irritation, concentration difficulty in school, (Heinrich, 2010); https://www.researchgate.net/publication/49636902_Association_between_exposure_to_radiofrequency_electromagnetic_fields_assessed_by_dosimetry_and_acute_symptoms_in_children_and_adolescents_A_population_based_cross-sectional_study

Source: Based on Gustavs K. 2017. *Current RF Exposure Limits.* www.buildingbiology.ca.
0.1 W/m² = 100 mW/m² = 100,000 μW/m² = 10 μW/cm²

and smart gas meters. Each of these smart meters increases exposure within the home to microwave radiation. Smart meters also generate dirty electricity, as do most energy efficient light bulbs. It is becoming increasingly difficult to avoid electrosmog even in one's homes.

During the oil crisis in the 1970s, energy efficient technology and more electronic devices came on the market. These electronic devices generate dirty electricity and, without adequate filtering within the device, the dirty electricity flows along electrical wires.

In the 1980s popularity of personal computers blossomed as they became smaller and more affordable. People now spend hours each day working at their computer or using it for recreation. Tasks that required a pencil and paper, a calculator, going to the library for a book, reading a newspaper, can all now be done without leaving the comfort of your home. Computers, tablets, and cell phones are used to listen to music and to watch videos. Indeed, cell phones have replaced the camera, video camera, calculator, radio, record player, television, newspaper, magazine, book, watch, calendar, and telephone. They tell you where you are and where your friends are. They provide maps for navigation, and applications for the latest weather and stock market report and they keep you occupied playing games when you have free time. Your exposure to microwave radiation from a cell phone depends on where, when, how, how often, and how long you use the device.

Concomitant with increasing exposure, more people are experiencing chronic ill health that appears to get worse in some environments or during certain activities. These symptoms include some combination of those provided in Table 22.2. Statements like, "Doctor I think my cell phone is making me sick," are often met with disbelief. After multiple tests that show no obvious problem, doctors recommend the patient visit a psychiatrist because the symptoms must be psychosomatic.

Research by Rubin (a psychologist) and his team in the U.K. have added greatly to this misunderstanding of electrohypersensitivity (EHS) (Rubin et al. 2006, 2010). They did blinded studies and found that individuals who claimed to be sensitive were unable to tell when a device was on or off as though detection of a signal was the same as sensitivity. An analogy is exposure to UV radiation. On a cloudy day, a person who is sensitive to the sun develops a sunburn whether they realize they are exposed to UV radiation.

In the Rubin et al. study (2006), some participants developed headaches and were unable to complete the testing. The authors state, "headache severity increased during exposure and decreased immediately afterwards" yet this was insufficient to proclaim sensitivity. The room with sham exposure was not shielded and it is difficult to achieve an electrosmog-free environment in most urban centers without shielding. Also, the device they used in the sham exposure had "minimal leakage" of the signal. To people with EHS, even low exposure can be harmful. Studies funded by the telecommunications industry almost invariably find results that are favorable to that industry.

In 2004, the WHO held a conference on EMF hypersensitivity in Prague. At that meeting EHS was defined as, "... a phenomenon where individuals experience adverse health effects while

---

TABLE 22.2
Typical EHS Symptoms

Auditory	Dermatological	Musculoskeletal	Ophthalmologic
Earaches, imbalance, lowered auditory threshold, tinnitus	Brown "sun spots," crawling sensations, dry skin, facial flushing, growths and lumps, insect bites and stings, severe acne, skin irritation, skin rashes, skin tingling, swelling of face/neck	Aches/numbness pain/ prickling sensations in: bones, joints and muscles in: ankles/anns/ feet/legs/neck/shoulders/ wrists//elbows/pelvis/ hips/lower back, cramp/ tension in: arms/legs/ toes, muscle spasms, muscular paralysis, muscular weakness, pain in lips/jaws/teeth with amalgam fillings, restless legs, tremor and shaking	Eyelid tremors/"tics," impaired vision, irritating sensation, pain/"gritty" feeling, pressure behind eyes, shiny eyes, smarting, dry eyes
Cardiovascular			**Other physiological**
Altered heart rate, chest pains, cold extremities especially hands and feet, heart arrhythmias, internal bleeding lowered/raised blood pressure, nosebleeds, shortness of breath, thrombosis effects	**Emotional** Anger, anxiety attacks, crying, depression, feeling out of control, irritability, logorrhoea, mood swings		Abnormal menstruation, brittle nails, hair loss, itchy scalp, metal redistribution, thirst/dryness of lips/tongue/ eyes
Cognitive	**Gastrointestinal**	**Neurological**	**Respiratory**
Confusion, difficulty in learning new things, lack of concentration, short/ long-term memory impairment, spatial disorientation	Altered appetite, digestive problems, flatulence, food intolerances	Faintness, dizziness, flu-like symptoms, headaches, hyperactivity, nausea, numbness, sleep problems, tiredness	Asthma, bronchitis, cough/ throat irritation, pneumonia, sinusitis
	Genito-urinary Smelly sweat/urine, urinary/bowel urgency		**Sensitization** Allergies, chemical sensitivity, light sensitivity, noise sensitivity, smell sensitivity

Source: Michael Bevington. 2010. *Electromagnetic–Sensitivity and Electromagnetic–Hypersensitivity (Also Known as Asthenic Syndrome, EMF Intolerance Syndrome, Idiopathic Environmental Intolerance–EMF, Microwave Syndrome, Radio Wave Sickness): A Summary.* Capability Books, UK. 43pp.

using or being in the vicinity of devices emanating electric, magnetic, or electromagnetic fields (EMFs)."

They went on to state, "... EHS is a real and sometimes a debilitating problem for the affected persons ... Their exposures are generally several orders of magnitude under the limits in internationally accepted standards." Despite this recognition that some people are severely affected by this condition, there was a push to call this phenomenon *idiopathic environmental intolerance* because many still refused to believe it was due to EM exposure.

WHAT IS ELECTROMAGNETIC POLLUTION?

Electromagnetic pollution refers to electromagnetic fields and electromagnetic radiation emitted by common household items that use electricity or emit radio frequency/microwave radiation. The pollution is classified by frequency and shown on the electromagnetic spectrum in Figure 22.2. It includes extremely low frequency (ELF) electromagnetic fields (EMF) and radio frequency radiation that consists of both intermediate frequencies (IF) and microwave (MW) radiation. The electromagnetic spectrum shows the different frequency categories along with the devices that generate these frequencies.

These frequencies are considered non-ionizing, which means they do not have enough energy to dislodge electrons and break chemical bonds. Ionizing radiation includes ultraviolet rays, x-rays, and gamma rays (Figure 22.2) and is known to be harmful. Consequently, the technology that exposes us to these ionizing frequencies is strictly controlled and highly regulated. The same cannot be said for non-ionizing radiation.

BASIC PROPERTIES OF ELECTROMAGNETIC ENERGY

Unlike sound waves, which require matter for transmission (knocking on wood, for example), electromagnetic (EM) energy can flow through a vacuum. As with sound waves, EM waves oscillate and this oscillation, waves, or cycles per second, is referred to as Hertz (Hz).

The electric field is measured in volts and the electrical potential difference between two objects is measured as volts/meter (V/m). The strength of the magnetic field (magnetic flux density) is measured as milliGauss (mG) or microTesla (µT). The equivalent of 1 mG is 0.1 µT.

In other chapters of this book that focus on light energy, the common way to characterize the light is by using its wavelength in nanometers (nm) rather than its frequency. The equation that relates wavelength and frequency for electromagnetic waves is:

$$\lambda \nu = c \qquad (22.1)$$

where λ is the wavelength (m), ν is the frequency (Hz), and c is the speed of light (ms^{-1}) or (299,792,458 ms^{-1}, often approximated to 300×10^6 ms^{-1}).

At the quantum level, EM waves also have properties that resemble particles leading to the wave/particle duality of electromagnetic energy.

WHAT ARE THE DIFFERENT TYPES OF NON-IONIZING RADIATION (NIR) THAT ARE OF CONCERN?

Research on the harmful effects of non-ionizing electromagnetic radiation (NIR) falls into four categories as follows (Table 22.3):

1. ELF electric and magnetic fields. Includes frequencies below 300 Hz (or 1000 Hz depending on the authority). This refers to electricity flowing along a wire and is often referred to as power frequency EMFs (60 Hz in North America and 50 Hz in the rest of the world).

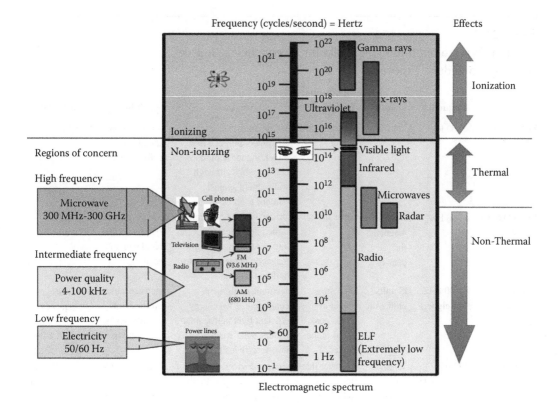

FIGURE 22.2 Electromagnetic spectrum showing areas of concern from a health perspective for non-ionizing radiation.

2. Intermediate frequencies (IF) in the kHz to MHz range are part of the radio frequency (RF) spectrum. Radio frequencies radiate through the air, hence the name radiation. IF falls at the lower end of the RF spectrum. Common terminology in the literature is "dirty electricity," as it is measured on electrical wires that include power frequencies and high frequency voltage transients (HFVT), which are short bursts of a high frequency (kHz to MHz) electric field. Another common name is "power surge."

3. Microwave (MW) radiation consists of the upper part of the RF spectrum from 300 MHz to 300 GHz. This is the part that is used in many wireless devices for short- and long-distance communication including cell phones and cell phone base stations with multiple antennas; smart meters and smart appliances; Wi-Fi for Internet access; Bluetooth for shorter distance communication between a cell phone and a laptop computer, for example; cordless phones; wireless baby monitors, computer games like Xbox, and in-home security systems that are not hard wired. The list of devices that use microwave radiation and that can communicate with cell phones is increasing rapidly and includes smart watches; health and fitness devices that monitor daily activity and night time sleep; light bulbs that can be turned on and off with a cell phone; soothers that monitor an infant's temperature; and diapers that alert a cell phone when the diaper needs to be changed. A smart home with smart appliances is a like a microwave oven constantly operating on low power.

4. Ground current (GC) may include all the frequencies mentioned above but this current flows along the ground rather than through the air or along wires. It has been shown to be a problem especially on dairy farms, where it interferes with milk production and adversely

TABLE 22.3

Different Types of Non-ionizing Radiation, Frequencies, Sources, and Ways to Reduce Exposure

	Frequency	Units	Monitoring Equipment	Sources	Solutions	Ideal Levels
ELF Electric Field	<300 Hz	V/m	Electric field meter	Electric wires, electric equipment plugged into outlet, indoor & outdoor electric wires although walls shield against outdoor sources	Distance, unplug equipment, easily shielded	≤5 V/m
ELF Magnetic Field	<300 Hz	mG or μT magnetic flux density	Gauss meter	Current, electric equipment turned on, indoor & outdoor electric wires, magnetic fields penetrate building material	Distance, turn equipment off, shield with mu metal	≤1 mG (≤0.1 μT)
IF Dirty Electricity	2–100 kHz (or higher)	GS units or |dV/dt|	Microsurge meter or peak–peak (p-p) scope meter	Electronic equipment, computers, TVs, energy efficient light bulbs, smart meters, solar panels, inverters, rheostats	Tuned capacitors can short out high frequency voltage transients	≤40 GS units, frequency dependent ≤0.01 V/m p-p at 10 kHz
RF & MW Radiation	30 MHz – 300 GHz	μW/cm² power density	RF meter that measures 8 GHz or higher	Wireless devices, mobile phone, Wi-Fi, Bluetooth, smart meter, cell towers, broadcast antennas, radar, microwave oven	Distance, shielded by metal, special carbon paint and special window film	≤0.1 μW/cm² outdoors and ≤0.01 μW/cm² indoors

Abbreviations: ELF, extremely low frequency; IF, intermediate frequency; RF, radio frequency; MW, microwave; Hz, Hertz (cycles per second); kHz, thousands of Hz; MHz, millions of Hz; GHz, billions of Hz.

affects the health of farmers and farm animals. This topic will not be discussed in this chapter, although it is becoming increasingly harmful and increasingly common in both rural and urban environments (Havas and Colling 2011, Stetzer et al. 2016).

BIOLOGICAL EFFECTS OF ELECTROSMOG

The scientific and medical evidence that electromagnetic exposure from ELF to MW radiation has serious biological and health effects includes epidemiological studies, *in vivo* and *in vitro* experiments. The effects fall into three categories: cancers, reproductive problems, and symptoms of EHS.

CANCER

Extremely low frequency magnetic fields. The scientific evidence includes epidemiological studies that document a statistically significant association between residential magnetic field exposure and childhood leukemia and between occupational electromagnetic exposure with adult leukemia, brain tumors, and breast cancer (see review by Havas 2000, Sun et al. 2013). Levels at which cancer risk increases range from 2.5–4 mG (0.25–0.4 μT) for childhood cancers (Wertheimer and Leeper 1979; Savitz et al. 1988; Ahlbom et al. 2001) and up to 10–12 mG (1.0–1.2 μT) for adult brain tumors (Savitz et al. 2000) and adult acute non-lymphocytic leukemia (Bethwaite et al. 2001). They include mammary gland tumors in *in vivo* studies with mice (Havas 2000), as well as *in vitro* studies with human breast cancer cells showing that magnetic fields at 12 mG (1.2 μT) promote cell division in estrogen receptor–positive human breast cancer cells and inhibit the chemotoxic effects of tamoxifen (Blackman et al. 2001). There is also some evidence that the effect is epigenetic for childhood leukemia and that magnetic fields (above 1.8 mG, 0.18 μT) that occur within 100 m of power lines or transformers involve the inhibition of the recovery gene, XRCC1Ex9 + 16A allele, in children with acute leukemia (Yang et al. 2008).

The Bonneville Power Authority (Lee et al. 1996) reviewed the literature related to health effects of power frequency electromagnetic fields. In one chapter they focused on cancer and reported that out of 212 studies, 101 studies (48%) found increased cancer risks while 8 studies (4%) found reduced cancer risks with low frequency EMF exposure. This type of report for a power authority (admitting that these frequencies are harmful) is most unusual. In another chapter, they reported on non-cancer health effects and found that 57 (51%) out of a total of 111 studies reported adverse effects mostly related to reproduction and mental health with only 6 studies (5%) showing beneficial effects. This is useful in weight of evidence reporting and shows that the weight of evidence strongly supports the concept that power frequency electromagnetic fields are biologically harmful.

Intermediate frequency EM fields have also been associated with cancer. Milham and Morgan (2008) found an association between dirty electricity and various cancers among teachers who taught in rooms with poor power quality (IF above 2000 GS units) in a Californian school. The 60 Hz magnetic fields in this school were not elevated and did not relate to the cancers among the teachers. Sixteen school teachers in a cohort of 137 teachers hired in 1988 through 2005 were diagnosed with 18 cancers. The observed to expected (O/E) risk ratio for all cancers was 2.78 (P = 0.000098). Increased risk ratios were documented for malignant melanoma (RR 9.8, P = 0.0008), thyroid cancer (RR 13.3, P = 0.0098), and uterine cancer (RR 9.2, P = 0.02) but not with breast cancer. A single year of employment at this school increased a teacher's cancer risk by 21%. Authors concluded that high frequency voltage transients (HRVT) or dirty electricity may be a universal carcinogen, similar to ionizing radiation.

Radio frequency and microwave radiation have been associated with cancer incidence and cancer mortality for people who live within 300–500 m of cell phone base stations in Germany, Israel, and Brazil (Wolf and Wolf 2004, Dode et al. 2011, Eger et al. 2004) and within 2 km of broadcast antennas in the U.K. (Dolk et al. 1997), Vatican City (Michelozzi et al. 2002), Australia (Hocking et al. 1996) and South Korea (Ha et al. 2007). For example, the odds ratio for children under the age of 15, for all types of leukemia was 2.15 (95% CI 1.00–4.67) among children who resided within 2 km of the nearest AM radio transmitter as compared with those who resided more than 20 km away (Michelozzi et al. 2002).

Studies with cell phones indicate that people who use them for more than 10 years have a higher incidence of developing ipsilateral gliomas (90% increased risk), salivary gland tumors (variable results), acoustic neuromas (60% increased risk), and possibly uveal melanomas (320% increased risk) (Sadetzki et al. 2008, Hardell et al. 2009, Cardis et al. 2011). The risk is greatest (400% increased risk) for those who began using a cell phone before the age of 20 (Hardell et al. 2009).

Police officers who use hand-held radar guns have a greater risk of developing testicular cancer (Davis and Mostofl 1993) and women who keep their cell phones in their bra for 10 years or more have a risk of developing breast cancer immediately under the phone (West et al. 2013).

Two large *in vivo* studies conducted by the U.S. Air Force (Chou et al. 1992) and the U.S. National Toxicology Program (NTP 2016) both documented a statistically significant increase in primary and/or metastatic tumors in rats/mice exposed for microwave radiation. In the U.S. Air Force study, rats exposed to 2.45 GHz (similar to Wi-Fi radiation) for 25 months had a 100% increase in metastatic tumors and a 260% increase in primary tumors. In the NTP study, rats were exposed for 2 years to 900 MHz and mice to 1900 MHz at cell phone modulations commonly used in the United States [Code Division Multiple Access (CDMA) and Global System for Mobile Communications (GSM)]. Increased incidence of malignant gliomas in the brain and schwannomas in the heart of male rats exposed to RFR was documented in a preliminary report.

Lai and Singh (1995) were among the first to document single-strand DNA breaks in rat brains exposed for 2 hours to either continuous or pulsed low level 2.45 GHz radiation either immediate or 4 hours post-exposure. They hypothesized that these effects could result from a direct effect of RF energy on DNA molecules and/or impairment of DNA-damage repair mechanisms in brain cells (Lai and Singh, 1996).

Despite these studies, the common mantra among health authorities is that only ionizing radiation has sufficient energy to break chemical bonds and thus cause cancer. While this may explain why ionizing radiation is a carcinogen, there is no reason to believe that the mechanism is the same for non-ionizing radiation. Indeed, both ionizing and non-ionizing radiation result in an increase in free radicals. The first generates free-radicals, while the second interferes with their neutralization (Havas 2017). The result is DNA damage and cancer in both cases. Numerous studies document oxidative stress in plants, animals, and humans exposed to non-thermal levels of RF and MW radiation and the beneficial effects of anti-oxidants (see Havas 2017).

REPRODUCTION

ELF Electromagnetic Fields

ELF electromagnetic fields have been associated with impaired reproductive health for both maternal and paternal exposure and also in *in vivo* laboratory experiments.

Adverse pregnancy outcomes that include miscarriages, still births, congenital deformities, and illness at birth, have been associated with occupational exposure during pregnancy to electromagnetic fields, especially video display terminals (VDT) (Goldhaber et al. 1988) and with residential exposure for women who used an electric blanket, heated water bed, or who had electric heating in the bedroom ceiling (Wertheimer and Leeper 1986, 1989, Hatch et al. 1998). These heating devices generate an elevated magnetic field that is near the body for hours each night.

Clusters of abnormal pregnancies associated with use of video display terminals (VDT) during pregnancy have been reported in Canada, the United States, Britain, and Denmark (DeMatteo 1986). Goldhaber et al. (1988) conducted a case-control study of 1583 pregnant women who attended one of three gynecology clinics in Northern California during 1981 and 1982. They found a significantly elevated risk of miscarriages for working women who reported using VDTs for more than 20 h each week during the first trimester of pregnancy compared to other working women who reported not using VDTs (OR 1.8, 95% CI: 1.2–2.8). While the risk with VDT was attributed to elevated magnetic fields, these terminals also generate dirty electricity as do most modern computers and this may have also contributed to the pregnancy outcomes.

Li et al. (2002) studied the effect of magnetic fields on the risk of miscarriage among women in the San Francisco area. Pregnant women wore a magnetic field monitor for a 24-hour period. A total of 969 subjects were included in the final analyses. Miscarriage risk increased with an increasing level of maximum magnetic field exposure. Women exposed to 16 mG (1.6 µT) or higher compared to those exposed to less than 16 mG had a rate ratio (RR) of 1.8 with a 95% confidence interval (CI) of 1.2–2.7. The association was stronger for early miscarriages (<10 weeks of gestation) (RR 2.2, 95% CI 1.2–4.0) and among "susceptible" women with multiple prior fetal losses or subfertility (RR 3.1, 95% CI 1.3–7.7). After including only women who indicated that their daily activity pattern during the measurement period was typical, the association was strengthened for maximum magnetic field exposure at or above 16 mG (RR 2.9, 95% CI 1.6–5.3); for early miscarriage (RR 5.7, 95% CI 2.1–15.7); and among the susceptible women (RR 4.0, 95% CI 1.4–11.5). The authors concluded that prenatal maximum magnetic field exposure above a certain level (possibly around 16 mG) may be associated with miscarriage risk and that this association is unlikely to be due to uncontrolled biases or unmeasured confounders.

Li et al. (2011) also reported that maternal exposure to magnetic fields during pregnancy increased the risk of asthma in offspring. Every 1 mG (0.1 µT) increase of maternal magnetic field exposure during pregnancy was associated with a 15% increased risk of asthma in offspring. Children whose mothers were exposed to high magnetic fields (>2 mG, 0.2 μT) had more than a 3.5-fold increased rate of asthma (95% CI 1.68–7.35), while children whose mothers had intermediate magnetic field exposure (>0.3–2 mG) had a 74% increased rate of asthma (CI 0.93–3.25).

Paternal occupational exposure to electromagnetic fields has also been linked to reduced fertility, lower male to female sex ratio in offspring, congenital malformations, and teratogenic effects expressed in the form of childhood cancer (Nordstrom et al. 1983, Spitz and Johnson 1985, Wilkins and Koutras 1988, Tornqvist 1998).

Nordstrom et al. (1983) did a retrospective study of pregnancy outcomes for 542 Swedish power plant employees working in high voltage (130–400 kV) substations. In Sweden, 400 kV transmission lines were introduced in 1952 and the pregnancies studied were from 1953 to 1979. Employees who worked on lines no higher than 380/220 V served as the reference group. During this period there were 880 pregnancies. Neither spontaneous abortions nor perinatal deaths differed between the two groups, but there was an increase of congenital malformations for high voltage switchyard workers, especially for those with wives aged 30 plus, compared with the reference group (OR~2.5). Couples also experienced some difficulty conceiving when the husband worked in a high-voltage switchyard (200 or 400 kV) (OR~2.5). In vivo studies with rats showed that exposure to high electric fields reduced plasma testosterone concentrations and reduced sperm viability (Free et al. 1981).

Li et al. (2010) conducted a population-based case-control study with healthy sperm donors to determine effects of magnetic fields on sperm quality. Participants wore a meter to document daily MF exposure. Those whose 90th percentile exposure was at or above 1.6 mG (0.16 μT) had a twofold increased risk of abnormal sperm motility and morphology (OR 2.0, 95% CI 1.0–3.9). Increasing duration of MF exposure above 1.6 mG further increased the risk (P < 0.03). The dose-response relationship was strengthened when restricted to those whose measurement day reflected a typical day during the previous 3 months (a likely period of spermatogenesis). There was an inverse correlation between magnetic field exposure and all semen parameters when adjusted for age. The authors concluded that magnetic field exposure may have an adverse effect on sperm quality.

Dirty Electricity and Intermediate Frequencies

To the best of my knowledge, there are no peer-reviewed publications on the adverse effects of dirty electricity on human reproduction. Most of the research in this area deals with other adverse biological effects. However, there is anecdotal evidence that women who have had difficulty getting pregnant become pregnant once the dirty electricity in their home or work environment is reduced (Stetzer, D. 2015. personal communication, www.stetzerelectric.com). Additional evidence comes from livestock, mostly dairy cows, on farms with dirty electricity carried along the wires and the ground.

RF/MW

Reproductive studies on the effects of RW/MW radiation include *in vivo* studies with test animals (mice, rats, etc.); with pregnant women occupationally exposed to microwave radiation and both *in vitro* and *in vivo* exposure of sperm. Studies report effects on sperm, increased miscarriages, and behavioral and/or health effects of prenatally exposed offspring.

Effects on Sperm

According to Friesen (2015), RFR has been implicated with abnormalities in sperm (motility, shape, cellular stress) in at least 20 studies and with DNA damage in at least 5 male reproductive studies. These have clear implications for male infertility and long-term genetic abnormalities to offspring with possible multigenerational effects.

Adams et al. (2014) reviewed the literature on effects of RF-EMR emitted by mobile phones on sperm quality. This meta-analysis included 10 studies and 1492 samples. Exposure to mobile phones was associated with reduced sperm motility (mean difference—8.1%, 95% CI—13.1 to −3.2) and viability (mean difference—9.1%, 95% CI—18.4 to 0.2), but the effects on concentration were more ambiguous. The authors concluded that pooled results from in vitro and in vivo studies indicate that mobile phone exposure adversely affects sperm quality.

La Vignera et al. (2012) reviewed the literature on the effects of RF-EMR on the male reproductive function in experimental animals (rats, mice, rabbits) and humans. Studies were conducted based on mobile phone RF exposure for different durations. Collectively studies show that RF-EMR decreases sperm count and motility and increases oxidative stress. Human spermatozoa exposed to RF-EMR have decreased motility, morphometric abnormalities, and increased oxidative stress; whereas men using mobile phones have decreased sperm concentration, motility and viability but normal morphology. These abnormalities appear to be related to duration of mobile phone use.

Adverse Pregnancy Outcomes

Just as with exposure to low frequency magnetic fields, women exposed during pregnancy to radio and microwave frequencies have a greater risk of miscarrying.

Physiotherapists are exposed to radio- and microwave-frequency electromagnetic radiation by operating shortwave ($\sim$27 MHz) or microwave ($>$300 MHz) diathermy units. In one study, Ouellet-Hellstrom and Stewart (1993) reported that pregnant physiotherapists who were exposed to microwaves 6 months prior to their pregnancy or during the first trimester were more likely to result in miscarriage (OR 1.28, 95% CI 1.02–1.59). The odds ratio increased with increasing level of exposure ($P < 0.005$). The highest exposure group (20 or more exposures/month) had a 1.59 OR. The overall odds ratio was slightly lower after it was controlled for prior fetal loss (OR 1.26, 95% CI 1.00–1.59), but remained statistically significant ($P < 0.01$). The risk of miscarriage was not associated with reported use of shortwave diathermy equipment.

Lerman et al. (2001) studied the association between shortwave diathermy use by pregnant physiotherapists and adverse pregnancy outcomes. The 434 women studied had 930 pregnancies of which 175 ended in spontaneous abortions, 45 had fetal malformations, 47 were delivered prematurely, and 33 infants had low birth weight. The remaining 630 normal pregnancies comprised the control group. Shortwaves were associated with a significantly increased odds ratio for congenital malformations (OR 2.24, CI 1.27–4.83, $P < 0.006$) and low birth weight (OR 2.99, CI 1.32–6.79, $P < 0.006$). This effect increased in a dose-related manner. However, after controlling for potential confounding variables, only low birth weight remained statistically significant (O.R. 2.75, CI 1.07–7.04, $P < 0.03$). The authors concluded that shortwaves have potentially harmful effects on pregnancy outcome, specifically low birth weight.

Effects on Offspring

Neurobehavioral disorders are becoming increasingly prevalent in children and an association between prenatal cell phone use and hyperactivity in offspring has been suggested. Aldad et al. (2012) tested the effect of in utero exposure to RFR from cellular phones on the behavior of mice. Mice exposed in utero were hyperactive and had impaired memory. These behavioral changes were due to altered neuronal development and neuropathology. The degree to which this is affecting behavior and development of human offspring exposed to RFR in utero remains to be determined.

Divan et al. (2008) reported on results from the Danish National Birth Cohort, which looked at prenatal and postnatal exposure to cell phone use and emotional and hyperactivity problems at age 7 years. Exposure to cell phones prenatally, and to a lesser degree postnatally, was associated with more behavioral difficulties. The original analysis included nearly 13,000 children who reached age 7 years by November 2006.

In a follow-up study with 28,745 children (Divan et al. 2012) the highest OR for behavioral problems were for children who had both prenatal and postnatal exposure to cell phones compared with children not exposed during either time period. The adjusted association was small but statistically significant (OR 1.5, 95% CI 1.4–1.7). These associations may be non-causal and due to confounders but—if they are real—they would be of public health concern given the widespread use of this and related technology.

Antennas and Reproduction

The effects are not restricted to Wi-Fi and cellular phones but also include RF radiation near antenna transmitters. In one study, 6 pairs of mice were exposed to RFR at an antenna park where the radiation ranged from 1.053–0.168 μW/cm^2 (Magras and Xenos 1997). Another 6 pairs served as controls. Both sets of mice were mated five times. Among the exposed mice, there was a progressive decease in the number of newborns per dam that ended in irreversible infertility by the fifth breeding.

Hormone profiles for people who lived near (20–100 m), at mid-range (100–500 m), and at greater distances (>500 m, reference) from mobile phone base stations were followed over a period of 6 years (Eskander et al. 2012; Eger et al. 2012). Significant decreases were noted among young (14–22 years) and older (25–60 years) participants in serum testosterone, progesterone, cortisol, T3, T4, and in plasma ACTH within 3 years that were even more profound after 6 years of exposure. The authors concluded that elevated RF exposure affected hormones in the pituitary–adrenal axis. Low progesterone during pregnancy may be implicated in miscarriages and low testosterone may result in reduced male fertility.

ELECTROHYPERSENSITIVITY (EHS)

At the end of the nineteenth century a mysterious illness emerged. The first people to be affected by it were the telegraph line installers and the telephone switchboard operators. The symptoms of this illness include nerve disorders, hence the name neurasthenia (nerves without strength). It was associated with depression, extreme anxiety, exhaustion, convulsions, unconsciousness, rashes, and a whole host of other malaise. The afflictions became so bad that in 1907, the Bell telephone switchboard operators in Toronto went on strike. They demanded much shorter working hours and better working conditions.

In the 1950s, with the invention of microwave frequencies, radar operators started suffering with similar symptoms that they called radio wave sickness or microwave syndrome.

Now at the turn of the twenty-first century with the introduction of personal wireless technologies the general population seems to be plagued with the same symptoms, which we call electrohypersensitivity (EHS) and which the WHO would like to call idiopathic environmental intolerance (IEI). My preferred name for it is rapid aging syndrome as the body appears to age abnormally rapidly.

What do these three "illnesses" have in common? The introduction of chronic overexposure to electromagnetic fields.

In the case of the telephone switchboard operators, the workers (mostly women) would manually place jacks into a switchboard panel to connect one telephone caller to another individual using a switchboard cable. Their proximity to the switchboard caused them to be chronically exposed to hundreds of live telephone connections for hours each day. They sat with electromagnetic fields on their head from the speakers in their headset and their bodies came in contact with voltage by the individual connections.

In the case of the radar operators, they worked near large radar antennas that were broadcasting and receiving microwave energy.

In the third case, a large population now lives within a sea of microwave radiation transmitted by smart phones, wireless tablets, Wi-Fi routers, cell phone base stations, smart meters, smart appliances, and so on.

So basically, neurasthenia, radio wave sickness, and electrohypersensitivity are one and the same. However, neurasthenia is classified as an illness in the WHO list of diseases and EHS is relegated to idiopathic environmental illness, which basically means we don't know the cause.

If you mention this to someone with EHS, they would disagree. We do know the cause—electrosmog exposure—and if the electrosmog exposure is avoided, the symptoms diminish or disappear.

Provocation Testing

While some believe EHS is psychosomatic (Rubin et al. 2010), others have documented physiological changes that can be monitored with changes in electrosmog exposure. Studies of EHS are difficult to design for a variety of reasons. Not everyone with self-proclaimed EHS has EHS. Testing needs to be done in an electrosmog-free environment. Some individuals do not respond immediately, and some continue to react once the source is removed. Pretesting exposure is important. The symptoms tested may not be the same as the symptoms experienced. Similarly, the frequencies tested may not be the ones that cause a problem. Statistical analysis that relies on combining the results for individuals with different and possibly no EHS will dilute the results and lead to false negatives. Despite these problems, several studies testing for EHS have been conducted that yield interesting results.

Rea et al. (1991) conducted one of the early studies. They started with 100 patients who believed they were electrically sensitive. By the end of the study, only 16 of the original 100 responded consistently to real exposure and not to sham exposure between 0.1 Hz and 5 MHz. Testing was done in an electrosmog-free environment, which is essential for this type of testing. Most of the reactions were neurological (such as tingling, sleepiness, headache, dizziness, and in severe cases unconsciousness) although a variety of other symptoms were also observed including pain, muscle tightness, spasm, palpitation, flushing, tachycardia, edema, nausea, belching, pressure in ears, and burning and itching of eyes and skin. Instrumental recordings of pupil dilation, respiration, and heart activity were also included in the study using a double-blind approach. Results indicated a 20% decrease in pulmonary function and a 40% increase in heart rate. Patients sometimes had delayed or prolonged responses. These objective recordings, in combination with the clinical symptoms, demonstrate that EHS individuals respond physiologically to specific EMF frequencies.

In another provocation study, Havas et al. (2010) exposed subjects to radiation from a cordless phone that generates 2.4 GHz when it is plugged into an electric outlet. In a double blind, placebo controlled study, with 25 volunteers, only some of which claimed to be EHS, 40% experienced some changes in heart rate variability (HRV) attributable to digitally pulsed (100 Hz) MW radiation. Maximum exposure was at less than 0.5% of the ICNIRP guidelines for 2.4 GHz frequencies and lasted only a few minutes (Table 22.1). Despite this "low" exposure, several volunteers experienced tachycardia; others mild to moderate changes in the sympathetic/parasympathetic balance; and some did not react to this provocation either because of high adaptive capacity or because of systemic adrenal exhaustion. The authors concluded that the orthostatic HRV combined with provocation testing may provide a diagnostic test for some EHS sufferers when they are exposed to electromagnetic emitting devices.

Electrosmog exposure affects blood viscosity in some individuals. Live blood analysis reveals that red blood cells become aggregated and stick together like rolled coins (rouleau formation) (Plate 22.1) making it more difficult for the cardiovascular system to distribute nutrients and get rid of waste products. Individuals with cardiovascular disease may experience more severe symptoms with the potential for heart attacks or strokes with highly viscose blood flowing through narrow or thin blood vessels.

Non-deliberate provocation occurs for people who live near cell phone base stations (cellular antennas) or experience other forms of chronic exposure. Those who live within 300 m of cell phone antennas tend to experience symptoms associated with EHS more often than those who live further away. This has been documented in Spain (Santini et al. 2002, Oberfeld et al. 2004); Netherlands (Health Council of the Netherlands 2004); Egypt (Abdel-Rassoul et al. 2007); and Austria (Hutter et al. 2006). The key symptoms are fatigue, pain (especially headaches), depression/anxiety, sleeping disorders, difficulty concentrating, cardiovascular problems, and dizziness. Symptoms have been documented well below ICNIRP guidelines (i.e., less than 1%) (Hutter et al. 2006).

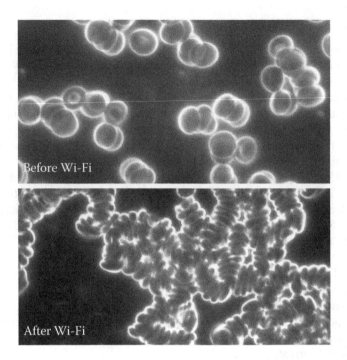

PLATE 22.1 Live blood before Wi-Fi exposure (top) and after 10 minutes of Wi-Fi exposure (bottom). Red blood cells aggregate in Rouleau formation following Wi-Fi exposure at 2.45 GHz.

Mitigation Testing

Another way to test sensitivity is to remove or reduce the electromagnetic pollutant and document whether symptoms improve. This type of testing was done in several schools with dramatic results. In one Wisconsin school that experienced "sick building syndrome," reducing the dirty electricity with special capacitors plugged into electric outlets resulted in fewer staff allergies, no more student migraines, and reduction of inhaler use by asthmatic students (Havas 2006a).

The dirty electricity was also reduced in three Minnesota schools (Havas and Olstad 2008). Thirty-four percent of the teachers improved and 64% of their symptoms improved when the capacitors were plugged in. This was a single blind study that used sham capacitors as well as real ones. The symptoms that improved include fatigue, mood, sense of well-being, dry eyes/mouth, flu-like symptoms, overall health, sense of satisfaction, coughing, sinus congestion, sense of accomplishment, sense of smell, dizziness, energy, headaches, ringing in the ears, anxiety, difficulty concentration, irritability, memory loss, facial flushing, and weakness. During this period, student behavior improved in 42% of the classes especially in the elementary grades. Without the capacitors, many of the behavior issues resembled ADD/ADHD.

Plugging capacitors in homes to reduce dirty electricity resulted in lower blood sugar among Type 1 diabetics requiring less daily insulin (Havas 2008) and improved muscular coordination among people with multiple sclerosis (Havas 2006b).

Exposure to electrosmog causes physiological stress in the body as measured by heat shock proteins (Blank and Goodman 2009). With prolonged exposure, the body depletes its energy reserves and stress hormones become activated and eventually depleted leading to adrenal exhaustion. The symptoms include chronic fatigue, poor sleep, anxiety or depression, cognitive dysfunction, and in some cases chronic pain, dizziness, nausea, and tinnitus. Some experience heart palpitations with pain or pressure in the chest resembling a heart attack. EHS diabetics experience elevated blood sugar and people with multiple sclerosis who are also EHS have a worsening of their symptoms. Indeed, some physicians may misdiagnose EHS for MS without an MRI scan as symptoms are similar.

WHAT DO AUTHORITIES SAY ABOUT ELECTROSMOG?

Most health authorities have yet to recognize the importance of electromagnetic hygiene and many nations have guidelines that are inadequate to protect public health (Table 22.1). While we have considerable evidence of the harmful effects of electrosmog, many health authorities denigrate these studies with non-scientific and highly subjective adjectives by claiming the evidence is insufficient, inconclusive, inconsistent, unconvincing, not replicated, controversial, and so on. As long as there are some scientists who question the science and continue to make these claims, policy makers have an excuse not to act. Indeed, it seems that science is used more to justify inaction than to take steps to remedy a potentially serious and expanding public health concern.

On May 11, 2015 a group of international scientists and medical doctors who do research related to electromagnetic energy sent an appeal to His Excellency Ban Ki-moon, Secretary-General of the United Nations Honorable Dr. Margaret Chan, Director-General of the World Health Organization, and U.N. Member States with the following recommendations (Blank et al. 2015):

Collectively we also request that:

1. Children and pregnant women be protected;
2. Guidelines and regulatory standards be strengthened;
3. Manufacturers be encouraged to develop safer technology;
4. Utilities responsible for the generation, transmission, distribution, and monitoring of electricity maintain adequate power quality and ensure proper electrical wiring to minimize harmful ground current;
5. The public be fully informed about the potential health risks from electromagnetic energy and taught harm reduction strategies;
6. Medical professionals be educated about the biological effects of electromagnetic energy and be provided training on treatment of patients with electromagnetic sensitivity;
7. Governments fund training and research on electromagnetic fields and health that is independent of industry and mandate industry cooperation with researchers;
8. Media disclose experts' financial relationships with industry when citing their opinions regarding health and safety aspects of EMF-emitting technologies; and
9. White-zones (radiation-free areas) be established.

More than 250 experts in the field from 41 countries signed this appeal and it continues to receive additional signatures. To date, neither the UN nor the WHO has responded to this appeal (www.emfscientist.org). It is one of the latest in international efforts to alert government officials about the serious consequence of EMF exposure. It follows on the back of numerous appeals and resolutions from scientists and medical doctors.

In 2011, the International Agency for Research on Cancer (IARC), a branch of the WHO, classified both ELF magnetic fields in 2002 and RFR in 2011 as a possible human carcinogen (Class 2b) (IARC 2002, 2012). Today, a growing number of scientists are requesting that classification be changed to either a Class 2a (probable carcinogen) or a Class 1 (carcinogenic to humans) (Morgan et al. 2015).

In 2016, the EMF working group for the European Academy for Environmental Medicine (EUROPAEM) published a document to help doctors diagnose and treat their patients with EMF-related health problems and illnesses (Belyaev et al. 2016). This document is a must read for physicians and health care professionals who want to improve their understanding of electrosmog, EHS, and related illnesses. The 35-page report has more than 300 references and topics that include current state of the scientific and political debate about EMF-related health problems from a medical perspective; worldwide statements of organizations regarding EMF; EMF and cancer, genotoxic effects, neurological effects, infertility and reproduction, electromagnetic hypersensitivity (EHS), and other diseases that require attention with respect to EMF exposure.

They also provide recommendations for action, treatment strategies, response of physicians to this development, and how to proceed if EMF-related health problems are suspected. They discuss when EMF exposures can be evaluated by questionnaires and when monitoring is required, and they recommend precautionary guidance values and EMF exposure values with information on how to reduce or prevent EMF exposure. They provide findings of medical examinations, recommended diagnostic tests, and provocation tests. They provide information about differences in individual susceptibility and they recommend that both the patient and the environment be treated. This is one of the most comprehensive documents on EHS designed specifically for health care practitioners.

WHAT CAN WE DO TO PROTECT OURSELVES FROM ELECTROSMOG?

Even though electromagnetic pollution is all around us, there is much we can do to minimize our exposure. Some of this involves blocking or filtering the unwanted frequencies; changing behavior and replacing some products with others that generate less or no electrosmog. The different parts of the electromagnetic spectrum require different types of technology to reduce and to monitor exposure.

ELECTROMAGNETIC HYGIENE: SPECIFIC RECOMMENDATIONS

ELF Magnetic Field

Magnetic fields have been associated with cancers and reproductive problems. Ideally, magnetic fields should be less than 1 mG (<0.1 μT). They are generated by electric devices and are associated with electrical wiring in the home and power lines, transformers, and substations outside the home (Table 22.3). Low frequency magnetic fields (those that we use for electricity) can penetrate walls, windows, doors, ceilings, and floors. Consequently, exposure in one room may be coming from an adjacent room. For this reason, it is important to spend as little time as possible near such sources even if they are on the other side of the wall. The bedroom environment is particularly important in this regard.

What to Do If Source Is Electric/Electronic Device

If the magnetic field is coming from electric/electronic devices (computers, photocopy machine, radio alarm clock, etc.) move the device further away from where people spend a lot of time. Even a few feet can make a big difference. This is particularly important at computer workstations and in the bedroom. If the device is an electric blanket, turn the blanket off and unplug it before getting into bed. Waterbeds also generate a high magnetic field because the water is heated.

What to Do If Source Is Wiring Inside a Building

If the magnetic field is coming from wiring inside the wall or under the floor or from electric heaters, move the bed, desk, and so on far enough away to reduce the magnetic field to less than 1 mG, if possible. In some cases, faulty wiring can lead to high magnetic fields in a room and this requires rewiring by a qualified electrician. Hence the need to measure the magnetic field. Knob and tube wiring used in older homes generates a high magnetic field and needs to be replaced (Riley 2012).

What to Do If Source Is External to Building

Electric fields are readily blocked by building material, but magnetic fields penetrate walls. If the magnetic field is coming from power lines, transformers, or substations outside the home/school/workplace, little can be done to reduce exposure within the building without expensive shielding. High voltage power lines should not be built near schools, homes, or hospitals. In Israel, homes cannot be sold if the magnetic field inside the home exceeds 10 mG.

Dirty Electricity

Dirty electricity refers to high voltage frequency transients (HVFT) or power surges that flow along electrical wires. It is generated by electronic devices (computers, plasma TV, dimmer switches, solar power, wind turbines, energy efficient light bulbs, smart meters) and has been associated with cancer, childhood asthma, impaired blood sugar regulation, neurological disorders, and symptoms of EHS (Table 22.3). Dirty electricity can be reduced with tuned capacitors and ideally levels should be below 40 GS units.

What to Do If Dirty Electricity Is Generated within Building

Dirty electricity can enter a building (home/school/workplace) at the service drop and can be generated within the building by electronic devices. Until electronic equipment is manufactured without producing dirty power, capacitors (referred to as filters) are needed to keep the levels of dirty electricity as low as possible. These filters need to be installed with proper monitoring (microsurge meter) to ensure levels are sufficiently low for maximum benefit. The electric utility recognizes the importance of power line filters to maintain power quality so that electronic equipment is not disrupted or damaged, but does not yet acknowledge the importance of good power quality from a health perspective. While filtering dirty electricity is one route, replacing devices that generate dirty electricity can also help. Energy efficient light bulbs can be replaced with incandescent light bulbs. Removing dimmer switches and replacing older computers and plasma TVs can reduce dirty electricity in the home.

What to Do If Dirty Electricity Is Generated External to Building

A certified electrician can reduce dirty electricity coming into a building with specially designed capacitors that are placed on or near the electric panel. However, if devices within the building also generate dirty power, this is insufficient to protect the occupants.

Radio Frequency and Microwave Radiation

Radio frequency and microwave radiation at levels below existing federal guidelines have been shown to have adverse biological and health effects (Table 22.1). This type of radiation can be generated within a building or it can penetrate the walls from nearby antennas or neighbors with Wi-Fi routers or cordless phones. It is much easier to control exposure from within home sources than those external to a building. Ideally, cell phone antennas should be at least 500 m from dwellings (homes, schools, hospitals) and broadcast antennas should be well beyond a 5-km radius depending on the strength of the transmitters. Radar antennas on a military base or near an airport or harbor emit microwave radiation that can travel for kilometers. People who live in the flight path of an airport will also have some radar exposure coming from the aircraft. Do not purchase a home that is near an RF/MW transmitter. For people who have already developed EHS, the distances mentioned above may not provide sufficient protection. Radio frequency radiation can penetrate walls and is blocked or reflected by metal objects that have the potential to generate hotspots. If you are in a location where there is a radio frequency (RF) source and metal objects (filing cabinet, frig, stove, sink, etc.), your RF exposure may be higher or lower depending on the location of the source, the metal, and your body.

What to Do If RF/MW Radiation Is Generated Outside Building

Sources external to a building are challenging to control. Ideally you want to maximize distance from the source although this might not be possible. RF shielding material is available but needs to be used with care as it can inadvertently increase your exposure if not properly installed. This material includes transparent film for windows; fabric (with metal fibers) for curtains, bed canopies, and clothing; carbon-based paint and wallpaper; as well as metal foil.

If antennas are near school property and radiation levels within the school are above 0.1 μW/cm², then special film can be placed on windows to reflect the radiation and special paint and shielding material can be put on walls and ceilings to keep the levels as low as possible. It is important not to renew licenses for antennas near schools and homes once they expire. However, if the school also uses Wi-Fi and wireless microphones, then the shielding on windows and walls may increase the levels within the buildings as this shielding material reflects the radiation back to its source.

What to Do If RF/MW Radiation Is Generated Inside Building

Replace wireless technology (cordless phones, wireless routers, wireless headsets, wireless printers, wireless games) with wired technology. Ethernet connects your computer to a router via wires and does not emit microwave radiation. Ethernet may still be available in schools that have transferred to Wi-Fi. Fiber optic technology is faster than Ethernet and Wi-Fi, and more secure than wireless routers and it does not emit microwave radiation. Fiber optics seem to be making a comeback in some communities.

HERE ARE A FEW THINGS YOU NEED TO KNOW ABOUT A FEW COMMONLY USED DEVICES

Cell Phones

Cell phones that have a data plan have multiple antennas. They have one for regular telephone calls, Wi-Fi connection, Bluetooth, and GPS. These emit radio frequency radiation (microwaves) when they are turned on. Airplane mode is not enough to eliminate these emissions and the Wi-Fi and Bluetooth also need to be turned off to ensure that your cell phone is not emitting microwave frequencies.

Cell phones detect the strength of the signal required to reach the nearest antenna and this signal strength is shown as bars. The further away you are from an antenna, the fewer bars on your cell phone and the stronger the signal has to be for your cell phone connection. If your cell phone is in roaming mode (trying to find a nearby antenna), it is going to emit the most microwaves. To minimize exposure, do not use your cell phone when it is roaming. Turn on airplane mode until you can get better reception.

Your cell phone tries to connect to a cell tower every few minutes when it is in standby mode. That means if you keep the cell phone near your body you are going to get a stronger "ping" from your cell phone. Best to keep your cell phone in airplane mode until you need it. This is especially important for children under the age of 18. Several national and international advisories are recommending that children under the age of 18 limit their cell phone use.

If you use a cell phone inside a space with lots of metal—like a car, bus, train, or elevator—some of that radiation is going to be reflected back inside the car because of the surrounding metal. If the vehicle is moving, the cell phone needs to connect with multiple antennas as the car moves from one cell zone to another. All of this is going to increase exposure in the car for all occupants.

Text instead of talk, and use the "speaker phone" option when talking and don't hold the cell phone next to your head. Do not keep the phone on your body (in a pocket, in your bra, or attached to a belt). When not using your cell phone, keep it in airplane mode (with Wi-Fi and Bluetooth turned off) so it does not radiate.

Cordless Phones

Cordless phones, whether they be 2.4 GHz or DECT (Digital European Cordless Telephony) phones, emit microwave radiation as soon as the base station is plugged into an electric outlet. The radiation generated by these phones is considerable with peak values over 500,000 μW/m² at a distance of 1–2 feet (Haumann and Sierck 2002). Levels drop with distance, but values can be higher in nearby rooms as this radiation passes through walls. The peak radiation values in the same room as a cordless phone are often higher than those encountered near cellular base stations located in residential communities. The best option for reducing RF exposure is to use a wired phone with no digital components.

In Europe it is possible to purchase cordless phones that are activated (i.e., emit microwave radiation) only when the handset is removed from the cradle (or base station). These phones cannot be purchased in North America nor can they be imported. The reason given by the European providers is that the Federal Communication Commission has not approved them because they interfere with military communications.

EcoDECT cordless phones are now available in North America and they have reduced emissions to "save battery power." These phones are better but ideally consumers should be able to purchase cordless phones that emit microwave radiation only when they are being used.

Internet Access: Computer, Wi-Fi Router, Tablets

Use an Ethernet cable for Internet access (not Wi-Fi). If you need to use Wi-Fi, ensure the wireless router is as far as possible from your body and turn it off when not in use. Ensure that you turn off the Wi-Fi on your computer (or any hand-held device) in addition to the router when not in use. Use a wired mouse and keyboard for both desktop and lap top computers. Unplug computer at night, particularly if it is in your bedroom. Use iPods/iPads/smart tablets in airplane mode with Wi-Fi and Bluetooth turned off and use a wired computer for Internet access.

Wireless Baby Monitors

As with cordless phones, wireless baby monitors also rely on microwave radiation for transmission. Baby monitors in North America emit constantly as long as they are plugged into an electric outlet. In Europe, sound-activated baby monitors that transmit microwaves only when a baby cries provide much lower exposure. However, they are not available in North America. Because infants and young children are more vulnerable to this radiation, placing a wireless baby monitor near a crib and exposing the child to microwave radiation is a bad idea. For parents who refuse to go without these wireless monitors it would be useful to cover (on all sides, on top, and beneath) the crib with MW shielding fabric to protect the infant. It is important to disconnect the baby monitor when not needed. These monitors are very powerful and can connect to the parent monitor well beyond 100 m and thus radiate the entire home as well as nearby neighbors.

Smart Meter

Smart meters allow the utility provider to get continuous data on power consumption and ultimately to charge higher rates for peak time electricity use. Smart meters are digital meters that are replacing the old analogue power watt meter. They emit bursts of microwave that last a few seconds, although the frequency of these bursts is a function of where a particular smart meter is in the grid or web of smart meters. Smart meters send messages to each other and the collector smart meter at the end of the line will emit the most radiation with fairly regular bursts of microwave radiation that is then sent to the utility.

Smart meters generate both microwave radiation and dirty electricity. The microwave radiation can pass through walls so a bedroom near the outer wall that is housing the smart meter is likely to have much higher levels of microwave radiation than other rooms in the home. In a condominium or apartment, multiple smart meters near an apartment are likely to provide a large blast of microwave radiation.

Smart meters also produce dirty electricity that runs along the wires inside the home. This poor power quality can be improved with capacitors. Several brands are now available along with meters that record the level of dirty electricity flowing along a wire. The capacitors short out high frequency voltage transients flowing along the wire. This improved power quality is much better for health and has the added benefit of protecting sensitive electronic equipment in the home and providing better sound quality on stereos for audiophiles. The capacitors are known by various names such as GS filters and power conditioners and are powerful surge suppressors. Ask your utility to have your wireless smart meter wired or use analog smart meters. If this is not possible, use dirty electricity filters to reduce the levels of dirty electricity generated by smart meters and do not sleep in a room adjacent to the smart meter. Shielding of the meter may be necessary if your smart meter emits frequent bursts of radio frequency radiation.

Smart Appliances

The original plan with smart meters was that they would ultimately be able to communicate with smart appliances. These are appliances that have a microchip that allows them to "talk" directly to the smart meter. The messages are transmitted wirelessly, and this provides yet another level of microwave radiation in the home. People who have purchased new appliances have become sick and the only resolution was to get rid of the appliance and replace it with one that isn't "smart." The chip cannot be removed without voiding the warranty of the appliance. Eventually the electric utility will be able to turn certain appliances on and off in your home during peak power consumption should they choose to do so. This also can be a health concern for those relying on keeping cool in the summer or warm in the winter and for those who require use of medical equipment for their survival.

Gaming Systems

Use only wired gaming systems such as the Play Station 3. Many gaming systems such as Xbox emit microwave radiation, even when not in use. Since these devices are often used for hours at a time and held close to the body it is imperative they are used with wired connections to connect the hand-held controllers.

Energy Efficient Light Bulbs

With concern about climate change and increasing carbon emissions, select governments around the world decided it was time to replace the incandescent light bulbs with energy efficient bulbs. The first bulbs that were commercially available were compact fluorescent light (CFL) bulbs. Today we also have light emitting diodes (LEDs). However, both forms of light generate dirty electricity. The amount of dirty electricity varies between bulbs and manufacturers and can differ between different batches of the same light bulb. There appears to be no standards of best practice.

Figure 22.3 shows the dirty electricity flowing along the wire and captured in the air from an incandescent light bulb and a CFL bulb. The more high-voltage frequency transients (HVFT) or spikes, the higher the level of dirty electricity. Installing capacitors can reduce dirty electricity but ideally these bulbs should be pre-filtered or replaced with incandescent lights.

CFLs also emit UV radiation and people should not sit close to an uncovered CFL bulb for hours at a time. Some of these bulbs now have an additional globe so they look like incandescent bulbs and this material filters out the UV radiation.

Both CFLs and LEDs emit flicker in the visible spectrum although the flicker may be too rapid for the eye to perceive. A light-noise detector converts the flicker frequency into sound, which enables rapid testing of these light bulbs. Remove CFL (compact fluorescent bulbs) from your work area. The best LEDs do not have transformers. To date we have not found an ideal light bulb that produces no flicker, no dirty electricity, and provides a full spectrum light ideal for health. In the meantime, use incandescent light bulbs, as these do not generate dirty electricity.

Lighting manufacturers are beginning to design lights that can communicate with a cell phone. The aim is that lights can be controlled from a distance. The lights we tested that can be paired with a cell phone emit high levels of microwave radiation as long as they are on, whether they are communicating with a cell phone or not. This is the wrong direction for the lighting industry and these light bulbs should be banned. They are analogous to shoe stores using x-rays to fit children's shoes. This is a frivolous and dangerous use of this technology and should not be allowed.

Bluetooth

Bluetooth is a way to connect a cell phone, tablet, or computer within a few feet of each other. Bluetooth also uses microwave radiation. Turn Bluetooth devices off when not needed. Use wired

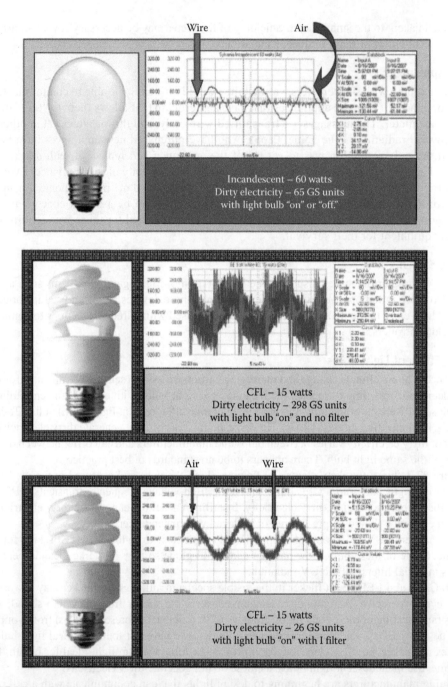

FIGURE 22.3 Spectrograph of wave form through the air and on wires measured with a fluke scope meter for an incandescent bulb (top) and a CFL bulb without (middle) and with (bottom) one dirty electricity filter. Incandescent bulb produces no dirty electricity and the waveform is identical with light bulb turned "on" or "off." CFL bulb (middle) generates dirty electricity (high frequency voltage transients) that can be measured on the wire (red) and in the air (blue). Note the 60 Hz sine wave has been removed with a Graham ubiquitous filter on the wire (red). One dirty electricity filter significantly improves power quality (bottom). (Data provided by Dave Stetzer, www.stetzerelectric.com.)

connections when possible. Avoid keeping a Bluetooth headset on your head. Use wired rather than wireless headphones and speakers.

Clock Radio

Clock radios emit electromagnetic fields that may affect sleep. It is important to move clock radios (and other electric equipment) at least 1 m away from your bed. Keep the bedroom as dark as possible as light also affects sleep.

Electric Equipment

Increase distance from electric cords and electric equipment. Move the power bar at least 1 m away from your feet at your desk. Use a wired extended keyboard to increase your distance from the computer screen, which will reduce the magnetic field.

Electrical Panel and Utility Room

Ensure that workers, students, or beds in your home are at least 3 m from an electrical panel and are not adjacent to a utility room as these generate high magnetic fields.

Electric Blanket and Waterbed

Avoid use of electric blankets and waterbeds. If you need to use an electric blanket, unplug it after it has warmed the bed. This eliminates the electric and magnetic fields generated by these blankets. If you turn the electric blanket off but leave it plugged in, it will generate an electric field. So, to reduce exposure unplugging the blanket is essential.

Turn Bedroom Power Off

Consider turning off the power (at the electrical panel) to your bedroom (and adjacent rooms) while you sleep.

Monitoring Your Exposure

You can use your computer to determine how many Wi-Fi hotspots are available in your area. Websites are available to determine your exposure to cell phone antennas (www.wigle.net global, www.antennasearch.com U.S.; and www.ertyu.org/steven_nikkel/cancellsites.html Canada).

To monitor your exposure, inexpensive meters are available. Ideally you require three different meters: one to measure RFR and MWR; another to measure dirty electricity (microsurge meter); and one to measure low frequency electric and magnetic fields.

ACKNOWLEDGMENTS

I would like to thank Sheena Symington for helping with the section on Electromagnetic Hygiene—Specific Recommendations.

REFERENCES

Abdel-Rassoul G, O Abou El-Fateh, XB Gao et al. 2007. Neurobehavioral effects among inhabitants around mobile phone base stations. *Neurotoxicology.* 28 (2): 434–440.

Adams JA, TS Galloway, D Mondal et al. 2014. Effect of mobile telephones on sperm quality: A systematic review and meta-analysis. *Environ Int.* 70: 106–112.

Ahlbom A, E Cardis, A Green et al. 2001. Review of the epidemiologic literature on EMF and health. *Environ Health Perspect.* 109 (Suppl. 6): 911–933.

Aldad TS, G Gan, XB Gao et al. 2012. Fetal radiofrequency radiation exposure from 800–1900 MHz-rated cellular telephones affects neurodevelopment and behavior in mice. *Sci Rep.* 2 (3): 12.

Belyaev I, A Dean, H Eger et al. 2016. EUROPAEM EMF Guideline 2016 for the prevention, diagnosis and treatment of EMF-related health problems and illnesses. *Rev Environ Health.* 31 (3): 363–397.

Bethwaite P, A Cook, J Kennedy, N Pearce. 2001. Acute leukemia in electrical workers: A New Zealand case-control study. *Cancer Causes Control.* 12 (8): 683–689.

Blackman CF, SG Benane, DE House. 2001. The influence of 1.2 microT, 60 Hz magnetic fields on melatonin- and tamoxifen-induced inhibition of MCF-7 cell growth. *Bioelectromagnetics.* 22: 122–128.

Blank M, R Goodman. 2009. Electromagnetic fields stress living cells. *Pathophysiology.* 16: 71–78.

Blank M, M Havas, E Kelley, H Lai, J Moskowitz. 2015. International appeal: Scientists call for protection from non-ionizing electromagnetic field exposure. *Eur J Oncol.* 20 (3/4): 180–182. www.emfscientist.org

Cardis E, BK Armstrong, JD Bowman et al. 2011. Risk of brain tumours in relation to estimated RF dose from mobile phones: Results from five Interphone countries. *Occup Environ Med.* 68: 631–640.

Chou C-K, AW Guy, LL Kunz et al. 1992. Long-term, low-level microwave irradiation of rats. *Bioelectromagnetics.* 13: 469–496.

Davis RL, FK Mostofl. 1993. Cluster of testicular cancer in police officers exposed to hand-held radar. *Am J Ind Med.* 24: 231–233.

DeMatteo B. 1986. *Terminal Shock: The Health Hazards of Video Display Terminals.* NC Press Ltd., Toronto, Ontario, 239pp.

Divan HA, L Kheifets, C Obel et al. 2008. Prenatal and postnatal exposure to cell phone use and behavioral problems in children. *Epidemiology.* 19 (6): S94–S95.

Divan HA, L Kheifets, C Obel et al. 2012. Cell phone use and behavioural problems in young children. *J Epidemiol Community Health.* 66: 524–529.

Dode AC, MMD Leao, F de AF Tejo et al. 2011. Mortality by neoplasia and cellular telephone base stations in the Belo Horizonte municipality, Minas Gerais state, Brazil. *Sci Total Environ.* 409: 3649–3665.

Dolk H, G Shaddick, P Walls et al. 1997. Cancer incidence near radio and television transmitters in Great Britain, I Sutton Coldfield transmitter. *Am J Epidemiol.* 145 (1): 1–9.

Eger H, KU Hagen, B Lucas et al. 2004. The Influence of Being Physically Near to a Cell Phone Transmission Mast on the Incidence of Cancer. Published in Umwelt Medizin Gesellschaft 17, 4 2004, as: 'Einfluss der räumlichen Nähe von Mobilfunksendeanlagen auf die Krebsinzidenz'.

Eger H, KU Hagen, B Lucas et al. 2012. How does long term exposure to base stations and mobile phones affect human hormone profiles? *Clinical Biochemistry.* 45: 157–161.

Eskander EF, SF Estefan, AA Abd-Rabou. 2012. How does long term exposure to base stations and mobile phones affect human hormone profiles? *Clin Biochem.* 45: 157–161.

Free MJ, WT Kaune, RD Phillips, HC Cheng. 1981. Endocrinological effects of strong 60-Hz electric fields on rats. *Bioelectromagnetics.* 2: 105–121.

Friesen M. 2015. Open Letter To: The Chair, Mr. Ben Hobb (Huron-Bruce, CPC), Standing Committee on Health (HESA), House of Commons, Federal Government, Canada, Information countering the statements of Dr. Demers, Mr. Adams and Dr. McNamee that there has been a full evaluation of the scientific literature for the review of Safety Code 6 (2015): Omission of hundreds of studies including over >90% showing potential harm to sperm and DNA. 4pp. See also, Male and Female Infertility, list of studies, http://archives.c4st.org/website-pages/hc-resolution-documents/male-and-female-infertility.html

Goldhaber MK, MR Polen, A Hiatt. 1988. The risk of miscarriage and birth defects among women who use visual display terminals during pregnancy. *Am J Ind Med.* 13: 695–706.

Gustavs K. 2017. *Current RF Exposure Limits.* www.buildingbiology.ca.

Ha M, H Im, M Lee et al. 2007. Radio-frequency radiation exposure from AM radio transmitters and childhood leukemia and brain cancer. *Am J Epidemiol.* 166 (3): 270–279.

Hardell L, M Carlberg, KH Mild. 2009. Epidemiological evidence for an association between use of wireless phones and tumor diseases. *Pathophysiology.* 16: 113–122.

Hatch EE, MS Linet, A Kleinerman et al. 1998. Association between childhood acute lymphoblastic leukemia and use of electric appliances during pregnancy and childhood. *Epidemiology.* 9: 234–245.

Haumann T, P Sierck. 2002. Nonstop pulsed 2.4 GHz radiation inside US homes. *World Health Organization, 2nd International Workshop on Biological Effects of Electromagnetic Fields,* 7–11 Oct 2002, Rhodes, Greece.

Havas M. 2000. Biological effects of non-ionizing electromagnetic energy: A critical review of the reports by the US National Research Council and the US National Institute of Environmental Health Sciences as they relate to the broad realm of EMF bioeffects. *Environ Rev* 8: 173–253.

Havas M. 2006a. Dirty electricity: An invisible pollutant in schools. *Feature Article for Forum Magazine, OSSTF.* Fall, 2006.

Havas M. 2006b. Electromagnetic hypersensitivity: Biological effects of dirty electricity with emphasis on diabetes and multiple sclerosis. *Electromagnetic Biology and Medicine*. 25: 259–268.

Havas M. 2008. Dirty electricity elevates blood sugar among electrically sensitive diabetics and may explain brittle diabetes. *Electromagnetic Biology and Medicine*. 27 (2): 135–146.

Havas M. 2017. When theory and observation collide: Can non-ionizing radiation cause cancer?. *Environ Pollut*. 221: 501–505.

Havas M, D Colling. 2011. Wind turbines make waves: Why some residents near wind turbines become ill. *Bulletin of Science Technology & Society*. 31 (5): 414–426.

Havas M, J Marrongelle, B Pollner et al. 2010. Provocation study using heart rate variability shows microwave radiation from 2.4 GHz cordless phone affects autonomic nervous system. *Eur J Oncol*. 5: 273–300.

Havas M, A Olstad. 2008. Power quality affects teacher wellbeing and student behavior in three Minnesota Schools. *Science of the Total Environment*. 402 (2–3): 157–162.

Health Council of the Netherlands. 2004. TNO study on the effects of GSM and UMTS signals on well-being and cognition. The Hague: Health Council of the Netherlands, publication no. 2004/13E, 55 pp.

Hocking B, IR Gordon, HL Grain, GE Hatfield. 1996. Cancer incidence and mortality and proximity to TV towers. *The Medical Journal of Australia*. 165: 601.

Hutter HP, H Moshammer et al. 2006. Subjective symptoms, sleeping problems, and cognitive performance in subjects living near mobile phone base stations. *Occup Environ Med*. 63 (5): 307–313.

IARC (International Agency for Research on Cancer). 2002. IARC monographs on the evaluation of carcinogenic risks to humans. *Non-ionizing Radiation. Part 1: Static and Extremely Low Frequency (ELF) Electric and Magnetic Fields*, Vol. 80. IARC Press, Lyon.

IARC (International Agency for Research on Cancer). 2012. IARC Monographs on the evaluation of carcinogenic risks to humans. *Non-ionizing Radiation, Part 2 Radiofrequency Electromagnetic Fields*. Vol. 102. IARC Press, Lyon.

International Commission on Non-Ionizing Radiation Protection. 1998. Guidelines for limiting exposure to time-varying electric, magnetic, and electromagnetic fields (up to 300 GHz). *Health Physics*. 74 (4): 494–522.

Kuhn TS. 1962. *The Structure of Scientific Revolutions*. University of Chicago Press, Chicago.

Kundi M. 2009. The Controversy about a Possible Relationship between Mobile Phone Use and Cancer. *Environmental Health Perspectives*. 117 (3): 316–324.

La Vignera S, RA Condorelli, E Vicari et al. 2012. Effects of the exposure to mobile phones on male reproduction: A review of the literature. *J Androl*. 33 (3): 350–356.

Lai H, NP Singh. 1995. Acute low-intensity microwave exposure increases DNA single-strand breaks in rat brain cells. *Bioelectromagnetics*. 16: 207–210.

Lai H, NP Singh. 1996. Single and double-strand DNA breaks in rat brain cells after acute exposure to radio-frequency electromagnetic radiation. *Int J Radiat Biol*. 69: 513–521.

Lee JM, KS Pierce, CA Spiering et al. 1996. *Electrical and Biological Effects of Transmission Lines: A Review*. Bonneville Power Administration Portland, Oregon.

Lerman Y, R Jacubovich, MS Green. 2001. Pregnancy outcome following exposure to shortwaves among female physiotherapists in Israel. *Am J Ind Med*. 39 (5): 499–504.

Li D-K, H Chen, R Odouli. 2011. Maternal exposure to magnetic fields during pregnancy in relation to the risk of asthma in offspring. *Arch Pediatr Adolesc Med*. 165 (10): 945–950.

Li DK, R Odouli, S Wi et al. 2002. A population-based prospective cohort study of personal exposure to magnetic fields during pregnancy and the risk of miscarriage. *Epidemiology*. 13 (1): 9–20.

Li DK, B Yan, Z Li et al. 2010. Exposure to magnetic fields and the risk of poor sperm quality. *Reprod Toxicol*. 29 (1): 86–92.

Magras IN and TD Xenos. 1997. RF radiation–induced changes in the prenatal development of mice. *Bioelectromagnetics*. 18: 455–461.

Michael Bevington. 2010. *Electromagnetic–Sensitivity and Electromagnetic–Hypersensitivity (Also Known as Asthenic Syndrome, EMF Intolerance Syndrome, Idiopathic Environmental Intolerance–EMF, Microwave Syndrome, Radio Wave Sickness): A Summary*. Capability Books, UK. 43pp.

Michelozzi P, A Capon, U Kirchmayer et al. 2002. Adult and childhood leukemia near a high-power radio station in Rome, Italy. *Am J Epidemiol*. 155 (12): 1096–1103.

Milham S, LL Morgan. 2008. A new electromagnetic exposure metric: High frequency voltage transients associated with increased cancer incidence in teachers in a California School. *Am J Ind Med*. 51 (8): 579–586.

Morgan LL, AB Miller, A Sasco, DL Davis. 2015. Mobile phone radiation causes brain tumors and should be classified as a probable human carcinogen (2A) (Review). *Int J Oncol*. 44 (5): 1865–1878.

Nordstrom S, E Birke, L Gustavsson. 1983. Reproductive hazards among workers at high voltage substations. *Bioelectromagnetics*. 4: 91–101.

NTP. 2016. Report of Partial Findings from the National Toxicology Program Carcinogenesis Studies of Cell Phone Radiofrequency Radiation in Hsd: Sprague Dawley® SD rats (Whole Body Exposures), Draft 6-23-2016, 87pp.

Oberfeld G, AE Navarro et al. 2004. The Microwave Syndrome – Further aspects of a Spanish Study, 3rd International Workshop on Biological Effects of Electromagnetic Fields, Oct 4–8, 2004, Kos, Greece, 9 pp.

Ouellet-Hellstrom R, WF Stewart. 1993. Miscarriages among female physical therapists who report using radio- and microwave-frequency electromagnetic radiation. *Am J Epidemiol*. 138 (10): 775–786.

Rea WJ, Y Pan, EJ Fenyves et al. 1991. Electromagnetic field sensitivity. *J Bioelectr*. 10: 241–256.

Riley K. 2012. *Tracing EMFs in Building Wiring and Grounding*. Create Space Independent Publishing Platform, USA, 96pp.

Rubin GJ, G Hahn, BS Everitt et al. 2006. Are some people sensitive to mobile phone signals? Within participants double blind randomised provocation study. *BMJ*. 332 (7546): 886–891.

Rubin GJ, R Nieto-Hernandez, S Wessely. 2010. Review idiopathic environmental intolerance attributed to electromagnetic fields (formerly 'electromagnetic hypersensitivity'): An updated systematic review of provocation studies. *Bioelectromagnetics*. 31: 1–11.

Sadetzki S, A Chetrit, A Jarus-Hakak et al. 2008. Cellular phone use and risk of benign and malignant parotid gland tumors—a nationwide case–control study. *Am J Epidemiol*. 167 (4): 457–467.

Santini R, P Santini, P Le Ruz, JM Danze, M Seigne. 2002. Study of the health of people living in the vicinity of mobile phone base stations: I. Influences of distance and sex. *Pathol Biol*. 50 (6): 369–373.

Savitz DA, H Wachtel, FA Barnes et al. 1988. Case-control study of childhood cancer and exposure to 60-Hz magnetic fields. *Am J Epidemiol*. 128 (1): 21–38.

Savitz DA, J Cai, E van Wijngaarden et al. 2000. Case-cohort analysis of brain cancer and leukemia in electric utility workers using a refined magnetic field job-exposure matrix. *Am J Ind Med*. 38 (4): 417–425.

Spitz MR, CC Johnson. 1985. Neuroblastoma and paternal occupation, a case-control analysis. *Am J Epidemiol*. 121: 924–929.

Stetzer D, AM Leavitt, CL Goeke, M Havas. 2016. Monitoring and remediation of on-farm and off-farm ground current measured as step potential on a Wisconsin dairy farm: A case study. *Electromagn Biol Med*. 35 (4): 321–36.

Sun J-W, X-R Li, H-Y Gao et al. 2013. Electromagnetic field exposure and male breast cancer risk: A meta-analysis of 18 studies. *Asian Pacific J Cancer Prev*. 14 (1): 523–528.

Tornqvist S. 1998. Paternal work in the power industry: Effects on children at delivery. *J Occup Environ Med*. 40: 111–117.

Wertheimer N, E Leeper. 1979. Electrical wiring configuration and childhood cancer. *Am J Epidemiol*. 109 (3): 273–284.

Wertheimer N, E Leeper. 1986. Possible effects of electric blankets and heated waterbeds on fetal development. *Bioelectromagnetics*. 7: 13–22.

Wertheimer N, E Leeper. 1989. Fetal loss associated with two seasonal sources of electromagnetic field exposure. *Am J Epidemiol*. 129: 220–224.

West JG, NS Kapoor, S-Y Liao et al. 2013. Multifocal breast cancer in young women with prolonged contact between their breasts and their cellular phones. *Case Rep Med*. 5.

Wilkins JR, III, RA Koutras. 1988. Paternal occupation and brain cancer in offspring: A mortality based case-control study. *Am J Ind Med*. 14: 299–318.

Wolf R, D Wolf. 2004. Increased incidence of cancer near a cell-phone transmitter station. *Int J Cancer Prev*. 1: 123–128.

Yang Y, X Jin, C Yan et al. 2008. Case-only study of interactions between DNA repair genes (hMLH1, APEX1, MGMT, XRCC1 and XPD) and low-frequency electromagnetic fields in childhood acute leukemia. *Leukemia Lymphoma*. 49 (12): 2344–2350.

23 Identifying Pharmaceutical-Grade Essential Oils and Using Them Safely and Effectively in Integrative Medicine

Joshua Plant and Scott Johnson

CONTENTS

The Primary Role of Essential Oils in Plants..552
The History and Advancement of Aromatics and Essential Oils 552
Pharmacological and Functional Evidence of Essential Oil Efficacy..554
Menthol (5-Methyl-2-(propan-2-yl)cyclohexan-1-ol) 554
Methyl Salicylate (Methyl 2 hydroxybenzoate)..555
Alpha-pinene (2,6,6,-Trimethylbicyclohept-2-ene) 556
Integrating Essential Oils into Medical Practice...556
Lavender Essential Oil for Anxiety..556
Peppermint Essential Oil for Irritable Bowel Syndrome 558
Blends of Essential Oils for Primary Dysmenorrhea...558
Blends of Essential Oils for Nausea...559
Essential Oil Best Practices and Safety 560
Methods of Administration 561
Inhalation 561
Transdermal Absorption/Topically...561
Oral Administration 562
Retention/Vaginal and Rectal Administration..562
Essential Oil Dosage 563
Essential Oil Safety..563
Essential Oil Application for Eyes and Ears 564
Phytophotodermatitis Potential of Essential Oils 565
Essential Oils and Epilepsy or Convulsive Disorders 565
Concomitant Use of Essential Oils and Medications and Health Contraindications.....................565
Pregnancy and Essential Oils...566
Essential Oil Therapy with Children..566
Conclusion 566
References...567

Medicines derived from plants have been an integral element of traditional medicine systems since the earliest recorded history. Indigenous cultures across the globe have used long-established and time-honored knowledge, skills, practices, and experiences with and of plants to prevent disease and maintain health. This tradition of relying on plants for health and healing continues today, and even modern Western medicine pursues healing molecules synthesized from plants to create novel pharmaceuticals.

More recently, the spotlight has been placed on one particular form of plant medicine—essential oils. These volatile, lipophilic compounds obtained from the leaves, seeds, flowers, twigs, resin, roots, fruits, and other parts of nature's most generous plants are experiencing a renaissance among patients and scientists alike. Essential oils represent a large and diverse group of plant extracts, most commonly extracted by distillation (steam or hydrodistillation) or mechanical processing (cold-pressing or expression). A small number of essential oils are also obtained through maceration or using carbon dioxide. Volatile extracts obtained by solvent extraction (with the exception of super-critical extracts obtained by carbon dioxide extraction) are not true essential oils, but concretes, absolutes, and resinoids.

THE PRIMARY ROLE OF ESSENTIAL OILS IN PLANTS

Out of an enormous number of plant species, only a few thousand are known to produce essential oils. After being produced by plant cells, essential oils (comprised of dozens of constituents) are stored in the glands of plants until they diffuse through the gland wall and evaporate to create a distinct aroma. The complete function of essential oils in a plant is not well understood, but scientists have learned some of the purposes they serve. For the plant, essential oil composition constantly adapts to the internal and external environment to serve three primary purposes:

1. **Defend** the plant from fungal and bacterial infections, parasites, and predatory insects and animals.[1–4] Production of essential oils comes at high metabolic cost to the host plant, so they are not typically produced in large quantities until required for plant survival.
2. Indirectly participate in the plant tissue **heal**ing process by increasing the release of volatile compounds in response to tissue damage, which reduces predation and pathogenic infection in the wound site to allow tissue repair to take place.[5–7] Volatile oleoresins produced by some trees after injury to the trunk is an example of how essential oils indirectly aid tissue healing in plants. Essential oil rich oleoresin serves to seal the wound against parasites and pathogens and prevent loss of sap.
3. Allow the plant to **thrive** by playing an important role in allelopathy, plant-to-plant communication, and the attraction of pollinators and animals to transfer pollen from flower to flower or disperse seeds, therefore creating offspring.[8–10] Essential oils can attract or deter insects and animals according to their survival needs, and some emit essential oils to influence the germination, growth, survival, and reproduction of competing plants.

Essential oils can be applied similarly to human health. It is well-established that many essential oils possess antimicrobial properties that **defend** humans against pathogens, aid wound **heal**ing both directly and indirectly (prevent pathogen adherence to dressings and reduce wound site infections), and encourage the human organism to **thrive** by aiding cellular communication and behavior.

THE HISTORY AND ADVANCEMENT OF AROMATICS AND ESSENTIAL OILS

Limited historical records and archaeological evidence suggests that the use of aromatic essences for medicinal, ritual, religious, food, beautification, and economic purposes dates back perhaps 6000 years. Ancient Chinese, Egyptian, and Indian civilizations reportedly used aromatic essences thousands of years ago, although their exact methods of extraction and precise uses remain somewhat mysterious. These ancient cultures likely used crude extraction methods—extraction of volatiles in vegetable or animal fat—and mainly relied on instinct and trial and error to determine the use of the aromatic essences they obtained from plants. This knowledge was then passed from one generation to the next orally.

It is not currently possible to determine which culture for sure was the first to use aromatic essences medicinally, but some experts give this credit to the Egyptians, based on analysis of residues on mummies and in jars collected from tombs.[11–13] The walls of Egyptian temples are adorned with hieroglyphics depicting the blending and use of aromatics and historical records suggest that Imhotep, the Grand Vizier of King Djoser (2780–2720 BC) promoted the use of aromatics for medicinal purposes.[14] The *Ebers Papyrus*, dating back to approximately 1534 BC but perhaps copied from a much earlier text from as far back as 3000 BC, is an Egyptian medical record containing hundreds of medicinal formulas, some of which utilize known aromatics.[15] In addition, the Egyptians were known to use aromatics and resins containing volatiles such as cedarwood, pine, myrrh, mastic, juniper, and cassia during the mummification process.

Another hypothesis is that the first use of aromatics may have occurred over 5000 years ago among the Indus civilization. This belief is based on equipment (distillation apparatus made of terracotta) and perfume containers discovered by Dr. Paolo Rovesti in 1975 at the foot of the Himalayas that date back to approximately 3000 BC[16] Scholars and historians speculate that this ancient equipment was used to extract and house volatile plant compounds. The *Vedas* is an ancient book of plant medicines originating in India that lists among the useful plant medicines the aromatic essences of cinnamon, coriander, ginger, myrrh, and sandalwood.

Surviving medical records from China, including the *Yellow Emperor's Classic of Internal Medicine* (dating back to at least 300 BC but some believe it originated in approximately 2600 BC) also references aromatics.[17] The ancient Chinese also reportedly burned incense to create harmony and balance. Other historical records suggest Hippocrates (460–~375 BC), Theophrastus (371–287 BC), Dioscorides (40–90 AD), and Galen (130–200 AD) each employed aromatics as medicines or to prevent illness.

It wasn't until the late tenth or early eleventh century that perhaps true essential oil distillation was popularized by the Arabian physician and alchemist Avicenna (980–1037 AD). He complied *The Canon of Medicine*, describing the medicinal use of over 500 plants, including aromatics.[18] However, this fact is also disputed, and some historians suggest the Arabians were primarily concerned with obtaining floral waters (the byproduct of essential oil extraction) rather than the essential oils.

There is little doubt that by the thirteenth century, essential oils were being distilled for medicinal purposes. Spanish physician Arnaldus de Villanova (1235–1311 AD) utilized distillation technology to produce essential oils like turpentine, rosemary, spike lavender, juniper (wood), clove, mace, nutmeg, anise, and cinnamon for therapeutic healing purposes.

European scientists continued to pave the way for essential oils to became viable therapeutic remedies throughout the fifteenth and nineteenth centuries. German physician Hieronymus Braunshcweig (c. 1450–1512 AD) wrote a number of texts regarding essential oils in the early 1500s. His works referenced 25 essential oils. Adam Lonicer (1528–1586 AD), a German botanist, peeked interest in essential oils as medicinals, particularly spice and seed essential oils. During the seventeenth and eighteenth centuries, French pharmacists distilled essential oils and began exporting lavender essential oil. Alchemists experimented with botanical extracts during the 1800s, which set the foundation for the discovery of the complex molecular chemistry of essential oils. This led to the breakthrough that essential oils possessed antibacterial and antiseptic properties during the nineteenth century, when some of the earliest studies (dating 1881 and 1887) were published.[19,20] The discovery of the medicinal and therapeutic qualities continued through the twentieth century throughout Europe.

Today, scientists and doctors continue to contribute to the knowledge and clinical use of essential oils through thousands of studies and documented practical application. The surge in essential oil use also creates unique challenges (demand greater than supply), which require stringent quality standards to ensure that essential oils destined for clinical use are pure, genuine, and possess the most desirable constituents profile to produce consistent and clinically relevant results. A pharmaceutical-grade essential oil must be extracted from the highest quality raw materials under pharma-grade standards, contain optimal levels of active and inactive volatile compounds, and more consistently and reliably produce therapeutic results.

PHARMACOLOGICAL AND FUNCTIONAL EVIDENCE OF ESSENTIAL OIL EFFICACY

As discussed earlier, essential oils have been used for thousands of years for their therapeutic and wellness benefits. Their wide-scale adoption across numerous cultures and thousands of years suggests strong efficacy, thereby withstanding the category of trends, wives' tales, and snake oils that usually find themselves adopted in a micro-culture for a short period of time.

Despite the resiliency of essential oils to overcome the stereotypes of snake oil and provide their benefit across numerous generations and civilizations, perhaps the strongest evidence of essential oil efficacy is found in their commonality of function with modern day pharmacological agents. In addition to providing benefit in health and wellness, essential oils in many ways provide an additional benefit to their pharmacological cousin, in that they are not synthesized from potentially toxic and deadly compounds, and they contain multiple constituents that buffer adverse effects and synergize positive effects. Essential oils contain natural biological compounds that are often readily consumed in the human diet, thereby eliminating any potential trace contaminants or toxic contributors. In this section, we will outline a few of the common active ingredients found in essential oils that are also accepted for use in today's widely accepted Western medicine philosophy.

MENTHOL (5-METHYL-2-(PROPAN-2-YL)CYCLOHEXAN-1-OL)

Menthol is one of the most widely used naturally occurring products with respect to health and wellness, and is widely accepted as a local anesthetic. Due to its effectiveness, pleasant taste, and commercial availability, it is found in many throat lozenges, pain creams, and drug delivery patches currently sold over the counter and works by delivering a "cooling" sensation (Figure 23.1).

Menthol utilizes numerous pathways of functionality, but primarily functions as a counterirritant and also as a local anesthetic. The mechanism of action of menthol acting as a counterirritant isn't greatly known, although it is known that menthol functions in the activation and subsequent desensitizing of epidermal nociceptors, which are often involved in the irritant pathways.[21]

In addition to functioning as a counterirritant through the polarization of epidermal receptors, menthol also delivers a pleasant physiological response (cooling of the skin) to function as a local anesthetic. The decrease in pain is noticed when the skin drops just 1°C from the surrounding tissue.[22] The discovery of menthol's mechanism of action on the cooling of skin was identified as recently as 2002, despite the use of menthol over thousands of years.[23] Menthol works through the TRPM8 (Transient Receptor Potential Cation Channel Subfamily M member 8) receptor, also

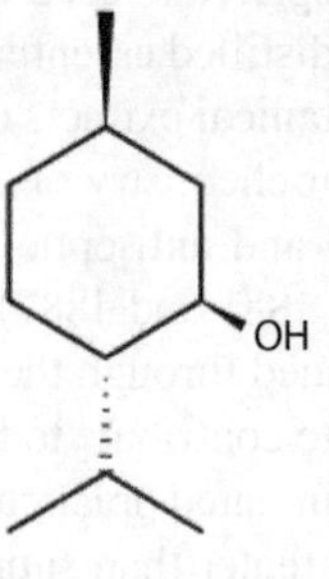

FIGURE 23.1   Menthol molecular structure.

known as the CMR1 (Cold and Menthol Receptor 1) receptor.[24] Interestingly, menthol functions as a local anesthetic by creating a robust membrane potential similar to that of when the same membranes are treated via cold at 6° below surrounding area.[25] This suggests that patients can receive the same pain-relieving benefits of applying ice to an area by applying menthol to the same area.

Natural Occurrence in Essential Oils:

- Menthol is found predominantly in your mint essential oils, most notably peppermint and corn mint, which contains approximately 35–55% and 60–80%, respectively.[26,86]

Notable Reagents Used in the Commercial Synthesis of Menthol:

- Zinc Bromide (ZnBr2): Zinc bromide is used for the cyclization of R-citronellal and is considered toxic at amounts less than 5 g.[27]

METHYL SALICYLATE (METHYL 2 HYDROXYBENZOATE)

One of the more common local anesthetics is methyl salicylate, which is found in nearly all over-the-counter muscle creams. With a functional concentration between 10 and 20% in pain creams, methyl salicylate has found itself to be the primary active ingredient in ameliorating pain (Figure 23.2).

The primary function of methyl salicylate is an anti-inflammatory. Though there are numerous pathways of inflammation, primary research of methyl salicylate analogs appear to work through the TNF-alpha pathway.[28] TNF-alpha is the pathway associated with inflammation found in arthritis and lupus, as well as necrotic cellular response. Though there are associations of methyl salicylate working to inhibit the macrophage directed response of the TNF-alpha pathway, due to the complexity and parallel pathways in which TNF-alpha functions downstream, little is known of the direct mechanism of action. However, evidence has shown methyl salicylate decreases inflammation across numerous disease models including arthritis,[29] acute lung injury,[30] and muscle pain management.[31]

Natural Occurrence in Essential Oils:

- Methyl salicylate is found to be the primary constituent in the common wintergreen essential oil, as well as the less common birch essential oil at levels greater than 90%.[86]

Notable Reagents Used in the Commercial Synthesis of Methyl Salicylate:

- Methanol is used to esterify salicylic acid and is considered toxic at levels greater than 80 mL, but poses problems including decreased vision and kidney failure at much lower concentrations.[32]
- Phenol is the beginning substrate for much of the methyl salicylate synthetically produced and is toxic even at vapor levels with a minimum lethal amount of 140 mg/kg.[33]
- Sulfuric acid is used for the acidification of the product and is one of the strongest and corrosive acids used in commercial production.

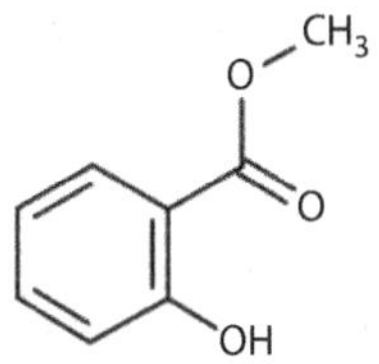

FIGURE 23.2   Methyl salicylate molecular structure.

ALPHA-PINENE (2,6,6,-TRIMETHYLBICYCLOHEPT-2-ENE)

Like menthol and methyl salicylate, alpha-pinene also functions as a mild anesthetic, but in addition functions as an antitussive. Alpha-pinene is used in many over-the-counter vapor rubs, throat lozenges, and other cough controlling agents (Figure 23.3).

The primary mechanism for alpha-pinene is likely by acting through the TRPV3 (Transient Receptor Potential Voltage 3) transmembrane ion channel. TRPV3 expresses itself along the epithelial tissue of the nose and tongue and has been implicated in the hyperalgesia in inflamed tissue thereby giving arise to a "cough." The evidence of alpha-pinene working through the TRPV3 channel has been mostly linked to the evidence of camphor, a cousin of alpha-pinene, acting as a functional ligand as determined through GFP fusion of the TRPV3 channels.[34]

Natural Occurrence in Essential Oils:

- Alpha-pinene is a major constituent in pine, rosemary, and eucalyptus essential oils at varying concentrations depending on harvest and sub-species (8–32%).

Notable Reagents Used in the Commercial Synthesis of Alpha Pinene:

- Phenol is the beginning substrate for much of the alpha-pinene synthetically produced and is toxic even at vapor levels with a minimum lethal amount of 140 mg/kg.[35]

INTEGRATING ESSENTIAL OILS INTO MEDICAL PRACTICE

According to the National Center for Complementary and Integrative Health, about 38% of adults use some form of complementary or alternative medicine for an array of diseases and conditions.[36] Some patients choose to use essential oils as an alternative to conventional medicine, while others use them concomitantly with prescribed treatment plans. An integrative approach to medicine uses both natural alternatives and conventional medicines, based on the available evidence for their safety and efficacy, placing patient outcome and safety as the highest priority. A great deal of *in vitro* and animal research and a growing body of clinical evidence has begun to validate the use of essential oils as integrative treatment options. We will briefly identify some of the prominent evidence-based essential oil therapies to consider implementing in practice.

LAVENDER ESSENTIAL OIL FOR ANXIETY

Lavender (*Lavandula angustifolia*) is one of the most widely researched essential oils in the published literature. This is particularly true in regard to clinical studies, with dozens of clinical studies completed to date. Lavender essential oil has a remarkable safety and efficacy performance record for subsyndromal anxiety or generalized anxiety disorder (GAD) when administered orally to patients. The essential oil used in the majority of clinical studies for anxiety complied with the European Pharmacopeia monograph (see Table 23.1).[37] A review reported that an anxiolytic effect is evident after two weeks of administration of 1–2 soft gels containing 80 mg each (1.5–2.5 drops depending on dropper size) of lavender essential oil (up to 160 mg total daily) for up to 10 weeks.[38]

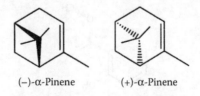

(−)-α-Pinene   (+)-α-Pinene

FIGURE 23.3 Alpha-pinene molecular structure, (+)- and (−)-enantiomers.

TABLE 23.1
Monograph Specifications European Pharmacopeia, Lavender Oil (5.0)

Linalyl Acetate	25.0%–46.0%
Linalool	20.0%–45.0%
Terpinen-4-ol	0.1%–6.0%
3-Octanone	0.1%–2.5%
1,8-Cineole	<2.5%
Alpha-Terpineol	<2.0%
Camphor	<1.2%
Limonene	<1.0%
Lavandulol	>0.1%
Refractive Index	1.455–1.466
Optical Rotation	$-12.5°$ to $-7.0°$
Relative Density	0.878–0.892

Given the potential for addiction and abuse and sedation effects of benzodiazepines, lavender essential oil is a much needed and viable evidence-based alternative.

A randomized, double-blind, placebo-controlled trial included 221 adults suffering from sub-syndromal anxiety disorder from 27 general or psychiatric practices. Patients were administered 80 mg/day of lavender essential oil preparation or placebo for 10 weeks. Lavender essential oil was superior regarding percentage of responders (76.9%) and remitters (42.6%), compared to placebo (49.1% and 42.6%, respectively).[39] The study authors noted that patients receiving lavender oil experienced significantly improved quality and duration of sleep, and improved mental and physical health without unwanted sedative or other adverse effects attributable to lavender.

The effectiveness of lavender essential oil preparations also compares favorably to standard anxiolytic medications. A randomized, double-blind, double-dummy trial divided 539 GAD patients into groups receiving (1) 80 or 160 mg of lavender oil, (2) 20 mg paroxetine, or (3) placebo once daily for 10 weeks. The Hamilton Anxiety Scale (HAMA) was used to measure efficacy. At the end of the 10-week trial, 60.3% of patients in the 160 mg lavender oil group showed a HAMA score of $\geq$50% of the baseline value and 46.3% of patients had a total score of <10 points at treatment end, compared to 51.9% and 33.3% for the 80 mg/d group, 43.2% and 34.1% for paroxetine, and 37.8% and 29.6% for placebo.[40] Interestingly, the study authors noted a pronounced antidepressant effect and improved mental health and health-related quality of life in the lavender oil groups. The antidepressant effect is noteworthy considering anxiety and depression are often comorbid.[41] Incidence densities of adverse events were 0.006 AEs/d for the 160 mg/d group, 0.008 AEs/d for the 80 mg/d group, 0.011 AEs/d for paroxetine, and 0.008 AEs/d for placebo. AE rates for lavender oil were comparable to placebo and lower than paroxetine, suggesting that oral lavender oil is very safe.

A multi-center, double-blind, randomized, placebo-controlled study compared lavender oil to the benzodiazepine Lorazepam for the treatment of GAD. Patients received 80 mg of lavender oil, or 0.5 mg of Lorazepam, or placebo for six weeks. The primary target variable was change in the HAMA scale, which is an objective measurement of anxiety severity. A decrease in HAMA was observed in both treatment groups (45% lavender oil, 46% lorazepam).[42] In addition, other subscores, such as Self-Rating Anxiety Scale, Penn State Worry Questionnaire, SF 36 Health Survey Questionnaire, Clinical Global Impressions of disorder severity, and sleep diary results were comparable for both treatment groups. No serious adverse events were reported during the study, with gastrointestinal complaints being the most commonly reported AEs in the lavender oil group, such as nausea (n = 4), eructation/breath odor (n = 3), and dyspepsia (n = 2). The Lorazepam group experienced nausea (n = 1) and fatigue (n = 6), which are known adverse reactions to the drug.

The same dosage of lavender essential oil proved effective for neurasthenia, post-traumatic stress disorder, and somatization disorder in a small open-label clinical trial that included 50 patients.[43] A significant number of study participants reported symptom amelioration of restlessness (57%), depression (51%), sleep disturbances (62%), and anxiety (72%) who were administered 80 mg/d lavender oil preparation. Half of patients reported 37 adverse events during the study (1848 days), corresponding to a frequency of 0.02 events per day. A causal relationship to the lavender essential oil could not be excluded for 21 of the adverse events, most of which were gastrointestinal in nature, notably eructation.

PEPPERMINT ESSENTIAL OIL FOR IRRITABLE BOWEL SYNDROME

Peppermint essential oil (*Mentha × piperita*) is a known smooth muscle relaxant, and an extensive database of clinical trials exists for the reduction of symptoms related to irritable bowel syndrome (IBS). It is most commonly administered in enteric-coated (EC), sustained/delayed release (SR), pH-dependent, or gastro-resistant (GR) capsules to reduce the risk of relaxing the hiatal sphincter—which can result in acid reflux—and to ensure compound dispersal in the small intestine. Common adult dosages include 180–200 mg t.i.d. for 2–4 weeks, with those presenting severe symptoms receiving 6 capsules daily (up to 20–40 drops daily depending on dropper size).[44,45] A systematic review and meta-analysis that reviewed 9 studies (726 patients total) concluded that peppermint oil is safe and effective for the short-term treatment of IBS.[46]

A placebo-controlled study evaluated the effectiveness of peppermint oil for IBS among patients with common presenting symptoms such as abdominal pain (88.3%), distension (86.7%), and flatulence (83.3%). Ninety patients were divided equally among the active and placebo groups, and administered 0.2 mL (187 mg, or 3–6 drops depending on dropper size) of peppermint oil (EC, SR, GR, capsules) or placebo, t.i.d. daily, 30 minutes before each meal for 8 weeks. After 8 weeks, peppermint oil significantly reduced abdominal pain and discomfort, and remarkably improved patient quality of life.[47] Reported AEs for heartburn (four in the peppermint oil group; five in controls), headache (six in the peppermint oil group; three in controls), and dizziness (three in the peppermint oil group; five in controls) were mild, transient, and well tolerated, suggesting the frequency of adverse events for peppermint is not significantly different than placebo.

Another double-blind study evaluated the effectiveness of 225 mg of peppermint oil b.i.d. for 4 weeks versus placebo. The study authors reported significant global improvement in IBS symptoms, with 75% of patients showing greater than 50% reduction of basal total IBS symptoms compared to 38% in the placebo group.[48]

pH-dependent, enteric-coated peppermint oil capsules also alleviated IBS in children better than placebo. As part of a randomized, double-blind controlled trial, 42 children received peppermint oil for IBS according to weight. Children weighing more than 45 kg received 0.2 mL (187 mg) t.i.d., whereas children weighing 30 kg to 45 kg received 0.1 mL t.i.d. for 2 weeks. After 2 weeks, patients receiving the peppermint oil experienced significant improvement in pain associated with IBS (71% of patients in the peppermint oil group vs. 43% in the placebo group).[49] The study reported no adverse effects of peppermint oil, but previous studies have reported mild and transient AEs, such as rectal burning, esophagitis, and allergic reactions.[50,51]

BLENDS OF ESSENTIAL OILS FOR PRIMARY DYSMENORRHEA

The prevalence of dysmenorrhea is estimated to be as high as 91% in women of reproductive age, making it a very common menstrual complaint with a major impact on quality of life, work productivity, and healthcare utilization.[52] Topical application of various combinations of essential oils has shown efficacy in reducing dysmenorrhea symptoms. Lavender and clary sage essential oils are frequently used with success.

A randomized, double-blind clinical trial determined the efficacy of an aromatic essential oil massage in 48 outpatients diagnosed with primary dysmenorrhea rating their pain greater than 5 on a scale of 1 to 10. Two 1-g spoonfuls of a combination of lavender (*Lavandula angustifolia*), clary sage (*Salvia sclarea*), and marjoram (*Origanum majorana*) essential oils (2:1:1 ratio) diluted to 3% in jojoba cream were massaged into the lower abdomen daily from the end of the last menstruation to the beginning of the next menstruation. The research showed that the essential oil massage significantly reduced the duration of menstrual pain from 2.4 to 1.8 days.[53] The study authors attributed the analgesic effect to the content of analgesic components (linalyl acetate, linalool, eucalyptol, and beta-caryophyllene) contained in the three essential oils, which accounted for as much as 79.3% of the blend.

Essential oil massage compared favorably to acetaminophen for relieving menstrual pain in high school girls. Thirty-two girls were included in the essential oil massage group and 23 in the acetaminophen group. A blend of clary sage (*Salvia sclarea*), marjoram (*Origanum majorana*), cinnamon (*Cinnamomum verum*), ginger (*Zingiber officinale*), and geranium (*Pelargonium graveolens*)—1:1:0.5:1.5:1.5 ratio diluted to 5% in carrier oil—was massaged into the lower abdomen for 10 minutes. The reduction of menstrual pain was significantly higher in the essential oil massage group versus the acetaminophen group; although the researchers were unable to determine if the benefit was achieved from the essential oils, the massage, or a combination of both.[54]

Other researchers controlled for the analgesic properties of massage by dividing 67 female college students into three groups: (1) an essential oil massage group (n = 25), (2) a placebo group that received massage with almond oil only (n = 20), and (3) a control group (n = 22). Subjects in the essential oil massage group received a lower abdominal massage with a combination of 2 drops of lavender (*Lavandula angustifolia*), 2 drops clary sage (*Salvia sclarea*), and 1 drop of rose (*Rosa damascena*) in 5 mL of almond oil. The essential oil therapy group experienced significant reductions in menstrual cramps levels and severity of dysmenorrhea compared to both placebo and control groups.[55]

A randomized, double-blind crossover study also demonstrated the effectiveness of essential oil combinations for primary dysmenorrhea. Forty-eight women received a once daily 10-minute abdominal massage for 7 days prior to menstruation as part of the first phase of the study. The treatment consisted of an essential oil massage with a blend of cinnamon (*Cinnamomum verum*), clove (*Syzygium aromaticum*), rose (*Rosa damascena*), and lavender (*Lavandula angustifolia*) essential oils (1.5:1.5:1:1 ratio) diluted to 5% in sweet almond oil. Group two (n = 47) received an abdominal massage with almond oil only during phase I of the trial. The two groups switched to the alternate regimen during phase II. During both treatment phases, the level and duration of menstrual pain and amount of menstrual bleeding was significantly reduced by the essential oil massage.[56] This study confirms that the efficacy is related to the essential oils and not simply the massage.

Lavender (*Lavandula angustifolia*) may be a key essential oil in the reduction of the severity and duration of menstrual pain according to another study. A quasiexperimental design with the subjects as their own control was utilized. Forty-four midwifery and nursing students with dysmenorrhea were followed through three menstrual periods. Participants documented their pain levels without any intervention during the first menstrual period. A placebo (liquid petrolatum) or lavender oil (2 mL) was massaged in a clockwise motion to the abdomen for 15 minutes during the second menstrual period. During the third menstrual period, the interventions were swapped so that those who received placebo received the lavender oil and vice versa. The results demonstrated that the lavender oil significantly reduced symptoms of dysmenorrhea when compared to placebo.[57]

BLENDS OF ESSENTIAL OILS FOR NAUSEA

Nausea can be caused by many factors, but one frequently observed by clinicians is post-operative nausea. Many essential oils, alone or in combination, have been administered to reduce varying causes of nausea, including post-operative nausea. A randomized trial of aromatherapy in 301 patients reporting post-operative nausea in a postanesthesia care unit was conducted. A blend of ginger (*Zingiber officinale*), spearmint (*Mentha spicata*), peppermint (*Mentha × piperita*), and cardamom (*Elettaria cardamomum*), or ginger alone, was placed on a gauze pad and inhaled through the nose followed by exhalation through the mouth for 5 minutes. Antiemetic medication requirements were significantly reduced in the aromatherapy group compared to the saline group, but not the alcohol (control) group.[58] The authors also pointed out that aromatherapy treatment is inexpensive, noninvasive, and can be controlled by patients as needed.

Other research has evaluated peppermint essential oil alone or in combination with lemon (*Citrus limon*) essential oil for post-operative nausea. Peppermint was inhaled through a personal plastic inhaler, or 2 mL of isotonic saline with 0.2 mL of peppermint oil added, or peppermint blended with lemon on an aromastick, inhaled as needed by the patient. Despite the varying methods of administration, a significant number of patients reported benefits of essential oil therapy (up to 82%) and almost half reported resolution of symptoms.[59]

Nausea and vomiting during pregnancy is experienced by up to 80% of all pregnant women, and treatment can be difficult due to various neuromuscular and metabolic factors implicated in its pathogenesis, as well as the uncertainty surrounding the full effects of potential drug treatments on the developing fetus.[60] The safety of essential oil inhalation makes it an ideal choice for pregnancy-associated nausea and vomiting. A randomized, double-blind, controlled clinical trial was conducted with 100 pregnant women experiencing nausea and vomiting. Participants in the experimental group (n = 50) applied 2 drops of lemon essential oil diluted in almond carrier oil to a cotton ball and placed the cotton ball about 3 cm from the nose while inhaling deeply three times through the nose whenever nauseated. Most participants inhaled the lemon essential oil 4–6 times daily. The placebo group (n = 50) inhaled almond oil colored with carrots to simulate the color of lemon peel oil. Of both groups, 50% of the experimental group were satisfied with their results, compared to only 34% in the control group.[61] The nausea and vomiting mean in the five intervals (1, 2, 3, and 4 days after and before intervention, and ANOVA with repeated measures) showed statistically significant differences between the lemon essential oil and placebo groups.

Essential oil inhalation has also been studied in hospice and palliative care patients. Twenty-five patients suffering from nausea in a hospice and palliative care program inhaled an essential oil blend containing: anise (*Pimpinella anisum*), sweet fennel (*Foeniculum vulgare* var. *dulce*), Roman chamomile (*Anthemis nobilis*), and peppermint (*Mentha* × *piperita*) in combination with other standard treatment options. Most patients receiving essential oil inhalation reported nausea relief.[62]

Nausea and vomiting is experienced by approximately 70%–80% of all cancer patients receiving chemotherapy, and it is ranked first on the list of troublesome symptoms experienced by chemotherapy patients despite drug interventions.[63,64] Oral administration of essential oils has been used to ameliorate chemotherapy-induced nausea and vomiting (CINV). Cancer patients preparing to receive chemotherapy (cancer naïve prior to study) were chosen to participate in a randomized, double-blind clinical study investigating the oral administration of peppermint and spearmint essential oils for CINV. Patients received a capsule filled with 2 drops of peppermint or spearmint essential oil (the rest of the capsule was filled with sugar) 30 minutes prior to chemotherapy (concomitant with normal antiemetic regimen) and again 4 hours after the first capsule, and finally 4 hours later at home. A significant reduction in CINV (intensity and number of emetic events) was observed during the first 24 hours for both the peppermint and spearmint groups when compared to placebo.[65] The study authors also reported that the essential oil intervention reduced the cost of treatment.

There are of course other essential oils that are viable candidates to use as an integrative approach to human health, but the scope of this text does not permit listing all possible evidence-based essential oil remedies. This text acts as an introduction to the evidence in support of regularly employing essential oils in health-care settings, both as an adjunct, or perhaps as alternatives to more invasive or risky treatment options.

ESSENTIAL OIL BEST PRACTICES AND SAFETY

Essential oils are unique remedies because they simultaneously influence psychological, biological, and cognitive health. The sense of smell—10,000 times more powerful than the sense of taste—is the only of the major senses that is directly connected to the brain (through the olfactory bulb). Airborne odor molecules enter the nostrils and dissolve in the nasal mucosa. Under the nasal mucosa, olfactory receptor neurons detect the odor molecules and transmit information to the olfactory bulb at the back of the nasal cavity. Sensory receptors of the olfactory bulb are part of the brain and send messages to the most primitive brain centers (limbic system structures) and the neocortex, which influence memory, emotions, and conscious thought. Therefore, the administration of essential oils produces a complete psychophysiological response that causes automatic adaptations by the central nervous system.

And this only considers one aspect of how essential oils influence human health. Beyond the olfactory processes involved, research demonstrates that essential oils influence hormone and neurotransmitter levels, organ function, antioxidant activity and defenses, immune function, the inflammatory response, and cellular behavior to name a few.[66-72]

METHODS OF ADMINISTRATION

Essential oils are normally administered in four ways:

1. *Inhalation.* Essential oils can be administered via diffuser, personal inhaler, direct inhalation from the bottle, steam inhalation, application to cotton, gauze, or a tissue, aromasticks, aromastones, or diffuser necklaces.
2. *Transdermal Absorption/Topically.* Direct application, usually diluted in a carrier oil, to a target area.
3. *Orally.* Preferably in a capsule, but mild oils can be administered in liquid (reduces dispersion and bioavailability; increases localized tissue irritation risk), or sublingually.
4. *Rectally or Vaginally.* Through a suppository, enema, syringe, or tampon insertion.

Although a common practice in animal studies is to administer essential oils via i.v., subcutaneously, or intramuscularly, human trials do not employ these administration methods currently. One case report outlines the percutaneous administration of essential oils for chronic MRSA osteomyelitis, but this is a rare exception.[73]

INHALATION

Inhalation is the safest way to administer essential oils, but it is still capable of producing remarkable psychophysiological outcomes. When volatile molecules from essential oils are inhaled, they travel up the nose and attach to olfactory cell-receptor sites. Once bound to the olfactory nerve receptor sites, odor molecules travel to the olfactory bulb via the glomerulus, where the odor is significantly intensified. The intensified odor stimulates the bipolar receptor to fire, and impulses are transmitted to the limbic system. In response to the odor molecules, the limbic system initiates physiological responses in the endocrine and nervous systems that trigger the release of hormones, chemicals, and neurotransmitters. These nervous and endocrine system responses influence myriad body functions: memory, learning, emotions, instinct, motivation, sleep, libido, appetite, thirst, heart rate, blood pressure, breathing, stress levels, hormone regulation, pain perception, appetite, metabolism, wakefulness, insulin production, body temperature, relaxation level, and sense of well-being.

TRANSDERMAL ABSORPTION/TOPICALLY

Transdermal absorption delivers essential oil molecules into the bloodstream without first being metabolized via the liver. Bypassing the stomach and liver means potentially a greater percentage of the active ingredient (rather than secondary metabolites with different therapeutic and toxic properties) directly enters the bloodstream. However, CYP enzymes in the skin may activate certain essential oil molecules (i.e., methyl chavicol [estragole], methyl eugenol, and safrole) making them more toxic during transdermal absorption, but the efficiency of dermal CYP conversion is unknown and relatively high concentrations are required for CYPs to contribute to bioactivation.[74,75] Transdermal, rectal, and vaginal delivery methods may help avoid potential side effects such as stomach upset due to the route of entry into the bloodstream.

Topical administration of essential oils requires care, and dilution in a carrier oil is strongly recommended for most applications due to the potentially irritating, sensitizing, and photosensitizing compounds contained in essential oils. Research suggests that compounds below 500–600 Daltons in molecular weight readily cross the skin layers and are absorbed by the body.[76] Since virtually all essential oil compounds are well below this threshold (typically 135–225 Daltons), penetration of and entrance into the bloodstream by these compounds is expected. Once applied to the skin, essential oil compounds penetrate through the epidermis into the blood vessel rich reticular layer of the dermis. Essential oil molecules enter and exit the bloodstream through the capillaries, pass through the arterioles and arteries, then enter general circulation. The circulatory system transports the lipophilic molecules to cells and tissues.

It is important to understand that essential oil absorption through the skin is somewhat limited due to their volatile nature. Studies suggest that only 4–10% of an essential oil is absorbed through the skin if applied without any covering. Occlusion after topical applications significantly increases absorption rates to an estimated 75%, which could dramatically increase therapeutic activity.[77,78] Essential oils are rapidly utilized, metabolized, dispersed, and excreted by the body and require frequent application to maintain therapeutic action. One study reported that peak serum concentration was achieved at 20 minutes, with zero lavender compounds detected 90 minutes post-application of a 2% dilution of lavender essential oil.[79] These factors must be considered for dosage requirements.

ORAL ADMINISTRATION

Essential oils can be administered orally, which allows for greater precision in dosing, increased convenience, and good bioavailability. Oral administration may also increase the risk of drug interactions and gastrointestinal complaints, and may decrease absorption due to degradation by stomach acid and enzymes when administered in liquids as opposed to capsules. The preferred oral delivery method for essential oils is in a capsule to improve compound dispersion and reduce side effects. A pH-dependent (delayed release) or enteric coated capsule is even better. The risk of gastrointestinal complaints can be reduced if the essential oil capsules are taken with food and a full glass of water. Eructation is commonly reported after oral administration, but it is usually mild and not serious.

Sublingual administration and the administration of essential oils in water or other liquids should be reserved for mild essential oils (lavender, chamomile, citrus oils, frankincense, copaiba, etc.) and used infrequently. These methods can increase the risk of localized mucous membrane irritation in the esophageal tract and stomach, initiates absorption in the buccal cavity, and may diminish compound dispersion (except sublingual administration, which has rapid access to the bloodstream prior to digestion and metabolism via the capillaries under the tongue).

Unless an enteric-coated or pH dependent capsule is used, capsule dissolution will begin in the stomach. Essential oil molecules travel to the small intestine and then to the liver via the portal vein for metabolism, processing, and dispersion. A portion of the essential oil molecules (now secondary metabolites) are released into the bloodstream while other molecules are sent back to the small intestine for additional metabolism to hydrophilic substances that are more easily excreted by the kidneys. Molecules released to general circulation are transported to cells and tissues throughout the body.

RETENTION/VAGINAL AND RECTAL ADMINISTRATION

Though rarely the first choice of compound administration, rectal and vaginal administration serves as an alternative to oral and parenteral administration. Retention is a very efficient method to deliver essential oils and produce localized benefits to the lower colon and the vagina, but is also capable of systemic therapy. This method bypasses the gastrointestinal system, avoiding the breakdown of essential oils during digestion. Bypassing the first phase of metabolism, vaginal administration releases essential oil molecules directly into the bloodstream. Partial avoidance of first pass metabolism occurs with rectal delivery. The absorptive membrane of the rectum allows for rapid absorption of low molecular weight compounds like essential oils.[80] In addition, highly lipophilic compounds (again like essential oils) have the potential for absorption into the lymphatic system because the rectum is extensively drained by the lymphatic circulation.[81] Lastly, the empty rectum presents a constant ad static environment as compared to the greatly varying environment of the gastrointestinal tract. Indeed, lipophilicity is perhaps the most important factor for increasing rectal membrane permeability.[82]

Vaginal administration delivers essential oil molecules mainly through the vaginal epithelium or through the vaginal mucosa to the uterus and then into general circulation. Absorption of compounds in the vagina occurs by dissolution in the vaginal space and across the membrane by permeability. Transport of lipophilic essential oil molecules occurs transcellulary via passive diffusion. Cyclic changes to the vaginal epithelium caused by hormones can drastically modify epithelial thickness and permeability, and therefore the absorption of essential oils. The vaginal epithelium is generally thinnest during days 19 through 24 of the menstrual cycle, except for in nonovulating women, which experience reduced epithelial cell layer count days 7 through 12.[83] Vaginal epithelium thickness peaks during reproductive years, and is at its lowest point during menopause, suggesting greater absorption of essential oils will occur in middle-aged to senior women. Vaginal permeability of low molecular weight lipophilic substances is significantly greater than hydrophilic substances.

ESSENTIAL OIL DOSAGE

The dosage used largely depends on the composition of the essential oil, the condition and severity of the condition being treated, the age, height, weight, and current health status of the patient, and the concomitant use of medications. For example, pennyroyal contains significant amounts of the toxic compound pulegone, which would require reduced dosage to avoid toxicity. On the contrary, lemon essential oil is predominantly d-limonene (a nontoxic and very safe compound) and can be administered at much higher doses. Alcoholics should generally receive one-half a standard dose of essential oil. Chronic alcohol use may limit essential oil availability and metabolism by competing for the same set of metabolizing enzymes, or potentially activate CYP enzymes (i.e., CYP2E1) that may transform essential oil compounds into toxic chemicals.[84] The CYP2E1 enzyme is involved in the hydroxylation of estragole to the proximate carcinogen $1'$-hydroxyestragole, which is further activated to the known hepatocarcinogen $1'$-sulfooxyestragole.[85] An evidence-based resource with detailed composition information, drug interactions, and health contraindications is recommended to guide proper usage and dosage. Table 23.2 provides dosage suggestions based on clinical study doses and practical clinical usage.

ESSENTIAL OIL SAFETY

Essential oils are very safe with few side effects when used reasonably and according to practical guidelines. Essential oil safety involves several factors including the age and current health of the patient, method of administration, dosage, length of administration, dilution ratio, concomitant medication use, and chemical composition of the essential oil. Essential oil composition is a key because some essential oils are known to have 12 or more chemotypes, which may each have different therapeutic properties, toxicity risks, and administration methods. The following are useful best practices and safety guidelines to follow based on the available evidence.[86]

TABLE 23.2
Dosage Guidelines

	Clinical Study Range	Recommended
Inhalation	• 20 mcL–3 mL; commonly 2–5 drops • Occasionally diluted in carrier oil or another substance • Inhalation time of 3 minutes to 24 hours; commonly 15–30 minutes	• Birth to 12 mos. (*up to 22 lb.*): 20 mcL–0.07 mL (0.5–2 drops) for 15–30 minute intervals, 2–4 hour breaks between • 1 to 5 years (23–*44 lb.*): 0.03 mL–0.13 mL (1–4 drops) for 15 to 30 minute intervals, 2 hour breaks between; • 6–17 years (45–*153 lb.*): 0.07 mL to 0.26 mL (1 to 8 drops) for up to 60 minute intervals, 60 minute breaks between • Adults (*154+ lb.*): 0.07 mL to 0.5 mL 92 to 15 drops), up to 120 minutes, 30-minute breaks between, or diffuser set to intermittent for up to 8 hours
Topical	• 0.25% to neat; commonly 1.5% to 5% • 10 mcL to 100 mL (diluted) • Almost always diluted; few neat applications	• Birth to 12 mos. (*up to 22 lb.*): 0.3% dilution (1 drop EO per 10–15 mL carrier oil) • 1 to 5 years (23–*44 lb.*): 1.5%–3% dilution (1.5–3 drops per 5 mL carrier oil); neat for certain conditions • 6–11 years (45–77 lb.): 1.5%–5% (1.5–7 drops per 5 mL carrier oil); neat for certain conditions • 12 to 17 years (78–153 lb.): 1.5%–20% dilution (1.5–30 drops per 5 mL carrier oil); neat for certain conditions; less than 10% dilution generally • Adults (154+ lb.): 1.5% to neat; less than 10% dilution generally
Oral	• 50 mcL/d to 1 mL t.i.d. • Occasionally diluted in carrier oil • Approximately 1 to 90 drops daily depending on dropper size	• Birth to 5 years (up to 44 lb.): Not recommended • 6 to 11 years (45–77 lb.): 0.03 mL to 0.25 mL/day; 1 to 2 drops for a typical dose unless otherwise indicated in a clinical study or evidence-based reference • 12 to 17 years (78–153 lb.): 0.03 mL to 0.5 mL/day; 1 to 3 drops up to 3 times daily for a typical dose unless otherwise indicated in a clinical study or evidence-based reference • Adults (154+ lb.): 0.03 mL to 1.5 mL/day; 1 to 5 drops up to three times daily for a typical dose unless otherwise indicated in a clinical study or evidence-based reference
Rectal	• 370 mL of water with 30 mL of peppermint preparation (16 mL of peppermint oil and 0.4 mL polysorbate made up to 21 mL with purified water) and an additional 10 mL of peppermint solution added to the enema tubing	• 0.33 mL to 0.70 mL of EO in 15 to 30 mL of carrier oil or solution, inserted into the lower portion of the rectum and retained for up to 8 hours q.d., up to twice weekly
Vaginal	• N/A	• 0.33 mL to 0.70 mL of EO in 15 to 30 mL of carrier oil or solution, inserted through the vagina and retained for up to 8 hours q.d., up to twice weekly; or soak tampon in above mixture, retain up to 8 hours, or replace t.i.d. to q.i.d. • Douche: 0.1 to 0.25 mL of EO in 1 L of distilled water, b.i.d., once weekly

ESSENTIAL OIL APPLICATION FOR EYES AND EARS

Keep essential oils away from the eyes. Essential oils should never be placed directly in the eye, and great caution should be exercised when applying near the eye. Always dilute essential oils before applying near the eye, and apply widely around the orbit of the eye. Direct administration in the eye may cause corneal tissue damage, corneal abrasions, vision loss, or chemical burns.[87] Administer a fatty substance (vegetable oil or milk) in the eye if accidental eye contact occurs. Pat the eye with a dry paper towel and repeat the fatty substance administration into the eye until relief is achieved.

Never administer essential oils directly in the ear canal. Some anecdotal reports suggest that this may result in a ruptured eardrum and, at the very least, will cause severe pain. If accidental ear administration occurs, add several drops of carrier oil to the ear, and continue to do so, until the pain is relieved. The preferred method for treating conditions of the ear is to place one to two drops of essential oil, diluted, on a cotton ball and insert the cotton ball into the ear with the cotton ball positioned as to not contact the flesh of the ear. Refresh the cotton ball approximately every 4 hours.

PHYTOPHOTODERMATITIS POTENTIAL OF ESSENTIAL OILS

A limited number of essential oils may cause chemically induced skin irritation when minor compounds present absorb energy from long-wave ultraviolet (UV-A 320–380 nm) radiation. When these compounds are present in the epidermis or dermis and exposed to UVA, activated derivatives are formed that induce cellular damage. The reaction typically begins approximately 24 hours after exposure and peaks at 48–72 hours.[88] Phytophotodermatitis reactions resemble an exaggerated sunburn, but have the potential to induce postinflammatory hyperpigmentation lasting weeks to months. Phytophotodermatitis can be avoided by preventing sun exposure for at least 12 hours following the application of photosensitive oils—angelica, bay laurel absolute, bergamot, bitter orange, cumin, grapefruit, khella, Mediterranean mandarin, neroli, lemon (expressed), lime (expressed), petitgrain, rue, and tagetes. These oils contain compounds known to induce phytophotodermatitis based on their concentration of phototoxic furanocoumarin compound(s), such as angelicin, bergamottin, bergapten, citropten, imperatrotin, isobergapten, isoimperatorin, methyoxsalen, and oxypeucedanin, and the duration of UVA exposure.[89–91]

ESSENTIAL OILS AND EPILEPSY OR CONVULSIVE DISORDERS

Some essential oils contain compounds (1,8-cineole, camphor, fenchone, methyl salicylate, pinocamphone, pulegone, sabinyl acetate, and thujones) that may reduce the seizure threshold of medications or exacerbate/trigger seizures and convulsions. Those with epilepsy or prone to convulsions should avoid the use of essential oils with significant quantities of these compounds.

CONCOMITANT USE OF ESSENTIAL OILS AND MEDICATIONS AND HEALTH CONTRAINDICATIONS

Essential oils have the potential to interact with medications if taken concomitantly, particularly orally administered essential oils. Some essential oil compounds are known to interact with antibiotics and antifungals (1,8-cineole, alpha-terpineol, bergamottin, carvacrol, (E)-cinnamaldehyde, (E)-cinnamic acid, citral (geranial + neral), citronellol, cuminaldehyde, eugenol, geraniol, menthol, methyl eugenol, terpinen-4-ol, and thymol); antidiabetics (ar-turmerone, carvacrol, carvone, (E)-cinnamaldehyde, citral, fenugreek oil (active compound not identified), geranium (active compound not identified), rosemary (active compound not identified), thymoquinone, and trans-anethole); or interfere with CYP450 enzymes (alpha-bisabolol, chamazulene, citral, frankincense lipophilic gum-resin terpene fractions, geraniol, menthol, menthyl acetate, and safrole); and so it is important to be knowledgeable of these interactions. Many other potential drug-essential oil interactions have been identified or are possible, therefore an evidence-based resource should be consulted.

In addition, some medical conditions require more cautious use of essential oils, due to the potential of essential oils to exacerbate the condition. One example is those with bleeding disorders that should avoid essential oils with antiplatelet or anticoagulant compounds (alpha-bulnesene, *ar*-turmerone, carvacrol, (E)-cinnamaldehyde, elemicin, estragole, eugenol, isoeugenol, lavandin (synergy of all main components), menthol, menthone, methyl salicylate, myristicin, safrole, thymol, trans-anethole, and verbenone). An evidence-based resource should be consulted to minimize contraindicated administration of essential oils.

PREGNANCY AND ESSENTIAL OILS

Many mild essential oils can be a vital part of pregnancy that can make the gestation period more pleasurable. The composition of the essential oil, method of administration, and patient risk for miscarriage or complications are factors that determine the level of risk for an essential oil being used during pregnancy. Oral administration has the greatest potential for adverse reactions, followed by rectal, vaginal, and topical administration. Diffusion poses little, if any, risk. The benefits to risks must be weighed by the patient and her healthcare provider.

According to *The Merck Manual*, most substances with a molecular weight of less than 500 Daltons readily cross the placenta and enter the fetus's bloodstream.[92] Since the most common essential oil molecules are less than 225 Daltons, it is logical to suspect that essential oil molecules diffuse across the placenta similarly to the way they cross other epithelial barriers. These molecules could positively or negatively influence fetal development and pregnancy outcome depending on the essential oil used. Common essential oils to avoid during pregnancy, but not exclusive, include pennyroyal, basil (estragole CT), thuja, tansy, wormwood, parsley, and mugwort (certain chemotypes). Others like those high in citral should be used cautiously until definitive safety research is concluded.

The greatest risk to a fetus from substances that transverse the placenta is during the first trimester. Substances that are known to be toxic, cause abortions, or cause birth defects should be strictly avoided during the first trimester. It is suggested that the internal use of essential oils be avoided during the first trimester. Topical or inhalation methods are preferred during gestation whenever practical. Topical application of dilutions no greater than 3% should be used during the first trimester, particularly among women with a prior history of miscarriage. Mild essential oils like balsam fir, citrus oils, cedarwood, chamomile, frankincense, copaiba, ginger, and tea tree are often used during pregnancy; but the decision of which, if any, essential oils are appropriate for use during pregnancy ultimately remains solely with the mother-to-be and her OB/GYN or healthcare practitioner.

ESSENTIAL OIL THERAPY WITH CHILDREN

The clear majority of essential oils are compatible with essential oil therapy in children. However, some essential oils should be avoided, particularly those with significant menthol, 1,8-cineole, camphor, myristicin, trans-anethole, pulegone, thujones, apiol, and methyl salicylate content. A very, very small minority of children may respond adversely to the use of essential oils depending on the method of administration and exposure level. Essential oils that contain high levels of these compounds, including central nervous system problems, respiratory distress (difficulty or labored breathing), premature thelarche, multiple organ dysfunction, and toxicity, and this reaction could occur from inhalation only with essential oils rich in menthol or 1,8-cineole. Essential oils high in 1,8-cineole, menthol, and camphor should be avoided through age 2, and used cautiously up through age 5. Essential oils with thujones should be avoided through age 5. Nutmeg (high in myristicin) should be avoided through age 5, and used cautiously through age 12. Parsley and dill oil (myristicin or apiol) should be avoided in children under age 12. Oral use of trans-anethole containing essential oils should be avoided through age 11. Wintergreen and birch (both high in methyl salicylate) should be avoided in children under age 12, especially during fever or viral illness.

CONCLUSION

Reasonable use of essential oils based on available evidence will result in few side effects and has great potential to improve human health. These complex essential oils, extracted from plants, have virtually unlimited potential, and science will continue to reveal the vast human benefits they provide. Practitioners searching for greater therapeutic effectiveness of essential oils can find it somewhere between the art of healing passed down from ancient traditions and the methodical study of the therapeutic action of essential oils, in terms of their known pharmacognosy and pharmacological functions.

As with other natural modalities, essential oil therapy is most effective when the totality of ancient traditions, patient results, clinical experience, pharmacognosy, and pharmacology are considered, along with the goal to create balance to the individual in physical, mental, emotional, and spiritual areas. This approach transcends typical treatments that separate the four areas of health (mental, physical, emotional, and spiritual) into separate modalities, and leads to better patient outcomes and more effective treatment. While some practitioners may be hesitant to venture into foreign realms of treatment modalities, the advantages, clinical results, and acquisition of a broader perspective that offers the greatest potential to meet the full depths of human health today far outweigh the temporary discomfort experienced. Essential oils are currently primed to make a significant impact on the healthy lifespan of human beings. The integrative physician, with a deep understanding of human anatomy, biology, pathology, pharmacology, and cytology, coupled with a meaningful awareness of essential oil therapy, can offer potential solutions to impending healthcare crises that lead to healing and greater patient satisfaction.

REFERENCES

1. Gonzalez-Lamonthe R, Mitchell G, Gattuso M et al. Plant antimicrobial agents and their effects on plant and human pathogens. *Int J Mol Sci.* 2009 Aug;10(8):3400–19.
2. Nazzaro F, Fratianni F, De Martino L et al. Effect of Essential Oils on Pathogenic Bacteria. *Pharmaceuticals (Basel).* 2013 Dec;6(12):1451–74.
3. Dudareva N, Negre F, Nagegowda DA et al. Plant volatiles: Recent advances and future perspectives. *Crit Rev Plant Sci.* 2006;25:417–40.
4. Sharma HC, Sujana G, Rao DM. Morphological and chemical components of resistance to pod borer, Helicoverpa armigera in wild relatives of pigeonpea. *Arthropod-Plant Interact.* 2009;3:151–61. doi: 10.1007/s11829-009-9068-5.
5. Paré PW, Tumlinson JH. Plant volatiles as a defense against insect herbivores. *Plant Physiology.* 1999;121:325–31.
6. War AR, Paulraj MG, Ahmad T et al. Mechanisms of plant defense against insect herbivores. *Plant Signal Behav.* 2012 Oct;7(10):1306–20.
7. Scala A, Allmann S, Mirabella R et al. Green leaf volatiles: A plant's multifunctional weapon against herbivores and pathogens. *Int J Mol Sci.* 2013 Sep;14(9):17781–811.
8. Gershenzon J, McConkey ME, Croteau RB. Regulation of monoterpene accumulation in leaves of peppermint. *Plant Physiol.* 2000;122:205–13.
9. Barney JN, Hay AG, Weston LA. Isolation and characterization of allelopathic volatiles from mugwort (Artemisia vulgaris). *J Chem Ecol.* 2005 Feb;31(2):247–65.
10. Caissard JC, Meekijjironenroj A, Baudino S et al. Localization of production and emission of pollinator attractant on whole leaves of Chamaerops humilis (Arecaceae). *Am J Bot.* 2004 Aug;91(8):1190–99.
11. Abdel-Maksoud G, El-min AR. A review on the materials used during mummification process in ancient Egypt. *Med Archaeology Archaeometry.* 2011;11(2):129–50.
12. Charrié-Duhaut A, Connan J, Rouquette N et al. The canopic jars of Rameses II: Real use revealed by molecular study of organic residues. *J Archaeological Sci.* 2007;34:957–67.
13. Colombini MP, Modugno Fr, Silvano Fl et al. Characterization of the balm of an Egyptian mummy from the seventh century Bc studies in conservation. 2000;45(1):19–29.
14. David, AR. 2007. Imhotep: Founder of medical science in ancient Egypt, In WF Bynum and H Bynum (eds.) *Biographical Dictionary of the History of Medicine.* Westport, CT: Greenwood Publishing Group.
15. Indiana University. Medicine In Ancient Egypt. Availabe at: http://www.indiana.edu/~ancmed/egypt. HTM.
16. Lawless J. 2013. *The Encyclopedia of Essential Oils: The Complete Guide to the Use of Aromatic Oils In Aromatherapy, Herbalism, Health, and Well Being.* Newburyport, MA: Conari Press.
17. Curran J. The yellow Emperor's classic of internal medicine. *BMJ.* 2008 Apr 5;336(7647):777.

18. Avicenna. (1025) The Canon of Medicine.
19. Bassolé IHN, Juliani HR. Essential oils in combination and their antimicrobial properties. *Molecules.* 2012;17:3989–4006.
20. Chamberlain M. Les essences au point de vue de leurs proprietes antiseptiques. *Ann Inst Pasteur* 1887;1:153–64.
21. Barkin RL. The pharmacology of topical analgesics. *Postgrad Med.* 2013 Jul;125(4 Suppl 1):7–18.
22. Campero M, Serra J, Bostock H et al. Slowly conducting afferents activated by innocuous low temperature in human skin. *J Physiol.* 2001 Sep 15; 535(Pt 3):855–865.
23. Patel T, Ishiuji Y, Yosipovitch G. Menthol: A refreshing look at this ancient compound. *J Am Acad Dermatol.* 2007 Nov;57(5):873–8.
24. Andersen HH, Olsen RV, Møller HG et al. A review of topical high-concentration L-menthol as a translational model of cold allodynia and hyperalgesia. *Eur J Pain.* 2014 Mar;18(3):315–25.
25. McKemy DD, Neuhausser WM, Julius D. Identification of a cold receptor reveals a general role for TRP channels in thermosensation. *Nature.* 2002 Mar;416:52–58.
26. Tsai ML, Wu CT, Lin, TF et al. Chemical composition and biological properties of essential oils of two mint species. *Trop J Pharm Res.* 2013 Aug;12(4):477–82.
27. Tohe DMM, Battersby RV, Wolf HU. Zinc Compounds. *Ullmann's Encyclopedia of Industrial Chemistry.* 2014 May.
28. Zhang X, Sun J, Xin W et al. Anti-inflammation effect of methyl salicylate 2-O-B-D-lactoside on adjuvant induced-arthritis rats and lipopolysaccharide (LPS)-treated murine macrophages RAW264.7 cells. *Int Immunopharmacol.* 2015 Mar;25(1):88–95.
29. Zhang X, Sun J, Xin W et al. Anti-inflammation effect of methyl salicylate 2-O-B-D-lactoside on adjuvant induced-arthritis rats and lipopolysaccharide (LPS)-treated murine macrophages RAW264.7 cells. *Int Immunopharmacol.* 2015 Mar;25(1):88–95.
30. Yang S, Yu Z, Yuan T et al. Therapeutic effect of methyl salicylate 2-o-b-d-lactoside on LPS-induced acute lung injury by inhibiting TAK1/NF-KappaB phosphorylation and NLRP3 expression. *Int Immunopharmacology.* 2016 Nov;40:219–28.
31. Higashi Y, Kiuchi T, Furuta K. Efficacy and safety profile of a topical methyl salicylate and menthol patch in adult patients with mild to moderate muscle strain: A randomized, double-blind, parallel-group, placebo-controlled, multicenter study. *Clin Ther.* 2010 Jan;32(1):34–43.
32. Kruse JA. Methanol and ethylene glycol intoxication. *Crit Care Clinics.* 2012 Oct;28(4):661–711.
33. Budavari S et al. *The Merck Index: An Encyclopedia of Chemicals, Drugs, and Biologicals.*
34. Billen B, Brams M, Debaveye S et al. Different ligands of the TRPV3 cation causes distinct conformational changes as determined by intrinsic tryptophan fluorescence quenching. *J Biological Chem.* 2015 Mar;290:12964–74.
35. Budavari S et al. *The Merck Index: An Encyclopedia of Chemicals, Drugs, and Biologicals.*
36. National Institutes of Health. National Center for Complementary and Integrative Health. The Use of Complementary and Alternative Medicine in the United States. Available at: https://nccih.nih.gov/research/statistics/2007/camsurvey_fs1.htm
37. European Medicines Agency. Lavandulae aetheroleum monograph. Available at: http://library.njucm.edu.cn/yaodian/ep/EP501E/16_monographs/18_monographs_l-p/lavender_oil/1338e.pdf
38. Kasper S. An orally administered Lavandula oil preparation (Silexan) for anxiety disorder and related conditions: An evidence based review. *Int J Psychiatry Clin Pract.* 2013 Nov;17(Suppl 1):15–22.
39. Kasper S, Gastpar M, Muller WE et al. Silexan, an orally administered Lavandula oil preparation, is effective in the treatment of 'subsyndromal' anxiety disorder: A randomized, double-blind, placebo controlled trial. *Int Clin Psychopharmacol.* 2010 Sep;25(5):277–87.
40. Kasper S, Gastpar M, Muller WE et al. Lavender oil preparation Silexan is effective in generalized anxiety-disorder—a randomized, double-blind comparison to placebo and paroxetine. *Int J Neuropsychopharmacol.* 2014 Jun;17(6):859–69.
41. Hirschfield RMA. The Comorbidity of Major Depression and Anxiety Disorders: Recognition and Management in Primary Care. *Prim Care Companion J Clin Psychiatry.* 2001;3(6):244–54.
42. Woelk H, Schlafke S. A multi-center, double-blind, randomised study of the Lavender oil preparation Silexan in comparison to Lorazepam for generalized anxiety disorder. *Phytomedicine.* 2010 Feb;17(2):94–99.
43. Uehleke B, Schaper S, Dienel A et al. Phase II trial on the effects of Silexan in patients with neurasthenia, post-traumatic stress disorder or somatization disorder. *Phytomedicine.* 2012 Jun;19(8):665–71.
44. Grigoleit HG, Grigoleit P. Peppermint oil in irritable bowel syndrome. *Phytomedicine.* 2005;12:601–6.

45. Quartero RL, de Wit AO, van der Heijden NJ et al. Bulking agents, antispasmodics and antidepressants for the treatment of irritable bowel syndrome. *Cochrane Database Syst Rev.* 2011;(8):CD003460.

46. Khanna R, MacDonald JK, Levesque BG. Peppermint oil for the treatment of irritable bowel syndrome: A systematic review and meta-analysis. *J Clin Gastroenterol.* 2014 Jul;48(6):505–12.

47. Merat S, Khalili S, Mostajabi P et al. The effect of enteric-coated, delayed-release peppermint oil on irritable bowel syndrome. *Dig Dis Sci.* 2010 May;55(5):1385–90.

48. Cappello G, Spezzaferro M, Grossi L et al. Peppermint oil (Mintoil((R))) in the treatment of irritable bowel syndrome: A prospective double blind placebo-controlled randomized trial. *Dig Liver Dis.* 2007 Jul;39(6):530–36.

49. Kline RM, Kline JJ, Di Palma J et al. Enteric-coated, pH-dependent peppermint oil capsules for the treatment of irritable bowel syndrome in children. *J Pediatr.* 2001 Jan;138(1):125–8.

50. Rees WDW, Evans BK, Rhodes K. Treating irritable bowel syndrome with peppermint oil: A multi-center trial. *Br Med J.* 1979;2:835–36.

51. Dew MI, Evans BK, Rhodes J. Peppermint oil for the irritable bowel syndrome: A multicenter trial. *Br J Clin Pract.* 1984;38:394–98.

52. Ju H, Jones M, Mishra G. The prevalence and risk factors of dysmenorrhea. *Epidemiol Rev.* 2014;36(1):104–13.

53. Ou MC, Hsu TF, Lai AC et al. Pain relief assessment by aromatic essential oil massage on outpatients with primary dysmenorrhea: A randomized, double blind clinical trial. *J Obstet Gynaecol Res.* 2012 May;38(5):817–22.

54. Hur MH, Lee MS, Seong KY et al. Aromatherapy massage on the abdomen for alleviating menstrual pain in high school girls: A preliminary controlled clinical study. *Evid Based Complement Alternat Med.* 2012;2012:187163.

55. Han SH, Hur MH, Buckle J et al. Effect of aromatherapy on symptoms of dysmenorrhea in college students: A randomized placebo-controlled clinical trial. *J Alt Complement Med.* 2006 Jul-Aug;12(6):535–41.

56. Marzouk TM, El-Nemer AM, Baraka HN. The effect of aromatherapy abdominal massage on alleviating menstrual pain in nursing students: A prospective randomized cross-over study. *Evid Based Complement Altern Med.* 2013;2013:742421.

57. Apay SE, Arslan S, Akpinar RB et al. Effect of aromatherapy massage on dysmenorrhea in Turkish students. *Pain ManagNurs.* 2012 Dec;13(4):236–40.

58. Hunt R, Dienemann J, Norton HJ et al. Aromatherapy as treatment for postoperative nausea: A randomized trial. *Anesth Analg.* 2013 Sep;117(3):597–604.

59. Lua PL, Zakaria NS. A brief review of current scientific evidence involving aromatherapy use for nausea and vomiting. *J Altern Complement Med.* 2012 Jun;18(6):534–40.

60. Lee N, Saha S. Nausea and vomiting of pregnancy. *Gastroenterol Clin North Am.* 2011 Jun;40(2):309–34.

61. Yavari Kia P, Safajou M, Shahnazi M et al. The effect of lemon inhalation aromatherapy on nausea and vomiting of pregnancy: A double-blinded, randomized, controlled clinical trial. *Iran Red Crescent Med J.* 2014 Mar;16(3):e14360.

62. Gilligan NP. The palliation of nausea in hospice and palliative care patients with essential oils of Pimpinella anisum (aniseed), Foeniculum vulgare var. dulce (sweet fennel), Anthemis nobilis (Roman chamomile) and Mentha × piperita (peppermint). *Int J Aromather.* 2005;15(4):163–67.

63. Lindley CM, Bernard S, Fields SM. Incidence and duration of chemotherapy-induced nausea and vomiting in the outpatient oncology population. *J Clin Oncol.* 1989 Aug;7(8):1142–9.

64. Molassiotis A, Saunders MP, Valle J et al. A prospective observational study of chemotherapy-related nausea and vomiting in routine practice in a UK cancer centre. *Support Care Cancer.* 2008 Feb;16(2):201–8.

65. Tayarani-Najaran Z, Talasaz-Firoozi E, Nasiri R et al. Antiemetic activity of volatile oil from Mentha spicata and Mentha × piperita in chemotherapy-induced nausea and vomiting. *Ecancermedicalscience.* 2013;7:290.

66. Martins DF, Emer AA, Batisti AP et al. Inhalation of Cedrus atlantica essential oil alleviates pain behavior through activation of descending pain modulation pathways in a mouse model of postoperative pain. *J Ethnopharmacol.* 2015 Dec 4;175:30–8.

67. Sinha S, Biswas D, Mukherjee A. Antigenotoxic and antioxidant activities of palmarosa and citronella essential oils. *J Ethnopharmacol.* 2011 Oct;137(3):1521–27.

68. Buch P, Patel V, Ranpariya V et al. Neuroprotective activity of Cymbopogon martinii against cerebral ischemia/reperfusion-induced oxidative stress in rats. *J Ethnopharmacol.* 2012 Jun 26;142(1):35–40.

69. Carrasco FR, Schmidt G, Romero AL et al. Immunomodulatory activity of Zingiber officinale Roscoe, Salvia officinalis L. and Syzygium aromaticum L. essential oils: Evidence for humor- and cell-mediated responses. *J Pharm Pharmacol.* 2009 Jul;61(7):961–67.

70. Šošić-Jurjević B, Ajdžanović V, Filipović B et al. Functional morphology of pituitary -thyroid and -adrenocortical axes in middle-aged male rats treated with Vitex agnus castus essential oil. *Acta Histochem.* 2016 Sep;118(7):736–745.

71. Srivastava JK, Pandey M, Gupta S. Chamomile, a novel and selective CoX-2 inhibitor with anti-inflammatory activity. *Life Sci.* 209 Nov;85(19–20):663–69.

72. LM Lopes C, Gonçalves e Sá C, de Almeida AA et al. Sedative anxiolytic and antidepressant activities of Citrus limon (Burn) essential oil in mice. *Pharmazie.* 2011 Aug;66(8):623–27.

73. Sherry E, Boeck H, Warnke PH. Percutaneous treatment of chronic MRSA osteomyelitis with a novel plant-derived antiseptic. *BMC Surgery.* 2001;1:1.

74. Jeurissen SMF, Punt A, Boersma MG et al. Human cytochrome P450 Enzyme specificity for the bioactivation of estragole and related alkenylbenzenes. *Chem Res Toxicol.* 2007;20(5):798–806.

75. Baron JM, Wiederholt T, Heise R. Expression and function of cytochrome p450-dependent enzymes in human skin cells. *Curr Med Chem.* 2008;15(22):2258–64.

76. Wiesenthal A, Hunter L, Wang S et al. Nanoparticles: Small and mighty. *Int J Dermatol.* 2011 Mar;50(3):247–54.

77. Francomme P, Penoel D. L'Aromatherapie Exactment. 1990, pg. 197. Roger Jolois, Editeur Limoges.

78. Jager W, Buchbauer G, Jirovetz L et al. Percutaneous absorption of lavender oil from massage oil. *J Soc Cosmetic Chemists.* 1992;43(1):49–54.

79. Jager W, Buchbauer G, Jirovetz L et al. Percutaneous absorption of lavender oil from massage oil. *J Soc Cosmetic Chemists.* 1992;43(1):49–54.

80. Lakshmi Prasanna J, Deepthi B, Rama Rao N. Rectal drug delivery: A promising route for enhancing drug absorption. *Asian J Res Pharm Sci.* 2012;2(4):143–49.

81. Jannin V, Lemagnene G, Gueroult P et al. Rectal route in the twenty first century to treat children. *Adv Drug Delivery Rev.* 2014 Jun;73:34–49.

82. Yamamoto A, Muranishi S. Rectal drug delivery systems: Improvement of rectal peptide absorption by absorption enhancers, protease inhibitors and chemical modification. *Adv Drug Delivery Rev.* 1997 Nov;28(2):275–99.

83. Patton DL, Thwin SS, Meier A et al. Epithelial cell layer thickness and immune cell populations in the normal human vagina at different stages of the menstrual cycle. *Am J Obstet Gynecol.* 2000 Oct;183(4):967–73.

84. Cederbaum AI. Alcohol metabolism. *Clin Liver Dis.* 2012 Nov;16(4):667–85.

85. Jeurissen SMF, Punt A, Boersma MG et al. Human cytochrome P450 enzyme specificity for the bioactivation of estragole and related alkenylbenzenes. *Chem Res Toxicol.* 2007;20(5):798–806.

86. Johnson S. 2015. *Evidence-Based Essential Oil Therapy: The Ultimate Guide to the Therapeutic and Clinical Application of Essential Oils.* Orem, UT: Scott A Johnson Professional Writing Services, LLC. Also: Johnson S. 2017. *Medicinal Essential Oils: The Science and Practice of Evidence-Based Essential Oil Therapy.* Orem, UT: Scott A Johnson Professional Writing Services, LLC.

87. Adams MKM, Sparrow JM, Tole DM. Inadvertent administration of Olbas oil into the eye: A surprisingly frequent presentation. *Eye.* 2009;23(1):244.

88. Smith E, Kiss F, Porter RM et al. A review of UVA-mediated photosensitivity disorders. *Photochem Photobiol Sci.* 2011 Dec 16;11(1):199–206.

89. Naganuma M, Hirose S, Nakayama Y et al. A study of the phototoxicity of lemon oil. *Arch Dermatol Res.* 1985;278(1):31–6.

90. Placzek M, Froemel W, Eberlein B et al. Evaluation of phototoxic properties of fragrances. *Acta Derm Venereol.* 2007;87(4):312–6.

91. Dugrand-Judek A, Olry A, Hehn A et al. The distribution of coumarins and furanocoumarins in Citrus species closely matches citrus phylogeny and reflects the organization of biosynthetic pathways. *PLoS One.* 2015 Nov;10(11):e0142757.

92. *The Merck Manual Professional Edition.* Available at: http://www.merckmanuals.com/professional/gynecology_and_obstetrics/drugs_in_pregnancy/drugs_in_pregnancy.html.

24 On the Sophistication of Herbal Medicines

Stephen Harrod Buhner

CONTENTS

Paradigm Conflicts...572
Self-Organization..573
Bacterial Intelligence 575
Plant Intelligence 578
Chemical Innovation in Plants 580
Resistance to Plants?...583
Stealth Pathogens 584
Borrelial Infections 585
A Few Comments on Dosages and Treatment Approaches 587
References..589

In the late 1940s, the successes of Waksman and Schatz (streptomycin) and Duggar (tetracycline) led many to believe that bacterial infections were basically conquered. That conceit led to widespread misuse and outright abuse of antibacterial agents. Nonetheless, we still neither fully understand nor appreciate resistance to antibacterial agents ... Many important advances in the practice of medicine are actually at serious risk. Multidrug resistant bacteria are compromising our ability to perform what are considered routine surgical procedures ... A ubiquitous phrase encountered in obituaries is "died from complications following surgery," but what is not well understood is that these "complications" are quite frequently multidrug resistant infections.

Steven J. Projan
Antibacterial Drug Discovery in the twentyfirst century, 2008, 417, 410

The advantages of natural compounds are fewer side effects in comparison to orthodox medical drugs and the production of synergistic effects for a more positive treatment outcome.

Kitazato et al.
Viral Infectious Disease and Natural Products with Antiviral Activity, 2007

Since birth, I have been, as most western peoples have, immersed in a twentieth-century, reductionist, and overly mechanical form of rationality and science. Being born in 1952, the scion of a powerful medical family which included a Surgeon General of the United States (Leroy Burney) and a President of the Kentucky Medical Association (David Cox), only exacerbated the condition. Indeed, physicians stretch back for more than two centuries in my family tree. Many of them were quite prominent; some contributed significantly to the development of modern medicine. It will then come as no surprise that from birth I was taught that plant medicines were simply a throwback to an earlier, more superstitious era of healing. I was told that they didn't work very well, that herbalism had, finally, been abandoned, overcome by the emergence of scientific medicine and healing. I was also taught that, because of pharmaceutical innovations, we were on the verge of a disease-free life for the first time in human history. As a later Surgeon General, William Stewart, put it when testifying to Congress, "It is time to close the book on infectious diseases" (Levy, 1992, 3). Unfortunately, the real world, as it often does, has had other plans.

My encounter with those "other plans" awakened me from my certitude, from the map of the world that a reductive medical science had instilled in me. It began, as these things often do, when I became seriously ill. The physicians I consulted could not diagnose what was wrong; nothing they suggested helped. So, I made a rather unorthodox decision. I abandoned technological medicine and began using a plant that grew near my home in the Colorado mountains. Within a few weeks the condition resolved and the picture of the world that I had been given began to crumble.

For the past 35 years I have been working intensively with herbal medicines. In the process I have learned that herbal medicines are not nearly so foolish and unscientific as I was taught they were. In fact, in nearly every country on earth research is overturning nineteenth- and twentieth-century biases about both plants and plant medicines. Plant medicines are, in actuality, not simply "raw drugs" but tremendously sophisticated interventives. They are especially good for treating resistant bacterial infections and what many researchers are now referring to as second generation bacteria, that is, stealth infections. These latter microorganisms include such things as the bacteria that cause Lyme disease (*Borrelia burgdorferi*) and others often associated with them such as babesial parasites. As Baud and Greub (2011) comment: "These emerging pathogens may represent the tip of the iceberg of a large number of as yet unknown intracellular pathogenic agents."

This section explores, to the limited extent possible in a single chapter, some of the sophistications of plant medicines and just why they exist. While I will share some of my personal experiences, most of the information I cite is taken from open-access, peer-reviewed journals and studies. To begin with, to grasp the sophistication of plant medicines, it is essential to understand just what bacteria and plants really are. They are not what the older, reductive paradigm has held them to be.

PARADIGM CONFLICTS

We live in a time when two fundamental perspectives about the nature of the reality matrix in which we are embedded are in conflict. One is the older, several-centuries-established, and somewhat reductive paradigm of seeing the world as a conglomeration of unrelated parts that can, by dissection, be understood and manipulated. Within this paradigm it is assumed that a human being can stand outside of the rest of nature and objectively study it. Nature is, in many respects, considered merely to be a static, unchanging background to the human world. In consequence, there is a widespread belief that we can tinker with that background as we will, that there will be no unexpected side effects if we do so.

In many respects we have, as a species, reached the limits of this paradigm. News reports of ecological instability are published daily. The rise of antibiotic resistant bacteria as a major worldwide problem is only one of the signs of that older paradigm's inaccuracy.

The second paradigm is quite different. Rather than being centered in the older Euclidian/ Newtonian/Cartesian (ENC) paradigm, this emerging paradigm is concerned with nonlinearity/ complexity/chaos theory and the related phenomenon of self-organization in biological systems. It is concerned with wholes rather than parts. Human beings are understood to be only one of many ecologically expressed life forms. They are, as are all life forms, inextricably embedded within that whole. Dissection of nature, while known to produce useful understandings, is recognized to be of limited value. Taking apart the watch to understand how it works, as any 8-year-old learns, doesn't mean that it can be put back together again.

This second paradigm is slowly supplanting that older paradigm as increasing numbers of negative environmental outcomes occur from the latter's use. Although much emphasis has been put on climate change, perhaps nothing has more significance to human beings than the rise of antibiotic resistant bacteria. Within the older ENC paradigm, considered foundational to both medicine and science, it is possible to create a pharmaceutical, apply it in practice, and sincerely believe that there will be no environmental repercussions from doing so. It is possible, as well, to believe that we can eliminate all disease. But the more accurate view, grounded in complexity theory and self-organization, reveals a much different picture of the world. Within that model it is obvious that bacteria would, of necessity, develop resistance to antibiotics, that their learning curve would be exponential not additive, and that, as David Livermore, one of Britain's primary bacterial resistance researchers puts it, "It is naive to think we can win" (Bosley, 2010).

I believe that deep explorations of both chaos theory and self-organization are crucial to really understand both microbial pathogens and the sophistication of plant medicines. Regrettably, a deep look is beyond the scope of this chapter. This touch on the subject is, of necessity, a light one.

SELF-ORGANIZATION

Nothing has undermined the older, more mechanical view of the world than spontaneous self-organization and nonlinearity in living systems. As mathematician Steven Strogatz (2003) comments ...

> In every case, these feats of synchrony occur spontaneously, almost as if nature has an eerie yearning for order. And that raises a profound mystery: Scientists have long been baffled by the existence of spontaneous order in the universe. The laws of thermodynamics seem to dictate the opposite, that nature should inexorably degenerate toward a state of greater disorder, greater entropy. Yet all around us we see magnificent structures that have somehow managed to assemble themselves. This enigma bedevils all of science today. Only in a few situations do we have a clear understanding of how order arises on its own.

Such synchrony always begins the same way. As researcher Scott Camazine (2001, 19) puts it, "At a critical density a pattern arises within the system." Thus, when a container is packed with increasing numbers of molecules, at a certain point, *which can never be predicted*, the random motions of the billions and billions of molecules will suddenly show an alteration in behavior. They will spontaneously synchronize, begin to act in concert, active cooperating, become tightly coupled together into one, interacting whole. The whole which comes into being at that moment of synchrony exhibits a collective, macroscopically ordered state of being. A unique more-than-the-sum-of-the-parts organism emerges of which the smaller subunits (the molecules) are now only a part. The molecules have *self-organized*. And ... it just happens. Like water turning to ice. From a simple decrease of 1° of temperature a phase change occurs. Something new comes into being.

And that new thing? Neither its physical nor its behavioral nature can be predicted from a study of its parts—an analysis of the prior state. As Camazine et al. (2001, 11) comment

> Complexity and complex systems generally refer to a system of interacting units that displays global properties not present at the lower level. These systems may show diverse responses that are often sensitively dependent on both the initial state of the system and nonlinear interactions among its components. Since these nonlinear interactions involve amplification or cooperativity, complex behaviors may emerge.

There is no linear, additive process that can be reductively analyzed and understood to have generated the total system that emerges at the moment of self-organization. Nor is the emerging system predictable in its shape or subsequent behavior. As physicist Paul Davies (1989) comments, nonlinear systems "possess the remarkable ability to leap spontaneously from relatively featureless states to those involving complex cooperative behavior." Or as Michael Crichton (1997) once put it ...

> It did not take long before the scientists began to notice that complex systems showed certain common behaviors. They started to think of these behaviors as characteristic of all complex systems. They realized that these behaviors could not be explained by analyzing the components of the systems. The time-honored scientific approach of reductionism—taking the watch apart to see how it worked—didn't get you anywhere with complex systems, because the interesting behavior seemed to arise from the spontaneous interaction of the components.

The emergent system, at the moment of self-organization, begins to *act*—to have behaviors. And just as a study of the parts of a self-organized whole cannot give a predictive idea of the larger whole's physical expression, so too the study of the smaller parts' behaviors cannot give an idea of the larger system's behavior. As Camazine et al. (2001, 8, 31), note, "an emergent property cannot be understood simply by examining in isolation the properties of the system's components. ... Emergence refers to a process by which a system of interacting subunits acquires qualitatively new properties that cannot be understood as a simple addition of their individual contributions." Or as systems researcher Yaneer Bar-Yam (1997) puts it, "A complex system is formed out of many components whose behavior is emergent, that is, the behavior of the system cannot be simply inferred from the behavior of its components. ... Emergent properties cannot be studied by physically taking a system apart and looking at the parts (reductionism)."

At the moment of self-organization, a *threshold* was crossed. On one side there was nothing but randomized molecular movements, on the other there is sudden self-organization and emergent behavior. All self-organized systems remain very close to this threshold, just barely on the self-organized side of the line. It is this dynamic balance point, near the edge of chaos, that makes the system so responsive to the interoceptive and exteroceptive inputs. It allows incredible innovations to occur in self-organized systems.

Michael Crichton (1997) described it impeccably...

> Even more important is the way complex systems seem to strike a balance between the need for order and the imperative for change. Complex systems tend to locate themselves at a place we call "the edge of chaos." We imagine the edge of chaos as a place where there is enough innovation to keep a living system vibrant, and enough stability to keep it from collapsing into anarchy. It is a zone of conflict and upheaval, where the old and new are constantly at war. Finding the balance point must be a delicate matter—if a living system drifts too close, it risks falling over into incoherence and dissolution; but if the system moves too far away from the edge, it becomes rigid, frozen, totalitarian. Both conditions lead to extinction ... Only at the edge of chaos can complex systems flourish.

At the moment of self-organization, the new living system enters a state of dynamic equilibrium. From that point on, the self-organized system retains an elegant sensitivity to that threshold point. It constantly monitors all inputs that touch it, for every input can potentially alter the self-organized state. The system then analyzes the nature of the input and crafts a response that will maintain self-organization. A very simple example of this is juggling.

First there are balls there, juggler here. But once juggling begins something more than the sum of the parts comes into being. The juggler and the balls become one tightly coupled unit. In that moment the juggler becomes highly sensitized to every tiny perturbation of the balance point. Much more quickly than linear thinking can accomplish, some deeper part of the juggler analyzes minute alterations in ball arcs, and crafts a response that keeps the balance point intact.

Every living system, phenomenon, and organism is like this. *Every* one of them exists close to the moment the balance point is found and every one works, at much greater degrees of complexity than juggling, to maintain the balance point. This is done through a tight coupling to both the internal and external worlds.

In self-organized systems, the information from the smaller subunit (in this example, the movement of the balls in space and time) travels to the larger whole. The larger system, what you might call the juggler/ball hybrid, remains highly sensitive to the balance point. It takes in information, analyzes it, and alters the juggler's behavior. In other words, the system alters its nature to incorporate the balls' movement changes (interoceptive inputs) so that it can keep its self-organizational state intact.

Information from the external world (exteroceptive inputs) is taken in similarly. Floor perturbations which alter how the feet are balanced, the flow of air in the room, comments from the audience, and so on, all affect his stance, orientation, and balance which, in their turn, affect his capacity to keep his balls in the air. So that exterior-to-the-system information is taken in and, again, below the level of conscious awareness, behavior is altered to keep self-organization—the homeodynamic balance—intact. This dynamic is ubiquitous in living systems. As James Lovelock (2003) comments, "No one doubts that humans are in thermostasis, yet our core temperatures range from 35 to 40°C and our extremities from 5 to 45°C". This may appear imprecise, but it serves us well.

All living organisms remain extremely sensitive to the environment in which they are embedded. They all engage in highly sophisticated analysis of inputs. Every one of them, when sensing an input that can affect homeodynamic balance, generates a suite of responses and from those responses they *choose* a course of action.

By any useful definition of the term, this *is* intelligent behavior. As *Merriam-Webster Dictionary* defines it: Intelligence is "the ability to learn or understand or to deal with new or trying situations [or] the ability to apply knowledge to manipulate one's environment."

One of the major problems with the older ENC model of the world is that it routinely defines *real* intelligence as something that humans alone possess. All other organisms are considered to be, in a pyramidal descending order, less intelligent. In many respects, most of the problems we are now facing as a species are being generated out of that inaccurate view of the world. Kevin Warwick (2001), a cyberneticist, observes succinctly that, "Comparisons (in intelligence) are usually made between characteristics that humans consider important; such a stance is of course biased and subjective in terms of the groups for whom it is being used."

I realize that to state that all self-organized systems are intelligent is problematical. To then assert that some are much more intelligent than human beings is to directly confront one of the most deeply held beliefs that we humans, and most scientists and physicians, possess. In and of itself, that will put many people off the content of this chapter. Nevertheless, it is root to the more holistic view of the world that is now emerging. It is also something that bacterial researchers have been saying for some time.

BACTERIAL INTELLIGENCE

Antibiotic resistant bacteria are now one of the (human) world's most serious emerging problems. Although most people have seen news reports about it one time or another, few realize that most if not all the world's bacterial researchers now assert that within our lifetimes antibiotics will become increasingly useless. Within the next few decades, we face, as many microbiologists have pointed out, the emergence of untreatable epidemic diseases deadlier than any known in history. The problem is that too many antibiotics in too large quantities have been expressed into the world's ecosystems.

In an extremely short period of geologic time, the Earth has been saturated with several *billion* pounds of non-biodegradable, often biologically unique pharmaceuticals designed to kill bacteria. Many antibiotics do not discriminate in their activity, but kill broad groups of diverse bacteria whenever they are used. The worldwide environmental dumping, over the past 65 years, of such huge quantities of synthetic antibiotics has initiated the most pervasive impacts on the Earth's bacterial underpinnings since oxygen-generating bacteria supplanted methanogens 2.5 billion years ago. As bacterial researcher Stuart Levy (1992, 75) comments, "It has stimulated evolutionary changes that are unparalleled in recorded biologic history."

What are these evolutionary changes? At the simplest level, it has stimulated the development of exceptionally sophisticated resistance mechanisms in *all* the planet's bacterial populations. Bacteria have literally begun rearranging their genomes. As those genomes shift, bacterial physiology and behavior alters, sometimes considerably. This kind of response is inevitable in any self-organized system. As Francisco Varela et al. (1989) observe, a self-organized biological network

> will reconfigure itself to an unspecified environment in such a way that it both maintains its ongoing dynamics and displays a behaviour that reveals a degree of inductive learning about environmental regularities.

As soon as bacteria encounter an antibiotic that can affect them, however minutely, they generate possible solutions. The variety and number of solutions they generate are immense, from inactivating the part of the bacterial cell that the antibiotic is designed to destroy, to pumping the antibiotic out of their cells just as fast as it comes in, to altering the nature of their cellular wall to make them more impervious. Some even go so far as learning to use the antibiotic for food.

The old-style, neo-Darwinian explanation for bacterial resistance is that when a person takes an antibiotic all the *susceptible* bacteria are killed off but ... there are always a few that are naturally resistant to the antibiotic. These survive to spread and thus resistance emerges. Occasionally you will also see statements that spontaneous mutations are arising that are naturally resistant to antibiotics; these mutated bacteria survive, have offspring, and thus spread. While there is some truth to that, a deeper look reveals a much different picture. Bacteria literally *remake* their genomes to alter their physical form. They then pass this innovation on to other bacteria as well as their own offspring.

Antibiotics entered general use in 1946. By 1953, after penicillin use was widespread, 6480% of the bacteria had become resistant; resistance to tetracycline and erythromycin was also being reported. By 1960, resistant staph had become the most common source of hospital-acquired infections worldwide. (By 1995 an incredible 95% of staph was resistant to penicillin.) In response to the 1960 outbreaks, physicians began using methicillin, a B-lactam antibiotic. Nevertheless, methicillin resistant staph (MRSA) emerged within a year. In 1968, the first severe MRSA outbreak in hospitals occurred in the United States. Inevitably, MRSA strains resistant to all clinically available antibiotics (except the glycopeptides vancomycin and teicoplanin) emerged. In 1999, 54 years after the commercial production of antibiotics, the first staph strain resistant to all clinical antibiotics had infected its first three people.

Bacteria are the oldest forms of life on this planet and they have developed great sophistication in responding to threats to their well-being. Among those threats are the thousands if not millions of antibacterial substances that have existed as long as life itself. The world is, in fact, filled with antibacterial substances, most produced by other bacteria, fungi, and plants. Bacteria learned how to respond to such substances a very long time ago. Or as Steven Projan (2008, 413) of Wyeth Research puts it, bacteria "are the oldest of living organisms and thus have been subject to three billion years of evolution in harsh environments and therefore have been selected to withstand chemical assault." Most of our antibiotics are actually just slight alterations of antibacterial substances already common in the world—substances that bacteria have long been aware of and are highly responsive to.

Bacteria share resistance information with other bacteria in many ways. They can do so directly, or simply extrude DNA containing the information from their cells, allowing it to be picked up later by roving bacteria. They often experiment, combining resistance information from multiple sources in unique ways that increase resistance, generate new resistance pathways, or even stimulate resistance forms that are not yet necessary. Even bacteria in hibernating or moribund states will share whatever information on resistance they have with any bacteria that encounter them. As bacteria gain resistance, they pass that knowledge on to *all* forms of bacteria they meet. They are not competing for resources, as standard evolutionary theory predicted, but rather, promiscuously cooperating in the sharing of survival information. "More surprising," one research group commented (Salyers, 2008), "is the apparent movement of genes, such as *tetQ* and *ermB* between members of the normal microflora of humans and animals, populations of bacteria that differ in species composition."

Irritatingly, bacteria appear to be generating resistance to antibiotics we haven't even thought of yet. For example, after placing a single bacterial species in a nutrient solution containing sub-lethal doses of a newly developed and rare antibiotic, researchers found that within a short period of time the bacteria developed resistance to that antibiotic *and* to 12 other antibiotics that they had never before encountered—some of which were structurally dissimilar to the first. Bacterial researcher Stuart Levy (1992, 101) observes, "It's almost as if bacteria strategically anticipate the confrontation of other drugs when they resist one."

In fact, they are acting in concert so well in response to the human "war on disease" that it has led Levy (1992, 87) to remark, "One begins to see bacteria, not as individual species, but as a vast array of interacting constituents of an integrated microbial world." Former FDA commissioner Donald Kennedy (Frappaolo 1986) echoes this when he states, "The evidence indicates that enteric microorganisms in animals and man, their R plasmids, and human pathogens form a linked eco-system of their own in which action at any one point can affect every other." Or as Lynn Margulis (and Dorian Sagan, 1997) once put it, "Bacteria are not really individuals so much as part of a single global superorganism."

Bacteria are, in fact, responding socially, as a community. As science writer Valerie Brown (2010) notes: "In a series of recent findings, researchers describe bacteria that communicate in sophisticated ways, take concerted action, influence human physiology, alter human thinking and work together to bioengineer the environment."

Bacteria are considered, by those who have deeply studied them, not only to be intelligent but also to possess a sophisticated language and a highly developed social capacity. They are, in fact, not all that different than us. As bacterial researchers Eshel Ben-Jacob et al. (2004) put it

> Bacteria use their intracellular flexibility, involving signal transduction networks and genomic plastic-ity, to collectively maintain linguistic communication; self and shared interpretations of chemical cues, exchange of chemical message (semantic) and dialogues (pragmatic). Meaning-based communication permits colonial identity, intentional behavior (e.g., pheromone-based courtship for mating), purposeful alteration of colony structure (e.g., formation of fruiting bodies), detection-making (e.g., to sporulate) and the recognition and identification of other colonies—features we might begin to associate with a bacterial social intelligence.

Colonies of bacteria, as Ben-Jacob (2003) observes, "have developed intricate communication capa-bilities, including a broad repertoire of chemical signaling mechanisms, collective activation and deactivation of genes, and even exchange of genetic materials. With these tools they can commu-nicate and self-organize their colonies into multicellular hierarchal aggregates, out of which new abilities emerge."

Each bacterium, as he goes on to say, "has internal degrees of freedom, informatic capabilities, and freedom to respond by altering itself and others via emission of signals in a self-regulated man-ner." In a later paper (Ben-Jacob 2006), he expands this considerably by noting that "each bacterium is, by itself, a biotic autonomous system with its own cellular informatics capabilities (storage, processing and assessment of information). These afford the cell plasticity to *select* its response to biochemical messages it receives, including self-alteration and the broadcasting of messages to initi-ate alterations in other bacteria."

Bacterial researcher James Shapiro (2007), at the University of Chicago, is particularly plain-spoken about how badly we have misunderstood bacteria.

> Forty years' experience as a bacterial geneticist have taught me that bacteria possess many cogni-tive, computational and evolutionary capabilities unimaginable in the first six decades of the twentieth century. Analysis of cellular processes such as metabolism, regulation of protein synthesis, and DNA repair established that bacteria continually monitor their external and internal environments and com-pute functional outputs based on information provided by their sensory apparatus.... My own work on transposable elements revealed multiple widespread bacterial systems for mobilizing and engineer-ing DNA molecules. Examination of colony development and organization led me to appreciate how extensive multicellular collaboration is among the majority of bacterial species. [Studies] show that bacteria utilize sophisticated mechanisms for intercellular communication and even have the ability to commandeer the basic cell biology of "higher" plants and animals to meet their own basic needs. This remarkable series of observations requires us to revise basic ideas about biological information process-ing and recognize that even the smallest cells are sentient beings.

Shapiro concludes his 23-page paper with this remarkable statement:

> The take-home lesson of more than half a century of molecular microbiology is to recognize that bacterial information processing is far more powerful than human technology. ... These small cells are incredibly sophisticated at coordinating processes involving millions of individual events and at making them precise and reliable. In addition, the astonishing versatility and mastery bacteria display in managing the biosphere's geochemical and thermodynamic transformations indicates that we have a great deal to learn about chemistry, physics, and evolution from our small, but very intelligent, prokaryotic relatives.

Bacteria, in fact, show just the same sorts of complex and sophisticated behaviors that humans do, from language, to sentience, to intelligence, to the creation of cities (i.e., biofilms), to cooperation in groups, to complex adaptation to their environment, to protection of offspring, to species memory handed down through the generations. And, if the definition of tool is extended, as it should be, to the creation of chemicals that are designed to produce specific alterations in their environment—or even the sophisticated, insulated, electrical cables that some bacterial communities use to heat their cities—their capacities include intelligent tool making.

That they don't have an organ, a brain, like the one in our heads, has misled us tremendously. As the molecular biologist Anthony Trewavas (2006, 6) comments ...

> Very early on, analogies were drawn between the connections that [bacterial] phosphorylation enables between bacterial proteins and the connections between neurone dendrites in higher animal brains. This led to their description as a phosphoneural network. The properties of these networks include signal amplification, associative responses (cross talk) and memory effects. Subsequent investigation indicated learning and the realization that these simple networks provide individual bacteria with informed decisions.

And as neuroscientist Peggy La Cerra (2003) relates:

> The hallmark of animalian intelligence systems is the capacity to predict likely costs and benefits of alternative paths of behavior. This logic is evident in our most ancient ancestors, bacteria. [As an example] E. Coli is a single-cell organism with a single molecule of DNA. This simplest of animals exhibits a prototypical centralized intelligence system that has the same essential design characteristics and problem solving logic as is evident in all animal intelligence systems including humans.

Neural networks are generated any time a biological self-organization event occurs. And "the computational capabilities" that we recognize as integral to intelligence, as Chakrabarti and Dutta (2002) note, naturally "emerge out of the collective dynamics of the network, which is nonlinear." From that comes, as Trewavas (2006, 8) observes, "Information processing, learning, memory, decision making, choice, predictive modeling, associating memory, sensory integration and control of behavior." These are, as he notes, "all aspects of biological intelligence."

Though the rise of bacterial resistance has begun to stimulate a moderately wide recognition among scientists that microbial intelligence exists—a recognition very much lacking among most physicians and the general populace—it is for the concept of plant intelligence that most scientists retain the greatest disdain.

PLANT INTELLIGENCE

The old paradigm about plants, which is very common and (unfortunately) still believed by most people, is that plants are "passive entities subject to environmental forces and organisms that are designed solely for accumulation of phososynthetic products." But as Baluska et al. (2006, 31) comment:

> The new view, by contrast, is that plants are dynamic and highly sensitive organisms, actively and competitively foraging for limited resources both above and below ground, and that they are also organisms

which accurately compute their circumstances, use sophisticated cost-benefit analysis, and that take defined actions to mitigate and control diffuse environmental insults. Moreover, plants are also capable of a refined recognition of self and non-self and this leads to territorial behavior. This new view considers plants as information-processing organisms with complex communication throughout the individual plant. Plants are as sophisticated in behavior as animals but their potential has been masked because it operates on time scales many orders of magnitude longer than that operation in animals. … Owing to this lifestyle, the only long-term response to rapidly changing environments is an equally rapid adaptation; therefore, plants have developed a very robust signaling and information-processing apparatus. … Besides abundant interactions with the environment, plants interact with other communicative systems such as other plants, fungi, nematodes, bacteria, viruses, insects, and predatory animals.

As with all self-organized systems, plants continually monitor their internal and external worlds for informational/functional shifts in the relevant fields. This includes such things as spatial orientation; presence, absence, and identity of neighbors; disturbance; competition; predation, whether microbial, insect, or animal; composition of atmosphere; composition of soil; water presence, location, and amount; degree of incoming light; propagation, protection, and support of offspring; communications from other plants in their ecorange; biological, including circadian, rhythms; and not only their own health but the health of the ecorange in which they live. As Anthony Trewavas (2006, 3) comments, this "continually and specifically changes the information spectrum" to which the plants are attending. Trewavas recognizes, as researchers in so many other fields are now doing, that the living organism, in this instance a plant, actually *chooses* the optimum response from a plethora of alternatives. As he says, potential "responses can be rejected; the numbers of different environments that any wild plant experiences must be almost infinite in number. Only complex computation can fashion the optimal fitness response."

Some plants, such as sundew, are so sensitive to touch, for example, that they can detect a strand of hair weighing less than 1 microgran (one millionth of a gram) to which they then respond. But what is more revealing is that they can determine with great specificity *what* is touching them. Raindrops, a common experience in the wild, produce no touch response. This kind of mechanosensitivity, which is, in plants, similar to our own, is used much as we use our own: The plants analyze what is touching them, determine its meaning, and craft a response. And that response can involve rapid changes in their genetics and subsequent physical form or phenotype. As McCormack et al. (2006) comment, "Plants perceive much more of their environment than is often apparent to the casual observer. Touch can induce profound rapid responses … in *Arabidopsis*, changes in gene expression can be seen within minutes after touch, and over 700 genes have altered transcript levels within 30 min."

Plants, in fact, possess a highly sophisticated neural system—as Charles Darwin noted long ago in his book, *The Power of Movement in Plants*. The "brain" of plants *is* their root system. More accurately, what we are talking about here is their neural network, not the place it is housed—an important distinction. Our neural network is housed in an organ, the brain, but it is the neural network housed in our brain that is important, not the organ that contains it. Plants don't need that organ; their neural network is housed in the soil in which they are rooted. As such there is no limit on the size of a plant's neural network as there is on our own. Some aspen root systems cover hundreds of acres and are many thousands of years old—their neural network dwarfs our own. Plants do have a "brain," and they always have. As Frantisek Baluska et al. (2004) comment…

Although plants are generally immobile and lack the most obvious brain activities of animals and humans, they are not only able to show all the attributes of intelligent behavior but they are also equipped with neuronal molecules, especially synaptotagmins and glutamate/glycine-gated glutamate receptors. Recent advances in plant cell biology allowed identification of plant synapses transporting the plant-specific neurotransmitter-like molecule auxin. This suggests that synaptic communication is not limited to animals and humans but seems widespread throughout plant tissues.

A specific part of the plant root, the root apex, that is, apices—the pointed ends of the root system—are a combination sensitive finger, perceiving sensory organ, and brain neuron. Each root hair, rootlet, and root section contains an apex; every root mass millions, even billions, of them. For example, a single rye plant has more than 13 million rootlets with a combined length of 680 miles. Each of the rootlets is covered with root hairs, over 14 *billion* of them, with a combined length of 6600 miles. Every rootlet, every root hair, has at its end a root apex. Every root apex acts as a neuronal organ in the root system. In contrast, the human brain has approximately 86 billion neurons, about 16 billion of which are in the cerebral cortex. Plants with larger root systems, and more root hairs, can have considerably more brain neurons than the 14 billion contained in rye plants; they can even rival the human brain in the number of neurons.

The numerous root apices act as one whole, synchronized, self-organized system, much as the neurons in our brains do. As Baluska et al. (2006, 28–9) comment: The root apices

> harbor brain-like units of the nervous system of plants. The number of root apices in the plant body is high, and all "brain units" are interconnected via vascular strands (plant neurons) with their polarly-transported auxin (plant neurotransmitter), to form a serial (parallel) neuronal system of plants. From observation of the plant body of maize, it is obvious that the number of root apices is extremely high ... This feature makes the "serial plant brain" extremely robust and the amount of processed information must be immense.

Plants remain extremely sensitive to environmental inputs. Plants analyze the inputs, then alter both form and behavior in response. As Trewavas (2003) observes ...

> Learning and memory are the two emergent (holistic) properties of neural networks that involve large numbers of neural cells acting in communication with one another. But, both properties originate from signal transduction processes in individual cells. Quite remarkably, the suite of molecules used in signal transduction are entirely similar between nerve cells and plant cells. ... Learning results from the formation of new dendrites, and memory lasts as long as the newly formed dendrites themselves. The neural network is phenotypically plastic and intelligent behavior requires that plastic potential. Plant development is plastic too and is not reversible; many mature plants can be reduced to a single bud and root and regenerate to a new plant with a different structure determined by the environmental circumstances.

In other words, if you take the cutting of a plant from one location and plant it in another, as the neural system of the new plant develops in the soil, analyzing its surroundings all the while, it alters, as it learns, the shape and formation of the plant body it develops. This, more effectively, fits it into the environment in which it is now growing. In short, plants possess a highly developed root brain which works much as ours does to analyze incoming data and generate sophisticated responses.

CHEMICAL INNOVATION IN PLANTS

To really understand why plant medicines are so effective in healing practice, it is crucial to understand that plants have been infected by pathogenic organisms for far longer than our species has been emergent on this planet. They can't run, they can't hide, they can't call the doctor. In consequence, they have become tremendously sophisticated at identifying the pathogenic organisms that attack them as well as the most effective responses to those attacks. They are the world's best chemists.

As an example, studies have continually found that when plants are being eaten by insect predators they release volatile compounds that will call the *exact* predator of that insect. As Ian Baldwin (2001) at the Max Planck Institute observes, "It's known that tobacco, corn, lima beans, tomatoes, cucumbers, oil seed rape—a whole bunch of different species—give off these signals when they're attacked by larvae [caterpillars]." As he continues, "Our study demonstrates that the volatile (airborne chemical) bouquet that is released after attack is very complex. Predators are attracted, and laying moths are repelled."

These volatiles are very specific in their chemical structure. They have to be in order to work, even a slight molecular rearrangement will make them ineffective. Plants, over hundreds of millions of years, have learned to create chemicals that perform very specific functions. Among these are the creation of a suite of complex compounds that are very specific for countering microbial infections. But they don't just create antibacterial substances to kill pathogenic microbes. They also create potent antiresistance compounds as well as synergists that make these other compounds more effective. Plants have never used the "silver bullet" approach in the treatment of their infections, presumably because, over time, it doesn't work.

Reductive approaches have, however, applied that "silver bullet" paradigm to the natural world. In consequence, a major thrust of twentieth-century research into plant medicines has been to identify what plant compounds produced the "active" effects. Pharmaceutical companies sponsored much of this research—they wanted to identify useful compounds from which to generate new drugs, including antimicrobials. One of the more famous findings, generated out of a desire to counter resistance in malarial organisms, is the compound artemisinin, found in *Artemisia annua*. Relatively recently, artemisinin was isolated, then semi-synthetic analogs were created and widely used to treat both resistant and nonresistant malarial infections. Unsurprisingly, within a short period of time, the malarial parasite began to develop resistance to these compounds, just as they have done with pharmaceuticals. The semisynthetic analogs were patentable, which artemisinin was not, but the molecular alterations also increased the bioavailability of the isolated compound. Artemisinin, by itself, is not all that bioavailable. But something quite different occurs when the whole plant is ingested, when the artemisinin is taken along with the other compounds in the plant.

Plants utilize a multicomponent approach to disease treatment rather than monotherapy and there are good reasons for this. When their antimicrobial compounds are examined *in situ,* more subtle elements of their response to infections begin to emerge. A crucial aspect of this is the importance of *context*—none of these constituents were developed by the plants in isolation. They were generated while the plant was immersed in an ecological scenario to which it was interactively responding. The "active" constituent is, *in reality,* the expression of a complicated chemical communication in which *none* of the other plant compounds are irrelevant. Unsurprisingly, artemisinin is more active (and more bioavailable) against malarial parasites if administered with the *Artemisia* flavonoids artemetin and casticin which are normally present in the plant.

Artemetin is a fairly strong anti-inflammatory, is hypotensive, modulates mitochondrial function, is antineoplastic, and is protective of endothelial function—primarily through antioxidant and antiapoptic actions. It, like casticin, appears to modulate apoptosis, protecting healthy cells from apoptosis and while stimulating apoptosis in damaged cells (such as cancer cells). Casticin is an immunomodulator (reducing a variety of overactive white blood cell responses), suppresses many cytokines (e.g., IL-1beta, IL-6, MCP-1), inhibits prolactin release (making it useful for treating hyperprolactinemia), is strongly anti-inflammatory, and is antineoplastic.

Neither of these compounds possess direct antiplasmodial actions. Comparatively little research, compared to artemisinin, has been conducted on the medicinal activity of flavonoids such as artemetin and casticin. As Ferreira, et al. comment (2010), "Based on what is currently known, or strictly based on the chemical structure of flavonoids, it is quite hard to predict the full spectrum of their biological activity." Speculation is that these flavonoids might, among other things, facilitate artemisinin interaction with heme, leading to the release of the artemisinin peroxide that generates its antimalarial effects. Still, no one knows for sure. As well, flavonoids chelate metals such as iron and copper as part of their antioxidant actions. Thus, these flavonoids might be producing their synergistic effects by reacting with iron and converting Fe $(+3)$ to Fe $(+2)$. Fe $(+2)$ is crucial to the bioactivity of artemisinin as it stimulates the release of (short-lived) toxic free radicals that produce some of the antimalarial actions of artemisinin. Further, these kinds of flavonoids strongly inhibit serine-threonine kinases. There is evidence that they might also inhibit *Plasmodium* kinases, in consequence hindering protozoal development and proliferation. But again, no one really knows why they are so synergistic with artemisinin.

There are other metabolically active flavonoids in *Artemisia annua* such as quercetin, chrysoplenetin, and chrysosplenol-D. These also have synergistic effects against plasmodial parasites. Quercetin has weak antiplasmodial activity but its stronger effects seem to occur from other actions. For example, it inhibits mammalian thioredoxin reductase release, an enzyme that is essential for the survival of the erythrocytic stage of *P. falciparum*. Chrysosplenol-D and chrysoplenetin are also weakly active against the malarial parasite but are highly synergistic with artemisinin *in situ*, significantly potentiating its effects. In mammals, these two compounds act as P-glycoprotein inhibitors. This facilitates the movement of artemisinin through the intestinal membrane and into the blood making it more bioavailable. The compounds act similarly within the plant body, facilitating the dispersal of artemisinin throughout the plant. They are also, like other flavonoids, anti-inflammatories. Additionally, these compounds exert a suppressive effect on the multidrug resistance pump common in *P. falciparum*.

And there are still more flavonoids, such as apigenin, lutiolin, and kaempferol, that themselves exert synergistic effects. In other words, there is a suite of "active" compounds in the plant which all work together to produce antimalarial effects. There is no one "active" constituent.

Interestingly, malaria infection itself potentiates the pharmacokinetics of artemisinin in the body. Plasma concentrations are *higher* when someone is infected and lower when they are not. Further, ingesting the properly prepared tea (made from the whole, flowering plant) results in a much faster absorption of artemisinin than taking the pure compound orally. As well, mice infected with a lethal dose of *P. falciparum* were found to survive only 5 days when treated with pure artemisinin but for 11 days when given the properly prepared tea.

The Chinese have used *Artemisia annua* for several thousand years and are very clear about proper preparation of the plant. While simple teas are sometimes used, the strongest preparations are made through two similar approaches. Both use the upper two-thirds of the plant in flower. (The flowering plant is much higher in both artemisinin and the flavonoids.) In essence, the fresh flowering plant is harvested, *soaked* in hot water for 4–12 hours (in a covered container), then the herb is wrung out (like a dishcloth), then pounded to express the plant juices. Alternatively, instead of hot water, hot milk is used. Milk (with its fats), if available, will extract 80% of the artemisinin from the plant, water extractions run from 25% with the dried herb to 60% in the fresh plant. (The plant is never boiled in the water as that significantly reduces the amount of artemisinin that is extracted.) Pounding will bring out approximately 20 times more artemisinin than soaking the dried plant and four times more than soaking the fresh plant. Pounded infusions produce between 18 and 27 mg/kg of artemisinin and suppress parasitemia 2.6 times better than pure artemisinin dosed at 30 mg/kg.

Examination of the "active" constituents in other plants also show this kind of sophisticated complex of synergistically acting compounds. For example, berberine, a strong plant antibacterial, is very active against many resistant and nonresistant bacterial organisms. It is considerably more active, however, if administered with another constituent, 5′-methoxyhydnocarpin (5′-MHC), which is common in goldenseal and other berberine-containing plants. This constituent, 5′-MHC, is a potent efflux pump inhibitor. It reduces or eliminates the ability of resistant *Staphylococcus* bacteria to eject, from inside their cellular membranes, antibiotic substances that might harm them.

In response to the bacterial generation of resistance to berberine (millennia ago), the plants created a new chemical, 5′-MHC, which has no known function other than to act as an efflux inhibitor, enabling the berberine to remain effective. If goldenseal were standardized for berberine content (which some people insist is important) and if, for some reason, the plant being standardized contained no 5′-MHC, its effectiveness as an antimicrobial would be significantly diminished. Yet 5′-MHC is not considered important enough as a standardization marker since it is not an "active" constituent.

Such complexities are hardly limited to the berberine plants. The anticonvulsant actions of the kava lactones in *Piper methysticum* (i.e., yangonin and desmethoxyyangonin) are much stronger when used in combination with other kava constituents that are generally considered irrelevant in any standardization missives. As well, concentrations of yangonin and another lactone, kavain, are much higher in the brain when the *whole plant* extract is used instead of the purified lactones themselves. In other words, some of the other constituents in kava help move the bioactive lactones across the blood/brain barrier and into the brain where they will do the most good. Blood plasma concentrations of kavain are reduced by 50% if the purified compound is used rather than an extract of the plant itself.

Plant compounds in *Isatis tinctoria*, a potent antiviral and anti-inflammatory herb are also highly synergistic. Tryptanthrin, a strong anti-inflammatory in the plant, possesses very poor skin penetration capacity. However, when the whole plant extract is applied to the skin, penetration of tryptanthrin is significantly enhanced. In other words, applying a salve of pure tryptanthrin to the skin, despite its anti-inflammatory nature, won't do you much good. But if you make the plant itself into a salve, the tryptanthrin moves rapidly into the skin and helps reduce skin inflammation. Tryptanthrin is, unfortunately, the only compound that is considered important to standardize in the plant.

Some additional sophistications can occur for those who wish to go even deeper. Among them are the *synergy* that occurs among the healing agents that are used. The use of healing agents (pharmaceuticals *or* herbs) always involves synergy between the agents used—though this is rarely addressed in a positive light. It's usually the side effects of drug combination or drug/herb combination that are highlighted. However, herbs *are* synergistic with each other and can be positively synergistic with pharmaceuticals as well. For example, Chinese skullcap root (*Scutellaria baicalensis*) and licorice (*Glycyrrhiza spp*) are synergists; they enhance the action of other herbs with which they are combined. Many herbs can, as well, enhance the action of pharmaceuticals. For example, Japanese knotweed (*Polygonum cuspidatum*) root, when used along with formerly ineffective antibiotics, can enhance the drugs' actions enough to make them effective.

Plants are complex, nonlinear, self-organized living systems. Neither they, nor their constituent elements, can be viewed, or understood, in isolation. This is because at the moment of self-organization complexities that can't be found by the reductive mind come into play. In other words, a complex synergy of interactions comes into play and it has nothing to do with "active" constituents. Every part is "active," every part is essential.

RESISTANCE TO PLANTS?

A common question is whether bacteria will develop resistance to antibacterial plants. The answer is that they already have ... multiple times over millennia. The important thing to keep in mind is that plants are living medicines. The plant we harvest this year is not the same as that from last year. Their constituent makeup is constantly in flux. If a pathogen develops a new resistance mechanism the plant will, quite rapidly, develop a response. This is another reason why standardization of plant medicines is a fool's errand. It places a static frame of reference on something that is never static. Evolution is an ongoing process. Plants move nearly in unison with resistance dynamics in bacteria—they continually develop new chemicals with which to counter them. As the comparative zoologist Richard Lewontin (2000) puts it, "The characteristic of a living object is that it reacts to external stimuli rather than being passively propelled by them. An organism's life consists of constant mid-course corrections." And plants are extremely sensitive to even the slightest alteration in the information spectrum they take in. Generation of new chemical responses occur extremely rapidly.

Chemical innovations flow into and out of the plant over time in response to environmental inputs. There is no such thing as a "standard" chemical profile of a plant medicine, a truth that is difficult for reductive medicalists. Every plant's chemical profile is different from season to season and from location to location. It's supposed to be that way. Evolution has not ended. The diseases we encounter are altering themselves all the time. They possess tremendous genetic flexibility. But, fortunately for us, so do the plants. They alter their genome and their chemical relationships right along with the bacteria. The alterations in plant chemical profiles are essential for them to remain functional medicines. As bacterial dynamics shift, the plants, *worldwide*, shift their chemical production and constituent spectrum in response.

STEALTH PATHOGENS

Plant medicines are exceptionally good for healing resistant infections. They are also very good at dealing with what is coming to be known as stealth infections such as the spirochete that causes Lyme disease. Stealth pathogens are very different than the bacteria (first-generation pathogens) for which antibiotics were created in the latter half of the twentieth century (such as *Staphylococcus*). At present, the major members of the Lyme group of infectious microorganisms are *Anaplasma, Babesia, Bartonella, Borrelia, Chlamydia, Ehrlichia*, and *Mycoplasma*. Rocky Mountain Spotted Fever and the other *Rickettsia* are a growing presence as are many *Wolbachia* organisms. At least 20 others, which are much less well known and generally, at this point, significantly less common, are beginning to be recognized as growing threats. Coinfection can occur with any of them.

The past several decades have seen a shift in the way many researchers are approaching disease treatment, nowhere more so than with these kinds of stealth pathogens that, due to their nature, often cause a wide range of symptoms. Researchers Ian Clark et al. (2004), for example, have done some marvelous work on the dynamics of cytokines specific to various disease conditions, especially malaria and its close relative babesia. They note …

> It is our view that focusing on malaria in isolation will never provide the insights required to understand the pathogenesis of this disease. How can the illnesses caused by a spirochete and a virus be so clinically identical: typhoid readily diagnosed as malaria and malaria in returning travelers so commonly dismissed as influenza? … Understanding why these clinical confusions occur entails appreciating the sequence of events that led up to the cytokine revolution that has transformed the field over the last 15 years.

Cytokines are small cell-signaling molecules released by cells that are damaged, cells of the immune system, and the glial cells of the nervous system. They are important in intercellular communications in the body. As it turns out, many disease organisms have learned to use cytokines for their own purposes.

In practical terms: when bacteria touches a cell, the cell gives off a signal, a cytokine, that tells the immune system what is happening and what that cell needs. This stimulates the innate immune system to respond; it sends specific immune cells to that location to deal with the problem. Those cells then initiate their own cytokine response to deal with the infection. Stealth pathogens subvert this process, enabling their successful infection of the body. As well, many stealth pathogens release, all on their own, many different types of cytokines, simply to jump start the process.

These kinds of microorganisms, once they enter the body, release an initial, and very powerful, cytokine—for example, tumor necrosis factor, aka TNF. That cytokine stimulates the infected cell to produce and release others, and those generate still others—all of which have potent impacts on the body. Thus, a *cascade* of cytokines occurs. This cascade (and any subsequent immune response) is carefully modulated by the pathogen to produce the exact effects it needs to facilitate its spread in the body. It modulates the cytokine dynamic in the body as expertly as an accomplished violinist plays a composition by Mozart. The microorganism uses the cytokines for a variety of purposes: to allow its entry into protected niches in the body (such as the brain), to facilitate its sequestration inside our body's cells (thus hiding it from the immune system), to break apart particular cells in order to get nutrients, and to shut down the parts of our immune response that can effectively deal with the infection. It is this cascade of carefully modulated cytokines that, in fact, create most of the symptoms that people experience when they become ill from a stealth infection. Even tiny alterations in the existing cytokine profiles inside our bodies can cause significant shifts in disease symptoms. Clark et al. (2004) comment, "In one IL-2 [interleukin-2] study, 15 of 44 patients developed behavioral changes sufficiently severe to warrant acute intervention and 22 had severe cognitive defects."

Many researchers are now insisting that the most important thing is not the microbial source of infection but rather the cytokine cascade that is generated. This is especially true during coinfections with multiple stealth pathogens. One of the better articles on this is Andrea Graham et al. "Transmission consequences of coinfection: cytokines writ large" that appeared in *Trends in Parasitology*, volume 23, number 6, in 2007. They comment, "When the taxonomic identities of parasites are replaced with their cytokine signatures, for example, it becomes possible to predict the within-host consequences of coinfection for microparasite replication" as well as symptom picture, treatment approaches, and treatment outcomes. As they also note, "The influence of cytokines on effector responses is so powerful that many parasites manipulate host-cytokine pathways for their own benefit," as is indeed the case with Lyme, the *Chlamydiae*, and Rocky Mountain Spotted Fever. Crucially, they continue, "the magnitude and type of cytokine response influence host susceptibility and infectiousness. Susceptibility to a given parasite will be affected by cytokine responses that are ongoing at the time of exposure, including responses to pre-existing infections." In other words, the bacteria can utilize inflammatory processes that are already occurring in the body (e.g., pre-existing arthritis) to facilitate successful infection.

BORRELIAL INFECTIONS

To give you an idea of how sophisticated this can be, here is a very brief look at a portion of the cytokine process that Lyme bacteria utilize during infection.

Borrelia bacteria are particularly fond of collagenous structures in the body. They, in fact, need to break these structures down into constituent elements to gain the nutrients they need to survive and reproduce. Thus, they are very sophisticated at modulating the body's cytokine responses to do so. Wherever the breakdown occurs is where symptoms emerge. If in the joints, arthritis. If in the heart, cardiac problems. If in the brain, neurological symptoms.

Borrelia utilize specific cytokine sequences to accomplish the breakdown. Commonly, they stimulate ERK, JNK, p38, and NF-kB in sort of that order. Once the bacteria attach themselves to the body's cells, the bacterial flagellin upregulates NF-kB. This is generally followed by the upregulation of interferon-alpha (IFN-α), Interleukin-10 (IL-10), IL-8, IL-1B, IL-6, tumor necrosis factor alpha (TNF-α), and metalloproteinases (MMPs). Again, sort of in that order. (Levels of these cytokines increase a minimum of 10 times as soon as the body's cells are exposed to *Borrelia*.)

However, the bacteria always utilize multiple, redundant processes to generate this cytokine cascade. The listed, linear, order-of-emergence outlined above does occur. So, too, does simultaneous emergence; so, too, does emergence in a different order (MMPs right after IL-8, for example). They utilize multiple, redundant processes to facilitate infection and circumvent the immune response. They are very good at what they do.

Other, more specialized cytokines emerge as the cascade continues. Still, these are the primary upstream cytokines that a Lyme infection stimulates. Interrupting their emergence, inhibiting them, is one of the most effective strategies for treating an infection, especially in people for whom antibiotics have not worked. This can turn the condition around, generally within a few months, sometimes within weeks. Herbal medicines are specific for modulating cytokine cascades—plants, when infected, experience them, just as we do.

I have done depth work on each of these cytokines and the plant medicines that can interrupt their emergence in many of my books—again, much too long for this chapter. Here is a brief look at only one of them, the matrixmetalloproteinases.

Matrixmetalloproteinases (MMPs) are, more accurately, metal dependent proteases (hence the "-metallo-"). They are a group of enzymes that are specific for degrading extracellular matrix (ECM) components and collagen. (Because of their action on the ECM, elevated MMPs facilitate the penetration of the spirochetes through extracellular matrix component barriers more deeply into the body.) MMPs are sometimes referred to as collagenases, in other words, enzymes that degrade collagen. They are also involved in many other functions, including cell proliferation, migration, adhesion, and differentiation. They help angiogenesis (new blood vessel formation) by breaking apart the ECM which allows passage through it for new vessels. Bone development, wound healing, learning, and memory are also dependent on healthy MMP function. During Lyme disease, the major impacts occur on collagen and ECM degradation *in every location where symptoms occur, from skin, to joint, to heart, to brain.* Malfunctions in MMP expression and behavior are linked to a wide range of pathologies, from arthritis, to neurological problems, to cerebral hemorrhage, to cancer and its metastasis, to vertebral disc problems, to atrial fibrillation and aortic aneurisms, to septic shock. They are especially damaging to the brain and CNS. (Most of these problems are commonly associated with borrelial infections.)

The type of MMPs that the spirochetes stimulate differs depending on many factors, including host immune strength, genospecies and strain type, and whether there are preexisting inflammatory conditions already present. (If, for example, you already have arthritic inflammation in any of your joints, the spirochetes take advantage of it, stimulating it even further for their own purposes.) The most common Lyme-stimulated MMPs are MMP-1, -3, and -9. (MMP-2, -8, -13, and -19 are sometimes present as well.) The spirochetes stimulate the monocytes and primary human chondrocytes (mature cartilage cells) in the synovial fluid to release MMP-1 and -3. The neutrophils that are called to locations of spirochete invasion release large quantities of MMP-9. Production of MMP-9 and 130 kDa gelatinase (aka MMP130) in the nervous system occurs through borrelial impacts on astrocytes and microglia. During neuroborreliosis, MMP-3 is common in the spinal fluid. The MMPs in the CNS break down the myelin sheaths that surround the nerves which is why the disease so closely resembles multiple sclerosis and other, similar, nervous system diseases.

MMPs are highly synergistic with, and need, plasminogen. The combination of these two compounds causes the most damage in infected sites. Lyme spirochetes possess a plasminogen-binding factor on their outer membrane. Plasminogen, in consequence, binds to their outer protein coats which raises plasminogen concentrations wherever spirochetes are located. Once MMPs are stimulated, they synergistically interact with the plasminogen causing significant glycosaminoglycan (GAG) and hydroxyproline release from affected structures. If the collagen being scavenged is in the joints, cartilage damage occurs. If in the heart, heart disease. If in the brain, neurological pathology. Once the GAGs are released, the spirochetes release *Borrelia* glycosaminoglycan binding protein (Bgbp). This binds GAGs to the spirochetes protein surfaces allowing them to more easily ingest them as a nutrient source.

MMP production, especially MMP-1 and -3, is stimulated through unique Lyme-initiated pathways, all involving mitogen-activated protein kinases (MAPKs). Specifically, the c-Jun N-terminal kinase (JNK), p38 mitogen-activated protein (p38), and extracellular signal-regulated kinase 1/2 (ERK ½) pathway. MMP-9 production occurs both through the JNK pathway and another, the protein kinase C-delta pathway.

While there are a number of herbs that can reduce the autoinflammatory conditions stimulated by MMP-1 and -3 (e.g., curcumin-containing herbs) the only herb that specifically blocks MMP-1 and -3 induction through this particular pathway is the root of *Polygonum cuspidatum,* also known as Japanese knotweed. Resveratrol (one of the plant's constituents) is also directly active in reducing MMP-9 levels through both the JNK and protein kinase C-delta pathways; it specifically inhibits MMP-9 gene transcription. Rhein, another constituent in the herb, inhibits the JNK pathway for all three MMPs: -1, -3, and -9. *Polygonum cuspidatum's* constituents also, rather easily, cross the blood–brain barrier where they exert specific actions on the central nervous system. They are antimicrobial, anti-inflammatory, and act as protectants against oxidative and microbial damage and as calming agents. The herb specifically protects the brain from inflammatory damage, microbial endotoxins, and bacterial infections.

After more than a decade of use, we have found this one herb to be foundational for stopping the damage that *Borrelia* cause, especially in the nervous system. Once the inflammation is stopped, rebuilding the damaged neural structures can occur, restoring function and quality of life. Often, the body's natural repair mechanisms can accomplish this on their own, other times herbs that facilitate the rebuilding of nerve sheaths and other damaged neural structures are necessary. (Some additional MMP-9 inhibitors are *Cordyceps*, EGCG, NAC, *Olea europaea, Punica granatum, Salvia miltiorrhiza, Scutellaria baicalensis. Cordyceps* is also a MMP-3 inhibitor; *Punica granatum* inhibits MMP-1 and -3.)

Inhibiting MMP production stops most of the breakdown of collagenous structures in the body, inhibits GAG releases, and will often halt the development of the disease. If the bacteria cannot break down collagen, they cannot feed. If they cannot feed, they cannot reproduce and spread.

A FEW COMMENTS ON DOSAGES AND TREATMENT APPROACHES

Plant medicines are quite different than pharmaceutical drugs. While safety and reliability are commonly said to be the major drive for standardization of plant medicines, there is also a desire to make them more amenable to standardized dosing regimens. Unfortunately, there is just too little understanding of the complexity of plant medicines and their interaction with the human body to accurately do so.

As an example: For the past 20 years, we have been suggesting the use of *Cryptolepis sanguinolenta* tincture for the treatment of MRSA infections that refuse to respond to antibiotics. Cryptolepis is a potent broad spectrum, highly systemic, antibacterial herb. We have found it to be specific for all Gram-positive bacteria, malarial and babesial parasites, and a few Gram-negative organisms. We have never seen it fail in treating MRSA. However, dosing can range considerably, from one teaspoon three times daily to one tablespoon six times daily depending on the severity of the infection and the individual's response to the herb. We generally start with one teaspoon three times daily, increase to six times daily, and so on, increasing as the situation demands. Other herbs, in other situations, may necessitate a much wider range of dosing.

Specifically, and counterintuitively, plant tinctures may produce sufficient healing effects when given in tablespoon doses *or in drop doses*. That is, for some people one tablespoon of the herbal tincture may be necessary to produce effects, for others three to four drops will do so. This is often hard to digest for people trained in a pharmaceutical mindset. Nevertheless, while rarely recognized, pharmaceuticals also possess that kind of range of action. Nothing has revealed this more than studies of pharmaceutical pollution in the world's waters.

Louis Guillette, a reproductive endocrinologist and professor of zoology at the University of Florida, is an expert in the study of endocrine-disrupting chemicals in the environment. He has often focused on pharmaceutical estrogens and estrogen mimics in water supplies and streams. Resultant male reproductive problems have been documented in panthers, birds, fish, alligators, frogs, bats, turtles, dogs, and humans. This includes, in some instances, complete feminization of males. His research has consistently found that androgen levels, ratios, and free testosterone levels are all significantly altered by these environmental pollutants.

Guillette (2000) has commented that the levels of chemical pollutants necessary to produce these effects are incredibly tiny. As he says: "We did not [test] one part per trillion for the contaminant, as we assumed that was too low. Well, we were wrong. It ends up that everything from a hundred parts per trillion to ten parts per million are ecologically relevant. … at these levels there is sex reversal … [The research] shows that the highest dose does not always give the greatest response. That has been a very disturbing issue for many people trying to do risk assessment in toxicology."

Because all life forms are nonlinear, self-organized systems, they are exceptionally susceptible to even tiny inputs, which explains, to a certain extent, why some homeopathic preparations work as they do. The grossest homeopathic preparations begin at six parts per trillion. Despite regular attacks on homeopathic medicines by mainstream medicalists, we have seen some homeopathic preparations produce significant alterations in disease conditions. Such *tiny* inputs, whether of homeopathics or herbal medicines, can cause physiology to shift, sometimes significantly.

Unfortunately for a reductive orientation, the inescapable truth is that medicinal plant dosages run along a rather broad spectrum. While suggested dosages for most plant medicines exist, I have found in practice that each person who is ill presents with unique disturbance of their body ecology. The cytokine cascade, even in people with the same disease (e.g., Lyme), can be subtly, or sometimes significantly different. The presence of existing conditions, the health of the immune system, the degree of fragility or robustness, life circumstances … all will have an impact on the effective dose. Therefore, healing, no matter whether one is pharmaceutically or herbally based, remains more an art than a science. I suspect this will always be true.

Ultimately, every herbal protocol can be more accurately compared to a bouquet of flowers than anything else. The individual flowers will possess a range of colors but when they are combined they become a unique entity possessing specific visual effects. I have found this a useful metaphor when creating a complex blend of plants for treating stealth pathogens. Even slight modulation of the herbs or dosages will produce an entirely different entity, with, sometimes, substantially different effects.

I may begin with an analytical understanding of what is happening and what I am attempting to create, but once a protocol is created for a particular person, there is the necessity to constantly adjust the blend to get the optimum outcome. Every time the patient enters my office, they are different. I must look closely enough to perceive that difference and compare it to where they were before to understand how the protocol must be altered in response. Further, I must constantly remind myself that each person has a slightly different form of infection, comprised, quite often, of multiple coinfectious agents.

Once I have a sense of the reality of that person's disease complex, I can begin to subtly modulate the process of its resolution. It is a *conversation* not a monologue that is occurring. I use the herbs to respond to what is being communicated. The body and the organisms respond to the intervention. I then take in and interpret what they are saying and generate a new response. In this it is crucial to see the person that is in front of me every time they enter the office. They are *not* the same person they were the last time I saw them. Nor is the disease complex.

While initial training, whether medical or herbal, may be analytical—a simple "if A then B" orientation—over time a much different approach to healing begins to emerge. Long exposure to a variety of people and disease conditions and sustained experience in treating them generates a *feeling* sense of the unique person/disease complex that enters the treatment room. This is often referred to as intuition, but I think it too inexact a term. A sense, much like that which occurs in a juggler, emerges. Some deeper part of the self senses the exact disturbance of the balance point that is in play and one begins, without reference to analytics, to *know* how to respond. It is not a *thinking* thing that occurs but a feeling thing. Analytical analysis remains tremendously useful, of course, but enters the process only when confusion arises about what is going on in the person or how to respond to it. Although this is rarely talked about, I have never met a competent physician who does not, eventually, approach healing in this way.

This is why true healing will always be more of an art than a science and why a combination of mind (thinking) and feeling are essential. Both are crucial in the process. Stealth infections need focus of mind, the ability to think deeply, to understand and treat them. But they also necessitate a well-trained and focused feeling sense as well. One without the other simply is not enough.

We are entering a time when the older models of healing are beginning to fail with increasing regularity. The world that exists outside our limited picture is intruding with greater frequency into our awareness. As frightening as this can be, we are being forced to confront the limitations of our thinking and actually do something new. Successful habitation of our planet means that we must adapt, just as the microbial populations of the world are doing. What better teachers could we ask for than the resistant and stealth pathogens that now plague us or the plants whose complexity can successfully treat them?

Stephen Harrod Buhner is Fellow of Schumacher College, a medical herbalist, and the author of 20 works of nonfiction which focus on medical herbalism, ethnobotany, plant ecology, and Gaian homeodynamis. He lives in New Mexico.

REFERENCES

Baldwin, I. Quoted in: Associated Press, "Plants Fend Off Predators, Study Suggests," *NY Times*, March 17, 2001; Will Dunham, "Plants' answer to bug attack: Call a predator," *LA Times*, March 26, 2001; Kessler et al., "Defensive function of herbivore-induced plant volatile emissions in nature." *Science* 2001;291:2141.

Baluska, F. et al. "Root apices as plant command centers: The unique 'brain-like' status of the root apex transition zone." *Biologia* 2004;59(Supplement 13):1–13.

Baluska, F. et al. "Neurobiological view of plants and their body plan." In *Communication in Plants: Neuronal Aspects of Plant Life* Baluska F., Mancuso S., and Volkman D. (eds) Berlin: Springer, 2006.

Bar-Yam, Y. *Dynamics of Complex Systems*, Reading, MA: Addison-Wesley, 1997, 10, 11.

Baud, D and Greub, G. "Intracellular bacteria and adverse pregnancy outcomes." *Clinical Microbiology and Infection* 2011;17(9):1312–22.

Ben-Jacob, E. "Bacterial self-organization: Co-enhancement of complexification and adaptability in a dynamic environment." *Philosophical Transactions* 2003;36(1807):1283–312.

Ben-Jacob, E. and Herbert L. "Self-engineering capabilites of bacteria." *Journal of the Royal Society Interface* 2006;3:197–214.

Ben-Jacob, E. et al. "Bacterial linguistic communication and social intelligence." *Trends in Microbiology* 2004;12(18):366–72.

Bosley, S. "Are you ready for a world without antibiotics?" *The Guardian*, August 12, 2010.

Brown, V. "Bacteria 'R' Us," Pacific Standard Magazine, December 2, 2010, online: [www]psmag.com/science/bacteria-r-us23628/, accessed 10/20/2012.

Camazine, S. et al. *Self-organization in Biological Systems*, Princeton, NJ: Princeton University Press, 2001.

Chakrabarti, B. and Dutta, O. "An Electrical Network Model of Plant Intelligence" *Conference Presentation, Bhagalpur University*, August 29, 2002.

Clark, I. et al. "Pathogenesis of malaria and clinically similar conditions." *Clinical Microbiology Reviews* 2004;17(3):509–39.

Crichton, M. *The Lost World*, London: Arrow Books, 1997, 2–3.

Davies, P.C.W. "The physics of complex organisation." In *Theoretical Biology: Epigenetic and Evolutionary Order from Complex Systems*, Goodwin B. and Saunders P. (eds) Edinburgh, Scotland: Edinburgh University Press, 1989, 102.

Ferreira, J. et al. "Flavonoids from Artemisia annua L. as Antioxidants and their potential synergism with artemisinin against malaria and cancer." *Molecules* 2010;15:3135–3170.

Frappaolo, P. "Risks to human health from the use of antibiotics in animal feed." In *Agricultural Use of Antibiotics*, Moats W. (ed) 102, Washington, DC: American Chemical Society, 1986.

Graham, A. et al. "Transmission consequences of coinfection: Cytokines writ large." *Trends in Parasitology* 2007;23(6):284–91.

Guillette, L. "Impacts of endocrine disruptors on wildlife." *Endocrine Disruptors and Pharmaceutically Active Compounds in Drinking Water Workshop, Center for Health Effects of Environmental Contamination, April 19-21*, 2000, 6. https://cheec.uiowa.edu/sites/cheec.uiowa.edu/files/endocrine_pharm.pdf, accessed Feb. 22, 2018.

Kitazato, K. et al. "Viral infectious disease and natural products with antiviral activity." *Drug Discoveries and Therapeutics* 2007;1(1):14–22.

La Cerra, P. "The first law of psychology is the second law of thermodynamics: The energetic evolutionary model of the mind and the generation of human psychological phenomena." *Human Nature Review* 2003;3:440–7, 442.

Levy, S. *The Antibiotic Paradox*, New York: Plenum Press, 1992, 3.

Lewontin, R. *The Triple Helix: Gene, Organism, and Environment*, Cambridge, MA: Harvard University Press, 2000.

Lovelock, J. "The Living Earth." *Nature* 2003;426:769–770.

Margulis, L. and Dorian S. *What Is Sex?* New York: Simon and Schuster, 1997, 55.

McCormack, E. et al. "Touch-responsive behaviors and gene expression in plants." In *Communication in Plants: Neuronal Aspects of Plant Life*, Baluska F., Mancuso S., and Volkman, D. (eds) Berlin: Springer, 2006:256–7.

Projan, S.J. "Antibacterial drug discovery in the twenty-first century." In *Bacterial Resistance to Antimicrobials*, Wax, R.G., Lewis K., Salyers A.A. and Taber H. (eds) Chapter 17. Boca Raton, FL: CRC Press, 2008.

Salyers, A. et al. "Ecology of antibiotic resistant genes." In *Bacterial Resistance to Antimicrobials*, Wax R.G., Lewis K., Salyers A.A. and Taber H. (eds) Boca Raton, FL: CRC Press, 2008, 11.

Shapiro, J. "Bacteria are small but not stupid: Cognition, natural genetic engineering, and sociobacteriology." *Studies in History and Philosophy in Biological and Biomedical Science* 2007;38(4):807–19; also: Exeter Meeting, 2006.

Strogatz, S. *Sync: The Emerging Science of Spontaneous Order*, New York: Hyperion, 2003, 1–2.

Trewavas, A. "Aspects of plant intelligence." *Annals of Botany* 2003;92:2.

Trewavas, A. "The green plant as intelligent organism." In *Communication in Plants: Neuronal Aspects of Plant Life*, Baluska F., Mancuso S., and Volkman D. (eds) Berlin: Springer, 2006.

Varela, F. et al. "Adaptive strategies gleaned from immune networks: Viability theory and comparison with classifier systems." In *Theoretical Biology: Epigenetic and Evolutionary Order from Complex Systems*, Goodwin B. and Saunders P. (eds) Edinburgh, Scotland: Edinburgh University Press, 1989, 112.

Warwick, K. *QI: The Quest for Intelligence*, London: Piatkus, 2001, 9.

25 Psychological Trauma
Integrating Somatic and Psychological Methods to Treatment

Leslie Korn

CONTENTS

The Biology of Traumatic Stress 593
The Stress Response 593
    Case 594
Group Stress and Trauma 595
Allostatic Load 596
Tend and Befriend: The Female Stress Response 596
Learned Helplessness 597
State-Dependent Memory, Learning, and Behavior 597
    Case 598
Somatic Symptoms of Trauma and Addiction 598
    Case 599
Self-Medication 599
Anxiety, Disordered Breathing, and Hyperventilation 601
Yoga and Breathing 601
    Mind Body Assessment 602
    Dissociation 603
Somatoform Behaviors, Eating Disorders, and Self-Injury 603
Addiction to Surgery 604
    Case 604
References 605

The experience of trauma is as old as humankind itself. One can only imagine the early hominid's evolutionary urgency to fight or take flight—the response that lies at the heart of the autonomic nervous system's response to trauma by increasing heart rate, blood flow, and oxygen levels. The emotion of fear primes the pump and energizes hormones like epinephrine, which clear the mind, sharpen the vision, and light the fire that excites the muscles to move quickly out of harm's way. Escape from trauma brings (temporary) victory; the alternative is to freeze in inaction, leading to injury or death. Some of the functions of the autonomic nervous system, so called because they are "automatic" and instinctual, include the pulses of heart and breath, the periodic flush of gastric acids, the electrical charges of the brain, and the eliminative waves of bowels, which open and close the ileocecal "gate." In health, these organs function rhythmically without conscious control, giving rise to the ebb and flow of life. The heart beats 40–220 beats a minute, depending on condition and activity. The breath cycle is completed 4 (yoga) to 20 times (aerobic) a minute, more or less. The brain emits electrical signals measured in cycles per second or hertz (Hz)—from approximately 2–3 cycles per second during deep sleep (delta), 4–7 Hz (theta), 8–12 (alpha), 13–18 (beta), and above 40 (gamma). Whether electroencephalographic (EEG) patterns actually drive the brain (Evans, 1986) or consciousness drives EEG, we have capacities to gain control over these processes. This forms the basis for self-regulation practices such as meditation or the modern technological equivalents, biofeedback, neurofeedback, or devices such as musical or electrical stimulation devices that entrain alphatheta brainwave patterns.

Posttraumatic stress disorder (PTSD) is the quintessential mind/body disorder that alters physiological, biological, and psychological homeostasis. Clinical observation and research point to a complex pattern of dysregulation that impairs physical, affective, and cognitive function. People who have been traumatized often present with distressing and frequently intractable psychosomatic symptoms, often without knowing consciously that the source of their symptoms is the trauma they experienced. This timely ebb and flow of natural rhythms—the polarized dynamic of opposites represented as sleep and wakefulness, inhalation and exhalation, systole and diastole, beta and delta—are severely compromised by trauma. An understanding of the methods that affect consciousness and brainwave function is useful for both the clinician and client in the treatment of trauma.

The healing of traumatic stress is rooted in the rhythms of reconciliation: forces that shift shapes as inner and outer, darker and lighter, hotter and colder, closer and farther. In Chinese tradition and many tribal cultures, the rhythms of the body are considered one with the natural world. Disease or illness results when one becomes out of balance with these forces. Practitioners of traditional Chinese philosophy and medicine refer to these dynamic polarities as yin and yang, mediated by a transitional third energetic phenomenon, called Tao or Balance. The reconciliation of opposing yet complementary forces has particular import for the treatment of posttraumatic stress. Trauma disrupts endogenous rhythmic cycles of function, and cyclic movement is replaced by a state of fixation. This is well established by conventional medicine as reflected in the concepts of autonomic hyperarousal and hyper/hypoactivity of the hypothalamic–adrenal–pituitary (HPA) axis. The autonomic nervous system is composed of three branches, the sympathetic, the parasympathetic, and the most recently identified, the ventral vagal complex or social nervous system (Porges, 2011). The restoration of balance within these forces—whether called yin and yang, ida and pingala, or parasympathetic and sympathetic—is at the heart of Eastern and Western medical traditions alike.

Rather than sustaining the natural flow of oscillating life force, trauma causes autonomic fixation and loss of the normal range of body regulation, including extreme, uncontrollable cycles of response characterized by opposing fluctuations of cognition, behavior, and kinesthetic perception. It is the restoration of flexible movement instead of fixation by balancing these extremes that poses the central dilemma for the integrated mind/body treatment of traumatic stress.

To understand more fully the disruption of rhythm and time perception caused by trauma, it is useful to explore briefly the role of circadian rhythm, light, chronic pain (fibromyalgia), and sleep problems, which are all characterized by circadian rhythm imbalance (Scaer, 2001). Circadian rhythm underlies the endogenous, 24-hour cycle of human function. The central nervous system regulates adrenal function via the hypothalamic–pituitary–adrenal axis, and stress disrupts the balance. Circadian rhythm is present each step of the way in this process. Circadian rhythm and the resulting secretion of endocrine hormones and neurotransmitters depend on the transmission of light through the eyes.

Time stops for the victim of trauma. The traumatic moment of the past becomes suspended like a still life that keeps flashing the same pictures before the mind's eye. These somatosensory images, called flashbacks, repeat themselves visually, aurally, and kinesthetically. They intrude on the present, making it difficult and often impossible for the sufferer to locate herself or himself in time. This inability to distinguish the present moment from the past is experienced simultaneously in a variety of ways. Often, the person feels as if it were the past but knows cognitively that it is the present. Yet the patient nonetheless shakes physically, in fear of the present or future. The experience of the past trauma is like a nagging, subcutaneous patch of poison that prevents the future from coming into focus. The future under normal circumstances is a vista filled with hope and plans; in trauma it is frozen by the past, for the future holds the ever-present fear that the past will be lurking. Thus, the victim lives in a timeless bardo, a netherworld of neither here nor there, what the Hindus call the world between worlds where the soul travels during its passage through the various stages of consciousness at death. Not actively participating in the rhythmic and changing course of life can lead to a sense of being swept along, as if out of control. Thus, it becomes apparent how a person's spirit can be crushed by trauma. The perception and experience of time provide the scaffolding about which meaning and purpose in life are constructed. Ordinarily, change is given coherence and meaning as we actively participate in the passage of time. This personal and collective creation of coherence and form refers to spirit, a word whose Greek derivation *respir* means "to breathe." In Hippocratic texts we read, "Breath is the rhythm of life" (Fried & Grimaldi, 1993). In trauma, the individual "holds the breath in fear" or "has the wind knocked out of him," as his spiritual scaffolding shakes and sinks under the burden of traumatic experience. Our individual rhythms and the perception of time are also interpenetrated with those of other human beings, animals, and the natural world.

THE BIOLOGY OF TRAUMATIC STRESS

Traumatic stress precipitates a condition of physiological and psychobiological imbalance in the nervous system and in the endocrine, immune, and neuropeptide systems. In response to trauma, the individual experiences two coexisting responses that are conditioned by a hyperaroused nervous system: one of overreaction (intrusion) and one of underreaction (avoidance/numbing) to actual or anticipated environmental stimuli. The victim must cope with conditioned responses that are psychophysiological in nature and if untreated are often impossible to control. These stimuli serve as reminders of the trauma through sensory cues: visual, auditory, and olfactory perceptions that trigger profound reactions that often perplex nontraumatized people who witness them.

Whatever the source of arousal, a response cycle of intrusive and avoidance symptoms are set in motion by the autonomic nervous system (ANS). ANS dysregulation is a major hallmark of posttraumatic stress. The traumatic battles that were experienced externally have now been recorded internally. These experiences are engraved semantically and somatically by a host of known and as yet undiscovered mechanisms. These include stress hormones that are believed to encode memory, learning, and behavior while an individual is in a particular state of consciousness. This is referred to as state-dependent memory, learning, and behavior (SDMLB), discussed later in more detail.

In addition to psychosomatic symptoms, a victim of trauma often copes with changes to self-identity resulting from the lifelong effects of direct assault on the physical body. This may include disabilities such as loss of a limb, loss of capacity to bear children, and chronic pain. Grief over loss of control, self-efficacy, and functional capacity will be a recurring theme in treatment. The constant state of hyperarousal is akin to always being "on edge" and results in a compensatory response that includes avoiding activities and numbing feelings and sensations. This overreaction to subsequent normal life events, as well as withdrawal from active participation, becomes a secondary loss—often a diminished or lost future. Successful treatment includes integrating approaches that enable the client to achieve better affective and somatic self-regulation. In order for one to do this, it is helpful to understand how the ANS responds to extreme stress.

THE STRESS RESPONSE

The stress response may be considered to exist along a continuum: eustress, stress, and traumatic stress. Eustress, a term coined by Dr. Hans Selye, refers to a positive stressful challenge, such as that occurring when one is training for a marathon or learning the skills required for a new job. It is the interaction between the normal daily stressors of life with the individual's personality that defines the way a person perceives and makes meaning of the event. This leads to the perception of the stress as positive or negative and determines the degree and type of response. For example, normal life events such as attending school, job changes, relocation, and marriage or partnerships all constitute normal life stressors that, when coupled with an individual's sense of control and purpose, determine the level of perceived stress. The perception of an event coupled with individual control, self-efficacy, and meaning influences psychological and physiological function. Stress traumatizes when stressors overwhelm the individual's capacity to cope. The idea that every person has a "breaking point" is based on the observations of the limits each person has to withstand stress. Traumatic stress is by definition an experience in which the survival of the whole organism is at stake, and it responds with the "fight, flight, or freeze" response. Selye first defined this general adaptation syndrome as a predictable psychophysiological response to stress. During experiments he began in the 1930s, Selye observed that after rats were exposed to toxic chemicals or frigid waters, they displayed a common psychophysiological reaction arising from the nervous system's response to overwhelming shock. Regardless of the type of stressor, he found a common generalized reaction in the animals. This included gastrointestinal, cardiovascular, and respiratory dysfunction as well as generalized depression and distress. Selye observed a three-stage response resulting in psychosomatic dysfunction: alarm, resistance, and exhaustion. In the first stage of alarm, stress results in ANS arousal and activation of the sympathetic response. The adrenal glands release the hormones epinephrine and norepinephrine, causing a rise in heart rate, blood pressure, and respiration, which enables the organism to fend off the threat. These stress hormones are considered to play an important role in the storage and consolidation of state-dependent memory, learning, and behavior.

CASE

Roger, a 45-year-old Iraq War veteran, illustrates the experience of hyperarousal and state-dependent memory learning and behavior: "I live near an auto mechanic and when I am in my yard gardening and hear a car backfire, I dive for the bushes. My wife finds me crouching and shaking and crying, afraid to come out because I am surrounded by mortar fire. When will this go away?" The hypervigilance and exaggerated startle response prevalent in PTSD occur because the "alarm" keeps going off and the patient is in a near constant state of alert to the perceived threatening environmental stimuli. Such a stimulus may take the form of a trigger that reminds the person of the original threat. For Roger it is the backfire of a car that sounds like mortar fire; for Joelle, it is seeing a man in daylight walking toward her, reminiscent of the man who raped her. Joelle, a 25-year-old student who was raped 2 years earlier, said: "Whenever I'm walking down a street and a man is walking towards me on the sidewalk, my whole body starts to shake uncontrollably. I tell myself this is the present, but at these moments my body is living in the past and the past rules my life."

However, a trigger may also be unrelated to the trauma and nonetheless stimulate a sensory response. It is theorized that stress hormones released as a result of arousal by an external reminder of the original threat are the biological substrates of the flashbacks experienced during the intrusive cycle. The alarm stage is followed by the resistance stage, in which the repetitive psychosomatic response to the stress leaves one "stuck in a groove" (Rossi, 1986) and unable to break free of the cycle. Following a period of hyperactivity, "fighting off" the stress, the individual may lapse into the third stage of exhaustion, which is associated with chronic unresolved symptoms. This stage includes symptoms such as the chronic tension and pain associated with whiplash months and years after an accident or chronic pain in the pelvic region years after a rape. Selye was the first researcher to demonstrate the relationship between exposure to stress, the subsequent release of hormones from the hypothalamic–pituitary–adrenal axis, and the development of psychosomatic symptoms. Building on Selye's work, researchers have determined that exposure to stress and violence during childhood adversely alters the normal development of the brain and nervous system. This results in enduring changes in psychophysiological and psychobiological function and leads to chronic health problems throughout adulthood.

GROUP STRESS AND TRAUMA

Exposure to chronic stress occurs among individuals but also in members of whole groups by virtue of their membership in those groups. Cultural trauma, historical trauma, and intergenerational trauma are among the concepts used to explain the response to chronic stress among whole groups of people and how this stress is "transferred" across generations. The roots of the terms historical trauma and intergenerational transmission of trauma derive from observations that the sociohistorical experience of cultural groups exposed to prolonged stress and suffering resulting from war, genocide, and interpersonal violence initiates the transfer of a psychobiobehavioral template of stress to offspring and subsequent generations. Seminal research conducted among survivors of the Nazi Holocaust (Nadler, Kav-Venaki, & Gleitman, 1985; Yehuda et al., 1998), the Khmer of Cambodia (Sack, Clarke, & Seeley 1995), American Indians (Brave Heart & DeBruyn, 1998; Whitbeck, Adams, Hoyt, & Chen, 2004) and aboriginal peoples (Gagne, 1998) of North America and Mexico (Korn & Rÿser, 2006) suggest identifiable patterns of trauma and health dysfunction. Historical trauma among American Indians refers to the legacy of colonization and genocide (Whitbeck et al., 2004) resulting from European contact in the United States, the effects of which persist today. The clinical significance of historical trauma and its interaction with exposure to lifetime traumatic events is unclear and has yet to be definitively elucidated. Recent attention has focused on the putative role of historical trauma in neurobiological function (Yehuda et al., 2005), and there is some evidence that these effects may be passed on at the neurobiological developmental strata via the HPA axis system (Gunnar & Donzella, 2002) in response to intergenerational trauma (Strickland, Walsh, & Cooper, 2006).

Yehuda et al. (2005) found that adult offspring whose parents had survived the Nazi Holocaust and developed PTSD had low cortisol levels, which reflects Selye's exhaustion stage discussed earlier. The intergenerational transmission of trauma is hypothesized to occur during the prenatal (Yehuda et al., 2005) and perinatal stages of neurobiological development (Schore, 2003), suggesting a theoretical basis for the predisposition to the development of PTSD, depression, anxiety, and vulnerability to substance abuse (Schore, 2003). Yehuda et al. (2005) report that infants born to mothers who were pregnant and developed PTSD following their witnessing of the 9/11 terrorist attack in New York City had significantly lower cortisol levels, suggesting the effects of HPA axis transmission on the fetus.

Persistent changes in HPA axis are also seen in subjects with a history of child sexual abuse and with current major depression. Findings from several studies suggest that chronic exposure to traumatic experiences reduces hippocampal volume and that hippocampal damage extinguishes the awakening cortisol response without affecting the rest of the cycle (Buchanan, Kern, Allen, Tranel, & Kirschbaum, 2004). Understanding how stress affects the 24-hour cortisol rhythm is central to making intervention decisions using nutritional and botanical medicine, which can restore cortisol rhythm and balance.

Acute stress can enhance immune function whereas chronic stress suppresses it (McEwen, 2000). Chronic stress produces cardiovascular reactivity, immunological, and endocrinological alterations (Kiecolt-Glaser, Malarkey, Cacioppo, & Glaser, 1994) and can negatively affect functional and structural changes in the brain (McEwen, 2000) and increase immune activation in patients with PTSD. For example, it is well known that stress can trigger autoimmune diseases such as rheumatoid arthritis and that people with PTSD are at higher risk for autoimmune function (Boscarino, 2004). In these cases, the body's immune system becomes hyperreactive, reflecting another level of systemic overreaction to perceived threat after the trauma events have passed. People with PTSD have increased levels of inflammatory markers and increased reactivity to antigen skin tests (Pace & Heim, 2011). The separation of nonhuman primate offspring from their mothers (grief) results in suppression of the immune system (Cohen, 1994). Widows and widowers are also found to be more susceptible to illness during the first year of the loss of their spouse. By contrast, high levels of social attachment behaviors appear to be protective against immunosuppression (Cohen, 1994).

The effects on health arising from traumatic stress experiences are amplified by the effects on immune function of actual exposure to chemical, biological, and waste products that occurred following the nuclear accident at Chernobyl in the Ukraine, the Gulf War, and the inhalation of toxic fumes and air by rescue workers following 9/11. These effects are further exacerbated by the delays or denial of the reality of exposure by government officials that affect victims. Of the psychological and physical trauma of radioactive exposure at Hanford nuclear reservation, which was built on Yakima Indian land, Russell Jim, director of the environmental restoration project, says:

> During the fifty years of Hanford's operation, especially when the [Columbia] river was highly contaminated by the reactors, the site managers knew full well that tribal people were being poisoned. But they simply ignored their own data and considered us to be expendable. (R. Jim, personal communication, September 12, 2004)

Environmental disasters are multifocal and not easily addressed in the short or long term (Goldstein, Osofsky, & Lichtveld, 2011). The mental and physical health effects of the stress of environmental contamination on Akwesasne Mohawk Indian land persist (Papadopoulos-Lane, 2010) and interact with historical trauma. The Exxon Valdez oil spill in Prince William Sound, Alaska, in 1989 ruined traditional fishing grounds and food sources for Alaska natives and nonnatives alike. Hurricane Katrina struck the southeastern United States in 2005, displacing thousands from their homes. The effects of such events are felt for years and often generations. The Deepwater Horizon oil spill of 2010 affects ways of life, with bodies, lands, seas, and wildlife exposed to neurotoxins. The stress does not end with the event but persists for years during attempts to receive reparations, which are often inadequate. PTSD is not limited to residents of these locales. First responders, both residents and visitors, are also vulnerable to high rates of secondary trauma. With the increasing contribution of climate change to adverse effects resulting from disasters, the trauma clinician will be called on to work with individual, social, and environmental causes of PTSD, which affect all aspects of individual and community function and induce extensive losses. Addressing loss and grief as a result of disasters is central to coping and surviving with trauma.

ALLOSTATIC LOAD

The observations that repeated exposure to stress, whether it begins in childhood or as an adult, accumulates and builds over time in life, affecting physical and mental health, has led to a model called allostatic load. This term refers to the price the body pays for being forced to adapt to the effects of chronic stress (McEwen & Seeman, 1999). Some evidence suggests that discrimination may constitute a stressor and contribute to a greater lifetime allostatic load. Cumulative stress across the lifespan is often associated with low socioeconomic status and chronic discrimination and may provide a psychophysiological model for minority health disparities. Conversely, social relationships mitigate the effects of allostatic load (Seeman et al., 2004). This intersects with a new model of stress response called "tend and befriend."

TEND AND BEFRIEND: THE FEMALE STRESS RESPONSE

Whereas Selye's model has dominated the concepts of stress response, Taylor et al. (2000) posit a female stress response model they call tend and befriend. This model adds a dimension to the fight or flight/freeze concept and suggests that women (and other female animals) respond to stress by engaging in activities of care and connection, that is, tending to the care of offspring and family and engaging in behaviors that support social connection, affiliation, and attachment. Oxytocin is considered to mediate this response biologically; it is the main neurohormone responsible for social behaviors and empathy. It is produced primarily in the hypothalamus and is associated with the thymus and immune function (Carter et al., 2005) and has been shown to promote trust and well-being while reducing fear and blood pressure (Ishak, Kahloon, & Fakhry, 2011; Olff, Langeland, Witteveen, & Denys, 2010). Dysfunction of the oxytocin system may be involved in the development of PTSD (Ishak et al., 2011), and combining nasal administration of oxytocin with cognitive behavioral therapy may be useful in reducing fear, enhancing safety and trust, and supporting social engagement (Ishak et al., 2011; Olff et al., 2010). Added to this, the role of touch therapies and massage and interaction with animal companions has many positive effects for treatment, including the increase of oxytocin levels. This research reinforces the importance of integrating psychological, biological, and physiological methods and their role in establishing and maintaining strong social connections for the recovery of physical and psychological health after trauma.

LEARNED HELPLESSNESS

What happens, however, when we cannot successfully fight or take flight or tend and befriend to ameliorate shock or stress? As clinicians, we often treat individuals who appear unable to act in their own best interest or to mobilize to make change, and we wonder how to help them. The research of Seligman and Beagley (1975) may illuminate the complex response to inescapable stress. During the 1960s, Seligman and Beagley conducted experiments on dogs that were exposed to stressors they could not escape. During the experiments, in order not to receive an electric shock to their paws, Seligman and Beagley trained the dogs to jump from one compartment in a shuttle avoidance box to an adjoining compartment. When the dogs had mastered this task, a barrier was put in place that prevented some of them from escaping the shock. Two-thirds of the animals could not escape and subsequently experienced depression, disruption of normal defecation, and generalized distress. More interestingly, when the barriers were removed and the animals were allowed to move to escape the shock, they remained passive. Seligman and Beagley's attempts to drag the animals across the grid to teach them that the cage was now safe were only partially successful: some dogs mastered the new task, but most remained helpless and passive. This loss of self-efficacy and the inability to mobilize change observed in the animals exposed to inescapable stress, which mimicked depression and posttraumatic stress in humans, led to the development of a behavioral analog called learned helplessness (Bremner, Southwick, & Charney, 1991).

The enduring somatic "tug of war" we so often see in traumatized people and the failed attempts to balance the extremes result from the original helplessness in the face of terror. Feeling helpless to change the present, the trauma survivor believes that there is no future. The persistent and pervasive effects of self-harming behavior, somatic dysfunction, and self-medication, however, only reinforce a sense of being out of control. Subsequent research reformulated the attributional theory of learned helplessness, hypothesizing that "mere exposure to an uncontrollable event is not sufficient to produce helplessness. Rather, it is the expectation that the future cannot be controlled that results in learned helplessness." Why some dogs were able to mobilize, relearn, and resist the development of learned helplessness is an important question to answer if we wish to understand the role of resiliency in the prevention of posttraumatic stress. Seligman's work evolved into "learned optimism" and "positive psychology," leading to the development of a program called "comprehensive soldier fitness," a resiliency training program.

STATE-DEPENDENT MEMORY, LEARNING, AND BEHAVIOR

Learned helplessness intersects with the central assertion of state-dependent memory, learning, and behavior: what we learn and remember is dependent on our psychophysiological state at the time of the experience (Rossi, 1986). The theory of state-dependent memory, learning, and behavior (SDMLB) includes the study of hypnosis, dissociation, information systems theory, and psychosomatic illness (Rossi, 1986). SDMLB refers to a complex system of mind/body communication that attempts to answer the following questions:

- What are the mechanisms of mind/body information exchange?
- How are overwhelming emotions transformed into physical symptoms?
- How does "broken" mind/body communication heal?

Conditions of intense sensory experience such as intense pleasure or pain underlie SDMLB. We are often transported back in time by a special song or the smell of perfume or aftershave that evokes in us the complexity of that personal historical memory. However, a sensory cue that triggers a traumatic memory may be overwhelming, intrusive, and painful. Recall that when Roger heard a car backfire, it brought back a state-bound memory of mortar fire. As one client who was violently beaten by her mother said to me, "When I walk into your office after your previous client, I get nauseous and feel like throwing up because she wears the same perfume as my mother."

How do physical symptoms express emotions and become reintegrated into adaptive modes of functioning? When stress is transduced into psychosomatic symptoms, Rossi (1986) refers to this process as information transduction: the conversion of information and/or energy from one form to another. He proposes that the limbic-hypothalamic-pituitary system is the major anatomical mechanism that acts as a mind/body transducer. This area of the brain is concerned with emotional experiences and reactions and includes the hippocampus, the amygdala, olfactory regions, and the hypothalamus. The hypothalamus controls the ANS, which integrates the basic regulatory systems of hunger, thirst, sex, temperature, heart rate, and blood pressure. SDMLB is rooted in the limbic-hypothalamic-pituitary system response (Rossi, 1999), and molecules of the body modulate mental experience and mental experience modulates the molecules of the body.

One task of all therapies is to help a client decondition from SDMLB, leading to the ability to:

- Exert control over "automatic" responses
- Decondition reactivity due to memories and experiences
- Change maladaptive behaviors acquired during a traumatic or altered (dissociated) state of consciousness

CASE

Laura experienced multiple childhood sexual and physical traumas and is now struggling to establish physical intimacy with her partner. She illustrates the difficulty of deconditioning from SDMLB:

> I learned how to use my mind to control the pain in my body. I would just leave my body. But now I want to stay in my body, to feel. Why can't I get my body to do what my mind says? I keep thinking that I should be able to—that it's a moral failure that I haven't succeeded by now.

Laura reveals feelings of futility, frustration, and shame that are common to people who have been victimized. Since many of the victim's functional difficulties arise out of dissociative symptoms that include amnesias and hyperamnesias, helping her to understand and decondition triggers, along with resymbolization, forms an important part of therapy. Rossi (1986) asserts that therapies work by accessing state-bound memories and reframing cognitive beliefs, and that "every access is a reframe."

SOMATIC SYMPTOMS OF TRAUMA AND ADDICTION

People with PTSD experience a nexus of symptoms that include somatization, depression, anxiety, and dissociation. They may experience musculoskeletal pain that alternates with lack of feeling and sensation, gastrointestinal problems, and heart, respiratory, and reproductive problems. Nightmares invade their sleep, and their waking life is affected by recurrent visual images of the trauma itself. They feel out of control. This perception, in turn, drives them to remain on guard—to be hyper-vigilant and overly controlled. Affective outbursts that include irritability, aggression, and fear lead to withdrawal and detachment from activities and interpersonal connections. Imbalances of neu-rochemicals in the brain contribute to the negative feedback loop of depression, irritability, self-mutilation, and eating disorders.

Because the causes of somatic symptoms cannot always be diagnosed, treating these conditions can be difficult for the general practitioner, who may lack knowledge of the extent of PTSD's effects on physical health. On the other hand, the practitioner may call these symptoms psychosomatic.

CASE

Sara, a 14-year-old young woman, had been sexually abused and had a diagnosis of oppositional defiant disorder. She abused drugs and alcohol, which brought her into treatment, and she was dis-ruptive, thus annoying her teachers and milieu therapists. She had very painful periods and kept complaining of pain in her pelvic region, but medical exams and testing revealed no precise cause. I told her that we were going to treat it and asked her to describe her pain in detail, to describe when it began, what she thought the cause was, and what she thought would help reduce the pain. She spoke in detail about the abuse she had experienced, and I asked her to touch the areas of her pain as she spoke. We limited these discussions to 15 minutes each session over a period of four sessions. I suggested that we move slowly and that each time the pain might have something new to reveal, so that as we discovered what the pain had to say, we would have more knowledge about how to treat it. Setting limits on the exploration of pain created safety for Sara, and this approach honored her focus on the physical pain, which was the story her body was telling about her experience. Simultaneously her "oppositional behavior" abated and she made progress. Together, we wrote a report to the physi-cian about the nature of the pain and its cause.

SELF-MEDICATION

In order to cope with somatic symptoms, trauma victims will often resort to self-medicating behav-iors. This contributes to the high rate of addiction among trauma victims: 75% of Vietnam War vet-erans with PTSD developed problems with alcohol, and 19%–59% of individuals seeking treatment for substance use disorders are estimated to have PTSD (Back, Sonne, Killeen, Dansky, & Brady, 2003). In one large study, one in three of the women with PTSD developed alcohol dependence; however, women who experienced trauma but did not develop PTSD also had similar rates, sug-gesting that it is the trauma and not the PTSD that leads to alcohol dependence (Sartor et al., 2010). One-third of female veterans met lifetime criteria for substance use disorder, with about half report-ing rape during their lives and one-quarter reporting rape within the military (Booth, Mengeling, Torner, & Sadler, 2011). Self-medicating behavior—like the use of alcohol and drugs, food fasts, binges, and self-injury, such as cutting and burning the body—reflects attempts to alter brain chem-istry and affect dysregulated by trauma.

Animals exposed to inescapable stress develop analgesia when exposed to another stressor shortly afterward. Stress-induced analgesia is due to the production of endogenous opioids and endocannabinoids. These contribute to complex cyclical patterns of affective and behavioral responses, including the addictions. Endogenous opioids are neuropeptides found in the brain and in receptors throughout the body. Their discovery has furthered our knowledge about the relation-ship of emotions to chemistry and has begun to illuminate some of the channels by which the brain, mind, and body communicate with each other. Dr. Candace Pert discovered the complex pathways of the endogenous opioids (endorphins, enkephalins) and suggests that they are the bio-chemical correlates of emotions. Endocannabinoids and their receptors exist in the brain, where they affect mood, pain, and behavior throughout the body; they are crucial modulators of the ANS and the immune system.

Chronic and persistent stress appears to decrease the effectiveness of the stress response and to induce desensitization. For many victims, this leads to the inability to react appropriately to danger and underlies the observation that people who have been repeatedly traumatized cannot utilize affective cues to activate the appropriate response.

Risk-taking behavior or reenactment is another type of addictive behavior.

Reenactment refers to behaviors where the individual reenacts and relives (unconsciously) parts of the trauma. This behavior suggests a biological analog to what Freud called the repetition compulsion. For example, a high percentage of female and male prostitutes also have histories of child sexual abuse. Most women begin prostitution as sexually abused adolescents. Veterans often return to war as mercenaries; for some, the Vietnam War did not end but just relocated to the jungles of Mexico and Hawaii.

Thousands of former veterans of the Iraq and Afghanistan Wars work throughout the world for private contract companies to carry out a range of war-related activities, and many have PTSD (Feinstein & Botes, 2009). Reenactment appears to arise in part from a psychobiological imperative to produce endogenous opiates that alleviate pain, numb feelings, and rage and have a tranquilizing effect. Researchers speculate that these naturally occurring opiates are chronically depleted in people with PTSD (Hoffman, Burges-Watson, Wilson, & Montgomery, 1989) and that chronic opioid depletion contributes to substance abuse, self-mutilation, eating disorders, and dissociation. Chronic stress exposure and PTSD likely lead to clinical endocannabinoid deficiency and the associated functional pain symptoms of fibromyalgia, migraines, and irritable bowel syndrome (Russo, 2008). Heroin, an exogenous opioid that temporarily reduces physical and emotional pain, supplants opioid production. This explains why recovering addicts are very pain sensitive and respond well to acupuncture, which stimulates the endogenous opioids and endocannabinoids. Painful states result in (unconscious) efforts by the victim to stimulate opioid/endocannabinoid production, either by reexposure to trauma, which activates brain opiate receptors in the same way as exogenous opioids like heroin, or by other self-harming behaviors, like cutting or burning the body. Prior to self-injury, victims report the overwhelming urge to feel and to relieve anxiety (Favazza, 1987; Villalba & Harrington, 2003).

There is some research on the efficacy of substituting acupuncture for cutaneous self-injuries like cutting and burning. One study demonstrated that acupuncture reduced self-injurious behavior (SIB) but not depression in adolescents (Nixon, Cheng, & Cloutier, 2003). Interestingly, researchers have identified SIB in nonhuman primates targeting known acupuncture analgesia points (Tiefenbacher, Novak, Lutz, & Meyer, 2005). Nixon, Cheng, and Cloutier (2003) suggest teaching self-acupuncture as an alternative to SIB. Combining these therapies with counseling links listening to oneself, the body-voice, and being heard by others to self-care activities and can be very effective. Machoian (2006) has worked extensively with teen girls with SIB, emphasizing the relational underpinning of self-harm: "the cry of not being listened to." Introducing therapies that pierce the skin, like acupuncture, or apply heat, like moxa, provide an alternative to self-harming behaviors. While these therapies stimulate similar sensations and psychobiological responses, they are enacted in the context of healing and self-awareness. They are easily integrated into cognitive-based mindfulness and provide a bridge to other self-regulation strategies. The patient learns new behaviors, is better able to manage affect, and develops new options for physical relaxation.

Traumatized people engage in reenactment behaviors both psychologically and biologically, and both aspects must be treated integratively. Helping clients to gain control over their behaviors requires both their ability to understand the psychobiology of their reactions and to substitute positive sources for the production of endogenous opioids. Therapeutic methods such as acupuncture, massage, exercise, and shamanic rituals are effective partly because they stimulate natural brain chemicals, including the endogenous opioids and endocannabinoids, and help people find healthy ritualized substitutes for unhealthy behaviors.

These methods also facilitate deep rest and engage the natural rhythms that restore health.

ANXIETY, DISORDERED BREATHING, AND HYPERVENTILATION

Disordered breathing is the physical manifestation of anxiety and is very common in PTSD. It exists along a spectrum of function; hyperventilation syndrome (HVS) is at one end of that spectrum. Disordered breathing often goes undiagnosed; most symptoms of hyperventilation are not the typical rapid, shallow breathing that occurs during panic attacks. People who over-breathe often complain of headaches, neck pain, jaw pain, leg and body cramps, and tension in the shoulder muscles. Posturally, such people may present with their jaws jutting out, as if gasping for air even as their shoulders slump forward. Unconscious attempts to restore posture by pulling the neck posteriorly, like a turtle pulling her head into her shell, results in a muscular "tug of war" in the neck and leads to chronic neck pain.

The postural changes that occur in HVS are as much emotional as they are physical, and we can often sense the oppression our clients feel by observing the patterns of their muscle contraction. Dysregulation of respiration may begin with birth trauma or can develop in response to chronic anxiety. Abuse affects posture and posture affects breathing. Women (more commonly than men) experience thoracic outlet syndrome, which may derive from a physical trauma, such as a car accident; an athletic injury, such as triceps pushups; or repetitive trauma due to computer work that strains ergonomics and thus posture.

Chronic scalene muscle tension in the neck, which co-occurs with associated breathing dysregulation (and asthma), exacerbates this syndrome. In hyperventilation, the neck muscles are often overdeveloped because they do most of the work, leading to chronic neck pain. The scalenes, through which the brachial nerve bundles pass, are often contracted from this overuse. Certainly many women have described receiving abusive attention to their breasts as children and have therefore undergone breast surgery. Many of these women also experience body dysmorphic disorder, which involves a preoccupation to the point of impairment with imagined or slight defects in appearance, resulting in surgeries that bring no relief (Didie et al., 2006). All of this occurs within the respiratory matrix of muscle and memory. In his analysis of the whiplash model of pain, Scaer (2011) suggests, I believe correctly, that the chronic pain syndrome often resulting from mild motor vehicle accidents does not correspond with the actual events—that it more likely represents dissociated memory that was laid down at the time of impact due to intense fear (Scaer, 2011).

With chronic hyperventilation or over-breathing comes brain hypoxia, which in turn contributes to depression and headaches. The occurrence of over-breathing, or HVS, is estimated in the general population at 10% and likely more, for it is often undiagnosed. Like dissociation, hyperventilation can be difficult to detect because, without the symptoms of a full-blown panic attack, the signs are often subtle. While the client is often aware of symptoms such as chest tightness, tingling, or excessive yawning or gasping for breath at times, he or he usually does not understand dysregulated patterns or why they occur. Over-breathing may develop as a conditioned fear response that occurs first at the time of trauma or it may occur later in life—for example, in latent PTSD. Asthma and PTSD are highly associated (Goodwin, Fischer, & Goldberg, 2007), and over-breathing commonly co-occurs with asthma, chronic bronchitis, and chronic laryngitis; indeed, these may be symptoms for many years before the causes are identified. Hyperventilation can occur without anxiety and anxiety can be caused by hyperventilation. In its chronic form, it is a conditioned behavior that responds to guided deconditioning, breathing retraining, and nutrition.

YOGA AND BREATHING

Pranayama exercises involve the alternation of breathing patterns to facilitate control of the ANS, brain hemispheric dominance, and thus states of consciousness, including mood. These methods may vary among different disciplines, including Hatha yoga, Kundalini yoga, and Kriya yoga; however, whatever discipline is used, the practice of pranayama leads to brain hemispheric synchrony in which neither hemisphere dominates but both function together. This contributes to trance states and integrated hypothalamic function (Rossi, 1986), the balanced state of healing. It is only dur-ing deep trance states or integrated right/left hemispheric function that both nostrils are fully open (Sansonese, 1994).

The nasal cycle marks physiological states. Greater airflow in the left nostril correlates with the resting phase, and greater airflow in the right nostril correlates with the activity phase. The hypo-thalamus integrates and regulates these two physiological states of rest and activity. With disruption of the HPA axis, the rest activity rhythms are also disrupted. This suggests that activities which reregulate these rhythms—such as specific breathing exercises associated with yogic pranayama, specifically forcing the breath through only one nostril—stimulate the contralateral hemisphere and ipsilateral sympathetic nervous system via the hypothalamus (Shannahoff-Khalsa, 2006). By ascertaining which hemisphere is dominant at any moment, we can also choose to change it through breathing exercises. By teaching these methods to clients, we can enable them to relax more easily or to focus attention. A more active left hemisphere is more conducive to intellectual activity. For example, lying on the left side of the body enhances intellectual or work-related activities. Lying on this side helps when people feel "spacey" or dissociated. Lying on the right side of the body opens the left nostril and hence activates the right side of the brain for inner work, creativity, relaxation, and sleep. Yoga breathing methods have shown significant efficacy for the treatment of PTSD and depression among people who experienced the 2004 Asian tsunami (Descilo et al., 2010).

The basic method of pranayama is taught in yoga classes and involves breathing through one nostril while holding the other closed.

Mind Body Assessment

Mental health clinicians do not routinely assess for physical symptoms; however, every effort should be made to assess for disordered breathing, especially where breathing retraining will be taught. Some of the signs of hyperventilation may be assessed while the therapist is sitting with clients and are obvious during the first session. These include repeated yawning, sighing or breath holding, irregular breathing cycles, noises related to breathing (Chaitow, Bradley, & Gilbert, 2002), and may also include complaints of not being able to take a deep breath or feeling tight in the chest. The inability to hold the breath for more than 30 seconds may be indicative of HVS; chronic hyperventi-lators can rarely hold the breath for more than 10 to 20 seconds (Chaitow et al., 2002). Speech may sound strained, particularly at the end of a sentence, which often cannot be finished without taking another breath, at which time in extreme cases gasping for breath or contraction of the vocal cords may be heard. Visually, clients may appear to take shallow breaths, have neck muscles that are tight, and have complaints of chronic fatigue or pain in the neck, particularly common in the trapezius and scalene muscles. The scalenes are respiratory accessory muscles and are often overused in people with both asthma and anxiety; shallow breathers benefit from stretching these muscles. The Nijmegen Scale (van Dixhoorn & Duivenvoorden, 1985) is a short survey that can be integrated into the initial intake to identify HVS and related symptoms.

Effective treatment of anxiety and disordered breathing incorporates the use of breathing exer-cises, cognitive-behavioral therapy, nutrition, and specific bodywork/massage techniques. Working with a professional to manually release the chronic contraction of the diaphragm and the acces-sory respiratory muscles such as the scalenes, sternocleidomastoid, and trapezius is very effective because it helps to make unconscious functional patterns conscious. Massage of these muscles also feels good, and the sense of pleasure where there had been pain reinforces the capacity to change and may enhance self-care compliance. Because HVS and anxiety always have a biochemical sub-strate, I address approaches to nutritional management (Korn, 2016). Breathing also has beneficial effects when done outdoors in the forest or next to moving bodies of water, like the sea or streams. A thousand years ago, the Greek physician Galen advised patients to breath by the sea to improve health. The positive effects of breathing at the ocean are believed to result from the high concen-trations of negative ions in the air. Air ions are either positively or negatively charged molecules surrounded by fewer than 10 water molecules (Fried & Grimaldi, 1993). Exposure to negative ions increases serotonin levels in the brain, which has a positive effect on mood, learning, performance, reaction time, and perception of pain (Fried & Grimaldi, 1993). Treatment with a high-density negative ionizer (and bright light) appears to act as a specific antidepressant for patients with major depression (Terman & Terman, 1995, 2005). Exposure to higher concentrations of negative air ions can be part of a holistic program for recovery.

DISSOCIATION

A traumatic event induces an altered state of consciousness called dissociation.

Dissociation at the time of a traumatic event appears to predispose a person to the development of PTSD, either subsequent to the event or later in life (Zatzick, Marmar, Weiss, & Metzler, 1993). Dissociation is defined as the disruption of the usually integrated functions of consciousness, memory, identity, sensorimotor control, and perception of the environment (Lewis-Fernández, 1994). It occurs as a natural protective response to trauma. Prolonged or repeated exposure to trauma creates lacunae in the fabric of consciousness, alters the construction of memory in response to the flood of neuropeptides and neurotransmitters, and adversely affects the healthy development and growth of the personality. Dissociation is part of a symptom matrix associated with PTSD. What is called somatization, self-injurious behavior, substance abuse, and eating disorders are really dissociative disorders.

Dissociation is a ubiquitous human capacity, varying by degree and manifestation, among people of all cultures. The experiences of dissociation occur along a continuum, ranging from absorption and imagination to the less common and more psychologically disruptive amnesia. Case studies of the dissociative disorders in the United States note histories of abuse in 72%–98% and 50%–75% of general psychiatric patients (Steinberg, 1994). Chu, Frey, Ganzel, and Matthews (1999) studied both the correlation between dissociation and early childhood sexual abuse and the corroboration of recovered memories, noting that elevated dissociative symptoms were correlated with early age of onset of physical and sexual abuse. They also found that the more frequent the sexual abuse, the more common partial or complete amnesia for the sexual abuse occurred.

Dissociative processes have both negative and positive effects on psychophysical health. Dissociation is linked to hypnosis, trance states, and metanormal experiences. However, it also has important distinguishing features. The similarities and differences of these various states of consciousness have implications for diagnosis and treatment. Gaining control over dissociative processes and finding a comfortable, person-specific zone of permeability between ego boundaries are two major tasks of treatment.

SOMATOFORM BEHAVIORS, EATING DISORDERS, AND SELF-INJURY

Persistent unresolved physical complaints for which there is no apparent cause form the backbone of physical medicine practice. Many of these symptoms are dissociative phenomena that manifest as chronic pain, somatization, self-injurious behavior, eating disorders, and other addictions. People who develop PTSD because of interpersonal trauma as children have higher rates of dissociation and affect dysregulation than do people traumatized as adults (van der Kolk, Roth, & Pelcovitz, 2005). The current concept of somatization (disorder) is rooted in what Freud called somatic compliance. This idea arose out of his observation that people with hysteria expressed physical symptoms of distress in a "language" that the psyche could not express in words. When the diagnostic category called hysteria was split into separate categories, the somatic symptoms of hysteria were termed conversion disorder: the conversion of psychological distress into physical symptoms. Chronic pain, headaches, and digestive and reproductive disorders are among the dominant modes of somatization in current traumatic nosology. This is understandable in the light of these organ systems' connections to autonomic innervation. Delineation and separation of these functions into psyche and soma, mind and body, is an artificial division. Somatization disorder is more appropriately classified as a trauma disorder. Increasingly, as the complexity of mind and body interrelationships is better understood, the somatization category will disappear and become integrated into a more comprehensive, interdisciplinary, and holistic approach that reflects the inseparability of mind and body. The association between PTSD, chronic pain, fibromyalgia, chronic fatigue, and depression is well documented (Raphael & Wilson, 1994). Most patients with fibromyalgia also have a significant history of early childhood stress or trauma. Fibromyalgia, like chronic fatigue syndrome, Gulf War syndrome, chemical sensitivity, and environmental illness is often considered a "somatized distorted belief" on the part of the patient or a displacement of trauma, much as hysteria was in the nineteenth century. For some individuals, other vague, multiorgan illnesses are a function of "belief," as Staudenmayer (1996) writes:

> Despite the significant therapeutic effort expended, some patients who are imprisoned by a closed belief system about the harmful effects of chemical sensitivities are resigned to travel down the path which ultimately leads to despair and depression, social isolation, and even death. (p. S100)

These are often the traumatized individuals who walk through our clinic door because no one has as yet either listened to or understood the causes of their multiple layers of illness. While dissociativity and somatization are both a response and a coping mechanism, they intersect with profound psychoneuroimmunological and hypothalamic–pituitary–adrenal axis dysfunction and together comediate the response that leads to illness complexes such as chemical sensitivity and other less than fully understood complaints. The chemicals or vaccines encountered in war and in the workplace of modern life serve as the "last straw" in which the HPA axis can no longer summon the energy to fight off yet another assault. Illness then progresses, especially when the liver can no longer detoxify, and the intestinal lumen can no longer prevent the passage of unmetabolized toxins into the bloodstream. Bell, Schwartz, Baldwin, and Hardin (1996) refer to this response as "neural sensitization," an autonomically mediated sensitivity to a variety of unrelated chemicals, drugs, alcohol, and stressors.

ADDICTION TO SURGERY

Because of living with chronic pain, the dissociated and traumatized client seeks out surgery, and when one surgery does not eliminate the pain, the surgeries multiply and the survivor is caught between needing help and the cultural imperative to cut. This can result in addiction to surgery.

CASE

Ruth described chronic, severe bulimia and self-injury that resulted in repeated hospitalizations. Severe pain in the region of her diaphragm led to several surgeries including removal of the gallbladder, a portion of her intestines, and several additional abdominal exploratory surgeries. She also experienced severe neck pain and had received several spinal fusions. Her surgeon began to believe that surgery might be a form of self-injury in her case, which precipitated his referral to me. When I began working with Ruth, I asked her what she felt would be helpful and what her goals were for treatment. She stated that she was considering gastric bypass surgery: she had already had her gallbladder removed and was planning plastic surgery to "tuck" the extra skin. Ruth requested that we do body-oriented psychotherapy, which would integrate touch and talk; she asked me to work in the central area of her body to release the tension in her diaphragm, which was, she said: "tight as piano wires." I gently applied pressure under her rib cage directly into the area of pain as she breathed deeply. As we worked, she had clear images of early life experiences when she felt terrified. During some of these sessions, she experienced some hyperarousal in response to the touch therapy, leading to both new and intensified memories of sexual abuse. We went slowly and gently, processing as we went along. During other sessions, she experienced deep relaxation, saying, "I haven't relaxed this much since I gave up recreational drugs. I didn't know it was possible." After five 1-hour sessions, Ruth said that her physical pain had decreased by 50%, but her memories felt overwhelming and interfered with her ability to work. She decided to take a break from the bodywork segments of our work together, and we spent several weeks discussing her memories and bolstering her self-care and self-regulation strategies through breathing and stretching. Ruth was able to release a lot of physical pain and to clarify somatic memories, which had previously seemed to her "like a dream" and prevented her from fully acknowledging the violence that had occurred in her early life.

Ruth's addiction to surgery is a form of self-harm or self-injury, and in this particular form the medical profession (often unwittingly) participates. People with chronic pain and depression are often desperate and seek help, care, and touch, to "cut the problem out." Self-injury, bingeing, purging, chronic pain, spinal fusions, and the (multiple) removal of organs are all efforts to express, eradicate, or at least endure the anxious speech of the body. These are cries for affiliation, for contact and communication with the first ego, in its own language of touch and holding. This protest against separation is the relentless nightmare of "borderline" patients. The cry goes unanswered as long as medicine withholds help. Injury through surgery allows the patient intimate contact with a healer. Surgeons cut, go inside, and (try to) make it right; for a sexual trauma survivor these surgeries may represent a reenactment of penetration. Rarely do the results address the underlying problem, and often they create additional, iatrogenic problems. How many sexual abuse survivors undergo gastric bypass surgery? How many of these individuals have psychiatric admissions postsurgery (Clark et al., 2007)?

How many people who have elective plastic surgery or liposuction have a history of trauma? Self-injury and addiction to surgery are included in criteria for the diagnosis of borderline personality disorder. There is a significant nonclinical or nonpsychiatric population who also self-injure, such as people who obtain tattoos and pierce their bodies.

There can be a tendency among health professionals to blame the victim. One otherwise sensitive writer notes "some patients 'trick' physicians and dentists into performing unnecessary surgery" (Favazza, 1987, p. 97). I believe that what occurs is not the trickery of patients but the failure of the professional to decipher the patient's story to truly address her or his needs along with the willingness of some surgeons to perform unnecessary surgery.

Since many of these clinicians are not trained to recognize the relationship among these symptoms and trauma and dissociation, this provides an opportunity for the therapist to educate the medical professional and facilitate a team approach. Surgery for chronic pain most often does not work simply because the trauma cannot be cut out. However, the alliance Ruth and I developed along with predesignated cues we agreed on allowed her to signal whether she wished to continue or end the session, and this provided a safety net for her. She was able to take the memories of her experiences and her feelings back into verbal psychotherapy to address them productively. At our last meeting, she said she felt proud and courageous and that she had caught a glimpse of her future—of reconnecting with her body and the pleasure and relaxation she would once again experience. She chose not to go ahead with surgery but to wait while she fully explored her other options.

Psychological trauma underlies extensive psychological and somatic distress. Substance abuse, self-injurious behaviors, chronic pain, mitochondrial dysfunction, autoimmune disease, insomnia, eating disorders, depression, anxiety, and hyperventilation are among the symptoms that co-occur at high rates among people who have experienced early life adversity, complex trauma, and PTSD. Effective treatment for individuals and families experiencing these complex disorders requires a tailored approach to everyone's needs that includes both somatic and psychological integration to help restore well-being.

REFERENCES

Back, S. E., Sonne, S. C., Killeen, T., Dansky, B. S., & Brady, K. T. 2003. Comparative profiles of women with PTSD and comorbid cocaine or alcohol dependence. *American Journal of Drug and Alcohol Abuse*, 29(1), 169–89.

Bell, I. R., Schwartz, G. E., Baldwin, C. M., & Hardin, E. E. 1996. Neural sensitization and physiological markers in multiple chemical sensitivity. *Regulatory Toxicology and Pharmacology*, 24(1 Pt 2), S39–S47.

Booth, B., Mengeling, M. A., Torner, J., & Sadler, A. G. 2011. Rape, sex partnership, and substance use consequences in women veterans. *Journal of Traumatic Stress*, 24(3), 287–294.

Boscarino, J. A. 2004. Posttraumatic stress disorder and physical illness: Results from clinical and epidemiologic studies. *Annals of the New York Academy of Sciences*, 1032, 141–153.

Brave Heart, M. Y. H., & DeBruyn, L. M. 1998. The American Indian holocaust: Healing historical unresolved grief. *American Indian and Alaskan Native Mental Health Research: The Journal of the National Center*, 8(2), 60–82.

Bremner, J. D., Southwick, S. M., & Charney, D. S. 1991. Animal models for the neurobiology of trauma. *PTSD Research Quarterly*, 2(4), 1–7.

Buchanan, T. W., Kern, S., Allen, J. S., Tranel, D., & Kirschbaum, C. 2004. Circadian regulation of cortisol after hippocampal damage in humans. *Biological Psychiatry*, 56(9), 651–656.

Carter, C. S., Ahnert, L., Grossmann, K., Hrdy, S. B., Lamb, M., Porges, S. W., & Sachser, N. (Eds.). 2005. *Attachment and Bonding: A New Synthesis*. Cambridge: MIT Press.

Chaitow, L., Bradley, D., & Gilbert, C. 2002. *Multidisciplinary Approaches to Breathing Pattern Disorders*. New York: Churchill Livingstone.

Chu, J. A., Frey, L. M., Ganzel, B. L., & Matthews, J. A. 1999. Memories of childhood abuse: Dissociation, amnesia, and corroboration. *American Journal of Psychiatry*, 156(5), 749–755.

Clark, M. M., Hanna, B. K., Mai, J. L., Graszer, K. M., Krochta, J. G., McAlpine, D. E., ... Sarr, M. G. 2007. Sexual abuse survivors and psychiatric hospitalization after bariatric surgery. *Obesity Surgery*, 17(4), 465–469.

Cohen, S. 1994. Psychosocial influences on immunity and infectious disease in humans. In R. Glaser & J. K. Kiecolt-Glaser (Eds.), *Handbook of Human Stress and Immunity* (pp. 301–319). San Diego, CA: Academic Press.

Descilo, T., Vedamurtachar, A., Gerbarg, P. L., Nagaraja, D., Gangadhar, B. N., Damodaran, B., ... Brown, R. P. 2010. Effects of a yoga breath intervention alone and in combination with an exposure therapy for post-traumatic stress disorder and depression in survivors of the 2004 South-East Asia tsunami. *Acta Psychiatrica Scandinavica*, 121(4), 289–300. doi: 10.1111/j.1600-0447.2009.01466.x

Didie, E. R., Tortolani, C. C., Pope, C. G., Menard, W., Fay, C., & Phillips, K. A. 2006. Childhood abuse and neglect in body dysmorphic disorder. *Abuse & Neglect*, 30(10), 1105–1115.

Evans, J. 1986. *Mind, Body and Electromagnetics*. Longmead, Great Britain: Element Books.

Favazza, A. R. 1987. *Bodies Under Siege: Self-Mutilation in Culture and Psychiatry*. Baltimore, MD: Johns Hopkins University Press.

Feinstein, A., & Botes, M. 2009. The psychological health of contractors working in war zones. *Journal of Traumatic Stress*, 22(2), 102–105.

Fried, R., & Grimaldi, J. 1993. *The Psychology and Physiology of Breathing in Behavioral Medicine, Clinical Psychology, and Psychiatry*. New York: Plenum.

Gagne, M. 1998. The role of dependency and colonialism in generating trauma in First Nations citizens: The James Bay Cree. In Y. Danieli (Ed.), *International Handbook of Multigenerational Legacies of Trauma: Group Project for Holocaust Survivors and Their Children* (pp. 355–372). New York: Plenum.

Goldstein, B. D., Osofsky, H. J., & Lichtveld, M. Y. 2011. The Gulf oil spill. *The New England Journal of Medicine*, 364(14), 1334–1348.

Goodwin, R. D., Fischer, M. E., & Goldberg, J. 2007. A twin study of post–traumatic stress disorder symptoms and asthma. *American Journal of Respiratory and Critical Care Medicine*, 176(10), 983–987.

Gunnar, M. R., & Donzella, B. 2002. Social regulation of the cortisol levels in early human development. *Psychoneuroendocrinology*, 27(1–2), 199–220.

Hoffman, L., Burges-Watson, P., Wilson, G., & Montgomery, J. 1989. Low plasma B endorphin in PTSD. *Australian and New Zealand Journal of Psychiatry*, 23(2), 269–273.

IsHak, W. W., Kahloon, M., & Fakhry, H. 2011. Oxytocin role in enhancing wellbeing: A literature review. *Journal of Affective Disorders*, 130(1–2), 1–9.

Kiecolt-Glaser, J. K., Malarkey, W. B., Cacioppo, J. T., & Glaser, R. 1994. Stressful personal relationships: Immune and endocrine function. In R. Glaser & J. K. Kiecolt-Glaser (Eds.), *Handbook of Human Stress and Immunity* (pp. 321–339). San Diego, CA: Academic Press.

Korn, L. 2016. *Nutrition Essentials for Mental Health: A Complete Guide to the Food-Mood Connection*. New York, NY: W. W. Norton and Company.

Korn, L., & Rÿser, R. 2006. Burying the umbilicus: Nutrition trauma, diabetes and traditional medicine in rural West Mexico. In G. C. Lang (Ed.), *Indigenous Peoples and Diabetes: Community Empowerment and Wellness* (pp. 231–277). Durham, NC: Carolina Academic Press.

Lewis-Fernández, R. 1994. Culture and dissociation: A comparison of ataque de nervios among Puerto Ricans and possession syndrome in India. In D. Spiegel (Ed.), *Dissociation: Culture, Mind, and Body* (pp. 123–167). Washington, DC: American Psychiatric Press.

Machoian, L. 2006. *The Disappearing Girl: Learning the Language of Teenage Depression*. New York: Penguin.

McEwen, B. S. 2000. The neurobiology of stress: From serendipity to clinical relevance. *Brain Research*, 886(1–2), 172–189.

McEwen, B. S., & Seeman, T. 1999. Protective and damaging effects of mediators of stress: Elaborating and testing the concepts of allostasis and allostatic load. *Annals of the New York Academy of Sciences*, 896, 30–47.

Nadler, A., Kav-Venaki, S., & Gleitman, B. 1985. Transgenerational effects of the holocaust: Externalization of aggression in second generation holocaust survivors. *Journal of Consulting & Clinical Psychology*, 53(3), 365–369.

Nixon, M. K., Cheng, M., & Cloutier, P. 2003. An open trial of auricular acupuncture for the treatment of repetitive self-injury in depressed adolescents. *Canadian Child and Adolescent Psychiatry Review*, 12(1), 10–12.

Olff, M., Langeland, W., Witteveen, A., & Denys, D. 2010. A psychobiological rationale for oxytocin in the treatment of posttraumatic stress disorder. *CNS Spectrums*, 15(8), 522–530.

Pace, T. W., & Heim, C. M. 2011. A short review on the psychoneuroimmunology of posttraumatic stress disorder: From risk factors to medical comorbidities. *Brain Behavior and Immunity*, 25(1), 6–13.

Papadopoulos-Lane, C. A. 2010. Cognitive appraisals, stress, and emotion about environmental contamination in the Akwesasne Mohawk Nation [*Doctoral dissertation*]. Albany, NY: State University of New York.

Porges, S. W. 2011. *The Polyvagal Theory: Neurophysiological Foundations of Emotions, Attachment, Communication, and Self-Regulation*. New York: Norton.

Raphael, B., & Wilson, J. P. 1994. When disaster strikes: Managing emotional reactions in rescue workers. In J. P. Wilson & J. D. Lindy (Eds.), *Countertransference in the Treatment of PTSD* (pp. 333–350). New York: Guilford.

Rossi, E. L. 1986. *The Psychobiology of Mind-Body Healing: New Concepts of Therapeutic Hypnosis*. New York: Norton.

Rossi, E. L. 1999. Sleep, dream, hypnosis and healing: Behavioral state related gene expression and psychotherapy. *Sleep and Hypnosis: An International Journal of Sleep, Dream, and Hypnosis*, 1(3), 141–157.

Russo, E. B. 2008. Clinical endocannabinoid deficiency (CECD): Can this concept explain therapeutic benefits of cannabis in migraine, fibromyalgia, irritable bowel syndrome and other treatment-resistant conditions? *Neuroendocrinology Letters*, 29(2), 192–200.

Sack, W. H., Clarke, G. N., & Seeley, J. 1995. Posttraumatic stress disorder across two generations of Cambodian refugees. *Journal of the American Academy of Child and Adolescent Psychiatry*, 34(9), 1160–1166.

Sansonese, J. N. 1994. *The Body of Myth: Mythology, Shamanic Trance, and the Sacred Geography of the Body*. Rochester, VT: Inner Traditions International.

Sartor, C. E., McCutcheon, V. V., Pommer, N. E., Nelson, E. C., Duncan, A. E., Waldron, M., ... Heath, A. C. 2010. Posttraumatic stress disorder and alcohol dependence in young women. *Journal of Studies on Alcohol and Drugs*, 71(6), 810–818.

Scaer, R. C. 2001. *The Body Bears the Burden: Trauma, Dissociation, and Disease*. Binghamton: Haworth.

Scaer, R. C. 2011. The whiplash syndrome: A model of traumatic stress. *Journal of Cognitive Rehabilitation*, 18(4), 6–15.

Schore, A. 2003. *Affect Regulation and the Repair of the Self*. New York: Norton.

Seeman, T. E., Crimmins, E., Huang, M. H., Singer, B., Bucur, A., Gruenewald, T., ... Reuben, D. B. 2004. Cumulative biological risk and socio-economic differences in mortality: MacArthur studies of successful aging. *Social Science & Medicine*, 58(10), 1985–1997.

Seligman, M. E. P., & Beagley, G. 1975. Learned helplessness in the rat. *Journal of Comparative and Physiological Psychology*, 88(2), 534–541.

Shannahoff-Khalsa, D. S. 2006. *Kundalini Yoga Meditation: Techniques Specific for Psychiatric Disorders, Couples Therapy, and Personal Growth*. New York: Norton.

Staudenmayer, H. 1996. Clinical consequences of the EI/MCS "diagnosis": Two paths. *Regulatory Toxicology and Pharmacology*, 24(1), S96–S110.

Steinberg, M. 1994. Systematizing dissociation: Symptomatology and diagnostic assessment. In D. Spiegel (Ed.), *Dissociation: Culture, Mind, and Body* (pp. 59–88). Washington, DC: American Psychiatric Press.

Strickland, C. J., Walsh, E., & Cooper, M. 2006. Healing fractured families: Parents' and elders' perspectives on the impact of colonization and youth suicide prevention in a Pacific Northwest American Indian tribe. *Journal of Transcultural Nursing*, 17(1), 5–12.

Taylor, S. E., Klein, L. C., Lewis, B. P., Gruenewald, T. L., Gurung, R. A. R., & Updegraff, J. A. 2000. Biobehavioral responses to stress in females: Tend-and-befriend, not fight-or-flight. *Psychological Review*, 107(3), 411–429.

Terman, M., & Terman, J. S. 1995. Treatment of seasonal affective disorder with a high-output negative ionizer. *Journal of Alternative and Complementary Medicine*, 1(1), 87–92.

Terman, M., & Terman, J. S. 2005. Light therapy for seasonal and nonseasonal depression: Efficacy, protocol, safety, and side effects. *CNS Spectrums*, 10(8), 647–663.

Tiefenbacher, S., Novak, M. A., Lutz, C. K., & Meyer, J. S. 2005. The physiology and neurochemistry of self-injurious behavior: A nonhuman primate model. *Frontiers in Bioscience*, 10, 1–11.

van der Kolk, B. A., Roth, S., & Pelcovitz, D. 2005. Disorders of extreme stress: The empirical foundation of a complex adaptation to trauma. *Journal of Traumatic Stress*, 18(5), 389–399.

van Dixhoorn, J., & Duivenvoorden, H. J. 1985. Efficacy of Nijmegen Questionnaire in recognition of the hyperventilation syndrome. *Journal of Psychosomatic Research*, 29(2), 199–206.

Villalba, V., & Harrington, C. 2003. Repetitive self–injurious behavior: The emerging potential of psychotropic intervention. *Psychiatric Times*, 20(2). Retrieved from http://www.psychiatrictimes.com/show-Article.jhtml?articleID=175802309

Whitbeck, L. B., Adams, G. W., Hoyt, D. R., & Chen, X. 2004. Conceptualizing and measuring historical trauma among American Indian people. *American Journal of Community Psychology*, 33(3–4), 119–130.

Yehuda, R., Engel, S. M., Brand, S. R., Seckl, J., Marcus, S. M., & Berkowitz, G. S. 2005. Transgenerational effects of posttraumatic stress disorder in babies of mothers exposed to the World Trade Center attacks during pregnancy. *Journal of Clinical Endocrinology & Metabolism* 90(7), 4115–4118.

Yehuda, R., Schmeidler, J., Elkin, A., Houshmand, E., Siever, L., Binder-Brynes, K., … Yang, R.K. 1998. Phenomenology and psychobiology of the intergenerational response to trauma. In Y. Danieli (Ed.), *Intergenerational Handbook of the Multigenerational Legacies of Trauma* (pp. 639–655). New York: Plenum.

Zatzick, D., Marmar, C., Weiss, D., & Metzler, T. 1993. Does trauma-linked dissociation vary across ethnic groups? *Journal of Nervous and Mental Disease*, 182(10), 576–582.

26 Anti-Aging and Regenerative Medicine

Adonis Maiquez

CONTENTS

Introduction 610
   Definition 610
   Definitions for Different Communities 610
      Anti-Aging for Scientific Community 610
      Anti-Aging for Medical and Reputable Business Community 610
      Anti-Aging for Business Community 610
   Anti-Aging versus Function Preservation 611
   Anti-Aging from a Functional Medicine Approach 611
   Current Research 611
      Calorie Restriction (CR) 611
      Orthomolecular Medicine 612
      Anti-Oxidants 612
      Plasmapheresis 613
History of Anti-Aging 613
   Blue Zones 613
   The Nine Common Traits of all Centenarians' Communities 614
      Move Naturally 614
      Purpose 614
      Down Shift 614
      80% Rule 614
      Plant Slant 614
      Wine @ 5 614
      Belong 614
      Loved Ones First 615
      Right Tribe 615
   Theories of Aging 615
      Short Overview of the History of the Theories of Aging 615
   Classification of Aging Theories 616
      Programmed Theories 616
      Programmed Longevity 616
      Neuro-Endocrine Theory 616
      Immunological Theory 617
      Damage Theories 617
      Wear and Tear Theories 617
      Oxidative Stress Theory of Aging/Free Radical Theory of Aging 617
      Inflammation-Based Theories 618
      Glycation 618
      Energy Metabolism and Aging 618
      Telomere Shortening 619

Other Theories—The Multi-Factorial Approach 619
Anti-Aging Interventions 620
Lifestyle Interventions 620
Nutrition/Foods 624
Nutraceuticals/Medications 624
Coenzyme Q10 625
Procedures 626
Addressing the Causes of Pre-Mature Death: Chronic Diseases 629
Kegel for Urinary Incontinence 630
Specific Exercises for Osteoporosis 630
Herbs for Diabetes Mellitus (DM) 630
Male Exercises for Prostate 630
Variety in Vegetables and Fruits 631
The Future of Anti-Aging 631
Epigenetics Influencers on Aging Genes 631
Genetic Therapy and Gene Manipulation 632
Heterochronic Plasma Exchange (HPE) 632
Tissue/Organ Cloning 632
Nanotechnology 632
Biomarkers of Aging (Detrimental Manifestation of Aging) 632
Summary 633
References 633

INTRODUCTION

DEFINITION

From time immemorial, the one thing that has kept humankind going is a quest for survival, a quest to increase the lifespan, the health span. Survival or anti-aging are but two sides of the same coin. However, anti-aging has diverse meanings and connotations for different groups. It is a blend of biotechnology and advanced clinical preventive medicine.

DEFINITIONS FOR DIFFERENT COMMUNITIES

Anti-Aging for Scientific Community

For the scientific community, anti-aging research refers to slowing and preventing, or reversing the process of aging. Although the future seems to be promising, currently there is no proven and available medical technology or therapy that slows or reverses aging in humans. The practice of calorie restriction and regular exercise is being assessed by the jury.

Anti-Aging for Medical and Reputable Business Community

In this community, anti-aging medicine refers to the detection, prevention, and treatment of age-related diseases. This differs from reducing the aging process itself. Several strategies and therapies are currently available, such as calorie restriction which is beneficial in lowering the risk of a wide range of age-related diseases.

Anti-Aging for Business Community

For the business community (which includes a great many fraudulent ventures), anti-aging is a valuable brand and a way to increase sales of their products. This has no bearing on how healthy you actually are or how long you live, and many of these products do not achieve the results claimed by them.

The real confusion lies between the first two connotations mentioned above: treating aging versus treating the disease of aging itself. Medical interventions can increase an individual's lifespan by preventing or curing age-related conditions that would otherwise prove fatal, thereby shortening life. For example, therapy for preventing heart disease or type 2 diabetes would help many people live relatively longer and healthier lives, but might have no effect on aging. There is conflict between the views of different groups whether this is anti-aging research. Some medical and business groups agree to it whereas scientists disagree. Is this anti-aging research? Scientists say no (Fightaging 2013, Hudziak, Schlessinger, and Ullrich, 1987).

ANTI-AGING VERSUS FUNCTION PRESERVATION

As discussed above, anti-aging has different definitions for different communities. Function preservation essentially means preserving the functions of a living thing and preventing it from declining into dysfunction. Though both terms seem to be similar, they both emphasize prevention of organs, organ systems, and organisms to dysfunction. However, there is a big difference in their mechanism. Anti-aging refers to slowing the process of aging where the organs deteriorate, but at a slower pace. In the case of function preservation, the functioning ability of organs is preserved or conserved without affecting the process of aging.

ANTI-AGING FROM A FUNCTIONAL MEDICINE APPROACH

Anti-aging medicine aims at slowing or reversing aging so as to extend the lifespan using various therapeutic interventions which include aesthetic medicine, bio-identical hormones, cosmetics and cosmeceuticals, complementary and alternative medical (CAM) therapies, nanotechnology, dietary supplements and herbal medicine, nutrition, physical fitness and lifestyle therapies, stem cell therapy, and traditional oriental medicine (Ciolac 2013b, Cousens 2009, Grossman 2005a, Heilbronn and Ravussin 2003, Kuhla et al. 2016, Liu et al. 2013b).

On the other hand, functional medicine is a science-based approach for treating the underlying causes of disease rather than treatment of symptoms. It implies a systems-oriented approach and engages both practitioner and patient in a therapeutic partnership. Functional medicine reviews interactions among environmental factors (environmental medicine), lifestyle factors, and genetic factors. Functional medicine considers the complex interaction between genes and environment and offers individualized therapies designed to restore balance, health, and improve function.

CURRENT RESEARCH

No therapy has yet been approved that can delay the aging process in humans. However, certain therapies have been able to delay some effects of aging. For example, avoiding skin exposure to the sun's ultraviolet (UV) rays can slow down skin's aging process, regular exercise can prolong lifespan. We will discuss the current therapies or diets being studied across the world.

Calorie Restriction (CR)

Extended lifespan with CR retards age-related chronic diseases in a variety of species, including mice, rats, fish worms, flies, and yeast; however, the mechanism causing the same is unclear. CR is known to reduce metabolic rate and oxidative stress, alters neuroendocrine signals and the sympathetic nervous system functioning, and improves insulin sensitivity in animals. Whether CR actually extends the lifespan in humans or improves biomarkers of aging is not known. The experiments involving humans conducted to date gave poor quality diet. Thus, there is lack of data on the effect of calorie-restricted diets of a good quality in non-obese humans. Further studies in non-obese humans aim at evaluating the effects of prolonged CR on metabolic rate, diverse biomarkers of aging, neuroendocrine adaptations, and predictors of chronic age-related diseases (Heilbronn and Ravussin 2003).

Orthomolecular Medicine

Orthomolecular medicine is the administration of adequate amounts of substances that are normally present in the body for the restoration and maintenance of health. This definition of orthomolecular medicine was given by Linus Pauling, Nobel Prize winner, who was one of the leading molecular chemists of the century in 1968. Orthomolecular therapy in addition to the treatment of health problems also focuses on reversing or slowing down the effect of factors which accelerate the aging process including frequent or chronic inflammation, free radical exposure, and toxic exposures (such as to industrial and agricultural hydrocarbons or heavy metals).

Several supplements that have been used as a part of medical therapy include coenzyme Q10, vitamins C and E, chromium, L-carnitine, alpha-lipoic acid, and quercetin. Several studies have confirmed the beneficial results of these supplements in cardiovascular disease, diabetes, congestive heart failure, hypertension, age-related deterioration of immune function, brain function, and vision as well as many other age-related health problems (Janson 2006).

Anti-Oxidants

A natural amino acid, carnosine, is a potent anti-oxidant. Recent studies have shown its benefits as an anti-aging agent. Carnosine possesses an ability to prevent glycosylation. Glycosylation is the cross linking of proteins with DNA molecules caused by sugar aldehydes that react with the amino acids on the proteins and form advance glycosylation end-products (AGEs). The anti-glycosylation potency of carnosine may be beneficial for cataracts, diabetes, neuropathy, skin conditions, and kidney failure (Kyriazis). Figure 26.1 shows that it possesses anti-oxidant properties, anti-neoplastic properties, wound healing properties, acts as an immune booster, and reduces gastric ulceration (Boldyrev 1993, Gariballa and Sinclair 2000).

In the lab, carnosine has been confirmed to increase longevity of human fibroblast cells, and might be a supplement of choice for longevity. It is used in an eye-drop form in Russia to treat

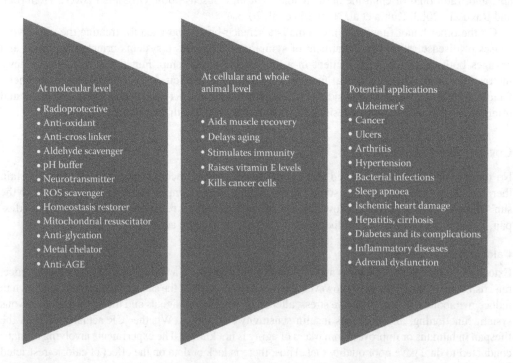

FIGURE 26.1 Mechanism of action and potential uses of carnosine. (Recreated from Hipkiss, A. R. 1998. Carnosine, a protective, anti-ageing peptide?. *The International Journal of Biochemistry & Cell Biology*, 30(8): 863–868.)

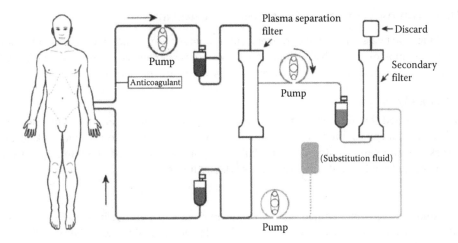

FIGURE 26.2 Plasmapheresis treatment. (Adapted from https://www.intechopen.com/books/understanding-the-complexities-of-kidney-transplantation/abo-incompatible-kidney-transplantation.)

glaucoma and has shown considerable success. It is thought that carnosine may possess important anti-aging eye functions. Carnosine supplement dosage of 50–100 mg per day is reported to be free of any side effects to date (Kyriazis).

Plasmapheresis

This procedure is being used to treat diseases in which metabolic waste starts to accumulate in the plasma (such as antibodies). It is already known that the blood transmits signals (hormones) for activities that need to be accomplished by different tissues. Harold Katcher, a professor of Biology at the University of Maryland, believed that the signals for aging of the tissues in old people are also transmitted by the blood. Plasmapheresis can be used to treat various age-related diseases by performing a heterochronic plasma exchange between young and old humans or other mammals. Experimental evidences supporting this procedure have already been established (Programmed-aging 2015). Plasmapheresis treatment has been depicted in Figure 26.2.

HISTORY OF ANTI-AGING

Research on human aging is aimed at finding a way to reduce the rate of morbidity and mortality in the elder population (Lonergan 1991). However, the majority of research being done involved dominant groups or mainstream people. The Baltimore Longitudinal Study of Aging (BLSA) initiated in 1958 had subjects that were white male, belonging to the upper middle class. No women were included in this study. The cross-sectional studies in the past would compare two groups with different characteristics such as older adults with college students, and very few studies include a single diverse group. However, it is worth noting that we need to include diverse groups in studies as they would affect the whole research results (Mehrotra and Wagner 2013).

BLUE ZONES

Blue zones are places in the world where people live healthier and longer than anywhere else on the Earth. Several Blue Zones exist on Earth where people with ages 90, or even 100 years are common. Along with a prolonged lifespan, these people appear to be living a very healthy life—without disability or medication. To date, five Blue Zones have been identified, and they are: the Italian island of Sardinia, Loma Linda (California), Okinawa (Japan), Ikaria (an isolated Greek island), and Nicoya Peninsula in Costa Rica (Barclay 2015).

THE NINE COMMON TRAITS OF ALL CENTENARIANS' COMMUNITIES

A team of medical researchers, demographers, anthropologists, and epidemiologists worked together to find out common evidence-based characteristics of these centenarian communities. They found nine characteristics shared by all these communities which are as follows.

Move Naturally

This trait suggested that the centenarians in blue zones don't pump iron, join gyms, or run marathons. They live in environments that constantly stimulate them to move without thinking about it. They work, nurture gardens, and do other daily living activities on their own to stay active. They don't have technology-based devices for yard work and house.

Purpose

Multiple studies have demonstrated that knowing your sense of purpose increases your lifespan by around seven years. The Nicoyans call it "plan de vida" and the Okinawans call it "Ikigai," which means, "why I wake up in the morning" (Buettner and Skemp 2016). Patricia Boyle, a researcher working on the "Rush Memory and Aging Project" at Rush University Medical Center, found that having a life purpose greatly reduces the risk of Alzheimer's and several other cognitive degenerative diseases (Bennett et al. 2012).

Down Shift

Even people living in the Blue Zones are affected with stress. Stress contributes to chronic inflammation which is known to be associated with major age-related disease. The people in Blue Zones have ways to shed the stress that they pursue routinely. For example, Okinawans remember their ancestors for a few moments each day, Sardinians do happy hour, Adventists pray, and Ikarians take a nap (Buettner and Skemp 2016).

80% Rule

The Okinawans have a rule of chanting a mantra "Hara hachi bu," which helps them memorize that when their stomachs are 80% full, they will quit eating. This 2500-year old Confucian mantra is chanted prior to meals. The 20% gap between not being hungry and feeling full helps them to take up less calories and thus gain less weight. These people have their smallest meal either in the late afternoon or early evening and then they don't eat anything else in the whole day (Babauta 2008).

Plant Slant

Beans, including black, fava, lentils, and soy are major consumptions by these centenarians. Meat (usually pork) is eaten on average only five times in a month. Serving sizes are 3–4 oz., about the size of a deck of cards (Barclay 2015).

Wine @ 5

People in all Blue Zones (except Adventists) are known to drink alcohol moderately and regularly. Moderate drinkers are known to live longer in comparison to non-drinkers. Usually, 1–2 glasses per day (mostly Sardinian Cannonau wine) is consumed with friends and/or with food (Barclay 2015).

Belong

Of the 263 centenarians interviewed, 5 belonged to some faith-based community. Denomination doesn't seem to matter. Research demonstrated that attending faith-based services four times in a month increases life expectancy by 4–14 years.

Loved Ones First

The centenarians in the Blue Zones were observed to put their families first, which means they keep their aging parents and grandparents in the same home or nearby, and this lowers disease and mortality rates of children in the home. Commitment to a life partner adds up to 3 years of life expectancy and they invest in their children both time and love.

Right Tribe

The research showed that the longest-lived people prefer to live or are born into social circles that follow healthy behaviors. Okinawans have a tradition to create "moais," which refers to groups of five friends who commit to provide any kind of help (emotional, financial) to each other for life. Research from the Framingham Studies showed that smoking, happiness, obesity, and even loneliness are contagious. The social networks of these long-lived people have shaped their health behaviors.

Most of the people have the capacity to make it well into their early 90s and that too without chronic disease. The Adventists reported that adopting a Blue Zone lifestyle can increase the average person's life expectancy by 10–12 years (Buettner 2014).

THEORIES OF AGING

Short Overview of the History of the Theories of Aging

The history of theories behind aging dates back to the nineteenth century when Darwin in 1859 proposed an evolutionary mechanics theory according to which "force of evolutionary selection is toward the longest possible lifespan and maximal reproductive capacity, that is, immortality." Whereas, the critics noted that the actual observation of limited lifespan varied from one species to another whereas according to Darwin's concept, natural selection favors individuals with maximal survival and reproductive capacity. To this criticism Darwin suggested that limited lifespan might offer an unknown benefit, but did not specify what it is.

In 1892, a programmed death theory was proposed by Weismann stating that the deaths of old individuals are beneficial for young individuals as it provides them space (Weismann 1891). Carrel in 1913 mentioned that Weismann's theory is unacceptable since cultivation of cell *in vitro* multiplied an unlimited number of times (Carrel 1913). Later in 1945, came the Modern Synthesis and neo-Darwinism codified traditional mechanics theory.

In the 1950s, theorists suggested that the evolutionary process has a neutral effect on aging and that Darwin's theory of survival of the fittest is only applicable to the young generation (http://www.programmed-aging.org/aging-theory-summary.html).

"Mutation accumulation theory" (1952) was based on Medawar's hypothesis and proposed that aging occurred due to random mutations which further lead to adverse aging characteristics (http://www.programmed-aging.org/theories/mutation_accumulation.html). William's (1957) theory called "Antagonistic pleiotropy theory" proposed that the combined effect of many pleiotropic genes leads to aging. Although, these genes had a beneficial effect when an animal is young, but leads to adverse effects in older age (http://www.programmed-aging.org/theories/antagonistic_pleiotropy.html).

In the early 1960s, two evolutionary mechanics theories were proposed. The British zoologist Vero Wynne-Edwards gave the "Group selection mechanics theory," suggesting that the behaviors that improved group survival could evolve despite an individual disadvantage (Wynne-Edwards 1986). Hamilton proposed the theory of "Kin selection" (Hamilton 1970). The list does not end here; the wide interest among the researchers to understand the process of aging has led to many other theories which will be discussed later in this chapter.

CLASSIFICATION OF AGING THEORIES

The traditional theories referred to as "non-programmed/non-adaptive" or "passive" theories contend that aging does not serve a valid "selectable" evolutionary purpose. Thus, no mechanism exists whose primary purpose is to cause aging or otherwise purposely limit lifespan, at least not in mammals. These theories suggested that aging is an unavoidable adverse side effect of some biological function in older age which is useful in young age. The other reason could be that organisms do not have an evolutionary need to live longer than some species-specific lifespan and therefore did not develop or lost the maintenance and repair capabilities needed for living longer. According to this concept, a lifespan longer than a species-specific value does not impose any disadvantage at all and gives little benefit (http://www.programmed-aging.org/theories/aging_theory_controversy.html).

The modern theories of biological aging in humans as well as others have been classified into two categories. They are Programmed Theories and Damage Theories.

Programmed Theories

Programmed theories are also known as adaptive or active theories. These theories imply that reproduction, aging, and death of an organism are all genetically programmed and follow a preset biological timetable. According to these theories, aging and limited lifespan serve an essential evolutionary purpose. Similar to the other biological functions, aging might be regulated by a complex system involving hormones, signaling, genes, sensing of external conditions, and other characteristics. According to this concept, a lifespan longer than the species-specific value is disadvantageous, thus produced evolutionary motivation to develop the aging aimed at purposely limiting the life span (http://www.bioidenticalhormonemd.com/anti-aging-functional-preventative-medicine.html). The programmed theories have been further divided into three sub-categories: Programmed Longevity, Endocrine Theory, and Immunological Theory.

Programmed Longevity

This theory of aging implies that aging is caused by sequential switching "on and off" of certain genes and shortening of telomeres throughout the lifetime, and that senescence is defined as the time when age-associated deficits are manifested (Jin 2010). The number of divisions of somatic cells are predetermined, after which the cells will not be able to replicate, which in turn will trigger apoptosis (cell death). The theory gained importance when Leonard Hayflick in 1961 found that normal human cells possess a finite capacity of cell divisions in tissue culture and then cease. He found that fetal cells replicate around 100 times whereas cells taken from a 70-year-old stopped replicating after only 20–30 divisions. This maximum number of divisions is referred as the "Hayflick Limit." However, when cancerous cells from a woman named Henrietta Lacks were cultured, they were found to replicate indefinitely and survive to this date, and were named "HeLa cells." Similarly, embryonic stem cells also have the potential to multiply indefinitely. Thus, the Hayflick concept of definite replication only applies to normal cells and excludes cancerous and embryonic stem cells (Shay and Wright 2000).

Neuro-Endocrine Theory

Biological clocks act through change in hormone secretions of the hypothalamic-pituitary feedback system to control the pace of aging. Changes in the endocrine glands (thyroid and adrenal glands), ovaries, and testes result in decline in the functional capacity of the person (Jin 2010). Zjačić-Rotkvić et al. in their review discuss how the neuroendocrine theory proposed by Dilman and Dean can be applied to the process of aging (Dilman and Dean 1992). Hypothalamic sensitivity loss leads to alterations in hormone concentrations, progressive loss of homeostasis, and reduction of signaling molecules and neurotransmitters. This theory suggested that decreased sensitivity of hypothalamus and peripheral receptors results in inadaptability, energy misbalance, and weakening of reproductive ability and the immune system. It explains how the metabolic changes such as hyperinsulinemia, decreased glucose tolerance, hyperlipidemia, with HDL cholesterol reduction result in gradual deterioration of health and, eventually, death (Jin 2010, Zjacic-Rotkvic, Kavur, and Cigrovski-Berkovic 2010). Studies have confirmed that aging is hormonally regulated and highlighted that the evolutionarily conserved insulin/IGF-1 signaling (IIS) pathway plays a key role in the hormonal regulation of aging (van Heemst 2010).

Immunological Theory

This theory hypothesized that there is a programmed decline in the function of the immune system which leads to increased susceptibility to infectious diseases, aging, and eventual death. The decrease in the function of two important immune system organs, thymus and bone marrow, is considered as the basis for the lack of general well-being that leads to aging. The thymus gland (also known as the gland of youth), reduces in size from infancy (250 gm) to adulthood (3 gm). It plays a role in the primary defense diseases. This age-related reduction in the size of the thymus signifies a reduction in our immune systems and suggests the role of the thymus in the aging process (Aronson 1993).

The decline in the immune system function can lead to several negative outcomes of many illnesses such as postoperative infections, urinary tract infections, pneumonia, and cellulitis in the elderly adult. With aging, T-cell functioning declines which eventually results in lowered resistance (Jin 2010). Although no direct evidence has been found, still dysregulated immune responses have been reported to be associated with inflammation, cardiovascular disease, Alzheimer's disease (AD), and cancer (Rozemuller, van Gool, and Eikelenboom 2005).

Damage Theories

Damage or error theories contend that environmental assaults to living organisms that induce cumulative damage at various levels are the cause of aging. The damage may occur either due to normal toxic by-products of metabolism or inefficient repair/defense systems. Damage theories include: wear and tear theory, rate of living theory, cross-linking theory, free radicals theory, and somatic DNA damage theory (Jin 2010, de Magalhães 2014).

Wear and Tear Theories

The wear and tear theory of aging was first proposed by German biologist Dr. August Weismann in 1882, and seemed to be perfectly reasonable to many people even today, because this is what happens to most familiar things around them. This category of damage theories proposes that biological aging in humans and other animals is caused by universal deteriorative processes that operate in any organized system. The theories contend that humans age for the same reasons and because of the same processes that cause aging in automobiles and exterior paint. Similar to the aging of car components, human body parts also wear out with continuous and repeated use, killing them and leading to death. It is important to note that in addition to mechanical wear, accumulation of oxidation and other chemical or molecular damage are included in the concept of "wear and tear." The example of how skin is damaged is good to explain the wear and tear concept and is a crucial evidence of aging. Exposure to ultraviolet radiations damages the skin, altering the cellular structure and affecting the production of collagen and elasticity which contributes to the youthful and hydrated appearance of the skin. The prolonged exposure to the environment over many years contributes to age-related changes (Jin 2010, http://www.programmed-aging.org/theories/wear_and_tear.html, http://www.who.int/uv/publications/proUVrad.pdf).

Oxidative Stress Theory of Aging/Free Radical Theory of Aging

Denham Harman proposed the free radical theory of aging more than 50 years ago, which postulates that aging occurs due to the accumulation of free radicals causing deleterious effects. An organism's lifespan is determined by its ability to cope with cellular damage caused by reactive oxygen species (ROS) (Harman 1955). Increased 8-oxo-dG content in the mtDNA and increased ROS production by mitochondria are commonly seen in aged tissues corroborating that continuous accumulation of oxidative DNA damage contributes to the aging process (Cui, Kong, and Zhang 2012). The association between increased oxidative damage in cells and aging has been demonstrated by several studies (Fraga et al. 1990, Hamilton et al. 2001, Oliver et al. 1987). A study in mice reported that in the absence of the anti-oxidant enzyme superoxide dismutase 1 (SOD1), there is a 30% decrease in its life expectancy (Elchuri et al. 2005). On the other hand, simultaneous over-expression of catalase and SOD1 increases the lifespan in Drosophila (Orr and Sohal 1994). Thus, all these studies demonstrate that interplay between protective anti-oxidant and ROS is a crucial factor in determining aging and lifespan.

Inflammation-Based Theories

Franceschi et al. coined the term "inflammaging," which denotes the upregulation of the inflammatory response with aging and the ensuing low-grade, chronic, systemic proinflammatory state that is associated with most age-associated diseases (Franceschi et al. 2000).

The association between the inflammation and the aging process has been recognized only recently. However, it is being considered as a keystone of the mechanisms that lead to the aging process. Acute as well as chronic inflammatory responses follow sequential phases and are controlled by hormonal and cellular stimuli (Kochman 2015). Cellular-molecular damage associated with inflammation is determined to be a major factor in aging. Several inflammatory factors have been recognized in mice and humans which include the innate immune response, adaptive immune response, and autogenous DNA damage (Finch 2010, Rodier et al. 2009). The acute phase response markers including C-reactive protein (CRP), interleukin-6 (IL-6), and tumor necrosis factor-α (TNFα) have been observed to increase with aging in humans as well as rodent models (Ferrucci et al. 2005, Panda et al. 2009).

The elevated blood CRP, IL-6, and other acute markers are risk indicators of cardiovascular diseases (Danesh et al. 2008, Ridker 2009) and in conjunction with low density lipoprotein (LDL) and other lipid risk indicators increase the risk further. Elevated level of IL-6 and LDL are demonstrated to increase the risk of cardiovascular events by 10 times (Luc et al. 2003). IL-6 elevations are reported to be the key risk indicators of cardiovascular events and mortality (Goldman et al. 2006, Sattar et al. 2009). Inflammatory processes are also known to be associated with atherosclerosis, Alzheimer's disease, cancer, and osteopenia (Finch 2010). Environmental factors accelerate aging, such as the airborne inflammogens, smoking and tobacco are associated with higher cardiovascular mortality, atherosclerosis, and some aspects of Alzheimer's disease (Finch 2010).

Glycation

This theory is based on Dr. Johan Bjorksten's cross-linking theory which suggested that many chemical reactions were based on free radicals (molecules with a highly reactive single electron). However, glycation occurs due to more basic chemical reactions and is a key process that causes aging of the organs (Kugler 2013). The destructive process of glycation involves cross-linking of proteins and sugars forming advanced glycation end products; it occurs in each body organ, for example, cataract in the eyes, reduced kidney functions, wrinkling of skin, aged pancreatic functioning causing diabetes, and so on. Fructose is reported to cause 7 times more glycation than glucose. Apart from protein glycation, this destructive process can also occur with lipids (fats), causing increased aging in people with type 2 diabetes. Glycation has also been linked with atherosclerosis, Alzheimer's, and other diseases affecting the kidney (Galkina and Ley 2009, Srikanth et al. 2011, Ulrich and Cerami 2001).

Energy Metabolism and Aging

In 1908, Max Rubner noted an association between metabolic rate, body size, and longevity. He hypothesized that animals are born with a limited amount of some substance, physiological capacity or potential energy, the duration of life depends on the expenditure rate of this energy. The faster they use it, the faster they will die. Later in 1928, Raymond Pearl proposed "the rate of living theory" based on Ruber's hypothesis suggesting that "the higher the metabolic rate, the higher will be the biochemical activity and the faster an organism will age" (Bennett et al. 2012, Pearl 1928).

Telomere Shortening

According to this theory, experimental evidences have proven that in cultured mammalian cells, the telomeres become shorter with consecutive cell divisions leading to cellular damage and cell senescence. The cells with too short telomeres are unable to replicate. Although the lifespan of continuously dividing cells is limited by telomere shortening, it appears unlikely to affect the aging process of post-mitotic cells. The aging process is not limited to dividing cells, but also includes non-dividing cells such as: in humans, both muscle cells and central nervous system neurons do not divide during adulthood, but exhibit morphological signs of age during senescence (Riddle et al. 1997).

Other Theories—The Multi-Factorial Approach

All existing theories of aging are based on the consideration of one or the other factor. However, aging is a complex process that occurs due to combination of multiple factors which include genetics (and epigenetics) environment, and stochasticity. The contribution of each factor differs in the overall phenotype. The multi-factorial approach hypothesizes that the contribution of each of the above-mentioned factors changes during the lifespan. Figure 26.3 explains the importance of genetics in old age as compared to its importance in the adulthood.

The multi-factorial process of aging not only implies at the organism level, but it also acts on each organ system, organ, tissue, and cell of the body, determining a different aging rate for each of them (Cevenini et al. 2010).

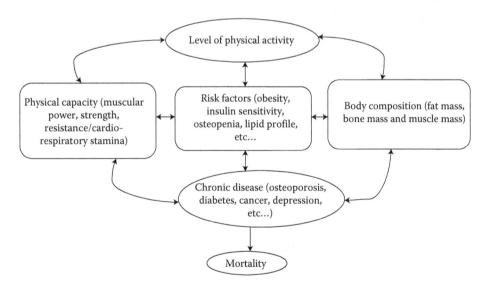

FIGURE 26.3 Schematic representation of the manner in which exercise and/or physical activity may influence disease incidence and, consequently, mortality during aging. Observe that most influences are bi-directional, indicating that the presence of a risk factor or chronic diseases may alter the exercise/physical activity level, increasing the effects of sedentary behavior on disease and mortality. (Adapted from http://www.ncbi.nlm.nih.gov/pmc/articles/PMC3654306/bin/cln-68-05-710-g002.jpg.)

ANTI-AGING INTERVENTIONS

Lifestyle Interventions

Exercise

As is already known, aging leads to functional as well as structural degeneration of the physiological systems in the body; which in turn results in increased susceptibility to chronic diseases among older people (Chodzko-Zajko et al. 2009, Ciolac 2013a). Figure 26.3 shows a schematic representation of the manner in which exercise and/or physical activity may influence disease incidence and, consequently, mortality and aging. It can be seen that most influences work bi-directionally, indicating that a risk factor or chronic disease(s) might alter the physical activity levels and increase the effect of a sedentary lifestyle on mortality.

Research has shown that regular physical activity and/or exercise can help prolong the lifespan and may also improve the quality of life (Ciolac 2013a). Exercise helps in improving the balance, muscle strength, glucose tolerance, metabolism, cardio-respiratory fitness, psychological health, and daily living activities of elderly people. Figure 26.4 highlights the consequences of sarcopenia and aging and its consequences. Again, noteworthy is that most influences are bi-directional.

Studies have shown that individuals with regular physical activity are at a lower risk of developing and consequently dying from musculoskeletal disorders (osteoarthritis, osteoporosis, and

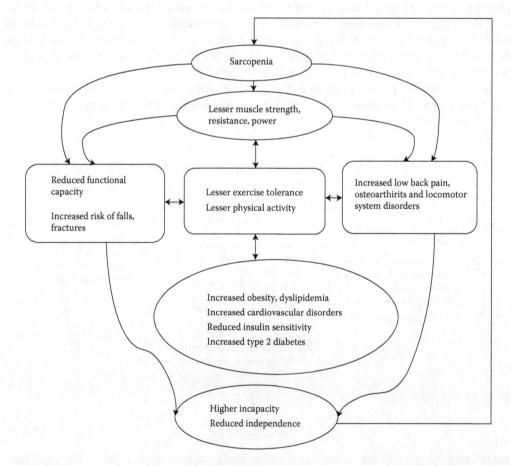

FIGURE 26.4 Schematic representation of the consequences of sarcopenia associated with aging and the feedback from its consequences. Observe that most of the influences are bi-directional. ↓ indicates reduction; ↑ indicates increase. (Adapted from http://www.ncbi.nlm.nih.gov/pmc/articles/PMC3654306/bin/cln-68-05-710-g001.jpg.)

sarcopenia) and several chronic diseases (type 2 diabetes, cardiovascular disease, obesity, and colon cancer) (Chodzko-Zajko et al. 2009, Haskell et al. 2007, Nelson et al. 2007).

A 22-year follow up study by Trappe et al. demonstrated that the young and middle-aged individuals who underwent aerobic training to maintain high levels of cardio-respiratory fitness had lower maximal oxygen uptake (VO_2max) decline in comparison to their untrained peers (Trappe et al. 1996). Ciolac in his review presented recommendations for exercises that can help prevent risk of chronic diseases and improve health (Ciolac 2013a). Exercise recommendations for better health and chronic disease prevention in older adults are shown in Figure 26.5.

Caution: Overtraining: In athletes, overtraining occurs when they undergo very high intensity training and take out little time for recovery or regeneration (Fry, Morton, and Keast 1991). There has not been much research on the relationship between the standardized overtraining and impaired recovery (i.e., whether increased in time for recovery occurs due to aging). However, several studies compared recovery patterns following acute exercise between younger and older individuals. Klein et al. (1988) compared a group of physically active young people (19–32 years) and aging persons (64–69 years) to assess the recovery pattern of the triceps surae muscle following muscle fatigue. The study showed that the recovery was slower in older individuals as compared to the young (Klein et al. 1988). But the studies assessing the impact of overtraining on aging included "recreationally active" or sedentary participants, so whether the findings of these studies could be applied to well-trained older individuals is still questionable (Fell and Williams 2008).

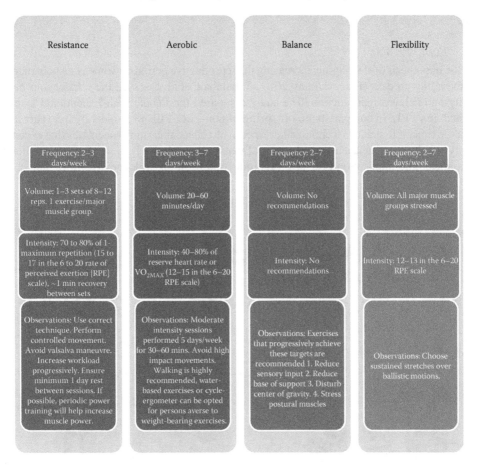

FIGURE 26.5 Exercise recommendations for promotion of health promotion and preventing chronic disease in older adults. (Redrawn from Table 1 of Ciolac, E. G. *Clinics (Sao Paulo)*. 2013 May; 68(5): 710–717. http://www.ncbi.nlm.nih.gov/pmc/articles/PMC3654306/table/t1-cln_68p710/.)

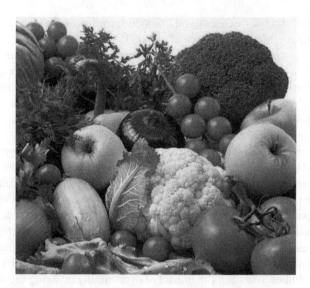

FIGURE 26.6 Fruits and vegetables are rich sources of anti-oxidants. Credit: By Olearys (Frutas e Vegetais) [CC BY 2.0 (http://creativecommons.org/licenses/by/2.0)], via Wikimedia Commons.

Delayed Reproduction

As per the hypothesis of slow-aging, increasing the reproductive period of women can help them slow down the aging process (Blagosklonny 2010). Tabatabaie et al. assessed the relationship between longevity and delayed reproduction. The study compared the People with Exceptional Longevity (PEL) and non-PEL. In comparison to off-spring of non-PEL, PEL were older by 2.5 years and 2.1 years at the time of first and last childbirth, respectively. Thus, this study speculates that exceptional longevity results from delayed reproduction (Tabatabaie et al. 2011). Several other studies have also supported the implication of delayed reproduction resulting in longevity (Korpelainen 2000, McArdle et al. 2006, Perls et al. 1997).

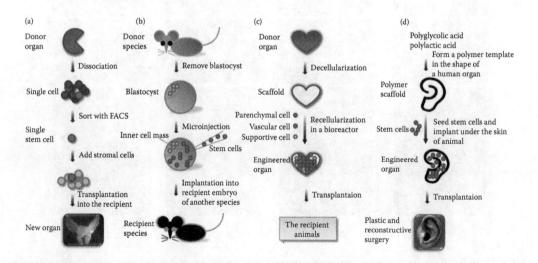

FIGURE 26.7 Approaches to generate functional organs using stem cell therapy. (Adapted from http://cellregenerationjournal.biomedcentral.com/articles/10.1186/2045-9769-2-1.)

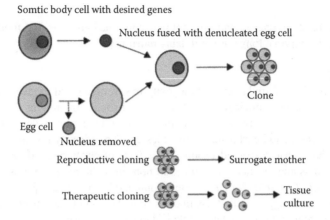

FIGURE 26.8   Somatic cell nuclear transfer. (Adapted from Cristen Conger "Could we clone our organs to be used in a transplant?" 16 September 2008. HowStuffWorks.com. <http://science.howstuffworks.com/life/genetic/cloned-organ-transplant.htm> 10 August 2017.)

Stress Management

Inflammation has been recognized as one of the important pathways that contribute to aging. Some of these inflammatory markers that can now be monitored are highly sensitive C-reactive protein, serum insulin, homocysteine, HgA1C, lipid acid profiles, triglycerides to high density lipoprotein (HDL) ratio, and ferritin. Stress is one factor that increases the secretion of these markers (Chauvin 2005). People who are under chronic stress experience premature aging which occurs due to higher oxidative stress, chronic glucocorticoid exposure, reduced telomere length, changes in cellular trafficking, thymic involution, steroid resistance, reduced cell-mediated immunity, and chronic low-grade inflammation (Bauer, Jeckel, and Luz 2009). Thus, stress management can help in reducing the secretion of these markers and consequently slowing down the aging process. Carnosine, a natural dipeptide, is reported to be a good anti-oxidating and anti-glycosylating age (Boldyrev, Gallant, and Sukhich 1999). It has been used in eye drops and found to offer anti-aging eye functions (Kyriazis). A study assessing the effect of Rhodiola, a traditional Chinese medicine, on the extension of longevity in Drosophila melanogaster found that it can help improve the health span and extend longevity by reducing oxidative stress (Jafari et al. 2007). Meditation, massage, and guided mental imagery are reported to be other methods of preventing or reducing the stress which helps in reducing the levels of cortisol (Epel et al. 2009, Khalsa 2002, Zhan, Wan, and Sun 2002).

Sleep

Sleep is an underutilized intervention for anti-aging. Studies have reported that women who either sleep less or sleep much longer then the normally suggested time limit experience accelerated signs of skin aging, decreased ability to repair the skin damage, and diminished skin barrier function (OyetakinWhite et al. 2013). Skin deprivation is also linked with several age-related diseases including high blood pressure, type 2 diabetes, obesity, and memory loss (Spiegel, Leproult, and Van Cauter 1999).

Social Practices

Social practices such as having a sense of purpose and family are determined to contribute to healthy aging. Hill and colleagues recently reported the results of a 14-year follow-up study which found that people of all age groups (young, middle-aged, and old) with a purpose in life have lower mortality rates (Hill and Turiano 2014). Another meta-analysis by Holt-Lunstad et al. also reported that people with less social support are likely to have higher mortality rates. It found that people in social groups (friends, family) have 50% reduced mortality rate (Holt-Lunstad, Smith, and Layton 2010).

Nutrition/Foods

Food is the prime source of energy and all vital nutrients. Various diets and foods have been used since ancient times to improve longevity and delay mortality.

Calorie Restriction

Calorie restriction has been found to extend longevity in several animal models. However, the exact mechanism behind the same is unclear. Few observational studies in humans that have assessed the effect of high-quality diet and/or reasonable quality diet found the rates of death due to malignancy, cerebral vascular disease, and heart diseases to be lesser. The infirmity was also reported to be less in participants of the calorie restricted group. The effects of chronic CR observed on markers of aging in animal models and predicted outcomes in non-obese humans are presented in a study by the *American Journal of Clinical Nutrition* (Heilbronn and Ravussin, 2003).

Another recent review suggested that CR in older rodents has not been effective. Thus, the use of CR as an anti-aging intervention in older people is dangerous (Morley, Chahla, and Alkaade 2010). More studies need to be conducted to assess the effect of CR on different age groups.

Whole Foods

Whole foods, the foods processed minimally, are associated with a lower risk of several chronic diseases and cancers and contribute to healthy aging. They are known to possess anti-oxidant properties. Foods such as blueberries, green tea, vitamin D, and blue green algae have been reported to extend longevity (Buono 2015). A recent *in vitro* study has reported the potential of blue green algae in promoting the proliferation of human stem cells which usually decline with age (Shytle et al. 2010). Another new study has reported the combined syngerstic effect of green tea extract, blueberry extract, carnosine, and vitamin D in stimulating the proliferation of hematopoietic stem cells. Blueberry extract is known to affect aging via its neuroprotective and neurorestorative effects and it also increase neurogenesis (Casadesus et al. 2004, Williams, Spencer, and Rice-Evans 2004).

Nutraceuticals/Medications

Nutraceuticals are food sources which in addition to providing basic nutrition, also offer several health and medical benefits (Meštrović 2015). They are phytoestrogens, coenzyme Q10, omega-3 fatty acids, and probiotics (all are anti-oxidants). Theories have suggested the role of free-radicals in accelerating aging. Thus, these nutraceuticals could be useful to intervene in the process of aging (Vranesic-Bender 2010). Anti-aging medicine is an emerging branch of science that aims to treat the process or mechanism causing aging; thus, reducing the risk of age-related diseases. Anti-aging medicines include bioidentical and synthetic hormones available as creams, injections, and tablets (Arora 2008). We discuss a few of the nutraceuticals and medications next.

DHEA

The hormone dehydro-3-epiandrosterone (DHEA) is secreted by the adrenal gland. Insufficiency of DHEA is associated with increased risk of aging, breast and ovarian cancer, and cardiovascular diseases (Johnson, Bebb, and Sirrs 2002). Thus, targeting DHEA replacement for anti-aging has gained attraction. However, studies conducted to date provide contradictory results with some stating it to provide positive effects (Arlt 2007), while others demonstrate that the replacement of DHEA has no beneficial effects in humans (Genazzani and Pluchino 2010, Nair et al. 2006). Thus, more studies with varying doses and longer durations need to be conducted. Most of the studies conducted in humans were short-term and used pharmacologic dosages (Dhatariya and Nair 2003).

Resveratrol, ASA, and Metformin

Resveratrol, a naturally occurring anti-oxidant is found to possess anti-aging effects. A recent study has found that resveratrol can extend longevity by increasing the production of SIRT1, a serum that could highly increase the energy production by mitochondria in cells and consequently block diseases (Cameron 2013). The topical application of resveratrol is reported to protect skin against aging (Aziz, Afaq, and Ahmad 2005, Goldfaden and Goldfaden 2011).

In the past decade, acetylsalicylic acid (ASA) has emerged as an effective anti-aging medicine. In 2004, Phillips and colleagues stated that aspirin (low dosage) with its anti-oxidant and anti-inflammatory characteristics could be used as supplementation to extend longevity (Phillips and Leeuwenburgh 2004). McIlhatton et al. found that as nitric oxide-donating (NO-ASA) at 10-fold lower dosage could increase the lifespan comparable to ASA (McIlhatton et al. 2011). More studies in animals and humans are being conducted to assess the long-term use and safety of this intervention. A recent study in animals has shown that metformin is useful to extend longevity and health span in mice models and is approved for a clinical trial to be conducted in humans with Alzheimer's disease and Parkinson's disease (Martin-Montalvo et al. 2013). The future for metformin as an anti-aging medicine looks promising.

Statins

Boccardi and colleagues (2013) reported that statins, in addition to lowering the age-related ailments such as cardiovascular disease and cholesterol level, can also extend longevity by reducing the rate of telomere shortening (Boccardi et al. 2013). Thus, this opens another option for anti-aging interventions. However, another recent study reported the contradictory results stating that statins could speed up aging (Izadpanah et al. 2015). Further research needs to be conducted to elucidate the use of statins for anti-aging.

Vitamin C and D

Vitamin C is a water-soluble anti-oxidant and has been shown to reduce the biomarkers of aging including isoprostanes (Fusco et al. 2007). It has been proven to be used in skin anti-aging formulations in concentrations between 5% and 15% (Ganceviciene et al. 2012). Vitamin D has come to be determined as one of the highly essential constituents of anti-aging medicine (Mitsuo and Nakao 2008). It has been reported to protect skin from ultraviolet radiation in animal studies (Reichrath 2012). Vitamin D supplementation studies in humans reported that it reduces the telomere shortening, too. Thus, it extends the lifespan (Liu et al. 2013a).

Coenzyme Q10

Studies have shown coenzyme (Co) Q10 possesses anti-aging effects. A study on an anti-aging skin moisturizer with CoQ10 as an ingredient demonstrated significant improvement in the appearance of the participants (Herndon et al. 2015). Another recent study in mice showed proniosomal (PN) gel formulation of CoQ10 to be a more effective anti-aging formulation in comparison to free CoQ10 (Yadav et al. 2016).

Alpha-Lipoic Acid

Alpha-lipoic acid is reported to extend longevity (Mahmoud and Hegazy 2016). A recent animal study suggests that long-term intake may lead to increased inflammation and hepatic steatosis (Kuhla et al. 2016). Thus, despite being a known anti-oxidant, it must be used with caution.

Chromium

McCarty was the first to assess the effectiveness of chromium picolinate on lifespan in rodents (McCarty 1994). Another study assessed the positive effect of a dietary supplement containing chromium picolinate in extending the lifespan of the mice (Lemon, Boreham, and Rollo 2005). Studies in humans have yet to be conducted.

L-carnitine

Animal studies have provided evidence for the use of L-carnitine as an anti-aging supplement (Hagen et al. 2002, Kira et al. 2006). However, conclusive human studies are yet to be conducted.

Quercetin

Chondrogianni reported that quercetin, a natural compound with anti-aging properties, could be used in anti-aging products to be applied topically (Chondrogianni et al. 2010). Further research needs to be conducted before recommending it for anti-aging purposes.

Carotenes and Flavanoids

They are known to be effective in preventing cutaneous aging by preventing facial wrinkles and elasticity. Some of the carotenoids used are β-carotene and Astaxanthin (Cho 2014, Jadoon et al. 2015). Flavonoids are known to be extracted from various plant sources and animal studies have reported that it possesses anti-oxidant activity. Thus, they can prevent formation of free radicals and extend lifespan (Jadoon et al. 2015, Sung et al. 2015, Zhou et al. 2011).

Melatonin

Evidence for the use of melatonin as an anti-aging component is provided by many animal studies (Hardeland 2013, Mattam and Jagota 2014), but its use in humans is yet to be studied clinically.

Enzymes

Enzymes are an essential part of our food that are usually lost in processed foods. A low level of enzymes is reported to be associated with several diseases including allergies, arthritis, cancer, and blood disorders (Lynn, http://www.oilsofthegods.com/www.oilsofthegods.com/YL_NUTRITION_files/Enzymes_TheEssentialTruth.pdf.). Enzyme levels decrease with age, thus, enzyme supplements should be taken that can help in slowing the aging process by their anti-oxidant activities (Cousens 2009).

Nicotinamide Adenine Dinucleotide [NAD(+)]

NAD(+) is an important coenzyme found in every cell. It has been established as an important cosubstrate for enzymes like sirtuins and polymerases. It essays a key role in many intracellular redox reactions. Concentrations of NAD(+) decline with aging, making it a focus for targeted anti-aging therapy (Verdin, 2015).

Biosynthesis of NAD(+) is mediated by SIRT1 and nicotinamide phosphoribosyltransferase (NAMPT), that jointly regulate circadian rhythm as well as metabolism. It has been seen that NAD(+) increase can mediate extension of health and lifespan. Similarly, reciprocal studies have also shown that defective NAD(+) levels maintenance and a decline in sirtuin activity might drive the normal process of aging. Supplementation of NAD(+) along with sirtuin activation is being researched as an effective method to reverse age-related pathologies (Imai and Guarente 2014).

Hot in anti-aging news is MIT's Leonard Guarente, who claims to have found the fountain-of-youth in his pill called Basis. One of the pioneers and global champions in anti-aging research, Guarente has discovered the single gene that is concerned with these sirtuins (Wallace 2016). Basis, using precursors for NAD(+), that is, nicotinamide riboside (250 mg) and pterostilbene (50 mg), tricks the body into thinking that it is starving, without the person actually feeling hungry. Anti-aging research already knows that starving or restricted-calorie diets lead to increased lifespans. Pterostilbene has shown reduction in markers of inflammation, cellular stress, and Alzheimer's disease (Chang et al. 2012). Elysium health, the company producing Basis, claims to be heavily evidence backed and is running a trial with 120 participants between the ages of 60 and 80. The firm insists to never make a claim that isn't substantiated by evidence, but the combination of anti-aging substances found in the pill doesn't seem to have any evidence.

PROCEDURES

Hormone Replacement Therapy

Hormone replacement therapy (HRT) is generally used for the administration of estrogen, or estrogen plus progestin, for women who have reached menopause. Estrogen is administered with progestin to women who still have a uterus, because estrogen taken alone increases the incidence rate of uterine cancer. To decrease this incidence rate, estrogen is administered with progestin.

HRT is very effective in alleviating the major symptoms of menopause, such as hot flashes, palpitations, insomnia, night sweats, emotional liability, frequent urination, and painful sexual intercourse. HRT is also recommended to those women who are at high risk of osteoporosis, because estrogen helps to decrease the osteoporotic hip fracture incidence rate by 25%–50% (Bluming and Tavris 2009, Gambrell 1987).

Osteoporosis and fractures are more common problems occurring after menopause, when the level of estrogen drops significantly. HRT restores the estrogen level and slows down the rate of bone loss, as well as helps in relieving the symptoms of menopause. Different studies have reported that HRT, even at low doses, reduces the rate of bone fracture and can significantly increase bone density. HRT is very useful for women who had early menopause (before 45 years of age) because these women are at a much greater risk of osteoporosis (Cousens 2009). Different forms of HRT (e.g., raloxifene and other designer estrogens) are now available which do not increase the risk of breast and endometrial cancer. Recently, the United States Food and Drug Administration (FDA) approved micronized progesterone, adding another hormone to the armamentarium for HRT (Fraga, Vojta, and Veloski 1999).

Bio-Identical hormones: Bio-identical hormones are similar to endogenously produced hormones but sourced from natural substances like yams and soy. In HRT, these hormones are replaced with natural hormones that include estrone (E1), estradiol (E2), estriol (E3), and progesterone (P4).

Estrogens: The body naturally produces three types of estrogen (estrone, estradiol, and estriol). Bioidentical estrogens are molecularly similar to these naturally produced estrogens but sourced from plants. Estradiol is the most physiologically active form of estrogen produced in the ovaries and metabolized in the liver. Increased serum estradiol level is associated with a high risk of endometrial and breast cancer (Kabuto et al. 2000). Estrone is obtained after reversible conversion of estradiol. The level of estrone increases after menopause when the adrenal glands play a major role in hormone synthesis as compared to ovaries (Miyoshi, Tanji, and Taguchi 2003, Ursin, Palla, and Reboussin 2004). Both estradiol and estrone are metabolized to estriol, which is the primary urinary metabolite. Due to its short duration of effect, estriol is considered as the weakest form of estrogen. The formulations of estriol, estrone and estradiol, or estriol and estradiol, are marketed with the name "Tri-Est," or "Bi-Est," respectively (Moskowitz 2006).

The FDA recommendations for adult growth hormone (GH) deficiency: Growth hormone deficiency (GHD) is a well-known clinical entity in the adult which causes abnormalities in body composition, substrate metabolism, and physical and psychosocial function. These abnormalities caused by GHD can be improved by GH replacement (Ho 2007). For adults diagnosed with GHD, the following criteria must be met to document medical necessity for growth hormone treatment:

1. The patient must have a documented diagnosis of somatotropin (growth hormone) deficiency alone resulting from hypothalamic-pituitary disease from known causes (e.g., damage from surgery, cranial irradiation, head trauma, or subarachnoid hemorrhage).
2. Before starting the somatropin therapy, the diagnosis for deficiency must be confirmed with appropriate testing to document the diagnosis.
3. The patient must have an abnormal response to one standard growth hormone stimulation test.
4. Adults with deficiencies of three or more other anterior pituitary hormones and a serum IGF-1 level below the age- and sex-appropriate reference range when off GH therapy, GHD is highly probable, the stimulation testing is not necessary in the absence of conditions that lower IGF-1 (Anonymous 2014).

Telomerase Therapy

Telomeres are DNA-protein complexes that cap the linear chromosome ends. In vertebrates, telomeres consist of tandem repeated sequences of TTAGGG and a number of telomere-associated proteins. Telomeres are considered to be more important for protecting chromosome ends from recombination and fusion and from being recognized as damaged DNA to maintain genomic integrity. Telomeres are also implicated in the cellular aging process (Argyle and Nasir 2003). Recent evidence confirmed that the short length of telomeres alone could lead to cancer. Telomerase is an enzyme that appears in some cell lines to overcome cellular senescence by extending the tips of the telomere's chromosomes. All the human cancers show activation of telomerase as a hallmark, most likely as a mechanism to facilitate unlimited tumor cell proliferation. The activation of telomerase is an early event in cancer. However, telomerase can stimulate progression of tumors by maintaining the length of telomeres above a critically short length, thus preventing the initiation of cellular senescence (Bernardes de Jesus and Blasco 2013). A large number of pharmaceutical companies and labs are developing telomerase-based therapies to fight against aging (Argyle and Nasir 2003, Bernardes de Jesus and Blasco 2013, Fossel 1996).

Astragalus

Astragalus is a traditional Chinese medicinal herb which improves the functioning of the immune system and boosts immune therapy for cancer (Programmed-aging 2015). Cycloastragenol is a compound obtained from astragalus and plays an important role in the activation of telomeres. It helps to kill cancer cells, heal burns and protects from heart disease. The researchers of the University of Texas, Anderson Cancer Center reported that astragalus improved the immune system. Patients having breast cancer showed a decline in mortality rate from 50% to 10%, when administered as a combination of astragalus with other compounds. The group of patients who received pure astragalus extracts showed double the chances of survival (Gupta, Pulapalli, and Srikanth 2015).

Calorie Restriction

Calorie restriction in some organisms delays the growth and development of different age-related diseases, for example, cancer, atherosclerosis, diabetes, and neuro-degenerative and respiratory failures, among others, thus increasing the lifespan. CR is reported to cause additional phenotypes, increases resistance to oxidative stress, enhanced damaged DNA repairing process, decreases levels of oxidatively damaged proteins, improves insulin sensitivity which leads to decrease in the fasting glucose, and protects from age-dependent metabolic syndrome, diabetes, and cancer (Kaeberlein et al. 2005, Vera et al. 2013).

Stem Cells

Stem cells have the potential to differentiate into cells with specific functions. There are two types of stem cells found in humans: embryonic and adult stem cells. Embryonic stem cells are pluripotent and thus able to differentiate into all other body cell types. Adult stem cells maintain and repair tissue (Schmid, Schürch, and Zülli 2008). The ability of stem cells to respond according to environmental demands may be diminished during aging.

The use of stem cells for therapeutic purposes has been recommended for various diseases. For reversing age-related effects, stem cell therapies and reprogramming of adult cells is being done by using pluripotent stem cells in *in vitro* systems for restoring the normal function (Upadhyay 2015). One stem cell-based therapeutic approach that has already proven effective in treating some forms of blood cell cancers (particularly leukemias) involves bone marrow transplantation, a procedure that replaces cancerous hematopoietic cells with normal hematopoietic donor cells (Rao and Mattson 2001).

Whole Foods and Nutraceuticals

Nutrition of stem cells is the best anti-aging system ever known. A viable alternative approach for stem cell transplantation is to stimulate endogenous stem cells which play an important role in healing and regeneration. Many natural food compounds and nutraceuticals have been shown to promote healing by stimulating endogenous stem cells, for example, blueberry, catechin, green tea, carnosine, and vitamin D_3 (Bickford et al. 2006).

Neupogen

Neupogen is the synthetic form of a protein which promotes the growth of white blood cells in the body. Neupogen is used to treat neutropenia which involves deficiency of white blood cells caused by cancer, after chemotherapy and bone marrow transplant (Mordini 2013, Sevinc et al. 2014).

Hyperbaric Oxygen Therapy

Hyperbaric oxygen therapy includes breathing of pure oxygen in a pressurized room. In a hyperbaric oxygen therapy chamber, the pressure of air is increased to three times higher than normal air pressure. Under these conditions, lungs get more oxygen than would be possible breathing pure oxygen at normal air pressure. During hyperbaric oxygen therapy, blood carries this oxygen to all the cells which helps fight against aging and stimulates the release of substances such as growth factors and stem cells, which promote healing (Buettner 2014).

Stem Cells Manipulations

Tissue-Specific Injection for Repair (Heart, Brain, Pancreas) and Intra-Articular It refers to intravenous injection and direct infusion of embryonic stem (ES) cells, or human adult bone marrow derived cells or mesenchymal stem cells into the coronary arteries. These stem cells are pluripotent, and can give rise to a variety of cell types that are instrumental in regenerating damaged myocardium, brain, and pancreas, including endothelial cells and smooth muscle cells (NIH Stem Cell Information Home Page 2016).

Intravenous Injection for "Frailty Syndrome" or Aging Frailty is a geriatric syndrome characterized by age-associated declines in physiologic function across multiorgan systems, leading to increased vulnerability for adverse health outcomes. Intravenous injection of mesenchymal stem cells is a potential treatment for frailty syndrome (Gonzalez, Woynarowski, and Geffner 2015).

Addressing the Causes of Pre-Mature Death: Chronic Diseases

There are different causes of premature death such as acute diseases, acute episodes of chronic diseases, and so on. Some chronic diseases may cause premature death such as myocardial infarction and stroke, cancer, diabetes, arthritis, obesity, and respiratory diseases. Addressing these conditions such that they are prevented, diagnosed earlier, managed better with a view to averting complications and improving lifespan should be the approach to anti-aging today apart from identifying means to stop or slow down the process of aging.

Preventive Tips

Although chronic diseases are a major health concern, they are also preventable. Lifestyle changes for example, diet and exercise, maintained weight, and daily physical exercise, maintained blood pressure and healthy blood cholesterol levels, screening on a regular basis, early diagnosis, and appropriate management go a long way in pushing back aging (Anonymous 2009).

As it is rightly said, *prevention is better than cure*. The complaints associated with aging should be averted or reduced by following some preventive measures. They include bringing exercises and herbs into your lifestyle.

Kegel for Urinary Incontinence

Kegel exercises help in strengthening the pelvic muscles, thereby help controlling urine flow. They are performed by tightening the pelvic muscles for a few seconds, followed by squeezing and lifting up the anal muscles. Subsequently, the pelvic muscles are strengthened. Kegel exercises can be performed 10–20 times a day (Pubmed Health, Chodzko-Zajko et al. 2009).

Specific Exercises for Osteoporosis

The minimal essential mechanical stress is important for bones which alters the bone architecture and leads to increase in osteoblast formation. However, the lack of stress gradually weakens the bones (Baechle and Earle 2008, Frost 2001). Anaerobic and aerobic exercises are important for the treatment of osteoporosis as they are helpful in providing essential strain required for promotion and maintenance of bone growth. A systematic review also supports the beneficial effects of exercise on bone mineral density by reversing/preventing bone loss in women. Many other studies support exercising as an intervention for patients with osteoporosis (Bonaiuti et al. 2002, Chaconas, Olivencia, and Russ 2013, Howe et al. 2011).

Herbs for Diabetes Mellitus (DM)

Diabetes mellitus is a progressive metabolic disease resulting from lack or insufficiency of insulin. Herbal treatment of DM is a reliable interventional strategy which involves low cost, fewer adverse effects, and maintains the quality of life of patients with DM. The herbs that are traditionally used for maintaining optimum glucose levels include *Allium sativum, Eugenia jambolana, Momordica charantia, Ocimum sanctum, Phyllanthus amarus, Pterocarpus marsupium, Tinospora cordifolia, Trigonella foenum graecum*, and *Withania somnifera*. The plants with anti-oxidant activity might prove more beneficial in treating diabetes (Modak et al. 2007). A new herbal formulation which is scientifically validated as anti-diabetic, that is, BGR-34, is prepared from a combination of natural plant extracts with no adverse effects (http://timesofindia.indiatimes.com/india/ Scientifically-validated-Rs-5-anti-diabetes-herbal-drug-launched-by-CSIR/articleshow/49531806. cms). Besides its anti-diabetic activity, it also improves immunity and acts as an anti-oxidant (https://www.functionalmedicine.org/about/whatisfm/).

Male Exercises for Prostate

The prostate, a vital part of the male reproductive system, is an organ that surrounds the urethra and is involved in the process of secretion of fluid into semen. As the age of a man advances, the prostate grows to an extent that it might become enlarged after the age of 50 years. This leads to interference with bladder function, causing urinary retention, and so on. It has been found that aerobics and resistance exercises play an important role in protecting men from prostatitis (inflammation of the prostate gland), benign prostatic hyperplasia (BPH), and prostate cancer. Aerobic exercises include walking, jogging, biking, tennis, rowing, jumping rope, dancing, hiking, and yard work. Resistance exercises work by protecting the health of the prostate gland. It helps in working of muscles by opposing a pulling or a pushing force. They include swimming, push-ups, and weight-lifting. Regular exercises might reduce testosterone level to control the prostate to reduce stress to ease severity of urinary problems (Buettner 2014, Segal et al. 2009).

Brain exercises and supplements: Advancing age results in gradual changes in the brain in terms of its size, vasculature, and cognitive function. With age, it shrinks and changes from molecular, hormonal to morphological levels. Risks of incidence of stroke, memory impairment, lesions, and dementia also increase with increasing age. However, all this can be avoided by following some protective factors that might reduce the chances of unhealthy aging (Peters 2006).

Exercise plays a beneficial role in maintaining a youthful brain. Previous studies suggest an increase in functioning of the brain along with maintenance of white and gray tissue density (Colcombe et al. 2003, Kramer et al. 1999).

A healthy, balanced, and nutritional diet is essential for a healthy brain, but intake of supplements is also warranted. A diet rich in energy, but poor in anti-oxidants might put the cognition and other functions at risk by enhancing biological aging (Otsuka, Yamaguchi, and Ueki 2002). As mentioned above that calorie/energy restriction might extend life and reduce oxidative stress, it also protects the body against cognitive dysfunction (Peters 2006). Consuming food that is rich in anti-oxidants is the key to healthy aging. It would also protect the brain from aging along with imparting good cognitive abilities and executive functioning (Jama et al. 1996, Yasuno et al. 2012). Hormones such as dehydroepiandrosterone, testosterone, estrogen, progesterone, melatonin, and pregnenolone are used as anti-aging agents. Various vitamin supplements such as B complex vitamins, folic acid, vitamin C, vitamin B6, vitamin E, and vitamin B12 could also be used. Anti-aging supplements such as coenzyme Q10, acetyl-L-carnitine, arginate, aspirin, carnosine, green tea extract, fish oil, L-alpha glycerylphosphorylcholine, pyrroloquinoline quinone (PQQ), resveratrol, *beta*-carotene, selenium, lycopene, and so on are useful to exhibit anti-aging effects (Jama et al. 1996, Larsen 1993, Ortega et al. 1997, Yasuno et al. 2012).

Variety in Vegetables and Fruits

The anti-aging property of fruits and vegetables results from their protective effects against cell oxidation. The bright colors of fruits and vegetables impart them their anti-oxidant properties where they scavenge harmful free radicals and avoid or prevent degenerative diseases such as atherosclerosis, cancer, diabetes, and arthritis as well as aging (Kaur and Kapoor 2001). Eating a rainbow of fruits and vegetables might help in prolonging the aging process (Figure 26.6).

3D Printing

Total knee replacement: 3D printing refers to replacement of tissue parts where total knee replacement is the most common and highly performed. It is also known as total knee arthroplasty (TKA). TKA has shown to improve joint function and reduce pain. It also results in better mobility and improvement in quality of life of patients with rheumatoid arthritis or osteoporosis as exercising and performing daily activities become easier (Janson 2006, Kane et al. 2003).

Stem cell therapy: Culturing of a patient's own stem cells to replace impaired organs with new and optimally functioning organs is another strategy to remove prosthetics from the life of scaffold patients. Stem cells are undifferentiated cells which can continuously divide, self-renew, and differentiate into various kinds of cells as depicted in Figure 26.7. Therefore, they are used for treatment of a wide variety of neurological diseases. Among all types of stem cells used, adult stem cells, a blastocyst complementation system coupled with a specific stem cell niche, a bio-scaffold decellularization and recellularization method, and a combinatorial tissue engineering-stem cells approach are used for organ transplantation as suggested by stem cell cloning in Figure 26.8 in cases of organ failure such as liver or kidney (Liu et al. 2013b).

Not only are anti-aging interventional studies tough to work on, they require several generations to prove their efficacy. The search for biochemical, physical, and psychological biomarkers which help in indicating a positive effect on the aging process might do wonders.

THE FUTURE OF ANTI-AGING

Epigenetics Influencers on Aging Genes

Epigenetics is an active participant which takes part in normal development and maintenance of gene expression patterns in mammalian tissues. It generally refers to the changes in gene expression which are unaffected by the primary DNA sequence-modifications (Sharma, Kelly, and Jones 2010). Aging of an organism is also influenced by epigenetic factors as epigenetic pathways significantly contribute to cellular senescence and age-associated phenotypes. Besides, it is also an aging determinant. Reversal of such age-associated epigenetic alterations might give rise to new interventional and therapeutic strategies, resulting in delaying of aging as well as many age-related diseases (Modak et al. 2007).

Genetic Therapy and Gene Manipulation

The best-validated and most promising gene therapy of the entire genetic experimental therapies is the direct delivery of telomerase. This was observed when ordinary laboratory mice were treated with a gene accompanied with an "extra" telomerase gene. The modified gene was spread to their cells by a genetically engineered adeno associated virus (AAV) of wide tropism expressing mouse telomerase reverse transcriptase (TERT). The results showed that the mice lived 13%–24% longer (as compared to the control group) with remarkable beneficial effects. They were fit and healthy. They also showed no signs of insulin sensitivity, osteoporosis, neuromuscular coordination, and several molecular biomarkers of aging. This formed evidence for TERT for imparting positive effects in delaying physiological aging and extending life in normal mice through a telomerase-based treatment (Bernardes de Jesus et al. 2012, Lonergan 1991).

Heterochronic Plasma Exchange (HPE)

According to Dr. Harold Katcher, plasmapheresis, a technique to replace one's own plasma cells with donor plasma cells, is a good method to perform HPE. The technique would be found beneficial if plasma of an old individual is replaced with the plasma of a young individual. This would result in reversal in aging signals, thus delaying the aging process in old patients. This would subsequently protect people from age-related diseases also. Besides, the procedure might help in determining the blood components specific for enhancing or inhibiting the aging process (Katcher 2013, 2015).

Tissue/Organ Cloning

Organ or tissue cloning is possible using the most talked about and common method of therapeutic and reproductive cloning, that is, somatic cell nuclear transfer (SCNT). In SCNT, the nucleus is removed from a donor egg, and replaced with the DNA obtained from the organism which has to be cloned. This method has been extensively used in cloning embryos by extracting stem cells from the blastocyst, followed by stimulation of stem cells and their differentiation into the desired organ. However, the mechanism of differentiation into specific cell types and the chemical or physical signals associated with it could be understood by reverse engineer cell differentiation processes (Bennett et al. 2012, Byrne et al. 2007, French et al. 2008, Wilmut et al. 2002).

Nanotechnology

Nanotechnology and its associated advances might lead to life extension by repairing many physiological processes responsible for aging and causing age-related diseases. Repairing of cells, use of biomedical nanotechnology for manufacturing prostheses and implants might allow people to live a better life (Schiavone and Tan 2006). As aging is mainly concerned with health and appearance, nanotechnology is acting as a novel drug delivery system in many cosmeceuticals and nutraceuticals (Sharma and Sharma 2012). The nanobiotic red blood cells (respirocytes) and white blood cells (microbivores) have been designed using nanotechnology where the former would increase the ability of person to live without oxygen and the latter would act by searching for and destroying unwanted foreign bodies/antigens such as bacteria, viruses, and other pathogens (Grossman 2005b).

Biomarkers of Aging (Detrimental Manifestation of Aging)

There is a heterogeneity observed in the lifespan of every individual human just as is in the aging rate (measurement of decline in functional capacity and stress resistance). Some biomarkers are potent enough to determine an individual's biological age as compared to chronological age. Basically, a biomarker of aging refers to a biological parameter of an organism which predicts the biological age which can be similar or different from chronological age. These markers change with advancing

TABLE 26.1

Aging Markers Which Could be Used for Predicting Biological Age

Aging Marker	Reason	References
Level of senescence associated β-galactozidase (SA-β-gal)	It is considered as main marker of aging. It is accumulated during aging in the lysosomes and cellular compartments. It is responsible for cleaving defective biomolecules.	Zhou et al. (2015)
Telomere length	After every cell division, telomere regions of DNA get shortened. The hayflick limit and depletion of proliferating capacity of cells during aging is associated with aging related diseases.	Aubert and Lansdorp (2008)
Telomerase activity	The number of cell divisions is proportional to telomerase activity. Its activation extends life by 10%.	Aubert and Lansdorp (2008)
Wound healing rate	It decreases with age.	Gosain and DiPietro (2004)

age. Therefore, they are targeted as a preventive or therapeutic strategy for various developing diseases (Baker and Sprott 1988, Hamilton 1970, Simm et al. 2008).

Table 26.1 explains some of the aging markers that could be used for predicting biological age.

SUMMARY

- The major target of clinicians in anti-aging research is to focus on improving and maintaining good health during aging.
- Preventive anti-aging measures involving exercise and intake of food/supplements rich in anti-oxidants are the best way to live a youthful life.
- The less calories, the better and longer the life.
- The use of stem cell therapy as a potent method for repair of wear and tear in tissues as well as development of new organs is stealing the limelight.
- Plasmapheresis might result in prediction, prevention, and treatment of various diseases associated with aging.
- Though effective, gene therapy and manipulation involve high cost and skilled clinicians; therefore, it is found to be cumbersome.
- Last, but not least, nanotechnology is a budding new therapeutic strategy in anti-aging processes. It might take time to establish, but its results would be a boon to society.

REFERENCES

Anonymous. 2009. The Power of Prevention Chronic disease. The public health challenge of the 21st century. National Center for Chronic Disease Prevention and Health Promotion.

Anonymous. 2014. Recombinant Growth Hormone. *Proprietary Information of UCare* 1:1–21.

Argyle, D. J., and L. Nasir. 2003. Telomerase: A potential diagnostic and therapeutic tool in canine oncology. *Vet Pathol* 40 (1):1–7.

Arlt, W. 2007. Can dehydroepiandrosterone or testosterone replacement effectively treat the symptoms of aging? *Nat Clin Pract Endocrinol Metab* 3 (6):448–9. doi: 10.1038/ncpendmet0502.

Aronson, M. 1993. Involution of the thymus revisited: immunological trade-offs as an adaptation to aging. *Mech Ageing and Develop* 72 (1):49–55.

Arora, B. P. 2008. Anti-aging medicine. *Indian J Plast Surg* 41 (Suppl):S130–3.

Aubert, G., and P.M. Lansdorp. 2008. Telomeres and aging. *Physiological Reviews* 88 (2):557–9.

Aziz, M. H., F. Afaq, and N. Ahmad. 2005. Prevention of ultraviolet-B radiation damage by resveratrol in mouse skin is mediated via modulation in survivin. *Photochem Photobiol* 81 (1):25–31. doi: 10.1562/2004-08-13-RA-274.

Babauta, L. 2008. The Two Okinawan Diet Rules (or How I'm Getting Leaner During the Holidays).

Baechle, T.R., and R.W. Earle. 2008. *Essentials of Strength Training and Conditioning* (3rd ed.). Champaign, IL: Human Kinetics.

Baker, G.T., and R.L. Sprott. 1988. Biomarkers of aging. *Experimental Gerontology* 23 (4–5):223–9.

Barclay, E. 2015. Eating to Break 100: Longevity Diet Tips From The Blue Zones. Retrieved from: http://www.npr.org/sections/thesalt/2015/04/11/398325030/eating-to-break-100-longevity-diet-tips-from-the-blue-zones. In.

Bauer, M. E., C. M. Jeckel, and C. Luz. 2009. The role of stress factors during aging of the immune system. *Ann N Y Acad Sci* 1153:139–52. doi: 10.1111/j.1749-6632.2008.03966.x.

Bennett, D. A., J. A. Schneider, A. S. Buchman, L. L. Barnes, P. A. Boyle, and R. S. Wilson. 2012. Overview and findings from the rush Memory and Aging Project. *Curr Alzheimer Res* 9 (6):646–63.

Bernardes de Jesus, B., and M. A. Blasco. 2013. Telomerase at the intersection of cancer and aging. *Trends Genet* 29 (9):513–20. doi: 10.1016/j.tig.2013.06.007.

Bernardes de Jesus, B., E. Vera, K. Schneeberger, A. M. Tejera, E. Ayuso, F. Bosch, and M. A. Blasco. 2012. Telomerase gene therapy in adult and old mice delays aging and increases longevity without increasing cancer. *EMBO Mol Med* 4 (8):691–704. doi: 10.1002/emmm.201200245.

Bickford, P. C., J. Tan, R. D. Shytle, C. D. Sanberg, N. El-Badri, and P. R. Sanberg. 2006. Nutraceuticals synergistically promote proliferation of human stem cells. *Stem Cells Dev* 15 (1):118–23. doi: 10.1089/scd.2006.15.118.

Blagosklonny, M. V. 2010. Why human lifespan is rapidly increasing: Solving "longevity riddle" with "revealed-slow-aging" hypothesis. *Aging (Albany NY)* 2 (4):177–82.

Bluming, A. Z., and C. Tavris. 2009. Hormone replacement therapy: Real concerns and false alarms. *Cancer J* 15 (2):93–104. doi: 10.1097/PPO.0b013e31819e332a.

Boccardi, V., M. Barbieri, M. R. Rizzo, R. Marfella, A. Esposito, L. Marano, and G. Paolisso. 2013. A new pleiotropic effect of statins in elderly: Modulation of telomerase activity. *FASEB J* 27 (9):3879–85. doi: 10.1096/fj.13-232066.

Boldyrev, A. A. 1993. Does carnosine possess direct antioxidant activity? *Int J Biochem* 25 (8):1101–7.

Boldyrev, A. A., S. C. Gallant, and G. T. Sukhich. 1999. Carnosine, the protective, anti-aging peptide. *Biosci Rep* 19 (6):581–7.

Bonaiuti, D., B. Shea, R. Iovine, S. Negrini, V. Robinson, H. C. Kemper, G. Wells, P. Tugwell, and A. Cranney. 2002. Exercise for preventing and treating osteoporosis in postmenopausal women. *Cochrane Database Syst Rev* 3 (3):CD000333.

Buettner, C. 2014. Power 9®. Reverse Engineering Longevity. Retrieved from: http://www.bluezones.com/2014/04/power-9/.

Buettner, D., and S. Skemp. 2016. Blue Zones: Lessons From the World's Longest Lived. *American Journal of Lifestyle Medicine* 10 (5):318–321.

Buono, connie dello. 2015. Anti aging plants and herbs. Retrieved from: https://clubalthea.com/2015/12/16/anti-aging-plants-and-herbs/.

Byrne, J, D Pedersen, L Clepper, M Nelson, W Sanger, S Gokhale, D Wolf, and Shoukhrat Mitalipov. 2007. Producing primate embryonic stem cells by somatic cell nuclear transfer. *Nature* 450 (7169):497.

Cameron, D. 2013. New Study Validates Longevity Pathway. Retrieved from: https://hms.harvard.edu/news/new-study-validates-longevity-pathway-3-7-13.

Carrel, A. 1913. Contributions to the Study of the Mechanism of the Growth of Connective Tissue. *J Exp Med* 18 (3):287–98.

Casadesus, G., B. Shukitt-Hale, H. M. Stellwagen, X. Zhu, H. G. Lee, M. A. Smith, and J. A. Joseph. 2004. Modulation of hippocampal plasticity and cognitive behavior by short-term blueberry supplementation in aged rats. *Nutr Neurosci* 7 (5–6):309–16. doi: 10.1080/10284150400020482.

Cevenini, E., E. Bellavista, P. Tieri, G. Castellani, F. Lescai, M. Francesconi, M. Mishto et al. 2010. Systems biology and longevity: An emerging approach to identify innovative anti-aging targets and strategies. *Curr Pharm Des* 16 (7):802–13.

Chaconas, E.J., O. Olivencia, and B.S. Russ. 2013. Exercise Interventions for the Individual with Osteoporosis. *Strength & Conditioning Journal* 35 (4):49–55.

Chang, J., A. Rimano, M. Pallas, A. Camins, D. Porquet, J. Reeves et al. 2012. Low-dose pterostilbene, but not resveratrol, is a potent neuromodulator in aging and Alzheimer's disease. *Neurobiol Aging* 33, 2062–2071. doi: 10.1016/j.neurobiolaging.2011.08.015

Chauvin, D. 2005. Anti-Aging Medicine...an Update. Retrieved from: http://www.cbass.com/Anti-AgingUpdate.htm.

Cho, S. 2014. The Role of Functional Foods in Cutaneous Anti-aging. *J Lifestyle Med* 4 (1):8–16. doi: 10.15280/jlm.2014.4.1.8.

Chodzko-Zajko, W. J., D. N. Proctor, M. A. Fiatarone Singh, C. T. Minson, C. R. Nigg, G. J. Salem, and J. S. Skinner. 2009. American College of Sports Medicine position stand. Exercise and physical activity for older adults. *Med Sci Sports Exerc* 41 (7):1510–30. doi: 10.1249/MSS.0b013e3181a0c95c.

Chondrogianni, N., S. Kapeta, I. Chinou, K. Vassilatou, I. Papassideri, and E. S. Gonos. 2010. Anti-ageing and rejuvenating effects of quercetin. *Exp Gerontol* 45 (10):763–71. doi: 10.1016/j.exger.2010.07.001.

Ciolac, E. G. 2013a. Exercise training as a preventive tool for age-related disorders: A brief review. *Clinics (Sao Paulo)* 68 (5):710–7. doi: 10.6061/clinics/2013(05)20.

Ciolac, E. G. 2013b. Exercise training as a preventive tool for age-related disorders: A brief review. *Clinics (Sao Paulo)* 68 (5):710–7.

Colcombe, S. J., K. I. Erickson, N. Raz, A. G. Webb, N. J. Cohen, E. McAuley, and A. F. Kramer. 2003. Aerobic fitness reduces brain tissue loss in aging humans. *J Gerontol A Biol Sci Med Sci* 58 (2):M176–80.

Cousens, G. 2009. *Conscious Eating*. Berkeley, CA: North Atlantic Books.

Cui, H., Y. Kong, and H. Zhang. 2012. Oxidative stress, mitochondrial dysfunction, and aging. *J Signal Transduct* 2012:646354. doi: 10.1155/2012/646354.

Danesh, J., S. Kaptoge, A. G. Mann, N. Sarwar, A. Wood, S. B. Angleman, F. Wensley et al. 2008. Long-term interleukin-6 levels and subsequent risk of coronary heart disease: Two new prospective studies and a systematic review. *PLoS Med* 5 (4):e78. doi: 10.1371/journal.pmed.0050078.

de Magalhães, J. P. 2014. Damage-based theories of aging. Reterived from: http://www.senescence.info/causes_of_aging.html.

Dhatariya, K. K., and K. S. Nair. 2003. Dehydroepiandrosterone: Is there a role for replacement? *Mayo Clin Proc* 78 (10):1257–73. doi: 10.4065/78.10.1257.

Dilman V., and Dean W. 1992. Neuroendocrine Theory of Aging. In *Neuroendocrine Theory of Aging*. Pensacola: The Center for Bio-Gerontology.

Elchuri, S., T. D. Oberley, W. Qi, R. S. Eisenstein, L. Jackson Roberts, H. Van Remmen, C. J. Epstein, and T-T. Huang. 2005. CuZnSOD deficiency leads to persistent and widespread oxidative damage and hepatocarcinogenesis later in life. *Oncogene* 24 (3):367–80.

Epel, E., J. Daubenmier, J. T. Moskowitz, S. Folkman, and E. Blackburn. 2009. Can meditation slow rate of cellular aging? Cognitive stress, mindfulness, and telomeres. *Ann N Y Acad Sci* 1172:34–53. doi: 10.1111/j.1749-6632.2009.04414.x.

Fell, J., and D. Williams. 2008. The effect of aging on skeletal-muscle recovery from exercise: Possible implications for aging athletes. *J Aging Phys Act* 16 (1):97–115.

Ferrucci, L., A. Corsi, F. Lauretani, S. Bandinelli, B. Bartali, D. D. Taub, J. M. Guralnik, and D. L. Longo. 2005. The origins of age-related proinflammatory state. *Blood* 105 (6):2294–9. doi: 10.1182/blood-2004-07-2599.

Fightaging. 2013. Fight Aging. Retrieved from: https://www.fightaging.org/archives/2002/11/what-is-antiaging/.

Finch, C.E.. 2010. Inflammation in aging processes: an integrative and ecological perspective. In, *Handbook of the Biology of Aging*. Edited by E. Masoro and S. Austad. 7th ed. San Diego, CA: Academic Press.

Fossel, M. 1996. *Reversing Human Aging*. New York: William Morrow and Company.

Fraga, C. G., M. K. Shigenaga, J-W. Park, P. Degan, and B. N. Ames. 1990. Oxidative damage to DNA during aging: 8-hydroxy-2'-deoxyguanosine in rat organ DNA and urine. *Proc Natl Acad Sci U S A* 87 (12):4533–7.

Fraga, P.D., C. Vojta, and C. Veloski. 1999. A Review of Hormone Replacement Therapy for Disease Prevention. *Hospital Physician* 17–30.

Franceschi, C., M. Bonafè, S. Valensin, F. Olivieri, M.de Luca, E. Ottaviani, and G. de Benedictis. 2000. Inflamm-aging: An evolutionary perspective on immunosenescence. *Ann N Y Acad Sci* 908 (1):244–54.

French, A. J., C. A. Adams, L. S. Anderson, J. R. Kitchen, M. R. Hughes, and S. H. Wood. 2008. Development of human cloned blastocysts following somatic cell nuclear transfer with adult fibroblasts. *Stem Cells* 26 (2):485–93.

Frost, H. M. 2001. From Wolff's law to the Utah paradigm: Insights about bone physiology and its clinical applications. *Anat Rec* 262 (4):398–419.

Fry, R. W., A. R. Morton, and D. Keast. 1991. Overtraining in athletes. An update. *Sports Med* 12 (1):32–65.

Fusco, D., G. Colloca, M. R. Lo Monaco, and M. Cesari. 2007. Effects of antioxidant supplementation on the aging process. *Clin Interv Aging* 2 (3):377–87.

Galkina, E., and K. Ley. 2009. Immune and inflammatory mechanisms of atherosclerosis (*). *Annu Rev Immunol* 27:165–97. doi: 10.1146/annurev.immunol.021908.132620.

Gambrell, R. D., Jr. 1987. Use of progestogen therapy. *Am J Obstet Gynecol* 156 (5):1304–13.

Ganceviciene, R., A. I. Liakou, A. Theodoridis, E. Makrantonaki, and C. C. Zouboulis. 2012. Skin anti-aging strategies. *Dermatoendocrinol* 4 (3):308–19. doi: 10.4161/derm.22804.

Gariballa, S. E., and A. J. Sinclair. 2000. Carnosine: Physiological properties and therapeutic potential. *Age Ageing* 29 (3):207–10.

Genazzani, A. R., and N. Pluchino. 2010. DHEA therapy in postmenopausal women: The need to move forward beyond the lack of evidence. *Climacteric* 13 (4):314–6. doi: 10.3109/13697137.2010.492496.

Goldfaden, R., and G. Goldfaden. 2011. Topical Resveratrol Combats Skin Aging. Retrieved from: http://www.lifeextension.com/magazine/2011/11/topical-resveratrol-combats-skin-aging/page-01. LifeExtension.

Goldman, N., C. M. Turra, D. A. Glei, C. L. Seplaki, Y-H. Lin, and M. Weinstein. 2006. Predicting mortality from clinical and nonclinical biomarkers. *J Gerontol A Biol Sci Med Sci* 61 (10):1070–4.

Gonzalez, R., D. Woynarowski, and L. Geffner. 2015. Stem Cells Targeting Inflammation as Potential Antiaging Strategies and Therapies. *Cell & Tissue Transplantation & Therapy* (7): 1–8.

Gosain, A., and L. A. DiPietro. 2004. Aging and wound healing. *World J Surg* 28 (3):321–6.

Grossman, T. 2005a. Latest advances in antiaging medicine. *Keio J Med* 54 (2):85–94.

Grossman, T. 2005b. Latest advances in antiaging medicine. *Keio J Med* 54 (2):85–94.

Gupta, P.K., S. Pulapalli, and Srikanth. 2015. Cycloastragenol(Telomeres Activator) and its relation with Cancer: A brief review. *Research and Reviews: Journal of Microbiology and Biotechnology* 4 (1):1–8. Available at: http://www.rroij.com/open-access/cycloastragenoltelomeres-activator-and-its-relation-with-cancer-a-brief-review.pdf

Hagen, T. M., J. Liu, J. Lykkesfeldt, C. M. Wehr, R. T. Ingersoll, V. Vinarsky, J. C. Bartholomew, and B. N. Ames. 2002. Feeding acetyl-L-carnitine and lipoic acid to old rats significantly improves metabolic function while decreasing oxidative stress. *Proc Natl Acad Sci U S A* 99 (4):1870–5. doi: 10.1073/pnas.261708898.

Hamilton, M. L., H. Van Remmen, J. A. Drake, H. Yang, Z.M. Guo, K. Kewitt, C. A Walter, and A. Richardson. 2001. Does oxidative damage to DNA increase with age? *Proc Natl Acad Sci U S A* 98 (18):10469–74.

Hamilton, W. D. 1970. Selfish and spiteful behaviour in an evolutionary model. *Nature* 228 (5277):1218–20.

Hardeland, R. 2013. Melatonin and the theories of aging: A critical appraisal of melatonin's role in antiaging mechanisms. *J Pineal Res* 55 (4):325–56. doi: 10.1111/jpi.12090.

Harman, D. 1955. Aging: A theory based on free radical and radiation chemistry.

Haskell, W. L., I. M. Lee, R. R. Pate, K. E. Powell, S. N. Blair, B. A. Franklin, C. A. Macera, G. W. Heath, P. D. Thompson, A. Bauman, Medicine American College of Sports, and Association American Heart. 2007. Physical activity and public health: Updated recommendation for adults from the American College of Sports Medicine and the American Heart Association. *Circulation* 116 (9):1081–93. doi: 10.1161/CIRCULATIONAHA.107.185649.

Heilbronn, L. K., and E. Ravussin. 2003. Calorie restriction and aging: Review of the literature and implications for studies in humans. *Am J Clin Nutr* 78 (3):361–9.

Herndon, J. H., Jr., L. Jiang, T. Kononov, and T. Fox. 2015. An Open Label Clinical Trial of a Multi-Ingredient Anti-Aging Moisturizer Designed to Improve the Appearance of Facial Skin. *J Drugs Dermatol* 14 (7):699–704.

Hill, P. L., and N. A. Turiano. 2014. Purpose in life as a predictor of mortality across adulthood. *Psychol Sci* 25 (7):1482–6.

Hipkiss, A. R.. 1998. Carnosine, a protective, anti-ageing peptide? *The International Journal of Biochemistry & Cell Biology* 30 (8):863–68.

Ho, K. K. 2007. Consensus guidelines for the diagnosis and treatment of adults with GH deficiency II: A statement of the GH Research Society in association with the European Society for Pediatric Endocrinology, Lawson Wilkins Society, European Society of Endocrinology, Japan Endocrine Society, and Endocrine Society of Australia. *Eur J Endocrinol* 157 (6):695–700. doi: 10.1530/eje-07-0631.

Holt-Lunstad, J., T. B. Smith, and J. B. Layton. 2010. Social relationships and mortality risk: A meta-analytic review. *PLoS Med* 7 (7):e1000316. doi: 10.1371/journal.pmed.1000316.

Howe, T. E., B. Shea, L. J. Dawson, F. Downie, A. Murray, C. Ross, R. T. Harbour, L. M. Caldwell, and G. Creed. 2011. Exercise for preventing and treating osteoporosis in postmenopausal women. *The Cochrane Library*.

http://timesofindia.indiatimes.com/india/Scientifically-validated-Rs-5-anti-diabetes-herbal-drug-launched-by-CSIR/articleshow/49531806.cms. Scientifically validated Rs 5 anti-diabetes herbal drug launched by CSIR. Accessed 4 May.

http://www.bioidenticalhormonemd.com/anti-aging-functional-preventative-medicine.html.

http://www.programmed-aging.org/aging-theory-summary.html.

http://www.programmed-aging.org/theories/aging_theory_controversy.html.

http://www.programmed-aging.org/theories/antagonistic_pleiotropy.html.

http://www.programmed-aging.org/theories/mutation_accumulation.html.

http://www.programmed-aging.org/theories/wear_and_tear.html.

http://www.who.int/uv/publications/proUVrad.pdf.

https://www.functionalmedicine.org/about/whatisfm/.

Hudziak, R. M., J. Schlessinger, and A. Ullrich. 1987. Increased expression of the putative growth factor receptor p185HER2 causes transformation and tumorigenesis of NIH 3T3 cells. *Proceed Natl Acad Sci USA* 84 (20):7159–63.

Imai, S. I. and L. Guarente 2014. NAD+ and sirtuins in aging and disease. *Trends in Cell Biology* 24 (8):464–71.

Izadpanah, R., D. J. Schachtele, A. B. Pfnur, D. Lin, D. P. Slakey, P. J. Kadowitz, and E. U. Alt. 2015. The impact of statins on biological characteristics of stem cells provides a novel explanation for their pleiotropic beneficial and adverse clinical effects. *Am J Physiol Cell Physiol* 309 (8):C522–31. doi: 10.1152/ajpcell.00406.2014.

Jadoon, S., S. Karim, M. H. Bin Asad, M. R. Akram, A. K. Khan, A. Malik, C. Chen, and G. Murtaza. 2015. Anti-Aging Potential of Phytoextract Loaded-Pharmaceutical Creams for Human Skin Cell Longevity. *Oxid Med Cell Longev* 2015:709628. doi: 10.1155/2015/709628.

Jafari, M., J. S. Felgner, Bussel, II, T. Hutchili, B. Khodayari, M. R. Rose, C. Vince-Cruz, and L. D. Mueller. 2007. Rhodiola: A promising anti-aging Chinese herb. *Rejuvenation Res* 10 (4):587–602. doi: 10.1089/rej.2007.0560.

Jama, J Warsama, L. J. Launer, J. C. M. Witteman, J. H. Den Breeijen, M. M. B. Breteler, D. E. Grobbee, and A. Hofman. 1996. Dietary antioxidants and cognitive function in a population-based sample of older persons The Rotterdam Study. *Am J Epidemiol* 144 (3):275–80.

Janson, M. 2006. Orthomolecular medicine: The therapeutic use of dietary supplements for anti-aging. *Clin Interv Aging* 1 (3):261–5.

Jin, K. 2010. Modern Biological Theories of Aging. *Aging Dis* 1 (2):72–4.

Johnson, M. D., R. A. Bebb, and S. M. Sirrs. 2002. Uses of DHEA in aging and other disease states. *Ageing Res Rev* 1 (1):29–41.

Kabuto, M., S. Akiba, R. G. Stevens, K. Neriishi, and C. E. Land. 2000. A prospective study of estradiol and breast cancer in Japanese women. *Cancer Epidemiol Biomarkers Prev* 9 (6):575–9.

Kaeberlein, M., D. Hu, E. O. Kerr, M. Tsuchiya, E. A. Westman, N. Dang, S. Fields, and B. K. Kennedy. 2005. Increased life span due to calorie restriction in respiratory-deficient yeast. *PLoS Genet* 1 (5):e69. doi: 10.1371/journal.pgen.0010069.

Kane, R. L., K. J. Saleh, T. J. Wilt, B. Bershadsky, W. W. Cross III, R. M. MacDonald, and I. Rutks. 2003. *Total Knee Replacement*: US Department of Health and Human Services, Public Health Service, Agency for Healthcare Research and Quality.

Katcher, H. L. 2013. Studies that shed new light on aging. *Biochemistry (Moscow)* 78 (9):1061–70.

Katcher, H. L. 2015. Towards an evidence-based model of aging. *Curr Aging Sci* 8 (1):46–55.

Kaur, C., and H. C. Kapoor. 2001. Antioxidants in fruits and vegetables–the millennium's health. *International Journal of Food Science & Technology* 36 (7):703–25.

Khalsa, D. S. 2002. Mind management for the 21st century. *Brain Longevity: An Integrative Medicine Approach*. Sep. 1-4. Available at: http://www.aboutpeople.com/PDFFiles/Brain%20Longevity.pdf.

Kira, Y., M. Nishikawa, A. Ochi, E. Sato, and M. Inoue. 2006. L-carnitine suppresses the onset of neuromuscular degeneration and increases the life span of mice with familial amyotrophic lateral sclerosis. *Brain Res* 1070 (1):206–14. doi: 10.1016/j.brainres.2005.11.052.

Klein, C., D. A. Cunningham, D. H. Paterson, and A. W. Taylor. 1988. Fatigue and recovery contractile properties of young and elderly men. *Eur J Appl Physiol Occup Physiol* 57 (6):684–90.

Kochman, K. 2015. New elements in modern biological theories of aging. *Folia Medica Copernicana* 3 (3):89–99.

Korpelainen, H. 2000. Fitness, reproduction and longevity among European aristocratic and rural Finnish families in the 1700s and 1800s. *Proc Biol Sci* 267 (1454):1765–70. doi: 10.1098/rspb.2000.1208.

Kramer, A. F., S. Hahn, N. J. Cohen, M. T. Banich, E. McAuley, C. R. Harrison, J. Chason, E. Vakil, L. Bardell, and R. A. Boileau. 1999. Ageing, fitness and neurocognitive function. *Nature* 400 (6743):418–9.

Kugler, H. 2013. An introduction to the theories of aging, and the logic of anti-aging thinking.

Kuhla, A., M. Derbenev, H. Y. Shih, and B. Vollmar. 2016. Prophylactic and abundant intake of alpha-lipoic acid causes hepatic steatosis and should be reconsidered in usage as an anti-aging drug. *Biofactors* 42 (2):179–89. doi: 10.1002/biof.1262.

Kyriazis, M. Carnosine, the new anti-aging supplement. Retrieved from: http://smart-drugs.net/info-carnosine.htm.

Larsen, P.L. 1993. Aging and resistance to oxidative damage in Caenorhabditis elegans, *Proceedings of the National Academy of Sciences of the United States of America*. 90 (19):8905–9.

Lemon, J. A., D. R. Boreham, and C. D. Rollo. 2005. A complex dietary supplement extends longevity of mice. *J Gerontol A Biol Sci Med Sci* 60 (3):275–9.

Liu, J. J., J. Prescott, E. Giovannucci, S. E. Hankinson, B. Rosner, J. Han, and I. De Vivo. 2013a. Plasma vitamin D biomarkers and leukocyte telomere length. *Am J Epidemiol* 177 (12):1411–7. doi: 10.1093/aje/kws435.

Liu, Y., R. Yang, Z. He, and W. Q. Gao. 2013b. Generation of functional organs from stem cells. *Cell Regeneration* 2 (1):1.

Lonergan, E.T. 1991. *Extending Life, Enhancing Life: A National Research Agenda on Aging.* U.S.: National Academies Press.

Luc, G., J. M. Bard, I. Juhan-Vague, J. Ferrieres, A. Evans, P. Amouyel, D. Arveiler, J. C. Fruchart, P. Ducimetiere, and Prime Study Group. 2003. C-reactive protein, interleukin-6, and fibrinogen as predictors of coronary heart disease: The PRIME Study. *Arterioscler Thromb Vasc Biol* 23 (7):1255–61. doi: 10.1161/01.ATV.0000079512.66448.1D.

Lynn, J. The essential truth bout enzymes. Retrieved from: http://www.oilsofthegods.com/www.oilsofthegods. com/YL_NUTRITION_files/Enzymes_TheEssentialTruth.pdf.

Mahmoud, Y. I., and H. G. Hegazy. 2016. Ginger and alpha lipoic acid ameliorate age-related ultrastructural changes in rat liver. *Biotech Histochem* 91 (2):86–95. doi: 10.3109/10520295.2015.1076578.

Martin-Montalvo, A., E. M. Mercken, S. J. Mitchell, H. H. Palacios, P. L. Mote, M. Scheibye-Knudsen, A. P. Gomes et al. 2013. Metformin improves healthspan and lifespan in mice. *Nat Commun* 4:2192. doi: 10.1038/ncomms3192.

Mattam, U., and A. Jagota. 2014. Differential role of melatonin in restoration of age-induced alterations in daily rhythms of expression of various clock genes in suprachiasmatic nucleus of male Wistar rats. *Biogerontology* 15 (3):257–68. doi: 10.1007/s10522-014-9495-2.

McArdle, P. F., T. I. Pollin, J. R. O'Connell, J. D. Sorkin, R. Agarwala, A. A. Schaffer, E. A. Streeten, T. M. King, A. R. Shuldiner, and B. D. Mitchell. 2006. Does having children extend life span? A genealogical study of parity and longevity in the Amish. *J Gerontol A Biol Sci Med Sci* 61 (2):190–5.

McCarty, M. F. 1994. Longevity effect of chromium picolinate--'rejuvenation' of hypothalamic function? *Med Hypotheses* 43 (4):253–65.

McIlhatton, M. A., J. Tyler, L. A. Kerepesi, T. Bocker-Edmonston, M. H. Kucherlapati, W. Edelmann, R. Kucherlapati, L. Kopelovich, and R. Fishel. 2011. Aspirin and low-dose nitric oxide-donating aspirin increase life span in a Lynch syndrome mouse model. *Cancer Prev Res (Phila)* 4 (5):684–93. doi: 10.1158/1940-6207.CAPR-10-0319.

Mehrotra, C., and L.S. Wagner. 2013. *Aging and Diversity: An Active Learning Experience.* New York: Taylor & Francis.

Meštrović, T. 2015. What are Nutraceuticals? Retrieved from: http://www.news-medical.net/health/What-are-Nutraceuticals.aspx.

Mitsuo, T., and M. Nakao. 2008. [Vitamin D and anti-aging medicine]. *Clin Calcium* 18 (7):980–5. doi: CliCa0807980985.

Miyoshi, Y., Y. Tanji, and T. Taguchi. 2003. Association of serum estrone levels with estrogen receptor-positive breast cancer risk in postmenopausal Japanese women. *Clin Cancer Res* 9 (6):2229–33.

Modak, M., P. Dixit, J. Londhe, S. Ghaskadbi, and T. P. Devasagayam. 2007. Indian herbs and herbal drugs used for the treatment of diabetes. *J Clin Biochem Nutr* 40 (3):163–73. doi: 10.3164/jcbn.40.163.

Mordini, S. 2013. The cuturiest. 9 Characteristics of a Culture that Determine Happiness, Longevity and Quality of Life. Retrived from: http://www.thecultureist.com/2013/06/06/9-characteristics-of-culture-that-determine-happiness-costa-rica/.

Morley, J. E., E. Chahla, and S. Alkaade. 2010. Antiaging, longevity and calorie restriction. *Curr Opin Clin Nutr Metab Care* 13 (1):40–5. doi: 10.1097/MCO.0b013e3283331384.

Moskowitz, D. 2006. Comprehensive Review of the Safety and Efficacy of Bioidentical Hormones for the Management of Menopause and Related Health Risks. *Alternative Medicine Review* 11 (3):208–23.

Nair, K. S., R. A. Rizza, P. O'Brien, K. Dhatariya, K. R. Short, A. Nehra, J. L. Vittone et al. 2006. DHEA in elderly women and DHEA or testosterone in elderly men. *N Engl J Med* 355 (16):1647–59. doi: 10.1056/NEJMoa054629.

Nelson, M. E., W. J. Rejeski, S. N. Blair, P. W. Duncan, J. O. Judge, A. C. King, C. A. Macera, and C. Castaneda-Sceppa. 2007. Physical activity and public health in older adults: Recommendation from the American College of Sports Medicine and the American Heart Association. *Med Sci Sports Exerc* 39 (8):1435–45. doi: 10.1249/mss.0b013e3180616aa2.

NIH Stem Cell Information Home Page. 2016. In Stem Cell Information [World Wide Web site]. Bethesda, MD: National Institutes of Health, U.S. Department of Health and Human Services [cited February 7, 2018] Available at https://stemcells.nih.gov/info/Regenerative_Medicine/2006Chapter6.htm.

Oliver, C. N., B-W. Ahn, E. J. Moerman, S. Goldstein, and E. R. Stadtman. 1987. Age-related changes in oxidized proteins. *J Biol Chem* 262 (12):5488–91.

Orr, W. C., and R. S. Sohal. 1994. Extension of life-span by overexpression of superoxide dismutase and catalase in Drosophila melanogaster. *Science* 263 (5150):1128–30.

Ortega, R. M., A. M. Requejo, P. Andrés, A. M. López-Sobaler, M. Elena Quintas, M. Rosario Redondo, B. Navia, and T. Rivas. 1997. Dietary intake and cognitive function in a group of elderly people. *Am J Clin Nutr* 66 (4):803–9.

Otsuka, M, K Yamaguchi, and A Ueki. 2002. Similarities and differences between Alzheimer's disease and vascular dementia from the viewpoint of nutrition. *Annals of the New York Academy of Sciences* 977 (1):155–61.

OyetakinWhite, P., B. Koo, M.S. Matsui, D. Yarosh, C. Fthenakis, K.D. Cooper, and E.D. Baron. 2013. *Effects of Sleep Quality on Skin Aging and Function.* University Hospitals Case Medical Center.

Panda, A., A. Arjona, E. Sapey, F. Bai, E. Fikrig, R. R. Montgomery, J. M. Lord, and A. C. Shaw. 2009. Human innate immunosenescence: Causes and consequences for immunity in old age. *Trends Immunol* 30 (7):325–33. doi: 10.1016/j.it.2009.05.004.

Pearl, R. 1928. *The Rate of Living.* Alfred A. Knopf, New York.

Perls, T. T., L. Alpert, and R. C. Fretts. 1997. Middle-aged mothers live longer. *Nature* 389 (6647):133. doi: 10.1038/38148.

Peters, R. 2006. Ageing and the brain. *Postgrad Med J* 82 (964):84–8. doi: 10.1136/pgmj.2005.036665.

Phillips, T., and C. Leeuwenburgh. 2004. Lifelong aspirin supplementation as a means to extending life span. *Rejuvenation Res* 7 (4):243–51. doi: 10.1089/rej.2004.7.243.

Programmed-aging. 2015. Programmed aging theories. Retrieved from: http://www.programmed-aging.org/theory-3/Katcher.html.

Pubmed Health. U.S. National Library of medicine. Pelvic Floor Training (Kegel Exercises). Available from: http://www.ncbi.nlm.nih.gov/pubmedhealth/PMHT0022366/.

Rao, M. S., and M. P. Mattson. 2001. Stem cells and aging: Expanding the possibilities. *Mech Ageing Dev* 122 (7):713–34.

Reichrath, J. 2012. Unravelling of hidden secrets: The role of vitamin D in skin aging. *Dermatoendocrinol* 4 (3):241–4. doi: 10.4161/derm.21312.

Riddle, D.L., T. Blumenthal, B.J. Meyer et al. 1997. C. elegans In *Theories of Aging.* Cold Spring Harbor, NY: Cold Spring Harbor Laboratory Press.

Ridker, P. M. 2009. Testing the inflammatory hypothesis of atherothrombosis: Scientific rationale for the cardiovascular inflammation reduction trial (CIRT). *Journal of Thrombosis and Haemostasis* 7 (s1):332–9.

Rodier, F., J-P. Coppé, C. K Patil, W. A. M. Hoeijmakers, D. P. Muñoz, S. R. Raza et al. 2009. Persistent DNA damage signalling triggers senescence-associated inflammatory cytokine secretion. *Nat Cell Biol* 11 (8):973–9.

Rozemuller, A. J., W. A. van Gool, and P. Eikelenboom. 2005. The neuroinflammatory response in plaques and amyloid angiopathy in Alzheimer's disease: Therapeutic implications. *Curr Drug Targets CNS Neurol Disord* 4 (3):223–33.

Sattar, N., H. M Murray, P. Welsh, G. J Blauw, B. M Buckley, S. Cobbe, A. JM De Craen et al. 2009. Are markers of inflammation more strongly associated with risk for fatal than for nonfatal vascular events? *PLoS Med* 6 (6):e1000099.

Schiavone, D. L., and W. Tan. 2006. In: *Biomedical Nanotechnology. Small.* N. H. Malsch (ed). 2: 288.

Schmid, D., C. Schürch, and F. Zülli. 2008. Stimulation of stem cells for real rejuvenation. *Mibelle Biochemistry*, Switzerland, August. www.ptpphytoscience.com.

Segal, R. J., R. D. Reid, K. S. Courneya, R. J. Sigal, G. P. Kenny, D. G. Prud'Homme, S. C. Malone, G. A. Wells, C. G. Scott, and M. E. Slovinec D'Angelo. 2009. Randomized controlled trial of resistance or aerobic exercise in men receiving radiation therapy for prostate cancer. *J Clin Oncol* 27 (3):344–51. doi: 10.1200/JCO.2007.15.4963.

Sevinc, A., M. Ozkan, A. Ozet et al. 2014. 1501pcomparison of the Efficacy of Filgrastim (Neupogen(R)) and Biosimilar Filgrastim (Leucostim(R)) in Patients with Chemotherapy-Induced Neutropenia: A Nationwide Observational Study. *Ann Oncol* 25 (suppl_4):iv525. doi: 10.1093/annonc/mdu356.22.

Sharma, B., and A. Sharma. 2012. Future prospect of nanotechnology in development of anti-ageing formulations. *Int J Pharm Pharm Sci* 4 (3):57–66.

Sharma, S., T. K Kelly, and P. A Jones. 2010. Epigenetics in cancer. *Carcinogenesis* 31 (1):27–36.

Shay, J. W., and W. E. Wright. 2000. Hayflick, his limit, and cellular ageing. *Nat Rev Mol Cell Biol* 1 (1):72–6. doi: 10.1038/35036093.

Shytle, D. R., J. Tan, J. Ehrhart, A. J. Smith, C. D. Sanberg, P. R. Sanberg, J. Anderson, and P. C. Bickford. 2010. Effects of blue-green algae extracts on the proliferation of human adult stem cells in vitro: A preliminary study. *Med Sci Monit* 16 (1):BR1–5.

Simm, A., N. Nass, B. Bartling, B. Hofmann, R-E. Silber, and A. N. Santos. 2008. Potential biomarkers of ageing. *Biological Chemistry* 389 (3):257–65.

Spiegel, K., R. Leproult, and E. Van Cauter. 1999. Impact of sleep debt on metabolic and endocrine function. *Lancet* 354 (9188):1435–9. doi: 10.1016/S0140-6736(99)01376-8.

Srikanth, V., A. Maczurek, T. Phan, M. Steele, B. Westcott, D. Juskiw, and G. Munch. 2011. Advanced glycation endproducts and their receptor RAGE in Alzheimer's disease. *Neurobiol Aging* 32 (5):763–77. doi: 10.1016/j.neurobiolaging.2009.04.016.

Sung, B., J. W. Chung, H. R. Bae, J. S. Choi, C. M. Kim, and N. D. Kim. 2015. Extract exhibits antioxidative and anti-aging effects via modulation of the AMPK-SIRT1 pathway. *Exp Ther Med* 9 (5):1819–26. doi: 10.3892/etm.2015.2302.

Tabatabaie, V., G. Atzmon, S. N. Rajpathak, R. Freeman, N. Barzilai, and J. Crandall. 2011. Exceptional longevity is associated with decreased reproduction. *Aging (Albany NY)* 3 (12):1202–5.

Trappe, S. W., D. L. Costill, M. D. Vukovich, J. Jones, and T. Melham. 1996. Aging among elite distance runners: A 22-yr longitudinal study. *J Appl Physiol (1985)* 80 (1):285–90.

Ulrich, P., and A. Cerami. 2001. Protein glycation, diabetes, and aging. *Recent Prog Horm Res* 56:1–21.

Upadhyay, R.K. 2015. Role of regeneration in tissue repairing and therapies. *Journal of Regenerative Medicine and Tissue Engineering* 4 (1):1.

Ursin, G., S.L. Palla, and B.A. Reboussin. 2004. Posttreatment change in serum estrone predicts mammographic percent density changes in women who received combination estrogen and progestin in the postmenopausal estrogen/ progestin interventions (PEPI) trial. *J Clin Oncol* 22:2842–8.

van Heemst, D. 2010. Insulin, IGF-1 and longevity. *Aging Dis* 1 (2):147–57.

Vera, E., B. Bernardes de Jesus, M. Foronda, J. M. Flores, and M. A. Blasco. 2013. Telomerase reverse transcriptase synergizes with calorie restriction to increase health span and extend mouse longevity. *PLoS One* 8 (1):e53760. doi: 10.1371/journal.pone.0053760.

Verdin, E. 2015. NAD+ in aging, metabolism, and neurodegeneration. *Science*, 350 (6265):1208–1213.

Vranesic-Bender, D. 2010. The role of nutraceuticals in anti-aging medicine. *Acta Clin Croat* 49 (4):537–44.

Wallace, B. 2016. An MIT Scientist Claims That This Pill Is the Fountain of Youth. The Cut. Available at https://www.thecut.com/2016/08/is-elysium-healths-basis-the-fountain-of-youth.html

Weismann, A. 1891. *Essays Upon Heredity and Kindred Biological Problems*. 2nd ed. Vol. I. UK: Oxford, Clarendon Press.

Williams, G. C. 1957. Pleiotropy, natural selection, and the evolution of senescence. *Evolution* 11, 398–411.

Williams, R. J., J. P. Spencer, and C. Rice-Evans. 2004. Flavonoids: Antioxidants or signalling molecules? *Free Radic Biol Med* 36 (7):838–49. doi: 10.1016/j.freeradbiomed.2004.01.001.

Wilmut, I., N Beaujean, PA De Sousa, A Dinnyes, TJ King, LA Paterson, DN Wells, and LE Young. 2002. Somatic cell nuclear transfer. *Nature* 419 (6907):583–7.

Wynne-Edwards, V.C. 1986. *Evolution through Group Selection*. Oxford: Blackwell.

Yadav, N. K., S. Nanda, G. Sharma, and O. P. Katare. 2016. Systematically optimized coenzyme q10-loaded novel proniosomal formulation for treatment of photo-induced aging in mice: Characterization, biocompatibility studies, biochemical estimations and anti-aging evaluation. *J Drug Target* 24 (3):257–71. doi: 10.3109/1061186X.2015.1077845.

Yasuno, F., S. Tanimukai, M. Sasaki, C. Ikejima, Y. Yamashita, C. Kodama, K. Mizukami, and T. Asada. 2012. Combination of antioxidant supplements improved cognitive function in the elderly. *J Alzheimers Dis* 32 (4):895–903.

Zhan, Q., P. Wan, and B. Sun. 2002. The effect of foot massage on the changes of old mouse T cell factor gene expression: A clinical and experimental study. *Modern Rehabilitation* 1:30.

Zhou, C., C. Sun, K. Chen, and X. Li. 2011. Flavonoids, phenolics, and antioxidant capacity in the flower of Eriobotrya japonica Lindl. *Int J Mol Sci* 12 (5):2935–45. doi: 10.3390/ijms12052935.

Zhou, D., D. Yin, F. Xiao, and J. Hao. 2015. Expressions of Senescence-Associated beta-Galactosidase and Senescence Marker Protein-30 are Associated with Lens Epithelial Cell Apoptosis. *Med Sci Monit* 21:3728–35.

Zjacic-Rotkvic, V., L. Kavur, and M. Cigrovski-Berkovic. 2010. Hormones and aging. *Acta Clin Croat* 49 (4):549–54.

27 Overcoming Chronic and Degenerative Diseases with Energy Medicine[1]

James L. Oschman

CONTENTS

Dedication 641
Introduction 642
From the Microscope to the Organism and Beyond 643
How Fast is the Nervous System? 644
Diffusing Signal Molecules versus Electromagnetic Fields 646
Lucretian Biochemistry 653
Biology of the Ultra-Fast and the Unconscious Mind 657
What is Light and What Medium Does It Travel Through? 662
Protection from Environmental Electromagnetic Fields 665
The Holistic Anatomical Perspective 667
Tensegrity 667
The Living Matrix 671
A Solid-State Tissue-Tensegrity Matrix System 673
A Vibratory Matrix 675
The Ground Regulation System 675
Views of the Living Fascia 676
Conclusions 676
DNA—An Alternative Perspective 678
Appendix I: Author's Academic Background 678
Appendix II: Molecular "Wires" 678
Acknowledgments 680
Notes 680
References 681

> It is not what you don't know that gets you into trouble.
> It's what you know for sure that just is not so.[2]

DEDICATION

This chapter is dedicated to Dr. Marco Bischof, Ph.D. to commemorate his 70th birthday. Marco (Figure 27.1) has long been one of the leading scholars in the frontier areas of the sciences and holistic medicine. His brilliant and inspiring essays cover the spectrum from cosmic to quantum. For example, see his articles entitled "Introduction to Integrative Biophysics" (Bischof 2003) and "Man as a Cosmic Resonator" (Bischof 2010). His multi-disciplinary scholarship spans several languages, enabling him to be one of the most broadly sophisticated scholars in the field of bioenergetic medicine alive today. Marco has pointed out how energy field and holistic approaches pre-date and

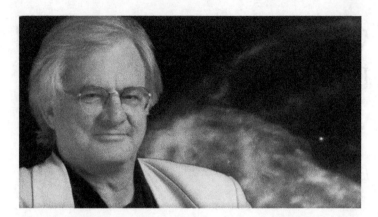

FIGURE 27.1   This chapter is dedicated to Marco Bischof, Ph.D. in celebration of his 70th birthday.

are fundamental to modern medicine, although this has been forgotten in many academic and clinical circles. For example, see his article entitled, "Field Concepts and the Emergence of a Holistic Biophysics" (Bischof 2000). Marco has done classic research on the emerging field of biophotonics and has published the most comprehensive text on the subject, *Biophotonen: Das Licht in unseren Zellen*; (*Biophotons—the Light in our Cells*, Bischof 1995). This is the most comprehensive treatise in the field of biophotonics and is based in part on his long relationship with the pioneers in the field, particularly the brilliant German biophysicist, Dr. Fritz Albert Popp, and the members of the International Institute of Biophysics in Neuss, Germany. Marco has served as President of that organization, as well as President of the International Light Association. Dr. Bischof and his colleagues have laid the foundation for an important medicine of the future—a medicine based on light. Marco's influence on the author's thinking will be noted throughout this chapter. On a personal level, he is a very warm and generous person, and a great dancer.

INTRODUCTION

All researchers need to consider the above admonition about what we think we know, that is just not so; this is vital if we are to progress beyond our current competence in biomedicine. There are many unsolved problems, and we do not understand the most serious medical conditions well enough to prevent them or to provide safe and cost-effective treatments.

Medical research is held back because academic scientists, including the author, have been taught many things that are either wrong or half-wrong. The "old school" half-wrong lessons are the most deceptive because they make sense at a superficial level, are easy to teach to our students, and can readily become incorporated into our thinking. They become axioms; positions we take for granted. Once they are implanted in our psyche they are always part of our logic. Getting beyond the limitations of our current medicine requires serious and continuous evaluation of what we think we know, of new methods that are available, and of new ways of thinking. In other words, if we keep thinking in the ways we have always thought, we will continue to do what we have always done, and that will get us the same results we have always gotten. This chapter discusses some concepts that will be unfamiliar to many readers, not because they have been proven to be incorrect, but because they are simply not part of the usual academic dialogue or research paradigm.

Disclaimer: This is a theoretical report and is not intended to provide any advice regarding diagnosis or treatment of diseases. Instead, it is meant as a summary of important ideas with the aim of stimulating research into important topics at the forefront of biomedical research.

Scientists are trained doubters, but the traditional bias against energy medicine has gone deeper than professional skepticism. Part of this is an ingrained but largely unjustified fear of energy, along with vested interests that benefit when the public is confused. Part of it is from a lack of understanding of what energy actually is, and failure to recognize the simple fact that we continually use the energies in our environment, light, sound, heat, smell, gravity, and touch to orient ourselves in space. In a sense, we are all energy experts but do not realize it. Basic physics is essential to understand energy medicine, but is given little attention in medical education. Hence, physicians who go into research do not know where to begin.

FROM THE MICROSCOPE TO THE ORGANISM AND BEYOND

After some 20 years of academic reductionist research, looking at the smallest particles of life with the world's most powerful electron microscopes, fascination with holism and holistic therapies led the author to "up periscope" and peek at the surrounding landscape. This led to many more years of inquiry that incorporated a whole systems perspective. It was realized that all the information on the detailed structure and function of cells and tissues, so carefully gathered over the past century, could be assembled into a systematic and systemic picture of life that encompasses all of the relevant sub-disciplines—physiology, biochemistry, cell biology, molecular biology, physics, biophysics, quantum chemistry, and quantum biology, to name a few. The result of multi-disciplinary investigations can lead to a merging of the extremes of holistic and reductionist science with the perspective that the whole arises from and is energized and informed by the behaviors of the smallest parts, such as the protons and electrons, and vice versa. And the observations of therapists who work from the holistic perspective every day are extremely valuable.

Modern thinking in physics and quantum physics suggests that electrons and protons and the stuff made of them, including living cells and tissues, are not actually things, but are condensations of energy; they are better described as fields of energy and information extending indefinitely into space rather than as isolated objects. This is a different way of looking at life than most of us have learned and become accustomed to. The situation is well summarized by the title and contents of a book edited by Stephen Hawking: *The dreams that stuff is made of: The Most Astounding Papers of Quantum Physics—and How They Shook the Scientific World* (Hawking 2011).

Crucial to the evolution of the author's career was a period in the late 1970s and early 1980s working as a staff scientist at the Marine Biological Laboratory at Woods Hole, Massachusetts in a laboratory across the hall from Albert Szent-Györgyi's Institute of Muscle Research, which later became the center of an international network of scientists known as the National Foundation for Cancer Research. After the loss of two of the beloved women in his life to cancer, Szent-Györgyi recognized that the persistence of chronic and degenerative diseases that cause so much suffering and financial stress world-wide meant that biomedicine was missing something vital about life. The existence of the often incurable conditions—meaning conditions we do not understand and therefore cannot treat—shows us that something profoundly important is missing from our thinking. He concluded that the missing piece was already known in every culture and in every medical tradition before ours, that is, healing can be accomplished by moving energy. This chapter is partly about defining what we mean by the healing effects of moving energy, with some specific examples of the application of energy medicine to resolve major health issues, including heart disease, cancer, and diabetes. These conditions are now epidemics on a global scale.

The author is grateful for experience in biophysics, a subject that is grounded in multi-disciplinary thinking, connecting biology and physics. But this was just a start. Details of the author's academic background are in an appendix.

Albert Szent-Györgyi was winner of the 1937 Nobel Prize in Physiology or Medicine for the synthesis of Vitamin C from Hungarian paprika, and for describing the components and reactions of the citric acid cycle (which was originally called the Szent-Györgyi cycle). In 1954, Szent-Györgyi received the Albert Lasker Award for Basic Medical Research for the isolation of the contractile proteins in muscle, a discovery that laid the foundation for modern muscle biochemistry. Always a pioneer, Szent-Györgyi, late in life, set out in a totally new direction for a biologist: quantum chemistry and quantum biology. His studies were very controversial and misunderstood, and for a long time he had difficulty obtaining financial support. To this day, many academic scientists are unaware that there are fields of quantum chemistry and quantum biology.

As a young investigator the author of this chapter seized on Szent-Györgyi's search for the "something missing" from our thinking. What could be more satisfying or important than filling in even one of the major gaps in our medical thinking and practice? One statement from Szent-Györgyi led to a lot of thought and exploration:

> Life is too rapid and subtle to be explained by slow moving nerve impulses and chemical reactions.

This statement, from a scientist who has been regarded as one of the most advanced thinkers of the twentieth century, is a suggestion for all of us to take a second look at the "sacred cows" of modern science. The title of a symposium in Szent-Györgyi's memory and honor, held at the Marine Biological Laboratory in Woods Hole, Massachusetts in July 1988: *To See What Everyone Has Seen, To Think What No One Has Thought* (Szent-Györgyi 1988). Many viewed that statement as characteristic of his adventurous and "out of the box" thinking.

> There are dominant ideas in every field. The brilliant thinker purposefully challenges those dominant ideas in order to think innovatively. If you can identify the standard viewpoint then survey the situation from a different viewpoint you have an excellent chance of gaining a new insight … When Jonas Salk was asked how he invented the vaccine for polio he replied, 'I imagined myself as a cancer cell and tried to sense what it would be like.'
>
> **Sloane undated**

What did Szent-Györgyi mean by his statement about the slow speed of nerve impulses and chemical reactions, and where did it come from? It came from watching his cat jump straight up in the air when it saw a snake in the grass. From an interview with Szent-Györgyi's colleague, Ron Pethig:

> The cat just suddenly shot up in the air because it had seen a snake, and Szent-Györgyi said there was no way that the whole reaction, that cat, everything in that cat, could jump all at once. This was not classical Newtonian physics. It had to be a sub-molecular event, a quantum leap.
>
> **Pethig 2004**

In other words, the reaction of the cat was far too fast to be explained by neural impulses traveling at meters/second and jumping across synapses in the neuro-matrix, and chemical messages rate-limited by random diffusion. Perhaps such rapid and subtle aspects of life are carried out by the systems we need to understand to cure the major health plagues of our times. What could these systems be? To find out, and to study quantum physics, in 1950 Szent-Györgyi went to the Institute for Advanced Studies in Princeton for a year to learn quantum theory. There he was able to talk with the great atomic physicists and mathematicians who had founded quantum physics. For example, Albert Einstein was a resident at the Institute at the same time.

HOW FAST IS THE NERVOUS SYSTEM?

One has to be impressed with what has been learned about the nervous system, as it has received abundant research funding and has preoccupied generations of neuroscientists. Some nerves conduct action potentials at velocities of 110 meters or 330 feet (more than the length of a football field) per second or faster. While this is impressive, the nerve networks that are thought to coordinate complex behaviors have many synapses, each producing a few milliseconds of transmission delay.

Study of the performances of elite athletes or dancers or musicians suggests that humans are capable of remarkably rapid and intricate movements and responses that often seem far too quick and well-coordinated to be explained by nervous processing, especially when one factors in multiple synaptic delays. Each synapse introduces a delay of 0.5–4 m sec, greatly limiting the speed with which neural circuits can transmit and process sensory information and produce meaningful actions (Katz and Miledi 1965).

A recent opinion article, entitled, "The Cerebellar Mossy Fiber Synapse as a Model for High-Frequency Transmission in the Mammalian CNS" discusses the limits on the speed of neural processing (Delvendahl and Hallermann 2016). The speed of neuronal information processing depends on neuronal firing frequency. The highest firing frequencies thus far have been observed at the cerebellar mossy fiber to granule cell synapse. High frequency was defined as frequencies well above 100 Hz. The article points out the obvious fact that the capacity for rapid information processing in the mammalian nervous system has been optimized by natural selection. However, the article also points out that the maximum firing frequency of neurons is still more than six orders of magnitude slower than the clock rate of modern computers. And the information processing rate of the brain may be limited to a millisecond timescale by its energy supply (Attwell and Gobb 2005).

The subject of clock rate may be of relevance to the problem articulated by Herbert Fröhlich:

An assembly of cells, as in a tissue or organ will have certain collective frequencies that regulate important processes, such as cell division. Normally these control frequencies will be very stable. If, for some reason, a cell shifts its frequency, entraining signals from neighboring cells will tend to reinstall the correct frequency. However, if a sufficient number of cells get out-of-step, the strength of the system's collective vibrations can decrease to the point where stability is lost. Loss of coherence can lead to disease or disorder.

Fröhlich 1978

If Fröhlich is correct, each cell in the body may have its own clock rate. From a regulatory/cybernetic perspective, this makes sense.

One would like to know the clock rate in the brain, and if other tissues have clocks. It appears that there are actually many clock rates in the brain. The oscillations occur on many different frequencies simultaneously and originate in many different parts of the brain. So if the oscillations have functional roles, the brain may be more of a "spread spectrum" computer than a single clock-based one (King 2011). If Fröhlich is correct, each cell in the body may have its own set of clock rates. From a cybernetic/regulation perspective, this makes sense.

One group of scientists, members of the International Neural Network Society, seeks to optimize computers on the basis of the latest neuroscience, and use advances in computer science to enhance understandings of brain function. We shall see later in this chapter that there is evidence that living tissues have semiconductor properties akin to those used in the integrated circuits such as those used to form clock circuits and information systems for computers. One feature worth looking for is solid state circuitry with local oscillators in the semiconductor fabric of the various cells and tissues. The reason this is important arises from a consideration of biological coherence.

Herbert Fröhlich is the scientist most closely associated with the topic of biological coherence. Fröhlich was a major participant in the development of quantum physics, and was nominated for the Nobel Prize in Physics in 1963 and 1964. In the late 1960s, Fröhlich predicted, on the basis of quantum physics, that the molecular fabric of cells and tissues must produce coherent or laser-like oscillations. His predication was confirmed in many laboratories (Fröhlich 1988). We now know that molecules can set up vibrations that travel about within an organism and that are radiated into the environment as biophotons. These vibrations or oscillations occur at many different frequencies, including visible and near-visible light frequencies. Cells and tissues are highly organized and are exceedingly sensitive to the information conveyed by coherent signals. These signals recognize no boundaries, at the surface of a molecule, cell, or organism—some of them are collective or cooperative properties of the entire organism. As such they are likely to serve as signals that integrate processes, such as growth, injury repair, defense, and the functioning of the organism as a whole. Each molecule, cell, tissue, and organ has an ideal resonant frequency associated with its functional activities.

Biological coherence will be discussed again when we look at the ways cells communicate with each other, and when we delve more deeply into biophotonics.

DIFFUSING SIGNAL MOLECULES VERSUS ELECTROMAGNETIC FIELDS

We are taught that hormones, neuro-hormones, cytokines, and other regulatory molecules are secreted by endocrine glands, immune cells, neurosecretory cells, or other sources and then diffuse randomly from their sites of origin to effector cells a distance away (Figure 27.2a). The signal molecule is then thought to fit into a receptor like a key fitting into a lock, to activate some cellular process. However, there are serious conceptual difficulties with the idea that our physiology is entirely coordinated by diffusing signal molecules and molecular keys fitting into molecular locks.

It should be obvious that slow and random diffusion is the exact opposite of what is needed to produce the rapid and subtle reactions that are the hallmark of life. Regulation by randomly diffusing signal molecules is an ancient "old school" concept, based in part on the "billiard ball" perspective

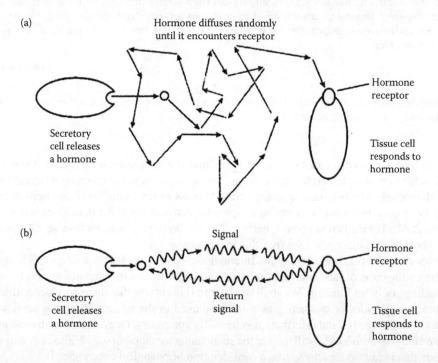

FIGURE 27.2   (a) It is widely thought that hormones, neuro-hormones, cytokines, and other regulatory molecules are secreted by endocrine glands, immune cells, neurosecretory cells, or other sources and then diffuse randomly from their sites of origin to effector cells a distance away. There the signal molecule is thought to fit into a receptor like a key fitting into a lock, to activate some cellular process. There are serious conceptual difficulties with this picture. (b) An energetic electromagnetic or biophotonic model solves many difficulties. This model is based on the idea that a molecule will emit a characteristic set of frequencies when it vibrates and these frequencies will resonate with receptor molecules. We know that molecules do, indeed, emit electromagnetic fields when they vibrate. This is the basis for the well-established technology of spectroscopy. Co-resonance between hormone and receptor provides feedback that the message has been received.

of indivisible atoms and their interactions. The idea dates to Lucretius (c. 99 BC–c. 55 BC) and his predecessors, Epicurus and Democritus. In more modern times, the picture was reinforced by the brilliant and accomplished British scientist, John Dalton (1766–1844) who applied these concepts to chemistry (Greenaway 1966). The unit of atomic mass, the Dalton, is named after John Dalton.

It should be obvious that slow and random diffusion is the exact opposite of what is needed to produce the rapid and subtle reactions that are the hallmark of life.

Lucretius must be credited with providing a concept that has had considerable longevity, even though we now know that the early picture of the hard indivisible atom was incorrect. We must ask why nature, with millions of years of trial and error, and countless physical processes to choose from, would select what is probably the slowest and most disorganized physical process available, namely random diffusion, to coordinate its vital processes, when much faster and much more specific physical processes were available. There has always been a strong selective pressure for high-speed responses. If the fight or flight response to a dangerous situation relied on adrenalin randomly diffusing from the adrenal cortex to produce the appropriate autonomic responses, many of our ancestors would not have survived long enough to reproduce (Figure 27.3). They would have been eaten! Of course, the problem has been solved in part by the development of the sympathetic nervous system, which delivers signals that can trigger vascular changes in different parts of the body almost instantaneously. For example, sympathetic stimulation can accelerate heart rate; widen bronchial passages; decrease motility (movement) of the large intestine; constrict blood vessels; increase peristalsis in the esophagus; cause pupillary dilation, piloerection (goose bumps), and perspiration (sweating); and raise blood pressure. But synaptic delays in the sympathetic nervous system and diffusion of catecholamines secreted into the circulatory system from the adrenal medulla are part of these regulations.

We must ask why nature, with millions of years of trial and error, and countless physical processes to choose from, would select what is probably the slowest and most disorganized process available, namely random diffusion, to coordinate its vital processes, when much faster and more specific methods were available.

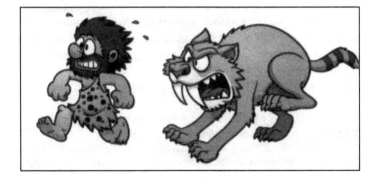

FIGURE 27.3 Given a choice from many possible physical processes, why would evolutionary selection prefer random diffusion of signal molecules—probably the slowest and least specific mechanism available—for its vital communications? There was a strong selective pressure for high-speed responses. If the fight or flight response to a dangerous situation relied on adrenalin randomly diffusing from the adrenal cortex to produce the appropriate autonomic responses, many of our ancestors would not have survived long enough to reproduce. They would have been eaten!

Another difficulty with the widely accepted random diffusion model is that it does not provide for feedback, which is important for the cybernetic aspects of regulation formalized by Norbert Wiener (1948). Specifically, feedback enables the source of a signal to recognize that the message has been received. Without such feedback, regulations would be chaotic rather than coordinated.

If the fight or flight response to a dangerous situation relied on adrenalin randomly diffusing from the adrenal cortex to produce the appropriate autonomic responses, many of our ancestors would not have survived long enough to reproduce. They would have been eaten!

An energetic electromagnetic or biophotonic model solves these and other issues (Figure 27.2b). This model is based on the idea that a molecule will emit a characteristic set of frequencies when it vibrates. We know from spectroscopy that molecules do, indeed, emit electromagnetic fields when they vibrate. Several lines of evidence, to be discussed next, support the concept that biophotons are involved in physiological regulations:

- Structural complementarity of signal molecules and their receptors
- Coherence or laser-like character of biophotons
- Electromagnetic resonance between molecules
- Studies of the shapes of photons reveal various ways they can encode information
- Well-documented existence of distant non-chemical communication
- Evidence from a variety of sources supporting the concept that biophoton emissions can coordinate events occurring in widely separated locations within a living organism
- Light provides a rapid means of communication as it operates at the speed of light
- Evidence that extremely weak electromagnetic fields can alter a wide variety of cellular processes with beneficial or harmful effects (Pall 2013)
- The existence of important biological processes that are very fast and are difficult to explain by conventional neural and molecular signaling concepts

It is known that signal molecules have structures that are complementary to the receptor molecules (this is what presumably enables the key to fit into the lock). This structural complementarity can likewise provide a basis for co-resonance. Electromagnetic signaling is fast (speed of light) and provides instantaneous feedback by co-resonance. This phenomenon is comparable to the tuning-fork effect in the realm of acoustics. In the case of molecule-to-molecule signaling, biological coherence can also be an important factor. Fröhlich and his colleagues demonstrated that if two large molecules are capable of large vibrations at certain frequencies and the medium separating them has appropriate properties, resonance-like interactions may take place even if the molecules are far apart. The mechanism involves longitudinal vibratory modes. Once a molecule becomes strongly excited, it may tend to continue to vibrate because it cannot lose energy by emitting radiation. In particular, there can be persistent long-range phase-correlated motions (coherent vibrations), especially in molecules that are strongly polar, as many biomolecules are (for references, see Oschman 2000, pp. 102 and 103). Cell membranes provide a specific example:

Cell membranes are highly ordered arrays of strongly polar phospholipid molecules (they are liquid crystals) and can support huge electric fields, on the order of 10^5 volts/cm. These huge fields keep the molecular arrays under a high degree of stress or tension; therefore the molecules tend to vibrate strongly and the vibrations last a long time, like the ringing of a huge bell. Oscillations of the membrane field have frequencies on the order of 10^{11} Hz, corresponding to far infrared light.

There is no doubt that vibrating molecules emit characteristic electromagnetic fields, and that these fields change frequency and other characteristics when a molecule undergoes a structural

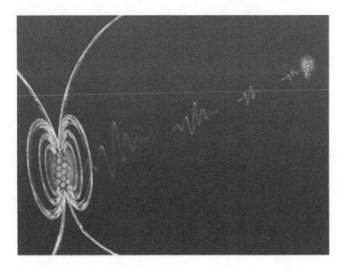

FIGURE 27.4 Recent work from the Max Plank Institute for the Science of Light and Department of Physics, University of Erlangen-Nuremberg in Germany has shown that a single photon from a single organic molecule can interact with another single molecule several meters away.

or chemical transformation of any kind. This is the basis for a widely used century-old technique, spectroscopy, used to identify the chemical composition of unknown substances as well as the chemical composition of distant stars and galaxies. Taken together, these discoveries raise the possibility that systemic regulatory processes such as sugar metabolism or the sympathetic fight or flight response could involve long-range coherence between specific populations of receptors on cells distributed throughout the body.

Electromagnetic resonance between molecules is extremely specific. Recent work from the Max Plank Institute for the Science of Light and Department of Physics, University of Erlangen-Nuremberg in Germany has shown that a single photon from a single organic molecule can interact with another single molecule several meters away with nearly 100% efficiency (Figure 27.4) (Rezus et al. 2012). And scientists at the Istituto Nazionale di Ottica in Florence, Italy have measured the shape of individual photons for the first time. Pulses of light can have almost any shape in space and time, depending on the amplitudes and phases of the pulse's frequency components. Much information can therefore be encoded in a single photon (Dumé 2012). The manner by which the fabric of the quantum information field may give rise to electric, magnetic, and electromagnetic fields and photons has been described by Marvin Solit, D.O. (1998) (Figure 27.5).

Distant non-chemical communication has been documented in a variety of biological systems. The classic example is provided by the work of the famous Russian embryologist and histologist Alexander Gurwitsch begun in the 1920s (Gurvitch 1926). He used two quartz capillaries containing onion roots. They were placed perpendicular to each other so that the growing tip of one root pointed toward meristem tissue of the other root. Gurwitsch and his colleagues performed hundreds of experiments and consistently found that actively dividing cells in the root tip stimulated a 35–40% increase in mitoses in the meristem tissue of the second root. When the onion roots were separated by a UV-opaque glass plate, the effect was absent. Therefore, Gurwitsch suggested that the growing tissue was emitting an ultra-weak ultraviolet UV light when the cells were dividing. He referred to this light as mitogenetic radiation (MR). Subsequent work by a variety of scientists in a number of countries documented and characterized MR emissions from dividing cells in microorganisms, embryos, culture tissues, regenerating organs, blood, neural, brain, and muscular tissues. These emissions were sharply increased by various toxic treatments (rapid freezing, narcosis, centrifugation, continuous and alternating electric current, and also in cancer).

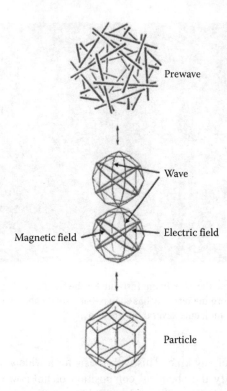

FIGURE 27.5 The manner by which electric, magnetic, electromagnetic fields and photons (as particles) may arise from the tensegritious fabric of the quantum information field has been described by Marvin Solit, D.O. The prewave is a tensegrity icosahedron with 30 struts in 15 directions. The electromagnetic wave arises from an icosidodecahedron with 60 struts that gives rise to the electric and magnetic fields at right angles to each other. The photon as a particle is a rhombic triacontahedron with 60 struts with a surface and a volume. This is referred to as a 3-phase model, prewave, wave and photon. For details, see Solit (1998).

Extensive research by Gurwitsch and many others has confirmed that all living systems are able to emit this type of radiation, laying the foundation for the modern field of biophotonics. Many experiments showed that the most appropriate candidates for the information signals were ultraviolet and infrared radiation. The extensive literature on this topic has been thoroughly and critically reviewed by Trushin (2004) and also by Sitizuraa, Taib, Abdullah and Yunus 2005; Kobayashi 2005; Van Wijk, Van Wijk, and Bajpai 2006; Özdemir and Kargi 2011; and Ignatov, Mosin, and Stoyanov 2014. An especially thorough review has been published by Cifra Fields and Farhadi (2011).

A series of studies led Popp and his colleagues and others to conclude that emitted biophotons are composed of coherent light. Specifically, the light appeared to decay in a hyperbolic way, in contrast to the exponential decay of non-coherent light (e.g., Popp 1994). However, an extremely thorough review of virtually all the literature on this subject (Cifra, Brouderb, Nerudová, and Kučera 2015) revealed a number of conceptual and mathematical errors and speculative interpretations on photocount statistics that led to a number of concepts that were uncritically accepted. The report concluded that the phenomenon of ultraweak photon emissions (UPE) from biological systems can be considered experimentally well established, but no reliable evidence for the coherence or non-classical nature of biophotons has actually been achieved. Cifra and colleagues indicated future directions for this research using methods of quantum optics. Detailed analysis of biophotons is quite challenging due to their extremely low intensity.

Direct evidence for molecule to molecule electromagnetic communication has been developed by Irena Cosic and her colleagues at the Royal Melbourne Institute of Technology (RMIT University) located in Melbourne, Victoria, Australia. In an extensive series of important and fascinating publications, Cosic has developed and applied a method she refers to as the Resonant Recognition Model (RRM) to predict electromagnetic resonances of macromolecules such as tubulin, microtubules, telomere DNA, and RNA macromolecules. The resonances are related to the free electron energy distribution along the macromolecule. The frequencies of these electromagnetic resonances depend on charge velocity. Using different velocities of charge transfer, Cosic and colleagues predicted resonant frequencies in a wide range of frequencies ranging from thousands of Hz to terahertz radiation—also known as submillimeter radiation. Terahertz waves have tremendously high frequencies ($1 \, THz = 10^{12} \, Hz$). Wavelengths of radiation in the terahertz band correspondingly range from 1 mm to 0.1 mm (or 100 μm). Terahertz radiation falls in between infrared radiation and microwave radiation in the electromagnetic spectrum, and it shares some properties with each of these. Like infrared and microwave radiation, terahertz radiation travels in a straight line and is non-ionizing (Cosic Lazar and Cosic 2015a,b).

> How do EMFs composed of low-energy photons produce non-thermal biological changes, both pathophysiological and, in some cases, potentially therapeutic, in humans and higher animals? It may be surprising that the answer to this question has been hiding in plain sight in the scientific literature. However, in this era of highly focused and highly specialized science, few of us have the time to read the relevant literature, let alone organize the information found within it in useful and critical ways.
>
> **Pall 2013**

Taken together, the evidence from a variety of sources and perspectives strongly supports the concept that biophoton emissions can coordinate events occurring in widely separated locations within a living organism by molecular resonance. Biophotons are the ideal means of communication for phenomena that require synchronous behavior among physically separate and independent biological units. Moreover, damaged or diseased tissues emit particular frequencies that can be used for diagnosis (Ives et al. 2014) and other frequencies can restore normal functioning (Karu 1999).

There is now good evidence that there are electromagnetic links between cells, tissues, and whole organisms (ever watch flocks of birds flying in formation, or schools of fish swimming synchronously?). Indeed, electromagnetic signaling is the most suitable kind of communication in various media, including the atmosphere, water, and living tissues.

Finally, in one of the most significant studies in recent years, Martin L. Pall (2013) has explained how exceedingly weak electromagnetic fields (EMFs) can have harmful or beneficial effects, essentially replacing another "old-school" concept that electromagnetic fields cannot affect cells and tissues unless they are ionizing or strong enough to produce heat.

Pall found twenty-three different studies showing that EMF exposures activate voltage-gated calcium channels, and that calcium channel blockers prevent such activation. The effects are produced by extremely low frequency fields, including 50/60 cycle exposures, microwave EMF range exposures, static electric fields, static magnetic fields and nanosecond pulses. Stimulation of the voltage-gated calcium channels leads to increased intracellular $Ca++$ which can act in turn to stimulate the two calcium/calmodulin-dependent nitric oxide synthases and increase nitric oxide which may act therapeutically by stimulating cGMP and protein kinase G. Nitric oxide may act in pathophysiological responses by acting as a precursor of peroxynitrite, producing both oxidative stress and free radical breakdown products. These interpretations are supported by two specific well-documented examples of EMF effects: EMF stimulation of bone growth, and EMF induction of single-stranded DNA breaks via the nitric oxide/peroxynitrite/free radical (oxidative stress) pathway.

The view that electromagnetic fields cannot affect cells and tissues unless they are ionizing or strong enough to produce heat is a classic example of something that many have learned that is just not so. It is an idea that may make sense at a superficial level, is easy to teach, and that can readily become incorporated into our thinking—it is an axiom that has been implanted in our psyche. It is a concept that is supportive to the vast and growing industries that utilize EMFs for cellular communications and Wi-Fi. However, Martin L. Pall has provided compelling evidence that safety standards for EMF exposure based on the thermal perspective are drastically in need of revision (Pall 2014).

> Many ignore the thousands of studies on this topic, but they should not be ignored. For example, voltage gated calcium channels have roles in the release of virtually every neurotransmitter in the brain. The brain is complicated and we cannot predict the results of exposure, hence it is not surprising that there are neuropsychiatric and neurodegenerative effects. Also, melatonin drops to zero, disturbing sleep. All of the evidence supporting the thermal paradigm is of the weakest kind. Eastern European countries have sensible and stringent safety standards. In other countries, the current exposure to EMF's is 10^{10} times what it was during evolution. This is ten thousand million times, and it keeps going up. To continue to do this without looking at the potential health effects makes no sense.

Professor Olle Johannson in Sweden reached a similar conclusion:

> Many people who worked in the electronics industry in Sweden, including an estimated 12% of the electrical engineers in that industry, became electrically sensitive, and helped form an organization called Föreningen för el-och bildskärmsskadade (Association for the Electrosensitive), or FEB. Due in part to the work of FEB and the research of Dr. Olle Johansson electrosensitivity is now a fully recognized disability in Sweden. "The world may be moving inexorably," Johansson warns, "toward one of those tragic moments that will lead historians to ask: 'Why did they not act in time?'"

Cellular Phone Taskforce, 2016

> The name, ultraweak photon emissions, brings up an important question. To whom are these emissions "ultraweak?" From the human perspective, the term "ultraweak" derives from the fact that they are difficult for us to detect. It was not until Fritz Albert Popp developed sensitive photon detectors that we were able to study these emissions. However, to a cell, these emissions are not ultraweak—they are the stuff of their ordinary conversations with other cells, and they have big effects on cell behavior.

Pall has solved two very important problems: why some people become sick from EMF exposure from distant sources, and how the minuscule fields projected from the hands of therapists and from healing devices can produce health benefits. His results help us understand how molecules and cells and their receptors can listen to the whispers coming from other molecules and other cells. And it provides a firm basis for biophotonics. Biophotons are often defined as ultraweak photon emissions (UPE), with a visibility 1000 times lower than the sensitivity of our naked eye.

The name, *ultraweak* photon emissions, brings up an important question. To whom are these emissions "ultraweak?" From the human perspective, the term "ultraweak" derives from the fact that the signals are difficult for us to detect. The intensity is about 10^{18} times lower than regular daylight. To study this phenomenon, Dr. Fritz-Albert Popp developed an instrument called a photon multiplier which could detect the glow of a firefly 10 miles away. However, to a cell, these emissions are not ultraweak—they are the stuff of their ordinary conversations with other cells, and they regulate cell behaviors.

Blank and Goodman (2011) summarized evidence that DNA responds to EMFs over a wide range of frequencies, from extremely low frequency (ELF) to radio frequency (RF). To accomplish this, it appears that DNA is a fractal antenna—an unusual kind of antenna that can transmit or receive electromagnetic fields at many different frequencies simultaneously. Hence, DNA in every cell has the potential to transmit and receive frequency information from every other cell, suggesting a feedback system with continuous communication with events taking place throughout

> DNA is a fractal antenna—an unusual kind of antenna that can transmit or receive electromagnetic fields at many different frequencies simultaneously. Hence, DNA in every cell has the potential to transmit and receive frequency information from every other cell, suggesting a feedback system with continuous communication with events taking place throughout the body, using light waves to encode and transfer information.

the body, using light waves to encode and transfer information. For active molecules, the emitted frequency changes with conformational changes.

Electromagnetic fields are generated by the movement of electromagnetic waves along a conductor—an antenna wire or a molecule. Every antenna has an optimal frequency, depending on its length. Ideally, the length of the antenna is the same as the wavelength of the signal being received or transmitted. This is called a full wavelength antenna. Half-wave and quarter-wave antennas also work but are less efficient than full wavelength antennas. Antenna length is more critical for transmitting than for receiving.

The fractal property of DNA is achieved by using a repeating design to maximize the length of the conductor that can receive or transmit electromagnetic waves. All subdivisions of the antenna have a geometry that is similar to the structure as a whole, that is, different sections of the antenna or molecule resemble the shape of the entire antenna or molecule.

Since DNA can interact with EMF over a wide range of frequencies, and does not appear to be limited to a single optimal frequency, it has the functional properties of a fractal antenna. The DNA molecule can conduct electrons within the double helix (Wan et al. 1999), so the DNA in the cell nucleus has the compacted structural properties of a fractal antenna. The ways molecules can act as conductors or "wires" are summarized in Appendix II.

While the concept is admittedly speculative, it has been proposed that spacetime may also be fractal and quantum coherent in the Golden Mean (Ho, el Naschie and Vitiello 2015). This conclusion comes from looking at spacetime from a wide perspective: from mathematics, quantum physics, far from equilibrium thermodynamics, biology, and neurobiology. If this is true, the conditions are optimal for resonance between space and DNA. Popp's Biophoton theory concerns DNA as the most probable source and receiver of biophoton emission that can coordinate all activities.

> We are still on the threshold of fully understanding the complex relationship between light and life, but we can now say emphatically, that the function of our entire metabolism is dependent on light.

Fritz-Albert Popp

LUCRETIAN BIOCHEMISTRY

Biochemistry texts usually ignore how substrates and enzymes come in contact with each other. One is more or less left to assume that dissolved reactants within the cell bounce around randomly until they accidentally bump into appropriate dissolved enzymes, which are also diffusing randomly, all on their own "random walks." In fact, the probability of correct encounters between free floating substrates and randomly diffusing enzymes within the volume of the cell has to be approximately zero. The fact that such reactions take place in test tubes containing solutions of molecules extracted from living tissue does not mean that it works that way in living cells.

Guenter Albrecht-Buehler has reached a similar conclusion about the chances of hormones or other signal molecules encountering receptors on cell surfaces. In a valuable article entitled "In Defense of Non-Molecular Cell Biology" he raised a major argument against the view that regulations take place by diffusion of signal molecules to receptor sites on cells, where they supposedly activate cellular processes (Albrecht-Buehler 1990). To this we have added the problem of cellular close packing in various epithelia (Figure 27.6). Albrecht-Buehler's conclusion: "Our usual concept of concentration is essentially meaningless."

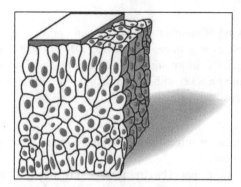 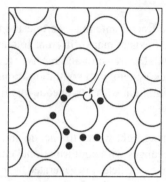

FIGURE 27.6 Cells in the body are generally packed closely together in layers called epithelia (left). Albrecht-Buehler in a valuable perspective entitled "In Defense of 'Non-molecular' Cell Biology" has raised a major argument against the view that regulations take place by diffusion of signal molecules to receptor sites on cells, where they activate cellular processes. While some epithelia are only one cell thick, others consist of many cells packed closely together (shown to the left). If one considers the average fluid volume around an individual cell, the actual space available is such that hormone molecules (black dots) with a concentration of 1 pM (6×10^{11} molecules/L) will have a concentration of approximately eight molecules in the space surrounding an individual cell. In the region around the receptor, the hormone concentration, for all practical purposes, is approximately zero. Albrecht-Buehler concluded that our usual concept of concentration is essentially meaningless.

A much more sensible concept for biochemical reactions is the metabolon, an orderly sequence of enzymes anchored on a structure such as a membrane or cytoskeletal filament (Srere 1985). A substrate molecule interacting with the first enzyme in the sequence is acted on and the reaction product is then quickly passed to the next enzyme, and so on. There is evidence for a Krebs cycle metabolon and for substrate channeling through the metabolon (Wu and Minteer 2014). While there is increasing evidence for this model, it is usually given only a footnote in biochemistry texts, which typically depict virtually all reactions as molecules more or less floating on the page, with no description of how they manage to find each other (examples are shown in Figure 27.7). Several books present organic chemistry more realistically, based on transfers of energetic electrons (Eberson 2011; Balzani 2001; Scudder 2013).

The lock and key model of ligand-receptor interaction is another example of a classic oversimplified "old school" model. It dates to Emil Fischer (1894). The model is deceptively easy to understand by anyone who has used a key to open a lock. Such images satisfy us that a problem has been solved, distracting us from further investigation. But a lot of progress has taken place since Fischer's report in 1894, and we urgently need to revisit the lock and key model from more recent perspectives, such as quantum electrodynamics. Modern science provides deeper and more thorough models worthy of consideration. In fact, this author believes these "old school" concepts are long-overdue for re-examination. Of course, we know that the scientific community is reluctant to revisit widely held beliefs, as evidenced by the violent reaction to Rupert Sheldrake's suggestions that some of our favorite ideas might be ready for another look (Sheldrake 2013).

> The diffusion of signal molecules and their interactions with receptors according to the random diffusion and lock and key models may be one of the main sources of confusion preventing us from understanding and treating major health problems, including cancer.

Two very different equations can be mentioned as fundamental to cellular regulations. Fick's law of diffusion, based on classical physics, derived by Adolf Fick (1855) describes the diffusion

Glucose

↓ 1

Glucose 6 phosphate

↓ 2

Fructose 6 phosphate

↓ 3

Fructose 1,6 biphosphate

↓ 4

Dihydroxyacetone
phosphate

↓ 5

Glyceraldehyde 3
phosphate

↓ 6

1,3 Diphosphoglycerate

↓ 7

3 Phosphoglycerate

↓ 8

2 Phosphglycerate

↓ 9

Phosphoenolpyruvate

↓ 10

Pyruvate

FIGURE 27.7 Biochemistry texts typically depict reactions as taking place between molecules more-or-less floating on the page, with no description of where they are located and how they manage to find each other. The diagram shows the 10 steps in glyicolysis, the conversion of glucose to pyruvate.

of substances. It postulates that the flux goes from regions of high concentration to regions of low concentration, with a magnitude that is proportional to the concentration gradient:[4]

$$J = -D \frac{d\varphi}{dx}$$

In dilute aqueous solutions, the diffusion coefficients of most ions, for example, are similar and have values that at room temperature are in the range of 0.6×10^{-9} to 2×10^{-9} m^2/s. For biological molecules, the diffusion coefficients normally range from 10^{-11} to 10^{-10} m^2/s (Crank 1980). This is very slow! Again, if the fight or flight response to a dangerous situation relied on adrenalin randomly diffusing from the adrenal cortex to produce the appropriate autonomic responses, many of our ancestors would not have survived long enough to reproduce. They would have been eaten (Figure 27.3)!

The time-dependent Schrödinger equation could replace Fick's law for understanding regulatory biology. We return to the work of Marco Bischof in collaboration with the brilliant quantum physicist, Emilio Del Giudice, for a modern treatment of this subject (Bischof and Del Giudice 2013).

$$i\hbar \frac{\partial}{\partial t} \Psi(\mathbf{r}, t) = \hat{H} \Psi(\mathbf{r}, t)$$

The Schrödinger equation predicts, on the basis of wave functions, how particles can form energetic standing waves, called stationary states (also called "orbitals" as in atomic or molecular orbitals). In essence, we cannot determine the exact position of a particle in space and time, but we can determine the probabilities of its properties. This quantum perspective is now being considered in relation to atoms or molecules in living systems. For example, recent research from the Fleming group at the University of California in Berkeley has revealed remarkable quantum processes taking place in the leaves of green plants:

> Wavelike electron energy transfer within the photosynthetic complex explains its extreme efficiency. It allows the excited electron to sample vast areas of phase space to find the most efficient path.

Engel, Calhoun, Read, Ahn et al. 2007

If wavelike electron energy transfer takes place in the chloroplasts of green plants, there is no reason it should not also take place in animals. The chloroplast is a virtual mirror image of the animal mitochondrion, so it would not be surprising to find wavelike electron energy transfer in mitochondria as well. This is quantum biology, a field pioneered by Albert Szent-Györgyi that is still in its infancy. He and his colleagues published some of the early reports in the field of quantum chemistry in the *International Journal of Quantum Chemistry and Quantum Biology* beginning with Szent-Györgyi (1977). Further investigations of electronic biology were published between 1957 and 1979 (Pethig 1979, Szent-Györgyi 1957, 1960, 1968, 1976, 1978). A modern film and book on quantum biology provides an excellent and clear introduction to the subject (McFadden and AI-Khalili, 2016).

The pioneering work on biological semiconduction is the basis for the modern field of nano-electronics. An article by Hush (2006), a major figure in the nano-electronics industry, credits Albert Szent-Györgyi (semiconduction in proteins) together with Robert S. Mulliken (molecular orbital theory) as the pioneers who laid the foundation for the entire field. Both were recipients of Nobel Prizes in the years 1937 and 1966, respectively.

Given the sophistication of molecular circuitry as developed in the electronics industry, one can speculate that the entire fabric of the body, termed the living matrix system (p. 631), could be an integrated semiconductor circuit reaching into every part of the organism (Figure 27.8a). Recent

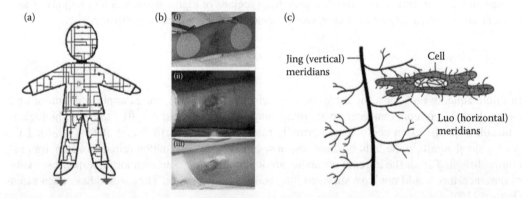

FIGURE 27.8 (a) On the basis of the semiconductor properties of many of the molecules comprising the living matrix and the successes from using organic molecules in the electronics industry, we can speculate that the bulk of the living organism may form a semiconductor network that reaches into every part. Like any other electronic circuit, optimal operation requires grounding. The rapid resolution of inflammation brought about by Earthing or grounding is consistent with this concept, as shown in (b), showing rapid recovery from a serious wound with minimal swelling and redness expected for such a serious injury. Cyclist was injured in Tour de France competition—chain wheel gouged his leg. (i) Grounding patches were placed above and below wound as soon as possible after injury. (ii) One day after injury (iii). There was minimal redness, pain, and swelling, and cyclist was able to continue the race on the day following the injury. In (c) we see the classical picture of the meridian system, with the vertical or Jing meridians and the horizontal meridians called Luo. Ancient teachings suggest that the Jing meridians have many branches, and it is suggested that these reach the surfaces of all cells in the body, contact the integrins, and connect to the cytoskeletons and nuclei.

work of Dr. Robert M. Metzger from the Lab for Molecular Electronics at the University of Alabama has shown how atoms and molecules can serve as circuit elements such as rectifiers (Metzger 2003). Experience with Earthing or grounding the human body is also consistent with the idea of electronic circuits within the body. The reason for this is the speed with which grounding can resolve chronic inflammation (Figure 27.8b). The most parsimonious explanation for this is that Earthing connects a barefoot person, via the point on the ball of the foot known as Kidney 1, with the entire continuously branching acupuncture meridian system that also extends throughout the body (Figure 27.8c). Hence, the phenomena involved in Earthing provide strong support for the concepts developed by Szent-Györgyi and others of electronic semiconduction within the body.

BIOLOGY OF THE ULTRA-FAST AND THE UNCONSCIOUS MIND

Over the years the author has followed up on Albert Szent-Györgyi's comment that slow moving nerve impulses and chemical reactions cannot account for the speed and subtlety of living processes. This has been a search for ultra-fast biophysical communication processes in the living body that might better explain *rapid and subtle phenomena*. One obvious place to find examples was in peak athletic and artistic performances, which led to a book *Energy Medicine in Therapeutics and Human Performance* (Oschman 2003). A turning point came while watching the 1989 World figure skating championships. One performer, Midori Ito, stood out because of her extraordinary and beautiful and relaxed performance. She was the first skater to perform a triple axel in the Olympics. A major concept introduced in that book is *systemic cooperation*, closely corresponding to the *Gestaltbildung* of Fritz Albert Popp. This is the process by which every cell in the body "knows" what every other cell is doing, so all cells and tissues can participate in any action. It became apparent to Popp and his colleagues that physiological integration and cooperation arise from the use of light as a communication medium within the organism. This led to the burgeoning field of biophotonics. For a concise and fascinating summary of that field, see an article by Marco Bischof published in the *Journal of Optometric Phototherapy* (Bischof 2005).

The author's exploration took a quantum leap from conversations with an eminent psychiatrist Maurie Pressman, MD, who had also studied sophisticated athletic performance. Pressman introduced hypnotism and psychoanalysis to the U.S. Olympic skating team and published several articles on the subject (Pressman 1977, 1979, 1980a,b). The result of the collaboration with Pressman was an article describing a number of processes that can conduct energy and information much faster than nerve impulses. The goal was to provide, for the first time, clues about the phenomena Sigmund Freud had speculated about a century earlier. Freud (1895/1957) had recognized that his "provisional ideas" in psychology would one day be based on some sort of organic substructures, but he had no idea at the time what these would be. Hence, the title of our report was *An Anatomical, Biochemical, Biophysical and Quantum Basis for the Unconscious Mind* (Oschman and Pressman 2014). In the article, we identified several biological processes that are hundreds or thousands of times faster than nerve impulses.

These high-speed processes include semiconduction in the living matrix. It is suggested that the living matrix/ground regulation system forms a semiconducting analog and digital network operating at hundreds or perhaps thousands of meters per second. A semiconductor is a material with electrical conductivity that is intermediate between that of an insulator and a conductor. Importantly, the conductivity of a semiconductor can be modified in precise ways by imposing small electric, magnetic, or photonic fields or by introducing impurities, in a process known in the electronics industry as "doping." The ability to control conductivity in small and well-defined regions of semiconductor materials has led to the development of a broad array of miniaturized electronic devices that have become the basis for nearly all modern electronics. This is mentioned because most if not all biomolecules have semiconductor properties (Pullman and Pullman 1958; Rosenberg and Postow 1969). This fact has been essential to the development of the flourishing molecular electronics industry (e.g., Cuevas and Sheer 2010). Research in this field is driven, in part, by the need to reduce the size and increase the efficiency of electronic technologies. Engineers are constantly looking for applications that take advantage of the extraordinary quantum properties of materials so they can develop and manufacture efficient circuits composed of atoms or molecules. Organic electronics uses organic (carbon-based) small molecules or polymers that show desirable electronic properties such as conductivity. Organic electronic materials are constructed using synthetic strategies from organic and polymer chemistry. A unimolecular rectifier is a single organic molecule which functions as a rectifier (one-way conductor) of electric current. The idea was first proposed in 1974 by Arieh Aviram, then at IBM, and Mark Ratner, then at New York University. Their publication was the first serious and concrete theoretical proposal in the new field of molecular electronics (UE). Perhaps the human body is a molecular electronic circuit. Note the grounding in Figure 27.8a.

Dr. Robert M. Metzger, Professor of Physical Chemistry Lab for Molecular Electronics at the University of Alabama, has pioneered the development of atomic and molecular transistors (e.g., Metzger 2003).

Moreover, the properties of organic semiconductors in living tissues can vary from place to place within cells and tissues, allowing for the possibility that the structural fabric of the organism, including the acupuncture meridian systems, can form a kind of biological electronic circuit with the ability to carry out processes that are analogous to those built into commercial transistors and integrated circuits. Specifically, the micro-circuitry of living cells and tissues may be capable of conducting, storing, and processing energy and information and transforming energy from one form to another, using efficient high-speed electronic and quantum processes comparable to those found in transistors, integrated circuits, computers, opto-electronic systems, cellular telephones, and other miniaturized technologies (see Oschman 1993).

Barnett (1987) described how molecules can act as string processors. The Primitive String Transformer (PST) is a computing device that can process analog or digital information algorithmically by transferring electrons from a donor to a polymer and switching a non-conjugated chain to a conjugated form, thereby delocalizing some of the electronic orbitals along the chain. This is a profound concept! If living tissues can accurately be described in terms of micro-circuitry, string processors, and integrated circuits comparable to those used in the electronics industry, new understandings of the nature of life and consciousness open up.

For example, Hameroff pointed out that individual neurons are at least as complex as nerve nets, and their cytoskeletons therefore have enormous capacity for intracellular information processing. A tiny neuron, a thousandth of an inch in diameter, has about 9 feet of cytoskeleton. Hence, there are close to a billion miles of semiconducting fibers in the brain. The microtubules, together with other semiconducting cytoskeletal structures, could form a sophisticated electronic communication network within neurons and other cells. According to Hameroff, nanosecond switching in microtubules predicts roughly 10^{16} operations per second, per neuron. This capacity could account for the adaptive behaviors of single-celled organisms such as paramecium, which elegantly swims, avoids obstacles, and finds food and mates completely without benefit of a nervous system or synapses. Since the human brain contains about 10^{11} neurons, nanosecond microtubule switching processes could accomplish about 10^{27} brain operations per second. This is 10 orders of magnitude more operations than can be achieved by synaptic switching. This means that the on-off switches known as synapses, which are obviously important components of neural networks, may not be the only place where information is processed and memories are stored. Hameroff stated that the "neuron doctrine" ignores the fact that neurons are living cells. The fact that many neurons are packed with microtubules opens up the possibility that the nervous system itself could have two parallel and distinct mechanisms for the transmission of information: a fast mechanism, involving waves of conformational change in microtubules and other cytoskeletal components, and a slower, classical mechanism, involving ionic currents, action potentials, and synapses (Hameroff 1999).

Another candidate for the ultra-fast biology is "wetware":

> In a book entitled *Wetware: A Computer in Every Living Cell*, Dennis Bray (2009) proposed that all cells are built of molecular biochemical circuits that process information from the environment and perform logical operations, comparable in sophistication to those taking place in electronic devices. Bray defines Wetware as the sum of all of the information-rich biochemical processes and "computations" taking place inside a cell—the interactions of dissolved molecules or arrays of molecules forming complex webs or circuits. Bray also suggested that the computational properties of cells provide the basis for the distinctive properties of living systems, including the ability to embody in their internal structures "images" of the world around them. This concept was supported by the work of Albrecht-Buehler who described a rudimentary form of cellular "vision" based on the light sensing properties of a cytoskeletal component known as the centriole. After some 30 years of observation, Albrecht-Buehler concluded that single tissue cells have their own data- and signal-processing capacities that help control their movements and orientation.

> **Albrecht-Buehler 1985, 1992**

Enzymatic products can move at very high velocities, as documented with techniques developed by Ahmed H. Zewail, who received the Nobel Prize in Physics in 1999 for creating the world's fastest camera. Using ultrafast lasers, Zewail (2003) was able to show that reactants can move at speeds of the order of 1000 m/second or 0.6 miles/second—about as fast as a rifle bullet. Hence, the biochemical "circuits" Bray described could allow for extremely fast flow of information and signal processing—one of the attributes of unconscious processing that has been difficult to explain in terms of neurophysiology.

Biological coherence, mentioned above in relation to the work of Herbert Fröhlich, offers another new frontier in biological regulations. For an elegant discussion of this topic, see a review by Bischof and Del Giudice (2013).

In his classic treatise entitled *Principles of Mental Physiology*, William Carpenter (1875) had suggested that our brains process information through two parallel tiers, one conscious and the other unconscious. Freud pointed out that much of our mental activity is unconscious. In the province of the mind, consciousness is the visible sentient tip of the iceberg (Figure 27.9). "Preconscious" is a term used in Freudian psychoanalysis to describe thoughts that are unconscious at a particular moment, but are not repressed and therefore are readily available for recall and easily "capable of becoming conscious"—a phrase attributed by Sigmund Freud to Joseph Breuer (Freud 1991).

The unconscious mind consists of dynamic mental processes that occur automatically and are not usually available to conscious introspection. They include, for example, thought processes, as opposed to thoughts, intuitive insights, and procedural knowledge that enables the highly skilled and rapid and virtually automatic aspects of peak human performance. An example described by Freud is our ability to express ourselves in speech. In his early years, Freud was an aphasiologist; he studied linguistic problems caused by brain damage. He noticed that we don't consciously pick the words and grammatical structures that we're going to use. All of that is done for us unconsciously and automatically, and we just speak. We know the gist of what we are going to say, but we do not know precisely what we are going to say until we say it.

The vast unconscious reservoir below the surface is functioning all of the time. In essence, one sees and interacts with the world through the "eyes" of their unconscious assumptions, usually without realizing it. The unconscious strongly influences the directions of our activities as well as our feelings and perceptions. Of course, biomedical researchers are not immune to being directed by unconscious axioms that can influence their logic. Nearly universal acceptance of regulations by diffusing molecules and the lock and key model are examples. A profound issue that we will discuss later is the image one has of the structure of cells. All beginning students of medicine or biology are introduced to a model of the cell that is completely outdated and incorrect. How can they be expected to research and understand cancer, for example, when their picture of cell structure is entirely obsolete?

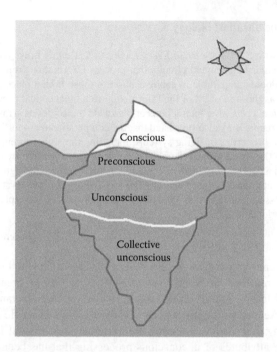

FIGURE 27.9   An iceberg is often used to represent Freud's theory that most of the human mind operates unconsciously. After fascinating introspection, Karl Jung added a deeper layer which he termed the collective unconscious.

Freud understood that the language of the unconscious is different from the language of consciousness, but did not appreciate that under many circumstances unconscious processes are vastly faster and more efficient at integrating sensory inputs and producing adaptive actions than conscious processes. The unconscious mind enables humans to survive in a world that requires massive information intake, rapid processing of that information, and rapid reactions.

Karl Jung added another, deeper layer, which he termed the collective unconscious:

> My thesis then, is as follows: in addition to our immediate consciousness, which is of a thoroughly personal nature and which we believe to be the only empirical psyche (even if we tack on the personal unconscious as an appendix), there exists a second psychic system of a collective, universal, and impersonal nature which is identical in all individuals. This collective unconscious does not develop individually but is inherited. It consists of pre-existent forms, the archetypes, which can only become conscious secondarily and which give definite form to certain psychic contents.

Jung 1996

The unconscious is rarely studied by biomedical researchers, even though it could involve the very systems that are disturbed in intractable chronic and degenerative diseases. A connection between emotional trauma and disease is well documented in the burgeoning field of psychoneuroimmunology (PNI), the study of how emotions impact our immune system, health, and well-being. PNI is an interdisciplinary subject, incorporating psychology, neuroscience, immunology, physiology, genetics, pharmacology, molecular biology, psychiatry, behavioral medicine, infectious diseases, endocrinology, and rheumatology. It is suggested that the problems of the intractable diseases will only be resolved by studies at the interfaces between these diverse disciplines. While multi-disciplinary studies may be challenging, it is possible that the key conceptual breakthroughs may render the problems far less difficult. For example, the properties of receptors, beyond the simple lock and key model, may disclose phenomena that will clarify many issues.

A main interest of PNI is the interaction between the nervous and immune systems and the relationships between mental processes and health. PNI studies, among other things, the physiological functioning of the neuro-immune system in health and disease; autoimmune diseases; hypersensitivities; immune deficiency; and the physical, chemical, and physiological characteristics of the components of the neuro-immune system *in vitro*, *in situ*, and *in vivo*.

When emotional trauma goes unhealed, the body remains in a constant state of heightened stress. Numerous studies have connected stress with lower immune function and higher incidences of disease in general. A recent report analyzed the findings of close to 100 other studies that showed how the sympathetic nervous system (SNS) can actually encourage metastasis when it is chronically activated. Dr. Douglas Brodie, MD, is a pioneer in understanding the connection between the emotions, the mind, and cancer. After almost three decades of research, he noted that the majority of individuals diagnosed with cancer have similar psychological traits. He calls this the "Cancer Personality Profile" (Brodie 1997).

The article with Dr. Pressman pointed out that techniques have been developed that could be employed to study high speed processes in real time and thereby provide a biophysical basis for ultrafast communications, including those thought to be involved in the subconscious mind. In the last few decades our knowledge in biology has increased explosively by development and application of new technologies and close cooperation with neighboring disciplines. Many new technologies are emerging that could be used to study the subconscious energy circuits in the human body. We need to know how gaps or blockages in these circuits can lead to chronic diseases, including cancer. Exciting and profoundly important discoveries await the investigator willing to go beyond current biomedical thinking. Biophotonics provides an important and revealing new window for biomedical research. Sadly the subject has attracted the attention of very few investigators in the United States.

To understand the significance of "moving energy for healing" we need to look at all of the energy systems in the human body, how they can be disrupted to cause health problems, and how they can be restored. Western biomedicine has only a superficial understanding of energy systems. In contrast, many complementary and alternative approaches validate the existence of a variety of energy systems that are unknown in conventional biomedicine. This is a new frontier topic that could very well revolutionize our biomedicine. Study of complementary and alternative and integrative approaches is both satisfying and revealing of aspects of human physiology that are simply missing in modern medicine. There is growing recognition that achieving an integrative multidisciplinary understanding of the cooperative and integrative interactions of molecules, cells, tissues, organs, and organisms is the next major frontier of biomedical science.

> Given a choice of physical processes, why would evolutionary selection prefer random diffusion of signal molecules—probably the slowest and least specific mechanism available, for its vital communications? Why would nature not utilize light for its vital regulations? Light has a great advantage over random diffusion because it travels at the speed of light and is exactly specific, that is, from molecule to molecule.

During the evolution of life, organisms had millions of years and a host of physical phenomena to "choose from." We can ask, "Given a choice of physical processes, why would evolutionary selection choose random diffusion of signal molecules—probably the slowest and least specific mechanism available?" Light has played many roles in the evolutionary process. Why would nature not utilize light for its vital regulations? Light has a great advantage over random diffusion because it travels at the speed of light and is precisely specific, that is, from molecule to molecule.

WHAT IS LIGHT AND WHAT MEDIUM DOES IT TRAVEL THROUGH?

Arthur M. Young was a brilliant scholar and inventor of the Bell Helicopter. In a remarkable book entitled *The Reflexive Universe*, Young asserted:

> Light, because it is primary, must be unqualified—impossible to describe—because it is antecedent to the contrasts needed to describe it ... The photon, having no bulk, can shrink any amount. It follows that a single photon can store unlimited energy and information by getting smaller ... This is one of the most surprising findings of quantum physics—that the smaller the photon, the more energy and information it contains ... All of the many-faceted properties of light point in one direction: to the ultimate centrality or primacy of light as the origin of everything.

Young 1999

Here it is suggested that the properties of space are antecedent to light and enable us to describe light and the effects of light. But how can we know about the properties of space? The fabric of space is some millions of millions of times smaller than an electron. No microscope can possibly resolve features at this dimension, which is known as the Planck scale.

However, we can take a clue from biology. It is found in the structure of the eye.

Vladimir B Ginzburg published 5 books on the vortical structure of space and electromagnetic fields, tracing the repeating cycles as such models went in and out of vogue over the centuries (Ginzburg 1996, 1999, 2002, 2006, 2013). James Clerk Maxwell and his friend, Michael Faraday, supported a vortex theory of electromagnetism with "potential fields" as the centerpiece. In his final classic paper on the electromagnetic field, Maxwell left out vortex models and used 20 quaternion equations. Two years after Maxwell's early death (he was only 48 years old), Oliver Heaviside and others replaced the quaternions with vector algebra, and eliminated the potential fields as "arbitrary" and unnecessary. By the end of the 1800s the Maxwell equations had been reduced from the original 20 to the 4 we find in physics texts today. Deleting the potentials deprived physics, biology, and medicine of important theoretical tools for nearly a century (Nahin 1988; Maret 2008).

For biology and medicine the forgotten potentials have important implications for regulatory physiology. The reason is that light is not simply light. There are other phenomena associated with light that are relatively difficult to detect at present, but that could be even more important than the light we can see and measure. The study of scalar fields, for example, is opening up new dimensions for our understandings of life and medicine.

We can trace the helical pathway followed by light through the vortically organized corneal stroma of the eye and the alpha-helical rhodopsin molecules in the outer segments of the retina. We have suggested that the alpha helical portions of membrane receptors are vortical "light pipes" that convey light into the cells. Adey and his colleagues have also discovered three examples of hormonal responses inside cells that can be triggered with electromagnetic fields, only, independently of the presence of the relevant hormones (Pilla et al. 2011). While this is a new idea for animal physiology, it is well known in plant physiology, where alpha helical membrane proteins are thought to function as light collectors that enable algae to survive in weak light environments.

The first helically organized structure that light must pass through is the corneal stroma (substantia propria) (Figure 27.10a and b). The stroma is about 500 μm thick and forms the bulk of the cornea. It combines optical transparency with mechanical resilience. These properties are possible because of an extracellular matrix containing narrow (36 nm diameter) parallel type I collagen fibrils spaced and organized uniformly into 200–250 sequential lamellae or sheets. Each sheet is arranged orthogonal to its neighbor and to the path of light through the cornea (Figure 27.10b and d) (Trelstad 1982; Holmes et al. 2000; Standring 2009). Strength arises from the plywood-like architecture. The collagen fibrils are much smaller than the wavelength of light, and their spacing is such that light they scatter is eliminated by destructive interference in all directions other than forwards into the retina.

Trelstad analyzed serial sections of corneas of birds, fishes, amphibians, and reptiles, cut perpendicular to the optical axis. The collagenous stroma is a cholesteric liquid crystal-like lattice which has

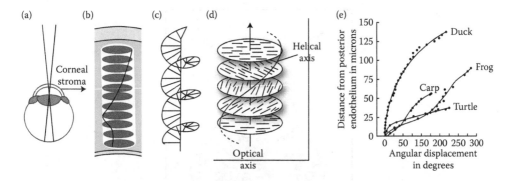

FIGURE 27.10 (a) The first helically organized structure that light must pass through to reach the retina is the corneal stroma (substantia propria) (a and b). The stroma is about 500 μm thick and forms the bulk of the cornea. It combines optical transparency with mechanical resilience. Its matrix consists of narrow parallel type I collagen fibrils spaced and organized uniformly into 200–250 sequential lamellae or sheets. Each sheet is arranged orthogonal to its neighbor and to the path of light through the cornea (b and d). Strength arises from the plywood-like architecture. Trelstad analyzed serial sections of corneas of birds, fishes, amphibians, and reptiles, cut perpendicular to the optical axis. The collagenous stroma is a cholesteric liquid crystal-like lattice which has the same right handedness in both eyes and is thus bilaterally asymmetrical (d).

the same right handedness in both eyes and is thus bilaterally asymmetrical (Figure 27.10d). Bilateral symmetry is the general rule for the heads of animals, with mirror symmetry in the sagittal plane dividing the body vertically into left and right halves, with one of each of the sense organs and limbs paired on either side. Why would this universal symmetry rule be broken for the corneal stroma? A logical answer is that the corneal stroma of both eyes must be transparent to light moving vortically in the same right-handed path (Figure 27.11). Different displacements between adjacent layers in different species (Figure 27.10e) may relate to matching of the index of refraction for life in different environments.

If biophotons from vibrating signal molecules follow vortical paths through the body, an interesting scenario arises at the receptors in cell membranes. Most if not all of the receptors on cell surfaces are composed of long proteins that snake back and forth across the membrane from 7 to 24 times. Seven-trans-membrane-helix (7TM) receptors (Figure 27.12) are responsible for transducing information initiated by signals as diverse as photons, odorants, tastants, hormones, and neurotransmitters. Several thousand such receptors are now known, and the list continues to grow. These are sometimes referred to as serpentine receptors because the single polypeptide chain "snakes" back and forth across the membrane. One of the most important receptor proteins is the voltage gated calcium channel because it regulates many cellular activities and responds rapidly to very weak electromagnetic fields (Pall 2013). This receptor protein traverses the cell surface 24 times.

Now to a key point: The receptor proteins crossing cell surfaces are right-handed alpha helices. What is the nature of the interaction between light, a right handed vortex, and the alpha helices in cell membranes, which are also right handed? The possibility arises that these alpha helical proteins at cell surfaces are actually "light pipes" that facilitate the entry of photonic messages into cells.

While this might at first seem to be a preposterous idea, there is abundant supporting evidence from the literature of plant physiology. Specifically, red and blue-green algae have intricate light-absorbing structures called phycobilisomes. These "antenna" complexes contain many alpha helical regions, and are described as "light pipes" funneling excitation energy (photons) into the reaction centers of chlorophyll a of photosystem II. Chlorophyll a, in turn, is another membrane protein with five trans-membrane helices (Deisenyhofer Michel and Huber 1985). It is thought that this arrangement enables the algae to survive in weak light environments. The arrangement permits 95% efficiency of energy transfer, as reviewed by Glazer (1985). Moreover, the light sensitive pigment in the human eye, rhodopsin, is also a seven-trans-membrane-helix. Finally, there is evidence for electromagnetic fields acting as first messengers for activating cellular processes without mediation of "second messengers"

Pilla et al. 2011. For further details, see Oschman and Oschman, 2015a,b.

These considerations lead us to a new possible model of regulations based on "messenger photons" interacting with both cell surface receptors and molecules within the cell.

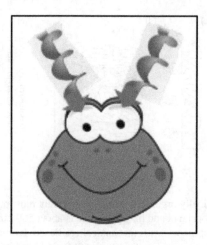

FIGURE 27.11 Bilateral symmetry is the general rule for the heads of animals, with mirror symmetry in the sagittal plane dividing the body vertically into left and right halves, with one of each of the sense organs and limbs paired on either side. Why would this universal symmetry rule be broken for the corneal stroma? A logical answer is that both eyes must accommodate to light moving vortically in the same right-handed path.

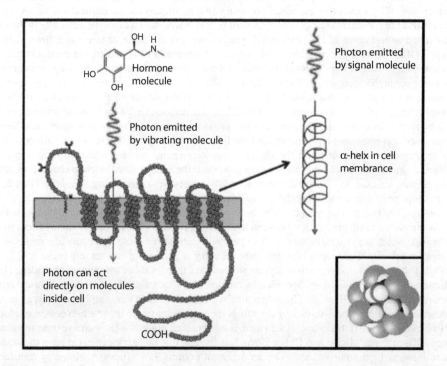

FIGURE 27.12 Most if not all of the receptors on cell surfaces are composed of long proteins that snake back and forth across the membrane from 7 to 24 times. Such seven-trans-membrane-helix (7TM) receptors are responsible for transducing information initiated by signals as diverse as photons, odorants, tastants, hormones, and neurotransmitters. These are sometimes referred to as serpentine receptors because the single polypeptide chain "snakes" back and forth across the membrane. Like the corneal stroma, the receptor proteins crossing cell surfaces are right-handed alpha helices. The possibility arises that these alpha helical proteins at cell surfaces are actually "light pipes" that facilitate the entry of photonic messages into cells.

PROTECTION FROM ENVIRONMENTAL ELECTROMAGNETIC FIELDS

Studies of the properties of light and space have practical implications for individuals who suffer from electromagnetic sensitivity. This is a definite medical condition that has been fully recognized in some countries (e.g., Sweden) as a disability attributed to the electromagnetic environment, specifically to increasing levels of radiation from cellular telephones and Wi-Fi, as was described above.

To understand these phenomena, it is of interest to determine the ways light and other kinds of electromagnetic fields traverse the skin to enter the body.

The technical issue is known as impedance matching. This is an electrical engineering term referring to the efficient transfer of energy from one medium to another, for example from air to the body. Impedance is the opposition of a system to the flow of energy from a source. In terms of electromagnetic fields and the human body, a valuable perspective is provided in a U.S. patent awarded to Charlene A. Boehm (2007). The patent provides methods for correcting for the fact that the electrical permittivity in living body tissue is not the same as for air. Permittivity is a measure of the resistance that is encountered when forming an electric field in a medium.

A valuable device for protecting sensitive individuals from electromagnetic pollution has been developed in Spain (Figure 27.13). Many devices claiming to protect from harmful electromagnetic fields can be found on the World Wide Web, but the PRANAN technology appears to have especially careful scientific research to support its safety and effectiveness. It is thought that the device converts potentially harmful environmental fields into fields that are normal and beneficial for the body. Evidence for this comes from many studies in leading Spanish university research departments showing improvements in physiological parameters while wearing the device (see Figures 27.14 and 27.15 from Escames 2011 and Alonso and Robayo 2012). Other studies analyzed cortisol, melatonin, lipid peroxidation, nitric oxide, pro-inflammatory and anti-inflammatory cytokines, the glutathione reduced/oxidized ratio, glutathione peroxidase, glutathione reductase, superoxide dismutase, and 6-Sulfatoximelatonin.[5] Taken together, the studies document that the Pranan Technologies provide an excellent defense against oxidative stress and inflammation caused by "electropollution." The results reported thus far have been obtained in a population of normal subjects, with no diseases or drug therapy. Thus, in subjects who present an oxidative stress/inflammatory condition, the beneficial effects of technology would be expected to be even more striking.

In designing the device, considerable effort was made in selecting the proper materials and defining the appropriate geometry for the front, back, and interior of the device to maximize effectiveness. One side of the device, shown to the left of Figure 27.13C, has an interesting pattern that corresponds to an ancient image found throughout nature, art, and architecture. Very early

(a) (b) (c)

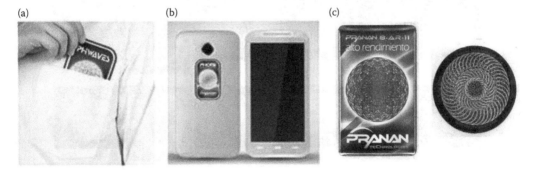

FIGURE 27.13 A valuable device for protecting sensitive individuals from electromagnetic pollution has been developed in Spain. Several studies support its safety and effectiveness. It is thought that the device converts potentially harmful environmental fields into fields that are normal and beneficial for the body. The evidence comes from studies in leading Spanish University research departments showing improvements in physiological parameters while wearing the device (Figures 27.14 and 27.15).

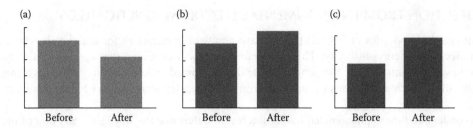

FIGURE 27.14 Examples of tests of the PRANAN device. All measurements taken from blood samples in 5 subjects before and after 30 days of daily use of PRNAN devices. (a) Lipid peroxidation index decreased by 33.47%. (b) Intracellular reduced glutathione increased by 16.28%. (c) Ratio of reduced/oxidized glutathione increased by 64.81%. These measures are considered important indicators of oxidative stress. (Adapted from Escames, G. 2011. Evaluation of neutralization of low intensity radiation harmful effects on five subjects cells redox markers. *Research Report to PRANAN* Dated June 3, 2011.)

representations of this design can be found in an ancient Egyptian temple (Figure 27.16a). More modern representations were produced to represent cosmological patterns recognized by the early astronomers Giordano Bruno and Johannes Kepler (see Figure 27.16b and c). This is a geometry that is thought to represent mathematical principles at work throughout nature (Goldstein Schappacher and Schwermer 2007). Many scholars have evaluated these patterns and concluded that they may relate to a fundamental geometric aspect of time and space (Calter 1998). For more information on this topic, see Oschman and Oschman (2015a,b).

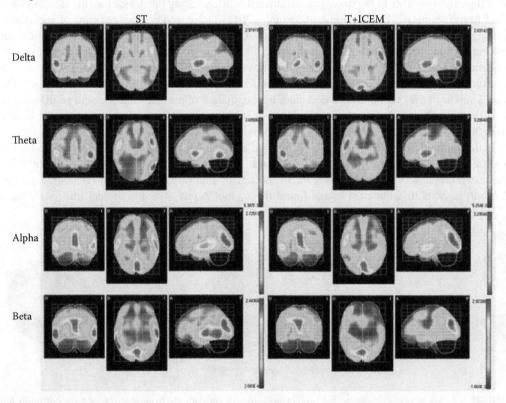

FIGURE 27.15 EEG brain bioelectrical activity in the phone only condition (left) and in the phone with PRANAN device (right). (Adapted from Alonso, T.O. and A.M.M. Robayo. 2012. Effect of external inhibition in electromagnetic exposures to radio frequencies emitted by mobile phones on the EEG brain bioelectrical activity. *Report to PRANAN* Dated July 24, 2012.)

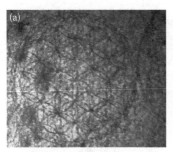 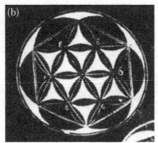 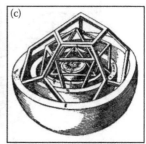

FIGURE 27.16   (a) The design on the face of the PRANAN device (Figure 27.11c) resembles an ancient relief found in the 6,000 year old Osirian Temple in Abydos, Egypt. The temple was a subterreanean complex thought to be the oldest of all the ancient Egyptian ruins. The symbol is carved with laser-like accuracy on huge granite blocks in the temple walls. (b) A more modern image created in a woodcut by Italian philosopher, mathematician, poet, and cosmologist, Giordano Bruno from Bruno's *Articuli centum et sexaginta adversus huius tempestatis mathematicos atque philosophos* (1588). (c) Inner section of German mathematician and astronomer Johannes Kepler's Platonic solid model of planetary spacing in the Solar system, from *Mysterium Cosmographicum* (1596).

THE HOLISTIC ANATOMICAL PERSPECTIVE

Next we introduce an anatomical perspective on the human body. When we refer to "anatomy" we consider all levels of scale, from the environment to the organism as a whole, organs, tissues, cells, membranes, organelles, molecules, atoms, and, finally, to the quantum level of organization, including the fabric of space that interpenetrates all of the parts—the same space that extends to and interpenetrates distant stars and galaxies.

In spite of much biomedical research, modern medicine has a limited perspective on anatomy because of its primary focus on biochemistry and pharmacology. In contrast, the so-called integrative therapies, which are rapidly growing in popularity world-wide, include a variety of anatomical and energetic concepts that can lead us to new perspectives on chronic and degenerative diseases. Some people rule out Energy Medicine because of an unfounded rumor that these approaches lack a scientific basis. Actually there is an abundance of scientific support for Energy Medicine (Oschman 2000, 2016) and study of energetics opens up many exciting new opportunities for further research and clinical progress. Holism can be studied holistically, that is, by bringing in and integrating as many perspectives as possible. We introduce next an over-arching anatomical concept known as tensegrity.

TENSEGRITY

A systemic perspective on energetic anatomy can begin with tensegrity (Figure 27.17) the structural concept developed by sculptor Kenneth Snelson and further advanced by the famous designer, architect, engineer, mathematician, philosopher, and poet, Buckminster Fuller (1895–1983):

> Fuller defined a tensegrity system as a continuous tensional network (tendons) supported by a discontinuous set of compressive elements (struts). Snelson preferred a highly descriptive term, "floating compression."

Tensegrity provides a universal set of building rules that guides the design of organic and human-made structures from simple carbon compounds to complex cells and tissues.

Discontinuous compression and continuous tension enable the construction of multi-story towers and large-scale exoskeletons of wire and steel, for example, geodesic domes. They are dramatic examples of the idea that tension and compression can be complementary elements in any structure.

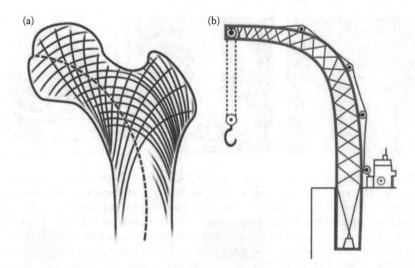

FIGURE 27.17 Tensegrity structures. (a) is the head of the femur. (b) is a crane. Both structures employ a combination of compression elements (called struts) and tension resisting elements (called tendons).

Great strength and economy in materials are achieved by relying on tension primarily, compression secondarily.

Tensegrity has a number of practical advantages and energetic features for the design of a living organism:

- The structure becomes stronger when under load.
- Potentially destructive forces, either impacts or stretches, are readily absorbed and conducted throughout the network, minimizing damage.
- Vibrations introduced at any point are conducted throughout the network.

Buckminster Fuller saw deep implications in Snelson's discovery for his evolving Energetic Geometry and coined the term "tensegrity" soon thereafter. In Buckminster Fuller's synergetics, tensegrity becomes a metaphor for how the Universe itself is constructed (Fuller 1982, 1983).

One of the "paradigm shifts" produced by the tensegrity perspective is that the human body is *not* supported in the Earth's gravity field by a set of weight-bearing bones, more or less stacked on top of each other, like bricks in a wall, each brick supported by the one below. Instead, a continuous web of soft tissues, the connective tissues and myofascia, actually *lifts* each bone off of the one below. This concept has profound therapeutic implications, and has been carefully documented by orthopedic surgeon, Stephen Levin, M.D., who has elaborated the concept of Biotensegrity.[6]

Tom Flemons, of Salt Spring Island, British Columbia, has made beautiful models that show how the soft tissues support the skeleton.[7] His model of the spine maintains its integrity without intervertebral discs (Figure 27.18, left). Flemons has made a remarkable complete tensegrity skeleton that can walk, sit, stretch, and contort. It will stand self-supporting, with all of the compression elements (bones) *floating* in the web of tension that is woven around them from top to bottom (Figure 27.18, right).

Harvard cell biologist and bioengineer Donald Ingber (1998) has extended the application of tensegrity concepts to the level of the cell and cell nucleus (Figure 27.19). In a series of brilliant papers, Ingber and colleagues have shown how cells sense mechanical forces and convert them into changes in intracellular biochemistry and gene expression—a process called "mechano-transduction."[8]

One energetic application of mechano-transduction is in explaining the effects of acupuncture needling as well as soft tissue therapies that stretch or flex or restore elasticity to connective tissue.

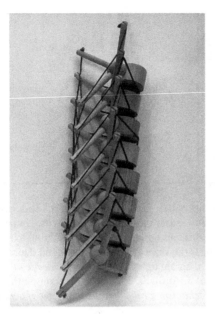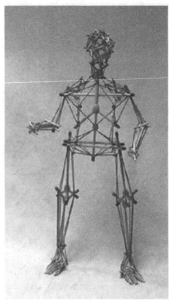

FIGURE 27.18 Tensegrity models constructed by Tom Flemons of Salt Spring Harbor, British Columbia. His model of the spine (left) maintains its integrity without intervertebral discs. The complete tensegrity skeleton shown at the right can walk (with support and guidance), sit, stretch, and contort. It will stand self-supporting, with all of the compression elements (bones) floating in the web of tension that is woven around them from top to bottom. Illustrations reproduced with the kind permission of Tom Flemons, Intesion Designs (http://www.intensiondesigns.com/bones_of_tensegrity.html). The illustration to the right is © 2006 by Tom Flemons.

Specifically, careful research by Helene Langevin and her colleagues has shown how the widespread practice of inserting and twisting an acupuncture needle actually causes the collagen fibers in the connective tissue to wind around the needle (Figure 27.20). This creates tensions that are conveyed through the extracellular matrix to fibroblast cells in nearby fascia. This changes the shape of the fibroblasts and their nuclei, thereby altering their functioning by mechanisms documented by the

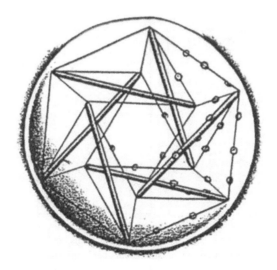

FIGURE 27.19 The cell, held together by tensegrity.

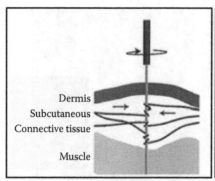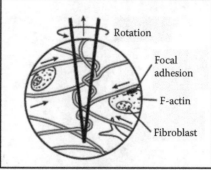

FIGURE 27.20 Research by Helene Langevin and her colleagues has shown how the wide-spread practice of inserting and twisting an acupuncture needle actually causes the collagen fibers in the connective tissue to wind around the needle (diagram on the left). This creates tensions that are conveyed through the extracellular matrix to fibroblast cells in nearby fascia. This changes the shape of the fibroblasts and their nuclei, thereby altering their functioning, as shown on the right. The diagram on the left is from *Evidence of connective tissue involvement in acupuncture*, published in FASEB J, April 10, 2002. The diagram on the right is from *Mechanical signaling through connective tissue: a mechanism for the therapeutic effect of acupuncture*, The FASEB Journal, October, 2001.

Ingber lab. This is one of the possible mechanisms by which acupuncture can beneficially stimulate the cellular processes needed for injury repair (Langevin et al. 2002). Hence, the tensegrity concept enables us to connect systemic functional anatomy with the energetic systems of acupuncture and bodywork.

Finando and Finando have described the correspondences between the location of meridians and particular lines of fascia as described by Myers (Finando and Finando 2011, 2012, Myers 2001) (Figure 27.21).

Brilliant research of Joie P. Jones, using ultrasonic microscopy, has shown that the acupuncture points are actually tensegrity structures (Figure 27.22a). Moreover, the points rotate spontaneously when a needle is inserted.[9] The acupuncture points are often located at places where several layers of fascia intersect (Figure 27.22b) (Langevin and Yandow 2003). Because of this, the rotations described by Jones have been interpreted as a process that enables acupuncture

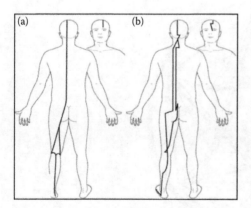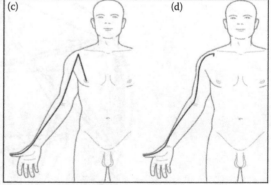

FIGURE 27.21 Correspondences between the location of meridians and particular lines of fascia described by Finando and Finando. Left: Comparison of superficial back line (a) and Bladder channel (b). Right: Comparison of deep front arm line (c) and Lung channel (d). (Based on Myers, T. 2001. *Anatomy Trains: Myofascial Meridians for Manual and Movement Therapists*. London: Churchill Livingstone.)

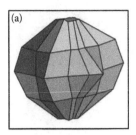 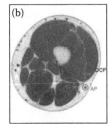 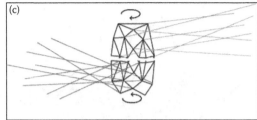

FIGURE 27.22 (a) The polyhedral or tensegrity structure of an acupuncture point as determined by ultrasonic microscopy of Joie P. Jones. (b) Langevin and Yandow mapped acupuncture points in serial gross anatomical sections through the human arm. They found an 80% correspondence between the sites of acupuncture points and the location of intermuscular or intramuscular connective tissue planes in postmortem tissue sections. (c) Ultrasonic imaging showed that the point (BL-67) rotates during needle insertion. Also, the upper half of the point rotates in the opposite direction to the lower half. One interpretation is that the two halves of the point are connected to different levels or planes in the fascia (b) and the twisting puts tension on both fascial planes.

needling to bring about tensions in two layers of fascia at the same time (Figure 27.22c) (Oschman 2016, Figure 14.2).

THE LIVING MATRIX

Detailed study of cell and tissue architecture has also led to the concept of the living matrix: a continuous molecular network that extends throughout the body and into every cell and nucleus. A key discovery was the presence of molecules, now called integrins, that connect the extracellular matrix across cell surfaces with the cytoskeleton, and other molecules that connect the cytoskeleton with the nuclear matrix. Termed "the living matrix" by Oschman and Oschman (1993), this is not only a continuous anatomical system, but it is also a continuous energetic system (Figure 27.23).

> The concept that the living matrix can transfer energy and information throughout the body evolved from Albert Szent-Györgyi's classic statement that proteins can be semiconductors (1941a,b). This concept was further documented in his books *Introduction to a Submolecular Biology* (1960) and *Bioelectronics* (1968) and his research papers.

Albert Szent-Györgyi and his colleagues provided a basis for the energetics of the living matrix by showing that most if not all the proteins and other molecules in the matrix are semiconductors (Gascoyne Pethig and Szent-Györgyi 1981). This controversial discovery will be discussed in more detail later in this chapter.

Key to the description of the living matrix was a discovery by Mark Bretscher from the Medical Research Council Laboratory of Molecular Biology in Cambridge, UK. While studying a protein associated with the membrane of red blood cells, Bretscher asked the question of whether the protein is embedded in the surface of the membrane, or is it sunken into the membrane interior, or, perhaps, it extends across the membrane from the outside of the cell to the inside (Figure 27.24)? Using radioactive tracers, Bretscher was able to show that the protein actually traverses the membrane (Bretscher 1971a,b). This was a revolutionary discovery and led to extensive study of the many roles of integrins. For example, SABiosciences has provided a diagram of the web of cellular pathways associated with the integrins (Figure 27.25).

Integrins are now known to coordinate a wide range of vital processes, including:

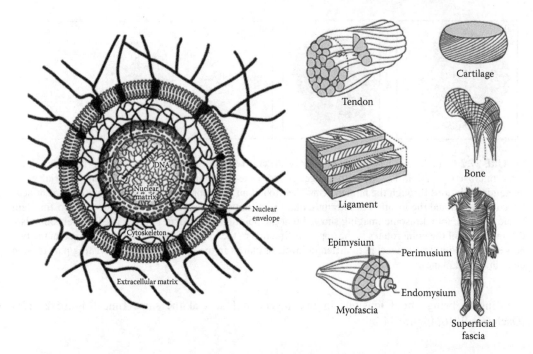

FIGURE 27.23 Detailed study of cell and tissue architecture has led to a concept of the *living matrix*: a continuous molecular network that extends throughout the body and into every cell and nucleus. A key discovery was the presence of molecules, now called integrins, that connect the extracellular matrix across cell surfaces with the cytoskeleton, nucleus, and genetic material, and other molecules that connect the cytoskeleton with the nuclear matrix. Termed "the living matrix" by Oschman and Oschman beginning in 1993, this is not only a continuous anatomical system, but it is also a continuous energetic system. Seldom-cited research of Nobel Laureate Albert Szent-Györgyi and his colleagues indicated that parts of the matrix could be semiconductors. This led to the concept that the components of the body could form a molecular electronic network. Some 15 years of inquiry into the benefits of Earthing or grounding the human body confirmed that electrons from the surface of the earth can ground the circuitry of the body, as in Figure 27.8a. The rapid benefits to the body's regulatory systems following contact with the surface of the earth confirm the bioenergetic nature of the living matrix, as discussed by Szent-Györgyi.

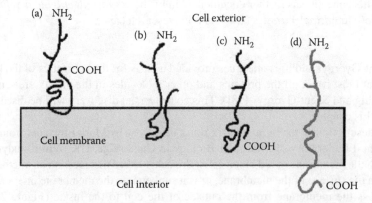

FIGURE 27.24 While studying a protein associated with the cell membrane of red blood cells, Cambridge UK scientist Mark Bretscher asked the question of whether the protein is embedded in the surface of the membrane, or is it sunken into the membrane interior, or, perhaps, does it extend across the membrane from the outside of the cell to the inside. Using radioactive tracers, Bretscher was able to show that the protein actually traverses the membrane. This was a revolutionary discovery and led to extensive study of the many roles of integrins.

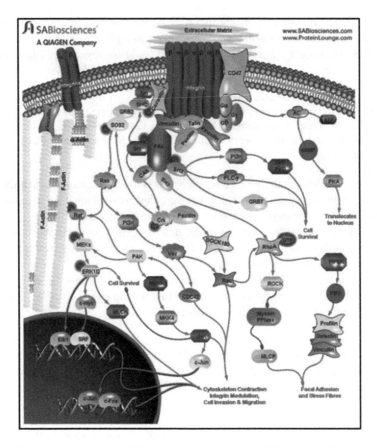

FIGURE 27.25 The intricate web of cellular pathways associated with integrins. Diagram reproduced with the permission of SABiosciences, a QAGEN Company, Frederick, MD, USA.

- Cell survival
- Growth
- Differentiation
- Cell migration
- Inflammatory responses
- Platelet aggregation
- Tissue repair
- Tumor invasion

Obviously, perturbing any of these coordinations can have serious consequences. Some that have been recognized include cancer-cell metastasis, angiogenesis, inflammatory disease, arthritis, and many other issues.

A SOLID-STATE TISSUE-TENSEGRITY MATRIX SYSTEM

At the time when we were beginning to see the systemic importance of Bretcher's discovery of trans-membrane proteins, we also became aware of the research of Albert Szent-Györgyi and his colleagues on the energetics of the protein fabric of the body. This line of inquiry began with Szent-Györgyi's historic presentation at the Korányi Memorial Lecture in Budapest. His talk was published in both *Science* (Towards a New Biochemistry 1941a) and *Nature* (The Study of Energy Levels in Biochemistry 1941b) at a time when his country and all of Europe was descending into the chaos of WWII. The remarkable insight that was the topic of his presentation was that proteins are semiconductors, rather than insulators, as had been thought previously. This idea explained how free electrons could occur naturally in proteins and could convey energy and information from place to place within an organism. He introduced these new ideas as follows:

> If a great number of atoms is arranged with regularity in close proximity, as for instance, in a crystal lattice, the terms of the single valency electrons may fuse into common bands. The electrons in this band cease to belong to one or two atoms only, and belong to the whole system ... A greater number of molecules may join to form such energy continua, along which energy, viz., excited electrons, may travel a certain distance.

This proved to be a prophetic statement, although it was not recognized as such at the time and led to much controversy. In retrospect, we can see that the concepts so eloquently stated in 1941 laid the foundation for many developments, some of which are becoming a major focus in modern research and in a global molecular electronics industry. The area where this shows up most clearly is in nano-electronics, which has developed into a world-wide search for ways of using atoms and molecules as miniature components of electronic circuits.

Szent-Györgyi's work focused on one of the central unexplored problems in biology and medicine: precisely what is it that brings about the unified functioning of an organism, and how does this orderly holistic process break down in chronic disease?

> Szent-Györgyi's work focused on one of the central unexplored problems in biology and medicine: precisely what is it that brings about the unified functioning of an organism, and how does this orderly holistic process break down in chronic disease?

These issues were on the agenda when the author moved to Woods Hole in the early 1970s with an interest in the possible science behind complementary and alternative medicine. Bretscher's research, the beginnings of the research on integrins, and Szent-Györgyi's work on energetic communications seemed to give some insights into the deeper meaning of a word that seemed to be disturbing to mainstream biomedicine: *holistic*. It had become clear that the integrins were providing a new insight into the systemic structure and function of organisms by showing how cellular activities could be influenced by the surrounding extracellular matrix, and *vice versa*. While the very existence of disciplines such as cell biology and membrane biology and physiology and biochemistry and molecular biology made the organism appear as a collection of separate compartments and parts and functions, to be studied individually, the integrins and the corresponding molecules traversing the nuclear envelope showed that all of these entities are continuously and intimately interconnected. The research on cell biology was showing that the cell interior was composed of a sort of fabric, the cytoskeleton, and that this fabric was interconnected with the extracellular fabric, the connective tissue. In 1984, the author published a paper that described how the ground substance materials histologists had identified in the nucleus, the cytoskeleton, and the connective tissues were really a continuous system composed of dissimilar but interconnected molecules (Oschman 1984).

At this time, it seemed that Szent-Györgyi's research was showing how the various proteins in this continuous ground matrix system could sustain a form of electronic and protonic communication that transcended the well-established nervous and hormonal communication systems.

Perhaps this was the same system Szent-Györgyi was referring to in his search for the control systems in cells that break down in cancer, and his search for systems that operate faster than nerves or chemical messaging.

During the author's tenure at the Marine Biological Laboratory, Szent-Györgyi's colleagues began to assemble a piece of equipment, an electron-spin resonance device that required a solid foundation and had to be set up in the basement of the building. To accommodate this device, the author exchanged his basement lab with one across the hall from Szent-Györgyi's main laboratory on the third floor. This placed the author in a position where he could see Szent-Györgyi come to and from work almost daily for a number of years.

It was during this period that the author was invited to visit the New England School of Acupuncture to explore Szent-Györgyi's concepts of energetics in relation to the ancient healing arts. Colleagues at the acupuncture school were exploring the ancient traditions by carefully translating a number of the classical texts. What they discovered was that the leading explorers and teachers of acupuncture, down through the ages, had all referred to fat, greasy membranes, fasciae, systems of connecting membranes; that through which the yang qi streams (Matsumoto and Birch 1988). Perhaps these shiny materials were actually semiconductors, and the electronic conduction Szent-Gyorgy was describing was one form of the elusive qi or Ch'I described in Oriental Medicine.

This was the background for a question that the author asked of Szent-Györgyi at the end of a symposium entitled *Search and Discovery: A Tribute to Albert Szent-Györgyi* (Kaminer 1975) held at Boston University School of Medicine. "Could these electronic processes he was describing take place in the extracellular fibrous protein systems of the human body?" Szent-Gyorgy did not have a good answer—he said he had enough to do in studying atoms and molecules, and something as large as a strand of connective tissue was far too large for him to consider from the perspective of quantum mechanics.

Szent-Györgyi's group was working at the level of quantum physics in an attempt to understand cancer and other chronic diseases at a subatomic level. At the time, the scientific community was completely disinterested in this research, and Szent-Györgyi was frustrated in his attempts to obtain financial support for the continuation of his studies. In retrospect, we can now see how disastrous this was for the search for solutions for chronic diseases, which still plague humanity.

A VIBRATORY MATRIX

In a classic report, Pienta and Coffey (1991) described the energetics of this system as follows:

> Cells and intracellular elements are capable of vibrating in a dynamic manner with complex harmonics, the frequency of which can now be measured and analyzed in a quantitative manner ... a tissue-tensegrity matrix system ... is poised to couple the biological oscillations of the cell from the peripheral membrane to the DNA ...

This statement emphasizes one of the important consequences of tensegrity—the ability to conduct vibrations.

THE GROUND REGULATION SYSTEM

Based on some 40 years of basic and clinical research, Alfred Pischinger, Hartmut Heine, and their colleagues in Austria and Germany referred to the matrix as the "ground regulation system" and the key to health and disease (Pischinger 2007). They viewed the fundamental unit life as a triad: capillary, matrix, cell, rather than the individual cell (Figure 27.26). In 1899 Andrew Taylor Still, the founder of the osteopathic profession, made a similar statement: "The fascia is the place to look for the cause of disease and the place to consult and begin the action of remedies in all diseases." This expands the "cell pathology" model of Virchow (1858), which has dominated western medicine for over 150 years. The cell pathology model states that all disease exists in cells and can be treated by agents that modify cell metabolism. The living matrix and ground regulation concepts shift the clinical focus to the cell environment. Yes, cells can become disturbed, but this is due to disturbances in their environment. Hence, another conceptual validation for the bodywork and movement therapies.

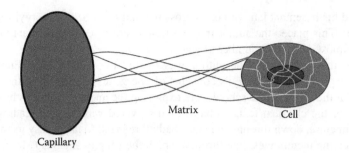

Capillary   Matrix   Cell

FIGURE 27.26 The ground regulation system proposed by Pischinger and Heine. The cell is not the fundamental unit of life. Instead, the fundamental unit is a triad, consisting of the capillary, matrix and the cell. Based on Pischinger, A. and Heine, H., The Extracellular Matrix and Ground Regulation. Berkeley, CA, North Atlantic Books.

VIEWS OF THE LIVING FASCIA

The detailed architecture of the fascial systems has been revealed by pioneering studies of a French hand surgeon, Dr. Jean-Claude Guimberteau, who has provided, for the first time, an intimate microscopic view of living connective tissue as revealed by high-resolution endoscopy. His remarkable explorations "under the skin" can be viewed in a book and a series of DVDs (Guimberteau and Armstrong 2015).

> From the DNA helix to the cytoskeleton, including the links to the integrins and neighboring cells, everything is in continuity, everything is connected, everything moves to fit, and everything moves and always comes back.

One of Guimberteau's findings is of special interest in relation to the "impedance matching" and geometrical issues described above in relation to the PRANAN device (see Figures 27.13 and 27.16). The geometric patterns Guimberteau identified under the skin may allow for resonance coupling between the microscopic architecture of the human body and geometry of space and the electromagnetic fields propagated through space. This is discussed in detail in Oschman (2016, Figure 13.9).

CONCLUSIONS

The kind invitation from Dr. Aruna Bakhru to write a chapter for this book has led the author to review the path that led to some new insights about bioenergetic medicine and the roles it can play in treating the so-called incurable diseases and disorders. This has involved re-examination of several widely agreed-upon concepts that seemed ready for further inquiry if we are to progress beyond our current understandings of the most significant unsolved issues in modern medicine. What remains to be discovered—what we don't know—probably dwarfs what we do know. And what we think we know may not be entirely correct or fully understood. Anomalies, which many researchers tend to sweep under the rug, should be actively pursued as clues to potential breakthroughs and new directions in science. The most important area in need of advancement is regulatory biology because most diseases and disorders arise from failures in regulation of the vital processes that maintain the integrity of the living system. One significant new insight is the living matrix/ground regulation/tissue-tensegrity matrix system that is both a well-defined anatomical feature of living organisms as well as a system-wide bioenergetic structure.

Regulatory biology has been dominated by ancient concepts such as billiard-ball biochemistry, random diffusion, and the lock and key model of hormone-receptor interactions. These concepts are in need of a second look, and this chapter summarizes the problems they present. Mechanistic and reductionistic approaches have involved separation of the living body into a variety of primary parts: organs, tissues, cells, organelles, molecules, atoms, and so on. In this process the vital connectedness has been lost. Habitual rejection of biofield hypotheses has exacerbated the connectivity issues. The living matrix, biophotonics, and bioenergetics provide us with opportunities to restore the elements of wholeness.

One of the author's key conceptual breakthroughs was the structure and functioning of the living matrix (see Figure 27.23). Rarely cited research of Albert Szent-Györgyi and his colleagues led to consideration of a bioelectronic role for this system, which extends throughout the entire organism, even into the nucleus of every cell. Confirmation of aspects of this concept has come from recent research on the important role of Earthing or grounding in stabilizing every physiological process we have measured.[11] The suggestion that the acupuncture meridian system/living matrix/ground regulation systems deliver antioxidant electrons to sites of inflammation is the most parsimonious explanation for the rapidity with which Earthing resolves chronic inflammation (Figure 27.8b). Perhaps chronic disease results when the semiconducting and biophotonic matrices of the body are not functioning properly, and the biochemical circuits are not stabilized by being grounded.

An essay on the scientific basis of the unconscious mind, in collaboration with Maurie Pressman MD, suggested many energy/information circuits in the human body that are hundreds or thousands of times faster than nerve impulses (Oschman and Pressman 2014). These circuits require further study to determine the roles they may play in health and disease. These may be the circuits Albert Szent-Györgyi was referring to when he said that the piece missing from modern medicine was already known in every culture and in every medical tradition before ours, that is, healing can be accomplished by moving energy. This chapter is partly about defining what we mean by the healing effects of moving energy. A logical question is the location of the interface between the living matrix/ground regulation systems and the brain and peripheral nervous system. The answer is that the interface is throughout the nervous system, since the nerves and the brain are actually components of the living matrix. We envision a continuous dynamic energetic movement or flow taking place within and between all of these systems, with light playing many key roles.

The chapter was not undertaken with the idea of building support for biophotonic models of regulation, but that is precisely what has emerged from considering the evidence for the conventional regulatory models that focus on the nervous system and diffusion of signal molecules.

Many of the hypotheses introduced here are speculative, but they are made with the confidence that emerging technologies will eventually be able to validate or refute them. For example, Pienta and Coffee (1991) discussed measuring the frequencies in the tissue-tensegrity matrix in a quantitative manner by Fourier analysis. In the decades since that statement was made, technologies have been developed that can characterize activities in the molecular fabric of the living matrix/ground regulation systems and wetware. One valuable resource is a series of symposia on ultrafast phenomena in semiconductors and nanostructure materials, including living tissues. For example, the development of powerful ultra-fast laser pulsing technologies has led to the use of terahertz scanning near-field infrared microscopy of biological materials (Schade et al. 2005). A second application of terahertz technologies involves spectroscopic methods for measuring the interactions between water and proteins at very small time scales (Havenith 2010). Atomic force microscopy can provide topographical information and measurements of mechanical stiffness, electrical conductance, resistivity, and magnetic properties at micro- and nano-scales in living materials (Darling and Desai 2012). The fascinating ideas of Bray (2009), that is, a biochemical basis for "a computer in every cell," may be testable by the use of the world's fastest camera developed by Zewail in 1999. Continuation of this inquiry with the modern research tools that have been mentioned could begin to identify local cellular and tissue changes produced by physical or emotional trauma. This is a key issue for all branches of therapeutics. For example, a widely cited article on the cause of cancer is entitled "Tumors: Wounds That Do Not Heal" (Dvorak 1986).

The living matrix and ground regulation systems are good candidates for part of the "organic substructure" of the unconscious mind referred to by Freud a century ago. We predict that measurable activities taking place in the matrix will eventually account for intuition and for the successes of programming intentions, as in the use of mental rehearsals in refining human performance. These measurable activities may also provide a substantive basis for the connections between emotional issues, body structure/function issues, and organic diseases.

Finally, it has been a privilege to dedicate this chapter to Dr. Marco Bischof, whose collaborations and inspiring writings provide the basis for suggesting that it is light, rather than diffusing signal molecules and nerve impulses, that orchestrates the myriad processes giving rise to life. For this author, Albert Szent-Györgyi's 1972 statement that life is too rapid and subtle to be explained by slow moving nerve impulses and chemical reactions began nearly half a century of inquiry that led inexorably to this chapter that concludes that light holds a vital key to the future of medicine.

DNA—AN ALTERNATIVE PERSPECTIVE

A dynamic web of light constantly released and absorbed by the DNA may connect cell organelles, cells, tissues, and organs within the body and serve as the organism's main communication network and as the principal regulating instance for all life processes.

The processes of morphogenesis, growth, differentiation and regeneration are also explained by the structuring and regulating activity of the coherent biophoton field ... and may also be basis of memory and other phenomena of consciousness, as postulated by neurophysiologist Karl Pribram and others.

Bischof 1995

For those who may be interested in following up on these ideas, an excellent way to begin would be to read all of the publications of Marco Bischof and also those of Herbert Fröhlich, the van Wijk's (e.g., Van Wijk, Van Wijk, and Bosman 2010) and Mae-Wan Ho (e.g., Ho 2008, 2012), as well as the other members of the International Institute of Biophysics from around the world. Marco Bischof prepared a Bibliography on Biophoton Research, Integrative Biophysics, and Related Subjects that can be found on the web page of the International Institute of Biophysics.[12] Also, see a new book by Anadi Martel (2016), *The Power of Light—Dawn of a New Medicine*, and the classic, by Jacob Liberman (1990), *Light: Medicine of the Future* (1990).

APPENDIX I: AUTHOR'S ACADEMIC BACKGROUND

The author has degrees in biophysics and biology from the University of Pittsburgh, and has conducted research in Cambridge, England, Case Western Reserve University in Cleveland, the University of Copenhagen and Institute of Biological Chemistry in Copenhagen, the Marine Biological Laboratory in Woods Hole, Massachusetts, and Northwestern University in Evanston, Illinois, where he served as a Professor of Biological Sciences. In the early 1980s he became interested in holistic medicine, and began teaching and lecturing on this subject from a scientific perspective. In 1996, he began a series of six articles on the subject, *What is Healing Energy?* for the *Journal of Bodywork and Movement Therapies* at the request of the editor, Dr. Leon Chaitow (Oschman 1996–1998). Because of the way these and subsequent articles were received by the holistic community, the publisher of the journal invited him to write a book on energy medicine, and *Energy Medicine: The Scientific Basis* was published in 2000 by Churchill Livingstone/Harcourt Brace. A second book entitled *Energy Medicine in Therapeutics and Human Performance* was published by Butterworth Heinemann/Elsevier in 2003. A second edition of the first book was published by Elsevier in 2016. Lectures and workshops on energy medicine have taken the author to cities throughout the United States and to dozens of countries in Europe, Asia, and South America.

APPENDIX II: MOLECULAR "WIRES"

Studies have shown that organic molecular "wires" can transfer charge by a variety of mechanisms, depending on voltage and temperature. Careful studies of the behavior of molecular wires and junctions between molecules have given rise to a variety of possible mechanisms of charge trans-fer that can be involved in many different physiological phenomena. Some of the phenomena are termed tunneling, vibronic coupling, and non-resonant Laudauer-type (coherent) coupling. In some cases, one mechanism may be operative in one direction while another mechanism operates in the opposite direction.

First, at this level of scale, quantum or wavelike properties dominate the behavior of electrons. One consequence is that the electron is never actually localized at a particular place on or in the molecular wire structure. Moreover, we often compare the flow of electricity through a conductor with the flow of fluids through pipes, with voltage being analogous to pressure and amperage cor-responding to the rate of flow. At the quantum level, charge transfer can occur from point A to point B without the charge actually moving through or being detectable in the intervening space.

Second, some charge transport mechanisms decay rapidly with distance along the wire while others do not. Mechanisms that decay more slowly can be dominant over longer distances. Another feature is that activation or amplification processes can be present, in which energy in the environ-ment is utilized to facilitate motion along the molecular strand in a hopping behavior that decays slowly if it all. This is sometimes referred to as polaronic transport.

Finally, there is a fascinating and unexpected paradox in the relationship between the speed of electron transfer reactions and the "driving force." Rudolph A. Marcus of the California Institute of Technology predicted a phenomenon that was completely unexpected by the chemist's intuition and that was initially difficult to accept and confirm. When the driving force increases beyond a certain level, electron transfer will begin to slow down instead of speed up, as we would expect. Odd as this may seem, the phenomenon was established experimentally and led to Marcus receiving a Nobel Prize in chemistry in 1992 for his contributions to the theory of electron transfer reactions in chemical systems (Marcus 1992).

The continuous living matrix system is also a water system that can be traced throughout the body, reaching into every part. In other words, electronic semiconduction via the protein fabric and proton transfer in the associated water network are not restricted by morphological boundar-ies. They can sustain vectorialized charge movements and oscillations ranging in velocity from the speed of light to less rapid but extremely fast protein conformation changes, to the slower biochemi-cal reactions and diffusive transport (Bender 1991; Burns 1989; Kaminura and Kaniya 1989; Bender 1991). The bound water forms electrets around many macromolecules. The activation energies and relaxation times of 10^5 s provide for charge transfer of both electrons and protons when donors and acceptors are present (Celaschi and Mascarenhaus 1977). Intrinsic membrane proteins (integrins) can guide charge transfer across the cell surface.

The study of charge transfer in biological polymers requires procedures that are different from those used in conventional biochemistry. This field has been referred to as solid-state biochemistry. The field encompasses the transfer of charge by a wide variety of mechanisms, including electronic, protonic, and hole conduction, to name a few. Other means of charge and energy transfer involve phonons, excitons, polarons, conformons, and solitons, which can have longitudinal or transverse modes.

One way to study charge transfers in protein matrices involves the creation of electron propaga-tion maps to show how the conformation of a protein will influence its ability to couple electron donors with nearby electron acceptors (Skourtis Regan and Onuchic 1994). While the conformation of the electron transfer protein is a key factor, there are others. These include separation distance, driving force and reorganization energy, and electron affinity of donor and receptor sites. A series of coupled oxidation/reduction reactions can pass electrons along a chain of molecules, the direc-tion and rate of transfer being determined by a variety of factors including the potential differences between the donor and acceptor sites and their relative affinities. With regard to the driving force, that is, the voltage or potential difference between a donor and an acceptor, it should be noted that the electron transfer process is governed by non-linear equations that give the counterintuitive result that larger driving forces can actually result in slower rates of transfer. As mentioned above, this surprising finding was made by Rudolph A. Marcus, and led to his award of the Nobel Prize in Chemistry in 1992.

Charge transfer may also involve quantum mechanical electron-tunneling pathways (Kraut and Pelletier 1992). Tunneling was also suggested by Chance and colleagues, based on the temperature independence of electron transfer in the range from 4 to 120 K (Chance and Nishimura 1960; DeVault and Chance 1966). Nakahara and colleagues confirmed that the electron carrier in the respiratory chain of sulfur bacteria is ohmic and electronic in nature (Nakahara Kimura Inokuchi and Yagi 1979). Others have suggested superconduction of electrons (Kinnaunen and Virtanen 1986).

Oxidation and reduction and reduction potential are frequently used but confusing terms in free radical chemistry. There are serious limitations to the use of oxidation/reduction concepts when looking at free electron interactions with free radicals in the human body. First, the chemical species in living systems are not isolated as they are when their reduction potentials are measured in a standardized *in vitro* system. Reaction conditions make a big difference. Moreover, the standardized reduction potentials are always measured at 25°C and corrected to pH = 7.0, but the actual pH and temperature in living tissues can be quite different from these values. The Nernst equation can be used to correct for the values of concentration and temperature. The resulting "effective" reduction potential can be used to predict which reactions are feasible, but this does not mean that those reactions will actually occur under the conditions present in a particular tissue (for a discussion of oxidation-reduction potentials as applied to free-radical chemistry, and the limitations of this approach, see Halliwell and Gutteridge 1999). Moreover, free radical reactions can be exceedingly fast, making it difficult to follow reaction rates based on changes in the concentrations of reactants and products.

A modern method for the direct study of free radical reactions is femtosecond spectroscopy, which makes it possible to observe what actually happens to a reacting molecule as it passes through its so-called transition state during which bonds are broken and formed. The transition state is as fast as the electrons and atoms in the molecule move—about 1,000 m/second—about as fast as a rifle bullet. The times involved are typically tens of femtoseconds (1 fs = 10^{-15} seconds). Ahmed Zewail developed a method for observing the transition state, giving birth to the new scientific field called femtochemistry. What is essentially the fastest camera in the world is used to film the molecules during a reaction and get a sharp picture of the transition states. The "camera" is a pulsed laser. The reaction is initiated by a strong laser flash and is then studied by a series of subsequent flashes to follow the events. The result is a slow motion image of how bonds are stretched and broken. Ahmed Zewail was awarded the Nobel Prize for showing the decisive moments in the life of a molecule—the breaking and formation of chemical bonds (Zewail 2003).

ACKNOWLEDGMENTS

I am indebted to Dr. Anadi Martel and Nora Oschman for valuable comments on the manuscript. Support for completion of the manuscript was provided by Maria Antonieta Riveros-Revello, in loving memory of her late husband, Raul Revello, MD, an outstanding pioneer in preventive medicine.

NOTES

1. From Chapter 26 in *Nutrition and Integrative Medicine: A Primer for Clinicians*, edited by Aruna Bakhru MD, Taylor & Francis Group, LLC, Boca Raton, FL.
2. Often mis-attributed to Mark Twain. Earliest source: *Revue Canadienne de Criminologie*, Volumes 5–6, Canadian Criminology and Corrections Association, 1963.
3. Interview with Ronald Pethig, August 20, 2004, http://profiles.nlm.nih.gov/WG/B/B/L/W/
4. In Fick's equation, J is the "diffusion flux," of which the dimension is amount of substance per unit area per unit time, so it is expressed in such units as mol m^{-2} s^{-1}. J measures the amount of substance that will flow through a unit area during a unit time interval. D is the diffusion coefficient or diffusivity. Its dimension is area per unit time, so typical units for expressing it would be m²/s. φ (for ideal mixtures) is

the concentration, of which the dimension is amount of substance per unit volume. It might be expressed in units of mol/m^3. x is position, the dimension of which is length. It might thus be expressed in the unit m. D is proportional to the squared velocity of the diffusing particles, which depends on the temperature, viscosity of the fluid, and the size of the particles according to the Stokes–Einstein relation.

5. http://www.pranan.co.uk/scientific-studies/
6. http://www.biotensegrity.com
7. http://tensegritywiki.com/Fiemons%2C+Tom
8. Ingber, D., https://apps.childrenshospital.org/clinical/research/ingber/publications.html
9. Oschman 2016, Chapter 14, page 232.
10. SA Biosciences, USA—QIAGEN Inc., 27220 Turnberry Lane, Valencia CA 91355, http://www.sabiosciences.com/
11. For references, see www.earthinginstitute.net.
12. http://www.panospappas.gr/bibliography1-1.htm

REFERENCES

Albrecht-Buehler, G. 1985. Is cytoplasm intelligent too? In: Shay J. (ed.) *Cell and Muscle Motility* vol. 6, pp. 1–21.

Albrecht-Buehler, G. 1990. In defense of 'non-molecular' cell biology. *Int. Rev. Cytol.* 120:191–241.

Albrecht-Buehler, G. 1992. Rudimentary form of cellular "vision." *Proc. Natl. Acad. Sci. USA*, 89(17): 8288–8292.

Alonso, T.O. and A.M.M. Robayo. 2012. *Effect of external inhibition in electromagnetic exposures to radio frequencies emitted by mobile phones on the EEG brain bioelectrical activity.* Report to PRANAN July 24, 2012.

Attwell, D. and A. Gobb. 2005. Neurpenergetics and the kinetic design of excitatory synapses. *Nat. Rev. Neurosci.* 6:841–849.

Balzani, V. ed. 2001. *Electron Transfer in Chemistry.* Hoboken, NJ: Wiley VCH Verlag GmbH.

Barnett, M.P. 1987. Molecular systems to process analog and digital data associatively. In: Carter, F.L., Siatkowski, R.E. and Wohltjen, H. (eds) *Proceedings of Third International Symposium of Molecular Electronic Devices.* Oct. 6–8, 1986, Arlington, Virginia. Amsterdam, The Netherlands: Elsevier, pp. 229–244.

Bender, M. 1991. In Interfacial phenomena. In: M. Bender (ed.) *Biological Systems.* New York: Dekker.

Bischof, M. 1995. *Biophotonen: Das Licht in unseren Zellen (Biophotons—the Light in our Cells).* Frankfurt: Zweitausendeins Publishers.

Bischof, M. 2000. Field concepts and the emergence of a holistic biophysics. In: Beloussov, L.V., Popp, F.A., Voeikov, V.L., and Van Wijk, R. (eds) *Biophotonics and Coherent Systems.* Moscow: Moscow University Press, pp. 1–25.

Bischof, M. 2003. Introduction to Integrative Biophysics. In: Popp Fritz-Albert and L.V. Beloussov (eds) *Integrative Biophysics.* Dordrecht: Kluwer Academic Publishers, pp. 1–115. https://www.academia.edu/13658751/Introduction_to_Integrative_Biophysics

Bischof, M. 2005. Biophotons: The light in our cells. *Journal of Optometric Phototherapy*, March issue: 1–5. http://www.rexresearch.com/biophotons/BiophotonsTheLightinOurCells6.pdf

Bischof, M. 2010. Man as a Cosmic Resonator. Re-imagining human existence in the field picture. *Conference paper: 11th Annual International Research Conference, Consciousness Reframed: Art and Consciousness in the Post-Biological Era, Making Reality Really Real*, Trondheim, Norway. https://www.researchgate.net/publication/280836340_Man_as_a_Cosmic_Resonator—Re-Imagining_Human_Existence_in_the_Field_Picture

Bischof, M. and E. Del Giudice. 2013. Review article. Communication and the emergence of collective behavior in living organisms: A quantum approach. *Hindawi Publishing Corporation, Molecular Biology International* Volume 2013, Article ID 987549, 19 pages http://dx.doi.org/10.1155/2013/987549

Blank, M. and R. Goodman. 2011. DNA is a fractal antenna in electromagnetic fields. *Int. J. Radiat. Biol.*, 87(4):409–415.

Boehm, C.A. 2007. United States Patent US 7,280,874—Methods for determining therapeutic resonant frequencies.

Bray, D. 2009. *Wetware: A Computer in Every Cell.* New Haven, CT: Yale University Press.

Bretscher, M. 1971a. Major human erythrocyte glycoprotein spans the cell membrane. *Nature New Biology* 231:229–232.

Bretscher, M. 1971b. A major protein which spans the human erythrocyte membrane. *J. Mol. Biol.* 59:351–357.

Brodie, D. 1997. *Cancer and Common Sense: Combining Science and Nature to Control Cancer.* White Bear Lake, MN: Winning Publications Inc.

Burns, R. 1989. Photoactive microtubule flux. *Nature* 340, 511–512.

Calter, P. 1998. Celestial Themes in Art & Architecture. *Dartmouth College.* http://www.dartmouth.edu/~matc/math5.geometry/unit10/unit10.html

Carpenter, W. 2013. *Principles of Mental Physiology: With Their Applications to the Training and Discipline of the Mind, and the Study of Its Morbid Conditions.* London, UK: Forgotten Books. (Original work published 1875).

Celaschi, S. and S. Mascarenhaus. 1977. Thermal-stimulated pressure and current studies of bound water in lysozyme. *Biophys. J.* 20(2):273–7.

Cellular Phone Taskforce, 2016. The work of Olle Johansson. http://www.cellphonetaskforce.org/?page_id=585

Chance, B. and M. Nishimura. 1960. On the mechanism of chlorohyll-cytochrome interaction: The temperature insensitivity of light-induced cytochrome oxidation in chromatium. *Proc. Natl. Acad. Sci. USA* 46:19–24.

Cifra, M., J.Z. Fields and A. Farhadi. 2011. Review: Electromagnetic cellular interactions. *Biophysics and Molecular Biology* 105:223–246.

Cifra, M., C. Brouderb, M. Nerudová and Kučera, O. 2015. Biophotons, coherence and photocount statistics: A critical review. *J. Luminescence* 164:38–51.

Cosic, I., D. Cosic and K. Lazar. 2015a. Is it possible to predict electromagnetic resonances in proteins, DNA and RNA? *EPJ Nonlinear Biomedical Physics* 3(5):1–8.

Cosic, I., Lazar, K., and Cosic, D. 2015b. Prediction of Tubulin Resonant Frequencies Using the Resonant Recognition Model (RRM). *IEEE Transactions on Nanobioscience* 14(4):491–496.

Crank, J. 1980. *The Mathematics of Diffusion.* Oxford, UK: Oxford University Press.

Cuevas, J.C. and E. Scheer. 2010. *Molecular Electronics: An Introduction to Theory and Experiment.* Singapore, China: World Scientific.

Darling, M. and H.V. Desai. 2012. Force scanning for simultaneous collection of topographical and mechanical properties. *Microscopy and Analysis* Issue 115, January/February issue.

Deisenyhofer, J.H. Michel, and R. Huber. 1985. The structural basis of photosynthetic light reactions in bacteria. *Trends. Biochem. Sci* 10:243–248.

Delvendahl, I. and S. Hallermann. 2016. The cerebellar mossy fiber synapse as a model for high-frequency transmission in the mammalian CNS. *Trends in Neurosciences* 39(11):722–737.

DeVault, D. and B. Chance. 1966. Studies of photosynthesis using a pulsed laser. I. Temperature dependence of cytochrome oxidation rate in chromatium. Evidence for tunneling. *Biophys. J.* 6(6):825–47.

Dumé, B. 2012. Photon shape could be used to encode quantum information. *Physics world.com.* http://physicsworld.com/cws/article/news/2012/aug/10/photon-shape-could-be-used-to-encode-quantum-information

Dvorak, H.F. 1986. Tumors: Wounds that do not heal. Similarities between tumor stroma generation and wound healing. *N Engl J Med* 315: 1650–9.

Eberson, L. 2011. Electron Transfer Reactions in Organic Chemistry (Reactivity and Structure: Concepts in Organic Chemistry) Softcover reprint of the original 1st ed. 1987 Edition. Springer; Softcover reprint of the original 1st ed. 1987 edition, November 22, 2011.

Engel, G.S., R.R., Calhoun, E.L., Read, T-K., Ahn et al. 2007. Evidence for wavelike energy transfer through quantum coherence in photosynthetic systems. *Nature* 446:782–786.

Escames, G. 2011. Evaluation of neutralization of low intensity radiation harmful effects on five subjects cells redox markers. *Research Report to PRANAN Dated June 3*, 2011.

Fick, A. 1855. On liquid diffusion. Poggendorffs Annalen. 94: 59—reprinted in *Journal of Membrane Science* 100: 33–38, 1995.

Finando, S. and D. Finando. 2011. Fascia and the mechanism of acupuncture. *J. Bodyw. Mov. Ther.* 15, 168–176.

Finando, S. and D. Finando. 2012. Qi, acupuncture and the fascia: A reconsideration of the fundamental principles of acupuncture. *J. Altern. Complement. Med.* 18(9): 880–886.

Fischer, E. 1894. Einfluss der Configuration auf die Wirkung der Enzyme. *Berichte der deutschen chemischen Gesellschaft.* 27:2985–2993.

Freud, S. 1957. Project for a scientific psychology. In Strachey J. (trans.), *The Standard Edition of the Complete Psychological Works of Sigmund Freud.* London, UK: Hogarth Press, vol. 1, pp. 283–397.

Freud, S. 1991. *On Metapsychology—The Theory of Psychoanalysis: Beyond the Pleasure Principle, Ego and the Id and Other Works.* London, UK: Penguin Books, pp. 175.

Fröhlich, H. 1978. Coherent electric vibrations in biological systems and the cancer problem. *IEEE Transactions on Microwave Theory and Techniques. TMTT* 26:613–617.

Fröhlich, H. ed. 1988. *Biological Coherence and Response to External Stimuli.* Springer-Verlag, Berlin.

Fuller, B. 1982, 1983. *Synergetics: Explorations in the Geometry of Thinking.* Volumes I and II. Macmillan Pub Co, 1982.

Gascoyne, P., R. Pethg and A. Szent-Györgyi. 1981. Water structure-dependent charge transport in proteins. *Proc. Natl. Acad. Sci.* 78:261–265.

Ginzburg, V.B. 1996. Spiral Grain of the Universe. In: *Search of the Archimedes File.* University Editions, Huntington, WV.

Ginzburg, V.B. 1999. *Unified Spiral Field and Matter. A Story of a Great Discovery.* Pittsburgh, PA: Helicola Press.

Ginzburg, V.B. 2002. *Unified Spiral Nature of the Quantum and Relativistic Universe.* Pittsburgh, PA: Helicola Press.

Ginzburg, V.B. 2006. *Prime Elements of Ordinary Matter, Dark Matter and Dark Energy.* Pittsburgh, PA: Helicola Press.

Ginzburg, V.B. 2013. *The Spacetime Origin of the Universe.* Pittsburgh, PA: Helicola Press.

Glazer, A.N. 1985. Light harvesting by phycobilisomes. *Annual Review of Biophysics and Biophysical Chemistry* 14: 47–77.

Goldstein, C., N. Schappacher and J. Schwermer. 2007. *The Shaping of Arithmetic after C.F. Gauss's Disquisitiones Arithmeticae*, New York, NY: Springer International, p. 235.

Greenaway, F. 1966. *John Dalton and the Atom.* Ithaca, NY: Cornell University Press.

Guimberteau, J-C. and C. Armstrong. 2015. *Architectue of Human Living Fascia. The Extracellular Matrix and Cells Revealed Through Endoscopy.* Edinburgh, U.K.: Handspring Publishing.

Gurvitch, A.G. 1926. *Das Problem der Zellteilung Physiologish Betrachtet.* Berlin: Springer- Verlag.

Halliwell, B. and J.M.C. Gutteridge. 1999. *Free Radicals in Biology and Medicine. Chapter 2, The Chemistry of Free Radicals and Related "Reactive Species.* Oxford, U.K.: Oxford University Press, pp. 36–104.

Hameroff, S.R. 1999. The neuron doctrine is an insult to neurons. *Behavioral and Brain Sciences* 22(5):838–839.

Havenith, M. 2010. THz spectroscopy as a new tool to probe hydration dynamics. In: Song J-J., K-T. Tsen, M. Betz, and A.Y. Elezzabia (eds) *Ultrafast Phenomena in Semiconductors and Nanostructure Materials XVI.* Proc. of SPIE 7600:1–5, Vancouver, WA.

Hawking, S. (ed.) 2011. *The Dreams that Stuff is Made of: The Most Astounding Papers of Quantum Physics— and How They Shook the Scientific World.* Philadelphia, PA: Running Press.

Ho, M-W. 2008. *The Rainbow and the Worm. The Physics of Organisms.* Singapore: World Scientific Publishing Company, 3rd edition.

Ho, M-W. 2012. *Living Rainbow H_2O.* Singapore: World Scientific Publishing Company.

Ho, M-W., Mohamed el Naschie, M., and Vitiello, G. 2015. Is spacetime fractal and quantum coherent in the golden mean? *Global Journals (US)* XV(1):1–21.

Holmes, D.F., C.J. Gilpin, C. Baldock, U. Ziese, A.J. Koster et al. 2000. Corneal collagen fibril structure in three dimensions: Structural insights into fibril assembly, mechanical properties, and tissue organization. *PNAS* 98(13):7307–7312.

Hush, N.S. 2006. An overview of the first half-century of molecular electronics. *Annals of the New York Academy of Sciences* 1006: 1–20.

Ignatov, I., O. Mosin and C. Stoyanov. 2014. Fields in electromagnetic spectrum emitted from human body. Applications in medicine. *Journal of Health, Medicine and Nursing* 7:1–22.

Ingber, D. 1998. The Architecture of Life. *Scientific American* 278:48.

Ives, J.A., E.P.A. van Wijk, N. Bat, C. Crawford, A. Walter et al. 2014. Ultraweak photon emission as a non-invasive health assessment: A systematic review. *PLoS ONE* 9(2):e87401.

Jung, C.G. 1996. *The Archetypes and the Collective Unconscious.* in US: Princeton University Press and London: Routledge, p. 43.

Kaminer, B. 1975. *Search and Discovery: A Tribute to Albert Szent-Györgyi.* New York: Academic Press.

Kaminura, S. and R. Kaniya. 1989. High-frequency nanometre-scale vibration in "quiescent" flagellar axonemes. *Nature* 340:476–478.

Karu, T.I. 1999. Primary and secondary mechanisms of action of visible-to-near IR radiation on cells. *J. Photochem. Photobiol. B: Biol.* 49:1–17.

Katz, B. and R. Miledi. 1965. The measurement of synaptic delay, and the time course of acetylcholine release at the neuromuscular junction. *Proc Royal Society of London Series B, Biological Sciences* 161(985):483–495.

Kinnaunen, P.K.J. and J.A. Virtanen. 1986. Some aspects of charge transfer in biological systems. In Gutmann, F. and Keyzer, H. (eds) *Modern Bioelectrochemistry.* New York: Plenum, pp. 177–197.

King, P. 2011. https://www.quora.com/What-is-the-clock-speed-equivalent-of-the-human-brain

Kobayashi, M. 2005. Two-dimensional imaging and spatiotemporal analysis of biophoton. In: X. Shen, R. Wijk (eds) *Biophotonics*. Springer, pp. 155–171.

Kraut, J. and H. Pelletier. 1992. Crystal structure of a complex between electron transfer partners, cytochrome c peroxidase and cytochrome c. *Science* 258:1748–1755.

Langevin, H.M. and J.A. Yandow. 2003. Relationship of acupuncture points and meridians to connective tissue planes. *Anat. Rec.* 269(6), 257–265.

Langevin, H.M., D.L. Churchill, J. Wu, G.J. Badger, J.A. Yandow, J.R. Fox, and M.H. Krag. 2002. Evidence of connective tissue involvement in acupuncture. *FASEB J.* 16(8):872–4. PMID: 11967233.

Liberman, J. 1990. Light: Medicine of the Future: How We Can Use It to Heal Ourselves NOW.

Marcus, R.A. 1992. *Electron Transfer Reactions in Chemistry: Theory and Experiment. From Nobel Lectures, Chemistry 1991–1995*, Bo G. Malmström (ed.) Singapore: World Scientific Publishing Co.

Maret, K. 2008. An Overview of Quantum Medicine: Presented at the 34th Annual U.S. *Psychotronics Association Conference*, July 18–20, Chicago, IL.

Martel, A. 2016. The Power of Light—Dawn of a new medicine. First published as Le pouvoir de la lumière, in French by Guy Trédaniel Éditeur.

Matsumoto, K. and S. Birch. 1988. *Hara diagnosis: Reflections on the sea*. Brookline, MA: Paradigm Publications.

McFadden, J. and J. Al-Khalili. 2016. *Life on the Edge: The Coming of Age of Quantum Biology*, Broadway Books; The Secrets Of Quantum Physics - Quantum Biology Theory Documentary, https://www.youtube.com/watch?v=gT22gRzyotA\

Metzger, R.M. 2003. Unimolecular rectifiers. In: Reed M.A. and Lee (eds) *Molecular Nanoelectronics*. Stevenson Ranch, CA: American Scientific Publishers, pp. 19–38.

Myers, T. 2001. *Anatomy Trains: Myofascial Meridians for Manual and Movement Therapists*. London: Churchill Livingstone.

Nahin, P.J. 1988. *Oliver Heaviside. The Life, Work, and Times of an Electrical Genius of the Victorian Age*. Baltimore, MD: The Johns Hopkins University Press.

Nakahara, Y., K. Kimura, H. Inokuchi and T. Yagi. 1979. Electrical conductivity of solid state proteins: simple proteins and cytochrome c3 as anhydrous film. *Chem. Lett.* 8(8):877–880.

Oschman, J.L. 1984. Structure and properties of ground substances. *American Zoologist* 24:199–215.

Oschman, J.L. 1993. A biophysical basis for acupuncture. *Proceedings of the First Symposium of the Society for Acupuncture Research held in Rockville*, MD on January 23–24, 1993.

Oschman, J.L. 1996–1998. A series of 6 articles entitled, What is healing energy. *Journal of Bodywork and Movement Therapies*, Edinburgh, U.K.: Harcourt Brace and Co. Ltd.

Oschman, J.L. 2000. *Energy Medicine: The Scientific Basis*. Edinburgh: Churchill Livingstone, Elsevier.

Oschman, J.L. 2003. *Energy Medicine in Therapeutics and Human Performance*. Edinburgh: Butterworth Heinemann.

Oschman, J.L. 2016. *Energy Medicine: The Scientific Basis*. 2nd edition, Edinburgh: Churchill Livingstone, Elsevier.

Oschman, J.L. and M.D. Pressman. 2014. An anatomical, biophysical and quantum basis for the unconscious mind. *International Journal of Transpersonal Studies* 33(1):77–96.

Oschman, J.L. and N.H. Oschman. 1993. Matter, energy, and the living matrix. October, 1993 issue of Rolf Lines, the news magazine for the Rolf Institute, Boulder, CO, 21(3):55–64.

Oschman, J.L. and N.H. Oschman. 2015a. The heart as a bi-directional scalar field antenna. *J. Vortex Sci. Technol.* 2:121. doi: 10.4172/2090-8369.1000121.

Oschman, J.L. and N.H. Oschman. 2015b. Vortical structure of light and space: Biological implications. *J. Vortex Sci. Technol.* 2:112. doi: 10.4172/2090-8369.1000112.

Özdemir, F. and A. Kargi. 2011. Electromagnetic waves and human health. In: *Electromagnetic Waves*, Vitaliy Zhurbenko (ed.), Vienna: InTech. Available from: http://www.intechopen.com/books/electromagnetic-waves/electromagnetic-waves-and-human-health

Pall, M.L. 2013. Electromagnetic fields act via activation of voltage-gated calcium channels to produce beneficial or adverse effects. *J. Cell Mol. Med.* 17(8):958–65.

Pall, M.L. 2014. *How WiFi & Other EMFs Cause Biological Harm*. Presentation at the Litteraturhuset, Oslo, Norway, October 18, 2014. Published on YouTube on Dec 1, 2014. https://www.youtube.com/watch?v=Pjt0iJThPU0

Pethig, R. 1979. *Dielectric and Electronic Properties of Biological Materials*. Chichester: Wiley.

Pethig, R.. 2004. Interview with Ronald Pethig in The Albert Szent-Gyorgyi Papers, National Library of Medicine, https://profiles.nlm.nih.gov/ps/accessNVGBBLW.ocr.

Pienta, K.J. and D.S. Coffey. 1991. Cellular harmonic information transfer through a tissue tensegrity-matrix system. *Medical Hypotheses* 34:88–95.

Pilla, A., R. Fitzsimmons, D., Muehsam, J., Wu, C., Rohde et al. 2011. Electromagnetic fields as first messenger in biological signaling: Application to calmodulin-dependent signaling in tissue repair. *Biochim Biophys Acta* 1810 (12): 1236–1245.

Pischinger, A. 2007. *The Extracellular Matrix and Ground Regulation: Basis for a Holistic Biological Medicine.* Berkeley, CA: North Atlantic Books.

Popp, F.A., Q. Gu, and K.H. Li. 1994. Biophoton emission: Experimental background and theoretical approaches. *Mod. Phys. Lett. B.* 8:1269–1296.

Pressman, M.D. 1977. Mind over figures. *Skating Magazine,* 54(3).

Pressman, M.D. 1979. Psychological techniques for the advancement of sports potential. In: Klavora, P. and Daniel, J. (eds.), Coach, athlete, and the sport psychologist.

Pressman, M.D. 1980a. Psychological techniques for the advancement of sports potential. In: Suinn, R. W. (ed.) *Psychology in Sports: Methods and Applications.* Minneapolis, MN: Burgess, pp. 291–296.

Pressman, M.D. 1980b. Psychodynamic experience in an Olympic skating camp. In: Straub, W. F. (ed.) *Sports Psychology: An Analysis of Athlete Behavior.* Ithaca, NY: Movement, pp. 373–380.

Pullman, B. and A. Pullman. 1958. Electron-donor and—acceeptor properties of biologically important purines, pyrimidines, pteridines, flavins, and aromatic amino acids. *Proc. Natl. Acad. Sci. USA.* 15;44(12):1197–202.

Rezus, Y. et al. 2012. Single-photon spectroscopy of a single molecule. *Phys. Rev. Lett.* 108, 093601.

Rosenberg, F. and E. Postow. 1969. Semiconduction in proteins and lipids-its possible biological import. *Ann. N.Y. Acad. Sci.* 158:161–190.

Schade, U., K. Holldack, M.C. Martin, and D. Fried. 2005. THz near-field imaging of biological tissues employing synchrotron radiation. In: Tsen, K-T., J-J Song, and J. Jiang (eds) *Ultrafast Phenomena in Semiconductors and Nanostructure Materials IX.* Proc. of SPIE Bellingham, WA: SPIE, 5725:46–52.

Scudder, P.H. 2013. *Electron Flow in Organic Chemistry A Decision Based Guide to Organic Mechanisms.* Hoboken, NJ: Wiley, 2nd edition.

Sheldrake, R. 2013. Science Set Free: 10 Paths to New Discovery, published by Deepak Chopra.

Sitizuraa, J., M.N. Taib, H. Abdullah and M.M. Yunus. 2005. Frequency Radiation Characteristic Around the Human Body. doi: 10.5013/IJSSST.a.12.01.05 online, 1473-8031 print.

Skourtis, S.S., J.J. Regan and J.N. Onuchic. 1994. Electron transfer in proteins: A novel approach for the description of donor-acceptor coupling. *J. Physical Chemistry* 98: 3379–3388.

Sloane, P. undated. *How to Think What Nobody Else Thinks.* http://www.lifehack.org/articles/lifestyle/how-to-think-what-nobody-else-thinks.html sport psychologist (pp. 133-143). Toronto, Canada: University of Toronto.

Solit, M. 1998. Holistic Geometry. http://www.fnd.org/pgs/geo/holistic_geometry.htm

Srere, P.A. 1985. The metabolon. *Trends in Biochemical Sciences* 10:109–110.

Standring, S. (ed.) 2009. *Gray's Anatomy.* 40th edition, Edinburgh: Churchill Livingston, 678–9.

Still, A.T. 1899. *Philosophy of Osteopathy,* Kirksville, MO, 86.

Szent-Györgyi, A. 1941a. The study of energy levels in biochemistry. *Nature* 148:157–159.

Szent-Györgyi, A. 1941b. Towards a new biochemistry? *Science* 93:609–11.

Szent-Györgyi, A. 1957. *Bioenergetics.* New York: Academic Press,.

Szent-Györgyi, A. 1960. *Introduction to a Submolecular Biology.* New York: Academic Press.

Szent-Györgyi, A. 1968. *Bioelectronics.* New York: Academic Press.

Szent-Györgyi, A. 1972. Electronic biology and cancer. *Tuesday Evening Lecture at the Marine Biological Laboratory.*

Szent-Györgyi, A. 1976. *Electronic Biology and Cancer.* New York: Marcel Dekker, Inc.

Szent-Györgyi, A. 1977. Welcoming remarks. *Int. J. Quantum Chem., Quantum Biol.* Symp.4;1.

Szent-Györgyi, A. 1978. *The Living State and Cancer.* New York: Marcel Dekker, Inc.

Szent-Gyorgyi, A. 1988. To see what everyone has seen, to think what no one has thought. *The Biological Bulletin* 174(3):191.

Trelstad, R.L. 1982. The bilaterally asymmetrical architecture of the submammalian corneal stroma resembles a cholesteric liquid crystal. *Dev. Biol.* 92:133.

Trushin, M.V. 2004. Distant non-chemical communication in various biological systems. *Rivista di biologia* 97(3):409–42.

Van Wijk, E.P., R. Van Wijk, and S. Bosman. 2010. Using ultra-weak photon emission to determine the effect of oligomeric proanthocyanidins on oxidative stress of human skin. *J. Photochem. Photobiol. B* 98:199–206.

Van Wijk, R., E.P.A. Van Wijk and R.P. Bajpai. 2006. Photocount distribution of photons emitted from three sites of a human body. *Journal of Photochemistry and Photobiology B Biology* 84:46–55.

Virchow, R. 1858. Die Cellularpathologie in ihrer Begründung auf physiologische und pathologische Gewebelehre.

Wan, C., T. Fiebig, S.O. Kelley, C.R. Treadway and J.K. Barton. 1999. Femtosecond dynamics of DNA-mediated electron transfer. *Proceedings of the National Academy of Sciences USA* 96:6014–6019.

Wiener, N. 1948. *Cybernetics: Or Control and Communication in the Animal and the Machine.* Paris, (Hermann & Cie) and Cambridge, MA: MIT Press, 2nd revised ed. 1961.

Wu, F. and S. Minteer. 2014. Krebs cycle metabolon: Structural evidence of substrate channeling revealed by cross-linking and mass spectrometry. *Angewandte Chemie International Edition* 54(6):1851–1854.

Young, A.M. 1999. *The Reflexive Universe. Evolution of Consciousness.* Cambria, CA: Anodos Foundation.

Zewail, A. H. 2003. Femtochemistry: Atomic-scale dynamics of the chemical bond using ultrafast lasers [Nobel lecture, December 8, 1999]. In I. Grenthe (ed.) *Nobel Lectures, Chemistry 1996–2000.* Singapore, China: World Scientific, pp. 274–367.

28 Non-Invasive Early, Quick Diagnostic Methods of Various Cancers (Part I) and Safe, Effective, Individualized Treatment of Cancer (Part II)

Yoshiaki Omura

CONTENTS

Part I: Introduction to General Background 689
The Case That Started It All 689
    The Bi-Digital O-Ring Test 691
    The Importance of the Thymus Gland 695
    Some Markers That I Use for Diagnosis and Evaluation of Therapeutic Effect Using BDORT 704
Part II: Clinical Implications of Human Papilloma Virus-Type 16 705
    Our Improved, Individualized, Safe, Effective Treatment Using Optimal Dose of
    Vitamin D3 and other Compatible, Synergetic, Beneficial Supplements 705
    Factors Promoting and Inhibiting These Anti-Cancer Effects 705
    Treatment Considerations 706
    Our Individualized Safe, Effective, and Affordable Cancer Treatment 707
    Factors Influencing Cancer Treatment 708
Bibliography 711

The research on highly sensitive Electro-Magnetic Field (EMF) resonance phenomenon between two identical molecules with identical weight performed at Pupin Laboratory of Graduate Experimental Physics, Columbia University became basis of new, non-invasive, early diagnostic method.

The diagnostic technique described herein takes inspiration from an elementary physical phenomenon called "resonance phenomenon." Every material has an intrinsic property known as its "resonant frequency." If a material is exposed to a mechanical wave that is oscillating at the material's resonant frequency, the material will begin to vibrate vigorously. For example, when a vocalist sings at particular frequency in the presence of a wine glass, the wine glass can shatter if the resonance frequency of the wine glass, is the same frequency of the singer and its intensity of the voice is very strong. This principle also applies to electromagnetic waves and is the foundation of radio communication. In radio communication, a transmitter emits a particular frequency of radio wave which propagates until it reaches a receiver (a type of electromagnetic field resonance circuit). If that particular wave has identical frequency as the receiver's resonant frequency, strong electromagnetic wave resonance phenomenon will be induced inside of L-C resonance circuit of the receiver. In fact, a tuner on a radio is actually altering the capacitance of the receiver inside the radio which in turn changes the resonant frequency of the radio. This is what allows a user to tune-in to different radio stations. In my initial experiments, I worked with two identical L-C electromagnetic field resonance circuits with identical coils and variable capacitors (Figure 28.1). If the capacitances of each L-C resonance circuits are tuned to match each other, and one of the L-C circuits are charged, because of the resonance phenomenon, the voltage response that one observes in the charged oscillator will also be observed in the uncharged oscillator even if it is located very far away. We performed our experiment on either end of the George Washington Bridge. One can measure this by using an oscilloscope to monitor the voltage across the capacitors in each L-C resonance circuit. The sinusoidal wave measured by the oscilloscope in each L-C resonance circuit will be identical. I discovered, however, that the human body could be used as a detector of the presence of electromagnetic field resonance between two identical L-C resonance circuits without using an oscilloscope. I noticed this phenomenon when uncharged L-C circuits resonating at the same frequency as the charged L-C resonance circuit was placed in a human's hand: the human's entire body would go weak. This happened when the two L-C circuits was in a parallel position to the charged oscillator at the end of the same room. I discovered this while spending 3 1/2 years at Columbia University Experimental Physics Department. I was concentrating my research on the electromagnetic field (EMF) resonance phenomenon. I was testing with one small L-C resonance circuit in my hand and the other identical L-C circuit at a distance. What I discovered was that when the variable capacitance of two identical L-C circuits became equal, suddenly the whole muscle strength of the person holding the second L-C circuit became extremely weak. I realized that when the muscle strength became very weak, this was detecting an electromagnetic field resonance phenomenon without using the oscilloscope. An oscilloscope is bulky, heavy, and expensive. I had found a method of detecting EMF resonance phenomenon without using oscilloscope. Now, I can find out immediately if there is electromagnetic field resonance phenomenon or not, using this method. The next question was, because I am a physician, since this study is using two electrical circuits, if I change to two identical molecules, then what will happen? Then I spent a few years repeating this experiment with two identical molecules with same amount and we discovered that we can detect similar electromagnetic field resonance phenomenon between two identical molecules with identical weight. Now we can detect any molecule in the human body without taking a biopsy or a blood test or any radiological test. We can detect any location if we have two identical molecules. When testing molecules, non-invasively, from a visible distance, it does not have to be in parallel position; any position will produce same resonance phenomenon as long as there is resonance. This can later be confirmed by the laboratory or radiological tests; however, these standard lab tests are not only expensive but also take much longer time and less sensitive for the detection of cancer (Figure 28.2).

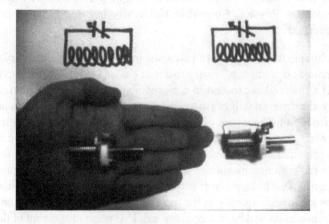

FIGURE 28.1   Two identical L-C resonance circuits used in my experiments.

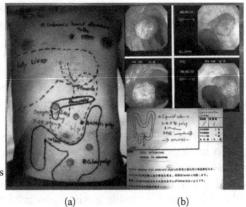

−Colon cancer found amongst seminar participants using BDORT (a).

−Bi-Digital O-Ring Test detected early colon cancer (image a) long before polyps were found in the same locations by colonoscopy (image b) about 2 years after it was detected by BDORT

(a)   (b)

FIGURE 28.2 Comparison between Bi-Digital O-Ring Test (a) and modern medical examination (b).

PART I: INTRODUCTION TO GENERAL BACKGROUND

1. We can detect electromagnetic field resonance phenomenon between two identical L-C circuits or between two identical molecules with identical weight.
2. If we have two identical molecules, one specific molecule inside of the body and the other one in the examiner's hand, we can detect any molecule inside the cells or the body non-invasively.
3. A U.S. Patent was given for this method in 1993 as a new concept known as Bi-Digital O-Ring Test which consists of four new concepts including highly sensitive EMF resonance phenomenon between two identical molecules with the same weight.

THE CASE THAT STARTED IT ALL

My first successful detection of cancer using this method (Bi-Digital O-Ring Test) to detect electromagnetic field resonance phenomenon between two identical cancer tissues (pancreatic cancer inside of abdomen and same cancer slide at the palm of examiner's hand).

My first patient happened to be the president of the New York State Board of Medicine. He had developed a severe backache which was continuing to worsen and he had seen all the well-known specialists, professors of pain, and no one was able to figure out the cause; there was no diagnosis, all the tests were negative. He had seen many top pain specialists in the world so finally he asked me to do acupuncture as he knew I was well-known acupuncturist. Normally when I perform acupuncture, the pain disappears and it often stays gone for a few days but in his case the pain came back in a few hours. I thought, this is something much more serious, so I suspected the possibility of pancreatic cancer. He was in his seventies and he was a psychiatrist and a neurologist. The reason for his pain, I finally figured out, was adenocarcinoma of the head of the pancreas. That evening when the pain came back, I went to his home to try to figure out why the pain came back. When I went to his home he was in bed but he was in bed in a half-sitting position, so I asked him what position did he sleep in and he replied that he slept in half-sitting position. At that time, I had completed a residency as a physician at the Cancer Institute of Columbia University. The patients with cancer of the head of the pancreas often told me that if they bent forward the pain diminished. All the patients used to sit or sleep in the same manner; if they bent forward instead of lying down, their pain diminished, so I felt he also had a possibility of cancer of the head of the pancreas. I went to examine him with a cancer slide of adenocarcinoma of the head of the pancreas. When he was tested using the Bi-Digital O-Ring Test, using the slide, suddenly there was resonance and his muscle strength went completely weak, so I said to him, "I am not sure but I think that it is possible you have adenocarcinoma of the head of the pancreas." This doctor was a graduate of Cornell Medical School; he immediately called Sloan Kettering Memorial Hospital and was admitted and all tests were done and all laboratory tests were negative. There was no change in blood chemistry and all x-rays and MRIs were negative. There was no radiological evidence of cancer; meanwhile the pain was getting worse, he was weak with no appetite, so they kept him in the hospital. At the end of two months, the MRI suddenly showed an abnormal area in the head of the pancreas; it took about two months from the time I told him that according to BDORT resonance phenomenon it looks like he has cancer of the head of the pancreas until MRI showed an abnormal area of the head of pancreas. The hospital at the time did not have a surgical expert in cancer of the head of the pancreas so they called MD Anderson in Houston where there was one specialist. When that specialist examined all the laboratory test results, he said it was too late, had you called me a month or two earlier he could have operated but now the cancer is inoperable. First when my patient was admitted at Sloan Kettering, he said to me, "You have made a misdiagnosis"; later when they found the cancer, they said chemotherapy or surgery is out of the question and the only thing they can suggest is palliative pain medication and let the patient die comfortably. They told his wife that the prognosis was a few months. At that point his wife called me every day, "Please save him." That weekend, I happened to go to a Japanese book store and saw an article in a famous Japanese monthly magazine called *Bungeishunjū* regarding a professor at Tokyo University who had developed stomach cancer and without surgery he was able to eliminate his stomach cancer. The professor was writing an unbelievable story, as he was a professor at Tokyo University. Our patient's wife asked me to call Professor Maruyama, who was treating the author of the article. I called Professor Maruyama, and he told me that he used the Maruyama vaccine at the medical school in Tokyo. When he was the head of the TB hospital at the medical school in Tokyo, he noticed that there were no cancer patients in the TB hospital. So, he established a new hypothesis: he thought that the TB bacillus creates some substance which inhibits cancer, so he made a vaccine and started treating cancer patients and he noticed that some patients got better but others saw no effect; he also noticed that the treatment had no side effects. Since the professor at Tokyo University recovered from stomach cancer, I called Professor Maruyama of Tokyo Medical College and he immediately sent the vaccine by overnight mail. I thought to myself that if I give the vaccine, I could lose my license, so the wife said she would give it and she started giving a combination of two vaccines daily. There was absolutely no effect after one week, so one possibility I considered was that the thymus gland function is reduced. The Tokyo University professor whose stomach cancer disappeared probably had better thymus gland function or he did something to stimulate the thymus gland. I performed the manual acupuncture technique to stimulate his thymus gland and suddenly, the next day my patient was better, he started standing and talking in combination with acupuncture and Maruyama vaccine, and he went to his office and started working. However, I asked his wife to continue the acupuncture with two needles horizontal on manubrium at both sides just above the bone parallel to the skin, three times daily. The patient went back to work. I recalled that during the Second World War in Japan, to make you healthy they taught you to stimulate your whole chest with a dry towel. I thought maybe the Tokyo University professor was doing this, but we never found out if he actually did. The acupuncture effect did not last for more than a few hours, 7–8 hours at the most.

Later a 24-hour nurse was hired. As she could not perform acupuncture, I changed my approach and asked her to use a portable vibrator on his manubrium and surrounding area. I showed the nurse how to use it and asked her to try hourly to stimulate the thymus. In a few days, my patient had no pain, good appetite, and could stand up by himself. He could do everything he was doing before, even go back to work. All in all, he survived 1 1/2 years. The reason he died, I found out later, was that his bile duct was occluded with cancer. The treating surgeon mechanically tried to open the bile duct; he tried to pass a tube through the bile duct, and that spread the cancer throughout the body. After that, suddenly he went downhill and cancer spread through his entire body. Shortly afterward he died. Before he died he told me to write about his story and said to me, "You have my special permission to use my name." He wanted people to know how he died. He wanted me to teach my method to others so that people would be saved. The diagnosis of cancer of the head of the pancreas was due to my clinical experience and that is how it all started. The non-invasive diagnosis of the pancreatic cancer had been done the same day I saw the doctor as a patient; at that time I suspected cancer of the head of the pancreas due to my clinical experience, so I only tested pancreatic cancer slide and it produced strong electromagnetic field resonance. Now, when I see new patients since I don't know what the cancer patient has, I have to screen for the presence of EMF resonance by examining all the well-known cancers using their corresponding tissue microscope slides.

I have a box of about 75 cancer slides of well-known/common cancers. The box is inside aluminum foil removable cover case that causes it to act like an antenna. In the beginning, I was testing with one slide at a time.

Now, if I examine a new patient without knowing absolutely anything about the patient's medical history, I can detect any cancer anywhere, in any part of the body. This method is based on the fact that each slide of specific cancer tissue is emitting a specific frequency of electromagnetic field, and this is in a plastic box; this box is almost like empty space because in between the molecules of the plastic box, the space is much bigger than the wavelength of the cancer information coming from the cancer slides. Each cancer cell has a specific frequency (vibration) so if I put the slides in the plastic box, this box is almost transparent because there is so much empty space between the molecules of plastic, and then when I put the aluminum foil over it, the vibrational information of all the 75 cancers is captured by the aluminum foil cover case antenna. So, when I check resonance, I can instantaneously check 75 cancers; if there is more than one cancer, I can detect all of them. So, this is a non-invasive, quick, accurate and economical diagnostic method. That is why the head of the European Parliament Anti-Cancer Committee invited me to give a lecture at the European Parliament at Brussels on February 8, 2017.

There are four new non-invasive methods that I have developed for detection of early stage or any stage of cancer which will be described later in this chapter.

THE BI-DIGITAL O-RING TEST

The BDORT or Bi-Digital O-Ring Test consists of at least two major components and major parts and is a technique for non-invasive semi-quantitative detection of most molecules existing in the human body. BDORT is an adjunct for non-invasive diagnosis, safe and effective treatment and clinical research which was developed by Yoshiaki Omura, MD, ScD, and U.S. Patent was given in 1993. This is the only U.S. Patent involving the human body; in the history of U.S. patents this is the only exception. The patent is for the method of diagnosis of diseases (Figure 28.3).

The main principle is based on the Electromagnetic Field Resonance phenomenon that exists between two identical molecules with identical weight. This invention was based on electromagnetic field resonance phenomenon between two identical L-C circuits which was discovered in the early 1910s at Pupin Laboratory of Graduate Experimental Physics Department of Columbia University, where Professor Pupin discovered that when there are two identical pairs of L-C electrical resonance circuits, if one circuit produces electrical oscillation with fixed frequencies which can be observed with an early oscilloscope but a second identical circuit is placed in a parallel location even at a distance as far as the eye can see, the second L-C resonance circuit also produces the same sinusoidal electrical oscillation, which can be measured and observed by an oscilloscope. While this author was performing this experiment, as mentioned before, I noticed that without using an oscilloscope, one of the oscillators touched a human hand, and the strength of the hand and fingers suddenly and drastically diminished. This caused the author to conclude that one can detect the presence of EMF resonance phenomenon by touching one of the identical L-C circuits without using an oscilloscope (Figures 28.4 and 28.5). The author thought that a similar phenomenon might take place between two identical molecules with identical weight and after years of research, this concept was confirmed to be true.

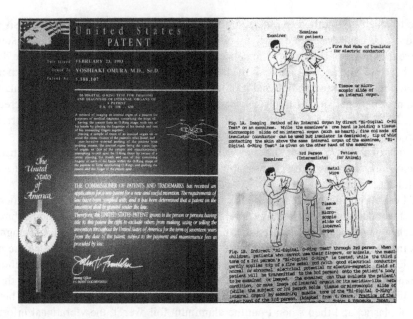

FIGURE 28.3   Patent for BDORT issued to Dr. Y. Omura.

The BDORT is performed using the O-Ring shape made by two fingers (thumb and one of the other fingers). The technique is based on the phenomenon of muscle weakness caused by resonance between two identical substances (Figure 28.6).

As other important principle of BDORT, an O-Ring made by two fingers also became weak and easily can open when the abnormal part of the body is touched, in the absence of EMF resonance phenomenon (with the exception of the thymus gland where abnormal part is touched, O-Ring became stronger).

According to my hypothesis of the mechanism of the first part of BDORT, molecular identification and localization method is due to an electromagnetic wave resonance phenomenon between two identical substances with an identical resonance frequency and separated by a visible distance. The information about the molecular structure and quantity of any molecule is contained in the

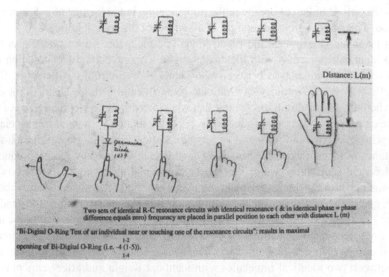

FIGURE 28.4   Principles behind the Bi-Digital O-Ring Test.

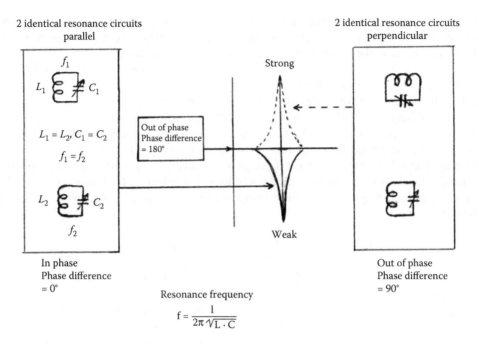

FIGURE 28.5 Principles behind BDORT.

specific electromagnetic field emitted by the particular molecule. These electro-magnetic waves, containing information about the particular substance, can be propagated through a metal wire, through a "concentrated electromagnetic field projector," or through a light beam with wavelength longer than green color (particularly a monochromatic, collimated light beam or soft laser beam). In the cases in which a light beam is used, the monochromatic light beam (including laser beam) acts as a very high frequency carrier of the electromagnetic waves emitted from a particular substance placed near the source of the light beam or near the end of the light beam, and information on the molecular structure and amount of the substance is carried by the light beam (including laser beam) in both forward and backward directions (bi-directional propagation of information). Even reflected light from any molecule or substance in the visual field that reaches the eyes carries information on the substance to the eye ground, particularly when the individual is gazing at the substance; simultaneously, information on a substance not normally existing in the body that happens to be in the body is sent out from the eye ground in electromagnetic waves to the object being gazed at by the individual.

What is Bi-Digital O-Ring Test (BDORT)?

The BDORT, or "Bi-Digital O-Ring Test" (Test of Bi-Digital O-Ring) is a technique for non-invasive diagnosis, safe and effective treatment, and clinical research, developed by Yoshiaki Omura, MD, ScD of New York.

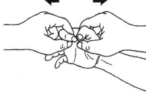

The technique is based on the phenomenon of muscle weakness caused by the resonance between two identical substances.

The BDORT is performed using O-Ring shape by 2 fingers (Thumb and other more fingers)

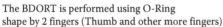

FIGURE 28.6 A diagrammatic representation of BDORT.

The reason why the human fingers are so sensitive is that the area of the fingers in the somato-sensory cortex of the brain has a disproportionately large representation compared to other parts of the body. This explains their sensitivity in relation to the rest of the body.

Your hands become your measuring device; hands can detect abnormal condition. It requires practice. You feel the energetic change, and the more you practice the better you get. It is a specific, unmistakable feeling of energy, sudden loss of muscle strength. An oscilloscope is bulky, expensive, and heavy to check if EMF resonance phenomenon exists or not to see on the oscilloscope if it is oscillating? I found that when the resonance is taking place, my hand becomes suddenly weak, every finger becomes weak, so we discovered a simple method of detection of the electromagnetic field resonance without using an oscilloscope. That is the biggest new discovery. Your hand acts as a tester. You are not supposed to give a patent on the human body but this is the only exception U.S. government made in the history of U.S. patents, the patent in relation to the human body.

The Bi-Digital O-Ring Test consists of following two main parts:

1. Simple method of quickly detecting electromagnetic field resonance phenomenon between 2 identical substances without using an oscilloscope.
2. When the abnormal part is touched or pointed at close range, the O-Ring suddenly becomes weak and how many O-Rings become weak and easily open determines the degree of abnormality. More abnormality means more O-Rings will open. The measuring system for an abnormal O-Ring opening is a -1 to -12 grading system or $+1$ to $+12$ for normal response. Anything over -7, you must suspect malignancy or strong viral or bacterial infection. When you suspect cancer, then you use the cancer slide. If specific cancer slide produces strong resonance, then you found correct cancer. If you check different cancer slides one by one it takes so much time. You can instantly check every slide in the box. You instantly check with the whole box of slides covered by removable aluminum cover case to see if there is resonance, then find out which slide is producing resonance. If there is no resonance with 75 common cancer slide screening kit, we can immediately tell the patient does not have any one of the 75 different cancers.

We systematically go through the list of slides—hematopoietic cancers, head, neck and so on. Using an organized box of cancer slides, first check the entire box of all the slides to see if there is resonance, then you can quickly go through the box checking with a finger pointing method to see which slide or slides produce resonance. Remove the cancer slide that produces resonance, then check again to see if it produces resonance. When the box is closed and covered with a removable aluminum foil cover case, it completely covers the slide box and the aluminum cover behaves as an antenna. It is receiving information from every cancer slide emitting different frequencies, and the aluminum cover box is catching all the frequencies because you are covering the entire slide box with the aluminum foil cover case. When the patient touches the aluminum cover case with slides inside the box that has all the cancer frequencies, we know immediately if there is resonance by examining of sudden openings of O-Rings of other hand of the patient. This is the basic principle of the BDORT. How do you know something is minus? The BDORT opens. If the BDORT is plus, it means it is normal and the ring does not open or tests strong (+).

Some additional findings—while comparing pathological tenderness by applying pressure with the thumb on the well-known organ representation areas in western and oriental medicine, we found that usually pathological tenderness requires 8200 g of force by 1 mm^2. However, by the time pathological tenderness is detected, often the disease has made significant progress. Our research indicated that if we touch over the skin of any abnormal part of the body by even touching one hair, the O-Ring can easily be opened without the creation of any pathological pain or tenderness. We found this to be a highly sensitive method of detection of pathology as the number of the openings

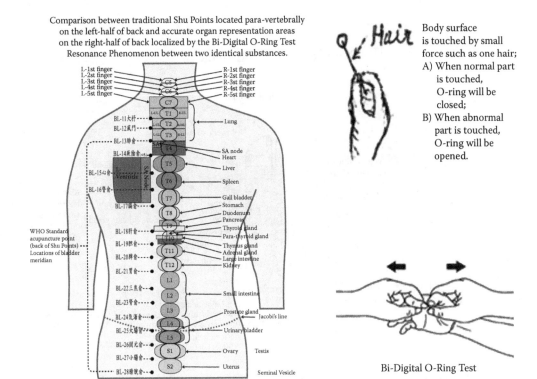

FIGURE 28.7 Sensitivity of BDORT vs. pathological tenderness over Shu points or other trigger points. (Copyright © 1999, 2001, 2002, and 2008 by Yoshiaki Omura, M.D., Sc.D. Information in parts or all of this chart in original form or modified form can not be reproduced without the author's written permission. Manufactured and distributed by ORT Life Science Research Institute, Inc., Kurume City, Japan.)

of the O-Ring was found to be proportionate to the degree of pathology. If the skin over normal tissue is contacted similarly, the O-Ring will not open but when there is pathology, the O-Ring will immediately open (Figure 28.7).

Before consuming any food, drink, medication or wearing clothes, accessories, bedding, and so on, BDORT can detect whether they will be beneficial, no effect, or harmful. When using medication, BDORT can determine the optimal dose at the outset. If the medication is not reaching the target organ to be treated, we can often enhance the drug effect by stimulation of the organ representation area of the corresponding pathological organ on the hands. If the patient is taking two or more drugs at the same time, using BDORT we can detect undesirable or harmful drug interaction before taking multiple medications.

THE IMPORTANCE OF THE THYMUS GLAND

The thymus gland is well known for its importance in the immunological aspects of the human body. It consists of two lobules and they are located in the upper chest cavity behind the manubrium sterni. Each gland consists of a cortex and a medulla.

Recently we suceeded in mapping different internal organs of the body on organ representation areas of the thymus gland (Figure 28.8). This new thymus gland representation area map can be used as a new method of detecting cancers and other serious medical problems. Also, they can be treated more effectively in conjunction with standard medical treatment plus thymus gland stimulation by combining the following six different approaches. thymus gland area stimulation by hand friction of the entire thymus gland alone gives us very significant, rapid improvement in

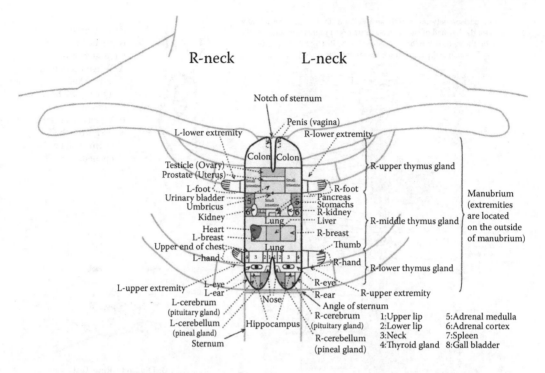

FIGURE 28.8 Thymus gland representation areas of right-handed person (Omura 2017). (Copyright © 1999, 2001, 2002, and 2017 by Yoshiaki Omura, M.D., Sc.D. Information in parts or all of this chart in original form or modified form can not be reproduced without the author's written permission. Manufactured and distributed by ORT Life Science Research Institute, Inc., Fukuoka, Japan.)

an emergency where no medicine or doctor is available. The following six approaches to improve thymus gland activities are as follows:

1. Keeping the body posture straight is the best way to maintain normal body condition.
2. Taking optimal dose of vitamin D3.
3. Use a long pillow which reaches upper half of the back while sleeping.
4. By the application of EMF neutralizer on the thymus gland representation area.
5. Vigorous stimulation of the entire thymus gland by repeated friction with the fingers of one hand (side to side) or repeated strong friction of the back of both hands to stimulate thymus gland representation areas on the back of hands.
6. Combination of optimal dose of vitamin D3 and 50 times manual pinching and rolling stimulation of skin of the thymus gland representation area on the back of L-hand or every 6~8 hours produced significant increase (about 15 times) of "Thymosin α_1" which has excellent anti-cancer effect, anti-inflammatory effects and significant increase (about 15 times) in "Thymosin β_4" which has significant improvment of circulation in cardiovascular system.

My diagnostic methods of non-invasive, quick diagnosis of cancers and related biochemical parameters were found by using: (1) visible or invisible changes at organ representation areas of face at eyebrows, alars of nose, lips, and so on, (2) one page "Mouth, Hand, and Foot Writing Form," (3) rapidly changing part of QRS complex and slowly changing, rising part of the T-wave of recorded ECGs, (4) thymus gland is the only organ in which its BDORT is (−) value when it is normal, but when it changes to (−) 1 or (+) value, one must suspect malignancy.

Within the past 15 years, we were able to make diagnosis of various cancers using visible or invisible changes appearing at organ representation areas of the face, eyebrows, alars of nose, lips, and so on. Particularly localized abnormal whitening of hairs of the eyebrows or disappearance of hair of the eyebrows often indicates potential malignancies and often-invisible abnormalities appear at the organ representation area at alars of nose for pancreatic cancers or the right-lower lip near the right corner of the mouth where the colon is represented. To screen cancer all over the body during the past 10 years, we have been successfully able to detect early stages of cancers at various parts of the body using "Mouth, Hand, and Foot Writing Form." When the abnormalities appear in all the 6 writings, it immediately indicates the existence of one of the bone marrow related malignancies, including various kinds of leukemia, multiple myeloma, Hodgkin's lymphoma and non-Hodgkin's lymphoma. These screenings of any cancer at any part of the body can be performed in less than 5 minutes using a cancer-screening kit containing about 75 of the most common cancers' microscope tissues and an additional ~200 rare cancer screening slide box is also used.

Since 2015, using maximum electromagnetic field resonance phenomenon between two identical molecules, we succeeded in detecting various malignancies from rapidly changing QRS complex of ECGs as well as slowly changing, rising part of the T-wave of ECGs corresponding to "vulnerable period for ventricular fibrillation." Using ECGs of more than 50 cancer patients without knowing which cancer each patient has, we were able to correctly diagnose 47 patients. The diagnoses of the remaining three patients were different from the ECG diagnosis, but eventually those different diagnoses were found to be incorrect and ECG diagnosis was found to be correct. One college professor was told that a colonoscopy did not show any cancer, but the ECG showed colon cancer. Multiple coexisting cancers can also be detected. Maximum accurate information on cancer from ECGs was found when dV/dt is maximum area of QRS complex of ECGs; to get the maximum biochemical information, usually QRS complex must have 1.2 mV. Drugs taken within 8–10 hours can often be detected from ECGs.

There are three systems I have developed for detection of early stage or any stage of cancer.

1. Accurate organ representation area map of the face, including eyebrows, nose, lips, tongue, and also hands and feet. This was mapped using the BDORT over the past 15 years. See Figures 28.9 through 28.12.

   We have successfully been able to use these organ representation area maps for non-invasive early diagnosis of cancer, cardiovascular and other medical problems as well as quick, non-invasive evaluation of therapeutic effects of any type of treatments.

   When you use this method, even before the patient explains their problem, often you can tell what the patient has by visible changes appearing on the face. For example, if somebody has no hair on the eyebrows at specific locations of the eyebrow we can always tell immediately that there is a problem with the corresponding organ, because we also discovered that the eyebrows represent every organ. The medial part of the eyebrow near the nose represents the heart. The first change is that the hair becomes white; later as time passes the hair disappears. When you see someone with no hair at a specific location, then you know that the corresponding organ has a serious abnormality. Pancreas is located at right alar of nose (nostril) represents the head of the pancreas. If anyone has −7 or higher (−) BDORT, we immediately suspect cancer. There are visible changes and invisible changes. Invisible changes are detected by the O-Ring test. It takes less than 1 minute to test. In the case of lip changes, left upper lip near middle of lip if it is −12 indicates strong very abnormal cardiovascular condition. A small area on the lower right of the lip corresponds to the pancreas. A deep crease on the cheek in the area adjacent to the lower half of the nasolabial fold corresponds to an area of the stomach and if I see a few deep creases and if it tests strongly negative of BDORT (−)7~(−)12, immediately I suspect stomach cancer, not the normal crease but deep creases in an abnormal stomach representation area with

① Thymus gland
② Left lung
③ Right lung
④ Esophagus
⑤ S-A node
⑥ Right atrium
⑦ Right ventricle
⑧ Left atrium
⑨ Left ventricle

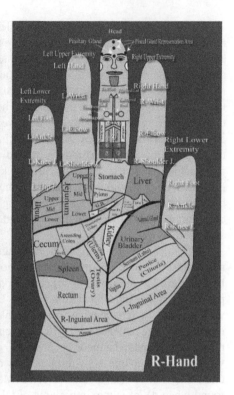

FIGURE 28.9 Accurate organ representation areas of the hands. (Copyright © 1999, 2001, 2002, and 2017 by Yoshiaki Omura, M.D., Sc.D. Information in parts or all of this chart in original form or modified form can not be reproduced without the author's written permission.)

strong (−) BDORT at right-upper lip next to middle of upper lip. These are typical of the cases of stomach cancer.

An optimal dose of vitamin D3 should be measured by BDORT. A range of vitamin D3 deficiency is between (−)1 and (−)12 BDORT. Even (−)12 BDORT changes to (+)12 when optimal dose of vitamin D3 is held in closed hand. If there is early stage of cancer, 800 IU makes (−) BDORT to (+)12 and optimal interval is about every 8 hours. If the condition is getting worse take four times a day. vitamin D3 is a panacea at optimal dose.

When specific part of eyebrow hair becomes white then you suspect something is wrong; when the hair disappears then it is much more advanced abnormality. If problem develops very recently, then there is not enough time for the hair to turn white or disappear. In that case, if upon testing some part of the organ representation chart area the BDORT suddenly opens, then that part has a problem. If one organ representation area shows a problem, then another organ representation area of the same organ also will show a problem.

When there is cancer, there is increase in human papilloma virus type 16 (HPV 16), they are usually highly infectious. Usually family members share the same HPV16 and have the same amount of viral infection. Only vitamin D3 at the optimal dose is what we found able to significantly reduce the viral infection and cancer risk. With commercially available vitamin D3, out of 10 bottles of 400 IU only 1 or 2 bottles are truly 400 IU and maybe 6 of them 800 IU and maybe 1 or 2 bottles have 1200 IU. So, check for optimal dose and you must take three or four times a day. From the patient's picture, you can tell if the patient has problems or not but cannot test the optimal dose of vitamin D3 except in person. In the picture, an abnormal deep crease in the stomach representation area, same

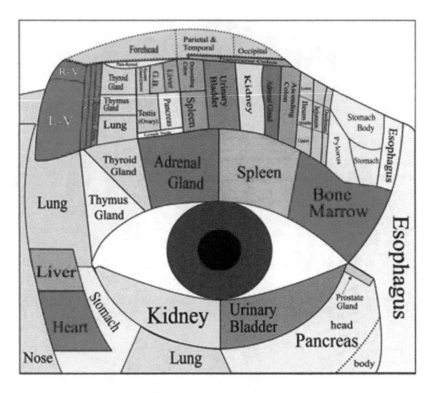

FIGURE 28.10 Accurate organ representation areas of left eyebrow, upper and lower eyelids. Some minor individual differences exist among different people. (Copyright © 2008 by Yoshiaki Omura, M.D., Sc.D. Information in parts or all of this chart in original form or modified form can not be reproduced without the author's written permission. Manufactured and distributed by ORT Life Science Research Institute, Inc., Kurume City, Japan.)

degree of abnormality can be found at right-upper lip just next to the mid-point of upper lip. To confirm, you should also check other areas corresponding to the same organ.

According to the first method based on organ representation areas, if anybody has a round projection on the chin, in the male it is testicular problem and in a female, it is an ovarian problem. It is divided into right and left sides, but even if one side is a problem, both sides usually protrude. When cancer is advanced, optimal dose of vitamin D3 is also increased. From the amount of optimal dose of vitamin D3 we can estimate abnormal degree of cancer.

When cancer is not visible, you need an O-Ring test. With an O-Ring test, we can quickly tell approximately if cancer is present (or not) and where it is located if cancer exists.

2. The second method is a one-page Mouth, Hand, and Foot Writing Form. See Figure 28.13. Using this method, we can make early diagnosis of any cancer in any part of the body and any stage of cancer without knowing any information of the patient. This is again due to resonance created by two identical molecules. We can find any molecule or bacteria, virus, fungi, or parasite inside the body without taking a biopsy or blood test provided the identical molecule or in the case of bacteria or virus, a monoclonal antibody or sample of the organism is available. Regarding cancer, as long as you have the unique identifiable molecule for the specific cancer or using specific cancer tissue slide, two identical tissues will always produce a strong EMF resonance and every O-Ring will open immediately.

Originally, about 15 years ago, I said to myself that the EKG contains information on the heart and EEG contains information on the brain, so what information do I have if I have the signature with the right hand or left hand of the patient? Do I have any medical

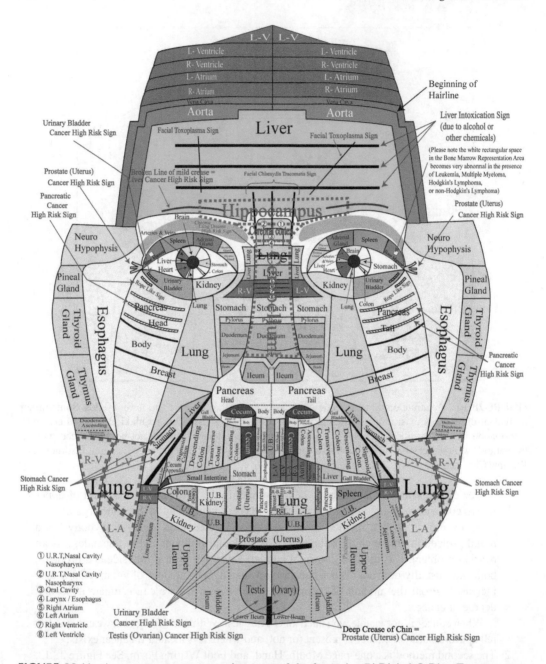

FIGURE 28.11 Accurate organ representation areas of the face using Bi-Digital O-Ring Test resonance phenomenon. (Copyright © 1999, 2001, 2002, and 2017 by Yoshiaki Omura, M.D., Sc.D. Information in parts or all of this chart in original form or modified form can not be reproduced without the author's written permission. Manufactured and distributed by ORT Life Science Research Institute, Inc., Fukuoka, Japan.)

information? Therefore, since I had been successful with cancer detection, now we know that we can detect any specific cancer and some other disease can also be detected. So, when I test with a right-handed signature, if they have cancer near the right chest, it can be detected very easily and any medical problems exist at the right part of the abdomen, we can pick up too. Then I said, "What will happen with the left hand?" And we found that left sided information can be picked up with the left hand. But we miss some of the medical

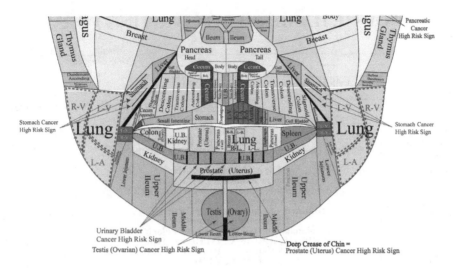

FIGURE 28.12   Organ representation areas of the upper & lower lips & surrounding areas. (Copyright ©
1999, 2001, 2002, and 2018 by Yoshiaki Omura, M.D., Sc.D. Information in parts or all of this chart in original form or modified form can not be reproduced without the author's written permission. Manufactured and
distributed by ORT Life Science Research Institute, Inc., Fukuoka, Japan.)

information at the lower part of the abdomen and the lower extremity. So, after doing many
experiments we ended up introducing foot writing. When I put a ball pen between the
right first and second toes, I write "RF" at space for Right Foot Writing. When I put a ball
pen deep in right side of the mouth and write "RM" then I get all the information above
the R-neck including right brain. After the right side, then do the left side of the mouth
by writing "LM." We started writing like this about 2005 and within the past 10 years we
improved everything.

In the form, write the chief complaint and symptoms. I don't need it for testing but it
helps with research to know the chief complaint and the symptoms, and also diagnosis if
available.

Hold the end of simplest ball pen in the mouth as far back as you can and write right
mouth writing with the pen on the right side of the mouth and repeat at the left side of the
mouth, without your hands touching any part of your body.

Then write RH with the right hand, LH with the left hand. For the foot writing, remove
shoes and socks, write RF and LF, and don't touch your body; you are not supposed to touch
any part of your body while you are doing this. Keep each writing in the one box on the form.

Currently, I have slides of viruses, fungi, bacteria, and neurotransmitters in addition to
cancer screening kits for diagnosis and research purposes. If there is cancer I can detect it
using cancer screening kit. Remember, if there is electromagnetic field resonance between
two identical molecules or between two identical cancer tissues, one inside of the body and
the other an identical cancer tissue microscope slide, we can now detect electromagnetic field
resonance. When you have resonance, strength of O-Ring made by thumb and other one finger
of the examiner's hand, suddenly O-Ring made by examinee became very weak and easily
opened.

Two warnings to bear in mind are:

a. The body is always producing cancer cells and the immune system is destroying them
   so do not get overwhelmed if you find multiple pre-cancers of very early stage which
   cannot be detected by standard lab test.

b. The EMF resonance method can pick up cancer frequencies long before they can be
   detected by standard radiological and laboratory tests.

MOUTH, HAND, & FOOT WRITING FORM

Name:_____ Age:_____ Sex:_____ Weight:_____ Height:_____
Address:_____ Date:_____ Time completed:_____ am pm
_____ Profession_____ Questions? Call 212-781-6262
Phone #:_____ Cellular Phone #:_____ Fax #:_____ E-mail:_____
Chief Complaint:_____

FAX TO DR. OMURA: 212-923-2279

Before Treatment: BP:_____ / _____ Pulse:_____ Resp. Rate:_____ Body Temp:_____

Left Mouth write L-M	: Telomere : : Sirtuin 1, longevity gene : : Integrin $\alpha_5\beta_1$ (or Oncogene C-fos Ab2): : 8-OH-dG : : Pb; Al; Hg; Cs ;Mg; Ca: : Chrysotile Asbestos; (Tremolite A.): : Acetylcholine; Dopamine; Serotonin; GABA : : β-Amyloid (1-42); Tau Protein: :Iodine;L- Homocysteine or CRP; TXB_2 : : Chlamydia T.; Borrelia B. : : Mycobacterium TB; Helicobacter Pylori; C.A. : : HPV-16, HPV-18, CMV; Herpes Type : : CA19-9 ;Substance P ;α-Fetoprotein : : DHEA ; Vit.D_3 :	**Right Mouth** write R-M
before treatment		before treatment
BDORT Grading: after treatment		BDORT Grading: after treatment
BDORT Grading:		BDORT Grading:
BDORT Grading:		BDORT Grading:
Left Hand write L-H	: Telomere : : Sirtuin 1, longevity gene : : Integrin $\alpha_5\beta_1$(or Oncogene C-fos Ab2) : : 8-OH-dG : : CEA; CA-125; DUPAN-2; CA15-3: : Pb; Al; Hg; Cs ; Mg: : Chrysotile Asbestos; (Tremolite A.): : Acetylcholine ; Ca: : Cardiac Troponin I; TXB_2; CRP : : Glucose ; Iodine : : Chlamydia T.; Borrelia B. : : Mycobacterium TB; Helicobacter Pylori; C.A. : : HPV-16, HPV-18, CMV; Herpes Type : : CA19-9; Substance P ;α-Fetoprotein : DHEA ; Vit.D_3 :	**Right Hand** write R-H
before treatment		before treatment
BDORT Grading: after treatment		BDORT Grading: after treatment
BDORT Grading:		BDORT Grading:
Left Foot write L-F	: Telomere : : Sirtuin 1, longevity gene : : Integrin $\alpha_5\beta_1$ (or Oncogene C-fos Ab2): : 8-OH-dG : : PSA;p CA-125; CEA ; CA15-3 : : Pb; Al; Hg; Cs ; Mg; Ca: : Chrysotile Asbestos; (Tremolite A.): : Acetylcholine ; TXB_2; Iodine : Chlamydia T.; Borrelia B. : : Mycobacterium TB; Candida Albicans; H.P. : : HPV-16, HPV-18, CMV; Herpes Type : CA19-9 ; Substance P ; α-Fetoprotein : DHEA ; Vit.D_3 :	**Right Foot** write R-F
before treatment		before treatment
BDORT Grading: after treatment		BDORT Grading: after treatment
BDORT Grading:		BDORT Grading:

After Treatment: BP:_____ / _____ , _____ / _____ Pulse:_____ , _____ Resp. Rate:_____ , _____ Body Temp:_____ , _____

FIGURE 28.13 Mouth, hand and foot writing form. (Copyright © 2012, 2013, and 2014 by Yoshiaki Omura, M.D., Sc.D.)

3. Recently, a third method of detecting cancer from the electrocardiogram was discovered by the author from the rapidly changing QRS complex and the slowly rising part of the T-wave, although this requires considerable knowledge of basic electrophysiology and the concept of advanced electromagnetic field theory and requires considerable training and practice. We can tell much more than what a regular cardiologist can detect via an EKG.

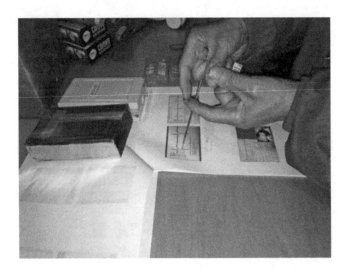

FIGURE 28.14 Cancer detection from EKGs. This author is holding colon cancer slide in the right hand and metal electrode (which is touching the cancer tissue slide) is touching rapidly changing QRS Complex to detect electromagnetic field resonance phenomenon.

4. Cancers can be rapidly suspected when part of the thymus gland representation area became (−)1 or (+)1, instead of Normal BDORT (−)2∼(−)10 for thymus gland. Under certain conditions when the magnitude of the QRS complex is over 1.2 mV, not only different cancers can be detected but cancer associated biochemical changes can also be identified. Therefore, it can also be used for evaluation of any cancer treatment to see if it is effective or harmful or not effective. Also, for example sometimes colonoscopic examination of the colon cannot find any visible cancer, but when cancer is growing under the mucus membrane, EKG can detect it and therefore when you do colonoscopy, EKG also should be performed at the same time. This method belongs to the future of medicine. See Figures 28.14 through 28.18. The head of the Anti-Cancer Committee of the European Parliament knows about my work. This was presented at the European Parliament Anti-Cancer Committee meeting on February 8, 2017 by the author.

Actually, all of the 4 methods described herein require considerable training and practice.

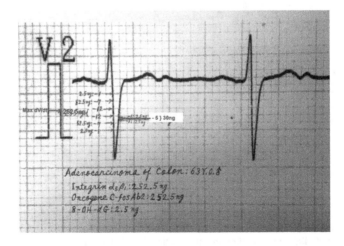

FIGURE 28.15 Detection of early stage of adenocarcinoma of the colon via EKG.

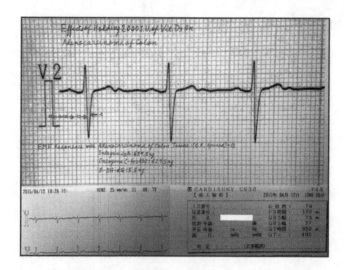

FIGURE 28.16 Effect of holding 2000 IUs of vitamin D3 on early stage of adenocarcinoma of the colon. Shift of BDORT from (−)8 to (−)12 due to overdose of vitamin D3 while optimal dose was about 400~600 IU.

Some Markers That I Use for Diagnosis and Evaluation of Therapeutic Effect Using BDORT

Telomere, Sirtuin I, Integrin $\alpha_5\beta_1$, 8-OH-dG (Eight Hydroxy Deoxy Guanosine), Lead, Aluminum, Mercury, Magnesium, Calcium, Chrysotile Asbestos, Acetylcholine, Dopamine, Serotonin, GABA, β-Amyloid (1–42), Iodine, L-Homocysteine, Chlamydia Trachomatis, Borrelia Burgdorferi, Mycobacterium Tuberculi, Helicobacter Pylori, HPV-16, HPV18, CMV, Herpes Simplex Type 1, Herpes Simplex Type 2, PSA, CEA, CA19–9, Substance P, Alpha-Fetoprotein, DHEA, vitamin D3. Toxoplasma Gondii, Thymosin α_1, Thymosin β_4, etc.

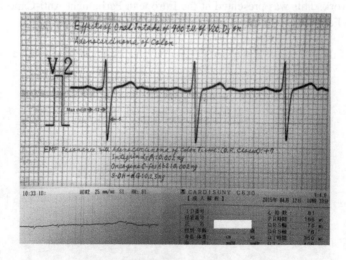

FIGURE 28.17 Effect of oral intake of 400~600 IUs of vitamin D3 on early stage of adenocarcinoma of the colon. BDORT (−)8 (indicating possibility of malignancy). Shift to (+)12 which indicates best effect (which corresponds to optimal dose). Please note Integrin $\alpha_5\beta_1$ and Oncogene C-fosAb2 = 627.5 ng (early stage of cancer) was inhibited to 0.002 ng (normal range) and 8-OH-dG = 5.5 ng (more than two times aggressive) was inhibited to 0.25 ng which is normal range.

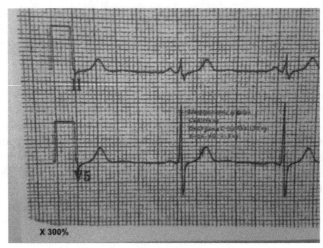

Although cancer was detected from ECG, colonoscopy
examination could not detect any colon cancer.

FIGURE 28.18 Adenocarcinoma of the colon was detected with BDORT from ECG of middle-aged male.

PART II: CLINICAL IMPLICATIONS OF HUMAN PAPILLOMA VIRUS-TYPE 16

Human Papilloma Virus Type 16 is often associated with the development of various cancers. Originally, it was thought to be associated with cervical, ovarian cancer, and breast cancer only, and thought to be sexually transmitted but we are finding out that it is much more than that. In families where one member has a strong HPV 16 infection, other family members seem to have the same degree of infection. Even cancer specialists are at risk as they come into frequent close contact with cancer patients carrying the virus on a daily basis. We found using BDORT that even if the patient does not develop a malignancy there is increased tendency to develop Alzheimer's and autism. Giving optimal doses of vitamin D3, Taurine, and pyrroloquinoline quinone (PQQ) was found to be extremely beneficial. They are even more beneficial when used in a compatible combination of all three.

OUR IMPROVED, INDIVIDUALIZED, SAFE, EFFECTIVE TREATMENT USING OPTIMAL DOSE OF VITAMIN D3 AND OTHER COMPATIBLE, SYNERGETIC, BENEFICIAL SUPPLEMENTS

Optimal dose of vitamin D3 was found to have safe and effective anti-cancer effect with additional significant excretion of bacteria, virus, and toxic substances through urine. Optimal dose of Taurine has similar but less effect. Overdose of these substances often resulted in cancer-promoting effects.

FACTORS PROMOTING AND INHIBITING THESE ANTI-CANCER EFFECTS

We found the optimal dose of vitamin D3, 400 IU for average adult has a safe and significant anti-cancer effect without side effects. However, widely used vitamin D3 doses of 2000–5000 or even higher doses have cancer-promoting effects. In the patient with liver and kidney problems, vitamin D3 could not be converted to the beneficial vitamin D3 receptor stimulant $1\alpha, 25(OH)_2D_3$. On the other hand, we found that one optimal dose of Taurine, 175 mg for average adults, three times/day for some patients also has a very significant, safe, effective, anti-cancer effect with equal or even better urinary excretion effect of bacteria, virus, and toxic substances. Taurine or optimal dose of DHEA often works even in cases where vitamin D3 does not work due to liver or kidney problems. We also found other safe, effective anti-cancer treatments by significantly increasing Telomere via the use of various methods. We found two most effective Telomere increasing substances: (1) Haritaki, which has been used in Ayurvedic and Tibetan medicine and (2) another substance with an equally strong Telomere increasing effect called Açaia which is originally found in the Amazon in Brazil. We also found Telomere increasing methods without using any medicine by 300 frictions between the palms of both hands. However, use of increasing Telomere without using any medicine will be highly desirable by repeating 300 frictions of the palms of both hands given three times/day for any cancer patient. We found in some patients a combination of these different beneficial substances can often cancel or reduce each other's effects. For example, the combination of Taurine and Açaia often reduces their anti-cancer effect, but the combination of Taurine and Haritaki often supplement each other, but without individually examining we cannot combine because some patients produce drug interactions and reduce effectiveness. Ginger by itself increases Telomere significantly, but will cancel the effect of Açaia and Taurine in some patients. Therefore, combining two desirable substances should be evaluated before giving them to the patient.

The unique 10 beneficial effects of optimal dose of vitamin D3 (also taurine or PQQ-pyrroloquinoline quinone has similar effects for some patients) found by this author are:

1. Marked anti-cancer effects without side effects, with marked decrease in Integrin $\alpha_5\beta_1$
2. Marked decrease in DNA mutation due to decrease in 8-OH-dG
3. Marked increase in urinary excretion of viruses, bacteria, fungi, and toxic substances such as asbestos and heavy metals
4. Marked increase in Acetylcholine in the brain, heart and the rest of the body
5. Marked increase in DHEA
6. Marked decrease in β-Amyloid (1–42)
7. Marked decrease in Cardiac Troponin I
8. Marked increase in Thymosin α_1 which has significant anti-cancer effect and anti-inflammatory effect
9. Marked increase in Thymosin β_4 which has significant improvement in circulatory system
10. Marked anti-allergy effects in some patients

TREATMENT CONSIDERATIONS

There are many treatments of cancer, but the most important thing is that treatment should not have any side effects. Current main accepted treatments consist of surgery, chemotherapy, and radiation treatment. When a tumor is discovered and the tumor is well localized, then surgery is performed, but during the surgery, using our sensitive Bi-Digital O-Ring Test examination often we find that a few cancer cells often spread to the surrounding areas and some of them get into the blood stream. However, standard laboratory tests cannot detect this until the cluster of cancer cells becomes at least a few millimeters in diameter. It can take several years, up to even 15 years, to become of detectable size and therefore there is no way you can detect early spread of cancer by standard laboratory testing. However, if the surgery involves complicated cancer which is more advanced and not well isolated, the chance of the cancer cells spreading to the surrounding area of the operation is much greater, but again to be able to detect any metastasis at least it takes a few months to a few years. But using BDORT, if there are enough cells metastasized, we can often detect them within a few weeks after surgery.

Chemotherapy is mainly aimed at killing cancer cells but in the process of attempting to kill cancer cells, because of its toxicity, often normal cells are also damaged and therefore there is always some side effect expected. Most significant side effect is on the brain and loss of recent memory and cardiovascular system.

Ideally to get optimal beneficial effect, the optimal dose which can provide maximum benefits with minimum side effects should be tested before giving chemotherapy, but unfortunately most of the chemotherapy is given without such evaluation. As a result, many patients die because of side effects and some of the side effects which are not seriously considered are side effects on the brain and memory as well as on the heart. Unfortunately, effects on the heart are not detected by standard EKG. Therefore, chemotherapy has a serious limitation unless an optimal dose is periodically determined rather than just giving the same amount each treatment. After each chemotherapy, some of our evaluation indicated that some of the patients immediately after treatment with cancer become even worse than before. We have a typical example of such a case: the patient was a physician working in one of the major hospitals in New York City and he attended our course for the first time. During the three-day weekend seminar and workshop for physicians we often screen for cancer using our first and second methods. This middle-aged male physician was a surgeon and anesthesiologist. By our early screening method, we detected early stage prostate cancer as well as pancreatic cancer, but cancer-related parameters were so low that standard laboratory testing did not confirm it. I advised him to periodically recheck by standard laboratory test. The following week he immediately tested for prostate cancer and pancreatic cancer, however standard tests could not detect any abnormality. He denounced our diagnostic method, but about six months later he again came back to our course. We asked, "Why did you come back?" and he said the annual hospital cancer screening test for the hospital staff found a positive test for prostate cancer because PSA was increased over 5 nanograms. Because of this, immediately after the meeting he went to one of the well-known major cancer hospitals in New York. He was admitted originally for a prostate cancer operation, but during the pre-op examination, they discovered that he had pancreatic cancer—a far more serious diagnosis than prostate cancer—and he was scheduled instead for chemotherapy for the pancreatic cancer. He wanted us to evaluate him before chemotherapy. First, we suggested that before chemotherapy he should ask for reevaluation of the laboratory test after the initial round of chemotherapy treatment, but the hospital refused. Only after completion of the entire series of chemotherapy, would they perform a reevaluation. Therefore, he asked us to evaluate before treatment and after treatment and so he made arrangements; his first chemotherapy treatment was scheduled during our 3-day weekend conference. To our surprise after the treatment, his cancer had become much worse than it was before his first chemotherapy treatment. His condition worsened over the subsequent two days and therefore we suggested that if he continued he would be dead pretty soon. This time, his wife came to our meeting and she saw what happened, but the doctor who received this chemotherapy insisted that Dr. Omura never mentioned that chemotherapy is making him sick and if he continues he will be dead. Originally, we could not understand why he was saying such a thing but eventually after seeing many cases like his case, we found out that after cancer treatment, the brain is influenced. Brain acetylcholine is markedly reduced and as a result the brain and memory are no longer functioning normally, but he refused to stop treatment despite our advice and his wife's insistence, and as predicted, he died in less than 6 months.

So now regarding the other approach of radiation therapy. Radiation therapy is often given together with chemotherapy before or after surgery, but the problem is that radiation therapy can also create side effects; x-rays often expose the normal tissue and sometimes can create damage and necrosis in normal tissue. A previously non-existent new problem can be created by unexpected exposure of strong x-rays to normal tissue which can damage the normal tissue and sometimes this side effect can become a more serious problem. Of course, radiation therapy will eventually improve by developing methods that will not expose normal tissue and that is being done right now.

We are not advocating replacing chemotherapy and radiation therapy with our method. Rather, we are advocating the integration of our technique to provide an improved outcome for the patient, but ideally only individually determined safe, effective treatment should be given by routinely evaluating optimal dose if they exist. If they cannot examine optimal dose at least they should examine changes in cancer marker and if it has no beneficial effects, harmful treatment should not be repeated.

Our Individualized Safe, Effective, and Affordable Cancer Treatment

We compared many cancers treatments before and after treatment performed by standard available techniques. The optimal dose of vitamin D3 is most safe, effective, and the most economical method and essential for every type of cancer as a fundamental treatment. We found using BDORT that most people have insufficient vitamin D3, and for a normal person vitamin D3 is obtained by two sources. One is from food including mushrooms and another source is exposure of the skin to ultraviolet frequency of sunlight, which opens up one of the rings of cholesterol and it becomes a precursor of vitamin D3. The required daily sun exposure time without exposing the whole body, just with regular clothes, is 15 minutes to 1 hour and often provides the sufficient daily requirement, but some people who are not exposed to the sun at all develop vitamin D3 deficiency. The most common deficiency can be solved by an optimal dose of vitamin D3 for each individual and the average adult optimal dose is average 400 IUs three times a day. If someone has an early stage of cancer, often the requirement increases to 800 IUs three times a day (average optimal dose) and if the patient has aggressive cancer or metastasis they require an average optimal dose of anywhere between 1200 and 3000 IUs three times a day; ideally, the optimal dose must be examined individually because if they take an overdose of more than two times of optimal dose and if the patient has cancer, it will promote the cancer.

There is a general tendency to believe that if you will take more doses of vitamin D3 it will be better but we found that in the presence of cancer, individualized optimal dose is the best treatment for any cancer and overdose often promotes the growth of cancer. Unfortunately, a problem is that in the United States and Canada many people believe you have to take a vitamin D3 minimum of 2000 IUs up to 5000 IUs. Some people believe that a high amount above 5000 IUs up to 10,000 IUs is beneficial. Our study showed that if a cancer patient takes over two times of optimal dose of vitamin D3, the cancer activity increases significantly. Even with 2000 IUs in most early stage of cancer patients, the cancer activity increases at least two times or higher and 5000 IUs or a higher dose is the most dangerous thing to take for a cancer patient because the cancer grows so rapidly that it is equivalent to committing suicide; one of the reasons why doctors and patients in the United States and Canada are using a minimum 2000 IUs of vitamin D3 is due to the finding that many people have a vitamin D3 deficiency which is completely factual, but the recommended minimum 2000 IUs is, according to my method, an overdose for early stage cancer. The cancer activity increases at least two times but because so many people are using this recommended 2000 IU, many companies make 2000 IU D3 in the form of tablets or capsules. When you go to the health store you can often find more products with higher doses such as 2000 IU or 5000 IU and it is more difficult to find 400 IU or 800 IU or commercially even 1000 IU. So, recently it has become more difficult to get the lower dose which is the most safe and effective dose. We also found a problem between the selection of tablet and capsule form containing liquid vitamin D3. We often found that the liquid form of vitamin D3 seems to change its effectiveness when it is exposed to high temperature more easily, but the tablet form is easier to cut for optimal dose and also is more stable than the liquid form. The other major problem with vitamin D3 is that few companies make vitamin D3 with 400 IUs but when we examine them, we found that even though the bottle says 400 IUs, the content is not always 400 IU. Some bottles contain 800 IU, some bottles contain 1200 IU, or even 2400 IU, as a result before using vitamin D3 you have to make sure that the amount you are getting is the real optimal dose as identified by doctors who are trained in BDORT. For those who supplement their diet with vitamin D3 by taking mushrooms, we noticed during the past few years that some mushrooms have very little vitamin D3 and we found the reason. Most of the mushrooms such as shitake were excellent sources of vitamin D3 but recently many shitakes are rapidly produced without sunlight exposed drying. Recently some companies produce shitake without sunlight exposure drying by using heat. These mushrooms have very little vitamin D3; therefore they are practically useless for that purpose.

FACTORS INFLUENCING CANCER TREATMENT

There are many factors contributing towards the growth of cancer. The following factors must be considered in order to treat cancer safely and effectively (Figure 28.19).

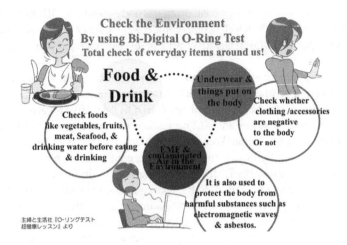

FIGURE 28.19 Cancer and environmental factors.

1. What you eat and what you drink—among the factors of eating and drinking—vitamin C beyond 180 mg inhibits 10 unique beneficial effects of vitamin D3; therefore when you are using optimal dose of vitamin D3, a large amount of vitamin C should not be taken. One cup of orange juice will be enough to inhibit vitamin D3 effect. 500 mg vitamin C will cancel most of optimal dose of vitamin D3 and reduce and Thymosin α_1, which has strong, anti-cancer effects, to less than 1/10 of normal value, while increasing Thymosin β_4 which improves circulation.

2. Often garlic and onions inhibit vitamin D3 effect. Also, some of the coffees as well as decaffeinated coffee can also inhibit vitamin D3 effect. Good quality green tea also contains a high amount of vitamin C, which can also inhibit vitamin D3 but cheap green teas often have less vitamin C; as a result they have less inhibiting effect on vitamin D3.

3. We found fish skin and animal skin promotes the growth of cancer; in particular, shiny white fish skin has more cancer promoting effects than bluish skin. When you eat fish, you should remove all the skin. On the other hand, fish such as salmon, tuna fish, and eels are excellent for inhibiting cancer activity provided they don't contain mercury or PCBs, and so on, and that can be easily detected by BDORT.

4. Almonds often contain asbestos, even organic almonds. Although generally most nutritionists think that almonds are one of the best nutritious foods and recommend them, unfortunately, most almonds contain chrysotile asbestos, which has a most undesirable BDORT of (−)12, and can promote cancer; chocolate containing almonds has the same problem. Cashews and dates are fine, and turmeric is good.

5. Lima beans, fava beans contain a kidney-shaped indented area (the hilum) which contains a highly toxic substance that tests (−)12 on BDORT, just this small area alone.

6. Most corn products are BDORT (−)12 and toxic. Most white rice available since 2016 is BDORT of toxic (−)12 but most of brown rice has BDORT (−)1∼(+)12 is much safe to eat. Any burned foods are (−)12, toxic, and carcinogenic.

7. Most of the vegetables—cauliflower, broccoli—head, the fuzzy part is all covered with chemicals. Even after washing with hot water, they still test toxic.

8. Sports drinks may contain a large amount of taurine. The optimal dose for taurine is 175 mg but one sports drink had 1000 mg of taurine. Also, some of them contain 1000 mg of vitamin C. We found one patient who developed some brain problems by drinking over-the-counter multivitamins every day. In a few months he developed neuromuscular and memory problems; they damaged the brain.

9. What you wear, everything ideally contacting the body should be BDORT positive but if a patient with cancer wears BDORT negative underwear, cancer will grow much quicker.

10. A lot of toilet paper is BDORT negative; also many women's tampons and sanitary pads are BDORT negative.

11. Many black colored underwear are often strongly BDORT negative and also if someone has colon cancer and prostate cancer, black things are often strongly negative for them.

12. For women who have breast cancer, their bra is BDORT negative regardless of color; more than 90% of bras sold in stores are −12 on testing, so cancer grows much faster. It is the equivalent of committing suicide. Wearing a necklace and earrings, metal zippers, and any metal in clothes, especially bras with underwire, are undesirable because metal functions like a special antenna attracting EMFs, interfering with brain function.

13. Many of the socks are negative on BDORT testing also some trousers, although not touching the body. However, even if a small part touches, it is negative.

14. Blue jeans, bra, and black underwear tests the worst on BDORT testing. Steve Jobs used to wear black shirt and blue jeans always; if he did not do that he would possibly have lived much longer.

15. Also, many shirts come with labels, and many labels are −12 on BDORT. Even if a small piece of the label touches the body, it is harmful. Many are −12; you need to cut them off before wearing.

16. Many people wear decorative metal, very harmful, navel rings, nose rings, tongue rings; all promote growth of cancer. Many tattoos have metal in the ink; also some women use nail polish acrylic and gels. Most lipstick especially red color is −12 on BDORT and lips represent all the organs, upper and lower lip.

17. Black eyeliner is the worst; it is a strong negative with BDORT.

18. Metallic surgical implants can also act as antennas for EMFs. Also, as mentioned earlier, any metal in clothes is undesirable as it functions as an antenna for strong EMFs.

19. One of the major sources of EMFs is a cellular phone; the higher the frequency, the more harmful it is, and using cell phone near the head is harmful. If a cancer patient holds a cell phone, cancer marker by BDORT increases, and that means it is promoting cancer. We can reduce the high frequency EMFs by using an EMF neutralizer, but we have to check and periodically change it as it does not last even one month. We have to change every 2–3 weeks. There are many products of EMF neutralization but many of them are not effective or last a short time; if you continuously use a cell phone without a protector, even if you stop talking after 1 minute, the cancer promoting effect lasts 10 minutes. If you have a neutralizer, as soon as you stop using it, no additional effects will develop. If you don't have a neutralizer, the side effect is while talking and 10 minutes after.

20. Water is very important; if you use water immediately upon opening the faucet, it is a strong (−)12, if you flush the water for 30 seconds or 1 minute, it becomes (+)7. Many bottled water tests strongly negative, but a few are strongly positive (+) of (+)7~(+)10.

21. If there is a visible antenna in your surroundings, you will get strong and dangerous effects and in that case, you have to put a ground wire or metal mesh and ground it. If you can see it from your window, cover the whole window with a wire mesh that is grounded.

22. Smart meter is one of the most dangerous things that influences the inside of the whole building and this can be reduced by putting a neutralizer near that instrument. Also, when there is no way to mitigate, do not sleep near the wall power source as they have a strong field; also routers are strongly negative.

23. Additionally, we found in cancer patients that by putting the neutralizer on the thymus gland, it reduced the cancer activity. Similarly, on the bone marrow representation area on the face neutralizer was helpful.

24. Cancer can develop in less than few months when the body is exposed to multiple cancer contributing factors. Important factors include frequent exposure to electromagnetic fields

such as high frequency electromagnetic field from cellular phones, eating (−)12 foods and drinking (−)12 waters and soft drinks, smoking, wearing (−)12 underwear and metal ring decorations which attract electromagnetic field and existence of strong viral infection of Human Papilloma Virus Type 16 (HPV-16) and so on. Most of egg yolk are infected by HPV-16 and rapidly developed cancer is often infectious.

BIBLIOGRAPHY

Omura, Y. "Role of Human Papillomavirus type-16 infection for various cancers as well as Alzheimer's disease and Autism, and safe, effective treatment of cancer by the combined use of optimal doses of Vitamin D3, Taurine, & PQQ when they are positively synergetic with additional advantage of significant urinary excretion of HPV-16 Virus and other bacterial and fungal infections." *2nd International Cancer Study & Therapy Conference, Published in Madridge Journal of Cancer Study & Research.* Vol. 2, No. 1, pp. 13, 2017.

Omura, Y. "Newly Discovered Organ Representation Areas of Various Organs of the Body on Thymus Gland Representation Area & Its Clinical Application for Non-Invasive, Early Diagnosis & Safe, Effective Treatment of Cancer & Other Serious Medical Problems." *Acupuncture & Electro-Therapeutics Research, The International Journal of Integrated Medicine.* Vol. 42, No. 2, pp. 65–96, 2017.

Omura, Y., Lu, D., Jones, M. K., Nihrane, A., Duvvi, H., Yapor, D., Shimotsuura, Y., Ohki, M. "Optimal Dose of Vitamin $D_3$400 I.U. for Average Adults has A Significant Anti-Cancer Effect, While Widely Used 2000 I.U. or Higher Promotes Cancer: Marked Reduction of Taurine & 1α, $25(OH)_2D_3$ Was Found In Various Cancer Tissues and Oral Intake of Optimal Dose of Taurine 175mg for Average Adults, Rather Than 500 mg, Was Found to Be A New Potentially Safe and More Effective Method of Cancer Treatment." *Acupuncture & Electro- Therapeutics Research, The International Journal of Integrated Medicine.* Vol. 41, No. 1, pp. 39–60, 2016. doi: 10.3727/036012916×14597946741564

Omura, Y. "Clinical implications of the HPV-16 infection & 7 beneficial effects of optimal dose of Vitamin D3 in safe, effective cancer treatment: Non-invasive rapid cancer screening using 'Mouth, Hand & Foot Writing Form' of 40 participants during 150-minute workshop on the Bi-Digital O-Ring Test, in the 1st day of European Congress for Integrative Medicine, September 9-11, 2016 in Budapest." *Acupuncture & Electro-Therapeutics Research, The International Journal of Integrated Medicine.* Vol. 41, No. 3–4, pp. 171–198, 2016.

Ducreux, M., Cuhna, A. Sa., Caramella, C., Hollebecque, A., Burtin, P., Goéré, D., Seufferlein, T. et al. "Cancer of the Pancreas: ESMO Clinical Practice Guidelines for Diagnosis, Treatment and Follow-Up." *Annals of Oncology.* Vol. 26, No. Supplement 5, pp. v56–v68, 2015.

Wu, L., Qu, X. "Cancer Biomarker Detection: Recent Achievements and Challenges." *Chemical Society Reviews.* Vol. 44, No. 10, pp. 2963–2997, 2015.

Omura, Y., Jones, M. K., Duvvi, H., Ohki, M., Rodriques, A. "Non-Invasive Quick Diagnosis of Cardiovascular Problems from Visible and Invisible Abnormal Changes with Increased Cardiac Troponin I Appearing On Cardiovascular Representation Areas of the Eyebrows, Left Upper Lip, etc. of the Face & Hands: Beneficial Manual Stimulation of Hands for Acute Anginal Chest Pain, and Important Factors in Safe, Effective Treatment". *Acupuncture & Electro-Therapeutics Research, The International Journal of Integrated Medicine.* Vol. 39, No. 2, pp. 135–167, 2014. doi: 10.3727/036012914×14054537750463

Hegyi, G., Szasz, O., Szasz, A. "Oncothermia: A New Paradigm and Promising Method in Cancer Therapies". *Acupuncture & Electro-Therapeutics Research, The International Journal of Integrated Medicine.* Vol. 38, No. 3–4, pp. 161–197, 2013.

Omura, Y. "Asbestos: Profound Evidence for Disease Associations (Including Cancer, Alzheimer's Disease, Autism, Failing Heart & Varicose Veins) and Novel Methods of Detection and Treatment." Chapter 41 In: *Advancing Medicine with Food and Nutrients,* Second Edition; I.Kohlstadt, MD, MPH, of Johns Hopkins University, CRC Press, pp. 777–798, 2012.

Omura, Y., Shimotsuura, Y., Fukuoka, A., Fukuoka, H., Nomoto, T. "Significant Mercury Deposits in Internal Organs Following the Removal of Dental Amalgam, & Development of Pre-Cancer on the Gingiva and the Sides of the Tongue and Their Represented Organs as a Result of Inadvertent Exposure to Strong Curing Light (Used to Solidify Synthetic Dental Filling Material) & Effective Treatment: A Clinical Case Report, along with Organ Representation Areas for Each Tooth." *Acupuncture & Electro-Therapeutics Research, The International Journal of Integrated Medicine.* Vol. 21, No. 2, pp. 133–160, 1996. doi: 10.3727/036012996816356915

MARUYAMA VACCINE INFORMATION

(This is not a complete reference but a start; the reader is recommended to do his or her own research.)

Alternative Oncology

An immune stimulant derived from the supernatant from a culture of tuberculosis (Aoyama B strain ofMycobacterium tuberculosis) is administered as one of two different vaccines, Z100 and the concentrated form, SSM. It may ameliorate the adverse effects of radiotherapy in cancer patients; some-believe it reduces the incidence of breast, lung and colon cancer.

An estimated 50,000 Japanese receive the vaccine each year; it is not approved by the Japanese Ministry of Health, but the cost is covered by insurance companies given with conventional chemotherapy in cancer patients. Source: Maruyama vaccine. (n.d.) Segen's Medical Dictionary. (2011). Retrieved August 25 2017 from http://medical-dictionary.thefreedictionary.com/Maruyama+vaccine

Chapman, W. Japanese Vaccine to Treat Cancer Stirs Controversy. The Washington Post, 1981. Retrieved from   https://www.washingtonpost.com/archive/politics/1981/07/24/japanese-vaccine-to-treat-cancer-stirs-controversy/551d398e-7632-4c8e-bc56-abedf71f045a/?utm_term=.f737da8dab0b

Kimoto, T. "Collagen and Stromal Proliferation as Preventive Mechanisms against Cancer Invasion by Purified Polysaccharides from Human Tubercle 8acillus (SSM)." *Cancer Detection and Prevention.* Vol. 5, pp. 301–314, 1982.

Kimoto, T. "Pathological Observations during Treatment with the Biological Response Modifier Maruyama Vaccine in Cancer: Implications for Collagen Production in the Prevention of Cancer Invasion and Metastasis." *Cancer Detection and Prevention.* Vol. 22, No. 4, pp. 340–349, 1998. doi: 10.1046/j.1525-1500.1998.cdoa33.x

Niwa, Y., Yamamoto, S., Maeda, M. "Effect of SSM (Maruyama Vaccine) on the Terminal Cancer Patients in Connection with Its Increasing Mechanism of AO Generation by Neutrophils." *Ensho.* Vol. 5, pp. 131–137, 1985. 10.2492/jsir1981.5.131

According to the Website "Forum for Maruyama Vaccine & Cancer," MARUYAMA (SSM, commonly called Maruyama Vaccine) has been playing a pioneering role in cancer immunotherapy. SSM awakens the immune system in humans and encourages production of cytokines such as interferon through activation of lymphocytes and other elements. SSM also increases collagen. By continuing to inject SSM, collagen fibers build up around cancer cells, encircling them and causing cancer cells to become dormant. Sometimes cancer is shrunk or reduced, which indirectly blocks cancer growth and causes it to self-destruct. With a history of over 45 years of use in medical practice, SSM's five characteristic effects have been confirmed through clinical studies and research. (1) No adverse side effects. (2) Superior survival prolongation. (3) Subjective symptoms relief. (4) Cancer shrinkage/disappearance. (5) Suppression of cancer growth/metastasis.

29 Low Doses Big Effects
Application to Pediatrics

Michel Bouko Levy

CONTENTS

Part 1: Think Homeopathy 714
Foreword 714
Natural Resonance 714
The Principles of Homeopathy 715
Homeopathic Remedies 716
Constitutions and Reactive Modes... 717
The Four Constitutions 718
    The Carbonic.. 718
    The Phosphoric.. 718
    The Natrum 718
    The Fluoric 718
The Four Reactive Modes 720
Skin Language 721
Homeopathic Drainage 722
The Wheel of Emunctories 723
The Line of Life 725
How to Prescribe 727
Part 2: Growth Disorders and Homeopathy 728
Part 3: E.N.T. and Homeopathy 728
Rhino Pharyngitis... 728
    Rhino Pharyngitis Discharge... 728
    Rhino Pharyngitis Cough 730
    Rhino Pharyngitis Drainage 730
    Rhino Pharyngitis Prevention.. 731
Otitis.. 731
    Five Main Remedies... 732
    Mastoiditis Threatened 732
    Eustachian Tube Drainage... 732
    Otitis Drainage to Accompany the Adenoids Drainage 732
Sinusitis... 732
    Suppuration Stage 732
    Sinusitis Discharge Remedies 732
    Ethmoidal and Frontal Sinusitis 733
    Maxillary Sinusitis 733
    Osteitis Remedies... 733
    Sinusitis Drainage 733
Nodes Drainage.. 733
Allergic Reactions.. 734

Part 4: Side Effects of Vaccination...735
   DTaP..735
   MMR...735
Detoxifying with Homeopathic Treatment 736
Part 5: Hyperactivity, Attention Deficit Disorders and Homeopathy.......................................738
Restless Child..738
   Anxiety..738
   Quarrelsome..738
   Screaming..738
Violent Child...739
   Cannot Bear to Be Approached, Touched, or Even Looked at...739
   Destructive..739
   Impatient 739
   Insolent...739
   Rejects Violently Things When Given 739
   Tears Clothes..739
   Rudeness 739
Whining..740
   Coward 740
Sleep Disorders 740
   Difficulty Falling Asleep after an Animated Conversation 740
   Night Anxiety...740
   Night Terrors 741
   Sorrows...741
   Nervous Drainage...741
Conclusion 741
Bibliography...742

PART 1: THINK HOMEOPATHY

FOREWORD

Once a doctor has learned how to best use his tools, he becomes able to work. He acknowledges the external world and knows how to function within this frame. Instructed by experience, he pursues his work with constantly renewed means. He practices with method and discipline, which ensures effectiveness. He respects the harmony of nature, which is essential to maintain it. Intrepid and determined, he protects the society that he has come to know and tries to meet its needs.

Healing is to both know and anticipate.

A doctor's conscience is animated by an invincible confidence in the future of humans and humanity, with freedom of thought, righteousness of judgment, honesty and integrity in all acts of life. He put his intelligence at the service of humanity, investigates natural laws and scientific rules. He keeps searching. His gift to himself is to defy ignorance rather than to renounce the search for truth. Condemned to the eternal torment of vacuum and incomprehension—heaps of questions occupy his mind. Find serenity in the love for goodness and in closeness with like-minded doctors.

Find peace of mind in obstinate work.

NATURAL RESONANCE

Nobel Prizes in Physics were awarded to Isidor Rabi in 1944 and to Felix Bloch and Edward Mills Purcell in 1952 for their studies on nuclear magnetic resonance. Nuclear magnetic resonance is a physical phenomenon in which nuclei in a magnetic field absorb and re-emit electromagnetic radiation. This energy is at a specific resonance frequency which depends on the strength of the magnetic field and the magnetic properties of the isotope of the atoms.

The Earth's magnetic field strength was measured by Carl Friedrich Gauss in 1835. It surrounds and protects the Earth. Magnetic field comes from the inside of the Earth to the level where it meets the solar wind. The sun stream is charged with particles which would strip away the ozone layer and expose the Earth to ultraviolet radiation. Above it is another magnetic field, the interplanetary. We live within these structures.

Homeopaths use substances diluted and dynamized. The rate of substance becomes quickly equivalent to physiological components of the body. The more diluted the substance, the smaller the phenomenon is to be considered in magnetic resonance: the cell, the molecule, the nucleus, the electrons, and the nano-chemical components for reaction.

The solvent used to prepare homeopathic remedies is based on H_2O, two molecules extremely reactive to nuclear magnetic resonance. Many molecules contain the ability to absorb specific radio frequency energy. The different atomic nuclei of a molecule resonate at different radio frequencies for the same magnetic fields. Homeopaths work on chemical and structural information of the molecule.

In 2015, a new study on "Transduction of DNA information through water and electromagnetic waves," conducted by a cooperative team of physicists and biologists led by Nobel Prize winner Luc Montagnier, demonstrated that:

1. Water is rewritable. It is an active medium for electromagnetic frequencies.
2. The information held in water remains fully intact after extreme dilutions and successions to decimal levels.
3. These frequencies will keep their effect when transferred and imprinted on pure water.

"This 10 years long collaborative work has yielded some scientific facts and concepts in a new domain of Science at the frontier of Biology and quantum field Physics."

Luc Montagnier

THE PRINCIPLES OF HOMEOPATHY

Twenty-four centuries ago, Hippocrates, the Father of Medicine, said:

- "Similia Similibus Curentur." The Law of Similar. This means "like cures like." The foundation of this reasoning requires the identification of an ANALOGY.
- Man must be considered within his surrounding world. He is an element of the cosmos and the duty of a physician is to help the patient in his adaptation to the surrounding world.
- Each human being has his own energy, which reflects his personality.
- Nature can bring out the spontaneous recovery from the disease through pathological alternations.

Hippocrates "Nature is the doctor of diseases."
The medical science of low doses was practiced from the beginning of the history of humanity. At the end of the eighteenth century, Doctor Samuel Hahnemann understood the importance of the Law of Similar studied by Hippocrates. His genius was to build an experimental system based on this natural resonance.

Samuel Hahnemann "I believe more in the experience than in my intelligence."
Healing is an art to which nature provides its essential principles. Our ancestors have systematically tested plants and insects from their environment and assessed their benefits and/or bad effects.

Principle	Remedy
The law of similar	**Dilution—potentization**
A substance which can cause a disease in a healthy subject can, when diluted in infinitesimal dilution, cure a similar disease.	The therapeutic effect of homeopathic remedies is linked to the dilution of the substances and to their potentization (dynamization) after each dilution.

Scientific method

Experimentation on the healthy subject—pathogenesis	Clinical study—observation, individualization
• With substances at allopathic and homeopathic dose • Brings out the sensitive subjects	• Describe the reactive forms: Constitution and reactive mode • Enriches the experimentation

Book of knowledge

Materia Medica

• Always updated by scientific method
• In harmony with the unity of the patient as a whole and the surrounding world

FIGURE 29.1   The principles of homeopathy.

Later, humans used substances from mineral and animal origin as well. It is the dosage which makes the poison or the medicine.

Samuel Hahnemann "Let's imitate nature."
The remedies are referenced in two manners: in a Materia Medica of the medicinal substances with a description of their toxic and therapeutic effects, such as Boericke Materia Medica, and a repertory of the symptoms, such as Kent Repertory. The remedies found in the repertory are checked in the Materia Medica and reverse (Figure 29.1).

HOMEOPATHIC REMEDIES

The three kingdoms of nature, mineral, vegetal, and animal, provide the substances used to manufacture homeopathic remedies. Between the more or less 4000 substances tested, plants play a critical role. Today we also use buds and young shoots which concentrate the whole energy of the plant. The animal kingdom has served humans since the beginning, either through the complete animal (FORMICA RUFA: crushed live ants), or with its secretion (LACHESIS: snake poison). Metals have a prominent role in the constitution of many essential molecules (i.e., iron in hemoglobin). They activate the enzymatic system when used in minute quantities as trace elements. Organotherapy uses healthy organs (OVARY) and their secretions (FOLLICULINUM) to stimulate or regulate biological disorders.

We are fortunate to have at our disposal remedies prepared by laboratories in accordance with pharmaceutical standards. The operations are strictly codified. Substances are diluted and dynamized (potentized). The Hahnemann Dilution System is the most common.

1. Hahnemann Dilution System:
   a. Decimal dilutions: 1 mL of Mother Tincture (MT) is added to 9 mL of solvent (alcohol and water). This solution is shaken to make the first decimal potency, 1DH or 1XH, where D or X stands for Decimal and H for Hahnemann.

      The 2DH contains 1 mL of the 1DH transferred into a new container. 9 mL of solvent is added, and the solution is succussed to obtain the second potency.

      This procedure is repeated 6 times to obtain the 6th potency, 6 DH, and 12 times for 12DH.
   b. Centesimal dilutions: 1 mL is added to 99 mL of solvent to make the first potency, or 1CH. The process applied to obtain these potencies is the same as used in the decimal system. Only the product ratio differs.

      This procedure is repeated 30 times to obtain the 30th potency, 30CH.
2. Korsakoff Dilution System: General Count Simon Nicolaievitch Von Korsakoff, 1788–1853, a Russian government official, was the first homeopath in Russia. He was responsible for preparing the homeopathic remedies for Tsar Nicholas I when he was travelling. He was a disciple, a correspondent, and a friend of Hahnemann, who esteemed him highly and, to a certain extent, approved his ideas. For practical reasons, Korsakoff developed a new method for diluting remedies. He simply emptied the vial in use and added 99 parts of water/alcohol to produce the next dilution. Observation had convinced him that at least the equivalent of one drop of the solution remained in the vial when emptied. This method was less expensive and less time-consuming, and worked well, particularly in the 200th dilution, and in the higher potencies. The potencies of remedies obtained through the Korsakoff method are differentiated from the potencies obtained with the Hahnemann system by the letter K.

Korsakoff studied, tried, examined, experimented, and made some successful discoveries. Involved with an early version of information technology, Korsakoff invented a dynamizer, one of the very first computers with punched card machines for information processing. He also wrote a book on artificial intelligence.

The remedies are most commonly delivered as granules, round pellets impregnated by the diluted remedy, and in liquid form. Other forms include tablets and powder, creams and syrups, and more recently sprays.

CONSTITUTIONS AND REACTIVE MODES

- The four constitutions describe the patient's framework; they determine the predisposition and sensitivity to develop specific pathologies.
- The four reactive modes direct the evolution of the chronic diseases; they show the development of the body and its functions.

The human edifice is a mosaic made of the four constitutions and four reactive modes. However, each person is characterized by 1 or 2 constitutions and reactive modes which evolve naturally throughout life. Some patients present one constitution that can be closely related to one reactive mode: Carbonic to Psora, Phosphoric to Tuberculinism, and Fluoric to Luesa.

The immune system has a hereditary program which must be studied during the first years of the infant and child through his diseases, their location, evolution, recurrence, periodicity, concomitant pathologies, and morbid alternations, and with the experience of his reactions to the therapeutics and the side effects appearing from the boosters. Examine and note the family background, mother and father, sisters and brothers, aunts and uncles; all help to analyze the pathology logic and to determinate the weight of the dominating constitution and reactive mode.

THE FOUR CONSTITUTIONS

THE CARBONIC

The Carbonic develops broadly. His skeleton is thick and resistant, his hands and teeth are strong and square, his joints are stiff. He is punctual, obstinate, likes discipline, and respects the law. He has a tendency to congestion, obesity, and sclerosis. See Figure 29.2.

THE PHOSPHORIC

The Phosphoric grows thin. His skeleton is long, fragile, and flexible. His teeth make the dentist's day. He is creative, artistic, and suffers from being oversensitive, with wide mood swings. He presents a tendency to decalcification, lymphatic system slowing down, chronic suppurations, and organ degeneration. See Figure 29.3.

THE NATRUM

The Natrum grows in a vague diamond shape. All of his tissues are bloated by water retention. His walk is slow and disturbed by an ineffective anxious restlessness and all kinds of tics. He is suspicious, introverted, secretive, and obsessional. His tendency is to develop chronic infections, and in particular warts and tumors of the genital system. See Figure 29.4.

THE FLUORIC

The Fluoric has a twisted growth. His skeleton presents with varied malformations and asymmetries with marked flexibility and hyperlaxity of the joints. He walks as though he is on a tight-rope.

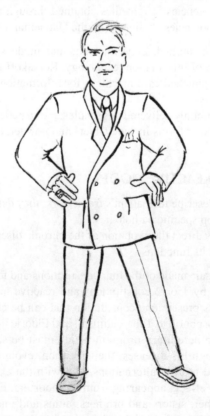

FIGURE 29.2 The Carbonic.

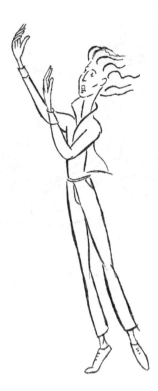

FIGURE 29.3 The Phosphoric.

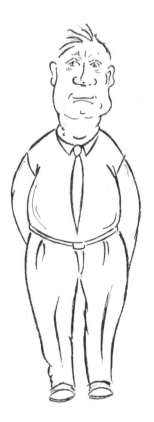

FIGURE 29.4 The Natrum.

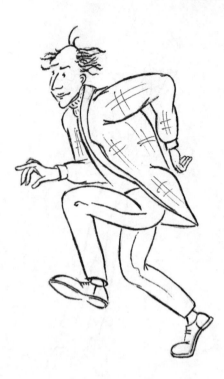

FIGURE 29.5   The Fluoric.

Intuitive or insensible, fast or slow, genius or mentally challenged, his nervous system is always involved. He will develop vascular disorders and ulcerative processes. See Figure 29.5.

THE FOUR REACTIVE MODES

The way one reacts to his surrounding influences is called reactive mode. Every one of the 4 reactive modes presents specific symptoms: etiological, modalities, mental, general, local, and so on. To each reactive mode corresponds an initial strain, the toxin root of the reactive mode. The logic of a patient's system, or reactive mode diseases, presents various images or symptoms:

- The Psoric: A centripetal dynamic from intestine to skin
- The Tuberculinic: Fragile and excessive, ups and downs, lungs
- The Sycotic: Water and toxin retention, fixed diseases and ideas
- The Luetic: Asymmetric and restless, nocturnal and vascular

The Psoric reactive mode (Earth element) has centrifugal reactions. His skin is talkative. He is improved by eliminations, which re-establishes his balance. The pathologies alternate periodically with allergies, urticaria, eczema, hay fever, asthma, piles, intestinal diseases, arthritis, parasitism, increased IgE, psoriasis, and so on. The eliminations, natural and pathological, are itching and ill-smelling. Between the periods of elimination, he feels well, but with functional aging he develops increased emotional and physical sensitiveness, thermoregulation disorders, fatigue, and abnormal hunger. Sedentary life, overabundance, lack of physical exercise, and allopathic suppression of his attempt to eliminate toxins will progressively break down the Psoric. All his diseases are attempts to balance his entries with his exits.

His reactive mode is to BALANCE.

The Tuberculinic reactive mode (Air element) evolves by sudden paroxysmal attacks according to his extreme sensitivity. Some Tuberculinics present with allergies while others with anergy, some with no specific defenses and others with increased IgG. The lymphatic, venous, hepatic, and respiratory systems are predominantly affected with a general exhaustion syndrome and nervous oversensitivity. His endocrine disorders are dominated mainly by the thyroid and suprarenal glands. He has a mineralization defect that is particularly aggravated during the growth periods of childhood and adolescence. Mentally and physically, this person is bounced up and down by cyclothymic rhythms, alternate excitement and depression. The chronic disease state might evolve quickly into a condition of cellular degeneration and necrosis such as hepatitis and pneumonia.

His reactive mode is to OVERREACT.

The Sycotic reactive mode (Water element) drags into conditions of progressive degeneration. Toxins, germs, vaccinations, and prolonged allopathic treatments aggravate the deceleration of his metabolic functions and the intoxication of his reticular-endothelial tissue by water retention. All of the symptoms are aggravated by dampness. He is like a garbage can that is maladjusted to his environment and cannot get rid of the toxic wastes that he accumulates. He usually develops persistent chronic infections, especially E.N.T. and genitourinary, obsessive ideas and tumors, which are the result of a failure of his immune system functions. The body is progressively invaded by overabundance diseases. The patient repeats the same disease sequence, the same behaviors and physical tics, and is always apprehensive.

His reactive mode is NO REACTION.

The Luetic reactive mode (Fire element) presents with a physical and mental disharmony that leads the patient to sclerotic and ulcerative processes. His target organs are the vascular walls, elastic tissue, bones, skin, mucus membranes, throat, and neuroendocrine system. He manifests unbalances of his entire system and, as a result of being dominated by the speed of life, pathologies related to environmental stress. He also develops cyclothymic instabilities, spasmodic disorders with insecurity syndromes, and growth disorders that can result in extreme conditions such as becoming either a midget or a giant. Restlessness and fears are aggravated during the night. These paradoxical behaviors and cellular mutations may drive his life to anarchy. He evolves with infection and necrosis, hardening and sclerosis, exostosis and decalcification, spots and ptosis.

His reactive mode is to live in UNBALANCE.

SKIN LANGUAGE

The skin is a mirror of the patient's general state; it represents the border between the individual and the world around him from which he continuously receives information. There is no doubt that it is a very expressive organ. The nervous system has the same embryological origin as the skin, and thus the skin is its natural emunctory. All diseases are cured from the inside to the outside. Before treating any skin disease, a perfect examination of the functional abilities of the inner emunctories must be evaluated as to their ability to eliminate toxins out of the body through drainage. Each reactive mode has a particular skin language. Sweating is one of the essential general symptoms, an extremely precious tool for the diagnosis of the correct remedy in acute diseases and some chronic cases. See Figure 29.6.

Psora (Psoric reactive mode):

- Recurrent and resistant eliminations alternate with quiet periods
- Dermatitis and eczema, periodical sweating
- Itching and suppuration, lymphatic overload
- Intestinal unbalance, discharge on connective tissue

Tuberculinism (Tuberculinic reactive mode):

- Decalcification, vasomotor disorders, venous congestion
- Recurrent night sweat during the demineralization periods

GEOMETRICAL SYNTHESIS

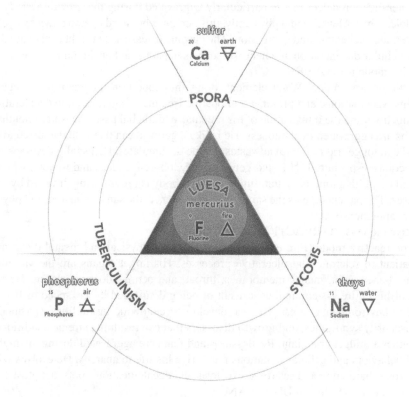

FIGURE 29.6 Geometrical synthesis.

- Hepatic insufficiency, neurovegetative sensitivity
- Tendency to profound lasting suppuration and convalescence

Sycosis (Sycotic reactive mode):

- Dirty and fat skin, all kinds of tumors, warts and colored spots
- Prolonged periods of sweat due to chronic internal infections
- Water retention in connective tissue with toxins, obesity
- Recurring infections, E.N.T. and genitourinary, immune defect

Luesa (Luetic reactive mode):

- Elastic tissue fragility of the vessel walls, arteries and veins
- Extreme states from dry to moist, worse at night
- Ulcerations, keloid, chronic itching, eczema
- Chronic skin pathology protects nervous and vascular systems

HOMEOPATHIC DRAINAGE

The disorders presented by a patient are superficial expressions reflecting the state of his internal organs. Each person is made of various layers and a doctor practicing homeopathy must eliminate them all carefully, one by one, to penetrate deep into the mechanism of the patient's functioning. At every stage of the process, the body needs assistance to detoxify and invigorate the affected organs and strengthen the canals of detoxification. The patient needs drainage of his essential "emunctories."

The key to chronic disease treatment is good detoxification. Drainage regulates the activity of the blocked or deficient organs and improves the quality of the essential emunctory functions. This is the first condition for a quick and complete healing. Of course, lifestyle and hygiene, associated to drainage, will contribute greatly in improving the functioning of the organs and maintaining good health.

How can we get good and quick results in acute and chronic diseases? An easy way to step into the homeopathic world and get immediate results is to use the techniques of drainage. This is the perfect field of action for homeopathic remedies. Homeopathic drainage is particularly effective in pediatrics for the treatment of diseases such as E.N.T., respiratory, and allergic pathologies.

1. *The organs and their canals.* The cleaning and the fortifying of the body are maintained by the organs of detoxification: the emunctories. A sick organ contains toxins and these toxins need to find a way out of body through a specific canal system. The toxins to be evacuated must be particularly directed to the sites where they tend to be, and through the proper canals, based on the location where nature points out it wants to operate the drainage of the toxins.

    The detoxifying system is made of two elements, the organ and its canals. Drainage consists of restoring the function of an organ and facilitating the elimination of toxins through its canals. The restoring of mute emunctories such as skin disease, mucus secretion or emotions, and the opening of new emunctories, show the pathway to healing.

    If a patient presents a pain at a certain site, it means this is the place chosen as emunctory by the chronic disease. The treatment must suppress the pain and canalize its source. It is necessary first to determine the patient's vitality and the quality of his emunctories. The treatment of any chronic disease also needs a nervous drainage to calm the excessive sensitiveness and irritability which puts an obstacle to the complete action of remedies.

2. *Central remedies and satellite remedies.* The action of central remedies involves the whole body. Satellite remedies are remedies that cover similar symptoms or have a limited but specific role. They facilitate the action of central remedies by improving the function of the affected emunctories. In acute and chronic pathologies, satellite remedies aid in the drainage of the patient. Any remedy can be considered as a satellite remedy when it has particular affinities with a specific tissue, organ, or function.

Some satellite remedies have a very specific action, such as LEMNA MINOR, for example, the satellite of THUYA OCCIDENTALIS and CALCAREA CARBONICA, which acts on nose mucosa. Others have a wide emunctory field of action, such as CHELIDONIUM, the satellite of several central remedies such as LYCOPODIUM and PHOSPHORUS, and act on several organs. A patient suffering from bronchiolitis will be treated with a lung tissue remedy, one dose of NATRUM SULFURICUM 15CH, assisted by a discharge remedy, 3 granules of ANTIMONIUM TARTARICUM 4CH as needed.

THE WHEEL OF EMUNCTORIES

The body's cleaning and fortifying abilities are naturally maintained by the Wheel of Emunctories. Two courses of emunctories treat and eliminate the stream of toxins along this wheel. See Figure 29.7.

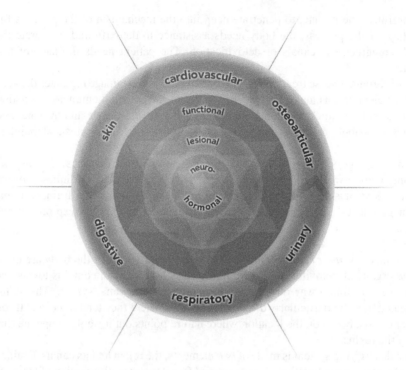

FIGURE 29.7   The Wheel of Emunctories.

The FIRST COURSE goes from the SKIN system to the DIGESTIVE system, then to the RESPIRATORY system. These three emunctories are OPEN emunctories, they have an ENTRY and an EXIT. The most open of all emunctories is the SKIN, which can be extremely talkative in some children. The DIGESTIVE system has an entry and an exit with, in between, many filters which accumulate toxins and need daily care. The RESPIRATORY system has an entry, but the exit is also the entry. Two points dominate this system, anxiety and immune system memorizing.

The SECOND COURSE evolves from the URINARY system to the OSTEOARTICULAR system, and finally to the CARDIOVASCULAR system. However, the URINARY system has an entry and an exit, it is an endocrine organ which filters the blood from the most toxic elements for the body. Each JOINT, each BONE, and each MUSCLE is a complete organ made of vessels and nerves, from liquid to solid, and easily becomes a jail for toxins. The most closed emunctory is the CARDIOVASCULAR system, made of muscle and labyrinth circuits, and impacted by emotions.

The ENDOCRINE and NERVOUS systems govern all the emunctories and must be considered at each stage of the treatment. Our Wheel of Emunctories turns according to our own constitution, reactive mode, and individual maturation. In the evolution of a chronic disease, the order in which the different organs are affected shows the treatment strategy to follow and the type of homeopathic drainage the patient needs.

In order to correctly analyze the patient's case, the doctor must be able to draw the patient's Line of Life. The course of the Line of Life shows the evolution of the reactive modes and a logic in the appearance of the different diseases that occurred during this particular life. With the Line of Life, the practitioner can locate the acute disease and build a strategy to heal chronic patients.

The reactive modes follow a NATURAL EVOLUTION along the life of a person; they are the dynamic elements of the organism and they govern the impulsions of the NATURAL CYCLES from birth to death. The same is valid for constitutions which also obey the natural evolution. They dominate and evolve in a certain order, during growth and maturity phases, and from infancy to old age, until death. An individual evolves through SEVEN NATURAL CYCLES.

The first cycle corresponds to intra-uterus life.

After birth, the Line of Life can be divided into six essential cycles:

- From birth until 7 years—BUILDS HIMSELF
- From 7 to 14 years—DISCOVERS HIMSELF
- From 14 to 21 years—LOOKS AT HIMSELF
- From 21 years to the menopausal period begins, for men and women
- The period of menopause, for men and women
- From then on, the endocrine system is stabilized until old age.

THE LINE OF LIFE

See Figure 29.8.

The first cycle, intra-uterus life:

- 0_1 corresponds to the first moment of birth, when the two germinal cells meet and combine producing the first embryonic cell which develops into a fetus in total darkness for 9 months. This is the first program that encodes hereditary information about the immune functions.

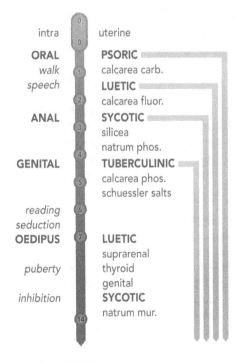

LINE OF LIFE
THE EVOLUTION OF
THE 3 FIRST CYCLES

FIGURE 29.8   The Line of Life.

- O_2 corresponds to the second birth, the discovery of oxygen and light.
- O_1 to O_2 contains the essential mystery of creation. Embryonic and fetal studies give very precious information to the doctor about the human body. The same type of cells produces the skin and nervous systems, another type of cell produces both the genital and urinary systems. All of the changes that take place in the mother during the pregnancy are extremely important for understanding the future health of the mother and her child.

The second cycle, the first seven years:

"It will be sufficient if you gave me the first seven years of life of a man, they contain all, and you can keep the rest."

Bruno Bettelheim

The second program is encoded from 0 to 7 years and will determine many of the disease patterns for the rest of a person's life. During the first cycle of 7 years, there is a natural evolution of the four reactive modes along the Line of Life which marks the development of any healthy child.

The infant is a PSORIC; he removes stresses through skin eruptions and digestive disorders. When these two emunctories are surpassed, pathologies of the respiratory system appear. The depth of the hereditary Psora can be precisely evaluated from these first moments of the child's life.

When the child starts walking and talking, he expresses his LUETIC reactive mode. He experiments with his center of gravity and the power of language, eventually becoming self-sufficient. This is the time for restlessness and night fears.

When the child discovers cleanliness, between the ages of 18 and 36 months, he becomes a SYCOTIC. His behavioral patterns are obsession, mentally and physically, with a lack of immune system response. He can repeat the same nose or ear infections over and over, never becoming completely healthy.

During growth accelerations, he is a TUBERCULINIC. He has sudden and violent pathologies such as fever, bronchitis, parasitism, arthritis, colic, and so on, with/or superimposed on chronic fatigue and decalcification. At this period the child must always take Doctor Schüssler tissue salts.

During the first seven years of life, this natural movement of the reactive modes can be disturbed by many factors such as diet, infectious diseases, epidemics, vaccinations, pollutions, stresses, and so on. The Line of Life shows the patient's individual sensitivity with one or two reactive modes dominating his history. The evolution of this second cycle corresponds to the visible maturation of his immune system and will express itself through similar pathologies for the rest of his life.

The other cycles are

- Seven years of age corresponds to the beginning of the OEDIPUS cycle. This period of time is dominated by the LUETIC reactive mode, just as when the child learned to walk. He then needed the same Luetic energy.
- During the THIRD cycle—from ages 7 to 14 years, the child develops into puberty. Growth periods drive him to the TUBERCULINIC reactive mode. The ENDOCRINE glands are stimulated and develop, starting with the suprarenal and then the thyroid gland. When the genital glands start maturing, puberty is established.
- During the FOURTH cycle, from age 14 to 21 years, these natural GENITAL and endocrine changes will orient the reactions of the person to the TUBERCULINO-SYCOTIC reactive mode which can remain with his entire life and provoke tumor pathologies when his fertility declines.

- During the FIFTH cycle, from 21 years of age to mature age, the different methods of adaptation turn around and show which of the 4 reactive modes the patient is operating in for that particular period of time. PSORIC centrifugal powers proceed by attempts of eliminating toxins until centripetal lesions take place, in particular on digestive organs, and SYCOTIC processes might take root. The pathologies of the second cycle return; each attack is followed by long lasting convalescence and morbid alternations.
- The SIXTH cycle, the period of menopause, for both men and women, is complex. The 4 reactive modes might be involved, particularly the PSORO-SYCOTIC and LUETIC, but also the TUBERCULINIC for the demineralization process. Here again, when the diagnosis is not clear, look at the second cycle of the Line of Life to orient your research.
- The SEVENTH cycle is dominated by elderly emunctories which are worn out with deep lesions of the VASCULAR and OSSEOUS systems. This patient should be given a prolonged drainage of his emunctory system. Respect the hierarchy of the natural Wheel of Emunctories.

The Line of Life indicates the dominant reactive modes of the patient and shows the correct order to follow with the homeopathic treatment. The strategy in front of chronic diseases lies in the precise analysis of the second cycle which points out the dominant general modalities of the person. When the natural development of the Line of Life does not occur, Luesa needs the support of remedies for the Tuberculinic reactive mode.

The infant with an immune dysfunction will present recurrent diseases. The skin is involved in most cases: color, sweating, heat/cold, rash, itching, eczema. The reactions precede and/or follow the acute elimination attempts and might replace them when the patient improves. The skin is the final step of toxins elimination; its reactivity testifies of the child's centrifugal energy power.

When the skin is not sufficient to canalize out the toxins, the first emunctory to be solicited is the digestive system: intolerance to milk and other foods, colic, diarrhea, constipation, parasitism, and so on. Digestive disorders will often accompany the main source of pathologies in the child: his respiratory system, from E.N.T. to bronchiole. The child might weaken progressively by losing weight, stunted growth, walk, talk, and psychomotor development, and an aggravation of the immune defects that he accumulates.

HOW TO PRESCRIBE

Each acute manifestation is a window of the chronic disease; the remedies correspond to the symptoms, the anatomic level, the way of reacting of mucosa membranes, and the specific toxins. An acute disease healed is a great step toward the understanding of the patient; it brings a security in case of attack, and it shows the direction to chronic disease healing.

For local symptoms, 3–5 granules in 4CH to 9CH are given as treatment, repeated as needed according to evolution of symptoms. The frequency of the intakes is spaced out as the symptoms improve. When the patient presents at least 2 general modalities or general symptoms, or concomitants, or a striking mind symptom, use central remedies to begin with: one dose in 15CH, then increase the potency in severe cases. Metals and metalloids have a deep and prolonged action; in most cases, they don't need to be repeated often, and should preferably be given in the evening.

Granules can be melted in a little water. Shake the bottle before each intake. In my experience, the best way is to put one granule by one, inside the cheek or inferior gum fold, and let it melt. Infants appreciate the sweet taste. A good way to use remedies in pediatrics is to give them in trituration form (powder) for chronic treatments. Drops in 2DH can be prepared alcohol free; gemmotherapy is very effective but it contains alcohol and has to be handled cautiously until the child weighs at least 60 lb.

PART 2: GROWTH DISORDERS AND HOMEOPATHY

The nutritional support with the constitution mineral is very beneficial for children.

- The plump healthy infant needs CALCAREA CARBONICA: his digestive system is very busy and the skin is talkative, respiratory disorders are recurrent from upper level to bronchiole, and the mucus membrane secretions are abundant.
- The thin nervous infant needs CALCAREA PHOSPHORICA: respiratory inflammation and fatigue periods follow one another, as well as spasmodic disorders, chronic fever and growth disorders.
- The premature or fearful puny infant needs SILICEA: he is skinny with a big sweaty head, long lasting infections, and food allergies starting with milk, gluten, and eggs.

Doctor Schüssler tissue salts are necessary during growth periods and have to be intensified when during convalescence and chronic diseases.

Doctor Schüssler mineral salts enter in the composition of blood and tissues and are necessary to their constitution and good functioning. During the chronic patient treatment, they are essential for the Tuberculinic, the infant, children, growth periods, and when the energy is worn out by long-lasting diseases. The mineral supply is prepared in 6DH, which corresponds to physiological quantities, and its assimilation in small rates is faster and deeper. It can penetrate into the cell, be recognized by it, so that the cell is able to use it for its metabolism and exchanges.

The main tissue salts are: CALCAREA FLUORICA, CALCAREA PHOSPHORICA, FERRUM PHOPHORICUM, KALIUM PHOSPHORICUM, NATRUM MURIATICUM, NATRUM PHOSPHORICUM, SILICEA. Give 5 granules or one tablet 1–3 times a day for periods of 1–3 months. Associate and alternate the different mineral salts for the best result. Start with the remedies specific of the injured organ, and consider constitution and reactive modes.

PART 3: E.N.T. AND HOMEOPATHY

RHINO PHARYNGITIS

Infants and children use three essential emunctories: the skin, digestive, and respiratory systems. Their pathologies go from one system to the other. Antibiotics create an artificial intestinal medium by modifying the natural flora. This complicates the case with digestive disorders, allergies, various bacteria and fungus sensitiveness. The nose is the sentinel of the respiratory system.

RHINO PHARYNGITIS DISCHARGE

Bland discharge, no burning:

- Bland watery profuse nose discharge, conjunctivitis, eyes and lids swollen, burning, violent cough with thick discharge, allergy, <(worse) mornings, warmth, indoors, from light: EUPHRASIA 4CH
- Watery copious discharge, from nose and eyes, paroxysmal sneezing, palate tickling, hay fever, <flowers, garlic odors and cold drinks, >(improved) by warm food and open air: SABADILLA 15CH
- Yellow thick abundant mucus, nose obstruction in the evening and fluent in the morning, cough dry at night and loose during the daytime, lymphatic and venous slowing down. Good to clear off the secretions, for beginning and ending discharges. Changeable mood, <warm room, night, >cold applications, open air, air conditioned, and consolation: PULSATILLA 15CH

Purulent discharge:

- Bleeding easy, painful, ulcerating: main remedy for purulent process, abscess. Ill-tempered, quarrelsome, impatient, does not want to be approached or touched, <least air draft, cold, contact, >warmth: HEPAR SULFUR 9CH to 30CH
- Main remedy for tonsillitis, with intense thirst and sweat, fetid thick purulent and yellow green discharge with ulcerated nostrils, cervical nodes inflamed, otitis, sinusitis, tonsillitis, bronchitis, all symptoms <night:
  - In acute cases: MERCURIUS CORROSIVUS 4CH to 9CH
  - In chronic cases: MERCURIUS SOLUBILIS 4CH to 30CH
- Posterior nares discharge, pressure and pain at the root of the nose, thick viscous yellowish, greenish discharge, tough elastic plugs which leave a rough bleeding surface, frontal sinusitis, polyps: KALIUM BICHROMICUM 4CH to 9CH
- Greenish and sticky, irritating, recurrent or chronic: HYDRASTIS, KALIUM BICHROMICUM
- Yellow and not irritating: KALIUM SULFURICUM, PULSATILLA

Watery burning discharge:
See: MERCURIUS SOLUBILIS

- Main remedy for otitis media, congested tympanum with dark blood, sudden aggravation, ill-looking and thinness. Exhaustion alternates with restlessness, extremely chilly, drinks often small quantities, burning pains, asthma, hay fever, alternations eczema/asthma, otitis/diarrhea, etc., <between midnight and 3 a.m., >warmth and warm hot applications: ARSENICUM ALBUM 4CH
- Main remedy for sneezing, hay fever-like, copious discharge with nose excoriation, red itching eyes, fluent intense sneezing, hoarseness, dry and spasmodic cough with headache, <morning: ALLIUM CEPA 9CH
- Corrosive nasal catarrh, otitis purulent and very painful, adenoids, constant desire to sneeze which aggravates, nodes swollen, recurrent fever with night sweat, ichthyosis, Tuberculinic, >by warmth: ARSENICUM IODATUM 4CH
- Eyes and nose inflammation, red swollen nostrils and conjunctiva, maxillary sinusitis, asthma, <night, seashore: KALIUM IODATUM 4CH
- Hoarseness, larynx and chest painful raw, laryngitis, extreme burning of nose and throat, constant nose itching until it bleeds, nose obstruction, Tuberculinic attack, <when weather suddenly changes to cold: ARUM TRIPHYLLUM 4CH

Watery burning discharge with important nose obstruction:

- Adenoids provoke nose obstruction, catarrhal deafness, good for drainage of chronic swollen posterior nares, sensitive to least cold: AGRAPHIS NUTANS 4CH
- Frontal headache with pressure at root of nose > when discharge appears, violent coryza with extreme nose dryness, dry painful teasing cough < at night and when lying down, ethmoidal sinusitis, allergy, adenoids: STICTA PULMONARIA 4CH
- Polyps in nose, posterior nares discharge thick yellow purulent, anterior nares watery, burning, hay fever, sinusitis, sneezing, <night, >local warmth: SANGUINARIUM NITRICUM 4CH to 9CH

Infant snuffles:

- Main remedy for infant snuffles, sudden suffocation around midnight, croupy cough, laryngitis, asthma, adenoids, profuse sweating before waking up, complete nose obstruction: SAMBUCUS NIGRA 3DH to 30CH

- Main remedy for spasms, nose obstruction < warm room, violent sneezing, hay fever, facial twitching, abdominal cramps, excessive flatulence, violent vomiting, constipation: NUX VOMICA 4CH to 9CH
- Constant nose obstruction, pain in the forehead > pressure and warm room, chest oppression and palpitations, <3 to 4 a.m.: AMMONIUM CARBONICUM 4CH to 9CH

Also see: BELLADONNA, CHAMOMILLA, DULCAMARA, HEPAR SULFUR, LYCOPODIUM, MERCURIUS, STICTA PULMONARIA, SULFUR FLAVUM

RHINO PHARYNGITIS COUGH

Hoarseness painful:
See: ARUM TRIPHYLLUM

- Main remedy of acute laryngitis, barking, suffocation, <before midnight: SPONGIA TOSTA 9CH
- Main remedy of whooping cough, much retching, painful hoarse voice, laryngitis, cervical and thoracic lymph nodes inflamed, Tuberculinic: DROSERA 4CH
- High fever without sweat, anguish, <before midnight: ACONIT NAPELLUS 15CH
- Paroxysmal fever, extreme dryness, destructive, nightmares, delusions and convulsions, fear of animals, <least jarring, air draft, cold, light, drinking: BELLADONNA 15CH
- Spasmodic hoarseness, inspiration provokes cough, asthma >at seashore: BROMUM 4CH

Spasmodic cough with difficult expectoration:

- Nausea and vomiting with cough, suffocation, asthma, violent coryza with intense sneezing, nose obstruction, easy bleeding of nose, lung, intestine, pale face, tongue clean: IPECA 4CH
- Whooping cough by laryngeal tickling, expectorates abundant thick viscous mucus from posterior nares, <night, 11:30 p.m., 3:30 a.m., and 6:00 a.m., and by warmth, >by open air: COCCUS CACTI 15CH
- Whooping cough, suffocating, coughs up abundant nasal catarrh from posterior nares, adenoids, <during sleep and just when waking up: CORALLIUM RUBRUM 4CH

Teasing cough from tickling throat:

- Incessant throat tickling provokes dry cough < inspiring the least cold air and lying down at night, preventing sleep, raw pain behind sternum: RUMEX CRISPUS 4CH
- Sore hoarseness > drinking cold water, <twilight and bed warmth, dry cold wind: CAUSTICUM 4CH

See: STICTA PULMONARIA

RHINO PHARYNGITIS DRAINAGE

Nose discharge drainage:

- Bland: AGRAPHIS NUTANS/CALCAREA SULFURICA/PULSATILLA/a.a.p. 4CH
- Burning: KALIUM BICHROMICUM/KALIUM IODATUM/MEZEREUM/a.a.p. 4CH

E.N.T. drainage, 1 or 2 homeopathic tsps of the trituration a day:

- Adenoids drainage:
  - Sycotic drainage, recurrent discharges especially in E.N.T. organs, nose obstruction and its reactional symptoms, centripetal reactions by adenoids, polyps and warts, lack of reaction to allopathic treatments, bacteria and fungus sensitizations: CALCAREA CARBONICA 8DH/TEUCRIUM MARUM 3DH/THUYA OCCIDENTALIS 8DH/a.a.p.
  - Cough drainage: CISTUS CANADENSIS/CORALLIUM RUBRUM/STICTA PULMONARIA/a.a.p. 4CH
- Eustachian tube drainage: HYDRASTIS/KALIUM MURIATICUM/MERCURIUS DULCIS/a.a.p. 4CH
  - Repeated fevers, boils and skin mycosis, yellow pus, urticaria, tonsillitis, chronic bronchitis, asthma, diarrhea, colitis: PENICILLINUM 15CH accompanied with CANDIDA 15CH

Rhino Pharyngitis Prevention

Start one month before critical season and continue one month after. The treatment is based on the satellite and central remedies of the individual. Mineral salts are to be maintained in infants and children. Associate oligotherapy to gemmotherapy for mild cases.

Oligotherapy, alternate one month course:

- 1st month:
  - Morning: COPPER GOLD SILVER TRACE ELEMENT
  - Evening: MANGANESE COBALT TRACE ELEMENT
- 2nd month:
  - Morning: MANGANESE COPPER TRACE ELEMENT
  - Evening: SULFUR TRACE ELEMENT
- Gemmotherapy, child over 60 pounds, 5 to 20 drops a day:
  - Morning: RIBES NIGRUM BUDS 1DH
  - Evening: ROSA CANINA YOUNG SHOOTS 1DH
- Tissue salts:
  - 1 to 2 homeopathic spoons of the trituration, or 3 to 5 granules: CALCAREA PHOSPHORICA/FERRUM PHOSPHORICUM/KALIUM MURIATICUM/NATRUM SULFURICUM/a.a.p. 6DH

OTITIS

Otitis media is one of the most frequent traumas of infancy, especially in the Tuberculinic and Sycotic reactive modes which are aggravated by early vaccinations. Tonsillectomies have been replaced in pediatric medicine by tubes in the ears. Only the otitis caused by bacteria may require the use of antibiotics. Most cases of otitis called "viral" or "allergic" are recurrent in spite of steroids and antibiotic. Antibiotic therapy has created systemic fungal disorders and provoked a weakening of the immune system reactions. This condition perverts the patient's response to his current daily stresses such as cold, heat, wind, fears, allergens, pathogens, and so on. Homeopathic medicine can cure acute, recurrent, and chronic cases, especially otitis related to Eustachian tube or adenoids obstruction. Ear pathologies are the most frequent side effects appearing after vaccination during the first year of life.

Five Main Remedies

See: ARSENICUM ALBUM, HEPAR SULFUR, PULSATILLA

- Main remedy for otitis with moderate fever, congested tympanum with bright blood, diarrhea, epistaxis, <night with exhausting sweat, Tuberculinic: FERRUM PHOSPHORICUM 7CH to 15CH
- Teething problems, one cheek red, irritating diarrhea with colic, restless and awkward, >being carried: CHAMOMILLA 15CH

Mastoiditis Threatened

- Main remedy for osteitis of facial bones, fetid otorrhea, septal and nasal ulcerations, oversensitive to noise. Authoritarian and awkward, tyrant, peevish and vehement at least contradiction, quarrelsome, screaming, <night, cold, Winter, >warm applications: AURUM METAL 9CH (not to repeat often)
- Burning pain <COLD and >heat: CAPSICUM 9CH

Eustachian Tube Drainage

- Every coryza ends with a bronchitis, chronic catarrh with deafness, laryngitis, asthma, all ailments < in damp weather, Tuberculinic: MANGANUM ACETICUM 4CH
- Itching, chronic catarrh with swollen nodes, snapping and noises in the ear, canker sores, thrush, chronic tonsillitis with recurrent grayish membranes: KALIUM MURIATICUM 4CH to 9CH
- Thickening and rigidity of tympanum, cavum and posterior nares drainage, diarrhea, ill-looking, chronic discharge: MERCURIUS DULCIS 4CH

Otitis Drainage to Accompany the Adenoids Drainage

- HYDRASTIS/KALIUM BICHROMICUM/KALIUM IODATUM/VIOLA ODORATA/ a.a.p. 4CH

SINUSITIS

It is one of the first pathologies a new homeopathic doctor can treat with homeopathy successfully. The results are excellent, fast, and long lasting.

Sinusitis is often related to allergic reactions. Psoro-sycotic disease includes periodicity, thermoregulation disorders, recurrences, and resistance to allopathic treatments. Use the rhino pharyngitis discharge remedies and the drainage remedies.

Suppuration Stage

- See: ARSENICUM ALBUM, HEPAR SULFUR, MERCURIUS SOLUBILIS

Sinusitis Discharge Remedies

- See: KALIUM BICHROMICUM, KALIUM IODATUM
- Neuralgia of face, ear, teeth when discharge is blocked, yellow pus tinged with blood excoriating nostrils, eczema, teething, burning pains <cold air, night, eating: MEZEREUM 4CH
- Tenacious excoriating discharge from posterior nares to throat, thick yellowish and ropy or watery, septum ulceration, Eustachian tube blockage: HYDRASTIS 4CH

Ethmoidal and Frontal Sinusitis

- See: ALLIUM CEPA, CORALLIUM RUBRUM, STICTA PULMONARIA

Maxillary Sinusitis

- See: CORALLIUM RUBRUM, HYDRASTIS, KALIUM BICHROMICUM
- Left side in particular: MEZEREUM
- Right side in particular: AURUM METAL

Osteitis Remedies

- AURUM METAL, MERCURIUS SOLUBILIS, PHOSPHORUS, PHYTOLACCA, SILICEA

Sinusitis Drainage

Alternate every other day 3 granules 1 to 3 times a day as needed:

- Even days: KALIUM BICHROMICUM/KALIUM IODATUM/STICTA PULMONARIA/ a.a.p. 4CH
- Odd days: CALCAREA CARBONICA/LEMNA MINOR/TEUCRIUM MARUM/a.a.p. 4CH

Intensify the frequency in case of beginning a new attack.

In case of suppuration: alternate HEPAR SULFUR 15CH/AURUM METAL 9CH every other week.

NODES DRAINAGE

Oligotherapy:

- Morning: COPPER GOLD SILVER TRACE ELEMENT
- Evening: MANGANESE COPPER TRACE ELEMENT

Organotherapy:

- LYMPHATIC GANGLION/SURRENINE/a.a.p. 4CH

Satellite remedies:

- Cervical nodes drainage:
  - CISTUS CANADENSIS/EUPHORBIUM/JUGLANS REGIA/a.a.p. 4CH
  - CALCAREA IODATA/CALCAREA PHOSPHORICA/SILICEA/a.a.p. 4CH

Thoracic nodes drainage:

- CISTUS CANADENSIS 4CH, DROSERA 4CH

Tonsils drainage:

- BARYTA CARBONICA/BARYTA IODATA/BARYTA MURIATICA/a.a.p. 9CH
- KALIUM BICHROMICUM/MERCURIUS SOLUBILIS/a.a.p. 4CH

Background treatment: one dose a week in the following order:

- High fevers with night sweats, healthy looking and fairly good appetite:
  - 1st week: SULFUR IODATUM 7CH
  - 2nd week: AVIAIRE 7CH
  - 3rd week: MERCURIUS SOLUBILIS 15CH
  - 4th week: CALCAREA CARBONICA 15CH
- Little or no fever, sick looking, irregular appetite:
  - 1st week: THUYA 15CH
  - 2nd week: PULSATILLA 15CH
  - 3rd week: AVIAIRE 7CH
  - 4th week: SILICEA 15CH
- Severe and recurrent tonsillitis, add: DIPHTEROTOXINUM 15CH
- Severe and recurrent otitis, repeat after each attack: AVIAIRE 9CH

Constitution:

- Stout, Carbonic:
  - 3 granules a day: BARYTA CARBONICA 9CH
  - Alternate every other 2 weeks one dose: CALCAREA CARBONICA 15CH/ GRAPHITES 15CH
- Thin, Phosphoric:
  - Alternate every other day 3 granules: ARSENICUM IODATUM 4CH/CALCAREA IODATA 4CH
  - Alternate every other 2 weeks one dose: CALCAREA PHOSPHORICA 15CH/ SULFUR IODATUM 15CH

ALLERGIC REACTIONS

- 3 granules 1 to 2 times a day: HISTAMINUM 4CH
- Alternate one dose every other week: APIS 15CH/HISTAMINUM 15CH

The best toxin root to prepare the remedy is the local one directly related to the individual allergy. Start one month before critical period and continue one month after, one dose a week of the toxic allergen in 15CH to 30CH.

Acute attacks require the same dosage, but more often. Results are excellent with botanicals.

- Indoor allergic reactions, dust and acaridans: BLATTA ORIENTALIS 30CH

Some of the most common botanicals:

- Ash: FRAXINUS AMERICANA
- Beech: FAGUS SYLVATICA
- Birch: BETULA
- Cedar: CEDRUS LIBANI
- Cypress: CUPRESSUS SEMPERVIRENS
- Elderberry: SAMBUCUS NIGRA
- Maple: ACER CAMPESTRIS
- Oak: QUERCUS PEDUNCULATA
- Plane: PLATANUS
- Pollens mixture: POLLANTINUM
- Poplar: POPULUS NIGRA
- Ragweed: AMBROSIA

Some of the most common insects and animals:

- Bedbug: CIMEX
- Bees: APIS
- Cat: CAT HAIR
- Flea: PULEX
- Hornets: VESPA CRABRO
- Horse: HORSE HAIR
- Mosquitoes: CULEX
- Seafood: HOMARUS GAMMARUS
- Wasps: VESPA VULGARIS

PART 4: SIDE EFFECTS OF VACCINATION

Note that the following stems from my personal clinical experience as a physician, and especially as a family doctor for a village and its school for many years. I have treated many children with adverse reactions to vaccination. Due to personal observation, I gave as little vaccines as I could, and never gave the MMR but treated children brought to me who had developed severe pathologies after being vaccinated for MMR. I treated them with homeopathic remedies and specific isotherapeutics and obtained great results.

The analysis of the Line of Life of the patient before and after the vaccinations might point out an aggravation of his chronic disease. The person with an immune dysfunction from a vaccination will present recurrent diseases most likely similar to the toxin effects. The Wheel of Emunctories might be disrupted, producing body eliminations, apart from the skin, at all digestive and respiratory levels first and with nervous sphere reactions.

Among all the vaccinations performed today, the longest scientific experience about the disease itself and its vaccination results is with DTaP and MMR. The first booster might open a Pandora's box. Side effects must be analyzed with meticulous care following the booster from the first minutes after the injection and up to 3 months later: local, general, mental, and periodicity.

The isotherapeutic of the vaccination must be used after homeopathic drainage: one dose in 15CH and going up to 30CH, MK, and XMK as needed. Note the reactions after the remedy. In most cases they happen around the 8th day. A skin rash augurs well, fever and physical symptoms are to be taken more seriously, and neurological reactions such as nightmares testify a deep imprint and sensitiveness for the toxin.

DTaP

About 50% of children have reactions in the first days following the booster: local inflammation, fever, loss of appetite, otitis, rhino pharyngitis, and cough. Some have severe symptoms such as local abscess, asthma, eczema, or even neurological with weeping and screaming, restlessness or sleepiness, twitching and spasms, nightmares and convulsions. The distant consequences are of the same order with a dominance of respiratory tract pathologies from E.N.T. to lung, chronic cervical adenitis, E.N.T. discharges, tonsillitis, recurrent spasmodic cough, but also intestines, colon, bacterial, fungal, and parasitic disorders. Vaccination aggravates the existing hereditary immune system weaknesses and provokes an immune blockage.

MMR

Measles dominates the MMR pathologies with allergies, conjunctivitis, rhinitis, spasmodic coryza, nose obstruction, cough, hay fever, asthma, physical and psychological growth disorders—essentially decalcification and language—and all the Tuberculinic anergic diseases.

Boosters might cause local abscesses, screaming, restlessness, sleepiness, nightmares, and fever. All children presenting "measles-like syndrome," called classical side effects, during the week following the booster need a specific homeopathic treatment. Distant consequences are recurrent E.N.T. inflammation, Eustachian tube chronic discharge, spasmodic cough, bronchitis, humid asthma, and eczema.

DETOXIFYING WITH HOMEOPATHIC TREATMENT

The treatment is composed of three levels:

- Homeopathic drainage of the sensitive emunctories
- Constitutional fortifying
- Reactive modes regulation with central remedies and satellite remedies

Adding tissue salts is always very beneficial for children. Oligotherapy is to be used for mild cases; organotherapy is helpful for severe recurrent pathologies.

1. One month before inoculation: Mineral salts can be used associated and/or alternated according to each individual.
   1 to 3 pills a day of the corresponding mineral salt of the infant:
   - Premature or ill-looking: SILICEA 6DH
   - Stout and healthy looking: CALCAREA CARBONICA 8DH
   - Thin and fragile child: CALCAREA PHOSPHORICA 6DH
   Immune system regulation:
   - One dose every 2 weeks: THYMUSINUM 7CH
     - Morning: COPPER GOLD SILVER TRACE ELEMENT
     - Evening: MANGANESE COPPER TRACE ELEMENT
   - In case of fragile child, recurrent pathologies, allergies
     - Morning: RIBES NIGRUM BUDS 1DH
     - Evening: ROSA CANINA YOUNG SHOOTS 1DH
2. After inoculation:
   - Just after the booster: ARNICA 15CH
   - The day after: SILICEA 15CH
   - 2 weeks later: THUYA OCCIDENTALIS 15CH
   Local inflammation with or without fever, abscess-like:
   - Alternate 3 granules as needed: ARNICA 4CH/BELLADONNA 4CH/LEDUM 4CH
   - Local treatment: wet compresses with CALENDULA MT and ECHINACEA MT
   Appearance of pathologies similar to the vaccination toxins:
   - Carbonic: one dose a month: CALCAREA CARBONICA 30CH
   - Phosphoric: one dose a week: CALCAREA PHOSPHORICA 30CH
3. Reactive mode regulation:
   a. Psoric drainage:
      - Rapid reactions to the booster, alternations of the pathologies from the outside to the inside and reverse, all kinds of skin reactions, itching, abscess, anorexia, vomiting, diarrhea, loss of weight, food allergies, especially milk, recurrent inflammatory fever, diseases start suddenly and patient recovers fast: ALOE/ CALCAREA SULFURICA/CINNABARIS/a.a.p. 4CH
      - One dose a week in the following order:
        - 1st week: NUX VOMICA 15CH
        - 2nd week: HEPAR SULFUR 15CH

- 3rd week: BELLADONNA 30CH
- 4th week: PSORINUM 7CH
- Adenitis chronic, repeated sudden short fevers, loss of weight, thinness, dermatitis, parasitism: PSORINUM 9CH and higher (not to repeat often)
- Diarrhea and fever after booster, recurrent gastroenteritis, food allergies, spasmodic colitis, long lasting bronchitis: PARATHYPHOIDINUM B 15CH
- Skin reactions: one dose a month as needed of SULFUR IODATUM 7CH to 15CH
- For itching eruptions, add 3 granules a day: APIS 4CH and HISTAMINUM 4CH

b. Tuberculinic drainage: For violent reactions and progressive loss of energy, when long-lasting fatigue follows each acute attack. Recurrent exhausting fever, respiratory system involved in most inflammations, lymph nodes recurrent and chronic, changing allergies, epistaxis, growth and endocrine disorders.
Drainage of lymph nodes:
- AGRAPHIS NUTANS/CISTUS CANADENSIS/MERCURIUS SOLUBILIS/ a.a.p. 4CH

For severe cases, add: LYMPHATIC GANGLION/SURRENINE/a.a.p. 4CH
- 1 or 2 homeopathic spoons of the trituration 1 to 3 times a day—12 TISSUE SALTS COMPOUND
- One dose a week in the following order:
  - 1st week: SULFUR IODATUM 7CH
  - 2nd week: PULSATILLA 15CH
  - 3rd week: AVIAIRE 7CH
  - 4th week: SILICEA 15CH

Severe tuberculinic reactions:
- Asthma, severe acute attacks during the night, see: ARSENICUM ALBUM 15CH
- Every cold provokes coughing, hoarseness <morning and >when lying: alternate MANGANUM ACETICUM 9CH/STANNUM IODATUM 9CH
- Loss of appetite and weight, ill-looking with profuse sweating of the head and soles, big skull on skinny body, obstinate: NATRUM MURIATICUM 15CH followed the day after by SILICEA 15CH
- Thinness, rapid loss of appetite, profuse sweating, slowed and difficult growth, headaches: CALCAREA PHOSPHORICA 15CH
- General symptoms of the toxin root, loss of energy and weight, extremely sensitive to cold, swollen inflamed tonsils and cervical nodes, morning watery diarrheas, profuse exhausting sweating in the evening, small boils, >by rest, open fresh air, mountain: TUBERCULINUM 7CH and higher

c. Sycotic drainage:
- CALCAREA CARBONICA 8DH/TEUCRIUM MARUM 3DH/THUYA OCCIDENTALIS 8DH/a.a.p.
- DULCAMARA/NATRUM PHOSPHORICUM/NATRUM SULFURICUM/ a.a.p. 4CH
- One dose a week in the following order:
  - 1st week: THUYA 15CH
  - 2nd week: NATRUM SULFURICUM 15CH
  - 3rd week: DULCAMARA 30CH
  - 4th week: SILICEA 15CH
- Bronchitis, bronchiolitis, asthma: alternate one dose every other week: NATRUM SULFURICUM 15CH/DULCAMARA 15CH
- Dust and acarian allergy: BLATTA ORIENTALIS 30CH

PART 5: HYPERACTIVITY, ATTENTION DEFICIT DISORDERS AND HOMEOPATHY

RESTLESS CHILD

All the physical symptoms concerning spasmodic reactions are noted according to anatomic location. (Also see Homeopathic and Drainage Repertory, ADHD in website blog: www. homeopathicdrainage.com.)

ANXIETY

- Main remedy for anxiety, to induce sleep. Sighing and sobbing, changeable mood and symptoms, weeping/laughter, spasms, from bad news, worries, mourning, divorce: IGNATIA 9CH
- Main remedy for apprehension, hides in his bed, claustrophobia, fear of lift, bridge, balcony, mall, hasty and impatient, horrible dreams of snakes, craves sweets and spicy foods, <heat, >open fresh air: ARGENTUM NITRICUM 15CH
- Main remedy for twilight anxiety, restless legs before going to bed, needs a light to fall asleep and a hand to hold, sympathetic and timid, easily worried and weeping, craves smoked foods: CAUSTICUM 9CH
- Anguished, cannot stay alone, suspicious, quarrelsome, destructive, craves acids, see: ARSENICUM ALBUM 15CH
- From mental overexertion, weak memory, insomnia, somnambulism: KALIUM PHOSPHORICUM 15CH
- Uncontrollable thinking, apprehension before examination and break down during, trembling, stuttering, vertigo, headache, frequent urination, nervous exhaustion: GELSEMIUM 15CH

QUARRELSOME

- Abdominal colic, from restrained anger, feeling of injustice, impatient, schooling: COLOCYNTHIS 4CH
- Capricious, kicks, bites, hits people and breaks things around, violent anger fits, whining, moaning because he cannot have what he wants, peevish, teething, colic, diarrhea, >being carried, car riding: CHAMOMILLA 15CH
- Cannot sleep after 3 a.m., cannot bear noises, odors, light, least touch, does not want to be touched, sullen, violent anger, fighting temper, destructive, see: NUX VOMICA 15CH
- Constant restlessness, legs, hands, fingers, head, runs, jumps, dances, violent, anger at least contradiction, suffocation, sexual excitement, delusions and nightmares: TARENTULA HISPANA 4CH
- Contradiction, anger, when child confuses day with night, impatient: STAPHYSAGRIA 9CH

Also see symptoms of remedies: ANTIMONIUM CRUDUM, ARSENICUM ALBUM, AURUM METAL, CAUSTICUM, CINA, HEPAR SULFUR, HYOSCIAMUS, IGNATIA, KALIUM PHOSPHORICUM, LACHESIS, LYCOPODIUM, MERCURIUS, NATRUM MURIATICUM, PLATINA, SEPIA, THUYA, TARENTULA HISPANA, VALERIANA, VERATRUM ALBUM

SCREAMING

- Teething, awkward and impossible to calm, the worst nights for the parents: JALAPA 15CH
- Does not want to be approached or touched, wants things and then throws them: CINA 15CH

Also see: APIS, AURUM METAL, CALCAREA PHOSPHORICA, CAUSTICUM, CICUTA VIROSA, CHAMOMILLA, CINA, CUPRUM, HELLEBORUS, HYOSCIAMUS, IGNATIA, LYCOPODIUM, PLATINA, STRAMONIUM, VERATRUM ALBUM

VIOLENT CHILD

CANNOT BEAR TO BE APPROACHED, TOUCHED, OR EVEN LOOKED AT

- Plump fat greedy child, extremely sensitive to cold bath, diarrhea, eczema: ANTIMONIUM CRUDUM 4CH to 15CH

Also see: AURUM, CHAMOMILLA, CINA, GELSEMIUM, HEPAR SULFUR, LYCOPODIUM, NATRUM CARBONICUM, NATRUM MURIATICUM, NUX VOMICA, SEPIA, SILICEA, SULFUR, THUYA

DESTRUCTIVE

- Delirium and delusions, fights and bites, mistrustful, suspicious, jealous, exhibitionist, varied phobia, fear of water just hearing it drop: HYOSCIAMUS 9CH and higher
- 2 other remedies for delirium:
  - High sudden fever: BELLADONNA 15CH
  - Night anguish: STRAMONIUM 9CH

Also see: ARSENICUM, CUPRUM METAL, MERCURIUS, NUX VOMICA, PLATINA, STAPHYSAGRIA, TARENTULA HISPANA, VERATRUM ALBUM

IMPATIENT

- ACONIT, ARGENTUM NITRICUM, CHAMOMILLA, COLOCYNTHIS, HEPAR SULFUR, IGNATIA, NATRUM MURIATICUM, NUX VOMICA, PULSATILLA, SEPIA, STAPHYSAGRIA, SULFUR

INSOLENT

- HYOSCIAMUS, LYCOPODIUM, NUX VOMICA, PLATINA, SULFUR, VERATRUM

REJECTS VIOLENTLY THINGS WHEN GIVEN

- CHAMOMILLA, CINA, IPECA, STAPHYSAGRIA

TEARS CLOTHES

- BELLADONNA, IGNATIA, STRAMONIUM, TARENTULA HISPANA, VERATRUM ALBUM

RUDENESS

- Fears and delusions, night restlessness, moaning and screaming, despaired and furious, prostration with icy coldness, vagotonia, fainting fits, violent vomiting and diarrhea with colic, anxious chest constriction: VERATRUM ALBUM 4CH

Also see: AURUM, HYOSCIAMUS, LYCOPODIUM, NUX VOMICA, STAPHYSAGRIA, STRAMONIUM

WHINING

- Awkward, throws and drops things given, rage, jealousy, fright, vexation, grief, fever: APIS 15CH
- Loquacity, jealousy, malicious, suspicious, commits underhanded actions, hysterical: LACHESIS 15CH
- Sullen mood, apprehensive and coward, afraid to be alone, incessant clinging, arrogant and quarrelsome, insolent and rude: LYCOPODIUM 15CH
- Fear being alone and of darkness, <in the evening and >by walking in open air, changeable mood, looks all the time for caresses, extremely emotional, melancholy, submissive, <by all kinds of heat, room, bed, weather, etc., and >by open air, see: PULSATILLA 15CH

Also see: AURUM METAL, CAUSTICUM, CHAMOMILLA, PULSATILLA, VERATUM ALBUM

COWARD

- Bashful, fear of strangers, hides when people come, slow understanding, tonsillitis recurrent and chronic: BARYTA CARBONICA 15CH and higher

Also see: ACONIT, BRYONIA, CHINA, GELSEMIUM, LYCOPODIUM, PULSATILLA, SILICEA, VERATRUM ALBUM

SLEEP DISORDERS

In the case of sleep disorders, homeopathy is of great help for the child and his family, especially when homeopathic remedies are introduced as soon as the disorders appear. Destabilizing of the metabolic rhythm metronome is to be analyzed through mind and general symptoms. Most patients share the same mind symptoms, such as anger, fatigue insomnia, sadness, and so on. A homeopathic diagnosis is always precise when it sticks to the Line of Life of the individual and to his reactive mode. In psychiatry, etiological factors must be taken into account with infinite care and the most reliable symptoms are general modalities. An easy start is to give JALAPA 15CH to the restless infant, or STRAMONIUM 9CH for night terrors.

DIFFICULTY FALLING ASLEEP AFTER AN ANIMATED CONVERSATION

- Cannot sleep from worries, must get up, emotional and timid, bashful and anxious, dread people, diaphragm spasms, palpitations, asthma, hysterical restlessness, loquacity: AMBRA GRISEA 9CH
- Joyful infant, wakes up during the night and wants to play, child oversensitive from school overwork, happy by pleasant thoughts, hyperactive and healthy: CYPRIPEDIUM 4CH

Also see: IGNATIA 9CH

NIGHT ANXIETY

- Nervous palpitations, hysterical reactions with numbness, asthma, delirium: SUMBUL 4CH
- Persistent insomnia, wakes up each night between 3 and 4 a.m., night sweat, excellent remedy for warts: THUYA OCCIDENTALIS 9CH

Also see: CAUSTICUM

NIGHT TERRORS

- Awakens terrified, delusions, violent painless muscle contractions, face, head, and limbs, convulsions, loquacity, incoherent talking, furious, fear of obscurity, needs a light all night, <in darkness and when alone, >by light and company: STRAMONIUM 9CH
- Restless hands and fingers, legs jerking, face twitching, moaning, stuttering, weeping fits, delusions, fears, horrible dreams, somnambulism, grinding teeth: KALIUM BROMATUM 9CH

Also see: BELLADONNA, HYOSCIAMUS

SORROWS

- Introverted and secretive, touchy and hateful, anger at trifles, checks if all the doors are correctly closed, fear of robbers, giggles/weeping, hysterical, palpitations, photosensitization, herpes, canker sores, hay fever, skinny with big appetite, craves salted foods and salt: NATRUM MURIATICUM 15CH and higher
- 2 satellite remedies of NATRUM MURIATICUM can be added:
  - Anxiety, sullen mood: IGNATIA 9CH
  - Physical symptoms, allergy: APIS 4CH

Also see: CAUSTICUM, IGNATIA

NERVOUS DRAINAGE

- Gemmotherapy: 5–20 drops in the evening: TILIA TOMENTOSA BUDS 1DH
- Oligotherapy: alternate MAGNESIUM TRACE ELEMENT/LITHIUM TRACE ELEMENT
- Satellite remedies:
  - Moderate anxiety: AVENA SATIVA/ASPERULA/ESCHSCHOLTZIA/PASSIFLORA/PISCIDIA/VALERIANA/a.a.p. 3DH
  - Severe anxiety, somatizations, delusions: HYOSCIAMUS/IGNATIA/STRAMONIUM/SUMBUL/a.a.p. 8DH

CONCLUSION

The practice of medicine and homeopathy gathers classical and modern knowledge. The symptoms expressed by the patient are the only solid base to first choose the remedies, and then perform an effective follow up after the patient started taking the remedies.

When you start practicing homeopathy, its power quickly manifests through results you might not have thought possible. When you heal an acute otitis media, rapidly and without side effects, with one dose of ARSENICUM ALBUM 15CH, you have an undeniable proof of the therapeutic effect of a low homeopathic dose. This same remedy is good for dry asthma attacks and can change the evolution of this chronic disease. After each acute manifestation treated with the correct homeopathic remedy, you can see the remission periods increase.

Some treatments can be very simple and yet the results are striking, such as giving 3 granules 2 times a day of THUYA 9CH for warts, APIS 4CH for allergic reactions, and IGNATIA 9CH for anxiety. In pediatrics, mental behaviors can be improved drastically. AMBRA GRISEA will help a timid child, and CINA 15 CH an awkward child. When physical symptoms are related to mental symptoms, and/or to concomitants and general modalities, homeopathy works at its best. For example, think about a patient suffering from otitis. He is aggravated by all kinds of heat and improved by cold applications, his weeping mood can change to a smile when comforted, he is never thirsty and runs a high fever. This patient will be treated successfully with PULSATILLA.

When I opened my first medical office at the beginning of my career, a young woman consulted me for a bad sinusitis. I gave her the appropriate allopathic treatment, but back she was, a week later, with stomach pains. According to the knowledge I acquired during my studies in medical school, I selected the appropriate allopathic treatment again but back she was, 3 weeks later, with terrible headaches and a severe cystitis. Disease was challenging me. I wanted to understand why the patient developed such a sequence of symptoms, and how I could help. I bought my first book on homeopathy. I have been practicing homeopathy ever since and never looked back.

BIBLIOGRAPHY

Allen H.C. *Keynotes and Characteristics with Comparisons.* Jain Publishing, New Delhi, reprint 1982.

Allen T.F. *Key and Characteristic Symptoms, Remedies of Fever, Materia Medica, Diseases and Therapeutics of the Skin.* Jain Publishing, New Delhi, reprint 1982.

Bach Ch. *Phytotherapie et matière médicale.* Lehning, 1982.

Barbancey J. *Pratique homéopathique en psychopathologie 1 and 2.* Similia, 1987.

Baur J. *L'enseignement du Dr Pierre Schmidt.* Similia, 1991.

Boericke W. *Materia Medica with Repertory.* Boericke ninth edition. 1927.

Boericke W., Dewey W.A. *The Twelve Tissue Remedies of Schüssler.*

Boger C.M. *Boenninghausen's Characteristics and Repertory, Synoptic Key of the Materia Medica.* Jain Publishing, New Delhi, reprint 1988.

Bouko L.M. *Homeopathy Everyday.* Bouko Levy, 1989, *Homeopathic and Drainage Repertory.* First edition. Similia, 1992, *Guide d'Homéopathie.* Adet Marseille 1993, *Homeopathic Drainage.* H.D.R.B. Publishing, 2015.

Bourgarit R. *Traiter votre enfant avec l'homéopathie, Thérapeutique homéopathique du nouveau-né et du nourrisson.*

Broussalian G. *Répertoire de Kent.* Broussalian, 1983, *Symptômes clés.* Broussalian, 1983, *Symptômes Mentaux.* Broussalian, 1983.

Burnett J.C. *Delicate, Backward, Puny, and Stunted Children, Enlarged Tonsil, Organ Diseases of Women, Diseases of Veins.* Jain Publishing, New Delhi, reprint 1982.

Coulter C.R. *Portraits of Homeopathic Medicines.*

Demangeat G. *Technique homéopathique, Cas cliniques.*

Denis M. *Homéopathie et dermatologie.* Similia.

Dufilho R. *Géographie homéopathique.* Coquemard Angoulème, 1965.

Duflo-Boujard O. *Ophthalmologie homéopathique.* Boiron, 1988.

Duprat H. *Matière médicale homéopathique.* JB Baillière, 1947.

Farrington E.A. *Comparative Materia Medica, Clinical Materia Medica, Lesser Writings.* Jain Publishing, New Delhi, reprint 1982.

Fortier-Bernoville, Renard L. *Comment guérir par l'homéopathie.* P.I.C., Paris, reprint 1954.

Hahnemann S. *Organon.* Hahnemann Foundation, 1982, Materia medica. Jain Publishing, New Delhi, reprint 1984, Chronic diseases.

Henry P. *Gemmothérapie.* Henry Pol, Belgium, 1982.

Herbert & Roberts. *Sensations as If.* Jain Publishing, New Delhi, reprint edition 1990.

Hippocrates. *Works, Aphorisms, Observation Method, Man, Nature, Disease Synthesis.*

Hodiamont G. *Homéopathie et physiologie.* J-B Ballière & Similia, 1983, *Plantes médicinales en homéopathie.* Debrus-Tensi, 1983, *Venins et remèdes du règne animal.* Brussels, 1957. Debrus-Tensi & Similia, 1984, *Nouvelles études d'homéopathie.* Brussels, 1960. Debrus-Tensi & Similia, 1984, *Matière médicale et remèdes végétaux.* Similia, 1985.

Julian O.-A. *Matière médicale homéopathique, Homéopathie et terrain, Micro-immunothérapie dynamisée.* Le François, Paris, 1977.

Jung C.G. *Symbolism of Body, Synchronicity and Paracelsia, Psychology and Alchemy.*

Kent J.T. *Materia Medica.* Jain Publishing, New Delhi, 1981, Repertory. Jain Publishing, New Delhi, 1981, *Lectures on homeopathic philosophy, Lesser writings.*

Kollitsch P. *Homéopathie: matière médicale, thérapeutique.* Helios, 1989.

Lathoud. *Matière médicale homéopathique.* Franche-Comté Impression Levier, 1981.

Lichtenthaeler C. *La médicine hippocratique.* A la Baconnière, Neuchatel, 1957, *La médicine hippocratique.* Les Frères Gonin Lausane, 1948.

Mendeleev D. Periodic table.

Missionary School of London. *Decachords.* Third edition. London, 1968.

Paracelsus. Medico-chemical works or Paradoxes.

Robert P. *Physiognomie.* Ferran Marseille, 1948.

Sananès R. *Homéopathie et language du corps.* Laffont, 1982, *Homéopathie et rhumathologie.* Similia, 1984, *Maux de tête et bleus de l'âme.* Laffont, 1986, *Insomnie Allergies, Digestif, Hormones et émotions.* Similia.

Schüssler W. Twelve Essential Mineral Salts.

Tyler M. *Homeopathic Drug Pictures.* Revised edition. The Homeopathic Publishing Company Limited, London, 1952.

Vallette A. *Homéopathie Infantile.* Maisonneuve, 1975.

Valnet J. *Aromathérapie.* Maloine, Paris, reprint 1975, *Phytothérapie, traitement des maladies par les plantes.* Maloine, Paris, reprint 1979.

Van Hellemont J. *Phytotherapy Compendium.* Belgium.

Vannier L. *Thérapeutique homéopathique.* Doin, 1977, La pratique de l'homéopathie, Typologie, Remèdes homéopathiques des cas aigus.

Vannier L., Poirier J. *Matière médicale homéopathique.*

Voisin H. *Matière médicale homéopathique.* Second edition. Maloine, Paris, 1976, *Répertoire homéopathique.* second edition Maloine, Paris, 1978.

Zissu R. *Matière médicale homéopathique constitutionnelle.* Le François, Paris, 1977.

30 Nutritional and Alternative Medicine
Legal and Ethical Considerations

Peter A. Arhangelsky, Esq.[1]

CONTENTS

Dual System of Government: State Boards and the FDA 746
FDA's Historical Bias against Alternative Products and Services 748
FDA's Regulation of Alternative Medicine 751
    FDA's Broad Definition of "Drug" 752
    FDA Regulation of Herbal Medicines, Dietary Supplements, Medical Foods, and Devices ... 753
        Herbal Products and Dietary Supplements 754
        Medical Devices 755
Specific Federal Regulatory Concerns for Alternative Practitioners 756
    Physician Dispensing and Compounding 756
    Telemedicine and Distance Consulting 758
    FTC Standards and Regulation 760
Changes to the Federal and State Regulations to Promote Health Freedom 761
    Changes to FDA Regulations 761
        Strengthen Laws That Permit Off-Label Use 761
        Broaden FDA's Expanded Access Regulations 762
        Lift Restrictions on Preventative or Wellness Advertising Related to Nutritional Products 763
    New Legislation to Promote Health Freedom 764
        Privatized Review for Alternative Medical Therapies 764
        Expand Freedom of Choice in Health Care by Expanding Access to Telemedicine 765
        Stronger Informed Consent Laws That Facilitate Medical Choice 765
Conclusion 765
End Notes 766

Practitioners who treat patients outside of the mainstream medical orthodoxy face risks peculiar to them that arise under federal and state law. Federal and state laws generally equate allopathic modalities with the expected standard of care. Nonetheless, complementary and alternative medicine has incrementally gained more protection in the law over time based on emerging legal doctrine, expanded protections at the state level, and broader medical education (particularly in the nutrition sciences). This chapter provides an overview of the federal legal systems that govern alternative medicine. It explains the legal difficulties and limitations confronting alternative medicine as it grows within a regulatory system designed around conventional care. Employing alternative medical therapies usually requires the purchase or sale of articles regulated by the U.S. Food and Drug Administration (FDA). This chapter describes the means by which practitioners can lawfully develop and use those regulated therapies in their practices and during patient care; the permissible scope of physician advertising; and the legal changes recommended to encourage medical innovation and growth in medical fields like alternative services and personalized medicine.

Each circumstance begets a potentially different legal analysis and, so, like the practice of medicine, there is no substitute for an evaluation based on the unique facts that define each case. We therefore caution at the outset that this chapter is educational and not meant to be applied in an individual case. Health care providers must act properly within the scope of state licensing laws. A comprehensive analysis of each state jurisdiction is impractical—each state employs schemes that differ in certain respects from other states. Practitioners must satisfy board regulations and, wherever questions arise concerning those regulations, regulated persons are well-advised to seek advice from legal counsel licensed in the state who have particular expertise in practice before the state's medical board and regulators.

DUAL SYSTEM OF GOVERNMENT: STATE BOARDS AND THE FDA

Health care practitioners are regulated at the state and federal levels. Operating with plenary authority over health and safety, each state has implemented a comprehensive regulatory scheme that governs the practice of medicine. Beyond statutes defining the practice of medicine in a state, medical boards adopt regulations and decisions that have the force of law to govern the intricacies of medical practice. Practitioners must understand not only statutory limits on medical practice but also the disciplinary rules, licensure requirements, continuing medical education requirements, and other generalized rules of ethics and professional conduct that govern their treatment choices and conduct. All states define the practice of medicine through statutes and regulations. Those statutes are broadly constructed to reach almost all healing arts and activities. For instance, California encompasses the following activities within the practice of medicine: "any system or mode of treating the sick or afflicted in this state, or who diagnoses, treats, operates for, or prescribes for any ailment, blemish, deformity, disease, disfigurement, disorder, injury, or other physical or mental condition of any person...".[2] Those definitional constructs are broad enough to encompass virtually every kind of treatment given to a patient or consumer. Under state law, practicing "medicine" without a license is a criminal offense.[3] The penalties for that conduct can be significant.

Once commonly condemned by medical boards, complementary and alternative medicine (CAM) has gained greater protection under state law. Most states have enacted formal regulatory models for nutritional practices and naturopathic practice. Novel regulatory approaches at the state level have opened access in previously unavailable or underserved areas. For instance, California allows certain nutritionists to practice without formal regulation provided the nutritionist maintains a narrow practice that avoids certain procedures or treatment otherwise reserved for licensed physicians.[4]

Operating a lawful practice still begins at the state level. Practices form under state law and follow standards of care established in local markets. Regulated practices (e.g., naturopaths, medical doctors, osteopaths, etc.) must apply for licensure through the supervising state board. Unethical or negligent practice is subject to disciplinary action at the state level through those governing boards.

Although the practice of medicine has historically (and exclusively) been regulated at the state level, federal agencies have increasingly encroached on areas previously regulated exclusively at the state level. State regulating boards have cited the failure to comply with federal law as a basis for disciplinary action. Some states have enacted licensure requirements that mandate compliance with all applicable laws, which include federal law.[5] The U.S. Food and Drug Administration (FDA) has routinely teamed with state investigators and law enforcement in gathering evidence from, or engaging in enforcement action against, practitioners and health clinics. Alternative medicine is particularly vulnerable at the federal level because medical devices and certain drugs, for example, certain compounded drugs such as bioidentical hormones, offered by practitioners may not be approved by the FDA. State regulators increasingly look to the federal government for guidance. The FDA gives regulators a uniform model applied across state borders for multijurisdictional issues. As FDA involves itself more in regulating compounding (including by physicians) and in policing drugs and devices in the market (including in medical practices), the principles of federalism that once shielded local practitioners and facilitated the development of novel, personalized patient care have increasingly given way to federal regulation.

The FDA has no statutory mandate to regulate the practice of medicine. Congress expressly limited the agency's ability to encroach on those historically state-regulated activities.[6] The federal courts have acknowledged FDA's limited powers over medical practice.[7] Yet, despite those strongly worded decisions, the FDA now exerts great influence and power over medical practices, in part, because the courts have failed to enforce the limitations of the Commerce Clause in Article 1, Section 8 of the U.S. Constitution. FDA's authority to regulate is largely coterminous with the Commerce Clause, meaning that FDA's reach into physicians' offices is now greater than ever.

The FDA regulates every tool, article, drug, or device that physicians use in their practices. Physicians rarely advertise services or treat patients without falling under an FDA regulation. The FDA boasts that it regulates "25 cents of every dollar spent by American consumers each year."[8] FDA laws and regulations therefore have a substantial reach, even at the local level. The Federal Trade Commission (FTC) regulates advertisements and promotions, including those by physicians and clinics for health care services. The Centers for Medicare & Medicaid Services (CMS) administers the Medicare programs. CMS regulations, policy decisions, Local Coverage Determinations (LCDs), and National Coverage Determinations (NCDs) directly influence the types of services offered to patients. The Drug Enforcement Administration (DEA) enforces laws and regulations related to controlled substances. DEA has the authority to schedule new substances under the Controlled Substances Act (CSA).[9] DEA also provides physician "registrations" that govern who may dispense or prescribe certain medications to patients.

Recent legal decisions at the federal level have affirmed the FDA's broad power over medicine. In 2012, the FDA regulated autologous stem cell procedures. As a medical procedure, the practice of transplanting stem cells had generally been within the ambit of state medical board regulation. The FDA argued that the administration of autologous cells was a new "drug" under the Federal Food, Drug, and Cosmetic Act (FDCA).[10] A Colorado laboratory had developed a procedure involving extraction of autologous stem cells that were later returned to patients following laboratory growth and expansion. Although the procedure largely concerned physical or surgical medicine, the FDA regulated the entire protocol under the "drug" standards, in part, because the laboratory had used FDA-approved drugs to preserve and encourage cell growth during the laboratory expansion process.[11]

More recently, the United States Court of Appeals for the Ninth Circuit issued a decision in September 2016 upholding the felony conviction of a Nevada urologist who had used a medical device in his practice for "off-label" uses.[12] Section 301(k) of the FDCA (21 U.S.C. § 331(k)) broadly prohibits "the doing of any ... act with respect to ... [a] drug [or] device ... if such act is done while such article is held for sale ... after shipment in interstate commerce and results in such article being adulterated."[13] Traditionally, the "held for sale" element never applied to physicians treating people directly within the doctor-patient relationship. The Ninth Circuit was asked to determine whether "a doctor's use of a device in the course of treating a patient [would] be considered a 'sale' under the [FDCA]?"[14] The court ultimately held that a regulated FDA article could be "held for sale" simply because the physician used the device in treating patients. The *Kaplan* case is a landmark decision, and one of first impression in the Ninth Circuit. The Ninth Circuit cited the *Regenerative* decision as support for its broad extension of FDA statutes into the physician-patient relationship. The rule from *Kaplan* is that physicians may not use "adulterated" products with patients; doing so now violates federal law.[15] The ruling also indicates that certain in-office treatments could be regulated as "sales" under the federal laws. The decision has major implications because most violations of the federal law result in "adulterated" product. For instance, the failure to follow current Good Manufacturing Practices in the preparation and sale of FDA products like dietary supplements renders those products "adulterated" under federal law.[16] The *Kaplan* decision suggests that physicians can be directly regulated by the FDA.

An understanding of federal law is therefore essential for any practitioner, and particularly for alternative practitioners. Successful practices advertise to local and out-of-state patients—a practice easily facilitated through the advent of information technologies (web-based conferencing, Internet marketing, etc.). Patients have incentives to reach beyond borders for innovative procedures that are not widely available.[17] The Internet connects patients with practitioners, but, unfortunately, also creates an interstate hook that enables the exercise of federal jurisdiction. As a consequence, the most relevant legal questions for CAM practitioners often in one way or another turn on interpretation of federal regulations.

FDA'S HISTORICAL BIAS AGAINST ALTERNATIVE PRODUCTS AND SERVICES

Nutrition science, herbal remedies, and food healing are common concepts in certain fields, including CAM. Foods and dietary supplements are generally not subject to premarket review under the federal law. That fact and FDA's statutory definition for the term "new drug" (which is based not on a substance's intrinsic characteristics or effects but on the intended use of it, i.e., anything intended for use in the treatment or prevention of disease is a "drug"), combined with aggressive protectionism in favor of approved drugs and against unapproved new drugs, lead invariably to a conflict between federal authorities and CAM practitioners. The FDA usually exercises strict control over regulated products. For almost all drugs, devices, biologics, and so on, the FDA requires premarket review (of some kind) before a product can proceed to market. FDA also delimits the indications for use of a drug, albeit a drug may be used by physicians for an off-label use (but may not lawfully be promoted by a physician or by the drug sponsor for that use). Under FDA's broad definition of "drugs,"[18] the agency can control any product that purports to affect any structure or function of the human body. The FDA receives substantial funding from the pharmaceutical industry, in part through "user fees," which are exorbitant application and facility registration fees paid into the FDA during the drug approval process. The FDA is an organization designed and staffed to accommodate orthodox, allopathic medical practices and the industries supporting same. The "drug approval" process is a costly process that few businesses can afford, which creates a government-sponsored oligopoly over certain therapeutic products. At present, to secure FDA approval of a "new drug," companies should expect to devote between $1.4 and $2.8 billion dollars to the effort.[19] A significant portion of that investment is earmarked for clinical studies sufficient to satisfy FDA standards. While few would question the need for safe, effective medicines, the FDA's approach to "drug" regulation generally shutters from the market alternative products that may not be patentable or may not fit squarely within the allopathic drug testing model. Most foods and dietary supplements cannot be marketed to consumers for therapeutic purposes of any kind.

Alternative medical practices rely on herbal medicines, energy-based concepts, natural medicine, and many similar modalities that are not subject to FDA premarket review, and also threaten the market for those pharmaceutical products already approved by the FDA. The lack of federal oversight has resulted in a biased administrative perspective against most alternative treatments. The FDA's consistent war on dietary supplements is just one example.

With heavy skepticism, the FDA has continually limited the market for dietary supplements promoted for therapeutic or preventative purposes. In the 1960s and 1970s, the FDA classified certain vitamins as over-the-counter (OTC) drug products. After Congress defeated those measures through the Proxmire/Rogers amendment, the FDA shifted to a "food additive" theory, under which the FDA blocked dietary ingredients from the market based on the premarket approval requirements unique to food additives. In 1993, Congress responded with the Dietary Supplement Health Education Act (DSHEA).[20] The DSHEA provided important safeguards that facilitate the free-flow of information to consumers concerning the health benefits of nutritional supplements, foods, and dietary ingredients. The FDA was infuriated. Then-acting FDA Commissioner David Kessler reportedly instructed FDA officials not to enforce the DSHEA.[21] Kessler was convinced that Congress would be forced to repeal the law if the public witnessed the worst elements of the dietary supplement industry.

Alternative practitioners must understand FDA's inherent bias against non-traditional medical practices. FDA's policies ultimately dictate whether CAM practitioners can develop and market the healing arts (and tools used to heal). Federal regulators have outwardly rejected CAM for lacking conventional "evidence-based" data or proof establishing the efficacy of those treatments. The FDA's approach to evidence-based medicine is problematic for many alternative systems, particularly those that rely on preventative measures that reduce risk of medical conditions or disease. FDA's and FTC's demands for exceptionally expensive long-term human clinical intervention studies have raised serious ethical and logistical questions for products that cannot fit neatly within the pharmaceutical model.

Both the FDA and FTC (and most interested federal agencies) follow an evidence-based scientific model that requires human clinical testing to demonstrate the efficacy of new therapies or treatments. For instance, companies or practitioners seeking to promote "health claims" for dietary supplements must satisfy FDA's rigorous review under the Evidence-Based Review System (the EBRS). Requiring credible scientific evidence is a well-justified position. But the FDA has interpreted those principles in ways that allow the agency to ignore evidence with which it disagrees. Thus, the FDA's review focuses only on a subset of politically favored clinical studies, while often disregarding reams of supportive science that the scientific community ordinarily accepts as relevant to an evaluation of the totality of publicly available evidence.

Under that system, the FDA generally will not approve a health claim for dietary supplements or foods without at least two randomized, placebo-controlled, double-blinded human clinical studies of high methodological quality (RCTs). The FTC backed FDA's interpretation by requiring, at minimum, two human clinical studies in support of promotional health claims.[22] And the standards for those clinical studies are set impossibly high. Thus, FDA and FTC have created a de facto baseline for establishing the efficacy of novel modalities offered at the consumer level and, perhaps, within the physician-patient relationship. Those FDA EBRS standards are borne from an antiquated system designed for pharmaceuticals.[23] For foods, dietary supplements, dietary ingredients, medical foods, and similar articles, the EBRS standards are impractical. Moreover, developing that level of substantiation is likely unethical for clinical investigators and physicians.

In 2013, the FTC targeted POM Wonderful's health claims associated with its pomegranate juice product. POM had sought to promote the general health benefits of pomegranate juice, including the cardiovascular benefits documented within POM's $34 million worth of supportive research.[24] FTC deemed some of POM's claims to be "drug" or "disease" claims under federal law. Operating under standards like the FDA's EBRS, the FTC's experts explained in litigation that POM would have needed two clinical studies of such breadth and scope that the total estimated cost *per study* was calculated at $600 million.[25] In other words, the FTC's experts testified under oath that POM would have required a research investment of $1.2 billion simply to promote the cardiovascular benefits of its pomegranate juice. Quite obviously, alternative practitioners and sellers of medicinal products that aid alternative health care cannot afford the pharmaceutical game, particularly where many naturally sourced products (e.g., dietary ingredients) are not patentable. These FTC and FDA policies encompass all regulated product categories. Because the standards are impossibly high, even reliable and efficacious therapies will likely not reach consumers if forced through the FDA's regime. To change how FDA perceives these products, and open channels for product development, the alternative medical fields need to focus on defending empirical endpoints commonly applied in each practice area.

Pharmaceutical agents are often designed to effect acute changes in body chemistry that address clearly defined abnormalities or biophysical dysfunction.[26] Alternative therapies, by contrast, often focus on preventative measures, overall wellness, and whole-body healing through natural mechanisms. Preventative therapies or wellness plans can be ill-suited to conventional "drug" intervention studies.

Unlike drug studies which often measure notable changes to acute conditions or endpoints over shorter durations, preventative and wellness medicine requires substantially more data over much longer durations. Foods, dietary supplements, energetic therapies, and herbal and homeopathic modalities often claim to reduce *risk* of experiencing certain adverse outcomes over time. Study design must confront the many confounding factors, variables, and impractically long durations necessary to prove positive outcomes under FDA's standards. Because we cannot predict with certainty who will experience certain outcomes, study population sizes must be substantial enough to include representative data that would also power statistically significant results. In preventative medicine or wellness studies, the durations would need to span decades at tremendous (if not impossible) costs to the sponsor. Longer study durations result in higher risk of confounders and protocol deviations. Maintaining protocol compliance becomes far more challenging. Drop-out rates increase substantially. Clinical investigators cannot control a subject's exact diet over 20 years. Data over longer durational studies in nutrition fields is almost always obtained through self-reported input from the test subjects—an element that FDA has rejected as imprecise. Ultimately, achieving a sound, pharmaceutical-grade clinical study for natural wellness and preventative therapies is near impossible because: (1) the cost to operate a methodologically sound study would be insurmountable; and (2) FDA could likely find enough bias to reject the data if the agency did not approve of the conclusion. Based on these concerns, "[s]everal nutrition researchers have, in recent years, raised concerns over what is perceived to be the misapplication of drug-based trials to assess nutrition questions, without taking into account the totality of the evidence or the complexities and nuances of nutrition."[27]

In the context of preventative therapies, the FDA and FTC have also ignored significant ethical issues in their demands for strict pharmaceutical-grade evidence.[28] Placebo-controlled studies may be unethical in preventative medicine that uses alternative or natural systems. Preventative approaches are offered to prevent or reduce the risk of disease onset in the first instance. If the hypothesis is that a preventative protocol would prevent disease, then providing placebo-controlled therapies to healthy subjects arguably denies those subjects important medical care. In reality the investigators have denied the control group a nutrient, therapy, or protocol that may reduce risk of a life-threatening condition over time. The status quo may, in hindsight, be unpalatable for researchers. If the study ultimately produces statistically significant results, that means the subjects in the control group actually developed disease conditions in higher frequencies.

Experts have thus condemned FDA's approach to evidence-based medicine in the nutrition context. "[M]edical interventions are designed to cure a disease *not* produced by their absence, while nutrients prevent dysfunction that would result from their inadequate intake..."[29] In other words, by withholding the nutrients from subjects in a food study, the investigators might actually cause the condition in otherwise healthy subjects:

> In order to conduct a RCT that adequately tests the efficacy of a nutrient for a specific chronic disease, it will usually be important to ensure an adequate contrast in intake between the intervention and the control groups. The control intake is an approximate analog of the placebo control in drug RCTs. However, since sufficiently low intakes are associated with significant disease in some body systems, doing so can lead to serious ethical problems, particularly if the disease outcome is serious and/or irreversible...[30]

In Blumberg et al., the authors discussed the contrasts between evidence-based *medicine* (EBM) and evidence-based *nutrition* (EBN):

> EBN thus departs from the situation of EBM, where, for most interventions, the use of a no-intake control group is usually quite appropriate. In EBM, the hypothesis is that adding an intervention ameliorates a disease, whereas in EBN it is that reducing the intake of a nutrient [or limiting that intake] causes (or increases the risk of) disease. This distinction is critical. No one proposes in EBM that a disease is caused by the absence of its remedy; whereas for nutrients the hypothesis is precisely that malfunction is caused by deficiency. A hypothesis about disease causation can rarely, if ever, be directly tested in humans using the RCT design. This is because in the RCT the disease/dysfunction occurs in at least some of the study participants, and the investigators must ensure that this will happen. Instead, where EBN must operate is with respect to two related, but different questions: (i) In addition to disease X, does the inadequate intake of nutrient A also contribute to other diseases? And (ii) at what level of intake of nutrient A is risk of all related disease minimized or all related functions optimized?[31]

In the drug model, investigators merely preserve the status quo in the placebo group. In nutritional studies, the investigators might contribute to the harm. Those same criticisms are equally applicable to alternative medical fields including, for example, Ayurvedic and Chinese medicine, which rely on nutritional or herbal products to promote wellness over time.

The FDA's EBRS is misguided as applied to alternative medicine and nutrition science. As a result, few companies or practitioners could ever satisfy those standards that are stacked in favor of large, financially endowed pharmaceutical interests. At a cost of $1.2 billion to develop an FDA-approved drug product, the game can be played only by pharmaceuticals that have patent rights in new chemical moieties (which permits them to recoup the heavy investment in research and development).

The unfortunate result is that alternative treatments appear to fail FDA's efficacy standards when those products cannot marshal the large-scale clinical studies that FDA expects in the drug context. FDA becomes highly skeptical of any product or treatment that lacks clinical trial proof of efficacy. Thus, historically, the FDA has disfavored alternative healing arts and products.

Because the FDA's standards now permeate all levels of medical regulation, CAM practitioners must appreciate the federal government's perspective on efficacy data, and understand the level of proof required by the FDA. CAM practitioners must strive to develop alternative endpoints in clinical research that, with sufficient support, can be advanced as "generally accepted" in the relevant medical community. An alternative evidence-based model must be advanced for preventative, wellness, and alternative medical systems; and the FDA must be legally compelled to accept those standards. Medical professionals need to revisit the FDA's Evidence-Based Review System (EBRS) as applied to nutritional products and alternative medicine. The FDA must begin to consider more concept-based data, including animal, in vitro, and mechanistic studies. Pressure from industry can help sway the FDA on these issues. The FDA should expand its EBRS to incorporate observational data as primary data (including cohort studies and case-control studies).[32] The agency should review *each* study for its scientific merit and weigh those studies against the actual risk to consumers from ingestion of the nutrient. Advancing medical innovation requires the FDA to consider all forms of reliable medical data. Rejecting data because it would not fit neatly within the FDA's concept of a large-scale clinical model is scientifically unreasonable.

But without change, the federal and state bureaucracies continue to funnel information through traditional medical paradigms. Accordingly, for alternative medical practices to flourish and grow within our modern administrative state, practitioners must develop generally accepted endpoints (or surrogate endpoints) that can translate within the administrative bureaucracy. For therapies involving energy medicine or mind–body medicine, workable quantitative and qualitative endpoints are essential to avoid adverse regulatory enforcement, and to expand the universe of available products and therapies at all levels in commerce.

FDA'S REGULATION OF ALTERNATIVE MEDICINE

When using FDA-regulated products in patient care, practitioners should fully understand how those products are regulated at the federal level. That knowledge is essential for any practitioner advertising services in interstate channels (including the Internet), or selling products to patients directly or indirectly. Practitioners who endorse specific products or dispense FDA-regulated articles are likely to be "regulated" persons under the federal law.

The FDA has generally divided "Complementary and Alternative Medicine" into several broad categories, including: biologically based practices; energy medicine; manipulative and body-based practices; mind–body medicine; and whole medical systems.[33] At the federal regulatory level, those medical practices are likely to involve the following regulated articles in various forms: drugs; foods, dietary supplements, or medical foods; homeopathics; medical devices; laboratory tests or diagnostics; and blood- or tissue-based products. Biologically based practices involve nutritional modalities that rely on foods, dietary supplements, and dietary changes that influence overall health.

Energy medicine often relies on the body's internal energy fields and the balancing of same. Energy medicine may involve "medical devices" to affect change where the practitioner uses a tool or device to alter the body's internal fields. Manipulative and body-based medicine encompass a wide range of physical techniques that might include reflexology, massage, chiropractic, and so on. Those practices face the least regulatory oversight at the federal level. But, where devices or equipment are used to assist the practitioner, the FDA will exercise jurisdiction. Similarly, mind–body medicine (e.g., yoga, biofeedback, etc.) is likely not subject to regulation at the federal level unless the practitioner uses devices to affect the body. Diagnostic tools and devices have been employed in certain settings, particularly in biofeedback techniques. Those devices (and thus the practice generally) become FDA- and FTC-regulated. "Whole Medical Systems" like traditional Chinese medicine and Ayurvedic medicine are also regulated to the extent practitioners administer external articles during patient care, including, for example, botanicals, dietary ingredients, nutritional products, devices, or any other regulated article.

A precise discussion of the FDA-regulated categories for relevant medical products follows with illustrative examples. A product will be regulated as a "drug" or perhaps something else entirely based on the intended use.

FDA's BROAD DEFINITION OF "DRUG"

In the federal Food, Drug, and Cosmetic Act (FDCA), Congress defined the term "drug" as follows:

A. Articles recognized in the official United States Pharmacopoeia, official Homoeopathic Pharmacopoeia of the United States, or official National Formulary, or any supplement to any of them; and

B. Articles intended for use in the diagnosis, cure, mitigation, treatment, or prevention of disease in man or other animals; and

C. Articles (other than food) intended to affect the structure or any function of the body of man or other animals; and

D. Articles intended for use as a component of any article specified in clause (A), (B), or (C).[34]

Because the statutory definition includes articles "intended for use" in treatment, or that affect any structure or function of the body, the term "drug" encompasses most therapeutic products that are ingested or applied to the skin. Under the FDA's "intended use doctrine," the agency considers all relevant information when determining how to classify a product. A product's "intended use" governs the regulatory status of that product. That intended use can be drawn from marketing statements, manufacturer brochures, sales pitches, convention lecture, and even social media commentary.

Under the intended use doctrine, therefore, a glass of orange juice can be regulated as a drug, food, dietary supplement, or cosmetic, depending on the intended use. If consumed as a beverage for taste and nutrition, FDA would regulate the product as a food. If consumed to increase the daily ration of Vitamin C, the product could be a dietary supplement. If used to alter the appearance or texture of hair, the product is a cosmetic. And if administered to reduce the duration of the common cold, the product would be a drug. The focus is on *how* the seller promotes the product to consumers or patients. Accordingly, any product (natural or synthetic) promoted for therapeutic purposes can be regulated as a drug under FDA law.

The consequences of "drug" regulation are significant. Prescription drugs can generally be marketed only with premarket approval through the FDA. Sales or use of "unapproved" new drugs expose individuals to steep penalties, including potential criminal action. The FDA has acted against health care clinics that provide access to so-called "unapproved" drug therapies. State laws have followed suit, adopting verbatim the FDA's "drug" definitions and often mirroring the FDA's network of drug regulations.[35]

A "new drug" can proceed to market under limited circumstances, generally through the drug approval process following a New Drug Application (NDA). Development of drug products first requires research under an Investigational New Drug Application (IND), followed by clinical studies. The estimated cost of drug approval for most drugs in the United States has now surpassed $2 billion.[36]

Certain over-the-counter drugs can be marketed under an FDA "monograph" system, whereby FDA has approved specific recipes and formulations for treatment of low-risk conditions. OTC drugs that fall beyond the FDA monographs must pass through the NDA process. The FDA has also adopted a process for generic drug applications that allows for the sale of bioequivalent formulations.

For many alternative practitioners, the definition of "drug" encompasses most natural remedies used with patients, including, for instance, herbal remedies. But most natural products will never proceed through the drug approval process. For that reason, practitioners depend on the FDA's tolerance of "off-label" use in patient care. The "off-label" use doctrine permits health care providers to use "approved" drugs for a so-called "unapproved" uses that are deemed medically appropriate. Off-label use is widespread in conventional medicine. For instance, when a physician prescribes an intravenous injection rather than oral ingestion, the different route of administration would be considered an "unapproved" use—but a use that physician may reasonably prescribe to suit a patient's needs if appropriate. Use of chemotherapy to treat certain kinds of cancers is considered an "unapproved" use in many instances. Chemotherapy has never been approved for use with children, although oncologists routinely prescribe same. Even a simple increase in dosage could be considered an unapproved, "off-label" usage. The most common unapproved uses relate to the prescription of FDA-approved drugs for intended uses that are not labeled. The field of mental health has depended on off-label uses. Researchers at Stanford recently found that of the top 14 drugs used for off-label purposes, the majority were mental health products like Zoloft and Celebrex, that were then administered off-label for other mental health conditions.[37] In some instances, the majority of prescriptions for certain drugs went to off-label uses.[38] Under conventional FDA law, those "unapproved" uses are strictly prohibited by law. While FDA historically condones the practice because of the agency's inability to directly regulate the practice of medicine, the agency has taken a more direct role recently in policing speech relevant to off-label use.

Now, recent legal decisions at the federal level have forced FDA to address the parameters of "off-label" practice. Courts have explained that "FDA[-]approved indications were not intended to limit or interfere with the practice of medicine nor to preclude physicians from using their best judgment in the interest of the patient."[39] In response, the FDA has announced official agency action that might lead to regulation in this pivotal area. The practice of medicine depends on broad "off-label" practices for unfettered innovation and individualized care. Restriction of the "off-label" doctrine is one of the most significant threats to the practice of alternative therapies in the 50 states. Alternative practitioners should advocate for an "off-label" doctrine that facilitates use of approved medications for off-label uses, but also "unapproved" therapies with established histories of safe use. Congressional action might be required to bolster physician autonomy within patient care. Subject to the laws and regulations of each state's regulatory board (which are adequate to protect patient safety), physicians and providers must have discretion to use any approved or "unapproved" therapy that falls within the standard of care. Intervention at the federal level with one-size-fits-all regulation unduly limits access to individualized medical care, and stifles innovation and creativity.

FDA REGULATION OF HERBAL MEDICINES, DIETARY SUPPLEMENTS, MEDICAL FOODS, AND DEVICES

To successfully market a product (or service that uses a product) under federal law, the product cannot be classified as an "unapproved" drug. The product must fall within the confines of another regulatory category. Products used in alternative care often fall within the definition of "dietary supplement," "medical food," or "medical device." For example, many biologically based therapies rely on botanical products, functional foods, probiotics, vitamins, or mineral products that could qualify as "dietary supplements" or "medical foods" under FDA regulations. The FDA has expressly rejected any suggestion that holistic or natural products within CAM practices would not be directly regulated: "the [FDCA] nor the PHS Act contains any exemption for CAM products. In other words, if a product meets the statutory definition of a drug, device, biologic product, food, etc., it will be subject to regulation under the Act and/or the PHS Act."[40]

Herbal Products and Dietary Supplements

Herbal products are frequently used as medicinal agents in alternative practices. Those products might be regulated under several categories. Products applied topically are likely considered "drugs." In most instances, where an herbal remedy is applied for therapeutic purposes, the FDA would classify the product as a "drug" unless an exemption applies. These products are often sold as "dietary supplements" on the open market. Practitioners later apply those dietary supplements for off-label uses in their medical practices. As discussed earlier (and throughout this chapter), a broad policy concerning off-label use is necessary to protect physicians using these products, particularly if those physicians advertise or promote the products themselves.

The term "dietary supplement" under federal law means "a product (other than tobacco) intended to supplement the diet that bears or contains one or more of the following dietary ingredients: (A) a vitamin; (B) a mineral; (C) an herb or other botanical; (D) an amino acid; (E) a dietary substance for use by man to supplement the diet by increasing the total dietary intake; or (F) a concentrate, metabolite, constituent, extract, or combination of any ingredient described in clause (A), (B), (C), (D), or (E)."[41] As relevant to this chapter, a dietary supplement is defined based on the product's "intended use," meaning that a supplement cannot be intended for use as a therapeutic agent. The supplement must also be "intended for ingestion" and cannot be represented as a conventional food.[42] Also, a dietary supplement generally cannot be an article approved as a drug or biologic by the FDA.[43] So, any product that contains an ingredient already approved by the FDA as a drug cannot then be marketed as a dietary supplement unless that ingredient was clearly marketed as a food or supplement before the FDA approved the drug application. Moreover, dietary supplements cannot consist of any article that was first *investigated* as a drug product (under an Investigational New Drug application) before that same article was sold to consumers as a food or dietary supplement.

FDA regulations governing dietary supplements are frequently at issue in naturopathic practices, where practitioners use herbal or botanical products and may wish to sell product to patients. Sales of product for wellness purposes are generally permissible. However, if the same product was sold for therapeutic purposes, the FDA would classify the product as a "drug," and that violates the federal Act through the sale of an unapproved drug product. For example, sales of supplements containing citric acid may be effective in treating urinary tract infections, preventing nephrolithiasis (kidney stone), or maintaining healthy bladder function. If sold for the general maintenance of healthy urinary tracts, a citric acid-containing product could theoretically be sold as a dietary supplement. But if sold to treat urinary tract disorders, FDA would regulate that same product as a drug. Through the Dietary Supplement Health Education Act (DSHEA) and the Nutrition Labeling and Education Act (NLEA), sellers of dietary supplements have a range of information that can permissibly flow to patients or consumers. But that information does not include "drug" claims according to the FDA.

Practitioners selling dietary supplements (including herbal products) must generally adhere to the regulations governing dietary supplements. Products sold for use with patients should bear suitable labeling under 21 C.F.R. Part 101.36, which governs dietary supplement labeling. Dietary supplements may never be used for topical purposes. Any therapeutic agent applied topically that purports to affect the structure or function of the body will be classified as a drug under federal law. Note that most states have food and drug laws that incorporate the federal act and, so, products improperly marketed at the federal level are usually unlawful on the state level as well. For example, California has enacted food and drug laws that mirror (and generally adopt) the federal laws verbatim.

Practitioners may also wish to apply herbal remedies through homeopathic tinctures. The FDA has exempted homeopathic products from the new drug regulations based on the agency's enforcement discretion. Under FDA guidance documents, homeopathic products should be limited to those appearing in the Homeopathic Pharmacopeia of the United States and its supplements.[44] The dividing line between homeopathic and unapproved drug can be difficult to discern for certain products, particularly those which have lesser dilutions. The FDA's policy on homeopathy should not be overextended to reach conventional drugs or drug products. For instance, the FDA recently acted against practitioners that sold diluted forms of HCG (human chorionic gonadotropin) claiming those agents were homeopathic based on dilution. Moreover, in late 2016, the FTC dramatically reduced the universe of potential homeopathic claims and products through an "enforcement policy" extending FTC advertising standards to all homeopathic products, regardless of the FDA's long-standing policies.[45] The FTC requires "competent and reliable" evidence, including human clinical studies, to support all homeopathic claims.[46] See *infra* Part IV.C (discussing FTC advertising standards). That position effectively rejects traditional "provings" under homeopathic principles. FTC based that decision on its belief that "homeopathic product claims are not based on modern scientific methods and are not accepted by modern medical experts."[47] The FTC will require substantial disclosures and qualifying language on homeopathic labels to avoid enforcement. Manufacturers, retailers, and practitioners marketing homeopathics must now consult counsel to determine how best to position products in the market following FTC's new and substantial limitations.

Medical Devices

A medical device is any "instrument, apparatus, implement, machine, contrivance, implant, in vitro reagent, or other similar or related article, including any component, part, or accessory which is—(1) recognized in the official National Formulary, or the United States Pharmacopeia, or any supplement to them, (2) intended for use in the diagnosis of disease or other conditions, or in the cure, mitigation, treatment, or prevention of disease in man or other animals, or (3) intended to affect the structure or function of the body of man or other animals, and which does not achieve its primary intended purposes through chemical action within or on the body of man or other animals, and which is not dependent upon being metabolized for the achievement of its primary intended purposes."[48]

Most regulated persons fail to appreciate just how broad the FDA's definition of "medical device" becomes when applied. Unlike dietary supplements, which have exemptions in the DSHEA that allow for structure/function claims, almost any product used to manipulate the body physically for treatment or diagnostic purposes will be a regulable device. Moreover, unlike foods and dietary supplements, medical devices usually require premarket approval or clearance before a practitioner can use the article with patients. To illustrate the breadth of FDA's device regulations, a tongue depressor is a regulable medical device, as are toothbrushes, and Q-Tip® cotton swabs.[49]

Before using or marketing a medical device in commerce, the product must proceed through the FDA's premarket approval process. That requires substantial data demonstrating that the device is safe and effective for a specific intended use. Premarket approval applications (PMAs) can require substantial evidence and data—the device version of a New Drug Application. FDA often requires human clinical studies to support the efficacy of a medical device at the PMA stage. Devices that are similar to existing products can pass through FDA's abbreviated premarket clearance process, otherwise known as the 510(k) pathway.[50] Under that procedure, the device must be "substantially equivalent" (SE) to a predicate device. If the new devices closely match a prior-approved device, then FDA will permit the subsequent device to be marketed under the same regulatory category as the predicate devices.

The FDA places devices into one of three categories based on risk to the patient. Class I devices have minimal risk and are generally easy for patients to self-administer. Class III devices involve invasive systems that present a high risk to patient safety, such as intravenous catheters, heart valves, and similar devices. Many Class I and II devices are now "exempted" by FDA regulation from the 510(k) clearance process. Therefore, devices like toothbrushes and tongue depressors can be marketed without FDA premarket approval or clearance, provided the product stays within the general parameters of the exempting regulations.

FDA's device regulations are broad enough to regulate medical software. Software systems that integrate physical devices or interpret medical data are regulated and must proceed through FDA. The FDA has also asserted jurisdiction over "mobile medical apps" that run on smartphones or similar devices.[51] According to FDA, "[w]hen the intended use of a mobile app is for the diagnosis of disease or other conditions, or the cure, mitigation, treatment, or prevention of disease, or is intended to affect the structure or function of the body of man, the mobile app is a device."[52]

The FDA has exempted many basic mobile applications. Wellness software and applications that facilitate the exchange of basic patient information or allow physicians and patients to interact have been excused by FDA (many similar applications do not meet the statutory definition of "device"). Applications intended for educational purposes or to permit communication with health care providers are generally not "devices" under the law. Moreover, apps that track general health information (weight, height) or those which keep track of medications are generally subject to FDA's "enforcement discretion," meaning FDA does not intend to enforce the device regulations. But applications intended to analyze patient data, test results, or make clinical decisions may be regulated under the FDCA, which requires premarket clearance and efficacy data. Similarly, applications intended to interface with or serve as accessories to other regulated devices are subject to the same form of regulation as the parent device.

FDA regulation of software-related devices is relatively recent and in the nascent stages. The legal contours of FDA policies are still emerging. The FDA is expected to publish guidance on the use of "Clinical Decision Support" (CDS) software systems within the next year. That guidance should reveal FDA's thinking on more complex devices that automate aspects of medical practice. For now, the FDA employs a pure risk-based approach to software devices. Where an application presents a significant risk to patients (i.e., if the device malfunctioned or was misused), the FDA will impose traditional regulatory standards and obligations.

Any practitioner relying on mobile software applications in daily practice should verify whether the applications themselves fall within FDA's device regulations. Recent federal decisions like *Kaplan*[53] indicate that physicians can be criminally liable for the use of unapproved medical devices with patients. Practitioners must also determine whether the use of any physical device is within the intended use cleared or preapproved by the FDA.[54]

SPECIFIC FEDERAL REGULATORY CONCERNS FOR ALTERNATIVE PRACTITIONERS

Building a successful business requires advertising and promotion. Most states govern the advertising activities of professionals at the local level, including lawyers, physicians, and other health care providers. Each practitioner should become familiar with the applicable laws and regulations within their local jurisdiction that are enforced by state-run licensing boards. Moreover, as the practice of medicine grows beyond borders through technology, alternative practitioners must also abide by federal regulations that govern commercial advertising. The following significant legal concerns are likely to impact most successful practices.

PHYSICIAN DISPENSING AND COMPOUNDING

Practitioners offering alternative medical services may rely on products or articles in their practices that are not commercially available, or are difficult to obtain. For example, herbal medications and specially formulated nutritional products may be custom-formulated for specific patients. Some practitioners may offer products during a patient visit or for in-office purchase. As with most aspects of medical practice, the laws and regulations governing physician dispensing of drug products vary significantly among the states. In general terms, state laws serve the following basic functions:

(1) narrowing the situations in which physicians can dispense product; (2) permitting state agencies and boards to license or identify dispensing physicians; (3) limiting profits derived from dispensed drugs; (4) guarding freedom of choice at the consumer level; and (5) mandating procedural controls like labeling and record-keeping requirements.[55] In certain states, the dispensing regulations are relaxed and allow dispensing under clearly defined circumstances.[56] California does not require a particularized license to dispense medication in-office. The statute permits dispensing by a range of practitioners, including licensed physicians or surgeons, naturopaths, optometrists, dentists, veterinarians, podiatrists, and so on.[57] Other states are not as lenient. Regardless, dispensing physicians must always comply with both state and federal laws—even where the practice of dispensing is permissible with limited controls.[58]

Federal law imposes limitations on in-office dispensing in a variety of circumstances.[59] Controlled substances under the Controlled Substances Act (CSA) are regulated by the Drug Enforcement Administration (DEA), which enforces detailed regulations concerning the prescription, storage, manipulation, record-keeping, and administration of controlled substances. Controlled substances can only be prescribed by practitioners holding a DEA registration. Practitioners require DEA registrations to prescribe any scheduled hormones (e.g., testosterone, HCG, GH, etc.). In certain states, naturopathic doctors are permitted to prescribe Schedule III-V controlled substances when operating under the supervision of a licensed Medical Doctor or Doctor of Osteopathic medicine. In states like California, an N.D. can affiliate with a licensed M.D. through a supervision agreement.[60]

The FDA also regulates dispensing and use of drugs within the physician-patient relationship. As discussed previously, the FDA's policies concerning "new drugs" generally prevent physicians from administering novel or "unapproved" therapies. The FDA's regulation of pharmacy compounding imposes restrictions on the use of existing drugs that are altered from their "approved" conditions. "Drug compounding is the process by which a pharmacist combines or alters drug ingredients according to a doctor's prescription to crease a medication to meet the unique needs of an individual patient."[61]

Following the Compounding Quality Act of 2013, the practice of "compounding" medications to support personalized medicine is narrowing. The FDA has imposed increasingly strict regulations on the art of compounding medications from approved drug sources.[62] Several of those FDA policies have impacted alternative practitioners.

Section 503A of the Act preserves the physician's ability to compound drug products for patients. The Act limits compounding practices to "licensed pharmacists in a State licensed pharmacy or a Federal facility" or "a licensed physician, on the prescription order for such individual patient made by a licensed physician or other licensed practitioner authorized by State law to prescribe drugs."[63] Practitioners who dispense medications to patients directly may need to alter product to accommodate specific patient needs. A compounded medication is an altered form of existing medications (or a mix of medications) in an exact strength or dosage designed specifically for a patient. By definition, however, a "compounded" medication is a "new" drug under the federal law, because any material change in the composition of an FDA-approved drug renders the article "new" and unapproved. The FDA has explained (and the federal courts have apparently accepted) that use of "unapproved" drug substances is not permissible. Thus, the compounding statute in Section 503A was intended to preserve practitioners' abilities to provide personalized medicine through compounded drugs, but only those drug substances that have been "approved" by the FDA.

The FDA wields its new compounding regulations under Section 503A to preclude the use of dietary supplements in compounding practice. In a move that narrows health freedom within the physician-patient relationship, the FDA recently deemed dietary ingredients beyond the realm of legitimate compounding practice. Section 503A(b)(1)(A)(i)(I) of the FDCA permits the compounding of ingredients (other than bulk drug substances) that comply with the standards of an "applicable USP or NF monograph, if one exists, and the USP chapters on pharmacy compounding."[64] In 2016 guidance documents, the FDA stated that it "does not consider USP monographs for dietary supplements to be 'applicable' USP or NF monographs within the meaning of section 503A..."[65] To the extent FDA would deem compounded dietary supplements on the USP Dietary Supplements compendium to be "new drugs" when prescribed by doctors, the FDA would prevent those doctors from prescribing and using nuanced medications with their patients, including, perhaps, certain herbal medications. The practice of compounding dietary ingredients is well-established. Alternative physicians should have authority to prescribe and administer patient-specific products in doses or formats that are not commercially available. Nonetheless, because the FDA's policies concerning compounded medications and dietary ingredients relate to all forms of compounding practice, physicians that prescribe or dispense alternative medications (e.g., herbals) must now exercise caution. Moreover, particular attention must be paid to advertising or promotional materials based on such medications (including services related to same). Breaching the FDA's compounding regulations results in the sale of an "unapproved new drug." The sale of adulterated or misbranded "new drugs" incurs substantial liability under federal law.

TELEMEDICINE AND DISTANCE CONSULTING

The number of websites providing medical and health care information has become limitless.[66] Many different forms of "telemedicine" exist in our technologically advanced environment. Physicians may communicate with patients in real-time through video conferencing. Websites can provide diagnostics and recommendations based on personalized medical data. Practitioners can connect with limitless numbers of patients through webinars or online services. Regardless of the medium, the provision of medical advice to specific patients can fall within the practice of "medicine" as broadly defined under state laws. Thus, physicians providing medical advice in foreign jurisdictions may unwittingly find themselves in violation of state laws barring the unlicensed practice of medicine.

Many states have enacted regulatory models for telemedicine practices. Those laws impose consent requirements and similar patient disclosures, or circumscribe the types of services that can be rendered. A hallmark of telemedicine practices generally requires patient-physician monitoring and contact—in other words, a legitimate personal relationship between practitioner and patient. Unsurprisingly, telemedicine-based practices are burgeoning, and the law has yet to catch up with technology. In 2016, 44 states introduced new legislature related to telemedicine.[67] With little interpretive case law and enforcement history, as of 2016, the law governing such practices is often unsettled and evolving.

Many states now have detailed regulatory schemes that govern the provision of health information, diagnoses, consultations, treatment, and so on, through interactive audio, video, or other similar communicatory mechanisms. Some of the states require the prior relationships with patients before embarking into a telemedicine relationship. Certain states, like Arizona, have comprehensive regulatory schemes. Other states, like New Jersey, have almost no enacted regulation governing the provision of medical services through telemedicine. Still others, like California, have regulated these practices on a more generalized level. States like New Mexico issue "telemedicine licenses" to providers licensed in good standing in other jurisdictions. Twenty-four states still require out-of-state physicians to apply for full licensure in the state wherein the services are being provided.[68]

The network of overlapping and conflicting state regulation of telemedicine practice can be convoluted and, so, practitioners are always encouraged to seek specific legal advice concerning their unique practices. Where a practitioner uses technology to expand the reach of their medical practice, they must determine whether that conduct would be permissible under applicable state laws. That concern is critical with the use of Internet services and video functions that reach potential patients across state lines. Practitioners will incur liability for the unlicensed practice of medicine in jurisdictions where "patients" are located. Thus, if a patient-physician relationship is formed through long-distance contact, or if the practitioner is providing medical advice to patients in other jurisdictions, that practitioner may create unintended liabilities.[69]

For CAM providers, a critical component to alternative healing may involve simply broadcasting the message that alternative treatment options are available. Some of those therapies or practices are not apparent or readily discoverable to the common patient. An educational component often accompanies wellness practices. That includes the transmission of information and research to patients searching for alternative, natural, or complementary medical care. With states interpreting the "practice of medicine" so broadly, practitioners are frequently confused as to the divide between educational speech and actual medical practice. Educational speech is usually protected by the U.S. Constitution, while the practice of medicine certainly invokes the various telemedicine regulations nationwide.[70] Confusion over medical speech has led medical boards to investigate practitioners speaking out against vaccines, or providing "medical advice" through interactive online forums. The critical question is when does a physician's advocacy or educational speech become regulable conduct? What kind of speech will render a practitioner liable under state laws? And can a practitioner be sanctioned or disciplined for medical information provided to online users?

The answers to those questions likely depend on how each state board governs the speaker directly. For instance, boards may determine that public statements regarding certain medical practices may rise to a violation of a practitioner's ethical obligations if the general advice is reckless or well below standards of patient care. In general, educational speech or advocacy is protected under the First Amendment to the United States Constitution. State and federal authorities face a steep burden to censor or prohibit non-commercial speech advocating for certain medical therapies or informing consumers of same. Trouble brews where the practitioner uses technology to reach patients with specific medical concerns in commercial settings (or in an environment that is promotional in nature). The commercial component may strip the speaker of constitutional protections (or significantly reduce those protections), making the speech directly reachable by government agencies. The use of Internet forums can also raise ethical concerns, including issues like solicitation of clients and informed consent. Moreover, because the existence and timing of a physician-patient relationship can be unclear during Internet relationships (see Dyer, supra), a practitioner must be careful not to incur liabilities for malpractice or similar tort theories.

A rule of universal application is impossible given the varied state regulatory regimes. But, in general, practitioners are likely protected (or incur little risk) when providing general medical information to a broad audience. Promotional messages broadly disseminated should not raise issues concerning unlicensed practice of medicine (and most malpractice concerns) absent a specific physician-patient relationship.[71] The turning point, therefore, is the direct provision of medical guidance to a specific individual or small group of individuals, within a purported physician-patient relationship. A practitioner could appropriately publish a subscription-based newsletter to a general patient list that included health recommendations and guidelines. That practitioner could likely host weekly call-in radio programs or webinars that involve the general provision of medical information to a wide group of individuals for educational purposes. A practitioner could likely not, however, provide direct and personalized medical counseling to a specific person located beyond state lines through email or video-conferencing programs without raising questions over the legal legitimacy of that contact.

The Ninth Circuit has held that practitioner statements outside of the patient practice are entitled to full protection under the First Amendment.[72] But note that practitioners can still be liable "for giving negligent medical advice to their patients, without serious suggestion that the First Amendment protects their right to give advice that is not consistent with the accepted standard of care."[73] The government is also limited from enacting content-based restrictions on speech based on the message conveyed to the public (rather than the means by which the message reaches individuals).[74] In *Pickup v. Brown*, the United States Court of Appeals for the Ninth Circuit carefully explained that government may not generally limit a practitioner from conveying information in his professional capacity outside of the patient relationship:

> At one end of the continuum, where a professional is engaged in a public dialogue, First Amendment protection is at its greatest. Thus, for example, a doctor who publicly advocates a treatment that the medical establishment considers outside the mainstream, or even dangerous, is entitled to robust protection under the First Amendment—just as any person is—even though the state has the power to regulate medicine. See Lowe v. SEC, 472 U.S. 181, 232, 105 S.Ct. 2557, 86 L.Ed.2d 130 (1985) (White, J., concurring) ("Where the personal nexus between professional and client does not exist, and a speaker does not purport to be exercising judgment on behalf of any particular individual with whose circumstances he is directly acquainted, government regulation ceases to function as legitimate regulation of professional practice with only incidental impact on speech; it becomes regulation of speaking or publishing as such, subject to the First Amendment's command that 'Congress shall make no law … abridging the freedom of speech, or of the press.'"); Robert Post, Informed Consent to Abortion: A First Amendment Analysis of Compelled Physician Speech, 2007 U. Ill. L.Rev. 939, 949 (2007) ("When a physician speaks to the public, his opinions cannot be censored and suppressed, even if they are at odds with preponderant opinion within the medical establishment."); cf. Bailey v. Huggins Diagnostic & Rehab. Ctr., Inc., 952 P.2d 768, 773 (Colo.Ct.App.1997) (holding that the First Amendment does not permit a court to hold a dentist liable for statements published in a book or made during a news program, even when those statements are contrary to the opinion of the medical establishment). That principle makes sense because communicating to the public on matters of public concern lies at the core of First Amendment values. See, e.g., Snyder v. Phelps, ––– U.S. –––, 131 S.Ct. 1207, 1215, 179 L.Ed.2d 172 (2011) ("Speech on matters of public concern is at the heart of the First Amendment's protection." (internal quotation markets, brackets, and ellipsis omitted)). Thus, outside the doctor-patient relationship, doctors are constitutionally equivalent to soapbox orators and pamphleteers, and their speech receives robust protection under the First Amendment.[75]

To avoid liability for public statements within the profession, practitioners should be careful to limit commercial components related to the speech itself. The speaker should impose clear barriers between public advocacy (or lecturing) and promotional speech that favors the commercial aspects of the practice. Receiving an honorarium for speaking engagements does not render speech "commercial" in nature. But receiving an interest in sales revenues for a dietary supplement promoted during a lecture likely would raise liability concerns.

FTC STANDARDS AND REGULATION

Beyond the discussion of First Amendment freedoms (*supra*), the commercial promotion, sponsorship, or endorsement of certain medical practices, products, or services will create risks under federal and state advertising laws. At the federal level, the Federal Trade Commission (FTC) regulates advertising of certain drugs, devices, dietary supplements, and general consumer goods or services.

All promotional claims (of any kind) must be supported or "substantiated" with evidence. The FDA and FTC have complementary jurisdiction over products like dietary supplements, over-the-counter drugs, medical devices, cosmetics, medical services, and almost all FDA-regulated products except prescription drugs. Under an agreement governing the division of responsibilities between the two agencies, the FDA has primary responsibility for labeling and FTC wields authority over advertising activities. The FTC has broad jurisdiction and claims primary authority over advertising interpretation. FTC also has greater enforcement powers than the FDA. It can disgorge profits and enter civil penalties far more punitive than the FDA. Any practitioner that promotes, endorses, or sponsors medical services or products is under the jurisdiction of the Federal Trade Commission. Those practitioners may also face liability from plaintiff attorneys in states with broad "consumer protection" laws that empower consumers to sue for false or misleading promotional activities.

The FDA requires that you have a "reasonable basis" for making any objective claim *before* disseminating the claim.[76] In other words, you must have substantiation in the form of scientific proof that your products or services do what you claim they do. Failure to have that reasonable basis for an objective claim, including claims made in the expert or medical endorsements and testimonials, is deceptive under Section 5 of the Federal Trade Commission Act (FTCA).

When the claims concern health, safety, and/or product efficacy, a "reasonable basis" means "competent and reliable scientific evidence." That standard will require tests, analysis, research studies, or other credible evidence supported by the expertise of professionals in the relevant area, that has been conducted and evaluated in an objective manner by persons qualified to do so, using procedures generally accepted in the profession to yield accurate and reliable results.[77] An advertiser is responsible for all claims present in an advertisement, including "implied" claims. Implied claims are drawn from the "net impression" of an advertisement. The FTC identifies and measures claims through the perspective of a "reasonable consumer."

Medical practitioners find themselves entangled with advertising law frequently. A practitioner might advertise a new service or therapy, and the FTC later deems those promotional materials false or misleading because the practitioner promised something that the science did not support. For example, advertising an HCG weight loss therapy in print or radio advertisements raises the specter of FTC enforcement. Practitioners may lend their name or identity to promotional materials designed by manufacturers or retailers. For instance, "Dr. Smith recommends HCG therapy." Regulated persons must understand that the latter circumstance creates the same measure of liability as the former. The FTC requires that all statements made by the "expert endorser" be truthful and not misleading based on the "competent and reliable" evidentiary standard. Significantly, the FTC has taken enforcement action against expert endorsers, holding them equally responsible as the manufacturer/advertiser.

Whether from an endorser or original advertiser, every advertisement should be supported by sufficient evidence to fend off administrative scrutiny. In recent years, the FTC has adopted a policy that requires at least two placebo-controlled, double-blinded human clinical studies to support therapeutic medical or health claims.[78]

As explained earlier, the First Amendment extends significant protections for educational or informational speech. But commercial speech has substantially less protection. To the extent speech carries a promotional or commercial purpose, all practitioners are advised to consult competent counsel to determine whether advertising campaigns are advisable.

CHANGES TO THE FEDERAL AND STATE REGULATIONS TO PROMOTE HEALTH FREEDOM

The realization of health freedom and patient choice depends on restriction of government censorship. Federal and state regulation of the medical professions must accommodate technological advancements. Federal regulation must be scaled back in favor of nuanced state models. Government policy must move beyond the stratified and antiquated FDA system of therapeutic taxonomy (i.e., drug, device, dietary supplement, cosmetic). The FDA's model lags behind where products like foods and supplements are frequently effective for multiple purposes. This chapter concludes by suggesting a series of general reforms that would significantly advance the availability of alternative and complementary medical systems for patients nationwide.

CHANGES TO FDA REGULATIONS

Strengthen Laws That Permit Off-Label Use

Congress should codify or strengthen federal laws that permit off-label advertising and promotion of medical products by licensed practitioners. The speed of research and innovation almost always outpaces the federal government's regulatory approval processes, which are inefficient at best. Modern medicine depends on the physician's ability to explore nuanced or innovative treatment options, particularly for products with a history of safe and effective use. "Off-label use is wide-spread in the medical community and often is essential to giving patients optimal medical care, both of which medical ethics, FDA, and most courts recognize."[79] In 2012, a landmark decision from the U.S. Court of Appeals for the Second Circuit recognized the importance of physician autonomy, and scrutinized the government's attempt to censor off-label information from pharmaceutical representatives.[80] Congress should expand these types of protections for off-label speech nationwide by extending the reasoning of that powerful *U.S. v. Caronia* decision into the Federal Food, Drug, and Cosmetic Act so that FDA cannot circumvent that decision through the broad intended use doctrine.

The FDA has threatened to regulate off-label speech more directly. FDA announced a public hearing on off-label communications held in November 2016.[81] "The purpose of [that] public hearing [was] to obtain comments on FDA's regulation of firms' communications about medical products, with a particular focus on firms' communications about unapproved uses of their approved/cleared medical products." The agency lodged eight broad questions for industry concerning the use of such off-label promotions. The agency sought information to determine how to regulate such speech in the future. FDA requested input concerning the appropriate forms of communication to consumer and patient audiences. FDA's sudden interest in that area likely foreshadows increased regulation.

The use of "off-label" speech should instead be broadened to allow physician-to-patient information concerning the beneficial health effects of all articles saleable under the FDA. Limiting "off-label" uses to "approved" FDA *drug* products may strip physicians of their right to apply nutritional therapies, dietary supplements, or medical foods for therapeutic means. If off-label speech cannot reach unapproved drugs, then the margin of safety narrows for physicians that regularly use dietary supplements for therapeutic use. Decisions like the Ninth Circuit's in *U.S. v. Kaplan* threaten to criminalize use of unapproved products within patient care, withering the same protections just given by decisions like *Caronia*. A national approach to medical speech within the physician-patient relationship should be a Congressional mandate. State medical boards and licensing bodies have shown themselves more than capable of regulating practitioners under local standards.

Put simply, FDA may regulate the means and instrumentalities of medical practice. But the federal government should otherwise remain out of medical offices.[82] To enforce those limitations, Congress should strengthen the limitations in 21 U.S.C. § 396, which imposes limits on FDA's authority. That statutory section states:

> Nothing in this chapter shall be construed to limit or interfere with the authority of a health care practitioner to prescribe or administer any legally marketed device to a patient for any condition or disease within a legitimate health care practitioner-patient relationship.

That section should be expanded to incorporate drugs and all FDA-regulated products that are "legally marketed" in commerce. Subject to board oversight, practitioners should have flexibility to prescribe or administer therapies that are consistent with emerging or evolving standards of care.[83]

Protecting patients from negligent, incompetent, and reckless practitioners is a primary goal for regulation at any level. Critics of federal reform often harp on potential harms to patients flowing from less oversight. Importantly, less federal regulation is not equivalent to less oversight. The state and federal actors retain plenary authority to discover and prosecute bad actors in the profession. Relaxing federal regulations allows those authorities to focus resources and better perform those supervisory tasks.

Broaden FDA's Expanded Access Regulations

FDA should permit expanded access (i.e., compassionate uses) for a wider variety of illnesses and conditions, and those uses should not be cabined to patients with "serious diseases or conditions" that impose life-threatening outcomes.[84]

"Expanded access" to FDA investigational drugs allows for the use of drugs outside of a clinical trial that is operating under a formal Investigational New Drug (IND) application for research purposes. According to FDA, investigational drugs have not yet been proven "safe and effective" for treatment purposes. Thus, the FDA categorically denies access to such articles unless the patient is enrolled in an FDA-sanctioned research trial. Many patients cannot qualify for these trials. Or the trials are closed or completed. In 21 CFR Part 310.300, *et seq.*, the FDA created an exemption for certain patients, allowing the use of investigational products under very specific circumstances.[85] FDA will approve an expanded access petition seeking use of an investigational drug only where the patient has a "serious or immediately life-threatening disease or condition, and there is no comparable or satisfactory alternative therapy to diagnose, monitor, or treat the disease or condition."[86] The FDA imposes a balancing test. The "potential patient benefit [must] justif[y] the potential risks of the treatment use and those potential risks [must not be] unreasonable in the context of the disease or condition to be treated."[87] The FDA has interpreted those elements narrowly. It has denied expanded access petitions for child cancer patients on grounds that chemotherapy (an unapproved drug when used in children) was first available. But with adequate disclosures and informed consent, the FDA's balancing approach between unapproved therapies and disease outcomes still functions for lesser diseases, particularly where the risk of adverse events from the unapproved medication is minimal. These changes promote innovation and expansion of off-label uses, and also encourage the development of potential alternative medical treatments that may exist only under narrowly defined clinical studies (because of low resources in research).

Patient autonomy in medical decisions demands that the expanded access criteria be revised and broadened. Informed consent and mandated disclosures can remedy any potential risk to patients choosing experimental therapies. Relaxing the criteria to include nonserious medical conditions imposes no significant risk to the public health or safety. The concept that a patient may have medical autonomy to use certain experimental drugs only in "life-threatening" situations seems at odds with the foundational moral principles that support the expanded access exemption even in life-threatening conditions. Personal choice and health freedom are unalienable concepts that apply universally across all medical decisions.

Lift Restrictions on Preventative or Wellness Advertising Related to Nutritional Products

Nutritional products are exponentially safer than FDA-approved pharmaceuticals. From 2008 through 2011, the FDA received just 6037 adverse event reports for dietary supplements.[88] Compare that number with the 873,945 adverse event reports for approved FDA drugs in 2011 alone.[89] Preventative medicine relies on lifestyle changes and proper nutrition. We should not apply pharmaceutical standards to those wellness regimes which rely on demonstrably safe products or systems. Yet the FDA has adopted impossibly high standards more akin to drug regulations for these products.

In 1990, Congress passed the Nutrition Labeling and Education Act (NLEA). Part of that legislation allowed for "health claims" in association with foods. The DSHEA expanded those provisions to dietary supplements in 1993. A "health claim" is a claim made on the label or in labeling of a food or supplement that expressly or by implication characterizes the relationship of any substance to a disease or health-related condition. Health claims are limited to claims concerning disease risk-reduction. In other words, health claims focus on disease prevention. A health claim cannot include language purported to diagnose, cure, mitigate, or treat disease. Under the NLEA, the FDA must preapprove any claim before it enters the market. Those limitations apply to all commercial statements concerning dietary supplements or foods. The failure to obtain FDA preapproval for a health claim would render any product bearing such a claim an "unapproved new drug."

Health claims can help advance preventative medicine and wellness programs. That type of information helps consumers and patients understand the types of dietary habits that may improve quality of life and reduce disease risk over time. But very few health claims have passed FDA review, largely because the agency insists on inflexible standards concerning the science required to support those claims. The FDA calls its system of scientific review the Evidence-Based Review System (EBRS).

Given the relative safety of dietary supplements, particularly under physician supervision, the FDA should broaden its standards to allow dissemination of speech based on a wider variety of scientific evidence, including animal models and observational data. Large-scale, double-blinded, placebo-controlled clinical studies should not be required for preventative claims, in part, because the financial limitations on such research are always impractical for food-based products. Consumers must receive more information, not less, and FDA's existing policy suppresses commercial speech for all but the most compelling scientific facts. Consumers and patients should be given more credit in their ability to process and understand the limitations on scientific research.

The FDA should broaden its restrictive policies that favor pharmaceuticals over natural products. It should expand the category of "medical foods" to encompass a wider array of nutritional products, and eliminate antiquated aspects of medical food regulation. Medical foods provide patients with specially formulated nutritional products designed to assist in the management of disease conditions. Medical foods therefore represent the rare instance where a nutritional product can be associated with a "disease" condition without also becoming a "drug." Medical foods do not treat disease; rather, they help manage those disease states. They are intended to meet distinctive nutritional requirements of a disease or condition, and used under medical supervision.

The FDA recently narrowed the qualifying criteria for medical foods. The most challenging limitation is FDA's requirement that medical foods cannot provide nutrition that can otherwise "be achieved by the modification of the normal diet alone."[90] The "normal diet," according to FDA, includes all products and articles in the food supply—including dietary supplements. In many instances, changes to diet are at least theoretically possible, but FDA does not consider the practicality of those changes. Thus, for example, if certain fish oils were helpful in the management of ADHD conditions, the FDA may not approve a medical food if a patient could theoretically consume 16 pounds of salmon daily. These policies should change. The medical food category is an emerging union of modern nutritional science with advanced medical understanding of disease management. Medical foods break through FDA's regimented (and antiquated) system of regulatory classification. The category should be expanded.

NEW LEGISLATION TO PROMOTE HEALTH FREEDOM

Congress has consistently recognized a need for alternative medical systems, but the federal government has, in turn, devoted very limited resources to the expansion of government-sponsored research. In 1991, the National Center for Complementary and Integrative Health (NCCIH) was established to explore complementary and alternative healing practices under scientific- and evidence-based standards. When compared with other government-backed research organizations, the NCCIH was underfunded and subject to consistent criticism. The path to innovation in alternative medicine proceeds through private practice—through those individuals actually connected with the patients they serve. Particularly for alternative practices that rely on the interpersonal connections between patient and practitioner, standardized government medicine will rarely capture the successes of patient care that CAM experience in their individualized practices. Promoting health freedom through legislative amendment empowers patients. The following changes to federal law would advance these goals.

Privatized Review for Alternative Medical Therapies

Shifting FDA's jurisdictional responsibilities onto third parties is a familiar concept. The FDA has successfully incorporated a privatized system in the medical device context for years. The "Accredited Persons Program" was established by the FDA Modernization Act of 1997 (FDAMA).[91] Under that system, the FDA permits third parties to conduct medical device premarket reviews for certain types and categories of medical device products. The FDA has also used third-party organizations to determine which food or feed ingredients can be marketed within animal products. The FDA formally accepts "ingredient definitions" published by the Association of American Feed Control Officials (AAFCO).

The FDA (through Congressional legislation) could implement a system permitting specialized third-party review of alternative medical systems and products. In context with permissible "off-label" uses for drugs and dietary supplements, a system of third-party certification bodies could help develop the conditions for use of articles commonly applied in complementary and alternative medicine. Those non-governmental organizations would be staffed with experts possessing substantially greater knowledge of and experience with alternative fields than FDA-salaried counterparts. Blinded reviews could be accomplished by research institutions, academia, or certification bodies that directly regulate the practices of medicine.

Expand Freedom of Choice in Health Care by Expanding Access to Telemedicine

Uniform policy is required to address more common cross-border or interstate medical practices. Each of the 50 states has begun to implement and enforce regulatory systems that address tele-medical practices. Clear laws concerning telemedicine would expand access to practitioners and innovative therapies. Those regulations could also resolve liability concerns for practitioners connecting with patients in other jurisdictions. For practitioners using telemedicine, the system needs uniformity. Until state licensing authorities can agree on methods to harmonize state telemedicine laws, the inconsistencies and burdens will threaten technological innovation.[92]

Stronger Informed Consent Laws That Facilitate Medical Choice

The Supreme Court has consistently held that more information is preferable to less in the marketplace.[93] Where a system of disclosures and notifications is sufficient to protect consumers, that sort of information-based system should be preferable to outright suppression or prohibition. The states can enact disclosure laws that inform consumers and patients of the limitations for certain medical therapies, while preserving access to those services and products. Those warning and disclosure systems promote consumer choice in health care. For example, California passed statutory laws that permit the practice of nutrition therapy and other alternative services by a wide range of practitioners, including those that cannot apply for licensure in other medical categories.[94] To provide services, the practitioner must first give clear information to the patient disclosing that: (A) the practitioner is not a licensed physician; (B) that the treatment is alternative or complementary to healing arts services licensed by the state; (C) that the services to be provided are not licensed by the state; (D) the nature of the services to be provided; (E) the theory or treatment upon which the services are based; and (F) the practitioner's education, training, experience, and other qualifications regarding the services to be provided.[95] The laws also include mandatory "Notice" postings at office locations for nutritionists.[96]

California's regulatory goal was to facilitate access to alternative therapies while giving consumers sufficient information to judge for themselves the credibility of each practitioner and the reliability of the services provided. California's legislation still prohibits the practice of many conventional services by unlicensed practitioners, including, for example, the use of certain diagnostics, the prescription of legend drugs or controlled substances, and so on.[97] Federal and state governments should explore similar "consent" or "disclosure" laws that permit the use of alternative services through non-traditional channels. For instance, the same "consent" regime could apply to the use of medical devices, certain drugs, healing services, or other therapeutic options that might otherwise remain "unapproved" and thus unlawful under existing law.

CONCLUSION

Governmental reform starts with a motivated electorate. The vast majority of all laws passed at the federal level come from unelected officials within an expanding administrative bureaucracy. American administrative law permits direct participation by individuals through citizen petitions, comments to proposed rulemakings or guidance documents, appeals of administrative decisions, and litigation. Direct involvement within that administrative process can spur positive agency action, and help assure that government regulators operate with full knowledge and understanding of the relevant issues. Constitutional and administrative law advocates depend heavily on CAM practitioners and patients to push against flawed regulations while promoting workable systems that benefit conscientious medicine and protect against unscrupulous practitioners. Please consider lending your voice to legal, administrative, and policy developments within the federal agencies.

END NOTES

1. Peter A. Arhangelsky is a Principal Attorney in the law firm Emord & Associates, P.C., Gilbert, Arizona, USA. He practices food and drug law, advertising law, and constitutional law. Mr. Arhangelsky has represented hundreds of FDA-regulated companies and practitioners in litigation, enforcement proceedings, and regulatory consulting matters.
2. Cal. Bus. & Prof. Code § 2052(a).
3. *See id.*
4. *See* Cal. Bus. & Prof. Code § 2053.5.
5. *See also* Federation of State Medical Boards. 2014. U.S. Medical Regulatory Trends and Actions (listing state regulations and medical practices acts). https://www.fsmb.org/Media/Default/PDF/FSMB/Publications/us_medical_regulatory_trends_actions.pdf (accessed Nov. 10, 2016) (summarizing state laws and medical practices acts in fifty states).
6. *See, e.g.,* 21 U.S.C. § 396 (West).
7. *See, e.g., United States v. Caronia,* 703 F.3d 149 (2d Cir. 2012).
8. U.S. Food and Drug Administration. 2016. Executive Summary: Strategic Plan for Regulatory Science. http://www.fda.gov/ScienceResearch/SpecialTopics/RegulatoryScience/ucm268095.htm (accessed Nov. 10, 2016).
9. *See, e.g.,* 21 U.S.C. § 811; 21 C.F.R. Part 1308.
10. *See United States v. Regenerative Scis., LLC,* 878 F. Supp. 2d 248, 261 (D.D.C. 2012), *aff'd,* 741 F.3d 1314 (D.C. Cir. 2014).
11. *See id.*
12. *See United States v. Kaplan, MD,* 836 F.3d 1199 (9th Cir. Sep. 9, 2016).
13. *See id.* at 1208 (quoting 21 U.S.C. § 331(k)).
14. *Id.*
15. *See Kaplan,* 836 F.3d at 1210-13.
16. *See* 21 U.S.C. § 342(g).
17. *See* MA Chirba, J.D., D.Sc., M.P.H. and SM Garfield, J.D. 2011. FDA Oversight of Autologous Stem Cell Therapies: Legitimate Regulation of Drugs and Devices or Groundless Interference with the Practice of Medicine? *J. Health & Biomedical L.* 7(233):244.
18. 21 U.S.C. § 321(g)(1).
19. JA DiMasi, HG Grabowski, RA Hansen. 2016. Innovation in the Pharmaceutical Industry: New Estimates of R&D Costs. *Journal of Health Economics* 47:20–33 (concluding that the true costs of pursuing and securing new drug approval through FDA was at $2.56 billion in 2013).
20. Pub. L. No. 103–417, 108 Stat. 4325 (1994).
21. PB Hutt 2009. The History & Future of the Dietary Supplement Health & Education Act. *Natural Products Insider,* http://www.naturalproductsinsider.com/articles/2009/09/the-history-future-of-the-dietary-supplement-health-education-act.aspx (accessed Nov. 10, 2016).
22. The FTC has routinely required at least two human clinical studies in support of promotional materials that include therapeutic claims. In demand letters and through enforcement, the FTC set the standard as follows:

> "at least two adequate and well-controlled human clinical studies of [product], or of an essentially equivalent product, conducted by different researchers, independently of each other, that conform to acceptable designs and protocols and whose results, when considered in light of the entire body of relevant and reliable scientific evidence, are sufficient to substantiate that the representation is true."

See In Re Nestle, FTC Docket No. C-4312, Order at Part II (emphasis added); *In re Dannon Company,* FTC Docket No. C-4313, Order at Part II; *see also FTC v. Iovate Health Sciences,* Case No. 10-CV-587 (W.D.N.Y), Stipulated Final Judgment and Order for Permanent Injunction at Part II.

23. *See* A Shao, PhD and D Mackay, ND. 2010. A Commentary on the Nutrient-Chronic Disease Relationship and the New Paradigm of Evidence-Based Nutrition. *Natural Medicine Journal* 2(12):10–18 (explaining that the use of human clinical trials to demonstrate nutrient-disease reduction relationships is often impractical or impossible).

24. *See In re POM Wonderful LLC and Roll Global LLC*, FTC Dkt. No. 9344 (2010).

25. *See* Initial Decision by ALJ D. Michael Chappell, *In re POM Wonderful LLC*, FTC Dkt. No. 9344 (2012), at 96 (explaining that FTC's expert "testified that studies of disease prevention should involve 10,000 to 30,000 men and that such studies are 'incredibly expensive' and in the range of $600 million").

26. *See* Shoa, *supra* note 20, at 10–11; J Blumberg et al., 2010. Evidence-based criteria in the nutritional context, *Nutrition Reviews*; 68(8):478–484; RP Heaney, MD, CM Weaver, PhD, and J Blumberg, PhD. 2011. EBN (Evidence-Based Nutrition) Ver. 2.0, *Nutrition Today* 46(1):22–26.

27. *See* Shoa, *supra* note 20, at 11–12 (explaining that the difficulties applying clinical intervention studies to the nutrition context lead experts to conclude that "[r]ecommendations, whether they be public health-based or practitioner-patient-based, should be developed from the totality of the available evidence, not on a single study or study design").

28. *See also* Federal Trade Commission. 1994. Enforcement Policy Statement re Foods and Food Advertising. https://www.ftc.gov/public-statements/1994/05/enforcement-policy-statement-food-advertising (accessed Nov. 12, 2016).

29. *See* J Blumberg et al. 2010. Evidence-based criteria in the nutritional context. *Nutrition Reviews* 68(8):478–484.

30. *Id.* at 480.

31. *Id.*

32. Although the FDA argues that observational data can support health claims, the agency has generally not approved dietary supplement health claims, or a human drug product, based on observational data alone.

33. *See* Food and Drug Admin. December 2016. Complementary and Alternative Medicine Products and Their Regulation by the Food and Drug Administration. http://www.fda.gov/downloads/RegulatoryInformation/Guidances/UCM145405.pdf (accessed Nov. 13, 2016).

34. *See* 21 U.S.C. § 321(g)(1).

35. *See, e.g.*, Cal. Health & Safety Code §§ 109925, 109975, 110080–135 (adopting federal regulations).

36. *See* DiMasi, *supra* note 19.

37. *See* SM Walton et al. 2008. Prioritizing future research on off-label prescribing: results of a quantitative evaluation. *Pharmacotherapy* 28(12):1443–1452.

38. *Id.* (noting that Seroquel, an antipsychotic approved by the FDA in 1997 to treat schizophrenia, was widely prescribed for other uses including bipolar conditions, and that such uses were prescribed despite an FDA "black box" warning resulting from safety concerns).

39. *Weaver*, 886 F.2d at 198–99; *United States v. Caronia*, 703 F.3d 149 (2d Cir. 2012).

40. *See* U.S. Food and Drug Admin. 2006. Guidance: Complementary and Alternative Medicine Products and Their Regulation by the Food and Drug Administration, at 7. http://www.fda.gov/OHRMS/DOCKETS/98FR/06D-0480-GLD0001.PDF (accessed Nov. 10, 2016).

41. *See* 21 U.S.C. § 321(ff)(1).

42. *See* 21 U.S.C. § 321(ff)(2).

43. *See* 21 U.S.C. § 321(ff)(3)(A).

44. *See* Food and Drug Admin. 1995 (updated 2015). CPG Sec. 400.400; Conditions Under Which Homeopathic Drugs May be Marketed. http://www.fda.gov/ICECI/ComplianceManuals/CompliancePolicyGuidanceManual/ucm074360.htm (accessed Nov. 12, 2016).

45. *See* Federal Trade Commission. November 2016. Enforcement Policy Statement on Marketing Claims for OTC Homeopathic Drugs. https://www.ftc.gov/system/files/documents/public_statements/996984/p114505_otc_homeopathic_drug_enforcement_policy_statement.pdf (accessed Nov. 16, 2016).

46. *Id.*

47. *Id.* at 1.

48. *See* 21 U.S.C. § 321(h).

49. *See* 21 CFR § 880.6025(a) (identifying regulated devices that consist of "absorbent tipped applicator[s] … intended for medical purposes that consist[] of an absorbent swab on a wooden, paper, or plastic stick. The device is used to apply medications to, or to take specimens from, a patient.").

50. *See* 21 U.S.C. §§ 360(k), 360(n), 360c(f)(1), 360c(i); *see also* U.S. Food and Drug Admin. 2014. Guidance: The 510(k) Program: Evaluating Substantial Equivalence in Premarket Notifications. http://www.fda.gov/downloads/MedicalDevices/.../UCM284443.pdf (accessed Nov. 10, 2016).

51. *See* U.S. Food and Drug Admin. February 2015. Guidance: Mobile Medical Applications. http://www.fda.gov/downloads/MedicalDevices/DeviceRegulationandGuidance/GuidanceDocuments/UCM263366.pdf (accessed Nov. 10, 2016).

52. *Id*. at 8.

53. *United States v. Kaplan*, No. 2:13-cr-377 (9th Cir. Sep. 9, 2016).

54. As with drug products, the use of medical devices "off-label" may also increase risk of liabilities that are uncovered by insurance contracts. Because certain policies may not cover for off-label practices, a careful review of insurance documentation is necessary before implementing new technologies or services.

55. *See* M Kvaal et al. May 1989. Physician Drug Dispensing. Office of Inspector General (white paper). https://oig.hhs.gov/oei/reports/oai-01-88-00590.pdf (accessed Nov. 10, 2016).

56. *See* Cal. Bus. & Prof Code §§ 4170-4175 (California's physician dispensing statute).

57. *See* Cal. Bus. & Prof. Cod § 4170(c).

58. R Hindmand and P Souter. 2013. Structuring Physician In-Office Dispensing and Compounding Arrangements. https://www.healthlawyers.org/Events/Programs/Materials/Documents/PHS15/u_hindman_souter.pdf (accessed Nov. 10, 2016).

59. *See* U.S. H.H.S., Office of Inspector General. May 1989. Physician Drug Dispensing: An Overview of State Regulation. https://oig.hhs.gov/oei/reports/oai-01-88-00590.pdf (accessed Nov. 10, 2016).

60. *See* Cal. Bus. & Prof. Code §§ 3640.2, 3640.5(f).

61. *Med. Ctr. Pharmacy v. Mukaskey*, 536 F.3d 383, 387 (5th Cir. 2008).

62. *See* U.S. Food and Drug Admin. 2012. The Special Risks of Compounding Pharmacies. http://www.fda.gov/downloads/ForConsumers/ConsumerUpdates/UCM107839.pdf (accessed Nov. 10, 2016).

63. *See* 21 U.S.C. § 353a(a)(1)(A)-(B).

64. *See* U.S. Food and Drug Admin. June 2016. Guidance: Pharmacy Compounding of Human Drug Products Under Section 503A of the Federal Food, Drug, and Cosmetic Act. http://www.fda.gov/downloads/Drugs/GuidanceComplianceRegulatoryInformation/Guidances/UCM469119.pdf (accessed Nov. 10, 2016).

65. *See* Food and Drug Admin. June 2016. Interim Policy on Compounding Using Bulk Drug Substances Under Section 503A of the Federal Food, Drug, and Cosmetic Act, at 2. http://www.fda.gov/downloads/Drugs/GuidanceComplianceRegulatoryInformation/Guidances/UCM469120.pdf (accessed Nov. 12, 2016).

66. *See* KA Dyer 2001. Ethical Challenges of Medicine and Health on the Internet: A Review. *Journal of Medical Internet Research* 3(2):e23. *PMC*. Web. 30 Oct. 2016.

67. *See* Center for Connected Health Policy. March 2016. State Telehealth Laws and Medicaid Program Policies, at 10. http://cchpca.org/sites/default/files/resources/50%20State%20FINAL%20April%20 2016.pdf (accessed Nov. 10, 2016).

68. *See* A Gupta and D Sao 2011. The Constitutionality of Current Legal Barriers to Telemedicine in the United States, *Health Matrix* 21:385.

69. *See also* TE Miller and AR Derse 2002. Between Strangers: The Practice of Medicine Online. *Health Affairs* 21(4):168–179 (articulating the regulatory and ethical considerations related to the online practice of medicine).

70. *See People v. Cantor*, 198 Cal.App.2d 843, 850 (1961) (broadly defining medical practice to include all therapies including hypnotism, etc.).

71. Although advertising regulations are always applicable to promotional statements.

72. *See Pickup v. Brown*, 740 F.3d 1208, 1227 (9th Cir. 2013).

73. *See id*. at 1228–29.

74. *See, e.g., Moss v. U.S. Secret Serv.*, 572 F.3d 962, 970 (9th Cir.2009) (viewpoint discrimination occurs "when the government prohibits 'speech by particular speakers,' thereby suppressing a particular view about a subject" (quoting *Giebel v. Sylvester*, 244 F.3d 1182, 1188 (9th Cir. 2001)); *Alpha Delta Chi–Delta Chapter v. Reed*, 648 F.3d 790, 800 (9th Cir.2011) ("Viewpoint discrimination is ... an egregious form of content discrimination, and occurs when the specific motivating ideology or the opinion or perspective of the speaker is the rationale for the restriction [on speech]." (quoting *Truth v. Kent Sch. Dist.*, 542 F.3d at 649–50) (internal quotations omitted); *Rosenberger v. Rector & Visitors of Univ. of Va.*, 515 U.S. 819, 828 (1995) (under the First Amendment, "government regulation may not favor one speaker over another"); *Perry Educ. Ass'n v. Perry Local Educators' Ass'n*, 460 U.S. 37, 46 (1983) (a restriction on speech is unconstitutional if it is "an effort to suppress expression merely because public officials oppose the speaker's view").

75. *Pickup v. Brown*, 740 F.3d 1208, 1227 (9th Cir. 2013).

76. *See Pfizer Inc.*, 81 F.T.C. 23, 86 (1972).

77. *See, e.g., Novartis Corp.*, 127 F.T.C. 580, 725 (1999).

78. *See, e.g., In Re Nestle*, FTC Docket No. C-4312, Order at Part II (emphasis added); *In re Dannon Company*, FTC Docket No. C-4313, Order at Part II; *see also FTC v. Iovate Health Sciences*, Case No. 10-CV-587 (W.D.N.Y), Stipulated Final Judgment and Order for Permanent Injunction at Part II.

79. *See* Beck & Azari, FDA. 1998. Off-Label Use, and Informed Consent: Debunking Myths and Misconceptions, *Food & Drug L.J* 53(71):72; *see also Buckman Co. v. Plaintiffs' Legal Comm.*, 531 U.S. 341, 351, 121 S. Ct. 1012, 1019, 148 L. Ed. 2d 854 (2001) (collecting authorities).

80. *See U.S. v. Caronia*, 703 F.3d 149 (2nd Cir. 2012) ("courts and the FDA have recognized the propriety and potential value of unapproved or off-label drug use").

81. *See* U.S. Food and Drug Admin., *Manufacturing Communications Regarding Unapproved Uses of Approved or Cleared Medical Products; Public Hearing; Request for Comments*, 81 Fed. Reg. 60299 (Sep. 1, 2016).

82. *See Amarin Pharma, Inc. v. U.S. Food & Drug Admin.*, 119 F. Supp. 3d 196, 200 (S.D.N.Y. 2015) ("the FDA does not regulate doctors").

83. *See, e.g., Sita v. Danek Med.*, 43 F. Supp. 2d 245, 262 n. 13 (E.D.N.Y. 1999) (explaining that "the FDA cannot regulate how doctors *use* approved drugs") (citing 21 U.S.C. § 396). The authority to regulate the doctor-patient relationship lies solely with the State and not the FDA. *See Whalen v Roe*, 429 U.S. 589, 603 n. 30 (1977) (it is "well settled that the State has broad police powers in regulating the administration of drugs by the health professions") (citations omitted); *Linder v. United States,* 268 U.S. 5, 18 (1925) ("direct control of medical practice in the states is beyond the power of the federal government"); *see generally Conant v. Walters*, 309 F.3d 629 (9th Cir. 2002) (holding that the government cannot punish a physician for recommending medical use of marijuana because that recommendation is protected by the First Amendment); *see also Denney v. Drug Enforcement Admin.*, 508 F. Supp. 3d 815, 827 (E.D. Cal. 2007) (explaining that "*Conant's* holding is premised on the notion that a physician's candid discussion of the advantages and disadvantage of medical marijuana with his or her patient is speech protected by the First Amendment").

84. *See* 21 C.F.R. Part 312 subpart I (outlining general requirements for expanded access use of unapproved new drugs).

85. *See* 21 C.F.R. § 312.305.

86. *See* 21 C.F.R. § 312.305(a)(1).

87. *See* 21 C.F.R. § 312.305(a)(2) (listing additional criteria).

88. *See* U.S. Government Accountability Office. March 2013. Dietary Supplements: FDA May Have Opportunities to Expand Its Use of Reported Health Problems to Oversee Products. http://www.gao.gov/assets/660/653113.pdf (accessed Oct. 24, 2016).

89. *See* U.S. Food and Drug Admin. Nov. 2015. Reports Received and Reports Entered into FAERS by Year. http://www.fda.gov/Drugs/GuidanceComplianceRegulatoryInformation/Surveillance/AdverseDrugEffects/ucm070434.htm (accessed Oct. 24, 2016).

90. *See* U.S. Food and Drug Admin. May 2016. Guidance, Frequently Asked Questions About Medical Foods; Second Edition. http://www.fda.gov/downloads/Food/GuidanceRegulation/GuidanceDocumentsRegulatoryInformation/UCM500094.pdf (accessed Nov. 10, 2016).

91. *See* U.S. Food and Drug Admin. Feb. 2001. Implementation of Third Party Programs Under the FDA Modernization Act of 1997; Final Guidance for Staff, Industry and Third Parties. http://www.fda.gov/downloads/MedicalDevices/DeviceRegulationandGuidance/GuidanceDocuments/ucm094459.pdf (accessed Nov. 10, 2016).

92. *See* CF Ameringer 2011. State-Based Licensure of Telemedicine: The Need for Uniformity but Not a National Scheme. J. *Health Care L. & Pol'y* 14(55):85.

93. *Central Hudson Gas & Elec. Corp. v. Public Serv. Comm'n of New York*, 447 U.S. 557 (1980); *In Re R.M.J.*, 455 U.S. 191 (1982); *Bates v. State Bar of Arizona*, 433 U.S. 350, 376 (1977); *Peel v. Attorney Registration and Disciplinary Comm'n of Illinois*, 496 U.S. 91 at 110 (1990); *Shapero v. Kentucky Bar Association*, 486 U.S. 466, 478 (1988).

94. *See* Cal. Bus. & Prof. Code §§ 2053.5, 2053.6.

95. *See* Cal. Bus. & Prof. Code §§ 2035.6(1)(A)–(F).

96. *See* Cal. Bus. & Prof. Code § 2068.

97. *See* Cal. Bus. & Prof. Code § 2034.5(a).

Index

A

AA, *see* Arachidonic acid
AAFCO, *see* Association of American Feed Control
    Officials
AAV, *see* Adeno associated virus
Abdominal obesity, 385
Abnormal O-Ring opening system, 694
ABO blood groups, 268
Absorption, 123–125
AC, *see* Attention control
Academia de Medicina Biológica de Los Robles, 48
Açaia, 706
ACC, *see* Anterior cingulate cortex
Accessory optic tract, 491
Accessory respiratory muscles, 602
Accredited Persons Program, 764–765
ACE inhibitors, *see* Angiotensin converting enzyme
    inhibitors
Acetylcholine, 507–508
Acetylcysteine, 72
Acetylsalicylic acid (ASA), 624–625
Acidogenic theory, 206
Acid reflux disease, *see* Gastroesophageal reflux disease
    (GERD)
Acne, 484, 485
ACP, *see* American College of Physicians
Acquired immunodeficiency syndrome (AIDS), 273
Acrodermatitis enteropathica (AE), 89
ACT, *see* Asthma Control Test
Actin filaments, 308
Action spectrum, 481, 482
Active theories, *see* Programmed theories
Active transport, 124
Acupuncture, 300, 303, 323–324, 360–361, 395
Acute dentoalveolar pathology, 244
Acute disease healed, 727
Acute elemental mercurialism, 143
Acute glyphosate poisoning, 517
Acute lesion, 211
Acute manifestation, 727
Acute psychological stress, 409
Acute stress, 595
Acutonic tuning forks, 462
AD, *see* Alzheimer's disease
ADA, *see* American Dental Association; American
    Diabetes Association
Adaptive posture, *see* Forward head posture
Adaptive theories, *see* Programmed theories
ADD, *see* Attention deficit disorder
Addiction
    somatic symptoms of trauma and, 598–599
    to surgery, 604–605
Adeno associated virus (AAV), 632
Adenocarcinoma of colon, 705
Adenoids drainage, 731
    otitis drainage to accompany, 732

Adenosine monophosphate-activated protein kinase
    (AMPK), 298
Adenosine triphosphate (ATP), 306, 477, 482–483, 502
ADHD, *see* Attention deficit hyperactivity disorder
Adiponectin, 273, 298
Adolescents, 369
Adrenal glands, 594, 627
Adrenalin, 504–505
Adult acute non-lymphocytic leukemia, 532–533
Adult respiratory distress syndrome (ARDS), 97
Adult stem cells, 628
Advanced glycation end-products (AGE), 65, 612
Adverse pregnancy outcomes, 536
Adverse reactions, 43, 128
AE, *see* Acrodermatitis enteropathica
Aerobic exercises, 367, 630
Aerobic/strengthening exercises (ASE), 375
Aerosol droplets, 441
Aerosol particles, 441
AF, *see* Atrial fibrillation
AGE, *see* Advanced glycation end-products
Age/aging, 177–178, 620; *see also* Anti-aging
    detoxification and, 160
    markers, 633
    variations in MBTs, 395–396
Aging theories, 615, 616; *see also* Anti-aging
    damage theories, 617
    energy metabolism and aging, 618–619
    glycation, 618
    history, 615
    immunological theory, 617
    inflammation-based theories, 618
    multi-factorial approach, 619
    neuro-endocrine theory, 616–617
    oxidative stress theory/free radical theory, 617–618
    programmed longevity, 616
    programmed theories, 616
    telomere shortening, 619
    wear and tear theories, 617
Agnisar Kriya, 368–369
AHA, *see* American Heart Association
AHR, *see* Aryl hydrocarbon receptor
AIDS, *see* Acquired immunodeficiency syndrome
Air, 331–332
    element, *see* Tuberculinic reactive mode
    ions, 602–603
    pollution, 265
Airway effect
    on cardiovascular system, 240–241
    on endocrine system, 242
    during infancy and childhood, 235–237
    on neurological system, 240
    on posture, 237–238
    on sleep, 233–234
    tongue function effect on facial growth and airway,
        232–233

Akkermansia muciniphila (A. muciniphila), 12
ALA-S, *see* 5-Aminolevulinic acid synthase
ALA, *see* Alpha linoleic acid; Alpha lipoic acid
Alcohol, 41, 79, 141–142, 267–268
ALES, *see* Ammonium laureth sulfate
Allergic/allergy, 51
    allergic-based lung disorder, 266
    interaction, 137
    otitis, *see* "Viral" otitis
    reactions, 734–735
    rhinitis, 232
    sensitization, 276
Allium sativum (A. sativum), 630
Allostasis, 170–171
Allostatic load, 163, 170–172, 405, 596
    index, 405
    principles, 167
Almonds, 709
Alochaka Pitta, 352
Alpha-linolenic acid, 271
Alpha-pinene, 556
Alpha linoleic acid (ALA), 27
Alpha lipoic acid (ALA), 45, 63–66, 95, 625
ALS, *see* Ammonium lauryl sulfate; Amyotrophic lateral
        sclerosis
Alternate nostril breathing (ANB), 387
Alternative medicine
    FDA's regulation of, 751–752
    privatized review for, 764–765
Alternative practitioners, federal regulatory concerns for,
        756–761
Alternative products and services, FDA's historical bias
        against, 748–751
Aluminum, 267
Alzheimer's disease (AD), 65, 178, 183, 190, 431, 617
    lifestyle interventions, 184
Āma, 344
    Āma dosha, 344
    origins in body, 344
    removal from tissues, 344–345
Amanita muscarina (A. muscarina), 132
Ambien, *see* Zolpidem
American College of Physicians (ACP), 360
American Dental Association (ADA), 217
American Diabetes Association (ADA), 23
American Dietetic Association, 270
American Heart Association (AHA), 429
American Journal of Clinical Nutrition, 91, 196, 624
AMH, *see* Anti-mullerian hormone
Amino acid(s), 71, 264–265, 754
    B-Ala, 75–76
    BCAA, isoleucine, leucine, valine, 74
    Choline, 77
    complexes to specific conditions, 77–78
    decarboxylase, 74
    Glycine, 75
    L-Arginine, 75
    L-carnitine, 74–75
    L-leucine, 74
    L-Lysine, 76
    L-ORN, 76
    L-PHE, 77
    L-taurine, 75
    L-Trp, 76

NAC, 72–73
    stimulating immune function, 73
    sulfur amino acids, 73–74
5-Aminolevulinic acid synthase (ALA-S), 80
Aminophylline, 266
Ammonium laureth sulfate (ALES), 222
Ammonium lauryl sulfate (ALS), 217, 222
AMPK, *see* Adenosine monophosphate-activated protein
        kinase
Amygdala activation, 402
Amyotrophic lateral sclerosis (ALS), 178, 513
ANA, *see* Antinuclear antigen
Anaerobic bacteria, 217
Anaerobic exercises, 630
Anaplasma, 584
ANB, *see* Alternate nostril breathing
Ancient sound healing
    for modern times, 457–458
    systems, 458
Anemia, 144
Angiotensin converting enzyme inhibitors (ACE
        inhibitors), 64, 128
Animal, 716
    pigment melanin, 304
    research models, 181
Animalian intelligence systems, hallmark of, 578
Animated conversation, difficulty falling asleep after, 740
Anise (*Pimpinella anisum*), 560
Ankylosing spondylitis, 68
Anorexia nervosa, 270
ANS, *see* Autonomic nervous system
Antacids, 124
Antagonistic pleiotropy theory, 615
Antenna, 653
Antennas and reproduction, 537
Anterior cingulate cortex (ACC), 429
Anthemis nobilis, see Roman chamomile
Anthropogenic sources, 525
Anti-aging, 486, 610; *see also* Aging theories
    addressing causes of pre-mature death, 629
    anti-oxidants, 612–613
    astragalus, 628
    biomarkers of aging, 632–633
    blue zones, 613
    for business community, 610–611
    coenzyme Q10, 625–626
    CR, 611, 628
    current research, 611–613
    definitions for different communities, 610
    effects, 11
    epigenetics influencers on aging genes, 631–632
    exercises for osteoporosis, 630
    from functional medicine approach, 611
    function preservation, *vs.*, 611
    future of, 631–633
    genetic therapy and gene manipulation, 632
    herbs for DM, 630
    history of, 613–633
    HPE, 632
    HRT, 626–627
    hyperbaric oxygen therapy, 629
    interventions, 620–626
    intravenous injection for "frailty syndrome"
            or aging, 629

Kegel for urinary incontinence, 630
lifestyle interventions, 620–623
male exercises for prostate, 630
for medical and reputable business
    community, 610
medicine, 610, 611, 624
nanotechnology, 632
neupogen, 629
nutraceuticals/medications, 624–625
nutrition/foods, 624
orthomolecular medicine, 612
plasmapheresis, 613
procedures, 626–631
for scientific community, 610
stem cells, 628, 629
supplements, 631
telomerase therapy, 628
tissue-specific injection for repair and
    intra-articular, 629
tissue/organ cloning, 632
traits of all centenarians' communities, 614–615
variety in vegetables and fruits, 631
whole foods and nutraceuticals, 629
wrinkles and, 486
Anti-angiogenic tumor-suppressing peptide, 506
Antibiotic(s), 490
adjunct therapies, 9
resistant bacteria, 575
Anti-cancer effects, 705–706
Anticholinergic syndrome, 132
Antidepressants, 252, 557
Anti-glycosylation potency of carnosine, 612
Anti-inflammatory processes, 434
Anti-mullerian hormone (AMH), 382
Antinuclear antigen (ANA), 217
Antinutritional factors, 83
Antioxidant responsive element (ARE), 57
Antioxidants, 51, 612–613; see also Intravenous
    orthomolecular therapeutic agents (IV
    orthomolecular therapeutic agents)
negative charge and, 445
precursors of antioxidant enzymes, 96
rich foods, 29
ALA, 63–66
CoQ10, 68–71
DMSO, 66–68
GSH, 56–63
vitamin C, 51–56
Antiviral effect of vitamin C, 49
Anxiety, 373–374, 408, 423, 428, 476, 601, 738
correction, 11
Lavender essential oil for, 556–558
Apana Vata, 351
Apigenin, 582
Apolipoprotein (Apo), 507
Apolipoprotein E (APOE), 188, 268–269
Apyrogenicity, 46
AQLQ, see Asthma Quality of Life Questionnaire
Arachidonic acid (AA), 266, 271
ARDS, see Adult respiratory distress syndrome
ARE, see Antioxidant responsive element
Arginase, 93
Aromatics, 552–554
Arsenic (As), 82

Ārtava, 333
Artemetin, 581
Artemisia annua (A. annua), 581, 582
Artemisinin, 581
Arthritis, 375–376
Artificial sweeteners, 222
Aryl hydrocarbon receptor (AHR), 7
ASA, see Acetylsalicylic acid
Asana yoga, 364
Ascorbate, 53
Ascorbic acid, see Vitamin C
Ascorbic acid, 80
ASD, see Autism spectrum disorder
ASE, see Aerobic/strengthening exercises
Ashi Point Puncture, 360
Ashtanga yoga, 364
"Asian"-style diet, 189
Aspartate aminotransferase (AST), 268
Aspergillus oryzae (A. oryzae), 136
Aspirin, 128
Association of American Feed Control Officials
    (AAFCO), 765
AST, see Aspartate aminotransferase
Asthi, 333
Asthma, 376–378
Asthma Control Test (ACT), 376
Asthma entails chronic inflammation, 376
Asthma Quality of Life Questionnaire (AQLQ),
    376, 378
Astragalus, 628
Atharvan Veda, 488
Atherosclerosis, 30, 55
Athletic performance and recovery, 486
Atmosphere, 441
AT nerve, see Auriculotemporal nerve
ATP, see Adenosine triphosphate
Atrial fibrillation (AF), 241
Attention control (AC), 384
Attention deficit disorder (ADD), 476, 738
restless child, 738–739
sleep disorders, 740–741
violent child, 739
whining, 740
Attention deficit hyperactivity disorder (ADHD), 236, 423,
    424, 427, 431, 476, 485
Auditory nerve, 450
Auriculotemporal nerve (AT nerve), 255
Autism, see Autism spectrum disorder (ASD)
Autism spectrum disorder (ASD), 387
Auto-immune conditions, nutritional treatment of selecting
    inflammatory and, 30–33
Autoimmune diseases/disorders, 275, 406, 407, 423
Autonomic nervous system (ANS), 190, 310–311, 489,
    591–593, 598
Auto-oxidative amino acid, 188
Autumn season, 341
Avalambaka Kapha, 353
Ayurveda, 319–320, 329
ayurvedic anatomy and physiology, 333
constitutional types, 334–335
five elements and three doshas, 331–333
history, 329–330
individual harmony and self-healing, 335–336
marma points, 333–334

Ayurvedic concept of disease, 344
  origins of Āma in body, 344
  removal of Āma from tissues, 344–345
Ayurvedic medicine, 320, 323, 705–706
  balancing doshas, 342–345
  doshas, 336–342

B

B12, methyl donor B vitamins, 188
B6, methyl donor B vitamins, 188
B9 (Folate), methyl donor B vitamins, 188
Babbitt, Edwin, 489
Babesia, 584
Bacillus subtilis (B. subtilis), 136
Bacterial-derived toxins, 12
Bacterial intelligence, 575–578
Bacteroidetes, 189
BAI, see Beck Anxiety Inventory
B-Ala, see Beta-Alanine
Balancing doshas, 342
  ayurvedic concept of disease, 344–345
  doshic imbalances, 342
  role of mind in health, 343–344
Baltimore Longitudinal Study of Aging (BLSA), 613
Barker hypothesis, 5
Bartonella, 584
Basicranium, 230
Basis, 626
Basophils, 445
Basti, see Bladder
BBC, see British Broadcast Corporation
BCAA, see Branched chain amino acids
B complex vitamins, 78
  cyanocobalamin, 81
  folic acid, 81–82
  neuroprotection, 81
  niacin, 80–81
  pyridoxine, 80
  riboflavin, 79–80
  thiamine, 78–79
BDI, see Beck Depression Inventory
BDNF, see Brain derived neurotrophic factor
BDORT, see Bi-Digital O-Ring Test
BDORT resonance phenomenon, 690
Beck Anxiety Inventory (BAI), 399
Beck Depression Inventory (BDI), 399
Behaviour Rating Inventory of Executive Function scale
    (BRIEF-ASR), 431
Behcet's disease, 298
Benign prostatic hyperplasia (BPH), 630
Beta-Alanine (B-Ala), 75–76
β-carotene, 188
Benveniste, Jacques (French immunologist), 445
Bezmialem Vakif University Medical Faculty in Turkey,
    52
Bgbp, see Borrelia glycosaminoglycan binding protein
BGR-34, 630
BH4, see Tetrahydrobiopterin
BHR, see Bronchial hyperresponsiveness
Bhrajaka Pitta, 353
Bi-Digital O-Ring Test (BDORT), 689, 691–695
  diagnosis and evaluation of therapeutic effect
      using, 704

Bi-Digital O-Ring Test method, 689
"Bi-Est", 627
Bifidobacterium spp., 13
  BB12 lactis, 195
  B. breve, 11
  B. lactis HN019, 12
Bilateral symmetry, 664
Bile, 126
Bilirubin, 305
Biochemistry, 674
Bioelectromagnetic body, 310, 312
  biofields and energetic medicine, 311–312
  life energy and holistic health, 312
Bioelectromagnetic communication, 311
Bioenergetic interconnectivity, 311
Biofields
  biofield-based therapy, 312
  medicine, 311–312
Biofilms, 12–13
Bio-identical hormones, 627
Biological coherence, 645, 648, 659
Biological effects of electrosmog, 532
  adverse pregnancy outcomes, 536
  antennas and reproduction, 537
  cancer, 532–534
  dirty electricity and intermediate frequencies, 535
  effects on offspring, 536–537
  effects on sperm, 535–536
  EHS, 537–539
  ELF electromagnetic fields, 534–535
  reproduction, 534
  RF/MW, 535
Biological medicine, 54
Biological semiconduction, 656
Biomarkers of aging, 632–633
Biophoton emission (BPE), see Biophotons
Biophotonic(s), 657, 661
  light, 303
  model, 648
  processes, 303
Biophotons, 299, 301, 310, 650, 651
  body's biophoton outputs are governed by solar and
      lunar forces, 306–307
  body's circadian biophoton output, 301–302
  cells and DNA using biophotons to store and
      communicate information, 301
  electromagnetic body and consciousness, 303–304
  human skin capturing energy and information from
      sunlight, 304–306
  medical applications of, 302–303
  meditation and herbs affect biophoton output, 303
  physical and mental eye emits light, 300–301
  theory, 653
Biophysics, 643
Bio-regulatory medicine, 71
Biorhythms, 495
BioSonic Otto 128 cps tuning fork, 466, 467
Biotin, 181
Biotransformation, see Drug metabolism
Bisphenol A (BPA), 154–156
Bladder, 347
Bland discharge, 728
Blastocyst complementation system, 631
Bleeding of gingival sulcus, 212

Blood
  filtering function of kidneys, 50
  flow, 124, 125
  glucose parameters, 372
  testing, 214, 267
Blood–brain barrier, 125
Blood pressure (BP), 50, 382, 387, 428
BLSA, see Baltimore Longitudinal Study of Aging
BLT, see Bright light therapy
Blueberry extract, 624
Blue light, 477
Bluetooth, 545, 547
Blue zones, 613
BMD, see Bone mineral density
BMI, see Body mass index
Bodhaka Kapha, 353
Bodies and nutrition, 267
  ABO blood groups, 268
  alcohol, 267–268
  APO E gene, 268–269
  genes, 267
  physiology, 269–270
Body mass index (BMI), 270, 282, 385
  cardiovascular disease, 271
  celiac disease, 275–276
  food allergy, 276
  hormones, 272–273
  hunger games, 273
  IBD, 275
  lactose and soy intolerance, 276
  malabsorption, 273–274
  post-bariatric surgery, 271
  sweat chloride, 275
Body's circadian biophoton output, 301–302
Bókkon's hypothesis, 301
Bone, 724
  growth, 229
  marrow, 278
Bone-based marmas, 347
Bone mineral density (BMD), 381–382
Bonneville Power Authority, 533
Boron (B), 82
Borrelia, 584, 585
Borrelia burgdorferi, 572
Borrelia glycosaminoglycan binding protein (Bgbp), 586
Borrelial infections, 585–587
Botanical oils, 223
Bottom-up model, 424
BP, see Blood pressure
BPA, see Bisphenol A
BPH, see Benign prostatic hyperplasia
Bradyarrhythmias, 241
Bradycardia, 517
Brain, 238
  and associated sensory organs, 230
  damage, 240
  exercises and supplements, 630
  hypoxia, 601
  waves, 454, 478
Brain derived neurotrophic factor (BDNF), 89
Branched chain amino acids (BCAA), 74, 264
Breast milk, 127
Breath cycle, 591
Breathing, yoga and, 601–603

BRIEF-ASR, see Behaviour Rating Inventory of Executive
    Function scale
Brief Resilience Scale (BRS), 405
Bright light therapy (BLT), 475, 487, 488
British Broadcast Corporation (BBC), 525
Bronchial hyperresponsiveness (BHR), 377
BRS, see Brief Resilience Scale
Bruises, 484
Bruxism, 231
Bulimia, 270
Bulimia nervosa, 270
Burnout, 400
Business community, anti-aging for, 610–611

C

C677 T MTHFR polymorphism, 159
CAARS-INV, see Conners Adults ADHD Rating Scale
CAD, see Coronary artery disease
Cadmium (Cd), 11, 73, 82
Caenorhabditis elegans (C. elegans), 512
Calcium (Ca), 82, 95, 210, 222
  oxalate kidney stones, 270
Calcium carbonate, 222
Calcium pantothenate, 80
Calculus, 213
Caloric restriction (CR), 297–298, 610, 611, 624, 628
  mimetics, 189
CAM, see Complementary and alternative medicine
Camera, 680
CAMS-R, see Cognitive and Affective Mindfulness
    Scale–Revised
Cancers, 246, 382–383, 406, 407
  cell, 691
  detection from EKGs, 703
  and environmental factors, 709
Cancer treatment; see also Chemotherapy
  factors influencing, 708–711
  individualized safe, effective, and affordable, 707–708
Candida, 142
C tuning forks, 463, 464
Canon of Medicine, 489, 553
Capacitors, 542
Capillaries, 441
Capillary blood glucose (CBG), 372
Carbohydrate-deficient transferrin (CDT), 268
Carbohydrate metabolism, 51
Carbomer, 223
Carbonic, 718
Carcinogen, 534
Carcinogen 1′-hydroxyestragole, 563
Cardamom (Elettaria cardamomum), 559
Cardiac arrhythmias, 517–518
Cardiac events, 366
Cardiology Division at Emory University School of
    Medicine, 64
Cardio-metabolic parameters
  endothelial function, 29–30
  modification of trimethyl-n-oxide levels, 30
  selecting mechanisms underlying food effect on, 29
Cardiovascular adverse events, 30
Cardiovascular disease (CVD), 55, 271, 423, 427–429
  nutritional intervention in, 21–23
Cardiovascular effects of meditation, 427–429

Cardiovascular function, 183
Cardiovascular health, 409–410
Cardiovascular system, 427, 482, 538, 724
   airway effect, 240–241
Caries-activity tests, 210
Caries-prone patient characteristics, 210
   fluid reversal, 210–211
Cariogenic, 208
Carnosine, 75, 612, 623
Carotenes, 626
Carrageenan, 222
Cartilage, 443
Casticin, 581
Catechol-O-methyltransferase (COMT), 158, 249
   phase II detoxification enzyme, 159
CB, see Chandra bhedana
CBC, see Complete blood count
CBG, see Capillary blood glucose
CCE, see Craniocervical extension
CD-RISC, see Connor–Davidson Resilience Scale
CDC, see Centers for Disease Control
CDMA, see Code Division Multiple Access
CDS, see Clinical Decision Support
CDT, see Carbohydrate-deficient transferrin
CE-Certification, 481
Celiac disease, 267, 275–276
"Cell pathology" model, 675
Cell phones, 525, 537, 543
Cell(s), 475, 645, 654, 715
   using biophotons to store and communicate
      information, 301
   division, 645
   interference with ion passage through, 128
   membranes, 648
   proliferation, 482
   regeneration, 482
   and tissue architecture, 672
Cellular debris, 238, 508
Cellular-molecular damage, 618
Cellular networks, 444
Centenarians' communities, traits of, 614
   belong, 614
   down shift, 614
   80% rule, 614
   loved ones first, 615
   move naturally, 614
   plant slant, 614
   purpose, 614
   right tribe, 615
   wine @ 5, 614
Centers for Disease Control (CDC), 34, 213
Centers for Medicare & Medicaid Services (CMS), 747
Centesimal dilutions, 716
Central nervous system (CNS), 59, 74, 76, 190, 238, 482,
      592
Central remedies and satellite remedies, 723
Central sleep apnea, 235
Centriole, 659
Cerebral vascular accidents (CVA), 241
Cerebrospinal fluid (CSF), 238
   posture effect on, 238–239
CF, see Cystic fibrosis
CFL, see Compact fluorescent light
CFQ-R, see Cystic Fibrosis Quality of Life instrument

CFS, see Chronic fatigue syndrome
CFU, see Colony forming units
C-G-F-A protocol for anxiety, 459
Challenge testing, 163–165
Chandra bhedana (CB), 387
Chandra nadi (CN), 387
Chaotrope, 511
Charge transport mechanisms, 679
Chelating agents, 96
Chemical
   alteration of extracellular environment, 128
   avoidance, 168
   chemical-free living space, 168
   incompatibilities, 44
   innovation in plants, 580–583
   toxicology, 132
Chemo-brain, 384
Chemokines, 484
Chemotherapy, 706; see also Cancers
   yoga during, 383–384
Chemotherapy-induced nausea and vomiting (CINV), 560
Chikungunya, 54
China's traditional medicine, 488
Chinese dietary therapy, 359
Chinese exercise system, 425
Chinese herbology, 358–359
Chinese manipulative therapy, 359
Chinese medicine, 319–320, 357
   acupuncture, 300, 303, 323–324, 360–361, 395
   in integrative way, 361
   modalities, 358–360
   philosophy, 357–358
Chinese skullcap root (Scutellaria baicalensis), 583, 587
Chlamydia, 584, 585
Chlamydiae, 585
Chlordane, 152–153
Chloride (Cl), 82
Chlorophyll, 512–513
Chlorophyll a, 663
Chloroplast, 656
Cholecystokinin, 273
Cholesterol, 505
   cholesterol-enriched mitochondria, 509–510
   cholesterol enrichment, 509–510
Cholesterol sulfate, 505, 507, 515–516
Choline, 77
Cholinergic syndrome, 132
Chromatic wheels, 489
Chromatothérapie, 494–495
Chromium (Cr), 82, 94–95, 625
Chromophores, 481, 488
Chromotherapy, 475, 476, 488, 490–492; see also
      Phototherapy
   chromatothérapie, 494–495
   and color importance, 488–491
   colorpuncture, 494
   lateral light therapy, 495
   Monocrom method, 496
   sample of chromotherapy methods, 492–493
   Sensora, 495
   spectro-chrome method, 493
   syntonic phototherapy, 493
   tools and methods, 492
   Van Obberghen color therapy, 495–496

Chromotherapy methods, sample of, 492–493
Chronic and degenerative diseases
    biology of ultra-fast and unconscious mind, 657–661
    diffusing signal molecules *vs.* electromagnetic fields, 646–653
    DNA, 678
    ground regulation system, 675–676
    holistic anatomical perspective, 667
    light and travels medium, 662–664
    living matrix, 671
    Lucretian biochemistry, 653–657
    from microscope to organism, 643
    molecular "wires", 678–680
    nervous system, 644–646
    protection from environmental electromagnetic fields, 665–667
    solid-state tissue-tensegrity matrix system, 673–675
    tensegrity, 667–671
    vibratory matrix, 675
    views of living fascia, 676
Chronic CR effects, 624
Chronic degenerative diseases, 39
Chronic diseases, *see* Noncommunicable diseases (NCDs)
Chronic diseases, 4, 5, 57, 621, 629
    preventive tips, 629
    treatment, 723
Chronic fatigue syndrome (CFS), 8, 190
Chronic glyphosate poisoning, 517
Chronic hyperventilation, 601
Chronic inflammation, 167, 401
Chronic obstructive pulmonary disease (COPD), 138
Chronic pain, 483, 592
Chronic renal insufficiency (CKD), 50
Chronic scalene muscle tension, 601
Chronic stress, 409, 410, 595
Chronic toxic encephalopathy (CTE), 153
Chronobiological applications of light, 486–488
Chronobiology, 486
Chrysoplenetin, 582
Chrysosplenol-D, 582
CI, *see* Confidence interval
Cigarettes, 265
Cinnamon (*Cinnamomum verum*), 559
CINV, *see* Chemotherapy-induced nausea and vomiting
Circadian rhythm, 486, 488, 592
Circulation and pain, 483
Circulatory flow, EZ water implications for, 308
Cisplatin, 62
Citrus limon, see Lemon
c-Jun N-terminal kinase (JNK), 586
CKD, *see* Chronic renal insufficiency
Clary sage (*Salvia sclarea*), 559
Climatic factors, 494
Clinical Decision Support (CDS), 756
Clinical implications of human papilloma virus-type 16, 705–711
Clinical indices, 32
Clinically standardized meditation (CSM), 425, 427
Clinician gender, 412
Clock radio, 547
Clock rate, 645
Clostridium difficile infections, 9, 282
    antibiotic adjunct therapies, 9
    protection against recurrent, 11

Clove (*Syzygium aromaticum*), 559
CMR1 receptor, *see* Cold and Menthol Receptor 1 receptor
CMS, *see* Centers for Medicare & Medicaid Services
CMV, *see* Cytomegalovirus
CN, *see* Chandra nadi
CNS, *see* Central nervous system
Cobalamin, *see* Vitamin B12
Cobalt (Co), 82
Code Division Multiple Access (CDMA), 533
Coefficient of variation (CV), 381
Coenzyme Q10 (CoQ10), 68–71, 625–626
    alpha-lipoic acid, 625
    carotenes and flavanoids, 626
    chromium, 625
    enzymes, 626
    L-carnitine, 625
    melatonin, 626
    NAD(+), 626
    quercetin, 626
Cognitive and Affective Mindfulness Scale–Revised (CAMS-R), 399, 400
Cognitive behavioral therapy, 432
Cognitive influence of color, 491
Coherent biophotons, 474
Coherent light, 479
Cold and Menthol Receptor 1 receptor (CMR1 receptor), 555
Cold quality, 332
Collagen, 506–507
Collagenases, 586
Collagenous stroma, 662–663
Collective unconscious mind, 660
Collier study, 85
Colloidal instability, 517–518
Colony forming units (CFU), 195
Colorpuncture, 494
Color(s), 476–477, 491–492; *see also* Chromotherapy
    circles, 489
    Goethe's chromatic wheel, 489
    monochromatic, 475
    pigments, 222
    polychromatic, 475
    test method, 496
    therapy, 494
Communication, 475
Compact fluorescent light (CFL), 545
Complementary and alternative medicine (CAM), 746, 751
    approaches, 397, 398, 406
    interventions, 300
    practice, 395
    therapies, 611
Complementary colors, 492
Complementary therapies, 8
    anti-aging effects, 11
    antibiotic adjunct therapies, 9
    correction of depression and anxiety, 11
    postoperative recovery, 9
    potential for infantile colic, 12
    protection against environmental toxicants, 11–12
    protection against recurrent *C. difficile* infection, 11
    protection against stress-induced dysbiosis, 9
    treating metabolic syndrome, 12
Complete blood count (CBC), 278, 279

Complex communication system, 190–192
    assessing function, 193–194
    dietary neuroprotection, 194–196
    from eubiosys to dysbiosis, 192
Complexity, 573
Complex sleep apnea, 235
Complex systems, 573, 574
Composite markers, 404–406
"Compounded" medication, 757
Compounding Quality Act, 757
Computed tomography (CT), 246, 252
Computer, 544
COMT, *see* Catechol-O-methyltransferase
COMT phase II detoxification enzyme, 159
Concentrated electromagnetic field projector, 693
"Concentrative" forms of meditation, 424
Conductivity of semiconductor, 657
Cone-beam maxillofacial CT, 252
Confidence interval (CI), 534
Conjugation, 57
    reactions, *see* Phase II reactions
Conjunctivitis, 143
Conners Adults ADHD Rating Scale (CAARS-INV), 431
Connor–Davidson Resilience Scale (CD-RISC), 405
Consciousness, 333, 343, 451, 455–456
    loss, 347
Constitutional types, ayurvedic medicine, 334–335
Constitutions, 717, 718
    carbonic, 718
    fluoric, 718, 720
    natrum, 718, 719
    phosphoric, 718, 719
Continuing Survey of Food Intakes by Individuals
        (CSFII), 82
Continuous living matrix system, 679
Continuous molecular network, 671
Continuous positive airway pressure (CPAP), 235
    therapy, 240
Contract research organizations (CROs), 58
Controlled Substances Act (CSA), 747, 757
Conventional modern therapeutics, 393
Conventional nutritional principles, 294
Convulsive disorders, 565
Cool color, 491, 492
COPD, *see* Chronic obstructive pulmonary disease
Copper (Cu), 82, 92–93
    enzymes, 92
CoQ10, *see* Coenzyme Q10
Cordless phones, 543
Cordyceps, 587
Coronary artery disease (CAD), 93
Coronary atherosclerosis, 366
Cortex, 695
Corticotropin-releasing factor system, 190
Cortisol, 400–401
Cosmetics, 137, 752
Cough, rhino pharyngitis, 730
Coward, 740
COX, *see* Cyclo-oxygenase
CPAP, *see* Continuous positive airway pressure
CPT, *see* Current procedural terminology
CR, *see* Caloric restriction
Craniocervical extension (CCE), 237
Craniofacial growth and development, 228–231

airway and sleep effect during infancy and childhood,
        235–237
cardiovascular system, airway effect on, 240–241
clinical evaluation, 249–252
craniofacial pain, 242–243
endocrine system, airway effect on, 242
eye and ear disorder, 244–246
management, 252–253
maxilla and mandibular disorders, 244
mouth breathing effect on facial growth, 231–232
neurological system, airway effect on, 240
nose and paranasal sinus disorders, 244
obstructive-SDB, 234–235
odontogenic pain, 243
oral mucous membrane disorders, 244
posture, airway effect on, 237–238
posture effect on CSF and energy flow, 238–239
salivary gland disorder, 244
sleep, airway effect on, 233–234
TMD, 246–249, 253–255
TMJ symptoms, 249
tongue function effect on facial growth and airway,
        232–233
tumors, 246
Craniofacial pain, 242–243
Craniomandibular complex, 237
C-reactive protein (CRP), 9, 170, 401, 618
Credible scientific evidence, 749
Crohn's disease, 90, 408, 433
CROs, *see* Contract research organizations
CRP, *see* C-reactive protein
Cryptolepis sanguinolenta (*C. sanguinolenta*), 587
CSA, *see* Controlled Substances Act
CSE, *see* Cystathionine γ lyase
CSF, *see* Cerebrospinal fluid
CSFII, *see* Continuing Survey of Food Intakes by
        Individuals
CSM, *see* Clinically standardized meditation
CSSH, *see* Cysteine persulfide
CT, *see* Computed tomography
CTE, *see* Chronic toxic encephalopathy
Cumulative stress load, 163
Cuproenzymes, 92
Curcumin, 189, 505
Current procedural terminology (CPT), 361
CV, *see* Coefficient of variation
CVA, *see* Cerebral vascular accidents
CVD, *see* Cardiovascular disease
Cyanocobalamin, 81
Cyclo-oxygenase (COX), 296
Cycloastragenol, 628
Cymatic(s), 451
    frequency in water, 454
    images, 455
    patterns mimic quantum entanglement, 455
CYP, *see* Cytochrome P450
CYP2D6 enzyme, 159
CYP2E1 enzyme, 160, 563
CYP3A4 enzyme, 162
CYP3A enzyme, 160
Cystathionine γ lyase (CSE), 512
Cysteine, 73
Cysteine persulfide (CSSH), 506, 511
Cystic fibrosis (CF), 275, 378–379

Cystic Fibrosis Quality of Life instrument (CFQ-R), 379
Cytochrome P450 (CYP), 6, 157, 505, 512–513
Cytokines, 484, 584, 646
Cytomegalovirus (CMV), 53
Cytoskeletal forces, 308
Cytoskeleton, 509

D

Damage theories, 617
Darkness hormone, 487
DARPA, *see* Defense Advance Research Project Agency
Darwin's concept, 615
DASH, *see* Dietary Approaches to Stop Hypertension diet
DB-PC trials, *see* Double-blind, placebo-controlled trials
DDE, *see* Dichlorodiphenyldichloroethylene
DEA, *see* Drug Enforcement Administration
Debris, 508
DECT, *see* Digital European Cordless Telephony
Deep breathing exercises, 393, 395
Deepwater Horizon oil spill, 596
Defense Advance Research Project Agency (DARPA), 485
Defensive reactions, 46
Deficiency, 40
Deficient DNA repair mechanisms, 304
Dehydration, 269
Dehydroepiandrosterone (DHEA), 210, 381, 505, 624
Delayed luminescence (DL), 302
Delayed-start trial design, 59
Delayed type hypersensitivity (DTH), 88
Delta waves, 234
Delusion, 343
Dementia, 431
Dengue fever, 54
Dental care, holistic approach to, 223
Dental connection to health
    anatomy of tooth, 207
    characteristics of caries-prone patient, 210–211
    dentinal tubules, 207
    DFT, 208–210
    materials used in dentistry, 214–223
    periodontal disease and oral systemic connection, 211–214
    reversal of dentinal fluid flow, 210
Dental fluid, 208, 209
Dental lymph, *see* Dental fluid
Dental materials, 215
Dental pain, 243
Dentin, 208
Dentinal fluid flow, reversal of, 210
Dentinal fluid transfer (DFT), 208–210
Dentinal fluid transport, 206
Dentistry, 205
    holistic approach to dental care, 223
    materials in, 214–216
    oral home care, 221–223
    root canal, 216–221
    tooth/body connection, 216
Denture materials, 215
Depletion of aromatic sulfate transporters, 514–515
Depression, 343, 373–374, 404, 423, 428, 431, 476; *see also* Stress

correction, 11
depression-related symptoms, 411
Depressive syndrome, 400
Depth of penetration, 477
DES, *see* Diethylstilbesterol
Desmethoxyyangonin, 582–583
Desulfovibrio desulfuricans (D. desulfuricans), 159
Detached observance, 460
Detoxification, 345, 723
    and age, 160
    and dose, 160
    enzymes, 170–172
    and gender, 160
    and genetic polymorphisms, 159–160
    with homeopathic treatment, 736–737
    pathways, 156–157
    phases, 157–159
    procedures, 168–170
    and route of administration, 160–161
    and suboptimal nutrient intake, 161–162
Detox reactions, 162
Detox remedies, 168–169
Detrimental manifestation of aging, 632–633
DFT, *see* Dentinal fluid transfer
DHA, *see* Docosahexaenoic acid
Dharana yoga, 364
Dhātu āma, 344
Dhātus, 333
DHEA, *see* Dehydroepiandrosterone
DHEAS, *see* Sulfated DHEA
DHLA, *see* Dihydrolipoic acid
Dhyana yoga, 364
Diabetes, 267, 272, 371–373
    nutritional interventions in, 23–24
    type 2, 183
Diabetes mellitus (DM), 89, 372–373, 630
Diabetic neuropathy, 64
Diabetic wounds, 484
Diagnostic studies, 252
Diarrhea, 88
Diazepam, 125
Dichlorodiphenyldichloroethylene (DDE), 152
Dietary approaches to hypertension, 25
    Dr. Walter Kempner and rice diet, 25–27
    medically supervised water-only fasting, 28
    nutrient dense plant-rich dietary protocol, 27
    selecting special foods, 27–28
Dietary Approaches to Stop Hypertension diet (DASH), 24–25
Dietary factors, 181
Dietary neuroprotection, 194–196
Dietary plant polyphenols, 194
Dietary prebiotics, 194
Dietary Supplement Health & Education Act (DSHEA), 359, 748, 754
Dietary supplements, 753–755
Diethylstilbesterol (DES), 155
Diet(s), 265
    fat-soluble vitamins, 280
    micronutrients and trace elements, 281
    and supplements, 277
    vitamins and minerals, 277–280
    water-soluble vitamins and micronutrients, 280–281

Diffusing signal molecules, 646
  DNA, 652–653
  EMFs, 651–652
  molecule electromagnetic communication, 650–651
  slow and random diffusion, 646–647
  vibrating molecules, 648–649
Diffusion
  capacity, 368
  of substances, 654–655
DIGESTIVE system, 724, 727
Digital European Cordless Telephony (DECT), 543
Dihydrofolate reductase inhibitors, 82
Dihydrolipoic acid (DHLA), 63, 65
Dimercapto-propane sulfonate (DMPS), 165, 167
Dimercaptosuccinic acid (DMSA), 165, 167
Dimethyl sulfoxide (DMSO), 45, 66–68
Dinācharya, 336
Dinshah Health Society, 493
Dinshah's Spectro-Chrome chromatic wheel, 490
Diphyllobothrium latum (*D. latum*), 279
Dirty electricity, 535, 542, 544
Disability-causing marmas, 348
Discharge, rhino pharyngitis, 728–730
Disease modifying treatment (DMT), 31
Disordered breathing, 601
Disruption of eNOS, 516
Dissociation, 603
Distance consulting, telemedicine and, 758–760
Distant non-chemical communication, 649
Distribution, 125
Disulfide bonds, 73
DL, *see* Delayed luminescence
DM, *see* Diabetes mellitus
DMPS, *see* Dimercapto-propane sulfonate
DMSA, *see* Dimercaptosuccinic acid
DMSO, *see* Dimethyl sulfoxide
DMT, *see* Disease modifying treatment
DNA, 178, 228, 652–653, 678
  using biophotons to store and communicate
    information, 301
  breakdown, 196
  DNA-damage repair mechanisms, 534
  methylation sequencing technologies, 404
DNA methyltransferases (DNMTs), 295–296
Docosahexaenoic acid (DHA), 183, 266, 271
Doctor Schüssler mineral and tissue salts, 728
Dopamine, 312, 504–505
Doping, 657
Dose/dosage, 477–478
  before and after light therapy, 479
  detoxification and, 160
  essential oils, 563
  importance, 122
Doshas, 331, 336
  air, 331–332
  doshic characteristics, 336–338
  Earth, 332–333
  effects of stress on different body types, 340
  ether or space, 331
  fire, 332
  food preferences, 339–340
  marma points on, 351–354
  personality and behavior according to doshic
    characteristics, 338–339

  seasons, 340–342
  water, 332
Doshic characteristics, 336
  kapha characteristics, 338
  pitta characteristics, 337–338
  vāta characteristics, 336–337
Doshic imbalances, 342
Double-blind, placebo-controlled trials (DB-PC trials), 74
Double-blind study, 558
Drainage, rhino pharyngitis, 730–731
Dreamless sleep brain wave frequencies, 478
"Driving force", 679
D-ribose, 96
Drug
  allergy, 129
  composition, 124
  compounding process, 757
  drug–receptor binding, 128
  excretion, 126–127
  factors affecting body's response to, 129
  FDA's broad definition of, 752–753
  metabolism, 125–126
  problem with existing, 5–7
  susceptibility, 130–131
  synergism, 130
  toxicity, 130
  undesirable responses to drug therapy, 128–129
Drug Enforcement Administration (DEA), 747, 757
Drums, 462
Dry quality, 332
DSHEA, *see* Dietary Supplement Health & Education Act
DTaP, 735
DTH, *see* Delayed type hypersensitivity
Dual system of government, 746–748
Dysbiosis, from eubiosys to, 192
Dysglycemias, 183

E

EAE, *see* Experimental autoimmune encephalomyelitis
Ear
  aches, 245
  disorder, 244–246
  essential oil application for, 564–565
Early behavior intervention, 387
Ear, nose, and throat (ENT), 358
  allergic reactions, 734–735
  and homeopathy, 728
  nodes drainage, 733–734
  otitis, 731–732
  rhino pharyngitis, 728–731
  sinusitis, 732–733
Earth, 332–333, 358
  magnetic field strength, 715
  Schumann resonance frequencies, 478
Earth element, *see* Psoric reactive mode
Eastern medicine, 319
  fulfills foundational criteria for science, 319–320
  music, resonance, and frequencies in, 320–321
Eastern modes of scientific thought, 321–322
Eastern science, 321–322
Eating disorders, 270, 374, 603–604
Ebers Papyrus, 553
EBM, *see* Evidence-based medicine

EBN, *see* Evidence-based nutrition
EBRS, *see* Evidence-Based Review System
EBV EA IgG, 53
EBV infection, 53
EBV VCA IgM, 53
EC, *see* Enteric-coated capsules
ECM, *see* Extracellular matrix
EcoDECT cordless phones, 544
Economic considerations for MBT, 411–412
ED, *see* Emergency department
EDCs, *see* Endocrine disrupting chemicals
EDTA, *see* Ethylenediamine tetraacetic acid
EEG, *see* Electroencephalogram
EES, *see* Electron excited states
"Effective" reduction potential, 680
EGCG, *see* Epigallocatechin gallate
EHP, *see* Endometriosis Health Profile
Ehrlichia, 584
EHS, *see* Electrohypersensitivity; Electromagnetic
        hypersensitivity
EIB, *see* Exercise-induced bronchoconstriction
Eicosapentaenoic acid (EPA), 183, 266, 271
EKG, *see* Electrocardiograms
Electrical energy, 331
Electrical panel and utility room, 547
Electrical systems, glyphosate's disruption of, 513–517
Electrical wires, 510
Electric blanket and waterbed, 547
Electric/electronic device, 541
Electric equipment, 547
Electricity, 530
Electrocardiograms (EKG), 216, 454–455, 699–700
    cancer detection from, 703
    detection of early stage of adenocarcinoma of colon
        via, 703
Electrodermal screening research, 216
Electroencephalogram (EEG), 216, 454, 462
    brain bioelectrical activity, 666
    patterns, 592
Electrohypersensitivity (EHS), 529, 537, 540
    mitigation testing, 539
    provocation testing, 538–539
Electrokinetic vascular streaming potential, 510–511
Electrolytes, 95
    calcium, 95
    Mg, 95
Electromagnetic (EM), 530
    body and consciousness, 303–304
    energy, 525
    phenomena, 322
    pollution, 524, 530
    properties, 530
    signaling, 648, 651
    spectrum, 530
    waves, 687–688
Electromagnetic fields (EMFs), 502, 530, 646, 651–652,
        687, 688, 710
    DNA, 652–653
    electromagnetic field resonance phenomenon, 691
    molecule electromagnetic communication, 650–651
    resonance circuit, 687–688
    slow and random diffusion, 646–647
    vibrating molecules, 648–649
Electromagnetic hygiene

authorities about electrosmog, 540–541
biological effects of electrosmog, 532–539
bluetooth, 545, 547
cell phones, 543
clock radio, 547
commonly used devices, 543
cordless phones, 543
dirty electricity, 542
electrical panel and utility room, 547
electric blanket and waterbed, 547
electric equipment, 547
electromagnetic pollution, 530
ELF magnetic field, 541
energy efficient light bulbs, 545, 546
gaming systems, 545
global distribution of Wi-Fi networks in 2006 and
        2016, 526
historical overview, 525
internet access, 544
monitoring exposure, 547
national and international radio frequency exposure
        guidelines, 527–528
NIR, 530–532
protect ourselves from electrosmog, 541–547
RF/MW radiation, 542–543
smart appliances, 545
smart meter, 544–545
specific recommendations, 541
turn bedroom power off, 547
typical EHS symptoms, 529
wireless baby monitors, 544
Electromagnetic hypersensitivity, *see*
        Electrohypersensitivity (EHS)
Electromagnetic resonance, 649
    oscillation, 509
Electromyography (EMG), 237, 252
Electron excited states (EES), 301
Electronic transition, 481
Electrons, 715
    transfer protein, 679
Electropollution, 665
Electrosmog, 524
    authorities about, 540–541
    biological effects of, 532–539
    electrosmog-free environment, 529, 538
    exposure, 538
    protect ourselves from electrosmog, 541
Elemental state, 143
Elettaria cardamomum, see Cardamom
ELF, *see* Extremely low frequency
EM, *see* Electromagnetic
Embryonic stem cells (ES cells), 616, 628, 629
Emergency department (ED), 411
EMFs, *see* Electromagnetic fields
EMG, *see* Electromyography
Emit radio frequency/microwave radiation, 526–527, 530,
        543
Emotional/emotions, 338–339, 343
    components, 248
    factors, 321
    trauma, 661
Emotional Transformation Therapy (ETT®), 495
Emphasis, 474
EMS, *see* Eosinophilia myalgia syndrome

Emulating nutrient synergies in Mediterranean diet model, 186–187
Enalapril, 128
Encephalopathy, 145
ENC paradigm, *see* Euclidian/Newtonian/Cartesian paradigm
Endeavor, 325
Endocannabinoids, 599–600
Endocrine
    airway effect on endocrine system, 242
    conditions, 272
    disorders, 242
    disruptors, 122–123
    "endocrine/hormonal" system, 209
    ENDOCRINE systems, 724
    health, 410
    society, 122, 271
Endocrine disrupting chemicals (EDCs), 122, 154
    mechanisms involved in creating impact, 155
    reproductive health, 155–156
Endocrine toxicity, 154
    other published research on, 154–155
Endogenous detoxification pathways, 151
Endogenous opioids, 599
Endogenous stem cells, 629
Endogenous toxins, 137–142
Endometriosis, 380
Endometriosis Health Profile (EHP), 380
Endothelial dysfunction, 29–30
Endothelial function, 29–30
Endothelial injury, 29
Endothelial nitric oxide synthase (eNOS), 56, 505–506
    disruption, 516
Endothelin, 23
Endotoxins, 46
Energetic
    electromagnetic model, 648
    exercises, 360
    healing modalities, 312
    influence of color, 491
    medicine, 311–312
Energy, 294–295
    efficient technology, 528
    harvesting, 442
    medicine, 667
    metabolism and aging, 618–619
    points, 333
    posture effect on energy flow, 238–239
    Qi, 216
Energy efficient light bulbs, 545
    spectrograph of wave form through air, 546
Enforcement
    discretion, 756
    policy, 755
Enlightenment, 449
eNOS, *see* Endothelial nitric oxide synthase
Enriched flour, 210
    on food labels, 78
ENS, *see* Enteric nervous system
ENT, *see* Ear, nose, and throat
Enteric-coated capsules (EC), 558
Enteric nervous system (ENS), 191
Enterocolitis, 88
Enterohepatic

cycling, 126
    recirculation, 158
Entrainment, 454
Environmental
    allergies and asthma, 266
    disasters, 596
    and lifestyle factors, 178
    medicine, 152
    pollutant, 524
    protection from environmental electromagnetic fields, 665–667
Environmental respiratory factors, 265
    air pollution, 265
    environmental allergies and asthma, 266
    tobacco, 265
Environmental toxicants, protection against, 11–12
Environmental toxins, 170–172
    administration, detoxification and route of, 160–161
    age, detoxification and, 160
    allostatic load and detoxification enzymes, 170–172
    assessment, 162–164
    bridging gap between academic publications, 150–152
    detoxification procedures, 168–170
    dose, detoxification and, 160
    endocrine toxicity, 154
    gender, detoxification and, 160
    genetic polymorphisms, detoxification and, 159–160
    heavy metals, 165
    history, 164
    immunotoxicology, 152
    and impact on health in high amounts, 152
    laboratory analysis, 164
    mechanisms involved in creating impact of EDCs, 155
    medications, detoxification and, 162
    molecular physiology, 156
    neurotoxicity, 152–154
    organic chemicals, 164–165
    pathways, detoxification, 156–157
    phases of detoxification, 157–159
    practical concerns, 167–168
    practical considerations, 162–166
    published research on endocrine toxicity, 154–155
    reproductive health, 155–156
    suboptimal nutrient intake, detoxification and, 161–162
    traditional approaches, 165–166
    traditional avoidance treatments, 166
    traditional treatments assisting in physical removal of toxins, 167
    traditional treatments improving ability of body, 166
Enzymatic oxidation, 511
Enzymes, 626
    COMT phase II detoxification enzyme, 159
    copper, 92
    CYP2D6, 159
    CYP2E1, 160, 563
    CYP3A, 160
    CYP3A4, 162
    glutathione S-transferase, 57
    inhibition or stimulation, 128
    methyltransferase, 157–158
    moonlighting, 505–506, 518
    salivary, 210
    SIRT, 185
Eosinophilia myalgia syndrome (EMS), 74

EPA, *see* Eicosapentaenoic acid; U.S. Environmental
    Protection Agency
Epidemiology of TMDs, 247
Epidermal nociceptors, 554
Epigallocatechin gallate (EGCG), 189, 587
Epigenetics, 296
    influencers on aging genes, 631–632
Epilepsy, 565
EPS, *see* Extracellular polymeric substance
ERK ½ pathway, *see* Extracellular signal-regulated kinase
    ½ pathway
ermB gene, 576
Erosion, 206
ERPs, *see* Event related potentials
Erythrism, 143
Erythrocyte sedimentation rate (ESR), 32
Erythrocytes, moment of acidification of, 60
ES cells, *see* Embryonic stem cells
Escherichia coli (*E. coli*), 513, 514
Esogetics™, 494
ESR, *see* Erythrocyte sedimentation rate
Essential nutrients, 161
Essential oils
    application for eyes and ears, 564–565
    best practices and safety, 560–561
    blends for nausea, 559–560
    blends for primary dysmenorrhea, 558–559
    composition, 563
    concomitant use of essential oils and medications,
        565–566
    dosage, 563
    and epilepsy or convulsive disorders, 565
    history and advancement, 552–554
    integration into medical practice, 556
    pharmacological and functional evidence of essential
        oil efficacy, 554
    phytophotodermatitis potential, 565
    pregnancy and, 566
    primary role in plants, 552
    safety, 563
    therapy with children, 566
Estradiol (E2), 158, 627
Estriol (E3), 627
Estrogens, 627
    receptor–positive human breast cancer cells, 533
Estrone (E1), 627
Ethanol, 222
Ethernet, 543
    cable for Internet access, 544
Ether or space, 331
Ethmoidal and frontal sinusitis, 733
Ethnic variations in MBTs, 396–397
Ethyl alcohol, 222
Ethylenediamine tetraacetic acid (EDTA), 167
Etiology of TMD, 247–249
Eubiosys to dysbiosis, from, 192
Euclidian/Newtonian/Cartesian paradigm
    (ENC paradigm), 572
Eugenia jambolana (*E. jambolana*), 630
European Academy for Environmental Medicine
    (EUROPAEM), 540
Eustachian tube drainage, 731–732
Event related potentials (ERPs), 430
"Evidence-based" data, 749

Evidence-based medicine (EBM), 750
Evidence-based nutrition (EBN), 750
Evidence-based practice, 423–424
Evidence-Based Review System (EBRS), 749, 751, 764
Evolutionary mechanics theories, 615
Evolution of life, 661
Excessive sympathetic syndrome, 132
Exclusion zone (EZ), 307, 440, 503, 509, 510
    water, 307–308, 441
Executive attention, 429
Exercise, 630
Exercise-induced bronchoconstriction (EIB), 377
Exercise training (EXT), 377
Exogenous toxins, 137
    alcohol, 141–142
    tobacco, 138–141
Exosomes, *see* Microvesicles
Experimental autoimmune encephalomyelitis (EAE), 79
Exposure parameters, 478
EXT, *see* Exercise training
Extensive metabolizers, 159
External qì gōng, 326
Extracellular matrix (ECM), 509, 585
    glycoproteins, 508
    structural defects, 93
Extracellular polymeric substance (EPS), 12
Extracellular signal-regulated kinase ½ pathway
    (ERK ½ pathway), 586
Extracellular tissues, 445
Extracranial tumors, 246
Extrapyramidal syndrome, 132
Extremely low frequency (ELF), 525, 530, 652
    electric and magnetic fields, 530
    electric/electronic device, 541
    electromagnetic fields, 534–535
    external to building, 541
    magnetic field, 532–533, 541
    wiring inside building, 541
Exxon Valdez oil spill, 596
Eyes
    disorder, 244–246
    essential oil application for, 564–565
    stimulation instruments, 493
EZ, *see* Exclusion zone

F

Facial and pharyngeal airway, 230
Facial growth
    and airway, tongue function effect on, 232–233
    mouth breathing effect on, 231–232
Facial systems, 676
FAP, *see* Functional abdominal pain
Fascia, 675
    living, 676
Fascination with yoga, 366
Fasting, 189
Fasting blood sugar (FBS), 372, 380, 410
Fat
    fat-soluble vitamins, 280
    tissue, 125
    vitamin E, 280
Fatal-death-if-pierced marmas, 348
Fatigue, 383

Fatty fish, 271
Favism, *see* Glucose-6-Phosphate Dehydrogenase
    Deficiency (G6PD-deficiency)
FBS, *see* Fasting blood sugar
FD&C, *see* Food, drug and cosmetic
FDA, *see* U.S. Food and Drug Administration
FDA Modernization Act (FDAMA), 764–765
FDCA, *see* Federal Food, Drug, and Cosmetic Act
Fecal calprotectin, 193
Fecal immunochemical tests (FIT), 277
Fecal microbiota transplantation (FMT), 8, 9
Federal and state laws, 745
Federal and state regulations to promote health freedom,
    761
    changes to FDA regulations, 761–764
    new legislation to promote health freedom, 764–765
Federal Food, Drug, and Cosmetic Act (FDCA), 747, 752
Federal legal systems, 745
Federal regulatory concerns for alternative practitioners,
    756
    FTC standards and regulation, 760–761
    physician dispensing and compounding, 756–758
    telemedicine and distance consulting, 758–760
Federal Trade Commission (FTC), 747, 760
    standards and regulation, 760–761
Female stress response, 596–597
Femtochemistry, 680
Femtosecond spectroscopy, 680
Fermentable, Oligo-, Di-, Mono-saccharides and Polyols
    (FODMAPS), 192
Ferritin, 278
FEV1, *see* Forced expiratory volume during first breath
Feynman, Richard, 442
FFMQ, *see* Five-Facet Mindfulness Questionnaire
FHP, *see* Forward head posture
Fibonacci number series/frequencies, 452
Fibromyalgia, *see* Chronic pain
Fibromyalgia Syndrome (FMS)
Fick's law of diffusion, 654
FICZ, *see* 6-Formylindolo[3,2-b] carbazole
Fight or flight response, *see* Stressful situations
Filters, 542
Fire, 332, 358
Fire element, *see* Luetic reactive mode
Firmicutes, 189
1st-pass effect, 47, 123
First Amendment protection, 760
Fish oil, 271
FIT, *see* Fecal immunochemical tests
Five-Facet Mindfulness Questionnaire (FFMQ),
    399, 400
Flame retardants, 156
Flavanoids, 504–505, 581, 582, 626
Flavoring, 222
FLAX effects in Peripheral Arterial Disease
    (FLAX-PAD), 27
Flax seed, *see* Linseeds
Flow mediated dilation (FMD), 29
Fluid reversal, 210–211
Fluoric, 718, 720
Fluoride (F), 82, 222
5-Fluorouracil, 128
FMD, *see* Flow mediated dilation
FMT, *see* Fecal microbiota transplantation

FODMAPS, *see* Fermentable, Oligo-, Di-, Mono-
    saccharides and Polyols
Foeniculum vulgare var. *dulce, see* Sweet fennel
Folate, 81
    trap phenomenon, 278
Folic acid, 80–82, 278
Follicle stimulating hormone (FSH), 381
Food, 294
    additive theory, 748
    allergy, 276
    calorie, 295
    as energy, 294–295
    healing, 748
    as information, 295
    as matter, 294
    microbiome, 297
    powerful implications for future, 299
    preferences, 339–340
    sociocultural meaning, 293
    supplements, 182
    timing and quality, 297–299
Food and Drugs Act and Regulations, 481
Food, drug and cosmetic (FD&C), 222
    color pigments, 222
Food protein-induced enterocolitis syndrome (FPIES), 276
Forced Expiratory Volume, 377
Forced expiratory volume during first breath (FEV1), 135,
    377, 378
Forced vital capacity (FVC), 135, 377, 378
Force of evolutionary selection, 615
Foreign bodies, 281–282
6-Formylindolo[3,2-b] carbazole (FICZ), 512–513
Forward head posture (FHP), 237, 254
Fossil fuel, 474
Fourth phase of water, 307, 439, 501
    applications in medical science, 443–444
    applications in natural science, 441–442
    future, 446–447
    implications, 439–440
    information in water, 445–446
    negative charge and antioxidants, 445
    pioneering paradigm, 309
    practical applications, 442–443
    water and healing, 444–445
    water transduce energy, 440–441
FPIES, *see* Food protein-induced enterocolitis syndrome
Fractures, 627
Frailty, 629
Free radical theory of aging, 617–618
Free sulfate, 504
Frequencies in Eastern medicine, 320–321
Fröhlich, Herbert, 645
Frontal sinusitis, 733
Fruits, variety in, 622, 631
    3D printing, 631
FSH, *see* Follicle stimulating hormone
FTC, *see* Federal Trade Commission
Full wavelength antenna, 653
Functional abdominal pain (FAP), 369
Functional foods, 189
Functional medicine approach, anti-aging from, 611
Function preservation, 611
Furchgott, Robert F., 482
FVC, *see* Forced vital capacity

G

G6PD-deficiency, *see* Glucose-6-Phosphate
    Dehydrogenase Deficiency
GABA, *see* Gamma-aminobutyric acid
GABAergic transmission, 11
GAD, *see* Generalized anxiety disorder
GAGs, *see* Glycosaminoglycans
Galactose, 276
Gaming systems, 545
Gamma-aminobutyric acid (GABA), 80
Gamma-glutamyl Se-methylselenocysteine, 86
Gamma glutamyl transferase (GGT), 268
γ-GCL, *see* Glutamate cysteine ligase
G tuning forks, 462–464
Gastric
    emptying, 124
    hormones, 282
Gastroesophageal reflux disease (GERD), 236, 368, 408,
    514
Gastrointestinal (GI), 41, 190
    absorption, 124–125
    disorder, 369
    dysbiosis, 189
    health, 408–409
    permeability, 190
    system, 309`
    tract, 124–125, 189, 341
Gastro-resistant capsules (GR capsules), 558
GC, *see* Ground current
GDP, *see* Gross domestic product
Gelled hexameric crystalline form, 501
Gender, detoxification and, 160
Generalized anxiety disorder (GAD), 556
Gene(s), 267
    expression, 433–434
    manipulation, 632
Genetic
    changes in health and disease, 432–434
    marker studies of genes, 249
    polymorphisms, 159–160
    therapy, 632
Genetotrophic disease, 295
GENOME project, 228
Genomic instability, 178–181
    AD, 183
    plus, 181–183
Genomic research, 403–404
Genomic stress, 178
Geranium (*Pelargonium graveolens*), 559
GERD, *see* Gastroesophageal reflux disease
GGT, *see* Gamma glutamyl transferase
GH, *see* Growth hormone
GHB, *see* Glycated hemoglobin
GHD, *see* Growth hormone deficiency
Ghrelin, 273
GI, *see* Gastrointestinal
Ginger (*Zingiber officinale*), 559
Gland of youth, *see* Thymus gland
Glaxo's Lovaza, 182
Glimpse, 255
Global System for Mobile Communications
    (GSM), 533
Glucose, 298

Glucose buffering, glycocalyx recycling as, 512
Glucose-6-Phosphate Dehydrogenase Deficiency
    (G6PD-deficiency), 50
Glucose tolerance factor (GTF), 94
Glutamate cysteine ligase (γ-GCL), 65
Glutathione, 48, 56, 196
    glutathione S-transferase enzymes, 57
    precursor, 73
    supplementation, 59
    tripeptide, 60
Glutathione-S-transferase M1 (GSTM1), 159
Glutathione disulfide (GSSG), 56
Glycated hemoglobin (GHB), 368, 380
Glycation, 618
Glycemic control, 373
Glycerin, 222
Glycine, 75
    glycine-rich ZNRF2, 516
    glycine-to-aspartate mutation, 513–514
Glycine receptors (GlyRs), 75
Glycocalyx, 502, 512
    recycling as glucose buffering, 512
Glycogen phosphorylase, 80
Glycosaminoglycans (GAGs), 502–503, 586
Glycosylated hemoglobin (HbA1c), 372–373, 410
Glycosylation, 612
Glycyrrhiza spp, 583
Glyphosate, 516
    cholesterol sulfate, PPAR γ, and liver, 515–516
    depletion of aromatic sulfate transporters, 514–515
    disruption of electrical systems, 513
    disruption of eNOS, 516
    sodium/potassium ATPase and heart, 516–517
    sulfate homeostasis, 513–514
GlyRs, *see* Glycine receptors
Goethe's chromatic wheel with six colors, 489
Government, dual system of, 746–748
Gram-negative bacteria, 46
Gray matter density, 401
GR capsules, *see* Gastro-resistant capsules
Green light, 477
Gross domestic product (GDP), 154
Ground current (GC), 531–532
Ground regulation system, 675–676
Group selection mechanics theory, 615
Growth disorders and homeopathy, 728
Growth hormone (GH), 75, 627
Growth hormone deficiency (GHD), 242, 627
GSH, *see* L-Glutathione
GSM, *see* Global System for Mobile
    Communications
GSNO, *see* S-nitrosoglutathione
GSSG, *see* Glutathione disulfide
GSTM1, *see* Glutathione-S-transferase M1
GTF, *see* Glucose tolerance factor
Guided imagery, 393, 395, 410
Gut–brain
    axis, 189–190, 514
    function, 193
Gut flora, *see* Gut microbiota
Gut microbiome, 11
Gut microbiota, 11, 190, 193, 189, 282
Gut motility, 124
Gut pH, 124

H

Hahnemann Dilution System, 716
Hahnemann, Samuel, 715–716
Half-wave antennas, 653
Hallucination, 343
HAMA, *see* Hamilton Anxiety Scale
Hamilton Anxiety Scale (HAMA), 557
Hans Jenny's high-speed photograph
    of sand vibrating on metal plate, 451, 452
    of water vibrating on metal plate, 452, 453
Haptene, 137
"Hard" class IV lasers, 477
Harmony, 450
Harmos, 450
HAT, *see* Histone acetyltransferase
Hatha yoga (HY), 365, 375, 601
Hayflick
    concept, 616
    limit, 616
HbA1c, *see* Glycosylated hemoglobin
HCV, *see* Hepatitis C
HCY, *see* Homocysteine
HD, *see* Huntington's disease
HDACs, *see* Histone deacetylases
HDG, *see* High-dose group
HDL, *see* High-density lipoprotein
HDL ratio, *see* High density lipoprotein ratio
HDMs, *see* Histone demethylases
Healing, 444–445, 450
    process, 552
    of traumatic stress, 592
Health; *see also* Nutrient(s)
    claim, 763
    process, 335–336
    professionals, 43
Health Canada, 481
Health care
    expand freedom of choice in, 765
    practitioners, 474, 481, 746
Health Enhancement Program (HEP), 432
Health Food Junkies, 167
Health-related quality of life (HRQoL), 375
Heart, 347, 516–517
    beats, 591
    disease, 23, 31
    of matter, 21
    nutritional intervention in cardiovascular disease, 21–23
    nutritional interventions in diabetes, 23–24
    nutritional interventions in hypertension, 24–28
    yoga and, 366–368
Heartburn, 408
Heart rate (HR), 372, 387
Heart rate variability (HRV), 400, 538
Heavy metals, 165, 277
    toxins, 165
HeLa cells, 616
Helicobacter pylori (*H. pylori*), 282
Heliotherapy, 474, 488
Hematomas, 485
Hemorrhage, 502
HEP, *see* Health Enhancement Program
Heparan sulfate, 506–507
    chains, 503

    molecules in matrix, 511
Hepatic detoxification, 157, 158
Hepatitis C (HCV), 53
Hepatocarcinogen 1′-sulfooxyestragole, 563
Herb(al)
    for DM, 630
    or botanical, 754
    products, 754–755
    remedies, 748
Herbal medicines, 277–281, 572
    bacterial intelligence, 575–578
    borrelial infections, 585–587
    chemical innovation in plants, 580–583
    dosages and treatment approaches, 587–589
    FDA regulation, 753–756
    paradigm conflicts, 572–573
    plant intelligence, 578–580
    resistance to plants, 583–584
    self-organization, 573–575
    stealth pathogens, 584–585
Heroin, 142
Herpes simplex virus (HSV), 53
    HSV1 or HSV2, 53
Hertz (Hz), 591
Heterochronic plasma exchange (HPE), 632
HF, *see* High frequency
HFVT, *see* High frequency voltage transients
HI, *see* Hypoxia-ischemia
Hibiscus, 28
Hidradenitis Suppurativa (HS), 13
High-density lipoprotein (HDL), 185, 502, 505
    ratio, 183
High blood pressure, 64, 240
High density lipoprotein ratio (HDL ratio), 623
High-dose group (HDG), 373
High dose IV vitamin C, 52
    antitumoral effect, 52
High-dose vitamin C, 47
High frequency (HF), 525, 645
High frequency voltage transients (HFVT), 531, 533
High voltage frequency transients (HVFT), 542, 545
Himalayan bowls, 461
Hippocampal volume, 402
Hippocrates, 715
Histone acetyltransferase (HAT), 295–296
Histone deacetylases (HDACs), 296
Histone demethylases (HDMs), 296
Histone methyltransferases (HMTs), 296
Histone modification analysis, 404
HMTs, *see* Histone methyltransferases
Hoarseness painful, 730
Holism, 667
Holistic
    anatomical perspective, 667
    approach to dental care, 223
    biomedicine, 674
    health, 312
Homeopathic/homeopaths/homeopathy, 714, 715
    constitutions, 718–720
    detoxifying with homeopathic treatment, 736–737
    drainage, 722–723
    E.N.T. and, 728–735
    foreword, 714
    growth disorders and, 728

homeopathic drainage, 722–723
homeopathic remedies, 716–717
hyperactivity, attention deficit disorders and, 738–741
line of life, 725–727
medicine, 731
natural resonance, 714–715
prescribe, 727
principles, 715–716
reactive modes, 717, 720–721
remedies, 716–717
skin language, 721–722
wheel of emunctories, 723–725
Homocysteine (HCY), 73, 188, 379–380
    acid, 279
Hormone replacement therapy (HRT), 626–627
Hormones, 272–273, 381–382, 631, 646
    diabetes, 272
    thyroid disease, 272–273
HPA axis, *see* Hypothalamic–pituitary–adrenal axis
HPE, *see* Heterochronic plasma exchange
HPV 16, *see* Human papilloma virus type 16
HR, *see* Heart rate
^{1}H-MRS, *see* Proton magnetic resonance spectroscopy
HRQoL, *see* Health-related quality of life
HRT, *see* Hormone replacement therapy
Hrudaya, see Heart
HRV, *see* Heart rate variability
HRVT, *see* High frequency voltage transients (HFVT)
HS, *see* Hidradenitis Suppurativa
HSV, *see* Herpes simplex virus
5-HTP, *see* 5-Hydroxy tryptophan
Huai Nan Zi, 326
Human
    blood, 502
    brain, 228, 658
    consciousness, 451
    consequences of EZ water for human health, 309
    edifice, 717
    genome, 297
Human body, 357, 501, 658
    emits, 299–307
Human papilloma virus type 16 (HPV 16), 698–699, 711
    anti-cancer effects, 705–706
    clinical implications of, 705
    factors influencing cancer treatment, 708–711
    individualized safe, effective, and affordable cancer treatment, 707–708
    individualized, safe, effective treatment, 705
    treatment considerations, 706–707
Hunger games, 273
Hunger hormone, 273
Huntington's disease (HD), 178
HVFT, *see* High voltage frequency transients
HVS, *see* Hyperventilation syndrome
HY, *see* Hatha yoga
Hyaluronic acid, 503
Hydrated silica, 223
Hydration, 269–270
Hydrazine, 159
Hydrocarbon-based compounds, 138
Hydrogen sulfide (H_2S), 159, 512
Hydronium ions, 443
Hydrophilic chromophores, 440
Hydrotherapy, 367

8-Hydroxy-2′-deoxyguanosine (8-OHGH), 184
4-Hydroxy-estradiol (4-OH-E_2), 158
25-Hydroxy D_3 (25OHD$_3$), 162
2-Hydroxyestradiol (2-OH-E_2), 158
1α-Hydroxylation, 162
Hydroxytirosol, 185
5-Hydroxy tryptophan (5-HTP), 74
Hyperactive brain wave frequencies, 478
Hyperactivity, 738
    restless child, 738–739
    sleep disorders, 740–741
    violent child, 739
    whining, 740
Hyperbaric oxygen therapy, 629
Hypercupremia, 92
Hyperglycemic excursions, 272
Hypersensitivity, 129
Hypertension, 24, 427–429
    dietary approaches to, 25–28
    dietary approaches to hypertension, 25–28
    nutritional interventions in, 24
    salt and dash, 24–25
Hypertonic presentations, 43
Hyperventilation, 601
Hyperventilation syndrome (HVS), 601
Hypnosis, 393
Hypnotism, 657
Hypoglycemia, 51
Hypothalamic–pituitary–adrenal axis (HPA axis), 141, 145, 170, 190, 241, 400, 592, 595
Hypothalamic–pituitary–adrenocortical axis, *see* Hypothalamic–pituitary–adrenal axis (HPA axis)
Hypothalamic sensitivity loss, 616
Hypothalamus, 209, 240–241, 598
Hypothyroidism, 385–386
Hypoxia-ischemia (HI), 75
Hysteria, 603

I

IARC, *see* International Agency for Research on Cancer
Iatrogenics, 34–35
IBD, *see* Inflammatory bowel disease
IBS, *see* Irritable bowel syndrome
Iceberg, 660
ICNIRP, *see* International Commission on Non-Ionizing Radiation Protection
Idiopathic environmental intolerance (IEI), 530, 537
IEI, *see* Idiopathic environmental intolerance
IF, *see* Intermediate frequencies
IFN-α, *see* Interferon-alpha
IFN–γ, 87
Ignarro, Louis J., 482
IIR, *see* Intestinal ischemia reperfusion
IIS pathway, *see* Insulin/IGF-1 signaling pathway
IL, *see* Interleukin
Illusion, 343
IM, *see* Intramuscular
Immediate-death causing marmas, 348
Immortality, 615
Immune dysfunction, 727
Immune function/system, 427, 617, 717
    improvements in health and disease, 432–434

Immune function/system (*Continued*)
   issues, 423
   stimulating, 73
Immunology, 482, 617
Immunosenescence, 88
Immunotoxicology, 137, 152
Impatient, 739
Impedance, 665
   matching, 665, 676
Impulsive behavior, 485
Incoherent light, 479
Incompatibility, 44–45
IND, *see* Investigational New Drug
In Defense of Non-Molecular Cell Biology, 654
Indian medicine, 319–320
Individual harmony and self-healing, 335–336
Individual toxic exposure, treatments and measures to
         reducing, 146
Industrial chemical melamine, 7
Industrial revolution, 474
Infant, 726
   snuffles, 729–730
Infantile colic, potential for, 12
Infections, 281
   foreign bodies, 281–282
   gut flora, 282
   H. pylori, 282
Inflammaging, 618
Inflammatory/inflammation, 53, 484, 517–518, 623
   disorders, 484
   factors, 618
   inflammation-based theories, 618
   link, 183
   nutritional treatment, 30–33
   parameters, 377
   processes, 618
Inflammatory bowel disease (IBD), 275, 408, 433
Infrared energy, 441
Inhalation, 561
Injectable ALA, 65
Injectable Coenzyme Q10, 70
Injectable route for orthomolecular supplementation, 42
Injectable solutions in clinical practice, 41
   application routes in parenteral nutrition, 42–43
Inorganic
   arsenic, 266
   salts, 143
   sulfate, 161
Inositol, 96
Insolent, 739
Insomnia, 386–387
Instability, 45–46
Institutional "procedures manual", 43–44
Instructor training, 412
Insufficiency, 40
Insulin/IGF-1 signaling pathway (IIS pathway), 617
Insulin imbalance, 210
Insulin resistance, 368
   syndrome, 242
Insulin signaling (IS), 183
Integrated Naturopathy and Yoga (INY), 373
Integrated Risk Information System (IRIS), 134
Integrative medicine, 361
Integrative therapies, 667

Integrins, 671, 679
Intelligence, 575
Intelligence quotient (IQ), 154
Intention, 451
   impact, 325–326
Interferon-alpha (IFN-α), 585
Interferon-gamma-driven signalling, 11
Interleukin (IL), 12
   IL-1β, 46
   IL-2, 87, 585
   IL-6, 46, 170, 401, 618
   IL-8, 46
   IL-10, 585
Intermediate filaments, 308
Intermediate frequencies (IF), 530, 531, 535
   EM fields, 533
International Agency for Research on Cancer (IARC),
         134, 540
International Commission on Non-Ionizing Radiation
         Protection (ICNIRP), 526
International Neural Network Society, 645
International Scientific Association for Probiotics and
         Prebiotics (ISAPP), 194
Internet access, 544
Intestinal immune response system, 190
Intestinal ischemia reperfusion (IIR), 72
Intracapsular disorders, 249
Intracranial tumors, 246
Intramuscular (IM), 49
   administration, 48
   injection, 43, 80
   route, 43
Intramyocellular lipid, 24
Intra-uterus life, 725
Intravenous (IV), 40
   CoQ10, 69
   for "frailty syndrome" or aging, 629
   GSH, 61
   infusion, 94
   intervention in cancer, 47
   magnesium, 50–51
   nutrients, 48–50
   nutritional deficiencies/insufficiencies supporting IV
         supplementation, 40–41
   route, 42–43, 86
Intravenous orthomolecular therapeutic agents (IV
         orthomolecular therapeutic agents), 51; *see also*
         Orthomolecular intravenous nutritional therapy
   amino acids, 71–78
   B complex vitamins, 78–82
   electrolytes, 95
   lipid-soluble vitamins, 82
   minerals and trace elements, 82–95
   multimineral preparations, 95–96
   others, 96–97
   precursors of antioxidant enzymes, 96
   vitamins, 78
Intravenous vitamin C (IVC), 47, 53
Intricate web of cellular pathways, 673
Intrinsically photoreceptive retinal ganglion cells
         (ipRGC), 486
Intrinsic membrane proteins, 679
Investigational New Drug (IND), 753, 763
In vitro studies, 532–533, 624

In vivo studies, 532–533
INY, *see* Integrated Naturopathy and Yoga
Iodine (I), 51, 82
Ion channels, 128
    and pumps, 507–508
Ionizing radiation, 530, 534
ipRGC, *see* Intrinsically photoreceptive retinal ganglion
       cells
IQ, *see* Intelligence quotient
IRIS, *see* Integrated Risk Information System
Iron (Fe), 82, 508–510
    deficiency, 277–278
    saturation, 278
Irritable bowel syndrome (IBS), 8, 192, 369–371, 408
    peppermint essential oil for, 558
Irritants, 136
    irritant-type contact dermatitis, 135
IS, *see* Insulin signaling
ISAPP, *see* International Scientific Association for
       Probiotics and Prebiotics
Isatis tinctoria (*I. tinctoria*), 583
Isoflavones, 504–505
Isoleucine, 74
IV, *see* Intravenous
IVC, *see* Intravenous vitamin C
IV orthomolecular therapeutic agents, *see* Intravenous
       orthomolecular therapeutic agents
Iyengar yoga program (IY program), 369

J

Japanese knotweed root (*Polygonum cuspidatum*), 583, 586
JNK, *see* c-Jun N-terminal kinase
Joint-based marmas, 347
Joint capsule, 308, 443
Jones–Ray effect, 504
Journal of Alzheimer's Disorders, 188
Journal of American Medical Association, 187, 361
Journal of Chinese Medicine, 325
Jumping genes, 512–513

K

Kaempferol, 582
Kalantara Pranahara, see Long-term death causing
      marmas
Kapalbhati, 369
Kapha, 331, 332, 333
    building material of body, 335
    characteristics, 338
    sub-doshas and marma points, 353
    symptoms, 342
Kaplan case, 747
Kashin-Beck disease, 85
Kefir grains, 195
Kegel for urinary incontinence, 630
Kelvin water dropper, 445
Keshan disease, 84
Kidneys, 126
    stones, 270
Kidney stones, 270
Kidscreen quality of life (KQoL), 369
"Kin selection" theory, 615
Kledaka Kapha, 353

Korean Constitutional Acupuncture, 324
Korsakoff Dilution System, 716
Kosmotrope, 511
KQoL, *see* Kidscreen quality of life
Kriya yoga, 601
Kundalini yoga (KY), 386, 601
KY, *see* Kundalini yoga

L

LA5, *see* Lactobacillus acidophilus
Laboratory analysis, detoxification of environmental
      toxins, 164
Lactobacillus acidophilus (LA5), 195
Lactobacillus spp., 13
    L. bulgaricus, 195
    L. paracasei, 11
    L. plantarum, 11
Lactose, 276
Lamina densa, 507
Landmark study, 168
L-Arginine, 75
Lasers, 214
    beam, 693
    therapy, 474
Lateral light therapy, 495
Lavandula angustifolia, see Lavender
Lavender (*Lavandula angustifolia*), 556, 559
Lavender essential oil for anxiety, 556–558
LBP, *see* Low back pain
L-Carnitine, 74–75, 625
LCDs, *see* Local Coverage Determinations
L-C resonance circuits, 688
L-Cysteine, 72
LD50 dose, 133
LDG, *see* Low-dose group
LDL, *see* Low density lipoprotein
Lead (Pb), 82, 144, 153
    effects on children, 145
    exposure to, 266
    paint, 144
"Leaky gut", integrative medicine practitioners, 190
Learning, holistic properties, 580
LED, *see* Light emitting diodes
Left nostril variations, 387–388
LEMNA MINOR, 723
Lemon (*Citrus limon*), 560
Length of stay (LOS), 374
Leptin deficiency, 273
Leucine, 74
Leukotrienes, 266
L-Glutathione (GSH), 56–63, 72
    GSH/glutathione disulphide ratio, 61
Licorice (*Glycyrrhiza* spp), 583
Life energy, 312
Lifestyle Heart Trial, 22, 29, 366
Lifestyle interventions, 620–623
    delayed reproduction, 622–623
    exercise, 620–622
    sleep, 623
    social practices, 623
    stress management, 623
Lift restrictions on preventative or wellness advertising,
      763–764

Ligament-based marmas, 347
Light emitting diodes (LED), 474, 477, 486, 492, 545
Light(ing), 474, 483, 661
    chronobiological applications, 486–488
    through eyes, 493
    light-on-skin modalities, 475
    manufacturers, 545
    modulation process, 495
    placement, 476
    quality, 332
    on skin, 493
    and travels medium, 662–664
Light therapy, 474–475, 481–483, 486
    chromotherapy, 490–492
    chromotherapy and color importance, 488–491
    chronobiological applications of light, 486–488
    healing with, 474
    living organisms, 474–475
    mechanisms of photobiomodulation, 481–483
    phototherapy, 475–481
    potential applications of photobiomodulation,
        483–486
    tools and methods of chromotherapy, 492–496
Like-likes-like cloud formation, 442
Like-likes-like principle, 442
Limbic-hypothalamic-pituitary system, 598
Line of Life, 725–727, 735
Linseeds, 27
Lipids, 298
    lipid-lowering drugs, 366
    lowering effect, 23
Lipid-soluble
    drugs, 125
    vitamins, 82
Lipofuscin, 510
Lipoic acid, 80
Lipopolysaccharides (LPS), 46, 192, 515
Liquid-crystalline phase, 441
Listening, 450
Lithium (Li), 82
Liver, 515–516
    function optimization, 74
Living matrix, 671–673
Living organisms, 474–475
L-Leucine, 74
LLLT, *see* Low-level laser therapy
L-Lysine, 76
Loading dose, 127
LOAEL, *see* Lowest-observed-adverse-effect-level
Local Coverage Determinations (LCDs), 747
Long-term death causing marmas, 348
Long-term IV nutrition, 90
Lorazepam group, 557
L-Ornithine (L-ORN), 76
LOS, *see* Length of stay
Low back pain (LBP), 360
Low-dose group (LDG), 373
Low-fat vegan diet, 23
Low density lipoprotein (LDL), 95, 185, 502, 505, 618
    cholesterol, 183
Low doses big effects
    E.N.T. and homeopathy, 728–735
    growth disorders and homeopathy, 728
    homeopathy, 714–727

    hyperactivity, attention deficit disorders and
        homeopathy, 738–741
    side effects of vaccination, 735–737
Lower maximal oxygen uptake (VO_2max), 621
Lowest-observed-adverse-effect-level (LOAEL), 133
Low fat diet, 22
Low-level laser therapy (LLLT), 475, 477, 479, 481, 484
L-Phenylalanine (L-PHE), 77
LPS, *see* Lipopolysaccharides
L-Taurine, 75
L-Tryptophan (L-Trp), 76
Lucretian biochemistry, 653–657
Luetic reactive mode, 721, 722
Luminal contents, 124
Lunar forces, 306–307
Lungs, 127
    functions, 368
Lutiolin, 582
LYCOPODIUM, 723
Lyme disease (*Borrelia burgdorferi*), 572, 584
Lymphatic system, 482
    functions, 238
Lymphocyte proliferation, 60
Lysine, 76
Lysosomes, 508–510
Lysyl oxidase, 93

M

MAAS, *see* Mindful Attention and Awareness Scale
Macrocytic anemia, 278, 279
Macro elements, 82
Macromolecules, 127, 651
    incorporation into, 128
Magnesium (Mg), 49, 82, 83, 95, 266
Magnetic fields, 541
Magnetic flux density, 530
Magnetic resonance angiography (MRA), 246
Magnetic resonance imaging (MRI), 246, 252, 429
Maintenance dose, 127
Majjā, 333
Major depressive disorder (MDD), 11, 431
Malabsorption, 87, 273–274, 281
Malas, 344, 345, 355
Malignant cancers, 246
Malignant hyperthermia, 132
Mammalian infants, 230
Mammary gland tumors, 532–533
Māmsa, 333
Mandibular disorders, 244
Mandibular motion, 249, 251
Manganese (Mn), 51, 71, 82, 83, 93–94, 183, 277
Mantras, 449, 451, 457–458
MAP, *see* Mean arterial pressure
MAPKs, *see* Mitogen-activated protein kinases
Marjoram (*Origanum majorana*), 559
Market authorization, 481
Marma chikitsā, 330
Marma meditation, 351
Marma points, 333–334, 347
    classification on doshas and sub-doshas, 351–354
Marma therapy
    benefits, 355
    clinical application, 354–355

marma areas, 347
marma meditation, 351
marma points anterior view, 349
marma points classification on doshas and sub-doshas, 351–354
marma points posterior view, 350
technique, 354
yogic marmas, 348
Maslach Burnout Inventory (MBI), 399, 400
Massage, 253, 395, 600, 602
body-based medicine, 752
essential oil, 559
stress prevention, 623
Masticatory muscle disorders, 249
Mastoiditis threatened, 732
Materially based model, 424
Material Safety Data Sheet (MSDS), 123, 135
Matrix glycoproteins, 502, 508, 511
Matrixmetalloproteinases (MMPs), 212, 585–587
Maxilla disorders, 244
Maxillary sinusitis, 733
Maximum Voluntary Ventilation (MVV), 377, 378
Maxwell's equation, 310
Mayo Clinic trial, 47
MB, see Mind–body
MBCT, see Mindfulness-based cognitive therapy
MBI, see Maslach Burnout Inventory
MBSR, see Mindfulness-based stress reduction
MBT, see Mindfulness Based Therapies
MBTs, see Mind body therapies
MCI, see Mild Cognitive Impairment
MCS, see Multiple chemical sensitivity
MCV, see Mean corpuscular volume
MDD, see Major depressive disorder
MDQs, see Menstrual Distress Questionnaires
Mean arterial pressure (MAP), 26
Mean corpuscular volume (MCV), 278
Meares–Irlen Syndrome, 474
Measles-like syndrome, 736
Mechanistic target of rapamycin (mTORC), 298
"Mechano-transduction" process, 668
Meda, 333
Medical
advice, 759
devices, 752, 753, 755–756
foods, 753–756, 764
interventions, 611
ozone therapies, 214
research, 642, 667
supervised water-only fasting, 28
toxicology, 131–132
Medical science, 715
water phase applications in, 443–444
Medical Subject Headings (MeSH), 475
Meditation, 406, 408, 423, 424–425; see also Yoga
cardiovascular effects, 427–429
detoxification and, 162
evidence-based practice, 423–424
historical context, 425–427
immune system improvements and genetic changes, 432–434
neurobiological effects of meditation, 429–432
pain pathways modulation by, 432
physiological effects, 427

Meditative state brain wave frequencies, 478
Meditative techniques, 451
Mediterranean diet, 184–186, 367
emulating nutrient synergies in Mediterranean diet model, 186–187
pathways modulated by resveratrol, 187
Mediterranean dietary pattern, 184–185
Mediterrasian diet, 188–189
Melanin, 304–305, 307, 309, 481
Melatonin, 185, 487, 514–515, 626
Membrane biology, 674
Memory, 580, 586
water, 446
Menkes syndrome, 92
Menopause, 380–381, 627
Menopause Strategies: Finding Lasting Answers for Symptoms and Health (MsFLASH), 381
Menstrual cycle, 269
Menstrual Distress Questionnaires (MDQs), 379
Mental āma, 344
Mental disorders, 411
Mental/emotional problems, 423
Mentha × piperita, see Peppermint essential oil
Mentha spicata, see Spearmint
Menthol, 161, 222, 554–555, 565
Merck Manual, The, 566
Mercury (Hg), 143–144, 153
amalgams, 214
Meridians, 216
MeSH, see Medical Subject Headings
Messenger photons, 663
Metabolic health, 410
Metabolic syndrome, 12
Metabolites, 125
Metallothionein (MT), 165
Metformin, 624–625
Methadone, 142
Methanol, 555
Methicillin resistant staph (MRSA), 576
Methionine, 73
Methionine residues, 74
2-Methoxyestradiol (2-MeO-E$_2$), 158
4-Methoxyestradiol (4-MeO-E$_2$), 158
5′-Methoxyhydnocarpin (5′-MHC), 582
5-Methyl-2-(propan-2-yl)cyclohexan-1-ol, see Menthol
Methyl 2 hydroxybenzoate, see Methyl salicylate
Methyl donor B vitamins, 188
Methylenetetrahydrofolate reductase (MTHFR), 159, 186
Methylmalonic acid, 279
Methylmercury, 153
Methyl salicylate, 555
Methylselenocysteine, 86
Methyltransferase enzymes, 157–158
MGR, see Mitogenetic radiation (MR)
5′-MHC, see 5′-Methoxyhydnocarpin
MI, see Myocardial infarction
Micorbiome, 142, 297, 514
biofilms, 12–13
complementary therapies, 8–12
examples of drugs efficacy and/or safety depend on microbiome status, 6
examples of microbiome rebiosis to treat diseases and conditions, 10
managing microbial ecology of patient, 7–8

Micorbiome (*Continued*)
  NCD epidemic, 5
  patient, 4–5
  problem with existing drugs, 5–7
  rebiosis to treat diseases and conditions, examples of,
    10
  role on human health, 4
Microalbumin, 272
Microarray technologies, 403
Microbes, 524
Microbial diversity, 193
Microbial ecology management, 7–8
Microbiota, 189–190
Micro elements, 82
Micronutrients, 280–281
  nutritional deficiencies, 275
  zinc, 86–92
Microorganisms, interference with metabolic processes
    of, 128
MicroRNAs (miRNAs), 296–297
Microtubules, 308, 658
Microvesicles, 296
Microwave (MW), 530, 531
  MW-frequency electromagnetic radiation, 536
  radiation, 525–526, 533, 544, 544
Mild Cognitive Impairment (MCI), 427, 431
Mind–body
  assessment, 602–603
  exercises, 375
  intervention, 432
Mind–body medicine, 393, 395; *see also* Ayurvedic
    medicine; Chinese medicine; Herbal medicines
  advances in research, 397
  age variations, 395–396
  barriers and facilitators of MBT uses, 412–413
  burnout, 400
  cancer, 406
  cardiovascular health, 409–410
  common MBTs, 394
  composite markers, 404–406
  economic considerations, 411–412
  epidemiology, 395
  genomic research, 403–404
  GI health, 408–409
  health outcomes, 406
  historical perspectives and development, 394–395
  mental health, 406–408
  metabolic and endocrine health, 410
  mindfulness, 399–400
  multi-factorial models, 397–398
  neuroimaging MBT studies, 401–403
  pain, neurological, and autoimmune disorders, 406
  physiological MBT research, 400–401
  psychosocial MBT research, 398–399
  side effects and risks of MBT, 410
  sociodemographic and ethnic variations, 396–397
Mind body therapies (MBTs), 393–395, 400, 401, 406,
    411, 423
Mind–brain continuum model, 424
Mindful Attention and Awareness Scale (MAAS),
    399, 400
Mindful listening, 451, 456–457
Mindful meditation, 393, 395
Mindfulness, 399–400

  training, 431
Mindfulness-based cognitive therapy (MBCT), 408, 425,
    426, 431, 432
Mindfulness Based Therapies (MBT), 432
Mindfulness-based stress reduction (MBSR), 395, 425,
    426, 432
Mind in health, 343–344
Mineral, 716, 754
  Chromium, 94–95
  Cu, 92–93
  Mn, 93–94
  Se, 84–86
  and trace elements, 82
  Zn, 86–92
Mine Safety Health Administration (MSHA), 131
Minimal essential mechanical stress, 630
MinTraz from OrthomoLab®, 48
miRNAs, *see* MicroRNAs
Mitigation testing, 539
Mitochondria, 510, 618
  cholesterol-enriched mitochondria, 509–510
Mitochondria DNA (mtDNA), 180
Mitochondrial dysfunction, 483, 605
Mitogen-activated protein kinases (MAPKs), 586
Mitogenetic radiation (MR), 303–304, 649
Mixed sleep apnea, *see* Complex sleep apnea
MM–16 Forte from HeilPro DKN®, 48
MMPs, *see* Matrixmetalloproteinases
MMR, 735–736
"Moais", 615
Mobile applications for MBT, 413
Mobile medical apps, 755
Mobile quality, 322
Modalities of Chinese medicine, 358
  Chinese dietary therapy, 359
  Chinese herbology, 358–359
  energetic exercises, 360
  Tui Na, 359
Modern cell biology, 441
Modern medical training, 450
Modern medicine, 456, 491, 642, 667, 761–762
Modern science, 306, 654
Modulation of light, 478–479
Molecular biology, 674
Molecular circuitry, 656
Molecular physiology of environmental toxins, 156
Molecular "wires", 678–680
Molecule-to-molecule signaling, 648
Molybdenum (Mo), 71, 82, 83, 92
Momordica charantia (*M. charantia*), 630
Monitoring exposure, 547
Monitoring of Side Effects Scale (MOSES), 59
Monoamine neurotransmitters, 504–505, 514
Monochromatic color, 475
Monochromatic light, 496
Monosaccharides glucose, 276
Monosodium glutamate (MSG), 33
Moonlighting enzyme, 505–506, 518
Moros' mineral constellations, 48
Morphine, 127
Morphogenetic field, 474
MOSES, *see* Monitoring of Side Effects Scale
Moss's theory, 231
Mother Tincture (MT), 716

Motor learning, 234
Mouth breathing
    effect on facial growth, 231–232
    etiology, 232
Movement-oriented practices, 425
Moxa, *see* Moxibustion
Moxibustion, 360
MR, *see* Mitogenetic radiation
MRA, *see* Magnetic resonance angiography
MRI, *see* Magnetic resonance imaging
MRSA, *see* Methicillin resistant staph
MS, *see* Multiple sclerosis
MSDS, *see* Material Safety Data Sheet
MsFLASH, *see* Menopause Strategies: Finding Lasting
    Answers for Symptoms and Health
MSG, *see* Monosodium glutamate
MSHA, *see* Mine Safety Health Administration
MT, *see* Metallothionein; Mother Tincture
mtDNA, *see* Mitochondria DNA
MTHFR, *see* Methylenetetrahydrofolate reductase
mTORC, *see* Mechanistic target of rapamycin
Multi-disciplinary investigations, 643
Multidimensionality of color effects, 491
Multidrug resistance-associated protein, 157
Multi-factorial approach, 619
Multi-factorial model, 397–398, 401
Multimineral preparations, 95–96
Multi-nutrient supplementation, naturally occurring model
    for, 184–186
Multiple chemical sensitivity (MCS), 58, 168
Multiple sclerosis (MS), 298, 433, 476
    nutritional treatment of, 30–31
Muscarinic pattern, 132
Muscle, 247, 248, 333, 724
    of mastication, 251
    muscle-based marmas, 347
    pain, 247, 341
    pelvic, 630
    relaxants, 252
    skeletal, 264
    symptoms, 152
    weakness, 692
Musculoskeletal disorders, 359, 620
Mushrooms, 123, 132, 708
Music, 450, 455, 461, 525
    in Eastern medicine, 320–321
    structured, 450
    therapy, 406
Mutation accumulation theory, 615
MVV, *see* Maximum Voluntary Ventilation
MW, *see* Microwave
Mycoplasma, 584
Myers' cocktail, 48
Myocardial infarction (MI), 241, 506

N

NAC, *see* N-acetylcysteine
N-acetyl-p-benzoquinoneimine (NAPQI), 160
N-acetylcysteine (NAC), 63, 72–73, 587
NAD(+), *see* Nicotinamide adenine dinucleotide
Nadi shuddhi (NS), 387
NAFLD, *see* Non-alcoholic fatty liver disease
Na-K pump, *see* Sodium-potassium ATPase pump

NAMPT, *see* Nicotinamide phosphoribosyltransferase
Nanobiotic red blood cells (respirocytes), 632
Nanotechnology, 611, 632
NAPQI, *see* N-acetyl-p-benzoquinoneimine
Narrow-band sources, 492
NaS1 sulfate transporter, 507
Nasal breathers, 231
Nasal light therapy, 476
National Center for Complementary and Alternative
    Medicine (NCCAM), 413
National Center for Complementary and Integrative
    Health (NCCIH), 357, 361, 413, 764
National Coverage Determinations (NCDs), 747
National Foundation for Cancer Research, 643
National Health and Nutrition Examination Survey III
    (NHANES III), 82
National Health Interview Survey (NHIS), 395
National Institute of Safety and Health Administration
    (NIOSH), 137
National Institutes of Health (NIH), 276, 357
Natrum, 718, 719
Natural amino acid, 612
Natural head posture (NHP), 237
Natural killer cells (NK cells), 433
    cytotoxicity, 60
Naturally occurring model for multi-nutrient
    supplementation, 184–186
Natural resonance, 714–715
Natural science, water phase applications in, 441–442
Nature (journal), 446
Nausea, blends of essential oils for, 559–560
NB, *see* Normal breathing
NCCAM, *see* National Center for Complementary and
    Alternative Medicine
NCCIH, *see* National Center for Complementary and
    Integrative Health
NCDs, *see* National Coverage Determinations;
    Noncommunicable diseases
NCGS, *see* Non-celiac gluten sensitivity
NCVD, *see* Neurocranio vertical distractor
NDA, *see* New Drug Application
Near infrared (NIR), 478
    energy, 440
    radiation, 475
Near ultraviolet radiation (NUV radiation), 475
"Negative acute phase reactant" proteins, 263
Negative charge and antioxidants, 445
Nephrotic syndrome, 263
Nernst equation, 680
Nerve disorders, 537
Nervous system, 644–646
Nervous systems, 561, 724
Neupogen, 629
Neural communication pathways, 191
Neuralgia, 483
Neural networks, 578, 580
Neural sensitization, 604
Neural therapy, 71
Neural therapy to Huneke (NTH), 96
Neural tube defects (NTDs), 81
Neurobehavioral disorders, 536
Neurobiological effects of meditation, 429–432
Neurocranio vertical distractor (NCVD), 254
Neurodegenerative diseases, 57, 59, 70, 178

Neuro-endocrine theory, 616–617
Neuro-hormones, 646
Neuroimaging, 240
    MBT studies, 401–403
Neuro-immune system, 661
Neuroinflammatory oxidative stress, 188
Neurological brain disorders, 476
Neurological disorders, 406, 407
Neurological system, airway effect on, 240
Neuromuscular responses, 232
Neuron doctrine, 658
Neuroprotective supplementary prescription, nutrients in,
    188
Neuropsychological symptoms, 143
Neurotoxicity, 152–154
Neurotoxicology, 136, 152
New Drug Application (NDA), 753
New legislation to promote health freedom, 764
    expand freedom of choice in health care, 765
    privatized review for alternative medical therapies,
        764–765
    stronger informed consent laws, 765
Newton's chromatic wheel, 489
NF-kB, see Nuclear factor-kappa beta
NHANES III, see National Health and Nutrition
    Examination Survey III
NHIS, see National Health Interview Survey
NHP, see Natural head posture
Niacin, 76, 78, 80–81, 277, 280
Niacinamide, 80–81
Nickel (Ni), 82, 145
Nicotinamide adenine dinucleotide (NAD(+)), 626
Nicotinamide phosphoribosyltransferase (NAMPT), 626
Nicotinamide riboside, 626
Nicotinic pattern, 132
NIF optic pathway, see Non-image-forming optic pathway
Night anxiety, 740
Night terrors, 741
NIH, see National Institutes of Health
NIOSH, see National Institute of Safety and Health
    Administration
NIR, see Near infrared; Non-ionizing radiation
Nitric oxide (NO), 56, 72, 379, 455, 482, 511, 651
    NO-ASA, 625
Nitric oxide synthase (NOS), 56, 482
Nitrogen balance, 264
Nitroglycerin, 123
Niyama (limb of yoga), 364
NK cells, see Natural killer cells
NLEA, see Nutrition Labeling and Education Act
N-methyl-D-aspartate receptor (NMDA receptor), 89
No-observed-adverse-effect-level (NOAEL), 133
NOAEL, see No-observed-adverse-effect-level
Nociceptive pain, 242
Nodes drainage, 733–734
Nogier frequencies, 479
Non-alcoholic fatty liver disease (NAFLD), 65
Non-celiac gluten sensitivity (NCGS), 192, 275–276
Noncariogenic diet, 208
Non-coding RNAs, 296
Noncommunicable diseases (NCDs), see Chronic diseases
Non-deliberate provocation, 538
Non-essential nutrients, 161
Non-healing wounds, 484

Non-image-forming optic pathway (NIF optic pathway),
    475
Non-invasive early, quick diagnostic methods
    BDORT, 691–695
    cancer cell, 691
    clinical implications of human papilloma virus-type
        16, 705–711
    comparison between BDORT, 689
    diagnosis and evaluation of therapeutic effect, 704
    importance of thymus gland, 695–704, 705
    L-C resonance circuit, 688
Non-invasive light therapy, 474
Non-ionizing radiation (NIR), 530–532, 534
Non-material realm, 321
Non-PEL, 622
Non-programmed/non-adaptive" theories, 616
Nonrandomized controlled trials (NRCTs), 370
Non-Rapid Eye Movement (NREM), 233
    stage 1, 233–234
    stage 2, 234
    stage 3, 234
Nonsteroidal anti-inflammatory drugs (NSAIDS), 31, 243
Non-stressed states, 400
Non-TMD problem, 249
Non-union bone fractures, 485
Non-visual optic pathway, 475
Non-visual receptors, 486
Noradrenalin, 504–505
Norepinephrine, 427
Normal breathing (NB), 387
Normal diet, 764
NOS, see Nitric oxide synthase
Nose discharge drainage, 730–731
Nose disorders, 244
NPC trial, see Nutritional Prevention of Cancer trial
n-3 polyunsaturated fatty acids (n-3 PUFAs), see Omega-3
    fatty acids
NRCTs, see Nonrandomized controlled trials
NREM, see Non-Rapid Eye Movement
NS, see Nadi shuddhi
NSAIDS, see Nonsteroidal anti-inflammatory drugs
NTDs, see Neural tube defects
NTH, see Neural therapy to Huneke
NTP, see U.S. National Toxicology Program
Nuclear factor-kappa beta (NF-kB), 296, 403, 515
Nuclear magnetic resonance, 714–715
Nucleus, 632, 715
Nutraceuticals, 629
    nutraceuticals/medications, 624–625
Nutri-AA-Pool, 78
Nutri-Brain®, 77
Nutri-Detox®, 77
Nutrient(s), 178; see also Health
    antagonistic, 43
    deficiencies in foods, 40
    in detoxification pathways, 161
    essential nutrients, 293
    IV, 50
    methyl donor B vitamins, 188
    micronutrients, 41
    minerals, 82
    in neuroprotective supplementary prescription, 188
    non-essential nutrients, 161
    orthomolecular, 40, 69–70

oxidizing, 502
selenium, 84
thiamine, 78
vitamin A, 188
zinc, 88
Nutrient dense plant-rich (Nutritarian) dietary protocol, 27
Nutrigenomics, 295, 296
Nutri-MINS from BioMolec®, 48
Nutrition, 25, 40, 262, 265–266
calorie restriction, 624
cerebral aspects of, 292
DHEA, 624
nutrition/foods, 624
resveratrol, ASA, and metformin, 624–625
science, 748
statins, 625
of stem cells, 629
vitamin C and D, 625
whole foods, 624
Nutritional and alternative medicine
dual system of government, 746–748
FDA regulation of herbal medicines, dietary
supplements, medical foods, 753–756
FDA's broad definition of "drug", 752–753
FDA's historical bias against alternative products and
services, 748–751
FDA's regulation of alternative medicine, 751–752
federal and state regulations to promote health
freedom, 761–765
specific federal regulatory concerns for alternative
practitioners, 756–761
Nutritional approaches to chronic illness
ethical aspects and Iatrogenics, 34–35
heart of matter, 21–28
nutritional treatment of selecting inflammatory and
auto-immune conditions, 30–33
selecting mechanisms underlying food effect, 29–30
summing up, 33–34
Nutritional assessment, clinical laboratory role in
bodies and nutrition, 267–270
body mass index, 270–276
diet and supplements and herbal medicine, 277–281
infections, 281–282
medical conditions, 270
traditional laboratory tests assessing nutritional status,
263–267
Nutritional deficiencies, 275
supporting IV supplementation, 40–41
Nutritional foodstuff values' tables of consumed foods, 40
Nutritional Prevention of Cancer trial (NPC trial), 86
Nutritional status, traditional laboratory tests assessing,
263
amino acids, 264–265
environmental respiratory factors and nutrition,
265–266
exposure to lead, mercury, and heavy metals, 266
nitrogen balance, 264
vegetarian and diets, 265
Nutritional supplements, 178
Nutritional therapeutic agents, 183; see also Antioxidants;
Intravenous orthomolecular therapeutic agents
(IV orthomolecular therapeutic agents)
emulating nutrient synergies in Mediterranean diet
model, 186–187

Mediterranean diet, 184–186
Nutrition health professionals, 182
Nutrition Labeling and Education Act (NLEA), 754, 763
NUV radiation, see Near ultraviolet radiation

O

OA, see Osteoarthritis
OAM, see Office of Alternative Medicine
Obesity, 385
Obligate nose breathers, 230
Observed to expected risk ratio (O/E risk ratio), 533
Obsessive compulsive disorder (OCD), 190, 423
Obstructive-SDB, 234–235
Obstructive sleep apnea (OSA), 234–235, 240, 241, 242
OSA/SDB-related mechanical effects, 241
Occidental medicine, see Western medicine
Occupational asthma, 136
Occupational Health and Safety Association (OHSA), 524
Occupational Safety and Health Administration (OSHA),
123, 267
Occupational toxicology, 134–137
OCD, see Obsessive compulsive disorder
Ocimum sanctum (O. sanctum), 630
Odontogenic pain, 243
O/E risk ratio, see Observed to expected risk ratio
Office of Alternative Medicine (OAM), 413
Offspring, effects on, 536–537
$1\alpha,25$ $(OH)_2D_3$, 162
25OHD₃, see 25-Hydroxy D₃
8-OHGH, see 8-Hydroxy-2'-deoxyguanosine
OHSA, see Occupational Health and Safety Association
"Old school" concept, 646, 651, 654
Olea europaea (O. europaea), 587
Oligotherapy, 731, 733
Omega-3
fatty acids, 266, 271
index, 271
Omega-6 fatty acids, 271
OP, see Organophosphorus pesticides
"Open-awareness" meditation, 424
Opiates, 142
Opioid analgesics, 243
Optic chiasm, 495
Optic nerve pathways, 487
Optimal dose of vitamin D3, 705
ORAC value, see Oxygen radical absorbance capacity
value
Oral administration, 562
Oral breathing, 231
Oral cancer, 246
Oral complex, 230
Oral Health in America (2000), 214
Oral home care, 221
artificial sweeteners, 222
calcium, 222
carbomer, 223
carrageenan, 222
detergents and surfactants, 222
ethanol, 222
FD&C color pigments, 222
flavoring, 222
fluoride, 222
glycerin, 222

Oral home care (*Continued*)
    hydrated silica, 223
    propylene glycol, 222
    triclosan, 222
    TSP, 222
Oral mucous membrane disorders, 244
Oral pharyngeal space, 233
Oral route, 39
Oral systemic connection, 211–214
"Orbitals", *see* Stationary states
Organic chemicals, 164–165
Organic electronics, 658
Organic molecular "wires", 678
Organic semiconductors, 658
Organic state, 143
Organophosphorus pesticides (OP), 152
Organotherapy, 716, 733
Organs and canals, 723
Oriental medicine, *see* Eastern medicine
"Oriental"-style diet, *see* "Asian"-style diet
Origanum majorana, see Marjoram
Ornithine (ORN), 76
Orthomolecular intravenous nutritional therapy; *see also*
            Orthomolecular parenteral nutrition therapy
    historical considerations, 47–48
    potential side effects considerations, 50–51
    specific products for use in, 47
    theoretical basis for therapeutic use of IV nutrients,
            48–50
Orthomolecular medicine, 41, 612
Orthomolecular mixtures
    apyrogenicity, 46
    incompatibility, 44–45
    instability, 45–46
    special care in preparation, 44
    sterility and modifications due to contamination, 46
Orthomolecular nutrients, 51
Orthomolecular nutrition, 40
Orthomolecular parenteral nutrition therapy, 42
    injectable solutions in clinical practice, 41–43
    mixture preparation for parenteral nutrition, 43–46
    nutritional deficiencies/insufficiencies supporting
            intravenous supplementation, 40–41
Orthomolecular supplements, 40
Orthopedic injuries, 483
OSA, *see* Obstructive sleep apnea
OSHA, *see* Occupational Safety and Health
            Administration
Osmosis, 443
Osteitis remedies, 733
Osteoarthritis (OA), 68, 72, 375
OSTEOARTICULAR system, 724
Osteoporosis, 384, 627
    specific exercises for, 630
Ostia, 244
OTC, *see* Over-the-counter
OTH, *see* Over-the-horizon
Otitis, 731
    drainage to accompany adenoids drainage, 732
    eustachian tube drainage, 732
    mastoiditis threatened, 732
    remedies, 732
Otto 128 tuning fork, 463
Over-breathing, 601

Over-the-counter (OTC), 748
Over-the-horizon (OTH), 525
Overtraining, 621
Oxidation, 445, 680
Oxidative stress, 51, 309
    theory of aging, 617–618
Oxygen molecules of water, 446
Oxygen radical absorbance capacity value (ORAC value),
            28
Oxytocin, 404
Ozone therapy, 71

P

P-a, *see* Pyropheophorbide-a
p38 mitogen-activated protein (p38), 586
PAA, *see* Phenylacetic acid
Pachaka Pitta, 352
Pãchana techniques, 345
PAH, *see* Polycyclic aromatic hydrocarbons
Pain, 242, 406, 407, 484
    circulation and, 483
    pain-causing marmas, 348
    pathways modulation by meditation, 432
PANAS, *see* Positive and Negative Affect Schedule
Panchakarma, 345
Pancha Kosha, 369
Paradigm shifts, 668
Paramecium, 658
Paranasal sinus disorders, 244
Parathyroid hormone (PTH), 94
Parenteral nutrition
    application routes in, 42–43
    mixture preparation for, 43
    special care in preparation of orthomolecular mixtures,
            44–46
Parenteral route, 42
Parkinson's disease (PD), 178, 190, 476
Parotid gland, 209
Passive diffusion, 124
Passive motion, 253
"Passive" theories, 616
Patanjali, 364
Pathogens, 20
Pathological aging, 193
Pathomechanics, 248
Pathway of phophate pentoses (PPP), 96
Pauling and Cameron's observations, 47
PBBs, *see* Polybrominated biphenyls
PBDEs, *see* Polybrominated diphenyl ethers
PBMC, *see* Peripheral blood mononuclear cell
PCBs, *see* Polychlorinated biphenyls
PCI, *see* Percutaneous coronary interventions
PCOS, *see* Polycystic ovarian syndrome
PCP, *see* Phencyclidine
PD, *see* Parkinson's disease
PDIs, *see* Peripheral decarboxylase inhibitors
PDT, *see* Photodynamic therapy
PEA, *see* Phenylethylamine
Peak expiratory flow (PEF), 377
Peak expiratory flow rate (PEFR), 378
Pecten, 305
PEF, *see* Peak expiratory flow
PEFR, *see* Peak expiratory flow rate

PEL, *see* People with Exceptional Longevity; Personal exposure limits
Pelargonium graveolens, see Geranium
Pelvic muscles, 630
PEMF therapy, *see* Pulsed electromagnetic field therapy
Penicillin, 128, 524, 576
People with Exceptional Longevity (PEL), 622
PEPID, 132
Peppermint essential oil (*Mentha × piperita*), 558, 559, 560
 for IBS, 558
Peptidylglycine monooxygenase hydroxylation (PHM), 92
Perceived stress, 398–399
Perceived Stress Questionnaire (PSQ), 399
Perceived Stress Scale (PSS), 398, 399
Percussive instruments, 462
Percutaneous coronary interventions (PCI), 34–35
Perfluorinated compounds (PFC), 156
Periarticular disorder, 483
Periodontal abscess, 211
Periodontal disease, 211–214
Peripheral blood mononuclear cell (PBMC), 404
Peripheral decarboxylase inhibitors (PDIs), 74
Peripheral nervous system, 482
Permittivity, 665
Pernicious anemia, 279
Perosis, 94
Peroxisome proliferator-activated receptors (PPARs), 296, 515
 PPAR γ, 515–516
Personal care products, 137
Personal exposure limits (PEL), 146
Personality and behavior to doshic characteristics, 338–339
Personalized lifestyle interventions, 367
Perspiration, 127
Pesticides, 156
PFC, *see* Perfluorinated compounds
P-glycoprotein, 157
 inhibitors, 582
pH
 of blood drops, 502
 of fluid, 209
 of intramuscularly injected products, 43
 of mixture, 44–45
Phagocytosis, 60
Pharmaceutical-grade essential oil identification, 552
 Alpha-pinene, 556
 blends of essential oils for nausea, 559–560
 blends of essential oils for primary dysmenorrhea, 558–559
 concomitant use of essential oils and medications and health contraindications, 565–566
 dosage guidelines, 564
 essential oil application for eyes and ears, 564–565
 essential oil best practices and safety, 560–561
 essential oil dosage, 563
 essential oil safety, 563
 essential oils and epilepsy or convulsive disorders, 565
 essential oils integration into medical practice, 556
 essential oil therapy with children, 566
 history and advancement of aromatics and essential oils, 552–554
 inhalation, 561

Lavender essential oil for anxiety, 556–558
 menthol, 554–555
 methods of administration, 561
 methyl salicylate, 555
 oral administration, 562
 peppermint essential oil for irritable bowel syndrome, 558
 pharmacological and functional evidence of essential oil efficacy, 554
 phytophotodermatitis potential of essential oils, 565
 pregnancy and essential oils, 566
 primary role of essential oils in plants, 552
 retention/vaginal and rectal administration, 562–563
 transdermal absorption/topically, 561–562
Pharmaceutical(s), 155
 agents, 749
 companies, 182
Pharmacodynamics, 127–128
Pharmacokinetics, 123
 absorption, 123–125
 distribution, 125
 drug excretion, 126–127
 drug metabolism, 125–126
 factors affecting drug absorption from gastrointestinal tract, 124–125
Pharmacological effects, 49
Pharmacology, 132–134
Pharmacotherapy, 372–373
Phase contrast microscope, 214
Phase I enzymes, 157, 162
Phase III transporter proteins, 157
Phase II reactions, 157
PHE, *see* Phenylalanine
Phencyclidine (PCP), 138
Phenol, 555, 556
Phenolic compounds, 80
Phenylacetic acid (PAA), 77
Phenylalanine (PHE), 77
Phenylethylamine (PEA), 77
Phenylketonuria (PKU), 267
Philosophy of Chinese medicine, 357–358
PHM, *see* Peptidylglycine monooxygenase hydroxylation
Phosphatidylethanol, 268
Phosphoric constitution, 718, 719
Phosphorus (P), 82, 83, 723
Photobiomodulation, 475
 ADHD, 485
 athletic performance and recovery, 486
 ATP, 482–483
 circulation and pain, 483
 inflammation, 484
 mechanisms, 481
 NO, 482
 potential applications, 483
 PTSD, 485–486
 wound healing, 484–485
 wrinkles and anti-aging, 486
Photodynamic therapy (PDT), 474
Photomelanometabolism process, 305
Photon multiplier, 652
Photosynthesis, human cells exploiting, 309
Phototherapy, 475; *see also* Chromotherapy
 before and after light therapy, 479
 color, 476–477

Phototherapy (*Continued*)
dosage, 477–478
exposure parameters, 478
light application, 475–476
light placement, 476
light source for photobiomodulation, 479, 481
light therapy, 475
medical devices and government acceptance, 481
modulation, 478–479
treatments applied to patients using LED lights, 480
Phthalates, 156
Phycobilisomes, 663
Phyllanthus amarus (*P. amarus*), 630
Physical alteration of cellular environment, 128
Physical medicine treatments, 253
Physical stress, 340
Physician dispensing and compounding, 756–758
Physiological effects of meditation, 427
cardiovascular effects, 427–429
immune system improvements and genetic changes in
health and disease, 432–434
neurobiological effects of meditation in health and
disease, 429–432
pain pathways modulation by meditation, 432
Physiological MBT research, 400–401, 402
Physiotherapists, 536
Phytic acid, 83
Phytonutrients, 161
Phytophotodermatitis potential of essential oils, 565
Pickup v. Brown, 759–760
Pimpinella anisum, see Anise
Pinocytosis, 125
Piper methysticum (*P. methysticum*), 582–583
Pitta, 331, 332
characteristics, 337–338
principle of heat and transformation, 335
sub-doshas and marma points, 352
symptoms, 342
Pittsburgh Sleep Quality Index (PSQI), 383
PKU, *see* Phenylketonuria
Placebo-controlled study, 558
Placental barrier, 125
Plain radiographs, 252
Plant(s), 306
chemical innovation in, 580–583
chloroplasts, 306
intelligence, 578–580
medicines, 587
primary role of essential oils in, 552
resistance to, 583–584
slant, 614
Plaque, 213
Plasma, 502
protein binding, 125
Plasmapheresis, 613, 632
Plasmodium kinases, 581–582
Plastic surgery, 330
PLoS Medicine, 58
PLP, *see* Pyridoxal 5-phosphate
Pluripotent stem cells, 628
PMAs, *see* Premarket approval applications
PMNs, *see* Polymorphonuclear granulocytes
PMR, *see* Progressive muscle relaxation
PMS, yoga and, 379

PN gel, *see* Proniosomal gel
PNI, *see* Psychoneuroimmunology
POEA, *see* Polyethoxylated tallow amine
Poisons, 122
Polarized-light therapy, 484
Polybrominated biphenyls (PBBs), 155
Polybrominated diphenyl ethers (PBDEs), 156
Polychlorinated biphenyls (PCBs), 154
Polychromatic color, 475
Polycyclic aromatic hydrocarbons (PAH), 152, 155, 161
Polycystic ovarian syndrome (PCOS), 382
Polyethoxylated tallow amine (POEA), 516
Polygonum cuspidatum, see Japanese knotweed root
Polymorphonuclear granulocytes (PMNs), 97
Polyphenolic compound, 505
Polyphenols, 185, 189
Polyunsaturated omega-3 (ω-3) fatty acids (PUFAs), 184
POMS scales, *see* Profile of Mood states scales
Porphyrins, 165
Positive and Negative Affect Schedule (PANAS), 405
Post-bariatric surgery, 271
Postinjury
metabolism, 74
swelling, 444
Post-mitotic neurons, 178
Postoperative recovery, 9
Postprandial blood sugar (PPBS), 410
Post-surgical injury, 483
Post-traumatic stress disorder (PTSD), 136, 386, 404, 476,
485–486, 592, 596, 600
Post-trauma wound healing, 484
Posture
airway effect on, 237–238
effect on CSF and energy flow, 238–239
Potassium (K), 82
Power frequency, 525
Power of Movement in Plants, The, 579
PPARs, *see* Peroxisome proliferator-activated receptors
PPBS, *see* Postprandial blood sugar
PPIs, *see* Proton pump inhibitors
PPP, *see* Pathway of phophate pentoses
PPRTVs, *see* Provisional Peer Reviewed Toxicity Values
PQQ, *see* Pyrroloquinoline quinone
Prakruti, 342
constitution, 334
Prana, cosmic life-force energy, 377
Pranan
device, 667
technology, 665
Prana Vata, 351
Pranayama, 378
exercises, 601
yoga, 364
Pratyahara yoga, 364
Prebiotics, 8, 194
Preconscious, 659
Prefrontal cortical damage, 240
Prefrontal–striatal–limbic circuit, 141
Pregnancy
and essential oils, 566
pregnancy-induced hypertension management, 50
Premarket approval applications (PMAs), 755
Pressure, 441
ulcers, 485

Prevention, rhino pharyngitis, 731
Primary BioSonic tuning forks, 462
Primary dysmenorrhea, blends of essential oils for, 558–559
Primitive String Transformer (PST), 658
Principle of non-locality, 455
Principles of Light and Color, 489
Principles of Mental Physiology, 659
Probiotics, 194, 195
Procaine, 96–97
    IV drip, 97
Profile of Mood states scales (POMS scales), 430
Progesterone (P4), 627
Programmed death theory, 615
Programmed longevity, 616
Programmed theories, 616
Progressive muscle relaxation (PMR), 395, 427
Proinflammatory cytokines, 401
Proliferation, 484
Proniosomal gel (PN gel), 625
Proof-of-concept study, 59
Propionibacterium acnes (*P. acnes*), 12–13
Propylene glycol, 222
Prostate, male exercises for, 630
Protein
    with cell membrane, 672
    kinase C-delta pathway, 586
    protein-calorie deficits, 263–267
Proton magnetic resonance spectroscopy (^{1}H-MRS), 59
Proton pump inhibitors (PPIs), 368
Provisional ideas in psychology, 657
Provisional Peer Reviewed Toxicity Values (PPRTVs), 134
Provocation testing, 538–539
Pruritic erythematous rash, 143
Psoriasis, 423, 484
Psoric drainage, 736–737
Psoric reactive mode, 720, 721
Psoro-sycotic disease, 732
PSQ, *see* Perceived Stress Questionnaire
PSQI, *see* Pittsburgh Sleep Quality Index
PSS, *see* Perceived Stress Scale
PST, *see* Primitive String Transformer
Psychiatric disorders, 514
Psychoacoustic of sound, 450
Psychoacoustics sound healing, 461; *see also*
            Vibroacoustic sound healing
    drums, rattles, percussive instruments, 462
    music, 461
    singing bowls and gongs, 461
    tuning forks, 462–465
    voice, 461
Psychoanalysis, 657
Psychological burdens, 408
Psychological distress, 411
Psychological trauma; *see also* Trauma
    addiction to surgery, 604–605
    allostatic load, 596
    anxiety, disordered breathing, and hyperventilation, 601
    biology of traumatic stress, 593
    group stress and trauma, 595–596
    learned helplessness, 597
    SDMLB, 597–598
    self-medication, 599–600
    somatic symptoms of trauma and addiction, 598–599

    somatoform behaviors, eating disorders, and self-injury, 603–604
    stress response, 593–594
    tend and befriend model, 596–597
    yoga and breathing, 601–603
Psychological variables, 428
Psychoneuroimmunology (PNI), 145–146, 660
Psychosocial components, *see* Emotional components
Psychosocial MBT research, 398–399
Psychosomatic disorders, 343
Pterocarpus marsupium (*P. marsupium*), 630
Pterostilbene, 626
PTH, *see* Parathyroid hormone
PTSD, *see* Post-traumatic stress disorder
PUFAs, *see* Polyunsaturated omega-3 (ω-3) fatty acids
Pulp, 208
Pulsation patterns, 478
Pulse(s)
    diagnosis, 322–323
    of light, 649
    structure, 478
Pulsed electromagnetic field therapy (PEMF therapy), 474, 478
Punica granatum (*P. granatum*), 587
Purine, 270
Purulent discharge, 729
Purusha, 324
Pyridimidine 5-nucleotidase, 144
Pyridoxal 5-phosphate (PLP), 80
Pyridoxine, 80
Pyridoxine hydrochloride, 80
Pyrogens, 46
Pyropheophorbide-a (P-a), 512
Pyrroloquinoline quinone (PQQ), 631, 705
Pyruvate carboxylase, 93

Q

Qi Gong, 360, 393, 395, 397, 410
Quality of life (QoL), 377, 378, 380, 381, 428
Quality trials, 433
Quantum
    biology, 644, 656
    chemistry, 644
    electrodynamics, 654
    entanglement, 455
    field, 455
    optics, 650
    physics, 643
    reality, 455
    theory, 455
    universe, 455
Quarrelsome, 738
Quarter-wave antennas, 653
Quasi-light body, 304
Quercetin, 296, 504–505, 582, 626
Quinalapril, 64

R

RA, *see* Rheumatoid arthritis
RADAR, *see* Radio Detection And Ranging
Radiant energy, 307, 441
    radiant energy-induced biological function, 442

Radio Detection And Ranging (RADAR), 525
 antennas, 542
 operators, 537
Radio frequency (RF), 525–526, 531, 533, 542, 652
 radiation, 525, 530
 radio-frequency electromagnetic radiation, 536
Radio frequency and microwave radiation (RF/MW
  radiation), 542–543
Rajas, 343
R-alpha lipoic acid, 65
Rakta, 333
Random diffusion model, 648
Randomized controlled trials (RCTs), 25, 360, 366, 370,
  373, 379, 386, 410, 427
Ranjaka Pitta, 352
Rapid and subtle phenomena, 657
Rapid eye movement sleep (REM sleep), 234
Rasa, 333
"Rate of living theory", 619
Rate ratio (RR), 534
Rattles, 462
RBCs, see Red blood cells
RCTs, see Randomized controlled trials
RDA, see Recommended Daily Allowance
RDW, see Red cell distribution width
Reaction time (RT), 387
Reactive modes, 717, 720–721
Reactive oxygen species (ROS), 57, 63, 66, 69, 72, 178,
  301, 306, 482, 618
"Reasonable basis", 761
"Reasonable consumer", 761
Rebiosis, 8–12
Receptor(s), 127
 on cell surfaces, 664
 proteins, 663
Recommended Daily Allowance (RDA), 40
Rectifiers, 657
Red blood cells (RBCs), 502
 traversing capillary, 503, 504
Red cell distribution width (RDW), 278
Red light, 477
Reduction, 445
 potential, 680
 reactions, 57
Reference dose (RfD), 133
Reflexive Universe, The (Young), 662
Regulatory molecules, 646
Regulatory toxicology, 137
Relative resonance, 326
Relaxation, 428
Relaxation Response (RR), 395, 426
Relaxation Response Resiliency Program (3RP), 404
Remedies, 732
Remodeling, 484
REM sleep, see Rapid eye movement sleep
Renal function tests, 269–270
Reproduction, 482
Reproductive health, 155–156
Reputable business community, anti-aging for, 610
Resilience, 404–405
Resilience Scale (RS), 405
Resilient Warrior, 404
Resistance
 exercises, 630

to plants, 583–584
Resonance
 in Eastern medicine, 320–321
 phenomenon, 687–688
Resonant frequency, 687–688
Resonant Recognition Model (RRM), 651
Respiratory
 burst, 60
 as method of meditation, 426
 system, 482, 724
Resting state functional MRI (rsfMRI), 81
Restless child, 738
 anxiety, 738
 quarrelsome, 738
 screaming, 738–739
Restoril, see Temazepam
Resveratrol, 586, 624–625
Retention/vaginal and rectal administration, 562–563
Retinohypothalamic pathway, 491
Retinoic acid signaling, 188
Retinotectal pathway, 491
Revisioning cellular bioenergetics
 "back to food itself", 293–294
 bioelectromagnetic body, 310–312
 biophotons, 299–307
 cerebral aspects of nutrition, 292
 food as information, 295–299
 food as thing, 294–295
 intention living force of physiology, 310
 sociocultural meaning of food, 293
 water as alternative cellular fuel source, 307–309
RF, see Radio frequency; Riboflavin
RfD, see Reference dose
RF/MW radiation, see Radio frequency and microwave
  radiation
RF/MW radiation, 535
Rheumatoid arthritis (RA), 31, 68, 298, 302, 375, 484
 nutritional treatment, 31–33
Rhinitis medimatosa, 124
Rhino pharyngitis, 728
 cough, 730
 discharge, 728–730
 drainage, 730–731
 prevention, 731
Rhodiola, 303
Rhythmic cycles, 454
Riboflavin (RF), 79–80
Rice diet, 25–27
Rickettsia, 584
Right nostril variations, 387–388
Rig Veda, 364
Riordan intravenous vitamin C, 47
RMIT University, see Royal Melbourne Institute of
  Technology
Rocky Mountain Spotted Fever, 584
Roman chamomile (Anthemis nobilis), 560
Root canal, 216–217
 evidence, 217–218
 tooth and organ connection, 218–221
ROS, see Reactive oxygen species
Rose (Rosa damascena), 559
Rotation diet, 169
Rough quality, 332
Route of administration, detoxification and, 160–161

Royal Melbourne Institute of Technology (RMIT University), 650
3RP, *see* Relaxation Response Resiliency Program
RR, *see* Rate ratio; Relaxation Response
RRM, *see* Resonant Recognition Model
RS, *see* Resilience Scale
rsfMRI, *see* Resting state functional MRI
RT, *see* Reaction time
Rubber-like "gutta percha", 217
Rudeness, 739
Rujakara, see Pain-causing marmas
Rush Memory and Aging Project, 614
Ryberg's method, 496

S

SAD, *see* Seasonal affective disorder; Standard American Diet
S-adenosyl-L-homocysteine (SAH), 158
S-adenosylmethionine (SAM), 158
Sadhaka Pitta, 352
Sadhya Pranahara, *see* Immediate-death causing marmas
"Safe IV infusions", 57
SAH, *see* S-adenosyl-L-homocysteine
Saliva(ry), 127
    bacterial DNA testing, 213
    DNA microbial testing, 213
    enzymes, 210
    gland disorder, 244
Salt, 24–25
Salvia miltiorrhiza (*S. miltiorrhiza*), 587
Salvia sclarea, see Clary sage
SAM, *see* S-adenosylmethionine
Samadhi yoga, 364
Samana Vata, 351
Sāma prakruti, 334
Samhitā, Charaka, 329–330
Sānkhya philosophy, 330
SAR, *see* Specific absorption rate
Sarod, classical Indian lute-like instrument, 323
Satchidananda, 366
Satellite remedies, 723, 733
Sattva, 343
SB, *see* Surya bhedana
"Scaling and root planing", 213
Scar tissue, 485
SCD, *see* Sickle cell disease
Schrödinger equation, 655
Science and Civilization in China, 320
Science Magazine, 3
Scientific basis of ayurvedic and Chinese medicine
    Eastern medicine fulfills foundational criteria for science, 319–320
    Eastern *vs.* Western modes of scientific thought, 321–322
    impact of intention, 325–326
    music, resonance, and frequencies in Eastern medicine, 320–321
    pulse diagnosis, 322–323
    return to original nature, 323–325
Scientific community, anti-aging for, 610
Scientific thought
    Eastern science, 321–322
    Eastern *vs.* Western modes, 321
SCN, *see* Suprachiasmatic nucleus

SCNT, *see* Somatic cell nuclear transfer
Screaming, 738–739
Scutellaria baicalensis (*S. baicalensis*), 587
SDB, *see* Sleep-disordered breathing
SDMLB, *see* State-dependent memory, learning, and behavior
SE, *see* Substantially equivalent
Seafood consumption, 144
Seasonal affective disorder (SAD), 487
Seasons, 340–342
Sedentary participants, 621
SeEnY, *see* Selenium-enriched yeast
SELECT, *see* Selenium and Vitamin E Cancer Prevention Trial
Selenite, 86
Selenium (Se), 82, 84–86, 161
Selenium and Vitamin E Cancer Prevention Trial (SELECT), 86
Selenium-enriched yeast (SeEnY), 86
Selenomethionine (SeMet), 86
Self-healing, 335–336
Self-injurious behavior (SIB), 600
Self-injury, 603–604
Self-medication, 599–600
Self-organization, 573–575
SeMet, *see* Selenomethionine
Semiconductor, 657
Sensora system, 495
Sensory receptors of olfactory bulb, 561
Serotonin, 312, 504–505, 514–515
    syndrome, 132
Serpentine receptors, 663
Serum
    proteins, 263
    sodium, 269–270
SES, *see* Socioeconomic status
Seventrans-membrane-helix receptors (7TM receptors), 663
Sex hormone-binding globulin (SHBG), 382
SF, *see* Slope factor
SHBG, *see* Sex hormone-binding globulin
Shira, see Head
Shodhana, 345
Shukra, 333
SIB, *see* Self-injurious behavior
Sick building syndrome, 539
Sickle cell anemia, 374
Sickle cell disease (SCD), 374
Side effect, 128
SIDS, *see* Sudden Infant Death Syndrome
Signal molecules, 646
Silicon (Si), 82
Silver-gray liquid, 143
"Silver bullet" approach, 581
Single nucleotide polymorphisms (SNPs), 157, 159, 186
SinoNasal Outcomes Test (SNOT-20), 59
Sinus disease, *see* Nasal disease
"Sinus headache", 244
Sinusitis, 732
    discharge remedies, 732
    drainage, 733
    ethmoidal and frontal sinusitis, 733
    maxillary sinusitis, 733
    osteitis remedies, 733
    suppuration stage, 732

SIRS, *see* Systemic inflammatory response syndrome
SIRT enzymes, *see* Sirtuin enzymes
Sirtuin enzymes (SIRT enzymes), 185
    SIRT1, 626
Skeletal muscle structure, EZ water implications for, 308
Skeletal system, 482
Skin, 11
    conductance, 400
    deprivation, 623
    hearing, 465
    language, 721–722
Sleep, 623
    effect of airway and sleep during infancy and
        childhood, 235–237
    airway effect on, 233
    apnea, 231, 234–235, 240
    deficiency, 240
Sleep-disordered breathing (SDB), 235, 236
Sleep disorders, 740; *see also* Eating disorders
    difficulty falling asleep after animated conversation,
        740
    nervous drainage, 741
    night anxiety, 740
    night terrors, 741
    sorrows, 741
Sleep effect during infancy and childhood, 235–237
SLES, *see* Sodium laureth sulfate
Sleshaka Kapha, 354
"Slipped tendon", *see* Perosis
Slope factor (SF), 133
Slow vital capacity (SVC), 378
Slow wave sleep (SWS), *see* Non-Rapid Eye Movement
        (NREM)—stage 3
SLS, *see* Sodium lauryl sulfate
Smart appliances, 526–527, 531
Smart meters, 525, 544–545
Smoking, 138
SN, *see* Surya nadi
S-nitrosoglutathione (GSNO), 511
SNOT-20, *see* SinoNasal Outcomes Test
SNPs, *see* Single nucleotide polymorphisms
SNS, *see* Sympathetic nervous system
Social factors, 321
Social media for MBT, 412
Social practices, 623
Society for Integrative Oncology, 406
Sociodemographic variations in MBTs, 396–397
Socioeconomic status (SES), 396
SOD, *see* Superoxide dismutase
Sodium-potassium ATPase pump (Na-K pump), 508,
        516–517
Sodium (Na), 82
Sodium laureth sulfate (SLES), 222
Sodium lauryl sulfate (SLS), 222
Solar forces, body's biophoton outputs governing by,
        306–307
Solid-state
    biochemistry, 679
    tissue-tensegrity matrix system, 673–675
Solvent exposure, 153
Somatic cell nuclear transfer (SCNT), 632, 622
Somatic symptoms of trauma and addiction, 598–599
Somatization disorder, 603–604
Somatoform behaviors, 603–604

Somatropin therapy, 627
Sonic entrainment, 455
Sonic intervals, 450
Sorrows, 741
Sound, 449, 455
    healers, 460
    mimics, 455, 456
"Sound bath", 461
Sound healing, 449–450, 456
    consciousness, 455–456
    Mantras, 457–458
    mindful listening, 456–457
    practice, 458–460
    psychoacoustics, 461–465
    theory, 451
    tools and instruments, 460
    treatment, 457
    vibration, 451–455
    vibroacoustic, 465–466
Soy intolerance, 276
Spacetime, 653
Spasmodic cough, 730
SPE, *see* Spontaneous photon emission
Spearmint (*Mentha spicata*), 559
Specific absorption rate (SAR), 526
Spectro-Chrome system, 489, 492, 493
Spermatogenesis, 535
Sperm, effects on, 535–536
Spiritual factors, 321
Spirochete, 584
Spitler's Syntonic physiological balance of ANS, 490
Spontaneous photon emission (SPE), 302
"Spread spectrum" computer, 645
Spring season, 341
SR capsules, *see* Sustained/delayed release capsules
Stained glass church window, 453
Standard American Diet (SAD), 211
Staphylococcus bacteria, 582
State-dependent memory, learning, and behavior
        (SDMLB), 593, 597–598
State boards, 746–748
Statins, 625
Stationary states, 655
Stealth
    infections, 584
    pathogens, 584–585
Stem cell(s), 628
    approaches to generating functional organs using, 622
    manipulations, 629
    SCNT, 622
    therapy, 631
Sterility and modifications due to contamination, 46
Sterilization process, 46
Stigma, 412
Stool testing, 193
Storage sites, 125
Streaming potential, 510–511
Streptococcus thermophilus (*S. thermophilus*), 195
Stress, 408
    effects on body types, 340
    hormone, 487, 593
    management, 406, 623
    physiology conceptual model, 396
    protection against stress-induced dysbiosis, 9

response, 241, 394, 593–594
    stress-induced analgesia, 599
    stress–inflammation relationship, 400
Stressful situations, 394
Stroke, 240
Stroma, 662
STSC, *see* Superfund Health Risk Technical Support
        Center
Sub-doshas, marma point classification on, 351–354
Sublingual administration, 562
Suboptimal nutrient intake, detoxification and, 161–162
Subspecialties of toxicology, 131
Substances, 451
Substantially equivalent (SE), 755
Substrate molecule, 654
Sudden Infant Death Syndrome (SIDS), 236, 517
Sugar, 210
Sulfalzine, 159
Sulfate
    gels water, 504
    homeostasis, 513–514
    ions, 502
    transport, 504–505
    transporters, 504
Sulfate, 508–510
Sulfated DHEA (DHEAS), 381
Sulfotransferases (SULTs), 515
Sulfur (S), 82
    amino acids, 73–74
Sulfuric acid, 508
SULTs, *see* Sulfotransferases
Summer season, 341
Sunlight, 474, 486
    human skin capturing energy and information from,
        304–306
Superfund Health Risk Technical Support Center (STSC),
        134
Super light, 496
Superoxide dismutase (SOD), 92, 93
    SOD1, 618
Suppuration stage, 732
Suprachiasmatic nucleus (SCN), 486, 487
Surface area, 124
Surfactants, 222
Surgery, addiction to, 604–605
Surgical incisions, 484
Surya bhedana (SB), 387
Surya nadi (SN), 387
Susceptibility, 130–131
Sushruta, 329–330
Sushruta Samhita, 334, 347
Sustained/delayed release capsules (SR capsules), 558
SVC, *see* Slow vital capacity
Swallowing process, 233
Sweat chloride, 275
Sweet fennel (*Foeniculum vulgare* var. *dulce*), 560
Swimming, 337
Sycotic
    drainage, 737
    reactive mode, 721, 722
Sympathetic nervous system (SNS), 395, 661
Sympathetic stimulation, 647
Synapses, 645, 658
Synergism, 130

Synergy, 583
Synovial membrane, 308
Syntonic phototherapy method, 489, 492, 493
Systemic candidiasis, 142
Systemic cooperation, 657
Systemic inflammatory response syndrome (SIRS), 97
Systemic regulatory processes, 649
Syzygium aromaticum, see Clove
Szent-Györgyi cycle, 643

T

Tablets, 544
Tachycardia, 517
Tai chi, 393, 395, 397, 410, 425
Tamas, 343
Tarpaka Kapha, 354
Taurine, 73
TBI, *see* Traumatic Brain Injury
TCA cycle, *see* Tricarboxylic acid cycle
TCM, *see* Traditional Chinese Medicine
TEA, *see* Triethanolamine
Tear(s), 127
    clothes, 739
Teasing cough, 730
Telecommunication technologies, 525
Telemedicine
    and distance consulting, 758–760
    expanding access to, 765
Telomerase reverse transcriptase (TERT), 632
Telomerase therapy, 628
Telomere(s), 628
    length, 404
    shortening, 619
Temazepam, 386
Temperature, 441
Temporomandibular disorders (TMD), 229, 246–247;
        see also Attention deficit disorders
    effects, 253–255
    epidemiology, 247
    etiology, 247–249
Temporomandibular joint (TMJ), 215, 246
    location, 250
    symptoms, 249
Temporomandibular joint dysfunction (TMJD), 481
Tend and befriend model, 596–597
Tensegrity, 667–671
Terahertz waves, 651
TERT, *see* Telomerase reverse transcriptase
tetQ gene, 576
Tetrahydrobiopterin (BH4), 56, 506
T helper subset 1 (Th1), 87
Theophylline, 266
Therapeutic
    agents, 178
    interventions, 611
    methods, 600
Thermography imaging techniques, 252
Thiamine, 78–79
    chloride, 80
    deficiency, 280
Thio-ethers, 217
Thoracic nodes drainage, 733
3-phase model, 650

Three doshas, 331–333
3D printing, 631
Threshold, 574
Thresholds levels (TLVs), 137
Thrombohemorrhagic phenomena, 517–518
Thrombosis, 502
Thymosin α1, 696
"Thymosin β4", 696
Thymus gland, 617, 692, 695
    accurate organ representation areas of face using
        BDORT, 700
    accurate organ representation areas of hands, 698
    accurate organ representation areas of left eyebrow,
        upper and lower eyelids, 699
    adenocarcinoma of colon, 705
    cancer detection from EKGs, 703
    detection of early stage of adenocarcinoma of colon
        via EKG, 703
    effect of holding 2000 IUs of vitamin D3, 704
    maximum EMF resonance phenomenon, 697
    mouth, hand and foot writing form, 702
    effect of oral intake, 704
    organ representation areas of upper & lower lips &
        surrounding areas, 701
    representation areas of right-handed person, 696
Thyroid
    disease, 272–273
    functioning, 410
    hormone, 305
Thyroid peroxidase antibodies (TPOAb), 85
Thyroid stimulating hormone (TSH), 380, 385
Thyroxine (T4), 84
TIBC, see Total iron binding capacity
Tibetan medicine, 705–706
Time-dependent Schrödinger equation, 655
Tin (Tn), 82
Tinospora cordifolia (T. cordifolia), 630
Tioctic acid, see Alpha Lipoic Acid (ALA)
Tissue-specific injection for repair and intra-articular, 629
Tissues, 645
    Āma removal from, 344–345
    tissue/organ cloning, 632
Tissue transglutaminase (tTG), 275
Titanium, 216
TLC, see Total leukocyte count
TLCO, see Transfer factor of lung for carbon monoxide
TLR4, see Toll-like receptor 4
TLVs, see Thresholds levels
TM, see Transcendental meditation
TMA, see Trimethyl anhydride
TMAO, see Trimethylamine-n-oxide
TMD, see Temporomandibular disorders
TMJ, see Temporomandibular joint
TMJD, see Temporomandibular joint dysfunction
7TM receptors, see Seventrans-membrane-helix receptors
TNF, see Tumor necrosis factor
Tobacco, 138–141, 265
Tocopherol, see Vitamin E
Tolbutamide, 125
Toll-like receptor 4 (TLR4), 46
Toluene, 153
Tonations, 489
Tongue function effect on facial growth and airway,
    232–233

Tonsils drainage, 733
Tooth
    and organ connection, 218–221
    tooth/body connection, 216
Total iron binding capacity (TIBC), 278
Total knee arthroplasty (TKA), see Total knee replacement
Total knee replacement, 631
Total leukocyte count (TLC), 376
Total parenteral nutrition (TPN), 90, 94
Total resonance, 326
Tourette's syndrome, 254
Toxemia gravidarum, 50
Toxic(ity), 130
    assessment process, 133
    chemicals, 524
    effects, 129, 133
    shock syndrome, 282
    substances, 137, 146
    treatments, 649
Toxic metals, 143
    Hg, 143–144
    lead, 144–145
Toxicology, 122
    basics, 123
    chemical, 132
    endocrine disruptors, 122–123
    exogenous and endogenous toxins, 137–142
    factors affecting body's response to drug, 129–131
    importance of dose, 122
    medical, 131–132
    occupational, 134–137
    pharmacodynamics, 127–128
    pharmacokinetics, 123–127
    and pharmacology, 132–134
    and psychoneuroimmunology, 145–146
    regulatory, 137
    selective toxic metals, 143–145
    subspecialties, 131
    toxic substances, 137
    treatments and measures to reducing individual toxic
        exposure, 146
    undesirable responses to drug therapy,
        128–129
TPN, see Total parenteral nutrition
TPOAb, see Thyroid peroxidase antibodies
Trace elements, 281
Traditional approaches, 165–166
Traditional avoidance treatments, 166
Traditional Chinese Medicine (TCM),
        300, 303, 324, 357, 491
Traditional medicines, 319
Traditional treatments
    assisting in physical removal of toxins from body, 167
    improving ability of body to metabolizing and
        elimination, 166
Trans-membrane proteins, 673
Transcendental meditation (TM), 303, 365, 427, 428
Transcriptomics, 403
Transdermal absorption/topically, 561–562
Transfer factor of lung for carbon monoxide
        (TLCO), 378
Transferrin saturation, 278
Transient Receptor Potential Cation Channel Subfamily M
        member 8 receptor (TRPM8 receptor), 554

Transient Receptor Potential Voltage 3 transmembrane ion channel (TRPV3 transmembrane ion channel), 556
Transition
    colors of chromotherapy, 492
    state, 680
Trauma, 483, 592
    group stress and, 595–596
    somatic symptoms of trauma and addiction, 598–599
Trauma Revised Injury Severity Score (TRISS), 85
Traumatic Brain Injury (TBI), 485
Traumatic brain injury, 476
Traumatic stress, 404, 594; *see also* Stress
    biology, 593
    healing, 592
Traumatic stress, 593
Tremors, 143
"Tri-Est", 627
Tricarboxylic acid cycle (TCA cycle), 79
Triclosan, 222
Tricyclic antidepressants, 252
Trier Social Stress Test, 432–433
Triethanolamine (TEA), 223
Trigonella foenum graecum, 630
Triiodothyronine (T$_3$), 84
Trimethyl-n-oxide levels modification, 30
Trimethylamine-n-oxide (TMAO), 30
Trimethyl anhydride (TMA), 137
2,6,6,-Trimethylbicyclohept-2-ene, *see* Alpha-pinene
Trisodium phosphate (TSP), 222
TRISS, *see* Trauma Revised Injury Severity Score
Trp, *see* Tryptophan
TRPM8 receptor, *see* Transient Receptor Potential Cation Channel Subfamily M member 8 receptor
Tryptanthrin, 583
Tryptophan (Trp), 76, 512–513
TSH, *see* Thyroid stimulating hormone
TSP, *see* Trisodium phosphate
tTG, *see* Tissue transglutaminase
Tuberculinic
    drainage, 737
    reactive mode, 720–722, 726
Tubular renal function, 144
Tui Na, 359
Tumor necrosis factor (TNF), 296, 584
    TNF-α, 12, 46, 212, 401, 515, 555, 585, 618
Tumor(s), 246
    cells, 509–510
Tuning fork
    effect, 648
    systems, 462–465
Turn bedroom power off, 547
Type 1 diabetes, 272
Type 2 diabetes, 190, 272, 371
Type 2 diabetes mellitus (T2DM), *see* Type 2 diabetes

U

Ubiquinol, *see* Coenzyme Q10 (CoQ10)
Ubiquinone, *see* Coenzyme Q10 (CoQ10)
Udana Vata, 351
Ulcerative colitis, 298, 408
Ultra-fast biology, 659
Ultrafast communications, 661

Ultrafast internal conversion, 305
Ultra-fast mind, biology of, 657–661
Ultrasonic microscopy, 670
Ultra-trace elements, 82
Ultraviolet light (UV light), 304
Ultraviolet radiation, 715
Ultra-weak photon emission (UPE), 302–303, 650, 652
"Unapproved" drug therapies, 752
UNB, *see* Uninostril breathing
Unbalanced detoxification, 162
Uncertainty
    factor, 133
    principle, 455
Unconscious mind, 659, 660
    biology, 657–661
UNICEF, *see* United Nations Children's Fund
Unified Parkinson's disease rating scale (UPDRS), 57
Unimolecular rectifier, 658
Uninostril breathing (UNB), 387
United Nations Children's Fund (UNICEF), 88
United States, yoga in, 365–366
UPDRS, *see* Unified Parkinson's disease rating scale
UPE, *see* Mitogenetic radiation (MGR); Ultra-weak photon emission
Uric acid, 270
Urinary
    kegel for urinary incontinence, 630
    porphyrin profiling, 165
    specific gravity, 269–270
    system, 724
U.S. Environmental Protection Agency (EPA), 123, 154, 267
U.S. Food and Drug Administration (FDA), 135, 222, 277, 361, 481, 483, 627, 745, 746–748
    broad definition of "drug", 752–753
    broaden FDA's expanded access regulations, 762–763
    changes to FDA regulations, 761
    expanded access regulations, 762–763
    historical bias against alternative products and services, 748–751
    lift restrictions on preventative or wellness advertising related, 763–764
    recommendations for adult GHD, 627
    regulation of alternative medicine, 751–752
    regulation of herbal medicines, dietary supplements, medical foods, 753–756
    strengthen laws permit off-label use, 761–762
U.S. National Toxicology Program (NTP), 533
UV light, *see* Ultraviolet light

V

Vaccination side effects, 735
    detoxifying with homeopathic treatment, 736–737
    DTaP, 735
    MMR, 735–736
Vagal afferent nerves (VAN), 191
Vāgbhata, 330
Vaikalyakara, see Disability-causing marmas
Valine, 74
Valproic acid, 82
VAN, *see* Vagal afferent nerves
Vanadium (Va), 82

Van Obberghen color therapy, 495–496
Vasculature, 504
Vasodilatation, 482
Vaso-occlusive crisis (VOC), 374
Vāta, 331, 332
    characteristics, 336–337
    principle of movement, 335
    sub-doshas and marma points, 351
    symptoms, 342
VDR, *see* Vitamin D receptors
VDT, *see* Video display terminals
Vedas, 553
Vedic tradition, 330
Vegetables
    3D printing, 631
    variety in, 622, 631
Vegetal kingdom, 716
Vegetarian diets, 265
Very high frequency (VHF), 525
Vessel-based marmas, 347
VHF, *see* Very high frequency
Vibration, 451
    cymatics frequency in water, 454
    sand vibrating on metal plate, 451, 452
    stained glass church window, 453
    top down view of DNA, 454
    water vibrating on metal plate, 452, 453
Vibrational blueprints, 451, 455
Vibratory matrix, 675
Vibratory signature, 451
Vibroacoustic of sound, 450
Vibroacoustic sound healing, 465–466,
            see Psychoacoustics sound healing
    vibroacoustic application of BioSonic 128 cps tuning
        forks, 467
Video display terminals (VDT), 534
Vikruti, 335
    in Ayurvedic medicine, 324
Violent child, 739
    destructive, 739
    impatient, 739
    insolent, 739
    plump fat greedy child, 739
    rejects violently things, 739
    rudeness, 739
    tears clothes, 739
"Viral" otitis, 731
Vishalyaghna, *see* Fatal-death-if-pierced marmas
Visible spectrum, 474, 475
Visual learning, 234
Vitamin B3, *see* Niacin
Vitamin D3, 698
    deficiency, 708
    optimal dose, 705
Vitamin D receptors (VDR), 162
Vitamin(s), 78, 754; *see also* Minerals
    folic acid, 278
    iron deficiency, 277–278
    supplements, 631
    Vitamin A, 188
    Vitamin B12, 279
    Vitamin B1, 280
    Vitamin B6, 266, 280
    Vitamin C, 47, 51–56, 78, 280, 505, 625

Vitamin D, 279–280, 505, 625
    Vitamin E, 280
VO$_2$max, *see* Lower maximal oxygen uptake
VOC, *see* Vaso-occlusive crisis
Voice, 461
Vyana Vata, 352

W

Walking, 337
Warfarin, 125
Warm color, 491, 492
Water, 332, 358, 444–445, 501
    as alternative cellular fuel source, 307
    centrality for health, 446–447
    consequences of EZ water for human health, 309
    EZ water implications for circulatory flow, 308
    EZ water implications for skeletal muscle structure,
        308
    human cells exploit photosynthesis, 309
    information in, 445–446
    memory, 446
    transduce energy, 440–441
    water-based energy conversion framework, 441
    water-loving surfaces, 307
    water-soluble vitamins, 280–281
Waterbed, 547
Water element, *see* Sycotic reactive mode
Water-only fasting, 28
Watery burning discharge, 729
Wave-particle duality, 455
Waveforms, 478
Wave shapes, 478
Wear and tear theories, 617
Weight of evidence (WOE), 133
Western biomedicine, 661
Western medicine, 319
Western modes of scientific thought, 321–322
Wetware: A Computer in Every Living Cell (Bray), 659
"Wetware", 659
Wheel of emunctories, 723–725
Whining, 740
White blood cells, 502, 507, 629, 632
White House, 142
WHO, *see* World Health Organization
Whole foods, 34, 624, 629
Whole Medical Systems, 752
Whole plant extract, 583
Wi-Fi, 525, 537
    hotspots, 547
    router, 544
Wine @ 5, 614
Winter season, 341
Wireless baby monitors, 544
Withania somnifera (*W. somnifera*), 630
WOE, *see* Weight of evidence
World Health Organization (WHO), 88, 134, 360
Wound(s), 483
    healing, 484–485
Wrinkles, 486

X

Xbox emit microwave radiation, 545

Y

YA, *see* Young adults
Yama yoga, 364
Yangonin, 582–583
Yellow Emperor's Classic of Internal Medicine, 553
Yellow light, 477
Yoga, 337, 364, 393, 395, 397, 406, 408, 410; *see also*
 Meditation
　and arthritis, 375–376
　and asthma, 376–378
　and autism, 387
　and breathing, 601–603
　and cancer, 382–383
　and CF, 378–379
　during chemotherapy, 383–384
　and depression and anxiety, 373–374
　and diabetes, 371–373
　dissociation, 603
　and eating disorders, 374
　and endometriosis, 380
　fascination with, 366
　and GERD, 368–369
　and heart, 366–368
　and homocysteine, 379–380
　and hormones, 381–382
　and hypothyroidism, 385–386
　and IBS, 369–371
　and insomnia, 386–387
　left and right nostril variations, 387–388
　and menopause, 380–381
　mind body assessment, 602–603
　and obesity, 385
　and osteoporosis, 384
　and PCOS, 382
　philosophy, 364–365
　and PMS, 379
　and post-traumatic stress syndrome, 386
　reverses arterial stiffness, 368
　and sickle cell anemia, 374
　sutras, 364
　therapy, 367, 380
　in United States, 365–366
　Vasistha's Adhi, 369
　yoga/meditation, 385
Yoga Skills Training (YST), 383
Yoga Sutras of Patanjali, 425
Yoghurt, 196
Young adults (YA), 369
YST, *see* Yoga Skills Training

Z

Zeta potential (ZP), 502
Ziegler's meta-analysis, 64
Zika viral infections, 54
Zinc (Zn), 82, 86–92
Zinc Bromide (ZnBr2), 555
Zingiber officinale, see Ginger
ZnBr2, *see* Zinc Bromide
Zolpidem, 386
Zonulin, 194
ZP, *see* Zeta potential

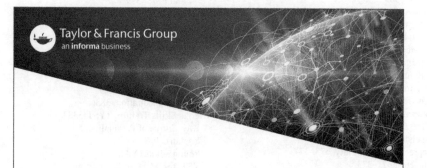